Clinical
Gastrointestinal
Endoscopy

Clinical Gastrointestinal Endoscopy SECOND EDITION

Gregory G. Ginsberg M.D.
Professor of Medicine
Gastroenterology Division
University of Pennsylvania School of Medicine
Director of Endoscopic Services
Hospital of the University of Pennsylvania
Philadelphia, PA, USA

Christopher J. Gostout M.D.
Professor of Medicine
Mayo Clinic College of Medicine
Consultant in Gastroenterology and Hepatology
Director of Endoscopic Research and Development
Mayo Clinic
Rochester, MN, USA

Michael L. Kochman M.D., F.A.C.P
Professor of Medicine
Co-Director, Gastrointestinal Oncology
Endoscopy Training Director
Gastroenterology Division
Hospital of the University of Pennsylvania
Philadelphia, PA, USA

Ian D. Norton M.B.B.S., Ph.D, F.R.A.C.P.
Director of Endoscopy
Department of Gastroenterology and Hepatology
Concord Hospital
Sydney, Australia

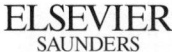

ELSEVIER
SAUNDERS

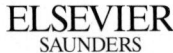
SAUNDERS

3251 Riverport Lane
St. Louis, Missouri 63043

CLINICAL GASTROINTESTINAL ENDOSCOPY   ISBN: 978-1-4377-1529-3
Copyright © 2012, 2005 by Saunders, an imprint of Elsevier Inc.

Library of Congress Cataloging-in-Publication Data

Clinical gastrointestinal endoscopy / [edited by] Gregory G. Ginsberg ... [et al.]. — 2nd ed.
       p. ; cm.
   Includes bibliographical references and index.
   ISBN 978-1-4377-1529-3 (hardcover: alk. paper)   1. Enteroscopy.   2. Gastroscopy.   I. Ginsberg, Gregory G.
   [DNLM: 1. Endoscopy—methods.   2. Gastrointestinal Diseases—diagnosis. WI 141]
   RC804.E64C56 2012
   616.3′407545—dc23
                                                                                    2011024705

Acquisitions Editor: Kate Dimock
Developmental Editor: Julie Mirra
Publishing Services Manager: Catherine Jackson
Senior Project Manager: Carol O'Connell
Cover Designer: Louis Forgione
Text Designer: Louis Forgione

Printed in the United States of America
Last digit is the print number: 9 8 7 6 5 4 3 2 1

Contents

Video Contents

Go to ExpertConsult.com to access the text, videos, and other supplemental materials online.

Section IV
Emerging Endoscopy

List of Contributors

James L. Achord, MD
Professor Emeritus
University of Mississippi Medical Center
Jackson, Mississippi
1: The History of Gastrointestinal Endoscopy

Matthew R. Banks, FRCP, PhD
Consultant Gastroenterologist
Honorary Senior Lecturer
Director of Endoscopy
University College London Hospitals
London, United Kingdom
7: Sedation and Monitoring in Endoscopy

David E. Barlow, PhD
Vice President, Research & Development
Olympus America Inc.
Center Valley, Pennsylvania
3: How Endoscopes Work

Todd H. Baron Sr., MD
Professor of Medicine
Consultant
Mayo Clinic
Rochester, Minnesota
47: Acute Pancreatitis and Peripancreatic Fluid

Juliane Bingener, MD
Associate Professor of Surgery
Mayo Clinic College of Medicine;
Consultant
Mayo Clinic
Rochester, Minnesota
55: Surgical Perspectives on Natural Orifice
Transluminal Endoscopic Surgery (NOTES)

Marco J. Bruno, MD, PhD
Professor of Gastrointestinal Oncology
University of Rotterdam;
Gastroenterologist, Director of Gastroenterology
& Endoscopy
Department of Gastroenterology and Hepatology
Erasmus Medical Center
Rotterdam, The Netherlands
51: Palliation of Malignant Pancreaticobiliary
Obstruction

Anna M. Buchner, MD, PhD
Assistant Professor
Division of Gastroenterology
University of Pennsylvania Perelman School of
Medicine
Philadelphia, Pennsylvania
58: Electronically Enhanced Endoscopic Imaging

Navtej S. Buttar, MD
Associate Professor of Medicine
Director, GI Bleed Team and Complex
Endoscopy
Division of Gastroenterology
Mayo Clinic College of Medicine
Rochester, Minnesota
13: Portal Hypertensive Bleeding

**David L. Carr-Locke, MD, DRCOG,
FRCP, FACG, FASGE**
Chief, Division of Digestive Diseases
Beth Israel Medical Center;
Professor
Albert Einstein College of Medicine
New York, New York
45: Infections of the Biliary Tract

Kenneth J. Chang, MD, FACG, FASGE
Professor of Medicine
Chief, Division of Gastroenterology and
Hepatology
Executive Director, H.H. Chao Comprehensive
Digestive Disease Center
University of California, Irvine
Irvine, California
42: Endoscopic Ultrasound-Guided Fine Needle
Aspiration of Pancreaticobiliary Lesions

Wei-Kuo Chang, MD
Associate Professor
Division of Gastroenterology
Department of Medicine
National Defense Medical Center;
Director of Endoscopy
Tri-Service General Hospital
Taipei, Taiwan, ROC
23: Techniques in Enteral Access

†Yang K. Chen, MD
Professor of Medicine
University of Colorado Health Sciences Center
School of Medicine
Denver, Colorado;
Director of Endoscopy
University of Colorado Hospital
Aurora, Colorado
33: Endoscopic Therapy for Gastric Neoplasms

Nicholas I. Church, MD, MRCP
Consultant Gastroenterologist
Royal Infirmary of Edinburgh
Edinburgh, United Kingdom
25: Diagnosis and Staging of Esophageal
Carcinoma

Nayantara Coelho-Prabhu, MD
Assistant Professor of Medicine
Senior Associate Consultant
Division of Gastroenterology and Hepatology
Mayo Clinic College of Medicine
Rochester, Minnesota
13: Portal Hypertensive Bleeding

Guido Costamagna, MD, FACG
Full Professor of Surgery
Catholic University;
Head, Digestive Endoscopy Unit
University Hospital
Roma, Italy
44: Benign Biliary Strictures and Leaks

Gregory A. Coté, MD, MS
Assistant Professor of Clinical Medicine
Division of Gastroenterology
Indiana University School of Medicine
University Hospital
Indianapolis, Indiana
57: Gastroduodenal and Colonic Endoprostheses

Sanford M. Dawsey, MD
Senior Investigator
Division of Cancer Epidemiology and Genetics
National Cancer Institute
Bethesda, Maryland
30: Screening for Esophageal Squamous Cell
Carcinoma and Its Precursor Lesions

Jacques Devière, MD, PhD
Professor of Medicine
Chairman, Department of Gastroenterology,
Hepatopancreatology and Digestive Oncology
Erasme Hospital
Université Libre de Bruxelles
Brussels, Belgium
53: Emerging Endoluminal Bariatric Techniques

James A. DiSario, MD
Monterey Bay Gastroenterology Consultants
Monterey, California;
Adjunct Professor of Medicine
Division of Gastroenterology, Hepatology and
Nutrition
University of Utah Health Sciences Center
Salt Lake City, Utah
43: Choledocholithiasis

Steven A. Edmundowicz, MD
Professor of Medicine
Chief of Endoscopy
Washington University School of Medicine
St. Louis, Missouri
57: Gastroduodenal and Colonic Endoprostheses

---

†Deceased.

Grace H. Elta, MD
Professor of Medicine
University of Michigan
Ann Arbor, Michigan
17: Benign Strictures

Gary W. Falk, MD, MS
Professor of Medicine
Co-Director, GI Physiology Laboratory
Co-Director, Swallowing Disorders Program
Division of Gastroenterology
University of Pennsylvania Perelman School of
Medicine
Philadelphia, Pennsylvania
26: Diagnosis and Surveillance of Barrett's
Esophagus

Arnaldo B. Feitoza, MD
Attending Surgeon
Digestive Endoscopy Unit
Department of Surgery
Hospital Aulino Feitosa
Telemaco Borba, Parana, Brazil
11: Postsurgical Endoscopic Anatomy

David E. Fleischer, MD
Professor of Medicine
Mayo College of Medicine;
Division of Gastroenterology
Mayo Clinic Arizona
Scottsdale, Arizona
30: Screening for Esophageal Squamous Cell
Carcinoma and Its Precursor Lesions

Evan L. Fogel, MD, MSc, FRCP(C)
Professor of Clinical Medicine
Director, ERCP Fellowship Program
Division of Gastroenterology/Hepatology
Indiana University Medical Center
Indianapolis, Indiana
37: Diagnostic Cholangiography
46: Sphincter of Oddi Dsyfunction

James T. Frakes, MD, MS
Clinical Professor Emeritus of Medicine
University of Illinois College of Medicine at
Rockford
Rockford Gastroenterology Associates, Ltd. (Ret.)
Rockford, Illinois
2: Setting Up an Endoscopy Facility

Shai Friedland, MD
Assistant Professor of Medicine
Stanford University
Stanford, California;
Staff Gastroenterologist
VA Palo Alto
Palo Alto, California
36: Colonoscopic Polypectomy, Mucosal
Resection, and Submucosal Dissection

Adam J. Goodman, MD
Assistant Professor of Medicine
Division of Gastroenterology and Hepatology
Director of Endoscopy
SUNY Downstate Medical Center
Brooklyn, New York
31: Extraintestinal Endosconography (including
Celiac Block)

Christopher J. Gostout, MD
Professor of Medicine
Mayo Clinic College of Medicine;
Consultant in Gastroenterology and Hepatology
Director of Endoscopic Research and
Development Unit
Mayo Clinic
Rochester, Minnesota
10: Small-Caliber Endoscopy
56: Emerging Intramural and Transmural
Endoscopy

Ian M. Gralnek, MD, MSHS, FASGE
Associate Professor of Medicine
Chief, Hospital-Wide Ambulatory Care Services
Head, GI Outcomes Unit and Senior Physician
Department of Gastroenterology—Rambam
Health Care Campus
Rappaport Faculty of Medicine, Technion-Israel
Institute of Technology
Haifa, Israel
15: Obscure Gastrointestinal Bleeding

Frank G. Gress, MD
Professor of Medicine
Chief, Division of Gastroenterology &
Hepatology
Department of Medicine
SUNY Downstate Medical Center
Brooklyn, New York
31: Extraintestinal Endosconography (including
Celiac Block)

Ian Grimes, MD
Fellow
Section of Gastroenterology and Hepatology
University of Wisconsin Medical School
Madison, Wisconsin
19: Ingested Foreign Objects and Food Bolus
Impactions

Naresh T. Gunaratnam, MD
Clinical Instructor
University of Michigan;
Director of Clinical Research
St. Joseph Mercy Hospital
Ann Arbor, Michigan
12: Nonvariceal Upper Gastrointestinal Bleeding

Kiyoshi Hashiba, MD
Director of Endoscopy
Hospital Sírio Libanês
Sao Paulo, Brazil
20: Kiyoshi Hashiba

Robert H. Hawes, MD
Professor of Medicine
Medical University of South Carolina
Charleston, South Carolina
49: Chronic Pancreatitis, Stones, and Strictures

Alberto Herreros de Tejada, MD, PhD
Consultant Gastroenterologist
Department of Gastroenterology
Puerta de Hierro University Hospital
Autonoma University School of Medicine
Madrid, Spain
32: Evaluation of Gastric Polyps and Thickened
Gastric Folds

Juergen Hochberger, MD, PhD
Professor of Medicine
Chief, Department of Gastroenterology
St. Bernward Academic Teaching Hospital
Hildesheim, Germany
39: Difficult Cannulation and Sphincterotomy

Marjolein Y.V. Homs, MD, PhD
Researcher
Department of Internal Medicine
University Medical Center Utrecht
Utrecht, The Netherlands
28: Endoscopic Palliation of Malignant
Dysphagia and Esophageal Fistulas

Douglas Howell, MD, FASGE
Associate Clinical Professor of Medicine
Tufts University School of Medicine;
Director, Advanced Interventional Endoscopy
Fellowship
Director, Pancreaticobiliary Center
Maine Medical Center
Portland, Maine
40: Endoscopic Retrograde
Cholangiopancreatography Tissue Sampling
Techniques

Maite Betés Ibáñez, MD, PhD
Associated Professor of Medicine
University of Navarra School of Medicine
Consultant Gastroenterologist
University Clinic of Navarra
Pamplona, Spain
16: Chronic Gastrointestinal Bleeding

Tonya Kaltenbach, MD, MS
Clinical Assistant Professor of Medicine
Stanford University School of Medicine;
Staff Gastroenterologist
Veterans Affairs Palo Alto Health Care System
Palo Alto, California
36: Colonoscopic Polypectomy, Mucosal
Resection, and Submucosal Dissection

David A. Katzka, MD
Professor of Medicine
Mayo Clinic College of Medicine
Rochester, Minnesota
18: Achalasia

Yakub I. Khan, MBBS, MD
Associate Gastroenterologist
Geisinger Medical Center
Geisinger Wyoming Valley Medical Center
Wilkes-Barre, Pennsylvania
12: Nonvariceal Upper Gastrointestinal Bleeding

Michael B. Kimmey, MD
Clinical Professor of Medicine
University of Washington;
President, Tacoma Digestive Disease Center
Tacoma, Washington
24: Acute Colonic Pseudo-obstruction

Richard A. Kozarek, MD
Clinical Professor of Medicine
University of Washington;
Director, Digestive Disease Institute
Virginia Mason Medical Center
Seattle, Washington
50: Pancreatic Duct Leaks and Pseudocysts

Glen A. Lehman, MD
Professor of Medicine and Radiology
Indiana University Medical Center
Indiana University School of Medicine
Indianapolis, Indiana
37: Diagnostic Cholangiography
46: Sphincter of Oddi Dsyfunction

Gary R. Lichtenstein, MD
Professor of Medicine
University of Pennsylvania Perelman School of
Medicine;
Director, Center for Inflammatory Bowel
Diseases
Gastroenterology Division
Department of Medicine
Hospital of the University of Pennsylvania
Philadelphia, Pennsylvania
21: Inflammatory Bowel Disease

David Lieberman, MD
Professor of Medicine
Chief, Division of Gastroenterology
Oregon Health and Science University
Portland, Oregon
35: Colorectal Cancer Screening and Surveillance

Jesse K. Liu, MD
Fellow
Division of Gastroenterology
Hospital of the University of Pennsylvania
Philadelphia, Pennsylvania
21: Inflammatory Bowel Disease

Takahisa Matsuda, MD
Staff, Endoscopy Division
National Cancer Center Hospital
Tokyo, Japan
36: Colonoscopic Polypectomy, Mucosal
Resection, and Submucosal Dissection

Johannes Maubach, MD
Department of Gastroenterology
St. Bernward Academic Teaching Hospital
Hildesheim, Germany
39: Difficult Cannulation and Sphincterotomy

Itay Maza, MD
Staff Physician
Department of Gastroenterology
Rambam Health Care Campus
Haifa, Israel
15: Obscure Gastrointestinal Bleeding

Stephen A. McClave, MD
Professor of Medicine
Director of Clinical Nutrition
Division of Gastroenterology, Hepatology, and
Nutrition
University of Louisville School of Medicine
Louisville, Kentucky
23: Techniques in Enteral Access

Lee McHenry, Jr., MD
Professor of Medicine
Indiana University Medical Center
Indiana University School of Medicine
Indianapolis, Indiana
37: Diagnostic Cholangiography
46: Sphincter of Oddi Dsyfunction

Detlev Menke, MD
Leading Consultant
Department of Gastroenterology
St. Bernward Academic Teaching Hospital
Hildesheim, Germany
39: Difficult Cannulation and Sphincterotomy

Klaus Mergener, MD, PhD, MBA
Director, GI Hospitalist Services
Digestive Health Specialists;
Clinical Medical Director, Gastroenterology
Multicare Health System
Tacoma, Washington
2: Setting Up an Endoscopy Facility

David C. Metz, MD
Professor of Medicine
Division of Gastroenterology
University of Pennsylvania Perelman School of
Medicine;
Co-Director, GI Physiology Laboratory
Director, Acid Peptic Disease Program
Co-Director, Swallowing Disorders Program
Hospital of the University of Pennsylvania
Philadelphia, Pennsylvania
18: Achalasia

Erica A. Moran, MD
Department of Gastroenterologic and General
Surgery
Mayo Clinic
Rochester, Minnesota
55: Surgical Perspectives on Natural Orifice
Transluminal Endoscopic Surgery (NOTES)

Marcia L. Morris, BA, MS
CEO
Genii, Inc.
St. Paul, Minnesota
6: Electrosurgery in Therapeutic Endoscopy

Miguel Muñoz-Navas, PhD
Professor of Medicine
University of Navarra School of Medicine;
Director, Department of Gastroentrology and the
Endoscopy Unit
University of Navarra Clinic
Pamplona, Spain
16: Chronic Gastrointestinal Bleeding

**V. Raman Muthusamy, MD, FACG,
FASGE**
Director of Interventional Endoscopy
Health Sciences Associate Clinical Professor of
Medicine
Division of Digestive Diseases/Department of
Medicine
David Geffen School of Medicine
University of California, Los Angeles
Los Angeles, California
42: Endoscopic Untrasound-Guided Fine Needle
Aspiration of Pancreaticobiliary Lesions

Douglas B. Nelson, MD
Staff Physician in Gastroenterology
Minneapolis VA Medical Center;
Associate Professor
University of Minnesota Medical School
Minneapolis, Minnesota
4: Cleaning and Disinfecting Gastrointestinal
Endoscopic Equipment

Nam Q. Nguyen, MBBS, PhD, FRACP
Senior Lecturer in Medicine
University of Adelaide;
Senior Consultant
Department of Gastroenterology
Royal Adelaide Hospital
Adelaide, South Australia
8: Patient Preparation and Pharmacotherapeutic
Considerations

Nicholas Nickl, MD
Professor of Medicine
University of Kentucky Medical Center
Lexington, Kentucky
29: Nonepithelial Tumors of the Esophagus and
Stomach

Ian D. Norton, MBBS, PhD, FRACP
Director of Endoscopy
Royal North Shore Hospital;
Associate Professor
University of Sydney
Sydney, Australia
6: Electrosurgery in Therapeutic Endoscopy
9: Reporting, Documentation, and Risk
Management

Ian D. Penman, MD, FRCP
Consultant Gastroenterologist
Royal Infirmary of Edinburgh
Edinburgh, United Kingdom
25: Diagnosis and Staging of Esophageal
Carcinoma

Bret T. Petersen, MD
Professor of Medicine
Division of Gastroenterology and Hepatology
Advanced Endoscopy and Pancreas Interest
Groups
Mayo Clinic
Rochester, Minnesota
38: Diagnostic Pancreatography

Patrick R. Pfau, MD
Associate Professor of Medicine
Chief of Clinical Gastroenterology
Section of Gastroenterology and Hepatology
University of Wisconsin Medical School
Madison, Wisconsin
19: Ingested Foreign Objects and Food Bolus
Impactions

Robert J. Ponec, MD, FACP, FACG
Salem Gastroenterology Consultants;
Medical Director
Salem Endoscopy Center
Salem, Oregon
24: Acute Colonic Pseudo-obstruction

Elizabeth Rajan, MD
Professor of Medicine
Consultant in Gastroenterology and Hepatology
Mayo Clinic
Rochester, Minnesota
52: Endoscopic Management of Post–Bariatric
Complications

Marvin Ryou, MD
Instructor in Medicine
Harvard Medical School;
Associate Staff Physician
Division of Gastroenterology
Brigham & Women's Hospital
Boston, Massachusetts
54: Gastroenterologic Perspectives on Natural
Orifice Transluminal Endoscopic Surgery
(NOTES)

Chang Beom Ryu, MD, PhD
Associate Professor of Medicine
Soon Chun Hyang University
Bucheon City, Republic of Korea
33: Endoscopic Therapy for Gastric Neoplasms

Michael K. Sanders, MD
Assistant Professor of Medicine
University of Pittsburgh Medical Center
Pittsburgh, Pennsylvania
48: Acute Relapsing Pancreatitis

Thomas J. Savides, MD
Professor of Clinical Medicine
University of California, San Diego
La Jolla, California
14: Lower Gastrointestinal Bleeding

Mark Schoeman, MBBS, PhD, FRACP
Senior Lecturer in Medicine
University of Adelaide;
Head of Gastrointestinal Services
Royal Adelaide Hospital
Adelaide, South Australia
8: Patient Preparation and Pharmacotherapeutic
Considerations

Kenneth W. Schroeder, MD, PhD
Associate Professor of Medicine
Mayo Clinic College of Medicine;
Consultant, Gastroenterology and Hepatology
Mayo Clinic
Rochester, Minnesota
9: Reporting, Documentation, and Risk
Management

Raj J. Shah, MD, FASGE
Associate Professor of Medicine
University of Colorado School of Medicine;
Co-Director, Endoscopy
Director, Pancreaticobiliary Services
University of Colorado Anschutz Medical
Campus
Aurora, Colorado
34: Endoscopic Management of Upper
Gastrointestinal Familial Adenomatous Polyposis
Syndrome and Ampullary Tumors

Stuart Sherman, MD
Professor of Medicine and Radiology
Director of ERCP
Clinical Director Gastroenterology and
Hepatology
Indiana University School of Medicine
Indianapolis, Indiana
37: Diagnostic Cholangiography
46: Sphincter of Oddi Dsyfunction

Peter D. Siersema, MD, PhD
Professor of Gastroenterology
Department of Gastroenterology and Hepatology
University Medical Center Utrecht
Utrecht, The Netherlands
28: Endoscopic Palliation of Malignant
Dysphagia and Esophageal Fistulas

Adam Slivka, MD, PhD
Associate Professor of Medicine
University of Pittsburgh;
Associate Chief, Division of Gastroenterology,
Hepatology, and Nutrition
University of Pittsburgh Medical Center
Pittsburgh, Pennsylvania
48: Acute Relapsing Pancreatitis

Roy Soetikno, MD, MS
Clinical Professor of Medicine
Stanford University School of Medicine;
Chief of Endoscopy
Veterans Affairs Palo Alto Health Care System
Palo Alto, California
36: Colonoscopic Polypectomy, Mucosal
Resection, and Submucosal Dissection

Kazuki Sumiyama, MD, PhD
Research Associate, Consultant Endoscopist
Department of Endsocopy
The Jikei University School of Medicine
Tokyo, Japan
56: Emerging Intramural and Transmural
Endoscopy

Hisao Tajiri, MD, PhD
Chairman and Professor
Division of Gastroenterology and Hepatrology
Department of Internal Medicine
The Jikei University School of Medicine
Tokyo, Japan
56: Emerging Intramural and Transmural
Endoscopy

Jason R. Taylor, MD
Clinical Lecturer
Division of Gastroenterology
University of Michigan
Ann Arbor, Michigan
17: Benign Strictures

Jennifer J. Telford, MD, MPH, FRCPC
Clinical Assistant Professor of Medicine
University of British Columbia
Vancouver, British Columbia, Canada
45: Infections of the Biliary Tract

Christopher C. Thompson, MD, MS
Director of Therapeutic Endoscopy
Brigham & Women's Hospital;
Assistant Professor of Medicine
Harvard Medical School
Boston, Massachusetts
54: Gastroenterologic Perspectives on Natural
Orifice Transluminal Endoscopic Surgery
(NOTES)

Mark D. Topazian, MD
Professor of Medicine
Consultant
Mayo Clinic
Rochester, Minnesota
41: Endoscopic Ultrasound of Pancreatic and
Biliary Diseases

Shyam Varadarajulu, MD
Associate Professor of Medicine
Director of Endoscopy
Division of Gastroenterology-Hepatology
University of Alabama at Birmingham School of
Medicine
Birmingham, Alabama
49: Chronic Pancreatitis, Stones, and Strictures

Charanjit Virk
Research Associate
Division of Gastroenterology and Hepatology
Mayo Clinic College of Medicine
Rochester, Minnesota
13: Portal Hypertensive Bleeding

Kenneth K. Wang, MD
Professor of Medicine
Director Advanced Endoscopy
Division of Gastroenterology and Hepatology
Mayo Clinic
Rochester, Minnesota
27: Endoscopic Treatment of Superficial
Esophageal Cancers

James L. Watkins, MD
Associate Professor of Clinical Medicine
Indiana University Medical Center
Indianapolis, Indiana
37: Diagnostic Cholangiography
46: Sphincter of Oddi Dsyfunction

Irving Waxman, MD
Professor of Medicine and Surgery
Director of The Center for Endoscopic Research
and Therapeutics (CERT)
University of Chicago
Chicago, Illinois
32: Evaluation of Gastric Polyps and Thickened
Gastric Folds

George J.M. Webster, BSc, MD, FRCP
Consultant Gastroenterologist
Honorary Senior Lecturer
Department of Gastroenterology
University College London Hospitals
London, United Kingdom
7: Sedation and Monitoring in Endoscopy

Liang H. Wee, BM, FRCA
Consultant Anaesthetist
Department of Anaesthetics
University College Hospital
London, United Kingdom
7: Sedation and Monitoring in Endoscopy

Wilfred M. Weinstein, MD
Professor of Medicine
Department of Medicine-Digestive Diseases
UCLA Center for The Health Sciences
Los Angeles, California
5: Tissue Sampling, Specimen Handling, and
Chromoendoscopy

C. Mel Wilcox, MD
Professor of Medicine
University of Alabama
Birmingham, Alabama
22: Infections of the Luminal Digestive Tract

Roy D. Yen, MD
Assistant Professor of Medicine
Division of Gastroenterology & Hepatology
Section of Therapeutic Endoscopy
University of Colorado
Aurora, Colorado
34: Endoscopic Management of Upper
Gastrointestinal Familial Adenomatous Polyposis
Syndrome and Ampullary Tumors

Kyo-Sang Yoo
Research Fellow
ERCP Service
Division of Gastroenterology/Hepatology
Indiana University Medical Center
Indiana University School of Medicine
Indianapolis, Indiana
37: Diagnostic Cholangiography

Preface

Welcome to the second edition of Clinical Gastrointestinal Endoscopy. This volume provides a comprehensive treatment of general and advanced gastrointestinal endoscopy and is prepared by leading authorities from around the globe. Authors were selected because of their personal contributions to the development of their assigned topics, acknowledged clinical prowess in the field, and proven track record as effective scientific writers. The result is a collection of the most authoritative and easily absorbed chapters available in endoscopy. The authors have taken the opportunity to design countless original diagrams, algorithms, and tables to precisely and easily display complex information. Each of the diagrams has been expertly redrawn to a consistent and attractive style. The authors have also lavished their exceptional collections of endoscopic photographs, EUS images, radiographs, and histomicrographs upon the book. Each of these stunning illustrations can be downloaded from the book's website so that you can use them in your presentations. Each of the world's leading contributors to this book has been asked to supply digital video demonstrating the diagnostic and therapeutic endoscopic procedures they cover. No other textbook offers real-time demonstrations of so many procedures from the world's experts—the reading experience has leapt from the page to the monitor. Each video clip, available on the accompaning website, expertconsult.com, has been meticulously edited to make the viewing experience efficiently educational.

These features make this volume essential reading for any fellow who is serious about endoscopy. This volume is also a vehicle for acquisition of new skills and an indispensable resource for practicing clinicians in both community and academic settings.

Clinical Gastrointestinal Endoscopy, second edition, is divided into four main sections covering Equipment and General Principles of Endoscopy, Luminal Gastrointestinal Disorders, Pancreaticobiliary Disorders, and Emerging Endoscopy (a glimpse into the future). The first section elegantly describes the history of gastrointestinal endoscopy and then provides primers on how endoscopes, endoscopic devices, and endoscopy units function. There are many real practice-changing pearls of wisdom in these pages. Section II: Luminal Gastrointestinal Disorders is divided into benign and malignant disorders. The benign disorders subsection devotes five chapters to endoscopic diagnosis and treatment of gastrointestinal bleeding followed by detailed coverage of endoscopic approaches to strictures, enteral access, ingested foreign objects, and gastroesophageal reflux disease. The chapters on malignant disorders give complete coverage of endoscopic approaches to management of inflammatory, infectious, and functional disorders of the luminal digestive tract. The chapters on neoplastic disorders are divided into esophageal, gastroduodenal, and colorectal subsections. Within each subsection, endoscopic diagnosis, staging, palliation, and curative therapies are comprehensively covered. The pancreaticobiliary section details simple and advanced techniques in ERCP and EUS for the diagnosis and management of benign and malignant disorders of the pancreaticobiliary systems.

The editors draw on their collective decades of clinical endoscopic experience to clearly represent the core of proven practice while energizing it with cutting edge innovations. They are themselves the products of some of the powerhouses of gastrointestinal endoscopic training and practice: Georgetown University, Indiana University, Mayo Clinic, University of Michigan, and the University of Pennsylvania. They have worked painstakingly to develop a user-friendly and, at the same time, authoritative product. The publishers are to be congratulated on thumbing their noses at convention, developing a creative and richly illustrated volume, further improved by the video demonstrations. The timelessness of most of the content will make this a "current" resource for many years.

Gregory G. Ginsberg, M.D.

Dedications

Developing and revising a book of this scope and detail is a considerable undertaking for all involved. It is made possible and even pleasurable when supported by people who evidence excellence in the quality of their work and their passion for the subject matter. Such is the case with the coeditors, authors, and publishers involved herein.

My coeditors are friends and professionals whom I admire. I thank them for their willing collaboration. A textbook is the sum of its parts, and I wish to express my sincerest appreciation to the individual authors for their personal investment in developing full, rich chapters. I am also appreciative of the organization, creativity, and professionalism on the part of the Elsevier publishing team.

Influencing the development of this book, I gratefully acknowledge those who have shaped my career. I am thankful for my teachers during fellowship at Georgetown, Stanley Benjamin, David Fleischer, Firas Al-Kawas, Jim Lewis, Lou Korman, and Tim Lipman. I am indebted to my divisional colleagues at Penn Medicine and to the many outstanding fellows with whom I have had the opportunity to interface.

I am fortunate enough to again be able to thank my exceptional wife, Jane, who supports my forays into projects like this in pursuit of professional satisfaction. Finally, I recognize my four lovely daughters, Jennifer, Kathleen, Elizabeth, and Meg, who remain unending sources of warmth and humor.

I hope this book will enhance your knowledge and abilities, enrich your professionalism, and enable you to provide the best possible care for your patients.

Gregory G. Ginsberg

This book is dedicated to my family: my wife, Mary, and my children, Elyse and Sidney. Without their indulgences, this book, and indeed my career, would not have been possible.

This second edition brings along with it an increasing responsibility to our patients, trainees, and colleagues; not only to ensure that the practice of gastroenterology is at the forefront of therapeutics and safety, but to also share our enthusiasm for the field and its continued relevance within the overall practice of medicine.

Over the years a number of key individuals sparked and nurtured my interest in gastroenterology and therapeutic endoscopy: Drs. Tom Layden and Jay Goldstein were critical early on in demonstrating to me the need for better diagnostics and additional effective therapies. Tachi Yamada, M.D., and Chung Owyang, M.D., had the foresight to allow me the specialized training, which I hope I have put to good use. Drs. Rick Boland, John DelValle, Grace Elta, Robert Hawes, Michael Lucey, Jim Scheiman, Peter Traber, and Maurits Wiersema were instrumental in helping me acquire and define my skill-set and in facilitating my clinical research and writing skills. My current colleagues at the University of Pennsylvania have been instrumental by challenging me and in providing critical insight and guidance.

Clifford G. Pilz, M.D., (1921–2005) deserves special mention. As my Chief of Medicine during medical school, residency, and chief residency, he clearly defined the epitome of the all-knowing physician; no question too small to deserve an answer, no sign or symptom too subtle to be ignored.

Michael L. Kochman

It has truly been a pleasure working on this project, and for that I must first thank Greg Ginsberg for his faith in spite of the "tyranny of distance" involved in working with me, as well as my coeditors, contributing authors, and everyone at Elsevier.

It is no understatement that my career was reinvented at the Mayo Clinic, and for that I will be eternally grateful for my many teachers and colleagues at Mayo, in particular Bret Petersen, Jonathan Clain, Gene DiMagno, Maurits Wiersema, and Todd Baron. I must especially thank Chris Gostout for his remarkable enthusiasm and mentorship.

Lastly, I must thank my wonderful wife, Stephanie, for her unwavering support and my beautiful children, Sophie, Michael, and Jack for all the joy they give me as well as reminding me what's really important.

I hope that this book is helpful in your day-to-day practice and maybe helps spark some of the enthusiasm for endoscopy that I have been privileged to experience.

Ian D. Norton

Endoscopy continues to evolve the diagnostic and therapeutic applications. It is important to document this growth and provide a resource for a continuing evolution in the field. We accomplish this, in part, by the creation of textbooks. On behalf of myself, my fellow coeditors, and, more importantly, the contributing authors of this text I have had the continuing pleasure to work with, we are able to provide you with an improved resource upon which to study the practice of endoscopy and better understand where endoscopy must go to better the care of our patients.

Christopher J. Gostout

Section I

Equipment and General Principles of Endoscopy

Ian D. Norton

Chapter 1

The History of Gastrointestinal Endoscopy

James L. Achord

Introduction

The role of the physician is to observe, detect anatomic abnormalities or disease, and conceive ways and means by which discovered deficiencies in function can be corrected or ameliorated. To extend the physical examination to areas hidden from external view, such as within body orifices, presents a problem of safe and effective access. In insatiable attempts to accomplish these goals, there is no human orifice along with its recesses that has not been inspected, probed, prodded, and otherwise examined over the centuries. It was a compelling necessity to develop safe, nonsurgical methods to accomplish this purpose. Before the 20th century, numerous attempts to access these hidden cavities were plagued by instrumentation that was inadequate and dangerous. The history of every science or technical development is invariably a series of small discoveries or innovations, often in fields remote from that under investigation. Small improvements, each resulting in incremental gains, lead toward the idealized goal. Often, changes that appear to be an advance are found to be an impediment by further discoveries, and we recognize that a different way is better. Therefore, the task is never ending.

The term *endoscopy* comes from the Greek prefix *endo-* ("within") and the verb *skopein* ("to view or observe"). In this chapter, we summarize major developments over the years in gastrointestinal (GI) endoscopy to the present. As in any summary, the contributions of some individuals inevitably are not cited, and I offer my apologies to these individuals.

Early Efforts

The visual exploration and examination of body orifices date to at least Egyptian and to later Greco-Roman times, during which mechanical specula for viewing the vagina and anus were developed and used to a limited extent. Further progress was delayed by lack of sufficiently strong metals and the ability to form them into usable instruments and the lack of adequate illumination. These initial efforts were directed at the genitourinary (GU) tract—with cavities that were only a short and relatively straight distance from the exterior.

Bozini is credited with the earliest known attempt to visualize the interior of a body cavity with a primitive endoscope (**Fig. 1.1**). He published his work in 1805.[1-3] Bozini devised a tin tube illuminated by a candle from which light was reflected by a mirror, a device he called a *lichtleiter* (light conductor). He used this device to examine the urethra, urinary bladder, and vagina, but it was an impractical instrument that never gained wide acceptance. Although there were multiple attempts to develop more usable instruments, all directed toward the GU tract, none were widely used. The most notable efforts were by Segalas in France in 1826 and Fisher in Boston in 1827,[2] both using straight metal tubes, but the lack of a satisfactory light source remained a major impediment.

The next significant development was the instrument of Desormeaux in France.[2] Desormeaux's contribution in 1855

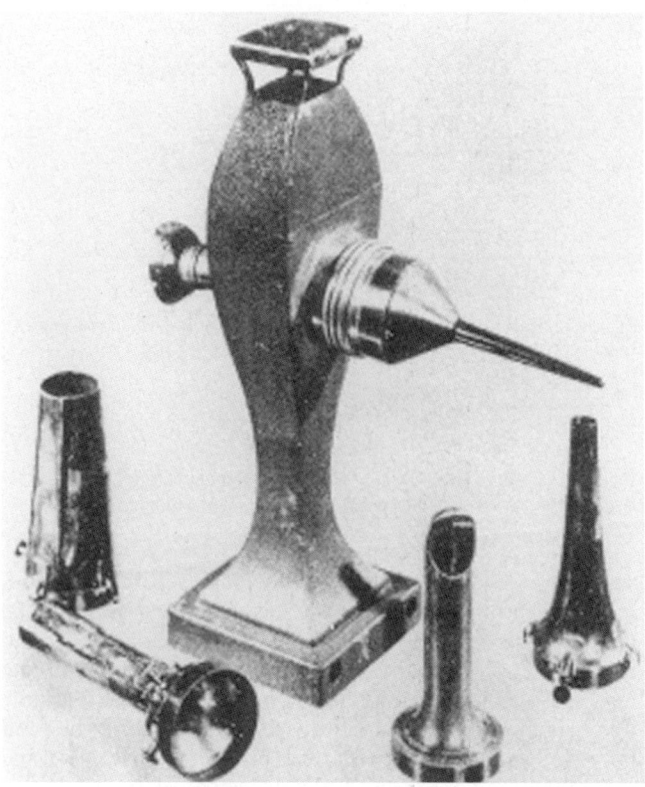

Fig. 1.1 Bozzini's lichtleiter, 1805. *(From Edmonson JM: History of the instruments for gastrointestinal endoscopy.* Gastrointest Endosc *37:S28, 1991.)*

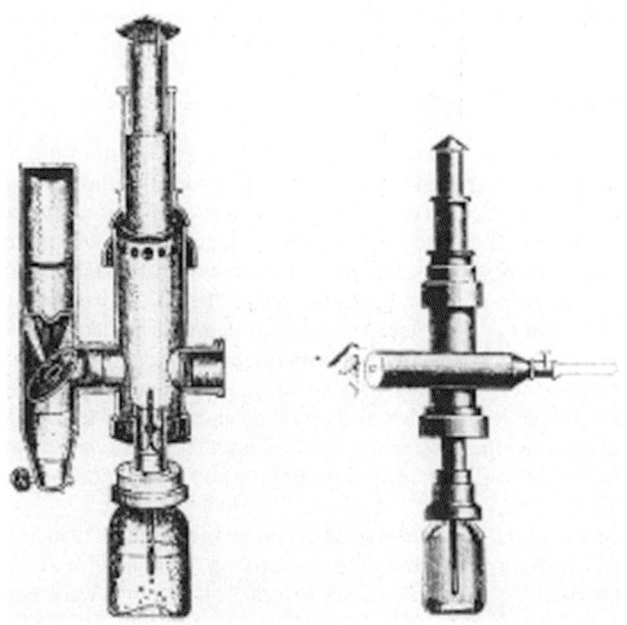

Fig. 1.2 Desormeaux's endoscope, 1853. *(From Edmonson JM: History of the instruments for gastrointestinal endoscopy.* Gastrointest Endosc *37:S29, 1991.)*

was a better, although still inadequate, light source using a lamp fueled with alcohol and turpentine ("gazogene") (**Fig. 1.2**). His instrument was based on that of Segalas. Others continued with efforts to improve the light source and the means to deliver it, but the devices were unsatisfactory for the more inaccessible areas of the GI tract.

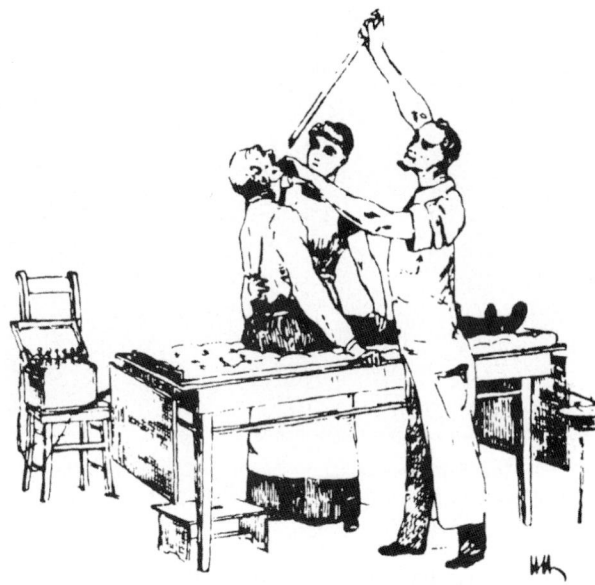

Fig. 1.3 Kussmaul's gastroscope, 1868. *(From Edmonson JM: History of the instruments for gastrointestinal endoscopy.* Gastrointest Endosc *37:S30, 1991.)*

Rigid Gastrointestinal Endoscopes

Kussmaul is credited as being the first to perform gastroscopy in 1868, using a straight rigid metal tube passed over a flexible obturator and a cooperative sword swallower (**Fig. 1.3**).[1-4] For a light source, he used a mirror reflecting light from the Desormeaux device but found it inadequate. He also quickly discovered that gastric secretions were a problem, despite using a flexible tube he had developed earlier to empty the stomach before the procedure. The value of his efforts was the demonstration that the curves and bends of the esophagus and esophagogastric junction could be traversed with careful manipulation and that the gastric pouch could be visualized. Kussmaul apparently demonstrated his "gastroscope" several times, but the illumination was too poor to allow a clinically useful image,[4] and he abandoned his efforts.

Encouraged by the efforts of Kussmaul, others switched their attention to developing esophagoscopes because the esophagus is much easier to visualize, and a less complex design than the gastroscope was required. The problems of perforation, at that time usually fatal, and of illumination remained major obstacles. Before the late 19th century, illumination of light reflected by a mirror into a straight metal tube continued to be used. As noted earlier, several light sources were developed, but the intensity left much to be desired. Several innovations were developed to solve this problem, including a burning magnesium wire, which produced a brilliant light but unacceptable heat and smoke. The most promising device seemed to be the brilliant light from a loop of platinum wire charged with direct current, introduced simultaneously by Bruck in Breslau and Milliot of Paris in 1882.[2] Although the illumination was good, major difficulties were encountered with the considerable heat generated, necessitating a water cooling system, and the cumbersome batteries used for a power source. Nevertheless, the platinum wire device was an encouraging development and was used in several instruments that saw relatively wide use.

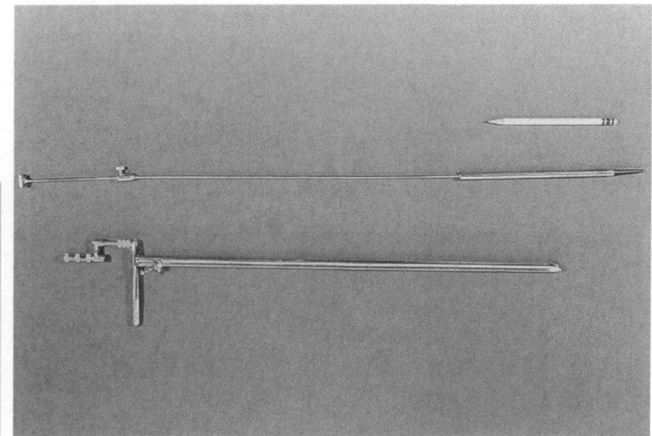

Fig. 1.4 Eder-Hufford esophagoscope, the result of multiple attempts to develop a clinically useful instrument, 1949.

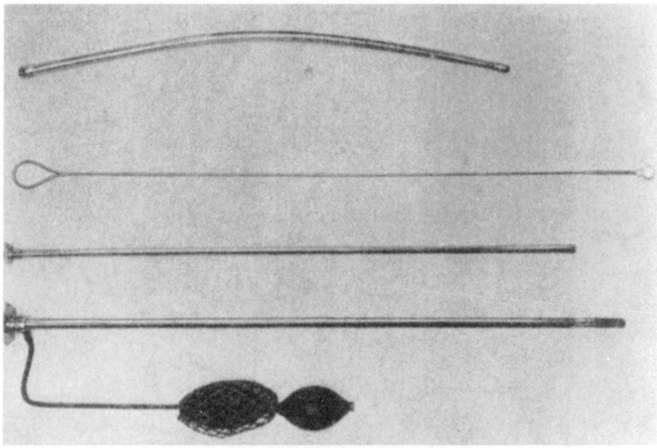

Fig. 1.5 Elsner's gastroscope, 1911. *(From Edmonson JM: History of the instruments for gastrointestinal endoscopy.* Gastrointest Endosc *37:S35, 1991.)*

These instruments were made obsolete just a few years later by Edison's incandescent electric light bulb introduced in 1879. In 1886, Leiter, an instrument maker, was the first to use the electric incandescent light bulb in a cystoscope just 7 years after Edison introduced it. With a few short-lived exceptions, all instruments used Edison's invention after 1886. Working with Leiter, von Mikulicz developed an unsuccessful gastroscope but a practical esophagoscope that he used extensively until distracted by his many other medical interests.

At the turn of the 20th century, Jackson, an otolaryngologist, also examined the esophagus and the stomach using a straight rigid tube and a distal electric light bulb, but few could match his talents in the GI tract. Under his influence, esophagoscopy was considered the exclusive province of ear, nose, and throat (ENT) departments in many community hospitals in the United States as late as the 1950s. The design of the esophagoscope remained a straight rigid tube, usually with a rubber finger–tipped obturator to make insertion safer. With the later addition of a 4× power lens on the proximal end and a distal incandescent bulb, various models were popular until the introduction of fiberoptics in 1961. The Eder-Hufford rigid esophagoscope (**Fig. 1.4**), introduced in 1949, was popular and still in use during my training in 1960–1962.

It was not until after 1900 that persistent efforts to develop a usable gastroscope were successful. All attempts to build a flexible instrument using a multiplicity of lenses were designed to be straightened after introduction and were fragile, easily damaged, and cumbersome. Straight tubes with simpler optics were useful, but perforations were still a problem.[1] In 1911, Elsner introduced a rigid gastroscope with an outer tube through which could be passed a separate inner optical tube with a flexible rubber tip and side-viewing portal (**Fig. 1.5**). The rubber tip, previously used in the esophagoscope obturator, was more crucial than it might appear, for it seemed to be, along with the later addition of a flexible metal coil proximal to it, the single feature that reduced the rate of perforation. Elsner's instrument worked as designed and was widely used, especially by Schindler, then in his native Germany, who called it the "mother of all instruments until 1932."[5]

In 1922, Schindler introduced his own version of the Elsner gastroscope, the major innovation of which was the important addition of an air channel to clear the lens of secretions. With the Elsner gastroscope, Schindler examined the stomachs of several hundred patients and meticulously recorded his findings in each procedure. He published *Lehrbuch und Atlas der Gastreoskopie* in 1923, with descriptions and remarkably accurate drawings. He trained others in the technique and was responsible for wide acceptance of gastroscopy. The procedure was first to empty the stomach with a nasogastric tube followed by sedation. The patient was placed on the left side, and an assistant held the head rigidly extended to produce a straight path into the esophagus and the stomach (the "sword swallower's technique"). The role of the assistant was crucial. Schindler's effort was impressive and convinced many of the value of an expert examination of the stomach.

Semiflexible Gastroscopes

It became apparent that straight, rigid tubes were not ideal for examination of the stomach. Fatal perforations continued to the detriment of acceptance of the procedure. Visualization of the surface of the stomach was incomplete at best, with many consistently blind spots. These problems stimulated investigation of methods to manufacture safer, "flexible" instruments. The use of the term *flexible* here is problematic in view of what we think of today as flexible instruments. Although these early instruments were not flexible by our standards, they were more flexible than the straight, rigid instruments that came before. *Semiflexible,* with passive angulation of the distal portion of 34 degrees and sometimes more, was a more appropriate term.

In 1911, Hoffman showed that an image could be transmitted through a curved line by linking several short-focus prisms. Using this principle, several instruments were constructed, but these were unsatisfactory or were not widely accepted. Schindler, working with Wolf, the renowned instrument maker, constructed a semiflexible instrument with a rigid proximal portion and a distal portion made elastic by coiled copper wire and terminating with first a rubber finger and later a small rubber ball. Illumination was with a distal incandescent light bulb. Air insufflation was made possible with a rubber bulb, expanding the stomach wall to beyond the focal length of the prisms, which were manufactured by Zeiss. In 1932, the sixth and final version was patented. This instrument, known as the Wolf-Schindler gastroscope, greatly

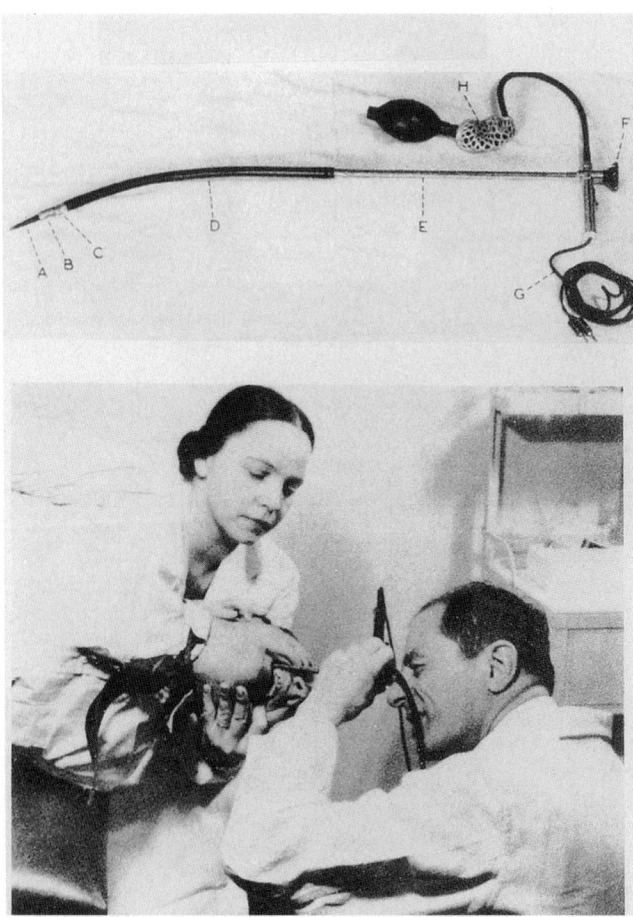

Fig. 1.6 Wolf-Schindler "flexible" gastroscope *(top)* being used by Schindler *(bottom)* with his wife as the head holder. *(From Edmonson JM: History of the instruments for gastrointestinal endoscopy.* Gastrointest Endosc *37:S37, 1991.)*

improved the safety and efficacy of gastroscopy and was used throughout the world (**Fig. 1.6**).

Thanks to the published meticulous work and enthusiasm of Schindler, whose designation as the "father of gastroscopy" is well deserved, the procedure was finally widely accepted as a valuable extension of the physical examination. The era of the semiflexible gastroscope from 1932–1957 has been called "the Schindler era." Schindler was chiefly responsible for transforming gastroscopy from a dangerous and seldom used procedure to one that was relatively safe and indispensable for evaluation of known or suspected disease of the stomach. He insisted that all clinicians who planned to use the instrument be properly trained and that "… no manipulation inside of the body is without danger; therefore no endoscopic examination should be done without reasonable indication."[6] In today's vernacular, the risk approaches infinity if the benefit approaches zero.

Schindler was born in Berlin in 1888. He gained considerable experience as an Army physician in World War I, where he became convinced that gastritis, then an often disparaged cause of symptoms, was a bona fide disease. His interest in gastritis lasted throughout his career and undoubtedly stimulated his interest in gastroscopy. The Wolf-Schindler endoscope of 1932 and Schindler's publications with drawings further enhanced what thereafter rapidly became a discipline.

His enthusiasm for and talent in using the gastroscope led to what has been called his "gospel of gastroscopy," which he and others spread throughout academia and to the community of practicing physicians. Because of his Jewish background, Schindler was put in "protective custody" by the Nazis, but with the help of the physicians Ortmeyer and Palmer and philanthropists in Chicago, he was able to immigrate to the United States in 1934.[1–4,7]

Chicago became the hub of GI endoscopy, and it was here, in Schindler's home, that the first discussions were held about forming a new organization for GI endoscopy, now known, after several name changes, as the *American Society of Gastrointestinal Endoscopy*. In 1943, just 9 years after his arrival in the United States, Schindler left Chicago for Loma Linda University. In 1958, he accepted an appointment as Professor of Medicine at the University of Minas Gerais in Belo Horizonte, Brazil. He came back to the United States in 1960 because of an eventually fatal illness of his wife and returned to his native Berlin in 1964, where he died in 1968 at the age of 80.[1] Despite his acclaim in endoscopy, Schindler insisted that one must be a physician first and an endoscopist second. He was very knowledgeable in the field of general gastroenterology and published, without coauthors, a synopsis of the entire field in 1957.[6]

The Wolf-Schindler endoscope was introduced into the United States by Benedict, Borland, and many others. Schindler's immigration to Chicago inspired a surge of interest in the United States, but with the outbreak of war in Europe, the German source of instruments disappeared. Several U.S. companies working with Schindler and others produced many popular gastroscopes that were significant variations on the Wolf-Schindler, including Cameron Co., which produced its first instrument in 1940.[8] The Eder-Hufford semiflexible gastroscope followed in 1946,[9] and American Cystoscope Makers, Inc. (ACMI) produced a gastroscope in 1950. A combination of the Eder-Hufford esophagoscope with a semiflexible gastroscope to be passed through it was the Eder-Palmer transesophagoscopic flexible gastroscope produced by the Eder Company in 1953. Each gastroscope had its proponents.

Biopsy

With the availability of instruments for visualization, it became apparent that tissue must be obtained to identify the nature of the observed abnormalities. Instruments for blind biopsies were used early on, but a device was needed that would allow the operator to obtain a biopsy specimen of abnormal tissue directly when seen at endoscopy. The Benedict Operating Gastroscope was produced in 1948 based on a 1940 model by Kenamore (**Fig. 1.7**).[10] The Benedict instrument, on which I was trained in 1960, was a popular instrument that was widely used. In the debates about the necessity for biopsy, Benedict, originally a surgeon who switched entirely to endoscopy, stated that gastroscopy was not a routine procedure and should be reserved for difficult problems in differential diagnosis, but "gastroscopic examination is not complete unless the gastroscopist has some means of biopsy readily available."[11] It soon became clear that the correlation between histology and a diagnosis based on visualization alone was often widely discrepant, and certain diagnoses could not be reliably

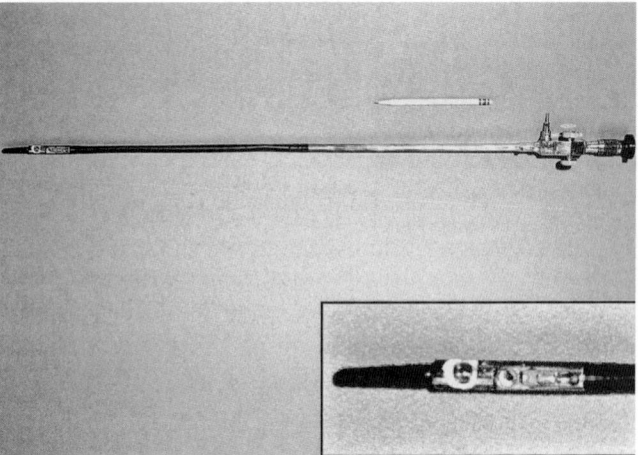

Fig. 1.7 Benedict operating gastroscope.

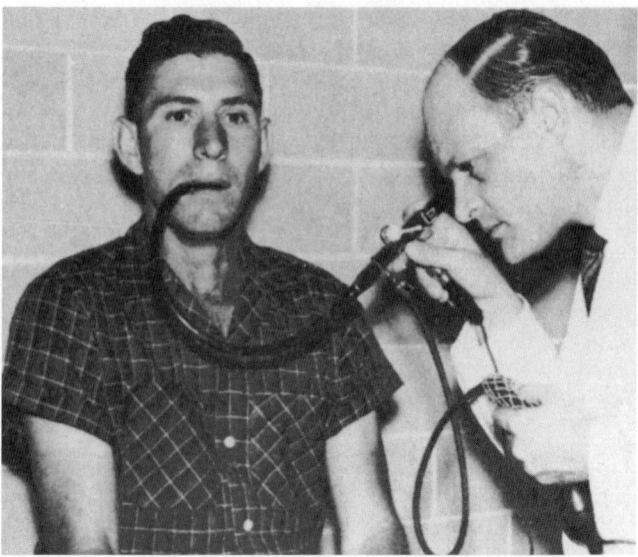

Fig. 1.8 Hirschowitz examining the stomach of an outpatient. *(From Hirschowitz BI: Endoscopic examination of the stomach and duodenal cap with the fiberscope. Lancet 1:1074–1078, 1961.)*

made without tissue examination. Efforts such as wash and brush cytology continued and have persisted in various forms to the present time.

Fiberoptics

By the 1950s, the ideal of a totally flexible GI endoscope with good visualization that could withstand the rigors of clinical use had not been realized, although the semiflexible instruments with their biopsy capabilities were satisfactory for most clinical purposes. In fact, these instruments were not rapidly abandoned by all with introduction of the remarkably flexible *fiberscope.* The development of the science of fiberoptics and its application to endoscopes (scopes) truly revolutionized the diagnostic and, later, the therapeutic abilities of endoscopy. Its importance in the development of this field cannot be overstated. A productive marriage of many areas of technology continues.

The principle of internal reflection of light along a conduction pathway was used by Lamm in October 1930.[1] The image was severely degraded by light escaping from the thin fibers of quartz he used, although the potential for total flexibility was present. Lamm could not interest Schindler or others in his efforts, and the experiment was discontinued. Almost 25 years later, in 1954, Hirschowitz, in fellowship training at the University of Michigan, visited Hopkins and Kapany in London to review their work[12] with glass fibers, which totally confirmed the work of Lamm and his predecessors. Hirschowitz became convinced that application of this principle could be used to develop a totally new and superior endoscope. He began work with a graduate student, Curtiss, who developed a technique of coating glass fibers with glass of a different optical density, preventing the escape of light and degradation of the image. This was the critical discovery that made the principle of internal reflection through glass fibers workable.

In 1957, Hirschowitz demonstrated his fiberscope, and he published his work in 1958 (**Fig. 1.8**).[13] His audience was not impressed, and it took another 3 years, working with ACMI, to produce a marketable scope, which he called the *Hirschowitz Gastroduodenal Fiberscope.* This was a very flexible side-viewing instrument with an electric light on its distal end, an air channel, and an adjustable focusing lens proximally. The

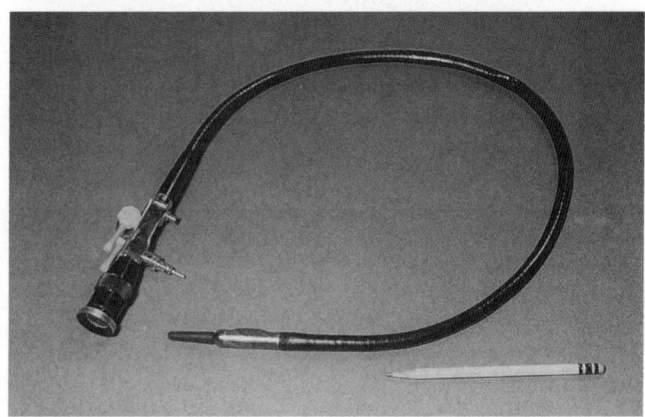

Fig. 1.9 ACMI fiberscope, 1962.

tip lacked what was by then the "obligatory" rubber finger, and this omission was a source of criticism; one was added on a later model. Although some individuals criticized the quality of the image, most believed the size and brightness were superior to the semiflexible scopes. This model, the ACMI 4990, was introduced to the market late in 1960 after being tested by Hirschowitz on himself and numerous patients. In 1961, I was in Gastroenterology fellowship at the Emory University Clinic with Schroder. I vividly recall his reaction when we first used our new fiberscope around March 1962 (**Fig. 1.9**). When he finished our first examination, he turned to me and said, "Anybody want to buy a used Benedict operating scope?" I don't think we ever used it again. The Hirschowitz Gastroduodenal Fiberscope was clearly superior in my young view, and I finished my training with that instrument.

There were problems with the fiberscope noted by us and by others. The distal light source would become so heated that thermal injury to the gastric mucosa was possible unless the tip was continuously moved. In prolonged procedures, protein in gastric secretions would coagulate on the bulb and the adjacent visualizing port, totally obscuring the lens. As the number of procedures with a single instrument increased,

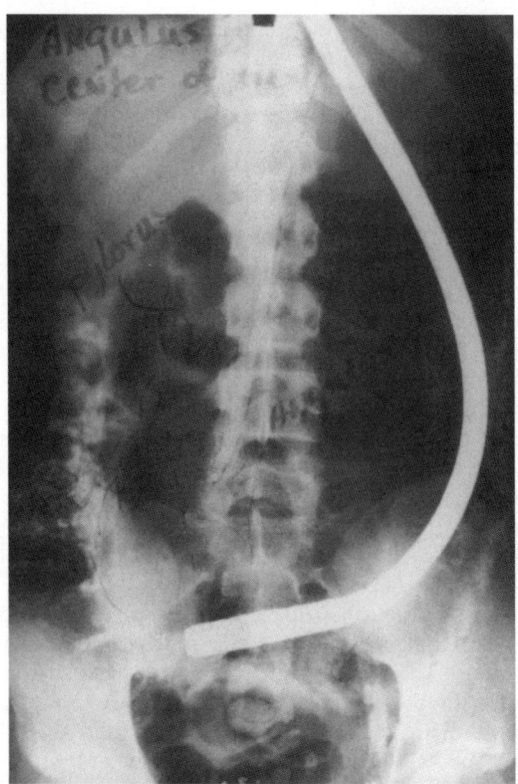

Fig. 1.10 Visualization of duodenum was sometimes obtained by over-inflating the stomach.

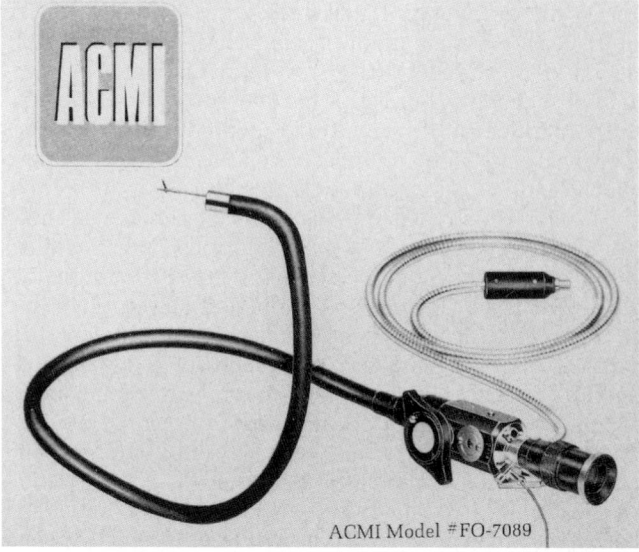

ACMI Model #FO-7089

Fig. 1.11 LoPresti forward-viewing esophagogastroscope. *(From advertisement in* Gastrointest Endosc *16:79, 1970.)*

some glass fibers would break, producing small black dots in the visual field. This was a persistent problem with fiberscopes during their entire history and especially apparent in training programs where a single scope was used by several trainees on many patients. The side-viewing lens prevented visualization of the esophagus, and the scope had to be passed blindly through the pharyngeal orifice. The previous semiflexible scopes in use shared this problem, and it was not considered a defect at the time. The flexibility itself resulted in some difficulty in advancing because attempts to push the instrument through the pylorus and into the gut resulted in more bowing in the gastric pouch (**Fig. 1.10**). Although one could sometimes visualize the duodenum, this was done by overinflating the stomach and looking through the pylorus without actually entering it. If one managed to introduce the tip into the duodenum, as occasionally happened, the visual field was inside the focal length of the instrument, and only a "red-out" was observed. Others had similar complaints.[4]

Many clinicians did not believe the additional expense of replacing the older, beloved instruments with which they had been successful for many years was warranted. Even ACMI officials did not see the fiberscope as totally replacing the instruments with lens systems.[2] Despite reservations, comparison and experiential studies showed the advantages of the new fiberscopes.[14–17] Following the flagship ACMI model 4990, several models of the fiberscope were introduced by ACMI and other companies, each with significant improvements, including the controllable tip in the side-viewing ACMI model 5004. Visualization of the gastric pouch, including retroflexed views of the cardia, was complete. The major objection to these instruments was the inability to pass the instrument

under direct vision and examine the esophagus; also, the area beyond the pylorus could not be consistently examined.

Most clinicians were already fully trained in use of the Eder-Hufford esophagoscope, and in the absence of a forward-viewing fiberscope, use of the Eder-Hufford esophagoscope continued. A forward-viewing scope was mandatory. LoPresti modified the tip of the fiberscope to create the foroblique fiberoptic esophagoscope in 1964.[18] Passing the instrument under direct vision was possible, and clinicians immediately discovered that they could examine not only the esophagus, but also a large portion of the proximal stomach. At a length of 90 cm, however, one could not reach the duodenum. Working with ACMI, LoPresti produced the longer *Panview Mark "87" gastro-Esophageal Endoscope* in 1970. By about 1971, the instrument had been lengthened to 105 cm with a four-way controllable tip capable of 180 degrees of deflection (**Fig. 1.11**).

The aptly named *panendoscope* was now a reality. Japanese and American manufacturers began to produce new models with such rapidity that endoscopists hardly had time to become thoroughly familiar with one before another, significantly improved (and more expensive) model was on the market. Patient comfort was greatly improved, and relative safety of the fiberoptic endoscopes rapidly became apparent. By 1970, most gastroscopic examinations were done with fiberscopes. The development of a "teaching head" fiberoptic bundle with a light splitter and attached eyepiece and attachment to the eyepiece of the scope allowed two people to visualize the image. Dividing the light from the endoscope considerably diminished the brightness of the image, however, to the operator and the observer. This device saw limited use and in primarily teaching institutions.

Endoscopic Retrograde Cholangiopancreatography (ERCP)

With access to the duodenum, the ampulla of Vater became visible. It followed that one should be able to inject contrast material into the bile and pancreatic ducts and increase diagnostic capabilities. Initial attempts in 1968 by McCune and associates[19] to modify an existing scope were only partially successful but did show that endoscopic visualization by injection of radiologic contrast agents into ducts was possible. In 1970, Machida and Olympus in Japan produced usable, side-viewing scopes with controllable tips and elevators to move the injection tube to the ampulla.

Japanese endoscopists[20] developed the technique of endoscopic retrograde cholangiopancreatography (ERCP) with an 80% success rate. Vennes and Silvis[21] showed the utility of ERCP in the United States and taught many physicians to use it.[4] It was immediately apparent that if clinicians could visualize the biliary and pancreatic ducts endoscopically (i.e., nonsurgically), they should be able to apply by some means long-established surgical techniques for treatment of choledocholithiasis and pancreatitis, such as sphincterotomy and stone removal. In 1974, just 4 years after the demonstration of the diagnostic utility of the new ERCP scopes, Kawai and colleagues in Japan[22] and Classen and Demling in Germany[23] independently developed methods of endoscopic electrosurgical sphincterotomy for extraction of biliary calculi in the common duct. This procedure requires great skill; in 1976, Geenen[24] reported only 62 operative procedures had been done by four endoscopists, and 7 of the procedures were failures. In 1983, Schuman[4] reported that several thousands of patients had undergone ERCP, and by now, hundreds of thousands of ERCP procedures have been done. Because of advanced radiologic techniques, ERCP is now seldom used for purely diagnostic purposes.

Photography

It is one thing to describe to others what one may see through any device and another to be able to show them. The large impact of Schindler's early publications was related, in part, to the excellent color drawings he presented. Early on, neither cameras nor photographic films were advanced enough to allow good color reproduction or sharp, accurate images in relatively poor lightening. Such documentation is essential for widespread appreciation of endoscopy by individuals who do not perform the procedure. The first clinically useful photography came with improvements in film by Kodak and the construction of an external integrated camera by Segal and Watson in 1948.[25,26] Although these authors reported that approximately 61% of the images were of good quality, this was not the experience of all clinicians.[4]

Although an intragastric camera was developed in 1848 by Lange and Meltzung, a clinically useful device was not available until 1950, when Uji, Sugiura, and Fukami, working with Olympus Corp.,[27] developed the Gastrocamera with synchronized flash that took good intragastric pictures and with a controllable distal portion. By following a prescribed pattern of rotation and flexion, a series of pictures was obtained that included the entire surface of the stomach. The big disadvantage was that the operator could not see through the instrument and had to await development of the very narrow (5-mm) film before the results could be seen. Photographs for demonstration required additional time in the photo laboratory while enlargements were made.

With the introduction of fiberoptic scopes in 1961, Olympus introduced a combination Gastrocamera fiberscope (GTF-A)

in 1964, but, as Schuman[4] commented, "it was *just* a gastroscope" and never attained popularity. Simultaneously, rapid development and physician acceptance of fiberscopes with the ability to use technically advanced 35-mm cameras with an external adapter made the Gastrocamera obsolete, and it was abandoned.

Sigmoidoscopy and Colonoscopy

The problems presented by examination of the anus and rectum were relatively easy. Straight metal tubes were used and found in the ruins of Pompeii.[2] The basic design of the anoscope has not changed in the past century or more except that it is now made of disposable plastic. It remains a tapering short tube with an obturator that is removed after introduction through the anal sphincter. Examination of the rectum and sigmoid required a longer tube, but no truly satisfactory device was available until 1894, when Kelly[28] at Johns Hopkins developed a 30-cm rigid tube with light reflected down the tube from a head lamp. Tuttle[29] incorporated a distal light source in his proctosigmoidoscope of 25 cm in 1903. These instruments have remained the basic design for the past 100 years. Within the past 15 years or so, disposable clear plastic tubes have been widely used. These are essentially a plastic version of the Kelly and Tuttle tubes with a distal electric light source, but visualization is possible through the clear plastic. With the application of fiberoptics to sigmoidoscopy in the late 1960s, examination of the sigmoid colon became not only satisfactory, but also much more comfortable to the patient.

Overholt,[30] who later went on to be the principal developer of colonoscopy using similar technology, presented his results of flexible sigmoidoscopy in 250 patients in 1968. Although early flexible sigmoidoscopes were made in variable lengths, the current length of 60 cm came to be the preferred one. Examination of the colon above the sigmoid presents obvious additional problems of multiple curves and angulations amenable only to highly flexible instruments and trained operators. Attempts, all unsuccessful, were made using semiflexible instruments, and these are reviewed by Edmonson.[2] Satisfactory examination of the length of the colon was impossible until the introduction of the flexible fiberscope. Attempts to use forward-viewing gastroscopes were not technically satisfactory, although several clinicians tried, including me. Turell[31] presented his attempts in 1967 using a modified gastroscope, but he concluded that the instrument was not ready for routine clinical use. By 1970, several manufacturers produced instruments specifically designed for colonoscopy, including ACMI working with Overholt in the United States and Olympus Corp. in Japan.

The primary problem with regularly completing examinations to the cecum was not the instruments so much as it was the techniques necessary for passage of the scopes into the more proximal portions of the colon. Earlier pioneers in developing successful techniques still in use include, among others, Overholt, Wolf, Shinya, and Waye in the United States; Niwa and colleagues in Japan; Salmon and Williams in England; and Dehyle in Germany.[4] Many of these early efforts were accomplished with the guidance of fluoroscopy to negotiate the more difficult turns and to identify the actual area being observed, but as experience was gained, fluoroscopy was no longer required. Learning under expert guidance and experience continues to be more necessary in colonoscopy (and ERCP) than in upper endoscopy. By 1971, the diagnostic advantage of fiberoptic colonoscopy over single-contrast barium enema was firmly established,[32] and the efficacy and safety of polypectomy were established by 1973.[33]

Digital Endoscopy (Videoendoscopy)

In 1984, barely 20 years after introduction of the endoscopic fiberscope, Welch Allyn, Inc., replaced the coherent fiberoptic image bundle in a colonoscope with a light-sensitive computer chip or charge-coupled device on which the image was focused by a small lens (see Chapter 3).[34] The digital signal was fed to a video processor, which generated an image to a television monitor. The image did not occupy the entire screen, leaving space for information to be typed in by a keyboard. The resolution of the image was at least equal to that of the fiberscope.

It was unnecessary to change the basic mechanics of the fiberscope. The fiberoptic light bundle remained unchanged, as did water, suction, and biopsy channels; also, the deflection and locking mechanisms were the same. The basic elements of the videoendoscope have not changed, although a magnified image is now available. Since the original introduction of the videoendoscope by Welch Allyn, which no longer produces the VideoEndoscope, the market has been dominated by Olympus Corp. and Pentax. The technology was rapidly adapted to all endoscopes—used in gastroenterology and in other fields.

Advantages of the electronic instruments include an image that can be seen not only by the operator, but also by anyone with access to a connected monitor in the same or another room. This feature greatly enhances the ability to teach others about the procedure and to inform other interested physicians about the findings in the individual patient. If desired, recording of procedures can be accomplished with videotape machines, and good-quality pictures of individual frames can be made immediately with externally integrated digital equipment. Individual endoscopists found that no adjustment of techniques was necessary when videoendoscopes were used, although they had to become accustomed to looking at the monitor screen rather than through an optical system with one eye (**Fig. 1.12**). This feature added to the useful length of the instrument because the whole scope could be held at the waist rather that brought to eye level.

More recent innovations in colonoscopy instruments by Olympus include the ability to make a portion less flexible to facilitate navigation of difficult bends and turns. In addition, an enlarged image is now available that is an improvement in vision and ease of manipulation. A major disadvantage of videoendoscopes is cost. Fiberoptic endoscopes, when they were still in use, could be purchased for less than $6000 and did not require processors or monitors, whereas the latest videoendoscopes are priced more than $20,000, and initial purchase of the entire package of endoscope, processing computer, monitors, and attachments may exceed $30,000. Initially, many questioned the wisdom of this added cost, which is passed on to the patient and their insurance companies.

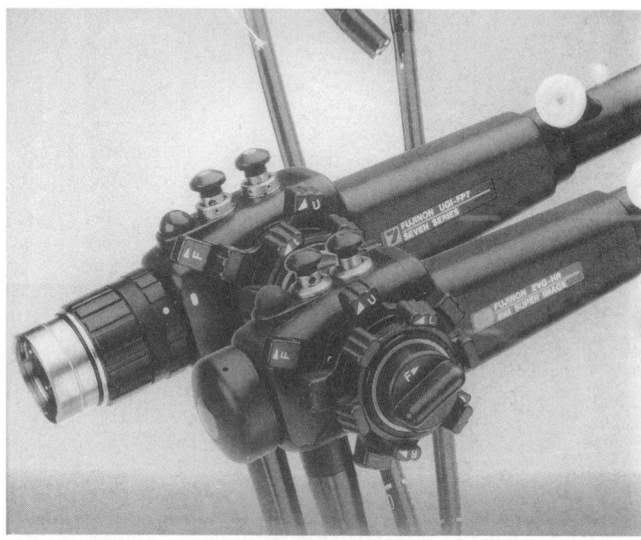

Fig. 1.12 Fujinon fiberoptic panendoscope *(top)* and its successor, the Videopanendoscope *(bottom)*, 1990, showing the two kinds of operating heads. *(From advertisement in* Gastrointest Endosc *36:240–241, 1990.)*

Endoscopic Ultrasonography (EUS)

Although the improvements in GI endoscopy are remarkable in the synthesis of diverse but complementary technologies, the information gained remains confined to what one can see from within the lumen of the gut. Simultaneous with these developments were those of computed tomography and external ultrasonographic tomograms. Conceptually, it was not only logical but also compelling to look beneath the mucosa of the gut by incorporating into GI endoscopes miniaturized models of ultrasonographic transducers already in use. The ability to explore noninvasively tissue and organs in proximity to the gut had exciting implications for diagnosis and therapy.

In Germany in 1976, working with Siemens Co, Lutz and Rosch[35] reported the use of a 1-cm ultrasonographic 4-MHz probe that could be passed through the biopsy channel of an Olympus TGF. They used it in two patients to differentiate successfully between pancreatic pseudocysts and tumors.[7] In 1980, Classen's group in Germany[36] and DiMagno and colleagues[37] at the Mayo Clinic reported EUS devices that were incorporated onto the tip of conventional fiberscopes, one using a 5-MHz transducer and the other using a 10-MHz transducer. These probes had good resolution at an acoustic focus depth of 3 cm. Others incorporated the transducer in the distal shaft of fiberoptic scopes and explored primarily the gut wall.[33,38] By 1985, ultrasonic transducers with variable frequencies incorporated into videoendoscopes were readily available, although expensive (>$100,000 for initial setup) (**Fig. 1.13**). It was immediately apparent that this procedure could accurately evaluate known or suspected intramural lesions of the gut,[39,40] and it was rapidly expanded to include the esophagus; problems of diagnosis and recurrence of neoplasia, especially in the pancreas; portal hypertension; the colon and rectum; and bile ducts.[41] In 1991, Wiersema and colleagues[42,43] showed that EUS could be used to obtain fine needle aspiration cytology of mediastinal nodes and of nodes and lesions of the upper and lower GI tract. The addition of Doppler technology has now made possible the study of the

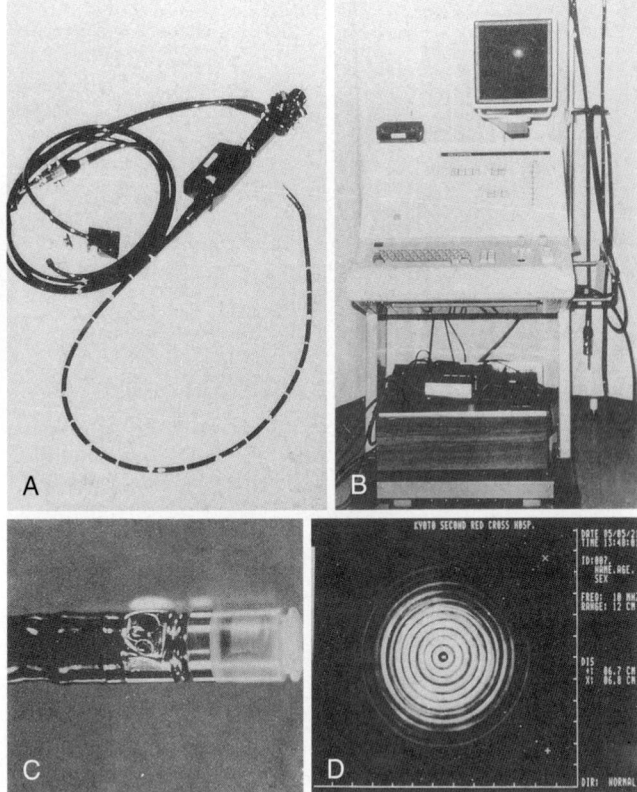

Fig. 1.13   Ultrasonic endoscope system, model IV, made by Olympus Corp., 1986. *(From Yasuda K, Mukai H, Fujimoto S, et al: The diagnosis of pancreatic cancer by endoscopic ultrasonography.* Gastrointest Endosc *34:1–8, 1988.)*

flow through various channels, including the thoracic duct and blood vessel anastomosis. The techniques of using EUS instruments differ only slightly from using videoendoscopes, but dedicated training is necessary to interpret the sonographic images obtained accurately. EUS is not amenable to self-instruction. EUS training centers have been established in academic centers, but retraining of practicing physicians is a problem.[44]

Capsule Endoscopy (Wireless Endoscopy)

In 2000, Iddan and colleagues[45] reported the development of a capsule containing a tiny CMOS camera that could be swallowed, take video (but slowed to 2 frames per second), and transmit the video over 7 hours to a receiving digital storage unit worn by the patient as he or she goes about their normal activities. These frames are downloaded to a computer from which they are projected onto a monitor at a rate that can be controlled by the observer. Pictures can be printed of areas of interest. Gastroenterologists in Israel conducted randomized trials comparing the wireless capsule efficacy with push enteroscopy and showed superior results with the capsule.[46–48]

Wireless capsule endoscopy caught the imagination of gastroenterologists over the world, and capsule endoscopy has been adopted as a part of standard practice for small bowel imaging. The findings are virtually unanimous in reporting

better results in identifying lesions in the small bowel compared with results from push enteroscopy.[49] The capsule avoids the discomfort and need for sedation inherent in push enteroscopy. In addition to lack of biopsy capability, a major disadvantage is the reported 4 hours of review time necessary, but this would likely be overcome by training of nonphysician personnel to screen the multiple images produced. Although the major use of the capsule to date has been elucidating the cause of occult bleeding from small bowel sources, where it seems to be superior to other methods, its future in other diseases, such as those in the colon, has already been investigated in large multicenter comparative studies. The future of wireless capsule endoscopy is bright. It will be interesting to see how the principle of wireless endoscopy is united to videoendoscopes with direct wireless connection between the camera and the computer processor.

Enteroscopy

The small intestine can be regarded as the final frontier of GI endoscopy. Although capsule endoscopy provides remarkable images of the small bowel mucosa, therapy with a capsule-based instrument is many years away. Surgically assisted small bowel enteroscopy may be performed via either the transoral or anal route or via a mid–small bowel enterotomy incision. The disadvantage of this technique is its invasive nature.[50] Endoscopic examination of the small intestine has remained technically difficult. The many loops of the small intestine prevent progression of the instrument tip by simple pushing. This problem was overcome initially with the use of the Sonde enteroscope,[51] which is a very fine, floppy instrument with a balloon at the tip. The Sonde enteroscope progressed through much of the small bowel under peristalsis, and then the proceduralist would slowly withdraw the instrument, assessing the mucosa while pulling back. This technique was thought to visualize 50% to 70% of the mucosal surface.[52] However, the procedure was uncomfortable, was time-consuming, and did not permit therapeutics, all of which limited its use.

The concept of small bowel enteroscopy was revolutionized by Yamamoto with the introduction of the double-balloon enteroscope in 2001.[53] This technique uses traction between a balloon at the tip of the enteroscope and another balloon on a flexible overtube to concertina the loops of small bowel and provide traction for forward movement. The procedure requires per oral and anal procedures to examine the entire small intestine, and even then only in a minority of Western patients is the whole small bowel visualized. Nonetheless, double balloon–assisted enteroscopy permits endoscopic therapeutics to most of the small bowel with the need for surgical assistance. A single balloon version is also available.

Natural Orifice Transluminal Endoscopic Surgery (NOTES)

The newest development in endoscopy is natural orifice transluminal endoscopic surgery (NOTES), in which the endoscope is inserted into the abdominal cavity via an incision in an accessible organ. The first report appeared in 2002. Incisions have been made in the stomach, vagina, and colon with successful tubal ligation, liver biopsies, biopsy of peritoneal metastases, oophorectomy, cholecystectomy, and nephrectomy. Most published articles report only experimental use in animals with the latest development being the simultaneous use of NOTES and laparoscopic techniques. Comparative studies are under way. A difficulty with the technique has been overcoming the lack of instrument "triangulation," that is, approaching a surgical site from two or more directions to create countertraction, tie sutures, and so forth. Although NOTES is an exciting surgical development, its remarkable potential will have to await the development of new instruments and expertise.

Summary

The development of endoscopy is a testimony to human ingenuity. Instruments have evolved from dangerous straight tubes illuminated by light reflected from candles, to more flexible and safer instruments with an image transmitted through a series of prism lenses and illumination by an electric light bulb, to images transmitted through fiberoptic bundles with illumination transmitted by fiber bundles from an external source, to our present remarkably safe electronic instruments with digital images transmitted to a video screen through wires and processed by computers. Most recently, we can visualize the lumen of the gut without touching the patient. Now we not only can visualize, biopsy tissue, and perform surgical procedures within the hidden cavities of the body, but also indirectly see beneath the mucosa and into immediately adjacent organs. This is really a remarkable story and "it ain't over yet"! To know and understand what has come before lends strength to efforts toward what is to be.

References

The complete reference list is available online at www.expertconsult.com.

Chapter 2

Setting Up an Endoscopy Facility

James T. Frakes and Klaus Mergener

Introduction

The safe and efficient performance of gastrointestinal (GI) endoscopy has the following requirements:[1]

- A properly trained endoscopist[2] with appropriate privileges to perform specific GI endoscopic procedures[3,4]
- Properly trained nursing and ancillary personnel
- Operational, well-maintained equipment
- Adequately designed and equipped space for patient preparation, performance of procedures, and patient recovery
- Cleaning areas for reprocessing endoscopes and accessories
- Trained personnel and appropriate equipment to perform cardiopulmonary resuscitation
- Robust quality improvement assurance program[5–7]

Many of the above-listed requirements for safe and efficient GI endoscopy depend on the careful development of endoscopy areas—specifically the setting up or planning and design of an endoscopy facility. This chapter describes that process, beginning with laying the groundwork, including the development of a business plan and review of regulatory issues; site selection; facility planning and design, including patient flow and space needs; equipment requirements; staffing needs; and

scheduling considerations. Some additional issues, such as endoscope cleaning and storage, tissue specimen processing and handling, record keeping and documentation, and quality assurance and improvement, are discussed briefly but are covered in more detail in subsequent chapters of this book (see Chapters 4, 5, and 9).

Exploring Possibilities

Type of Facility

There are numerous types of endoscopy facilities, including hospital endoscopy units, single-specialty or multispecialty ambulatory surgery centers (ASCs), and office endoscopy suites. Each model has a unique set of advantages, disadvantages, and regulatory issues. The hospital and ASC environments are highly regulated by state and federal agencies and by third-party accreditation bodies. In the United States, these include the Joint Commission on Accreditation of Healthcare Organizations (JCAHO), the Accreditation Association for Ambulatory Healthcare (AAAHC), and the American Association for Accreditation of Ambulatory Surgery Facilities (AAAASF). Private payers sometimes impose their own specific requirements. Office endoscopy suites, previously less regulated, have been subjected to more controls by state and federal agencies in recent years.

The decision regarding which type of facility to establish is affected by the practice environment (solo practitioner, small or large group, single-specialty or multispecialty group, independent or hospital-based) and local economics and politics. Regardless of the service location, high quality must be maintained. The American Society for Gastrointestinal Endoscopy (ASGE) has stated that the "standards for out-of-hospital endoscopic practice should be identical to those recognized guidelines followed in the hospital."[1] In an insurance-based environment, the hospital-based unit poses the fewest financial risks and demands for the endoscopist during the early phases of operation, and its use avoids alienating hospital administration by preserving hospital case volume. The hospital-based unit affords the endoscopist little control over operations, however, and offers him or her the lowest total financial return. Office endoscopy offers control and convenience with better financial return for the physician, but it poses some safety and liability concerns.[8,9] A single-specialty endoscopic ambulatory surgery center (EASC) provides the best of control, efficiency, convenience, and reimbursement for the physician owners and is extremely popular with patients, referring physicians, and payers.[10,11] At the time of this writing, a major ASC payment reform is being implemented by the Centers for Medicare and Medicaid Services (CMS), which is resulting in drastic cuts of facility payments for endoscopic services. How this reform will affect efforts to provide beneficial GI services to patients at a reasonable cost remains to be seen. More information about this payment reform is available elsewhere.[12] Regardless of the type of facility being developed, formulating a business plan and understanding various regulatory issues are usually the first steps in the process.

Business Plan

The decision to set up an endoscopy facility should be made only after detailed data gathering and the formulation of a business plan (e.g., market analysis, financial pro forma, implementation time line).[13–15] For a hospital-based unit or academic medical center, facility planners and accountants often perform these functions. For an office-based suite or an EASC, the tasks fall to the physician owners, aided by numerous consultants, contractors, or corporate partners. Even with skilled help, however, development of an accurate and reliable business plan and pro forma are highly dependent on physician estimates, insights, and work habits. Physician input into the business plan makes the difference between a perfunctory exercise and an accurate predictor of future performance. Endoscopy facilities represent small to medium-sized investments requiring substantial financial resources and staff. Procedure volume must be sufficient to produce adequate revenue to cover the costs of building and running the facility and to generate a profit on investment. Generally, three or four busy endoscopists performing 1200 to 1800 total procedures per year are required to offset the financial risk of the facility.[16]

Many factors influence the financial performance of an endoscopy facility, including initial investment, expected volumes of service, revenue per unit of service, fixed operating costs, and variable costs per unit of service. The initial investment includes the cost of construction, equipment, and working capital for the first few months of operation. Strategic planning is important to anticipate group growth and demand for services in the coming 5 to 10 years.[13,15] The impact of managed care plans or other major health plans on the practice must also be anticipated. In addition, competition, new technology, population changes, and demographics might affect case volume for the practice and the endoscopy facility.

A pro forma is a calculation examining the financial feasibility of a project based on anticipated investment and operating costs and revenues. The purpose of the pro forma is to predict reliably cash flows and profitability for the project. Initial investment costs have been defined previously. Also incorporated in the pro forma are estimated total costs per case based on estimated fixed and variable costs and expected case volume. Fixed costs are costs that remain constant regardless of the number of procedures performed and include rent, interest, depreciation, taxes, insurance, amortization, and management fees. Variable costs, which account for the largest component of the average cost per case, include salaries and benefits, medical supplies, medications, equipment, maintenance and repair, administrative supplies, utilities, and accounting and legal fees. Break-even volumes can be determined by subtracting the variable expense per procedure from the average payment per procedure to indicate the contribution available to be used for overhead and profit. Dividing fixed costs by the contribution margin per procedure indicates the number of procedures needed to pay the fixed costs, also known as the break-even point. Additional service units above that level constitute profit. Vicari and Garry[13] provided a simple example of a pro forma. The business plan and pro forma are mandatory in assessing the financial feasibility of the proposed endoscopy unit before construction. They further aid discussions in obtaining financing and help the architect design the unit for anticipated volumes.

Regulatory and Certification Issues

Before planning and designing the facility, one must understand the relevant regulatory and certification issues. As with the business plan, units developed in a hospital or academic medical center usually benefit from administrators and planners familiar with these complex issues. Physician owners of an office endoscopy suite or EASC must gain their own understanding. Various agencies provide myriad rules and regulations concerning endoscopy facilities.[17–23] Legislation can come from federal, state, or local authorities. Regulations may come from federal agencies, state departments of health, and third-party accreditation organizations and private payers. Although these rules and regulations can seem excessive and needlessly costly, their intent is to ensure safe and successful outcomes for patients. Regulations and certification issues for endoscopy facilities can be divided into six main categories, as follows:[17]

- General federal regulatory laws and rules
- Facility state licensure
- Medicare certification
- Third-party accreditation
- Physician credentialing
- Private payer requirements

General Federal Health-Related Laws

Federal regulatory laws and rules include Fraud and Abuse Statutes (also known as antikickback laws), which are laws designed to prevent excessive or inappropriate payments. Endoscopy centers typically fall into a specific "safe harbor," a designation that protects EASC investors or shareholders from allegations of fraud or abuse. The safe harbor applies if the physician participants are surgeons or specialists engaged in the same surgical or medical practice specialty, including gastroenterology. These physicians can refer patients directly to their center and perform procedures on them as an extension of and significant part of their practices.

Additional requirements of the safe harbor apply. Ownership of the facility, or remuneration from it, cannot be related to volume of referrals, services furnished, or the amount of business otherwise generated from that physician to the EASC. The amount of payment to physician owners from facility revenues must be directly proportional to the amount of each owner's capital investment. There must be no requirement that a passive investor make referrals to the EASC, and the EASC or any investor cannot make loans or guarantee a loan for a physician, if these funds are used to purchase ownership in the EASC. Each physician must agree to treat Medicare and Medicaid patients. Finally, the physician owner must derive at least one-third of his or her medical practice income from the performance of procedures that require an EASC or hospital endoscopy unit setting.

Other general federal health-related laws and rules relevant to endoscopy facilities include the False Claims Act and copayment waivers, Stark provisions, Health Insurance Portability and Accountability Act (HIPAA) provisions, and labor and employment issues. The False Claims Act was designed to prevent false billings, claims that are medically unnecessary, and billings for inappropriately high payment. Copayment or deductible waivers may also be illegal if the government suspects such waivers are likely to induce referrals. Stark provisions stem from the Ethics in Patients Referrals Act. They are closely related to Fraud and Abuse Statutes but are civil rather than criminal laws. The regulatory body overseeing Medicare has ruled that a physician does not make an illegal referral for a procedure when he or she either personally performs the service or refers a patient to a partner to perform the service. HIPAA provisions are rules and regulations covering patient health information disclosed by any covered health care entity, provider, or facility. Regarding labor and employment issues, numerous rules and regulations cover discrimination, harassment, protection of the disabled, and workplace safety. The Occupational Health and Safety Act (OSHA) of 1970 seeks to protect employees from recognized work hazards that might cause death or serious harm. For endoscopy centers, OSHA requirements of major importance cover cleaning of endoscopic equipment, disinfection, and appropriate ventilation.

State Licensure

The state department of health licensing authority is interested in several features of a potential endoscopy facility. First, before any design and construction is undertaken, a careful review of the state's certificate of need (CON) requirements is needed. Some states do not allow construction of new facilities unless need is demonstrated. This process can be difficult, and prospective physician owners of endoscopy facilities may encounter opposition from hospitals, fearing competition and seeking to maximize use of their own facilities. Regarding specific construction guidelines, state regulators are most often interested in the flow of the facility, cleanliness, and control of infection within the procedure areas. Many states have adopted specific room sizes, acoustic regulations, door and hall size requirements, handicapped access provisions, requirements for exhaust systems, and specific fire codes. The state fire marshal would be concerned with emergency exits. Building codes from the National Fire Protection Association generally apply to endoscopy facilities built as new centers or as centers built in existing buildings. Many states also follow guidelines from the American Institute of Architects and the U.S. Department of Health for design and construction of health care facilities.

Medicare Certification

Medicare certification is usually sought after obtaining state licensure and is required for any facility seeking reimbursement for Medicare and Medicaid work. Medicare regulations and requirements are usually more extensive than regulations of the state and address governance of the facility, transfer agreements with a nearby hospital, continuous quality improvement activities, Medicare architectural requirements, and medical records. Additional standards concern organization and staffing, administration of drugs, and procurement of laboratory and radiology services. Two other requirements warrant special attention as they relate to EASCs. First, the facility must be used exclusively for providing "surgical" services, a definition that includes GI endoscopies. This requirement mandates a separation from other health care activities, separate staffing, and maintenance of special medical and financial records. Finally, the facility must comply with state licensure laws,[20] which is potentially difficult in some states because of restrictive CON requirements.

Third-Party Accreditation

After state licensure and Medicare certification have been obtained, some states or specific payers may require a third-party accreditation before authorizing payments to an endoscopy facility. This accreditation can be provided by inspection from JCAHO, AAAHC, or AAAASF. Although these accreditations are typically achieved after state licensure, sometimes they can be pursued simultaneously with Medicare inspection. Under certain circumstances, Medicare accepts accreditation from one of the third-party accreditation authorities in lieu of its own survey; this is known as attaining "deemed status," and it obviates an additional inspection. These third-party accreditations focus on patient-related and organizational functions and, in the case of an EASC, concentrate on the "environment of care" or "facilities and environment."

Third-party inspection of a facility can be challenging and demands that the owners and operators fully understand the standards of each specific accrediting organization. A JCAHO survey scrutinizes five patient-focused functions and six organization-focused functions. Patient-related functions include patient rights and organization ethics, assessment of patients, care of patients, education of patients and family, and continuity of care. Organization functions include standards dealing with organization improvement; leadership;

management of the environment of care; human resources; information; and surveillance, prevention, and control of infection. AAAHC and AAAASF inspections assess similar functions, although these may be grouped under different organizational headings.

Physician Credentialing

Credentialing and privileging of physicians using an EASC may be mandated by federal, state, local, or third-party organizations and include a formal application process, verification of licensure and drug enforcement administration status, malpractice history, admitting privileges, advanced cardiac life support (ACLS) status, and documentation of training.

Payer Requirements

Individual health plans or insurers may have their own requirements, and these may vary significantly from payer to payer. Careful attention to local payer mix and any special requirements is necessary before designing and building an endoscopy facility to ensure qualification for payment. As outlined previously, the regulatory and certification issues for endoscopy facilities are "complex, detailed, and broad."[17] Any physician wishing to develop an endoscopy facility must understand these rules of regulation and certification. Appropriate legal counsel should be considered essential.

Choosing a Site

For hospital-based endoscopy facilities, the location of the facility is usually determined by the hospital's own planners. Although some hospitals have developed separate units for outpatient and inpatient endoscopies, most hospitals operate a single endoscopy unit. Choosing its location requires careful consideration of patient transport issues; the flow of inpatients and outpatients in and out of the unit; and the proximity to radiology, emergency department, intensive care units, and inpatient wards. With office-based endoscopy or EASCs, physician owners choose the site. The site size and location require careful consideration because most office-based facilities or ASCs later expand to accommodate more physicians and patients. Preliminary land requirements are determined from space estimates (discussed later), parking requirements, appropriate landscaping or "green areas," and anticipated expansion. For an office endoscopy suite or EASC, proximity to a hospital is desirable to minimize travel for patients requiring hospital transfer and for physician convenience. The site should be near but perhaps not on a major street to ease patient parking. Many patients coming to an ASC or office-based facility are elderly or may be anxious about their upcoming procedures. Access should be easy. Locating the physician offices adjacent to the ASC should be strongly considered because it may be very efficient for staff and patients.

Facility Planning and Design

After forming a realistic business plan and acquiring an understanding of relevant regulatory and certification issues, attention turns to the planning and design of the facility. Although the remainder of this chapter includes some remarks about issues specifically related to hospital units, the main focus of the

discussion is on the development of an outpatient endoscopy facility, details of which are equally applicable to hospital units. Objectives must be articulated to the design professionals to ensure that the facility meets the needs of patients, endoscopists, and staff. Some points to keep in mind are the following:[24]

- Allow adequate time for planning.
- Set aside a regular block of time for discussion, review, and program development.
- Choose experienced design professionals who communicate well.
- Involve staff to ensure attention to their needs and wishes.
- Prepare a statement of needs and goals to aid the architect in preparing a detailed program.
- Prepare an inventory of equipment that will be used.
- Visit other facilities to gather ideas worth incorporating.
- Use flow studies to evaluate placement of functional elements.
- Review preliminary drawings carefully.
- If questions arise about the size or shape of a space, lay it out with tape on the floor and simulate work practices.

Planning and design of the facility is a team project. The team mainly involves a physician representing the endoscopists who will use the facility; two staff people, including the nurse responsible for patient care activities within the unit and the appropriate administrator; the architect; and the builder. The responsible physician must be given adequate time away from clinical duties to devote to planning, design, and oversight of the construction of the facility. Designated time must be set aside because the process is ongoing and cannot be relegated to lunch hours and brief sessions whenever time can be stolen from clinical activities. The architect is the primary professional involved in overseeing the entire project. It is wise to select an architect who specializes in medical buildings, particularly one who has experience in designing endoscopy facilities. Similarly, selection of a contractor who has experience in medical construction, particularly construction of endoscopy facilities, is important. Both the architect and the contractor must thoroughly understand the requirements of regulatory and certifying bodies and local and state building codes. Sometimes the design and contracting can be provided by one company with both design and building capabilities.

Although the physician representative, designated staff persons, architect, and contractor compose the major elements of the planning and design team, additional input may be needed from a mechanical engineer, electrical engineer, telephone contractor, information technology expert, and attorney.[25] Consideration might also be given to involving a layperson or "patient" to ensure sufficient attention to issues of patient comfort, dignity, and privacy.

Planning

The planning stage is concerned with deciding what activities will be conducted in the facility, what equipment will be needed, and how space will be allocated.

Scope of Activities

The first consideration is which endoscopic procedures and other services will be performed in the facility.[19] The type of facility will, to a great extent, answer this question. For a hospital unit that must provide a wide range of endoscopic services, one or more rooms must be large enough and appropriately equipped to accommodate the special equipment required for complex procedures (e.g., endoscopic retrograde cholangiopancreatography [ERCP], endoscopic ultrasound [EUS], balloon enteroscopy, laparoscopy, anesthesia cart). In some community hospitals, endoscopy units are shared with other specialties, such as cardiology or pulmonology, and have to accommodate procedures such as transesophageal echocardiography or bronchoscopy. If the hospital is part of an academic medical center, the unit may serve additional purposes, including teaching and research, requiring further modifications in space, equipment, and staffing.

For an office suite and EASC, services offered will be based on logistics and reimbursement ramifications. In these out-of-hospital facilities, procedures usually are limited to "routine" high-volume procedures having predictable turnaround times and minimal recovery times and requiring standard equipment and less expensive accessories. In an EASC, it is crucial that all procedures done be on the Medicare approved list to qualify for facility reimbursement. For both the office suite and the EASC, procedures usually are limited to upper GI endoscopy, esophageal dilation, and colonoscopy including polypectomy. Predictably, rapid turnaround time is crucial for an efficiently functioning EASC or office facility. Prolonged procedures or procedures that are unpredictable in duration, such as ERCP, are best done in the hospital. Procedures requiring prolonged recovery times, such as liver biopsy, are also best left for the hospital environment. Finally, procedures that require numerous and expensive accessories are best scheduled at the hospital because neither office suites nor EASCs can recover the costs of these accessories.

The question sometimes arises whether it is better to have a multispecialty or single-specialty ASC. From the standpoint of services offered and equipment, a single-specialty EASC has the advantage of being the "focus factory."[27,28] In this environment, endoscopists, skilled GI nurses, and administrative staff maximally use equipment of relatively low cost, performing predictably timed procedures with a rapid turnaround. A single-specialty EASC avoids the problem of a multispecialty facility in which highly specialized equipment lies idle much of the time while physicians from differing specialties are performing their individual procedures.

Equipment

The greatest capital expense after the basic construction is equipment. Some tabulation of the equipment needed is necessary in the early planning stages and facility design. The basic equipment needed for an endoscopy unit is listed in **Box 2.1**.[1,26,29] A detailed discussion of individual items is not presented here, but a few points are useful in integrating the equipment needs into planning and design. Generally, examining or procedure tables have been replaced by height-adjustable, rolling procedural stretcher carts that allow patients, once properly gowned for endoscopy, to mount the movable cart and not leave it until ready to leave the facility. These useful carts allow patients to be shuttled from preparation areas to procedure rooms and back to recovery areas and serve as procedure tables. This capability is very important to

---

Box 2.1 Endoscopy Facility Equipment List

I.   Major endoscopic and electrosurgical equipment
   A. Endoscopes, light sources, videoprocessors, and monitors
   B. Electrocautery units and accessories
   C. Hemostasis unit (e.g., Heater Probe, Gold Probe)
   D. Physiologic monitoring devices including pulse oximetry, blood pressure, and cardiac monitoring
II. Catheters, snares, forceps, and brushes
   A. Polypectomy snares
   B. Forceps
     1. Biopsy
       a. Regular or needle
       b. Hot biopsy
   C. Brushes
     1. Cleaning
     2. Cytology
   D. Graspers
   E. Retrieval baskets
III. Photo generator and image manager
IV. Esophageal dilators
   A. Wire-guided (Savary or American)
   B. Balloon
V.   Rolling procedural stretcher carts with adjustable heights
VI. Suction equipment
VII. Pharmaceuticals
   A. Sedation and analgesia agents
     1. Benzodiazepines
     2. Narcotic analgesics
     3. Miscellaneous preference
   B. Benzodiazepine antagonists
   C. Narcotic antagonists
   D. Glucagon
   E. Atropine
   F. Topicals
VIII. Intravenous equipment, solutions, needles, and syringes
IX. Chemicals
   A. Formalin
   B. Disinfection solutions
X.   Emergency cart, resuscitation equipment, supplies, and medications
XI. High-level disinfection equipment (cleaning trays, sinks, automatic endoscope washers, and autoclave)
XII. Instrument storage cabinets
XIII. Blanket warmer
XIV. Radios and audio compact disc players
XV. Eyewash station

From references 1, 18, and 21.

---

overall system efficiency and adds to patient safety by avoiding transfer to and from a procedure table.

Another major determinant of overall system speed and efficiency is the availability of endoscopes. Adequate numbers of endoscopes, high-level disinfection systems ("scope washers"), and adequate storage for extra endoscopes are required. Adequate numbers of endoscopes must be available to prevent inefficient downtime in the unit. In most endoscopy suites, variable costs account for 80% or more of the total costs of providing endoscopic services, and 50% to 60% of this is attributable to staff salaries, wages, and benefits.[14] It is inefficient and fiscally unwise to have highly paid physicians and staff waiting for endoscopes. One of the most efficient scenarios is for one endoscopist to work out of two rooms so that he or she can move from room to room without major downtime. This scenario typically requires that each unit have three colonoscopes and three upper endoscopes for every two rooms in the facility. This allows two rooms always to be equipped for either upper endoscopy or colonoscopy with one endoscope always available to restock the next room during turnaround.

The luxury of additional endoscopes per two rooms allows for the inevitable loss of an endoscope resulting from breakage and repair time. A high-volume, efficient endoscopy unit cannot afford to be penny wise and endoscope foolish when it comes to the number of endoscopes available. Regarding esophageal dilators, the decision of whether to use a Savary or American dilator system versus balloons can have major economic consequences. This is less of an issue in the hospital where some device costs can be separately billed. However, in an office suite or an EASC, use of balloons and other expensive accessories such as hemoclips may be problematic, particularly with Medicare or Medicaid patients, for whom the facility fee is set by regulation and extra costs for accessories cannot be passed on. Finally, with the growing use of propofol or anesthesia services for endoscopic procedures, additional medications and equipment are often required for this service.[30,31]

Physical Environment

Before beginning specific planning and design, some issues affecting space efficiency should be considered. It is the goal for physicians and staff to work as quickly and efficiently as possible while giving the patient the assurance that he or she is receiving appropriate care. System speed in the endoscopy facility usually comes from the following three delivery components:

1. Preparation and recovery of the patient
2. Reprocessing and return of endoscopes to the procedure room
3. Physician work habits

If the first two components operate properly, the number of procedure rooms available is not as important as the practice habits of the physician in performing procedures, talking to patients and their families, completing medical records, and returning to the procedure room.[30] In an efficient facility, physician discipline is needed because room turnover and equipment reprocessing time can be rapid. Scheduled times for one physician operating out of two rooms with adequate staff and equipment can be easily allotted at 30 minutes for colonoscopies and 20 minutes for upper GI endoscopies (Rockford Gastroenterology Associates, Ltd., Rockford, IL, unpublished data).

Flow

Architects use flow diagrams to plan movement patterns in arranging space before actual design plans. Physician and nurse input is crucial in arranging the flow relationships

within the endoscopy facility to maximize efficiency, minimize travel distance, and achieve economy of movement. A basic flow diagram showing the components for a simple endoscopy unit is shown in **Fig. 2.1**. The patterns of movement in a more complicated facility are conceptualized in **Fig. 2.2**. Simple flow diagrams such as these can be elaborated into a functional relationship diagram as shown in **Fig. 2.3**. Although this diagram suggests a floor plan, it is not a true floor plan. The sizes of the areas within the diagram are not proportional to the actual relative sizes of the rooms they represent. This type of functional relationship diagram shows the way that patients, staff, physicians, and equipment move through the facility.

For hospital-based units, specific patient flow issues must be considered. Separate entrances for sick, bedridden patients and ambulatory individuals should be considered. The monitoring and treatment requirements for sick inpatients must be taken into consideration. Separation of inpatients and outpatients in waiting or holding areas, preparation areas, and recovery areas may also be helpful. In the example of an ambulatory endoscopy center shown in **Fig. 2.3**, an endoscopy facility and an adjacent clinic facility are shown. The endoscopy facility on one side of the firewall can qualify as an ASC if the rules and regulations are followed and the endoscopy facility is separated from the clinic building by a required 1-hour fire rated wall-door construction system. This construction is usually achieved by using a wall with two layers of fire-rated gypsum board on either side of the structural wall supports and having the wall extend through the ceiling to the roof of the structure above.[32]

A functional relationship diagram can be turned into a floor plan by assigning actual space requirements to the rooms that are represented. **Fig. 2.4** shows a sample architectural space program worksheet that can be used to turn a functional relationship diagram into a floor plan. A 40% circulation allowance must be added at the end of the tabulation to account for wall thicknesses, corridors, and so forth.[32,33]

Designing the Endoscopy Facility

The *Guidelines for Design and Construction of Health Care Facilities (AIA Guideline)*, published by the American Institute of Architects (AIA) and the Academy of Architecture for

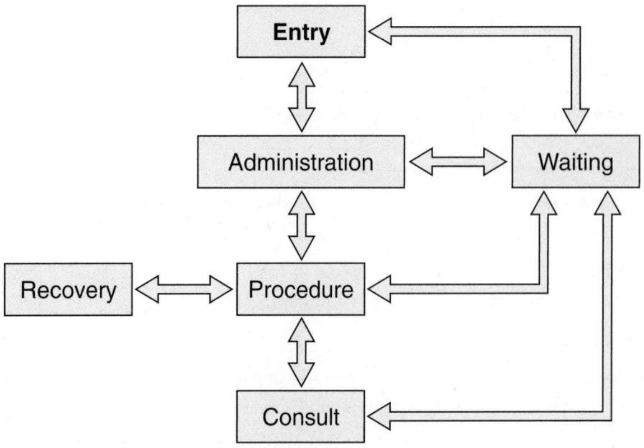

Fig. 2.1 Flow diagram for simple endoscopy unit. *(From Rich ME: Office layout and design. In Overholt BF, Chobanian SJ, editors: Office endoscopy, Baltimore, 1990, Williams & Wilkins.)*

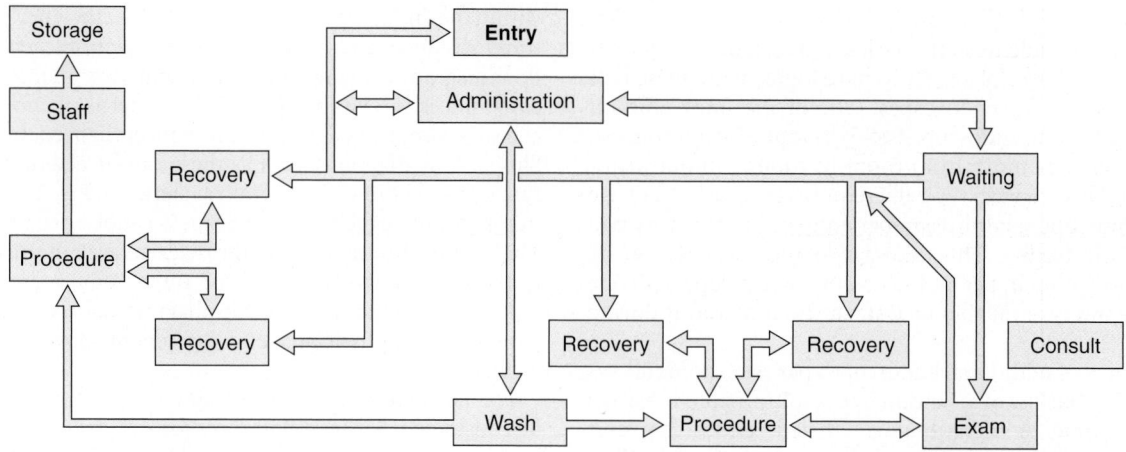

Fig. 2.2 Flow diagram for larger endoscopy unit. *(From Rich ME: Office layout and design. In Overholt BF, Chobanian SJ, editors:* Office endoscopy, *Baltimore, 1990, Williams & Wilkins.)*

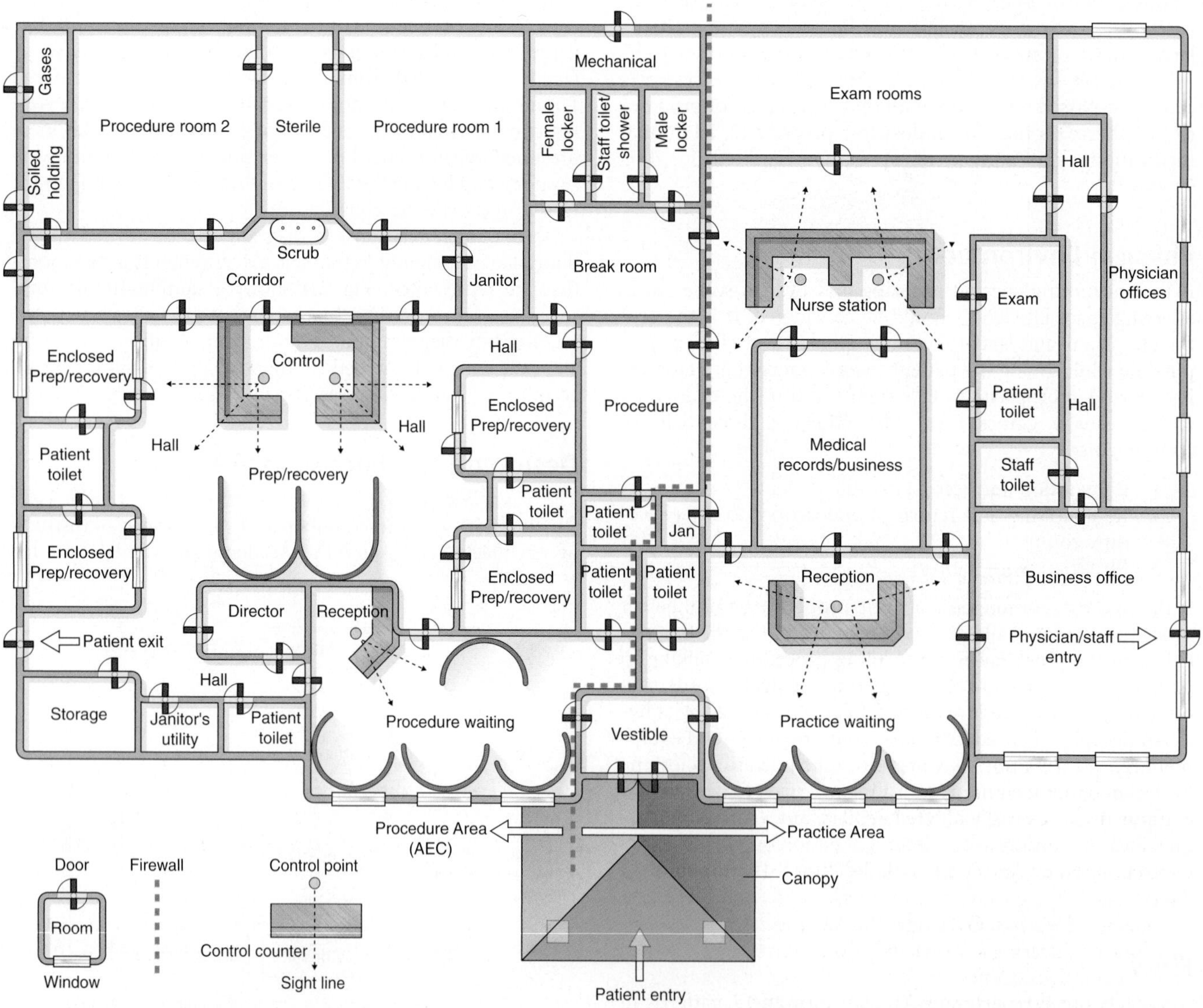

Fig. 2.3 Functional relationship diagram of ambulatory endoscopy center. *(From Marasco JA, Marasco RF: Designing the ambulatory endoscopy center.* Gastrointest Endosc Clin N Am *12:193, 2002.)*

ROOM	DESCRIPTION	AREA
A Waiting Module		SF
1. Seats	☐ 2.0 to 2.5 x # of patients in building at once @ 18 SF/seat	___ SF
2. Nourishment/TV	☐ 1 @ 10 SF =	___ SF
3. Waiting room toilet	☐ 1 @ 55 SF =	___ SF
4. Family room		SF
B. Business Reception Module		SF
1. Reception area	☐ 50 SF/position	___ SF
2. Billing		___ SF
3. Transcription		___ SF
4. Director		___ SF
5. Files	☐ # of patients/year x 3 years divided by 100 patients/lineal feet = lineal feet @ 1.75 lineal feet per square feet	___ SF
C. Control Module		SF
1. Control station	☐ 18 to 120 SF	___ SF
2. Storage	☐ 20 to 30 SF	___ SF
3. Dictation area	☐ 20 to 30 SF	___ SF
D. Prep/Recovery Module		SF
1. Enclosed stations	☐ 2 per procedure room @ 100 SF =	___ SF
	☐ Glassed enclosed procedure room side	___
2. Recovery lounge	☐ 2 per procedure room @ 65 SF =	___ SF
	☐ Recliner	___
3. Toilet/dressing	☐ 1 per 2 prep/recovery stations @ 65 SF	
E. Operating Rooms (Procedure Room) Module		SF
1. See utilization chart for number		___
2. Procedure rooms	☐ 270 SF	___
	☐ Procedure room could be as little as 180 SF - discuss with state	
3. Scrub area	☐ See state regulations	
	☐ Could be inside room - if not then 10 SF	
F. Utility Module		SF
1. Sterilization	☐ 80 to 100 SF	___ SF
	☐ Discuss with state	
2. Clean storage	☐ 10 to 40 SF	___ SF
3. Dirty storage	☐ 20 to 50 SF	___ SF
4. General storage	☐ 80 to 180 SF	___ SF
5. Janitor's closet	☐ May need 2 - 15 to 20 SF	___ SF
6. Gas storage	☐ 30 to 50 SF	___ SF
7. Uninterruptible power source	☐ 20 to 40 SF	___ SF
G. Staff Dressing Module		SF
1. Check state to see if separate male and female ☐ dressing rooms are needed		___ SF
2. Check state to see if separate toilet and/or shower is needed for male and female		
3. Dressing (male and/or female)	☐ 10 SF per locker - minimum 60 SF	___ SF
	☐ 55 SF per toilet	___ SF
	☐ 70 SF for shower and toilet	___ SF
4. Break room	☐ Could be in practice area	___ SF
	☐ 80 to 100 SF	
TOTAL NET AREA	**Sum of A through G**	SF
40% CIRCULATION	**40% of Total Net**	SF
TOTAL GROSS AREA	**Total Net + Circulation**	SF

Fig. 2.4 Architectural space program worksheet. *(From Marasco JA, Marasco RF: Designing the ambulatory endoscopy center.* Gastrointest Endosc Clin N Am *12:194, 2002.)*

Health, includes a section on the design and construction of GI endoscopy facilities. The document is updated on a 4- to 5-year revision cycle with the latest edition published in 2006 and a new version anticipated for 2010. The *AIA Guideline*, which is referenced by many federal and state jurisdictions, was originally conceived as minimum construction requirements for hospitals. Over time, the document has evolved to include engineering systems, infection control, and safety and architectural guidelines for design and construction of hospitals and other types of health care facilities. It provides an invaluable resource for the construction of a new ambulatory endoscopy center, the construction of a hospital-based endoscopy unit, or the renovation of existing units. The *AIA Guideline* can be purchased through the Facility Guidelines Institute (FGI) at http://www.fgiguidelines.org/about. For existing hospital facilities, many considerations are subject to limited space and resources and require a compromise between optimal choices and the realities of the existing building. Marasco and Marasco[32,33] suggested designing the endoscopy facility in modules. The modules to be designed include the following:

- Waiting module
- Business-reception module

- Preparation-recovery module
- Procedure room module
- Utility module
- Staff dressing module

Each of the above-listed modules is discussed separately because there are rules, regulations, and practical points to be kept in mind during design.

Waiting Module

There has been a marked shift toward outpatient-based endoscopy since the mid-1980s. This shift has major implications for the design and operation of the endoscopy facility. The patient's experience of the endoscopy facility often begins outside of the building in the parking lot. Patients arriving for endoscopy are often anxious and sometimes frightened. Maps with careful driving instructions and signs posted in the vicinity of the endoscopy facility can minimize confusion and offer reassurance. An all-weather canopy and automatic opening doors are helpful to elderly, ill, or disabled patients. The reception and waiting room area provides an early impression of the endoscopy facility and should project efficiency and friendliness. Wheelchair storage should be available in this area, with wheelchairs stored out of sight. There must be adequate room for patients' escorts because one or two people usually accompany each patient scheduled for endoscopy. It is good to have a sub-waiting room for the endoscopy facility if there is an adjacent clinic area. A separate waiting area might be required under rules and regulations; even if not required, it might prove useful because waiting times for the clinic may be quite different from waiting times for patients undergoing endoscopy. The waiting areas should be well appointed and equipped with a television set, DVD player, and reading material. A toilet should be available near, but not directly off of, the waiting room. A small refreshment station near the reception area is also appreciated by escorts. The number of seats required is generally 2.5 times the number of patients in the building at any given time. The general waiting area for Rockford Endoscopy Center, Rockford Gastroenterology Associates, Ltd., Rockford, Illinois, is shown in **Fig. 2.5**.

Business-Reception Module

The business-reception module includes reception area, billing stations, transcription, space for a director, files, and computer banks. Medicare requires that separate medical records be stored for the EASC portion of any facility that shares space with or adjoins a clinic building. Careful attention to these storage requirements is important to ensure eligibility for Medicare certification. The records required by Medicare may be very limited and can be duplicated from the main records of the combined clinic/endoscopic facility. Often the practice and endoscopy areas can share a common business-reception module, but variances may be required from the state or the certifying body.

Preparation-Recovery Module

The preparation-recovery area of the endoscopy facility requires constant patient surveillance from the nursing staff. This area usually contains a nursing control station (**Fig. 2.6**), which allows unobstructed viewing of patients during the preparation and recovery stages of their visit. The most efficient arrangement for preparation and recovery is to have them occur in the same place. Patient clothing can be stored in a locked cabinet in the preparation-recovery area or can accompany the patient during transport to the procedure room and back, stored underneath the rolling procedural stretcher cart. Patients can be rolled into procedure rooms on properly designed rolling carts that are also used as procedure tables. In this way, patients can move from preparation to procedure and back to recovery requiring no mounting or dismounting from wheelchairs or carts.

Generally, at least two preparation-recovery rooms or curtained bays are required per procedure room. Some patients who need additional recovery time after they are able to dismount the procedure cart can recover in recliner chairs. A few curtained recliner chair areas can provide this extra recovery space. The number and type of recovery bays may vary depending on the type of sedation used. Corridors between procedure areas and preparation-recovery spaces should be wide enough to provide easy patient cart movement. Toilets

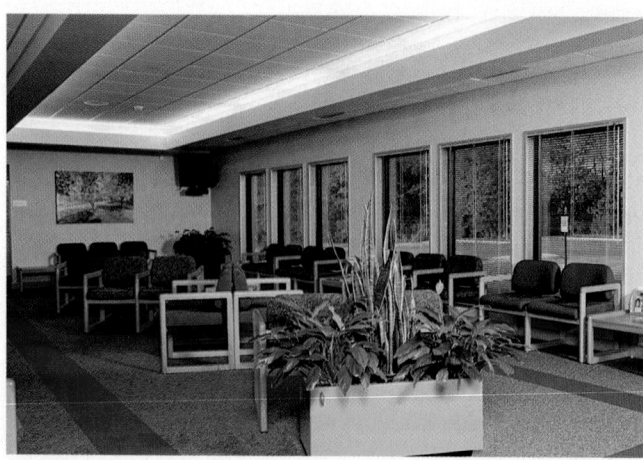

Fig. 2.5 General waiting area for Rockford Endoscopy Center, Rockford Gastroenterology Associates, Ltd., Rockford, Illinois. *(Photograph by David Friedrich, Media Production, OSF Saint Anthony Medical Center, Rockford, IL.)*

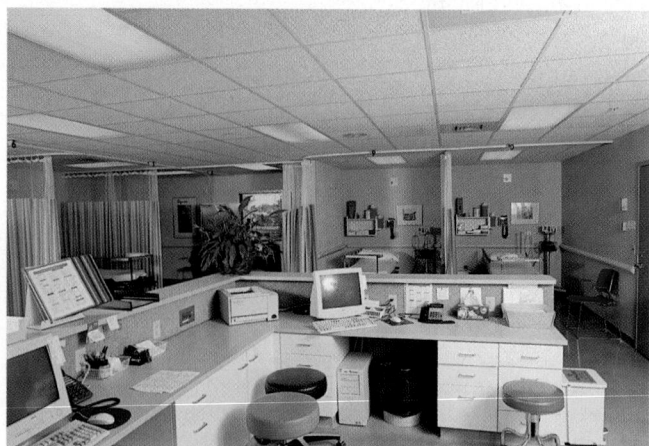

Fig. 2.6 Nursing control station for preparation-recovery area, Rockford Endoscopy Center, Rockford Gastroenterology Associates, Ltd., Rockford, Illinois. *(Photograph by David Friedrich, Media Production, OSF Saint Anthony Medical Center, Rockford, IL.)*

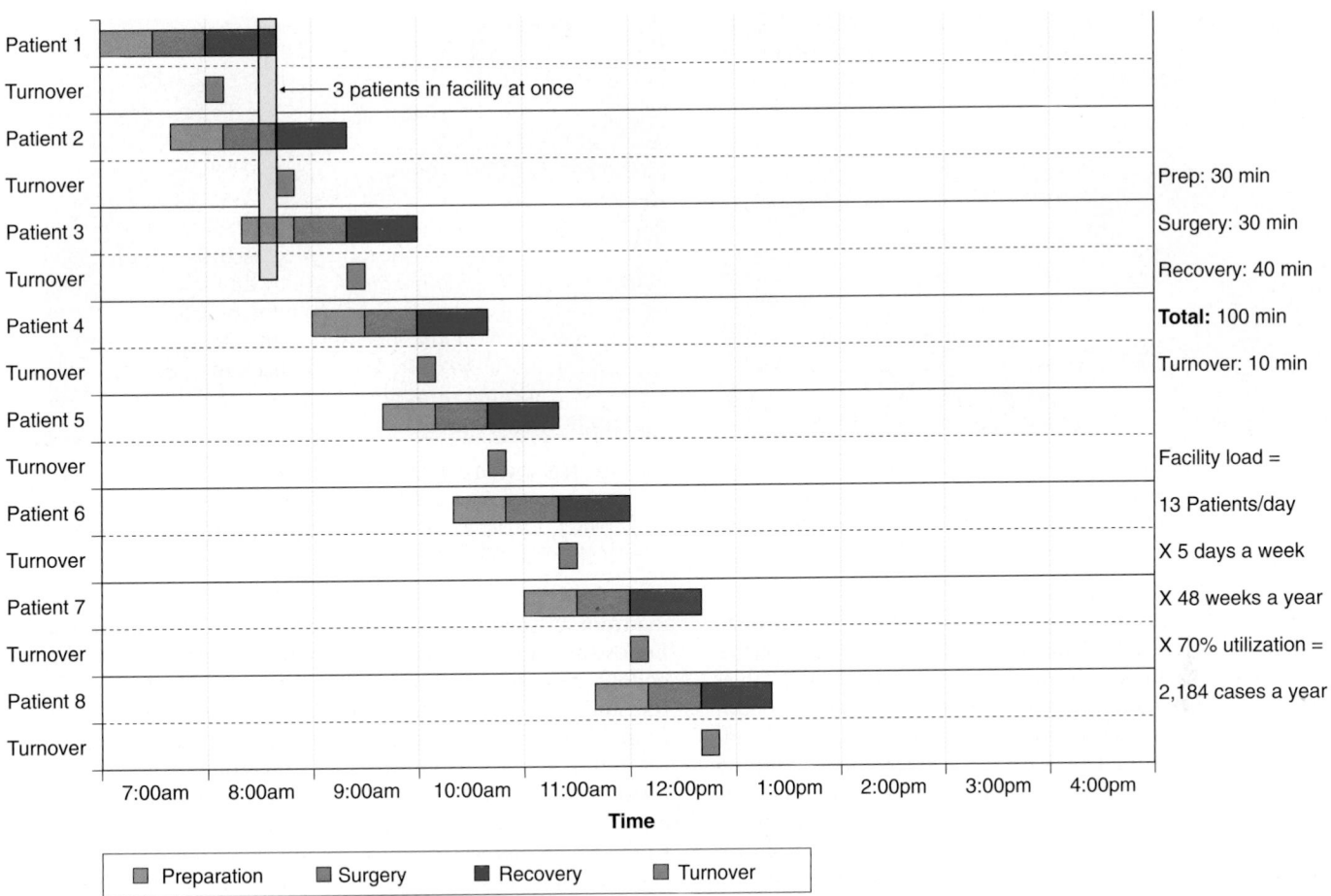

Fig. 2.7 Sample procedure room utilization analysis. *(From Marasco JA, Marasco RF: Designing the ambulatory endoscopy center.* Gastrointest Endosc Clin N Am *12:199, 2002.)*

should be close to both preparation-recovery and procedure areas.

Procedure Room Module

The number of procedure rooms is determined by the caseload of the endoscopy facility. This number is often overestimated. Much more important than the number of procedure rooms is the amount of recovery space available. In an efficient facility where turnaround time is quick, the number of procedure rooms can be minimized. It is most efficient for one endoscopist to have two rooms available so that turnaround between cases can be very rapid. Using procedure rooms for recovery compromises efficiency by tying up a specialized procedure room. Block scheduling of a single endoscopist with two rooms offers maximum efficiency. To determine the required number of procedure rooms, Marasco and Marasco[32] recommended using a utilization chart, an example of which is shown in **Fig. 2.7**. By filling in the time of each of the time segments required in the endoscopy facility and adding the anticipated patient load, the number of procedure rooms needed can be estimated. Allowances should be made for growth in numbers of physicians and patients over the subsequent 5 years. Generally, annual caseloads increase 10% to 15% per year. By using the patient load anticipated 5 years hence and dividing this load by the

number of procedures per room per year, the number of required rooms can be calculated. By examining vertically on the utilization chart, one can estimate the number of patients who will be in various stages within the endoscopy facility. This information can help predict the number of seats needed in the waiting room, the number of necessary procedure rooms, and the number of preparation-recovery bays and recliner chairs needed.

The minimum size for an endoscopy room is probably 200 square feet,[1,24] but this is often inadequate to accommodate newer, larger videoendoscopy equipment, video monitors, and additional equipment for anesthesia services, if used. Approximately 300 square feet is more appropriate for the modern endoscopy room.[1,32] Sometimes state licensing departments or Medicare mandates a minimum size for an "operating room" that is inappropriately large for an endoscopy room. In that instance, a variance can be requested, but it is not automatically granted.

In an endoscopy procedure room layout, placement of the light source, videoprocessor, dual video monitors, and electrocautery must be considered carefully. Many variations are possible to fit the preferences of the endoscopists and nursing staff. Rooms should be planned with equipment and supplies integrated into the layout and positioned strategically around the site of the patient on the procedural stretcher cart. The floor should be free of cables and wiring; these can be arranged

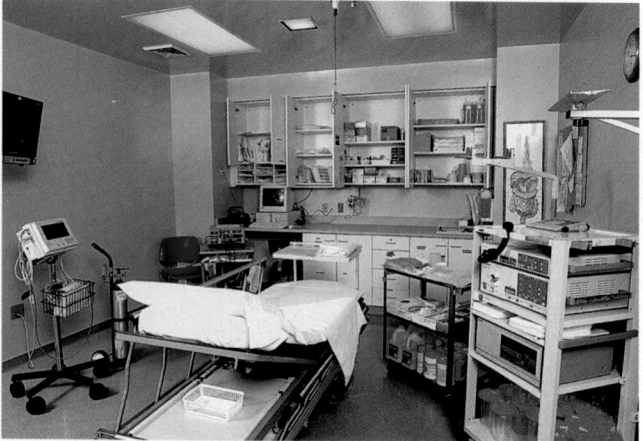

Fig. 2.8 Typical endoscopy procedure room, Rockford Endoscopy Center, Rockford Gastroenterology Associates, Ltd., Rockford, Illinois. *(Photograph by David Friedrich, Media Production, OSF Saint Anthony Medical Center, Rockford, IL.)*

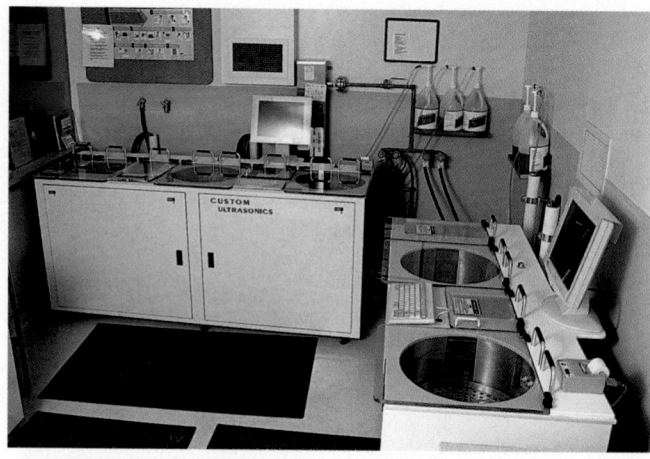

Fig. 2.9 High-level disinfection unit for multiple endoscopes, Rockford Endoscopy Center, Rockford Gastroenterology Associates, Ltd., Rockford, Illinois. *(Photograph by David Friedrich, Media Production, OSF Saint Anthony Medical Center, Rockford, IL.)*

along the perimeter of the room or preferably above a dropped ceiling or in the walls. This arrangement allows physicians, staff, and equipment to move unfettered by cords and cables and avoids damaging these sensitive components. All endoscopic accessories, suction, oxygen, supplies, and all resuscitation equipment should be at hand. An emergency call button should be included in each procedure room, and an emergency (crash) cart should be stored nearby. A typical endoscopy procedure room (Rockford Endoscopy Center) is shown in **Fig. 2.8**. A more detailed discussion of basic clearances and human dimensional requirements is provided by Waye and Rich.[34]

Utility Module

Efficient equipment turnover time can be achieved by having appropriate equipment for rapid cleaning and high-level disinfection. In this scenario, the speed of the endoscopy facility is determined by the efficiency of the physician between procedures rather than by the number of procedure rooms.[32] Instrument cleaning and high-level disinfection can be accomplished by strategically placing the cleaning area between two procedure rooms or having an efficient large cleaning area within a short distance of several procedure rooms. Adequate numbers of endoscopes stored properly and reprocessed efficiently ensure that the most expensive cost elements of the endoscopy facility—the physicians and nursing staff—are not kept waiting for equipment.

Cleaning rooms should be large and adequately ventilated with ample plumbing and power provisions for future changes. Oversized sinks are required, and there should be a place for soiled instruments to hang while waiting to be cleaned. Automated endoscope washers with multiple scope compartments, such as that shown in **Fig. 2.9**, provide an efficient way of reprocessing endoscopes. Different instrument reprocessing units vary in their cleaning time, which has an impact on the number of scopes required by a busy unit. A "pass through" window from soiled to clean utility areas should be available to maintain separation of "clean" and "dirty" areas.

A closed cabinet for the storage of clean endoscopes is preferred to open storage to protect instruments and to prevent inadvertent sightings of instruments by anxious patients. Endoscope storage cabinets that circulate air through the endoscope channels provide added protection against moisture and bacterial growth within channels. A storage unit with channel air circulation is shown in **Fig. 2.10**. Exhaust fans in the cleaning area are a must, as are provisions for disposal of toxic chemicals. Also included in the utility module are storage areas. General storage for supplies must be readily accessible to the preparation-recovery areas and the procedure rooms. There must be locked cabinets for storage of drugs. Biohazardous waste and gases such as oxygen must also be stored. An alternative power source, such as a battery backup system or generator, is necessary to ensure uninterrupted power.

Staff Dressing Module

Requirements for dressing room spaces are different in regulated and unregulated endoscopy facility environments. Rules for the ASC or hospital may be quite different from the office. It is wise to know the regulations from the state department of health and from certification agencies. Male and female locker areas are generally required, but variances can be requested to eliminate the need for unnecessary shower facilities. An additional part of the staff dressing module is the break room. Some state departments of health or certification bodies require a break room within the confines of the endoscopy facility. Careful attention to state and federal regulations is warranted to ensure that licensure and certification requirements are met.

Summary of Planning and Design

The design of an efficient endoscopy facility is facilitated by a functional relationship diagram showing the flow of patients through the facility. An architectural space program is developed by tabulating the areas necessary and assigning space required. This architectural space program determines the size of the facility. A procedure room utilization calculation determines the number of procedure rooms and other areas necessary to handle the patient caseload, and provisions should be made for caseload growth. Careful attention to planning and

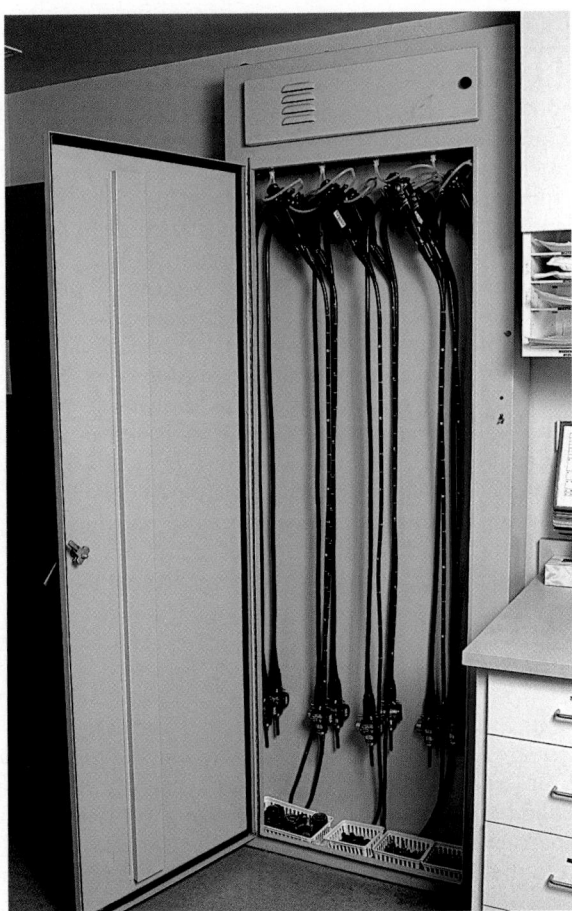

Fig. 2.10 Endoscopy storage cabinet providing air circulation through endoscopy channels, Rockford Endoscopy Center, Rockford Gastroenterology Associates, Ltd., Rockford, Illinois. *(Photograph by David Friedrich, Media Production, OSF Saint Anthony Medical Center, Rockford, IL.)*

design results in the construction of a pleasant, efficient endoscopy facility that meets the needs of patients, physicians, and staff.

Staffing and Scheduling

Decisions regarding staffing and scheduling are critical to the safe and efficient operation of the endoscopy facility, have a major impact on patient outcomes, and affect the financial viability of the endoscopy unit.

Staffing

Decisions regarding staffing hinge on regulatory requirements, volumes of procedures, and case mix (disease acuity). Numerous federal and state regulations affect staffing decisions, and a thorough knowledge of these requirements is necessary to ensure compliance with state licensing requirements, Medicare certification regulations, and third-party accreditation standards.[35,36]

Medicare guidelines stipulate that a registered nurse (RN) must be available on site during all hours of operation of a hospital or ASC endoscopy facility. The nurse practice act of each individual state also affects staffing decisions. A state nurse practice act defines the scope of practice for RNs, licensed practical nurses (LPNs), and other assistants or technicians. These nurse practice acts may limit who can start intravenous (IV) lines, administer IV medications, or provide other clinical services. To determine the number of full-time equivalents (FTEs) needed for staffing, one must quantify the time needed to care for a single patient, multiply this by the number of procedures scheduled daily, and divide by the work hours per day of a full-time employee. One current industry standard suggests an average time of 3 hours per procedure to admit, treat, and discharge a patient in an endoscopy facility (AMSURG Corporation, unpublished data).[35] Some factors that influence the decision to use RNs versus LPNs versus technicians include scope-of-practice regulations, salary costs, and availability. Regardless of the mix, care should always be directly supervised by an on-site RN.[37]

A typical two-room endoscopy facility might be staffed as follows:[35]

- Procedure room number 1: one RN or LPN
- Procedure room number 2: one RN or LPN
- Cleaning room: one endoscope technician
- Preparation-recovery area: two RNs and one LPN, or one RN and two LPNs or technician (the LPN or technician should also be used to float between procedure rooms)

Each endoscopy facility requires at least one receptionist and perhaps a second clerical person. The use of dedicated endoscope technicians to perform cleaning and high-level disinfection and instrument setup promotes strict adherence to endoscope reprocessing guidelines and endoscope durability.

Scheduling

Most facilities use block scheduling to maximize efficiency and convenience.[35,36] Block scheduling of one physician with two endoscopy rooms allows efficient movement of the endoscopist from one room to the next without delays caused by other endoscopists. It is possible for that individual to intermingle daily tasks such as telephone calls or chart review during any downtime. Block scheduling also allows for time allotments based on the performance characteristics of individual endoscopists. Examples of block scheduling and tools for use in block scheduling have been published by McMillan.[35] Equipment availability can affect scheduling. An ample number of endoscopes and rapid, efficient cleaning and high-level disinfection facilitate a more efficient schedule.

The first patient of the day can be prepared in the procedure room if an additional procedural stretcher cart is available for each procedure room at the beginning of the day. Time allotments for procedures vary from facility to facility. Reportedly, most facilities allow 45 minutes for colonoscopy and 30 minutes for upper GI endoscopy.[35] Other facilities schedule more tightly, allowing 30 minutes for colonoscopy and 20 minutes for upper GI endoscopy, including procedures with dilations (Rockford Gastroenterology Associates, Ltd., Rockford, IL, unpublished data). The tighter scheduling can be accommodated by efficient endoscopists, good staffing, adequate equipment, rapid turnaround time, and ample preparation-recovery space (two to three preparation-recovery bays per procedure room). Careful staffing and scheduling are imperative to ensure high-quality care, good patient outcomes, and optimal fiscal performance of the endoscopy facility.

Documentation and Information Technology

An accurate and complete medical record for each patient and a log of the unit's overall activities must be kept (see Chapter 9).[1] The endoscopy report and nursing notes should include date, patient identification data, endoscopist, specific instruments used, endoscopic procedure, indications, informed consent, extent of examination, duration of procedure, findings, notation of tissue sampling, therapeutic interventions, complications, and limitations of the examination. Photographs, electronic images, and biopsy reports should also be part of the record. Quality indicators and patient outcomes should be tabulated, and a method of regular peer review should be developed.[7] Information management in an endoscopy facility affects all aspects of the operation, including scheduling, billing and reimbursement, patient medical record, procedure reports, clinical laboratory and anatomic pathology reports, imaging, pharmacy, patient education, performance improvement data, financial management, materials management and inventory, budgeting and forecasting, payroll and personnel, and staffing and scheduling.[38] Modern information technology may allow more efficient and effective operations within the facility. Information technology is changing medical practice at a rapid pace and may allow more efficient and effective operations within the endoscopy facility.

To minimize repetitive data entry and difficulties with sharing and analyzing data across different systems, the modern endoscopy unit should plan ahead and consider installing an information technology system that provides compatibility between the office electronic medical record (EMR), the endoscopic facility, the billing department, and possibly the local hospital. The interface should allow prompt transfer of demographic data and pertinent components of the medical history and physical examination. Bidirectional transfer of information ensures that the procedure report and billing information are transmitted to the individuals who need access to it. Even further increases in functionality can be envisioned. For example, the use of wireless networks and voice-recognition software for endo-writers and EMRs may be possible. Electronic systems can also be used to enhance service offering to patients and families. The system could generate automatic reminder letters or offer educational material and resources for the patient and family if a new diagnosis has been made. The pathology request, endoscopy report, referral letter, discharge instructions, plans for follow-up, and billing information can be generated from the base examination and completed before the patient leaves the facility. Many of the documents can be sent electronically.

Quality Measurement and Improvement

Increasing health care costs, constrained resources, and evidence of variations in the quality of care rendered have triggered a renewed emphasis on quality measurement and improvement. Two reports by the Institute of Medicine advocate widespread changes in health care, including paying for performance as a means of achieving the delivery of high-quality care.[39,40] Medicare regulations and third-party accreditors require endoscopy facilities to engage in an ongoing comprehensive self-assessment of the quality of care provided. This process includes quality improvement efforts directed toward numerous facets of the operation of the facility. Reasons for quality improvement activities include ensuring that patients receive the highest quality of care possible; providing a competitive edge when seeking contracts; and addressing the recent emphasis of legislators and regulators on quality improvement activities as part of the licensure, certification, and accreditation process. Johanson[41,42] described continuous quality improvement in the ambulatory endoscopy center. The philosophies and tools presented in this article provide a framework for quality improvement activities in all endoscopic facilities. A 2006 publication by a joint task force from the American College of Gastroenterology (ACG) and the ASGE provides an excellent resource with recommendations and ranking of quality indicators that can be used as a starting point in quality measurement and improvement efforts.[7]

Summary

Since its introduction into clinical use in the early 1960s, GI endoscopy has developed as a crucial tool in the management of disorders of the GI system. Endoscopy has transformed the discipline of gastroenterology. The growing use of increasingly complex endoscopic procedures and the evolution of endoscopy to the outpatient setting have fostered the careful development of endoscopy facilities that enable the delivery of endoscopic services in a safe, efficient manner that is reassuring to the patient and produces good outcomes.

The process of setting up an endoscopy facility begins with exploring the types of facilities, developing a business plan, and researching relevant regulatory and certification issues. With those objectives accomplished, attention turns to planning the facility, including site selection, choosing equipment, and planning the physical environment and flow of patients and staff. Finally, the general plans for the facility are turned into specific architectural designs, which form the basis for construction of a pleasant, efficient facility. Once the facility is constructed, careful attention to appropriate staffing, scheduling, documentation, and quality improvement activities promotes efficient and effective care, good patient outcomes, and responsible physical performance of the facility.

Acknowledgments

The authors thankfully acknowledges Brenda Juhlin, Executive Secretary for Rockford Gastroenterology Associates, Ltd., for her help in preparing the manuscript.

References

The complete reference list is available online at www.expertconsult.com.

How Endoscopes Work

David E. Barlow

Overview

The flexible videoendoscope embodies more than 3 decades of refinements in solid-state imaging and mechanical design. Many different models are available, each having slightly different features and each optimized for the portion of the gastrointestinal (GI) tract that it is designed to examine. Although alternative designs for the control section of the endoscope have been proposed (e.g., "pistol-grip"), the basic shape and layout of the instrument are relatively unchanged since flexible endoscopes were first introduced. The basic components and controls of all flexible videoendoscopes are quite similar (**Fig. 3.1**).

The instrument is designed to be held and operated by the endoscopist's left hand. Some physicians use their left index finger to control alternately the suction and air/water valves, while the remaining fingers grip the instrument. Others use their left index finger for the suction valve, the middle finger for the air/water valve, and the ring and small fingers to grip the instrument. The up-and-down angulation knob is manipulated by the physician's left thumb. The left-and-right angulation knob is controlled either by the thumb and first two fingers of the left hand or by the right hand. The endoscopist's right hand is primarily used to control the insertion tube—pushing, torquing, and withdrawing as necessary.

Insertion Tube

The insertion tube of the endoscope is a major differentiating feature among endoscopes designed for gastroenterology. Although obvious differences exist depending on the application of the endoscope (e.g., the extra long length of the enteroscope, the thinness of a transnasal esophagoscope), the subtler differences between endoscope models are just as important. This is especially true for colonoscopes; although endoscopists may prefer using a particular colonoscope model for various reasons, the instrument's insertion tube characteristics more than anything else likely cause an endoscopist to pick a particular colonoscope as the instrument of choice. If any single specification of the instrument can determine the speed and ease with which the endoscopist can insert the instrument, it is the mechanical characteristics of the insertion tube.

Endoscope manufacturers have put significant effort into refining the construction of the insertion tube and selecting ideal materials. **Fig. 3.2** shows the internal components of a typical colonoscope. The insertion tube usually contains (1) tubes for suction (biopsy), air, and water feeding; (2) often an additional tube for a forward water jet; (3) four angulation control wires; (4) fine electrical wires connecting the charge-coupled device (CCD) image sensor at the distal tip of the endoscope to the videoprocessor; and (5) delicate glass fibers

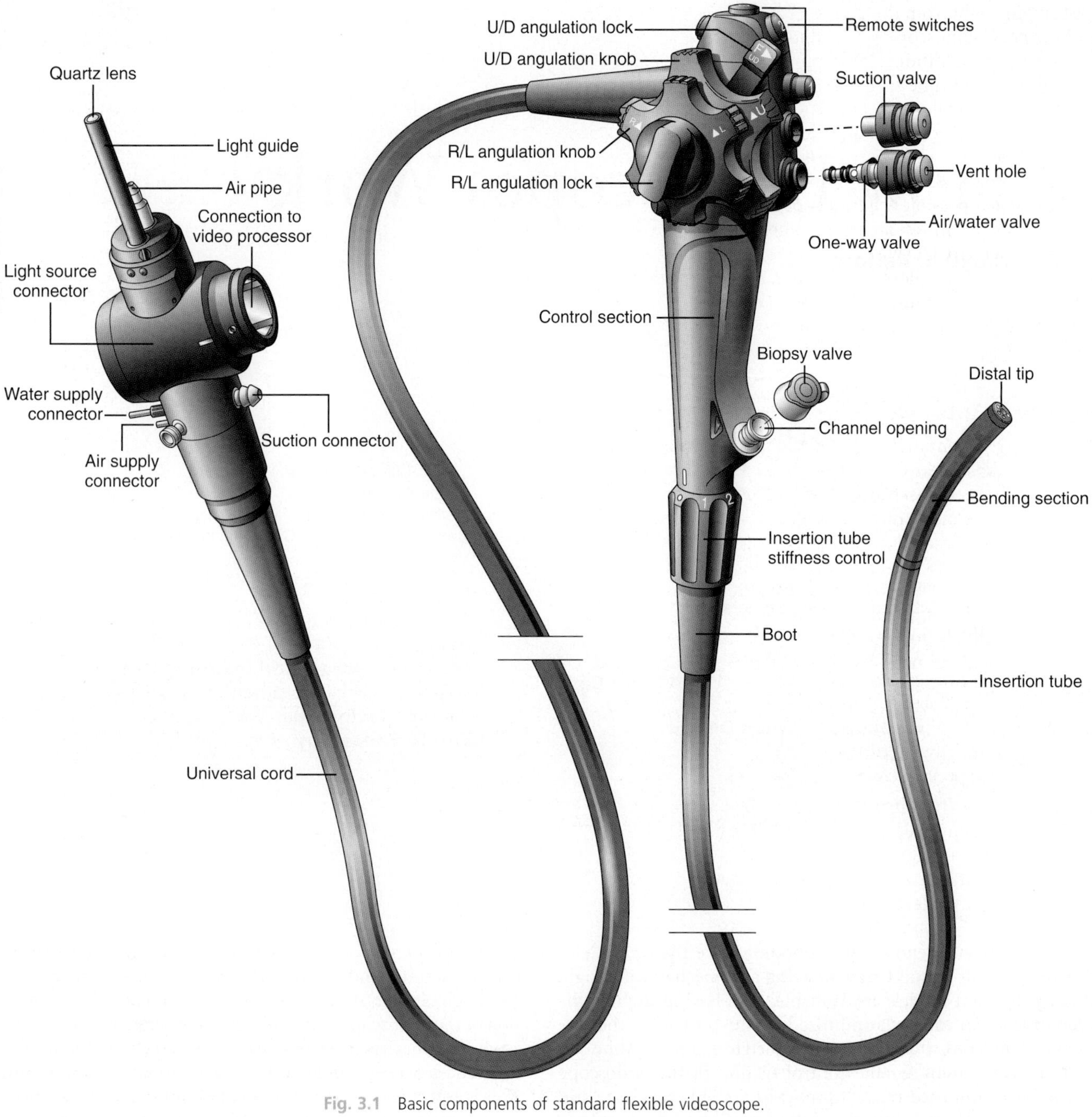

Quartz lens

Light guide

Air pipe

Connection to video processor

Light source connector

Water supply connector

Air supply connector

Suction connector

Universal cord

U/D angulation lock

U/D angulation knob

R/L angulation knob

R/L angulation lock

Remote switches

Suction valve

Vent hole

Air/water valve

One-way valve

Control section

Biopsy valve

Channel opening

Distal tip

Bending section

Insertion tube stiffness control

Boot

Insertion tube

Fig. 3.1   Basic components of standard flexible videoscope.

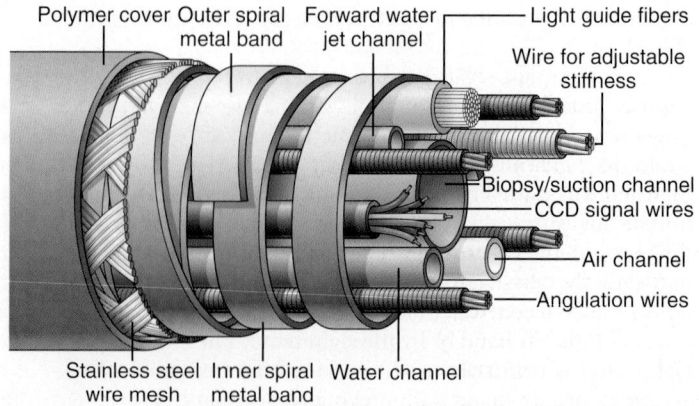

Polymer cover

Outer spiral metal band

Forward water jet channel

Light guide fibers

Wire for adjustable stiffness

Biopsy/suction channel

CCD signal wires

Air channel

Angulation wires

Stainless steel wire mesh

Inner spiral metal band

Water channel

Fig. 3.2   Internal components of variable-stiffness colonoscope.

for bringing light from the light source to the distal end of the endoscope. Colonoscopes with adjustable insertion tube flexibility have an additional component—a tensioning wire to control insertion tube stiffness. Duodenoscopes also have an additional wire/coil sheath running the length of the insertion tube for controlling the up-and-down position of the forceps elevator (see later discussion). It is the task of the endoscope designer to pack all of these individual components into the smallest space possible while still providing freedom for the components to move about without damaging the more fragile elements (CCD wires, fiberoptic strands) as the instrument is torqued and flexed during use. A dry powdered lubricant is applied to all internal components to reduce the stress that they place on each other during manipulation of the insertion tube.

Insertion Tube Flexibility

As previously mentioned, the handling characteristics of the insertion tube are extremely important, particularly for colonoscopes. For easy insertion, the instrument must be capable of accurately transmitting all of the subtle movements and torque applied by the endoscopist. Any rotation that the endoscopist applies to the proximal portion of the shaft (torque) must be transferred to the distal tip of the instrument in a 1:1 ratio, although this capability is lost when the instrument is looped. The torquing ability of the instrument is facilitated by flat, spiral metal bands that run just under the skin of the insertion tube (see **Fig. 3.2**). Because these bands are wound in opposite directions, they lock against one another as the tube is torqued, accurately transmitting rotation of one end of the tube to the other. At the same time, gaps between these spiral bands allow the shaft to flex freely. The bands also give the insertion tube its round shape. Their stiffness prevents the internal components of the insertion tube from being crushed by external forces. These spiral bands are covered by fine strands of stainless steel wire, braided into a tubular mesh. A plastic polymer layer, typically black (or dark green on colonoscopes), is extruded over this wire mesh to create the smooth outer surface of the insertion tube. The polymer layer provides an atraumatic, biocompatible, and watertight surface for the insertion tube. It is usually marked with numbers to gauge the depth of insertion.

Experience has shown that a more rigid insertion tube is optimal for examining the fixed anatomy of the upper GI tract. The colon, with its tortuosity and freely moving loops, is best examined by a more flexible instrument. The instrument should be sufficiently floppy (nonrigid) to conform easily to the tortuous anatomy of the patient and to exert minimum force on the colon wall and attached mesentery. The instrument also should have sufficient column strength to prevent buckling when the proximal end of the instrument is pushed. In addition to its flexibility, the colonoscope should have sufficient elasticity to pop back into a straightened condition when it is pulled back; this aids in removing loops.

Obtaining the best combination of flexibility, elasticity, column strength, and torquing ability is the art and science of insertion tube design. Improvements in one of these characteristics often negatively affect one or more of the others. The final design is usually a compromise between these ideal characteristics, confirmed by months of clinical testing. To improve insertion further, the flexibility of both gastroscope

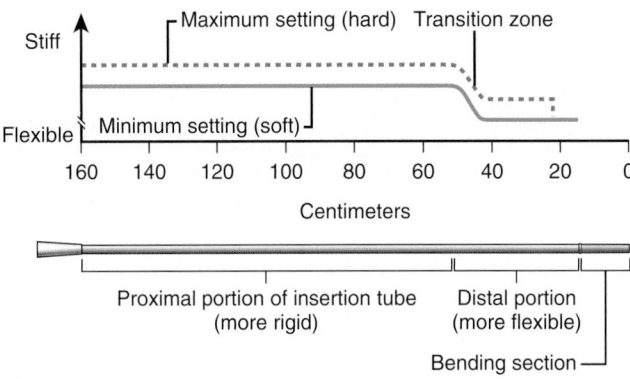

Fig. 3.3 Graphic representation of insertion tube stiffness. Note the variation—the distal 40 cm is more flexible. Note extra stiffness when the instrument is in the "stiff" setting *(dashed line)* versus in the "soft" setting *(solid line)*.

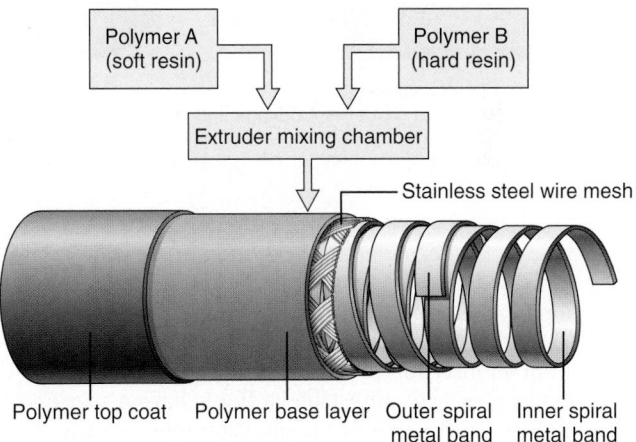

Fig. 3.4 Composition of insertion tube cover.

and colonoscope insertion tubes typically varies from end to end. As **Fig. 3.3** illustrates, the distal 40 cm of a colonoscope insertion tube is significantly more flexible than the proximal portion. This variation in flexibility is achieved by changing the formulation of the tube's outer polymer layer as it is extruded over the wire mesh during manufacturing. As **Fig. 3.4** illustrates, the extruder contains two types of resins, one significantly harder than the other. Initially, as the distal end of the insertion tube passes through the machine, a layer of soft resin is applied to the distal 40 cm of the wire mesh. This soft resin is gradually replaced by the hard resin within a transition zone near the middle of the tube. The proximal portion of the insertion tube (50 to 160 cm) is constructed of only the hard resin.[1] The end result is an insertion tube that has a soft distal portion for atraumatically snaking through a tortuous colon, with a stiffer proximal portion that is effective at preventing loop reformation in the portions of the colon that have already been straightened by the colonoscope.

Adjustable Flexibility

Clinical experience has shown that endoscopists often disagree over what constitutes the ideal insertion tube. This disagreement may be due to differences in training, insertion

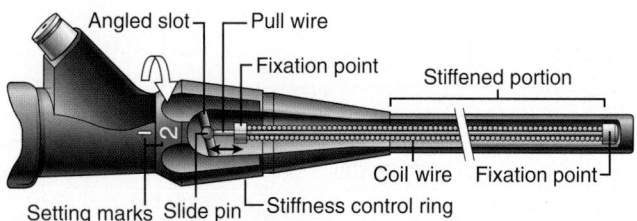

Fig. 3.5 Mechanism for stiffening a variable-stiffness colonoscope.

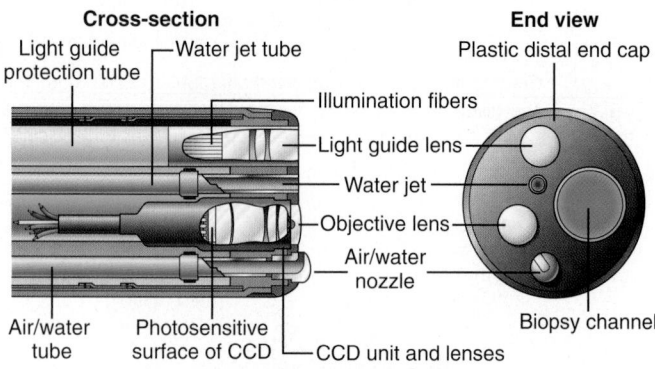

Fig. 3.6 Colonoscope distal tip assembly.

technique, or past experience. In addition, some endoscopists have expressed a desire to change the characteristics of the insertion tube during the procedure, based either on insertion depth or on the patient's anatomy, which has led to the development of an insertion tube with adjustable stiffness.[2]

Colonoscopes with adjustable stiffness have a tensioning wire that runs the length of the insertion tube (see **Fig. 3.2**). The amount of tension in this wire is controlled by rotating a ring at the proximal end of the insertion tube, just below the control section (**Fig. 3.5**). When the pull wire in this stiffening system is in the "soft" position, the stiffening system provides no additional stiffness to the insertion tube beyond that provided by the wire mesh and polymer coat. As **Fig. 3.5** illustrates, when the control ring is rotated to one of the "hard" positions, an angled slot in the control ring pulls on the slide pin at the end of the pull wire, stretching the pull wire and placing it under heavy tension. This tension stiffens the coil wire that surrounds the pull wire and adds significant rigidity to the insertion tube. As **Fig. 3.3** illustrates, although the base stiffness of the insertion tube is established by varying the mixture of hard and soft resins in the polymer base layer, the insertion tube can be stiffened further at will during the procedure by rotating the stiffness control ring. The variable stiffness mechanism does not run the entire length of the insertion tube so that the distal portion of the endoscope is not affected.

Distal Tip

Fig. 3.6 illustrates the components found in the distal tip of a typical end-viewing endoscope, such as a gastroscope or colonoscope. The larger of the circular glass lenses on the distal tip is the objective lens. This lens focuses a miniature image of the GI mucosa on the surface of a solid-state CCD image sensor. The image sensor sends a continuous stream

of images back to the videoprocessor via a collection of very fine electrical wires. The objective lens and CCD unit are tightly sealed to prevent condensation from fogging the image and to protect the imaging system from damage if fluid were to enter the instrument accidentally. Light to illuminate the interior of the body travels through the instrument via fiberoptic illumination fibers. This light is evenly dispersed across the endoscope's field of view via a light guide lens system.

Some endoscopes have a single illumination system (as shown in **Fig. 3.6**). Other endoscope models have two fiberoptic bundles and two light guide lenses to improve illumination on both sides of the biopsy forceps (e.g., snare) and to facilitate the packing of components within the insertion tube. The channel used for biopsy and suction exits close to the objective lens on the distal tip. The position of the biopsy channel relative to the objective lens determines how accessories appear in the image as they enter the visual field. On some instruments, the snare or biopsy forceps appears to emanate from the lower right corner of the image; on other instruments, these accessories enter the visual field from the lower left corner, and so forth. When planning difficult procedures, such as piecemeal polypectomy or hemostasis, it is crucial that the endoscopist know where the accessories will enter into his or her field of view.

The insertion tube also contains small tubes that carry air and water through the instrument (see **Fig. 3.2**). These tubes typically merge into a single tube a few inches from the distal tip (see **Fig. 3.9** further on). This combined air/water tube connects to the air/water nozzle on the tip of the instrument. Under control of the endoscopist, water can be fed across the objective lens to clean it, or air can be fed from the nozzle to insufflate the GI tract. Some gastroscopes and colonoscopes have an additional water tube and a water-jet nozzle on the distal tip for washing debris from the mucosa (see **Fig. 3.6**).

Fig. 3.7 illustrates the components found in the distal end of a typical duodenoscope. **Fig. 3.7A** is a schematic cross section through the optical and illumination systems found in the distal tip of the duodenoscope. The objective lens for viewing the tissue is now located on the side of the distal end rather than on the very tip of the instrument. A prism is used to deflect the angle of view 90 to 105 degrees and to convert the instrument into a side-viewing endoscope. The illumination fibers are likewise steeply bent at the tip of the instrument, directing the light to emanate from the side. As in end-viewing instruments, an air/water nozzle positioned near the objective lens directs water across the lens to clean it, followed by air to blow away any remaining water droplets. Air from this nozzle is also used to insufflate the patient. All duodenoscopes have a forceps elevator to deflect actively the tip of any accessory passed through the channel. The elevator mechanism is shown in **Fig. 3.7B**. This elevator normally lies in a recess within the tip of the endoscope (lowered position). When the endoscopist wishes to raise the accessory up into the field of view, he or she operates a thumb control on the control section of the instrument (not shown). This thumb control pulls on the elevator wire, lifting the elevator out of its recess into a raised position, deflecting the tip of the accessory up into the field of view. In some instruments, such as the V-scope (Olympus Corp, Melville, NY), this elevator has a small groove that

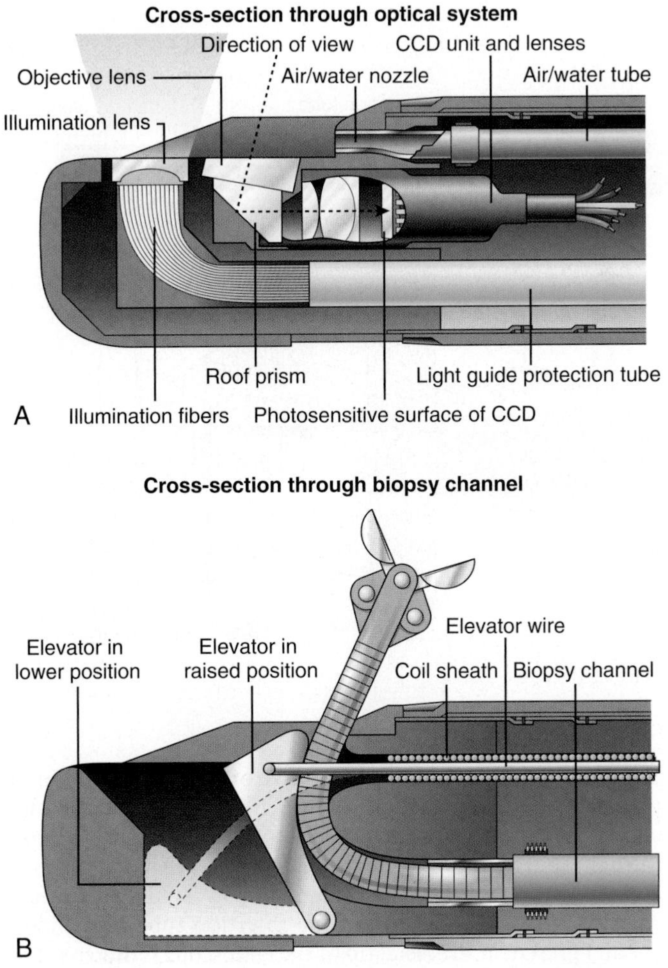

Cross-section through optical system

Objective lens

Illumination lens

Direction of view

Air/water nozzle

CCD unit and lenses

Air/water tube

Roof prism

Light guide protection tube

Illumination fibers   Photosensitive surface of CCD

A

Cross-section through biopsy channel

Elevator in lower position

Elevator in raised position

Elevator wire

Coil sheath Biopsy channel

B

Fig. 3.7   **A** and **B,** Duodenoscope distal tip assembly.

entraps a 0.035-inch guidewire to aid in wire stabilization during accessory exchanges.

Bending Section and Tip Angulation

The distal tip of the insertion tube of the endoscope can also be manipulated by the endoscopist. The deflectable portion, referred to as the bending section, is constructed differently from the rest of the insertion tube. As **Fig. 3.8** illustrates, the bending section is composed of a series of oddly shaped metal rings, each one connected to the ring on either side of it via a freely moving joint. These joints are constructed using a series of pivot pins, each one displaced from its neighbors by 90 degrees. One set of pivots allows the bending section to curl in the up-and-down direction. A second set allows the bending section to curl in the right-and-left direction. Together, they enable the bending section to curl in any direction. The direction of the curl is controlled by four angulation wires that run the length of the insertion tube (see **Fig. 3.2**). These four wires are firmly attached to the tip of the bending section at the 3 o'clock, 6 o'clock, 9 o'clock, and 12 o'clock positions. Pulling on the wire attached at the 12 o'clock position causes the bending section to curl in the up direction and achieves what endoscopists refer to as "*up* tip deflection." Pulling on the wire attached at the 3 o'clock position causes *right* tip deflection. Pulling the other two wires causes *down* and *left* deflection. The endoscopist is able to pull on each of these wires in turn by rotating either the up-and-down or right-and-left angulation knobs. (For simplicity, **Fig. 3.8** illustrates only the up-and-down angulation system.) Rotating the up-and-down and right-and-left knobs together produces a combined tip movement (e.g., upward and to the right) and allows the endoscopist to sweep the tip of the endoscope in any direction.

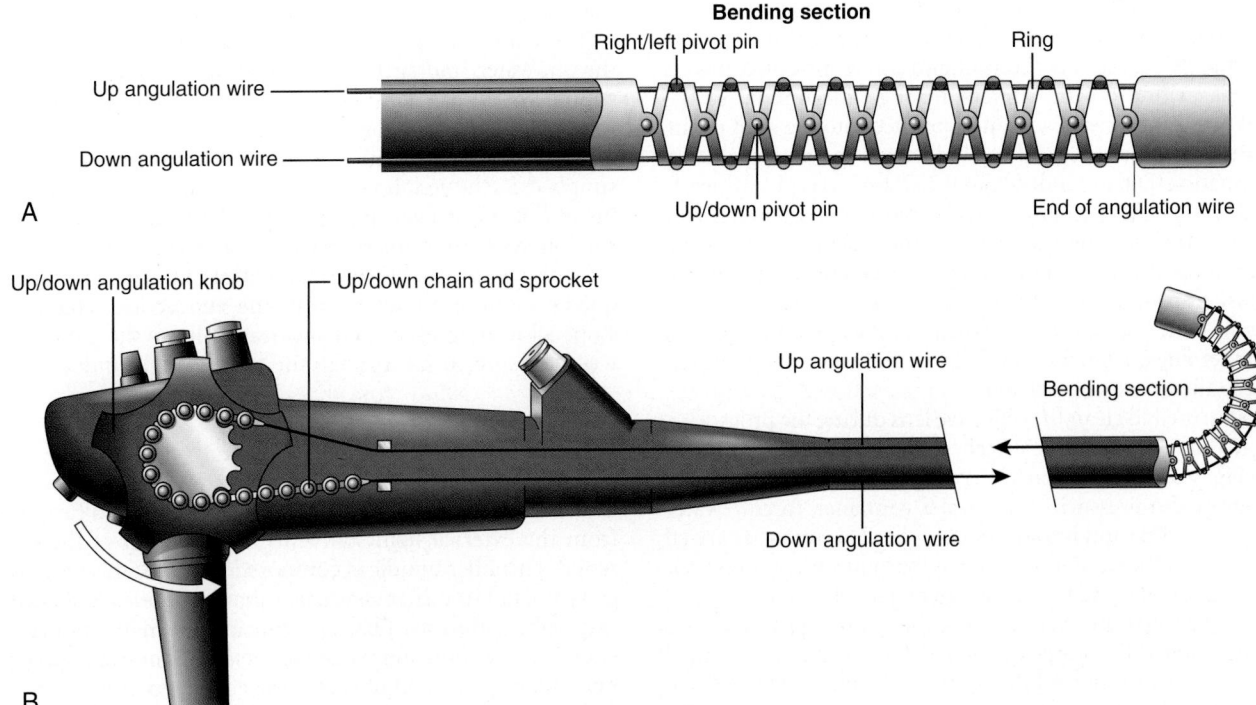

Bending section

Right/left pivot pin

Ring

Up angulation wire

Down angulation wire

Up/down pivot pin

End of angulation wire

A

Up/down angulation knob

Up/down chain and sprocket

Up angulation wire

Bending section

Down angulation wire

B

Fig. 3.8   **A,** Construction of bending section. **B,** Rotation of angulation knob caused deflection of bending section.

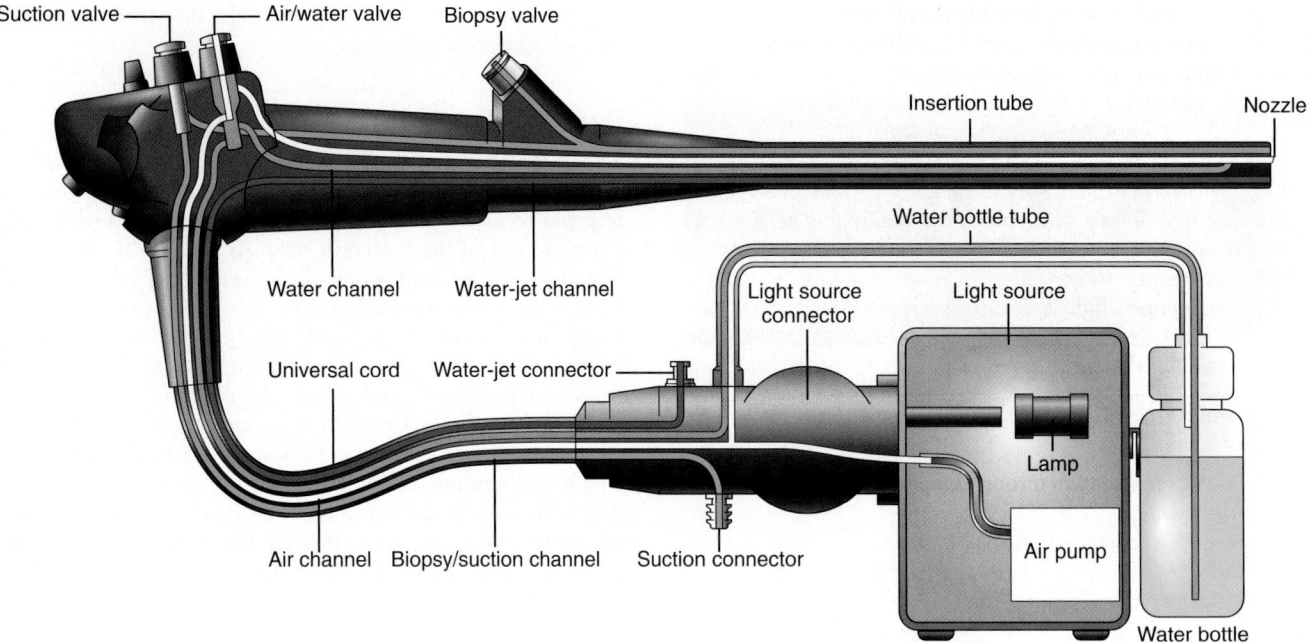

Fig. 3.9 Configuration of air, water, and suction systems.

Air, Water, and Suction Systems

A schematic of a typical endoscopic air, water, and suction system is shown in **Fig. 3.9**. An air pump in the light source provides air under mild pressure to a pipe protruding from the light source connector of the endoscope. This air is carried by an air channel (tube) to the air/water valve on the control section. If this valve is not covered, the air simply exits from a vent hole in the top of the valve (see **Fig. 3.1**). This vent hole allows the air pump to pump freely when air is not needed, reducing wear and tear on the pump. If the endoscopist wants to insufflate the patient, he or she covers the vent hole with a fingertip; this closes off the vent and forces air down the air channel, exiting the instrument through the nozzle on the distal tip. A one-way valve is incorporated into the shaft of the air/water valve (see **Fig. 3.1**) to hold air in the patient during examination. During endoscopy, the GI tract is typically insufflated to a pressure slightly above atmospheric pressure. If it were not for this one-way valve in the system, air from the organ under examination would flow back into the nozzle on the distal tip, up the air channel in the insertion tube, and out the hole in the air/water valve whenever the operator removed his or her finger from the valve. The antireflux valve is required to keep the patient insufflated.

Water, used to clean the objective lens during the procedure, is stored in a water bottle attached to the light source or cart (see **Fig. 3.9**). In addition to feeding air for insufflation, the air pump also pressurizes this water container, forcing water out of the bottle and into the endoscope. This water is carried via a tube on the water bottle cap to the light source connector of the endoscope and then by a water channel up the universal cord to the air/water valve. When the endoscopist depresses the air/water valve, water continues down the water channel in the insertion tube and flows out of the nozzle at the distal tip. The nozzle directs this water across the surface of the objective lens, cleaning it.

Suction is also controlled by a valve on the control section of the endoscope. A suction source, either the hospital's wall suction system or a portable suction pump, is connected to the light source connector of the endoscope. When the endoscopist depresses the suction valve, suction is applied to the suction/biopsy channel within the insertion tube. Any fluid (or air) present at the distal tip of the endoscope is drawn into the suction collection system. A channel-opening valve (also called a biopsy valve) closes off the proximal opening of the biopsy channel and prevents room air from being drawn into the suction collection system.

There are several inherent safety features in the design of the air, water, and suction system shown in **Fig. 3.9**. The air supply system has no moving parts and no mechanical valves that could stick in a continuously "on" position, resulting in accidental overinsufflation of the patient. Instead, the air simply exits the vent hole in the valve, unless the physician has his or her finger over this opening, and in the event that the suction system becomes obstructed and the endoscopist has difficulty with possible overinsufflation, he or she simply can quickly remove all valves from the endoscope. This action stops all feeding of air and water and allows the patient's GI tract to depressurize through the open valve cylinders.

Illumination System

Endoscopes use an incoherent fiberoptic bundle to carry light from the external light source to the distal tip of the endoscope. This fiber bundle is composed of thousands of hairlike glass fibers (30 μm in diameter) that are optically coated to trap light within the fiber and to transmit light from end to end via a phenomenon known as *total internal reflection*. Light rays entering one end of such a fiber reflect off of the walls of the fiber many thousands of times before exiting the opposite end of the fiber. The types of glass used to make the core and cladding of the fiber and the thickness of the core and cladding all are carefully chosen to enable the fiber bundle to carry as much light as possible (see Kawahara and Ichikawa[3] for a more complete discussion of fiberoptics).

Endoscopic light sources typically use 300-W xenon arc lamps to produce the intense, white light needed for videoendoscopy. These lamps also produce considerable heat. Heat sinks, infrared filters, and forced-air cooling systems within the light source prevent the fiber bundle of the endoscope from overheating and burning. A close inspection of the tip of the endoscope's light guide reveals a burn-resistant quartz lens that serves to collect light from the light source lamp and to direct it into the endoscope (see **Fig. 3.1**). At the other end of the endoscope, the light guide lens at the distal tip of the instrument spreads this light uniformly over the visual field (see **Fig. 3.6**). An automatically controlled aperture (iris) in the light source controls the intensity of the light emitted from the endoscope tip.

When the endoscope is in a large cavity such as the stomach and significant light is required, the aperture in the light source opens up, allowing the endoscope to transmit maximum light. When the endoscope tip is very close to the mucosa and illumination is bright, the aperture in the light source automatically closes down to reduce the amount of light exiting the light source. If the illumination is too low, the video image on the monitor is dark and grainy. If the illumination is too strong, the image on the monitor is washed out (i.e., "bloom"). The videoprocessor automatically keeps the brightness of the illumination within a range that is acceptable for the CCD image sensor by carefully controlling the amount of light produced by the light source.

Solid-State Image Capture

The image sensors used in videoendoscopes are typically referred to as CCDs. These sensors are solid-state imaging devices constructed of silicon semiconductor material. The silicon on the surface of the sensor is responsive to light. When a photon of light strikes the photosensitive surface of the CCD, it displaces an electron from a silicon atom at the surface. A free, negatively charged electron is produced in the silicon material along with a corresponding positively charged "hole" in the crystalline structure of the silicon where the electron was previously bound. This action is referred to as the *photoelectric effect* and is illustrated in **Fig. 3.10**. As additional photons hit the surface of the sensor, additional free electrons and additional corresponding holes are created. The charges built up in the sensor are directly proportional to the amount of light falling on the CCD. Also, these charges are created regardless of the color of the light falling on the sensor.

Although a single photosensitive element is useful for measuring the brightness of light falling on a surface (as in a light meter), it cannot reproduce an image. To reproduce an image, the photosensitive surface must be divided up into a matrix of thousands of small, independent photosites. When an image is focused on the surface of such a sensor, the brightness of the image is automatically measured at each individual photosite within the matrix. Knowing the brightness of every point in the image allows a vision system to reproduce the image accurately. The CCD is a common component of such a solid-state vision system. The surface of a CCD image sensor

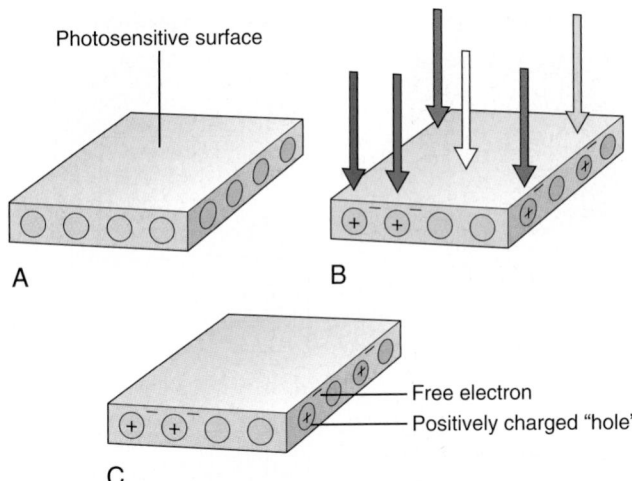

Fig. 3.10 Photoelectric effect. **A,** Photosensitive surface. **B,** Photons hitting the surface liberate electrons, generating a buildup of charges within the material. **C,** After exposure to light ends, the charges remain.

is divided into a rectangular array of discrete photosites, individually referred to as picture elements, or *pixels*. **Fig. 3.11** illustrates a CCD sensor with such an array. In a video image endoscope, the CCD is located in the distal tip of the instrument directly behind the objective lens (as shown in **Fig. 3.6**). The objective lens focuses a miniature image of the observed mucosa directly on the surface of this sensor. The pattern of light falling on the CCD (i.e., the image) is instantly converted into an array of stored electrical charges because of the photoelectric effect previously described. Because the charges stored in each of the individual pixels are isolated from neighboring pixels, the sensor faithfully transforms the optical image into an electrical replica of the image.

This electrical representation is processed and sent to a video monitor for reproduction. As **Fig. 3.11** illustrates, pixels in dark areas of the image develop a low voltage because of the generation of fewer charges. Pixels in brighter areas of the image develop a proportionately higher voltage because of the creation of more electron/hole pairs. Each pixel is able to develop any level of charge, from some minimum to some maximum, depending on the brightness of the incident light. The conversion process from light to electrical charges is linear. Doubling the number of photons falling on a pixel doubles the number of charges generated at the pixel, until the storage capacity of the photosite is full.

Reading the Image Created on the Charge-Coupled Device

After the CCD is exposed to the image, the charges developed in the CCD must be "read out" in an orderly manner and processed to reproduce the original optical image. The manner in which the charges are moved about within the CCD as they are read out depends on the configuration of the CCD. The three most common types of CCDs are the line transfer CCD, the frame transfer CCD, and the interline transfer CCD.[4] Each of these CCD types has specific advantages in terms of sensitivity of the CCD to light (i.e., the brightness required of the

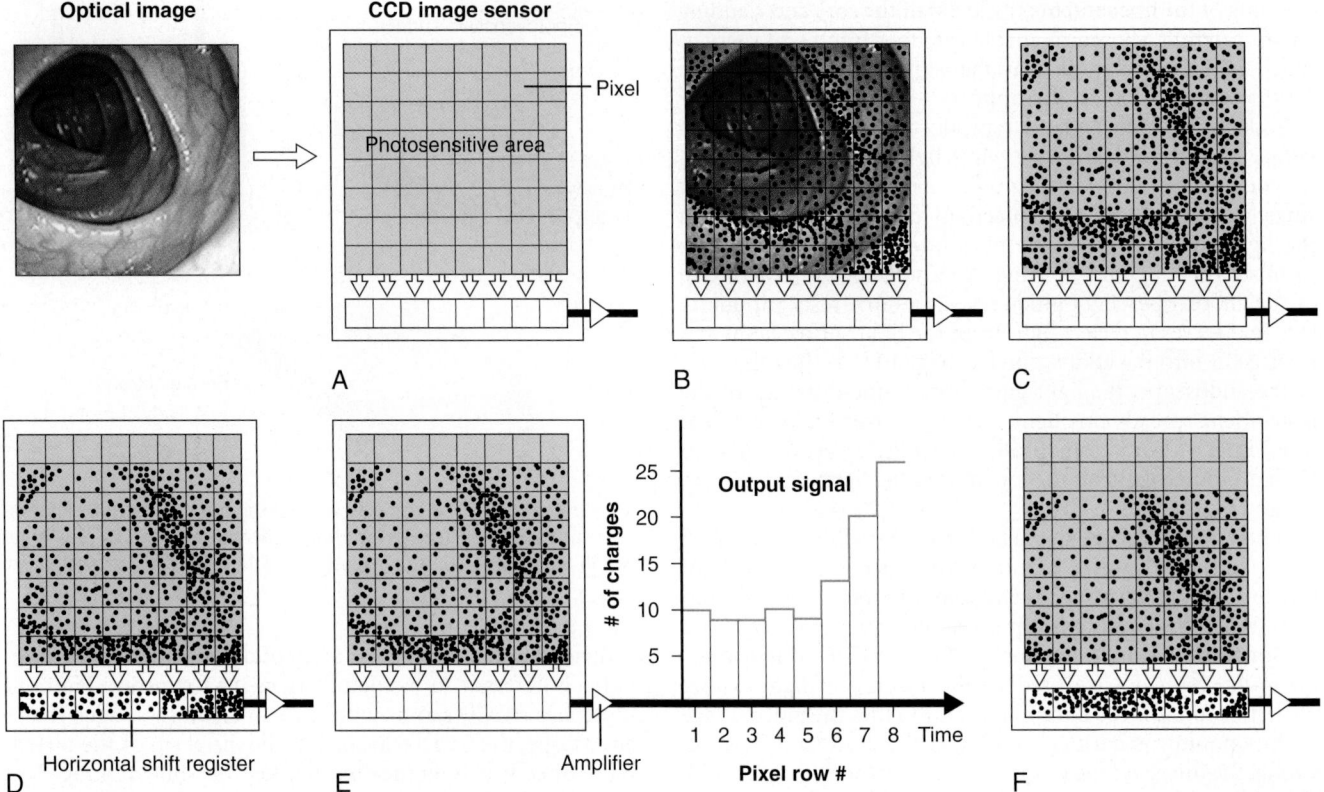

Fig. 3.11 Image capture and readout with line-transfer charge-coupled device (CCD). Although an actual endoscopic CCD contains several hundred thousand pixels, for simplicity, the array illustrated contains 64 pixels arranged in an 8-row × 8-column matrix. **A,** Image of mucosa is projected on the photosensitive surface of CCD. **B,** Electrical replica of image is created because of the photoelectric effect. **C,** Electrical replica remains when shielded from light. **D,** Replica is shifted down one row pushing data from the bottom row into the horizontal shift register. **E,** Shift register is emptied, creating an output signal. **F,** Replica shifts down another row. The process repeats.

endoscope's illumination system), the type of light source required (strobed vs. nonstrobed), the size of the CCD (which affects the size of the endoscope's distal tip), and the speed at which the charges can be transferred out of the CCD. The CCD schematically illustrated in **Fig. 3.11** is a line transfer CCD. **Fig. 3.11A** illustrates the projection of an optical image onto the photosensitive surface of the CCD. Electrical charges are developed at each photosite in the array after brief exposure to the image (**Fig. 3.11B** and **C**). For simplicity, **Fig. 3.11** illustrates an array with only a very few pixels and only a very few resulting charges. These charges are represented by small dots within the photosites.

The charges within each pixel are controlled and shifted over the surface of the CCD via electrodes adjacent to each photosite (these electrodes are not shown in **Fig. 3.11**). By varying the voltages applied to these electrodes, the electrons within individual pixels are transferred as charge packets from one pixel to another. Sequential voltage changes on these electrodes march the charges toward the bottom edge of the CCD and into a horizontal shift register (see **Fig. 3.11D**). The charges in the horizontal shift register are passed through an output amplifier and are converted into an output signal. The output signal fluctuates in direct proportion to the number of charges stored in each pixel. At the point in the process illustrated in **Fig. 3.11E**, the charges in the bottom row of the original image have been read out and passed through the output amplifier and sent to the videoprocessor for reconstruction.

The electrical representation of the entire image has shifted down one row on the CCD. Once the horizontal shift register has been read out and cleared (emptied), the charges in each pixel of the array are sequentially transferred down to the pixel below, resulting in a second shift of the image replica. This transfer fills the horizontal shift register with the charges that were originally in the second-to-the-bottom row of the array, as shown in **Fig. 3.11F**. The charges in the horizontal shift register are again read out, resulting in an output signal that is representative of the brightness of the image falling on the second-to-the-bottom row of the original image.

The processing of the image replica continues, in a similar step-by-step fashion, until the entire CCD has been read out. Once the CCD is read and cleared, it is ready for another exposure. The charge-coupling process—the transfer of charges from pixel to pixel as packets—gives the CCD its name (*charge-coupled device*). The charges in the furthermost corners of the CCD are moved sequentially through several hundred photosites before they reach the horizontal shift register. In current videoendoscopes, the CCD is exposed, read out, and reexposed 60 to 90 times each second. To maintain image fidelity during these repetitive transfers, it is essential that these charge packets remain intact with no loss or gain in charge quantity in the process of undergoing hundreds of thousands of transfers per second as the CCD is being read out. The photosensitive array of a line transfer CCD must be shielded from light during the entire time that the image is

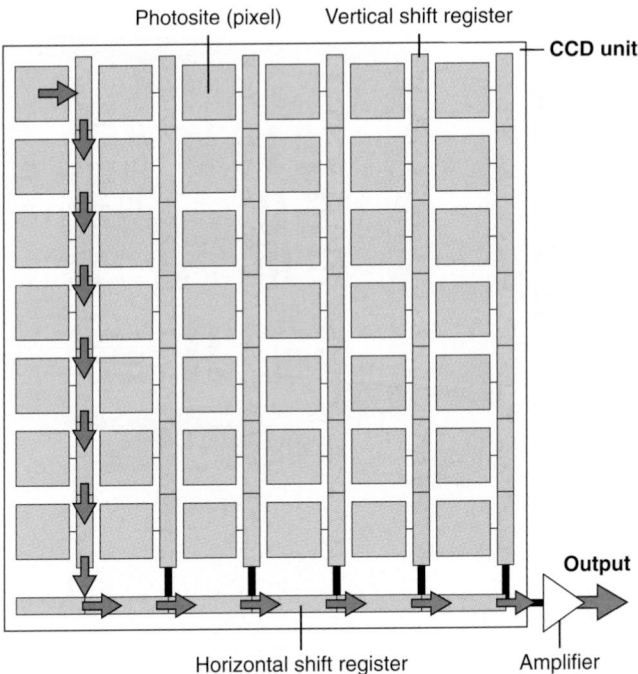

Fig. 3.12 Schematic of interline-transfer charge-coupled device (CCD).

charges created in the upper left corner pixel.) The vertical shift registers are shielded from light, allowing them to be emptied as the CCD is continuously exposed to light. The CCD collects a second image as the first image is being read. When the vertical shift registers are finally empty, the newly created image replica in the sensor array is instantly transferred from the photosites to the vertical shift registers, and the process repeats.

A big advantage of the interline transfer CCD is that it does not require strobing of the illumination. Because the entire sensor array is cleared to the vertical shift registers in one step, the sensor array is immediately ready to capture the next image. So-called color chip endoscopes that use continuous, nonstrobed light sources are examples of interline transfer CCD systems.

Image Resolution

Image resolution is a key component of endoscopic image quality. Resolution is commonly measured using a test method similar to that illustrated in **Fig. 3.13**. A test chart consisting of sharply printed black and white lines is positioned at a measured distance from the tip of the endoscope. This test chart contains a series of increasingly closely spaced lines. The image of this chart (**Fig. 3.13C**) as reproduced on the video monitor of the endoscope is carefully studied. The more widely spaced lines are clearly distinguishable as individual line pairs. The more closely spaced lines typically blur together, however, and are unrecognizable as distinct lines.

The limit of resolution of the endoscope is defined as the distance between the closest set of line pairs that can still be distinguished as lines before the image becomes so blurred that the lines simply blend together. As the test chart is moved closer to the tip of the endoscope, the image of the test chart has increased magnification, and the endoscope is able to resolve smaller and smaller line pairs. **Fig. 3.14** illustrates a typical plot of endoscope resolving power as a function of distance. As the endoscope is moved closer and closer to the test chart, finer and finer line pairs are resolved by the endoscope, until at point *A* the endoscope reaches its maximum resolving power. At this point, the endoscope is also at its point of closest focus. Moving the test chart closer to the endoscope degrades the image because of increasing loss of focus. Limited by image blur, the working range of the typical standard colonoscope illustrated in **Fig. 3.14** is 7 to 200 mm (as depicted by the solid purple line).

A few videoendoscopes available on the market have an optical zoom feature. These endoscopes typically have a control on the endoscope's body that adjusts the lenses in the distal tip of the endoscope for sharp focus when the endoscope is very close to the target tissue. As illustrated in **Fig. 3.14**, these endoscopes can resolve line pairs that are perhaps four times smaller than a standard endoscope; this is accomplished by allowing the endoscope to focus at a distance of only a couple of millimeters from the tissue. This fourfold increase in resolving power comes at a price, however. Similar to microscopes, these instruments have a very limited depth of field—in the range of 1 or 2 mm. If the endoscope moves too close or too far from the tissue, the image quickly goes out of focus, and image quality deteriorates. As depicted by the solid blue line in **Fig. 3.14B**, the working range of a zoom

being moved and read out (the steps illustrated in **Fig. 3.11C** and following). This shielding is necessary to prevent mixing information from the image under transfer with new charges being generated at the photosites by the light still falling on them. To preserve the original image, the photosites must be completely dark while the image replica is read out. One method of doing this in an endoscopic application is to strobe, or momentarily interrupt, the light emitted by the endoscope as the CCD is being read; this creates a momentary burst of light to expose the image sensor, followed by a brief period of darkness as the CCD is read out and cleared. Endoscopists who have used a red, green, and blue (RGB) sequential endoscopy system (typically called a black and white CCD system) are familiar with the concept of strobed endoscopic light sources.

Interline Charge-Coupled Device

Although strobed video systems are in common use in endoscopy, they have several disadvantages, particularly with the smooth reproduction of motion. An alternative to a line transfer CCD with a strobed light source is an interline transfer CCD with a continuous (nonstrobed) light source. As illustrated in **Fig. 3.12**, an interline transfer CCD has a series of vertical shift registers placed adjacent to each column of photosites. Immediately after light exposure, the charges developed at the photosites are transferred in one quick step to the adjacent vertical shift registers. Because of the rapid, one-step transfer of charges to the vertical shift registers, it is unnecessary to interrupt illumination of the CCD during the read-out process. In the meantime, the charges in the vertical shift registers are transferred, step-by-step, down to the horizontal shift register, where they are read out in a conventional manner. (The *red arrows* in **Fig. 3.12** illustrate the read-out path of the

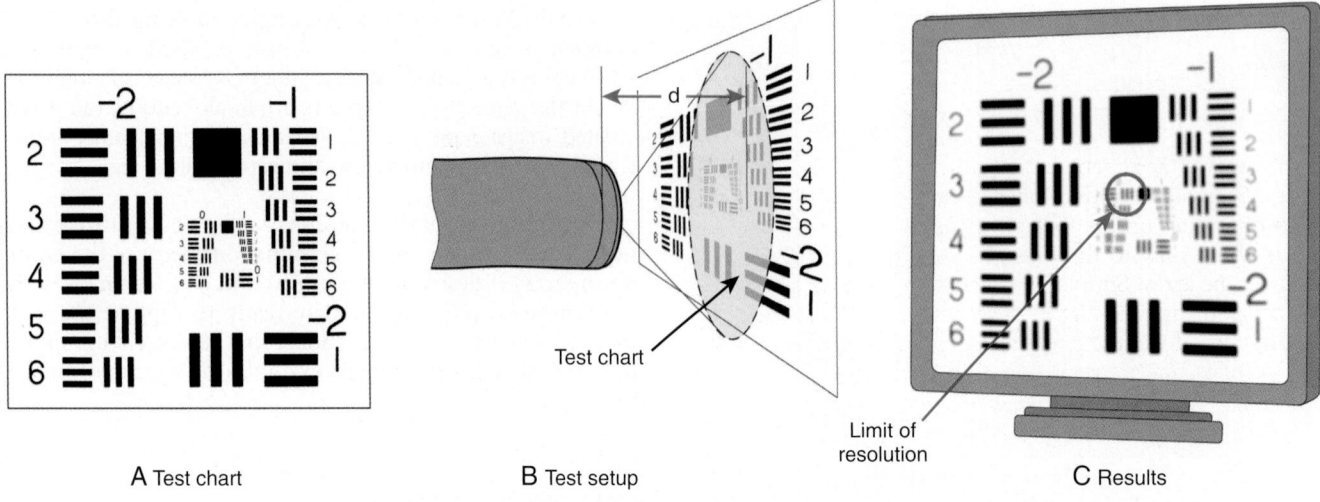

A Test chart   B Test setup   C Results

Fig. 3.13   Test setup for quantifying resolving power.

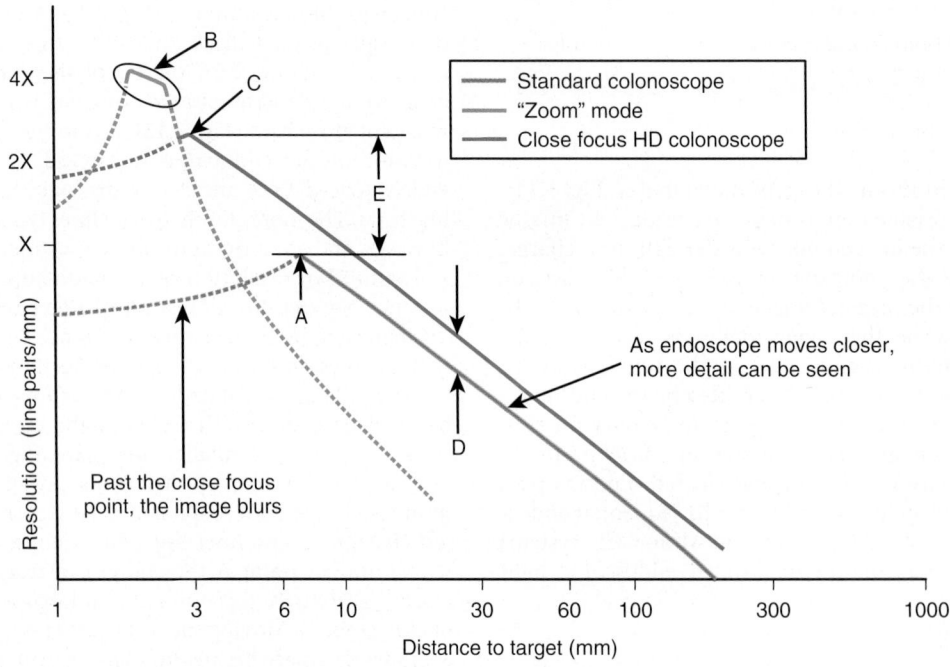

Fig. 3.14   Resolving power of standard, zoom, and close-focus colonoscopes.

endoscope in its "zoomed" mode is very limited, and the endoscope is very difficult to keep in focus.

More recently, close focus high-definition (HD) endoscopes have been introduced that offer advantages over standard and optical zoom endoscopes. Overall, the HD endoscope has increased resolving power because it has a greater number of pixels in its image sensor versus a standard endoscope (see **Fig. 3.14D**). In addition, the optics on close focusing endoscopes allow them to approach the observed tissue much more closely before going out of focus. The close focus HD colonoscope illustrated in **Fig. 3.14** is able to come within 3 mm of the test chart before going out of focus, resulting in threefold greater resolving power (**Fig. 3.14E**) compared with a standard colonoscope. Although its resolving power is still less than that of an optical zoom colonoscope, the fact that

this close focusing colonoscope has a very broad depth of field (3 to 200 mm, as depicted by the solid green line) makes this colonoscope as convenient to use as any standard endoscope.

The foregoing discussion of zoom endoscopes refers to endoscopes that have an *optical zoom* function. This is in contrast to the *electronic zoom* function found on most videoendoscopes. Electronic zoom does not increase the actual resolving power of the endoscope. Electronic zoom simply takes the information captured by the central portion of the CCD and enlarges its display on the monitor. Electronic zoom does not add any new image information to the monitor image and does not change the endoscope's resolving power as measured in the above-described test. Optical zoom does add significant image detail because of the ability of the endoscope to approach the tissue more closely and to obtain a true magnified image.

Reproduction of Color

All solid-state image sensors are inherently monochromatic devices. They can reproduce only black and white images. The silicon photosites on the surface of the CCD develop charges in proportion only to the intensity (brightness) of the light falling on the array. Simple image sensors cannot distinguish the color of the incident light. As shown in **Fig. 3.10**, a photon of red light produces the same charge as a photon of blue light. For an endoscope to reproduce the necessary attribute of color, the system must have an additional means to analyze the color (wavelength) of the light falling on the sensor.

Trichromatic Vision

It has been discovered that nearly any color to which the human eye is sensitive can be matched by mixing light of three colors—red, green, and blue (RGB). If three light projectors are fitted with RGB filters and the projected spotlights are overlapped, the resulting image would appear similar to that shown in **Fig. 3.15**. The color resulting from the overlap of the red and green projectors is indistinguishable from monochromatic yellow light. Likewise, light from the overlapping green and blue projectors produces the mental sensation of looking at pure cyan light. The overlap of red and blue produces magenta. Surprisingly, where all three of the projectors overlap in the center, the observer sees an area of pure white, with no hint of the three component colors. If the intensities of each of the three projectors are accurately controlled and varied, it is possible to reproduce virtually any spectral color in the central area of the overlap.

All video images are reconstructed using the three component colors of RGB. Because these three colors can be additively combined to mimic all other spectral colors, they are commonly referred to as the three *additive primary colors.* These three colors, RGB, are the colors of the phosphors used to create full color images on the face of a video monitor (**Fig. 3.16**). The colors yellow (Ye), cyan (Cy), and magenta (Mg) also play an important role in video imaging and are referred to as *complementary* colors. Commercial videoendoscopes currently use two different systems for recreating color. The first commercial video image endoscope, the VideoEndoscope introduced by Welch Allyn in 1983, was based on an RGB sequential imaging system.[5] Many current instruments continue to use this system. The second system, the so-called color-chip endoscope, has now become the predominant system worldwide. Each color reproduction system has its own advantages and disadvantages, as explained later.

Red, Green, and Blue Sequential Imaging ("Color Wheel")

The components of an RGB sequential videoscope system are schematically illustrated in **Fig. 3.16**. The endoscope has a monochromatic (black and white) CCD mounted in its distal tip. The objective lens at the tip of the endoscope focuses a miniature image of the endoscope's field of view on the photosensitive surface of this CCD. This image is illuminated via a fiberoptic bundle running through the endoscope. This fiberoptic bundle carries light from a lamp within the light source to the distal tip of the endoscope. In contrast to the light used for fiberoptic endoscopes or the light used for color-chip endoscopes, this light is not continuous but is strobed or pulsed. The high-intensity xenon lamp within the light source emits continuous white light with the approximate color temperature of sunlight. A rotating filter wheel with three colored segments (RGB) is placed between this lamp and the light guide post of the endoscope. This filter wheel chops and colors the light falling on the light guide bundle into alternating bursts of red, black (no light), green, black, blue, and black. When observed at the distal tip of the endoscope, this illumination appears to the eye to be a flickering white light, rather than the actual sequential bursts of RGB. Rotating at 20 to 30 revolutions/sec, these three primary colors appear to merge, creating white illumination when observed with the unaided eye.

The purpose of this unique illumination system is to produce three separate monochromatic images, each obtained when the field of view is sequentially illuminated by the three primary colors in turn. During the fraction of a second when the red filter is in the light path, the GI mucosa is illuminated only by red light. The CCD image sensor captures a monochromatic (black and white) image of the mucosa as it appears under this red illumination (**Fig. 3.17**). Tissue that is naturally reddish in color reflects heavily under red light and appears to be bright. Areas of the tissue with less red reflect red light weakly and appear dark under red illumination. After a monochromatic image of the mucosa is obtained under red illumination, the filter wheel rotates to the adjacent opaque area of the wheel. At this point, the endoscopic illumination goes momentarily dark, and the image on the CCD is read out, directed through a processing and switching circuit, and stored in the "red image" memory bank of the videoprocessor (see **Fig. 3.16**). After the red image is stored, the filter wheel rotates to place the green filter in the light path. A monochromatic

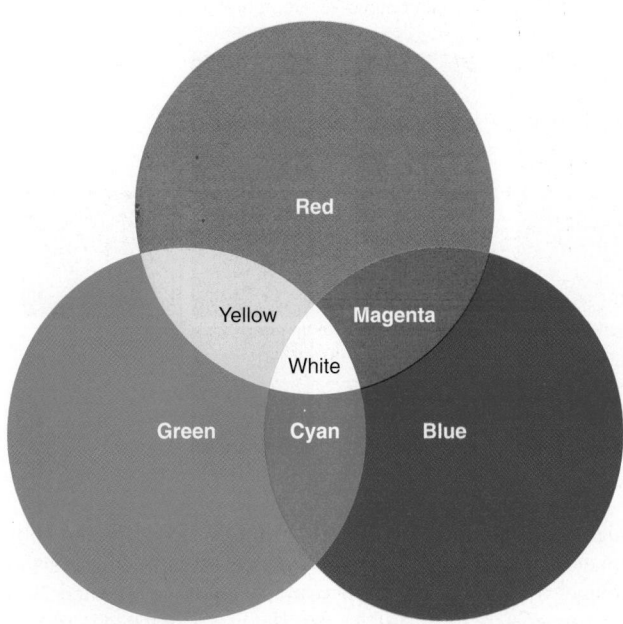

Fig. 3.15   Illustration of additive primary colors.

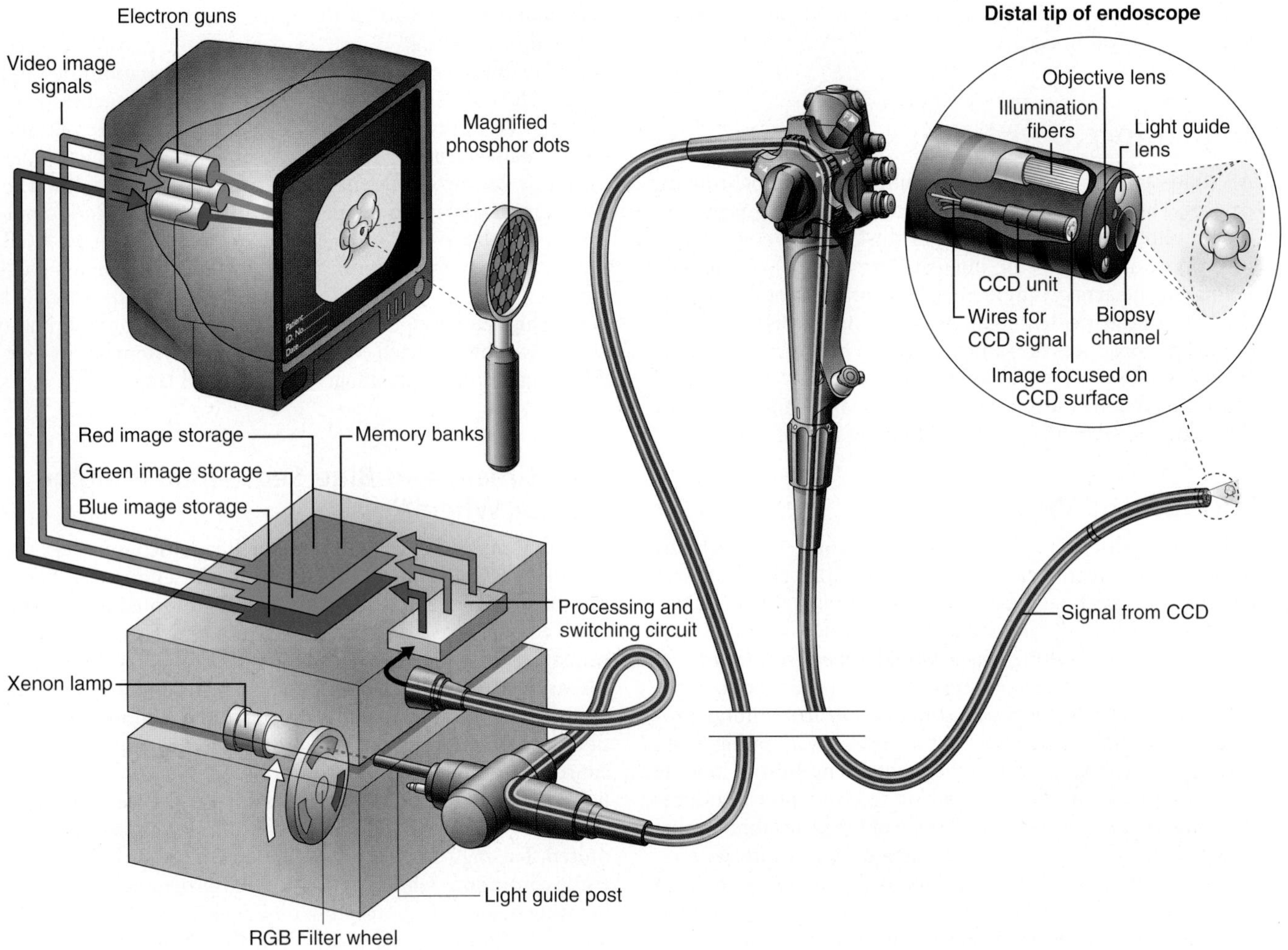

Video image signals

Electron guns

Magnified phosphor dots

Red image storage

Green image storage

Blue image storage

Memory banks

Processing and switching circuit

Xenon lamp

Light guide post

RGB Filter wheel

Distal tip of endoscope

Objective lens

Illumination fibers

Light guide lens

CCD unit

Wires for CCD signal

Biopsy channel

Image focused on CCD surface

Signal from CCD

Fig. 3.16 Schematic of red, green, and blue (RGB) sequential endoscope imaging system.

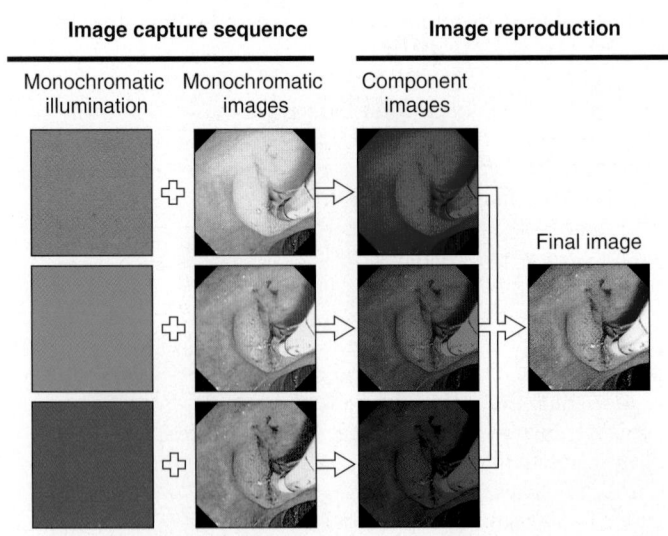

Image capture sequence

Monochromatic illumination

Monochromatic images

Image reproduction

Component images

Final image

Fig. 3.17 Image capture with red, green, and blue (RGB) sequential illumination.

image of the mucosa as it appears under green illumination is obtained by the CCD (see **Fig. 3.17**). This image is read out and sent to the videoprocessor for storage in the "green image" memory bank. In a similar manner, a third monochromatic image is obtained when the filter wheel rotates to the blue segment. This image is correspondingly stored in the "blue image" memory bank. This sequence of capturing a set of images for each of the three primary colors is repeated 20 to 30 times each second—the precise speed being determined by the specifications of the videoprocessor. Synchronization

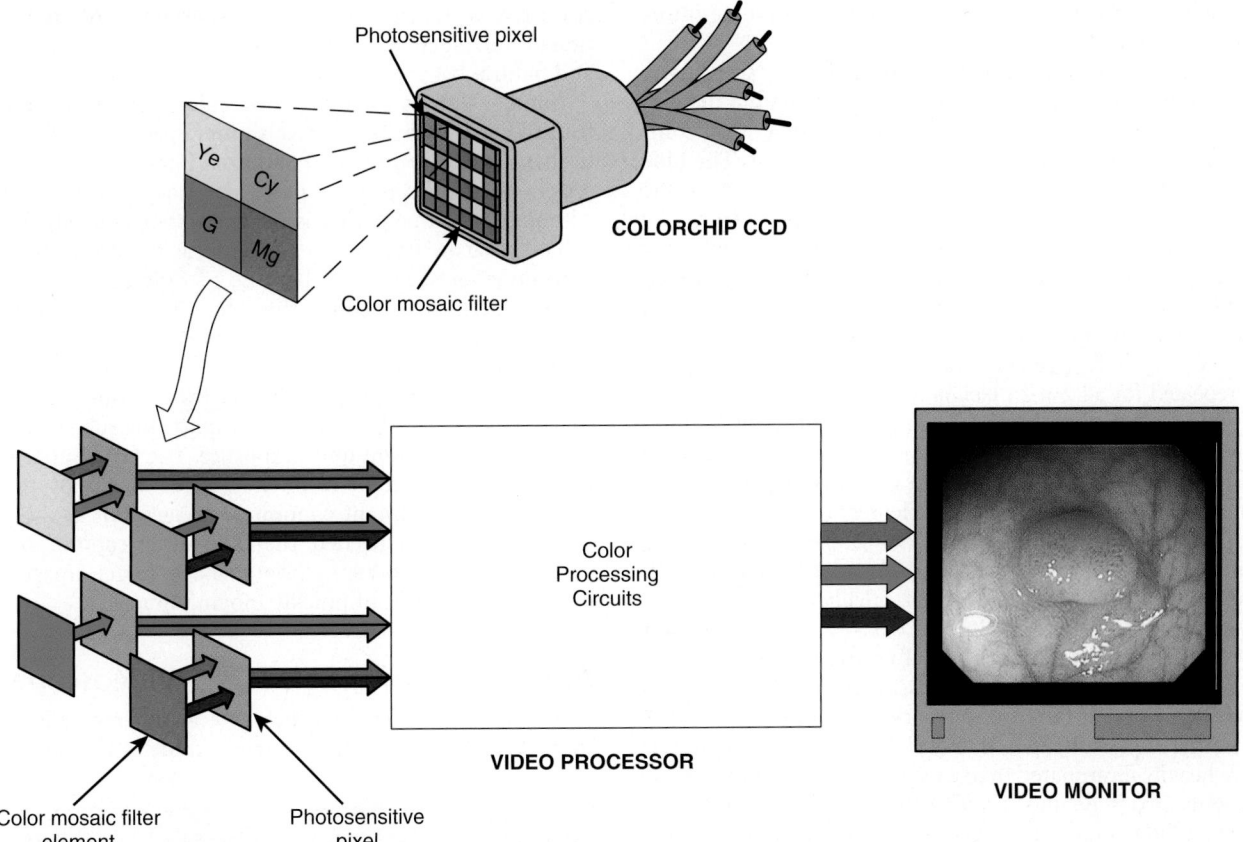

Fig. 3.18 Color mosaic filter matched to the pixels in a color-chip charge-coupled device (CCD) allows the image sensor simultaneously to capture full color information from the image projected on its photosensitive surface.

circuitry matches the rotation of the filter wheel with the readout of the CCD and sequences the switching circuit to direct each new image to the proper memory bank.

Color-Chip Imaging

As an alternative to the RGB sequential imaging system, some videoendoscopes use a color-chip imaging system. A color-chip CCD is essentially a black and white image sensor with a custom-fabricated, multicolored microfilter bonded to its surface. This filter allows the CCD to resolve directly and simultaneously the component colors of the image. The term *instantaneous single-plate CCD* is sometimes used for this device to emphasize that all three color components are obtained concurrently by a single "plate," or CCD. A color-mosaic filter of the type shown in **Fig. 3.18** is commonly used in color-chip CCDs. It is possible to design a mosaic filter with myriad different color configurations; however, the color choices shown in **Fig. 3.18** are very common. The colors used in this mosaic filter are yellow, cyan, magenta, and green (Ye/Cy/Mg/G). These segments are arranged in a 2 × 2 pixel box pattern that regularly repeats over the face of the CCD.

Because the final output signals sent to the video monitor must be the standard RGB component images, the image produced behind this Ye/Cy/Mg/G filter must be converted into its primary RGB components before display. This conversion is done by adding and subtracting information from neighboring pixels until the specific values for RGB are calculated for each pixel in the sensor. As **Fig. 3.19** illustrates, yellow filter

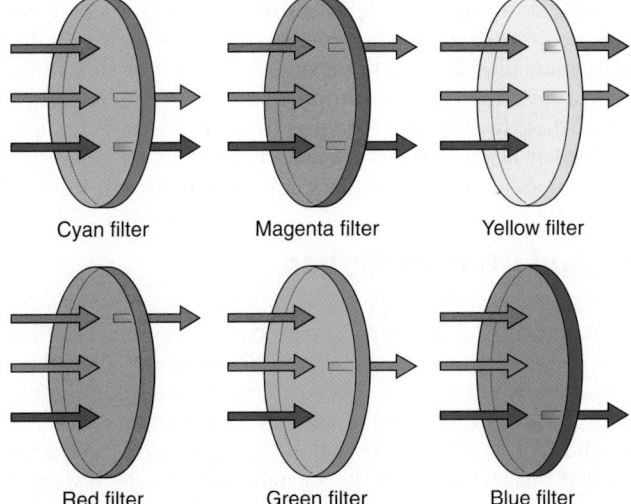

Fig. 3.19 Effect of filter color on transmission of red, green, and blue (RGB) light.

elements absorb blue light but pass red and green light; this enables the pixels behind all yellow filter elements to receive both red and green information. **Fig. 3.19** also shows that pixels behind cyan filter elements receive both blue and green portions of the color spectrum. Magenta pixels receive both red and blue light. In a representative block of four Ye/Cy/Mg/G pixels, two pixels receive red information, three pixels receive green information, and two pixels receive blue information (see **Fig. 3.18**).

By adding and subtracting the information obtained from adjacent pixels using an appropriate algorithm within the videoprocessor, it is possible to derive the individual RGB component values for each block of Ye/Cy/Mg/G pixels. The blue component value can be determined by subtracting the number of charges generated in the green pixel from the number of charges generated in the cyan pixel (B = Cy − G or B = [B+G] − G). The red component value can be determined by subtracting the number of charges generated in the green pixel from the number of charges generated in the yellow pixel (R = Ye − G or R = [R+G] − G). Calculations such as these are repeated for all 2 × 2 pixel blocks across the entire face of the CCD. When the process is completed, all required RGB component values for each pixel block in the matrix will have been calculated. One may question why it is desirable to use a mosaic filter composed of complementary colors (Ye, Cy, and Mg) and to employ a processing algorithm if using primary RGB filters to cover the pixels would yield the RGB component values directly without calculation. The answer lies in the fact that a Ye/Cy/Mg/G mosaic filter has a significant advantage in brightness over an RGB mosaic filter.

When RGB filter segments are used, each pixel is filtered to receive only one of the three primary colors (see **Fig. 3.19**). A cyan-filtered pixel is exposed to both blue and green light. It is more heavily illuminated than a pure blue or pure green pixel. Likewise, pixels behind a yellow filter (red + green) or a magenta filter (blue + red) receive more photons (light) than pixels behind a pure RGB filter. Because of the increased light intensity passing through a Ye/Cy/Mg/G mosaic filter, a CCD with this construction exhibits far greater light sensitivity. The clear advantage of complementary colored mosaic filters is that because of the increased light sensitivity, these filters allow the videoscope designer to construct an endoscope with a smaller light guide fiber bundle, to maximize the angle of view of the endoscope and to increase the depth of field of the endoscope. All of these features improve performance, but each requires additional light. For this reason, all commercial color-chip endoscopes use complementary color mosaic CCDs.

Reproduction of Motion

The color-chip videoscope has an inherent advantage over the RGB sequential videoscope in reproducing motion. The filter wheel in RGB videoprocessors typically rotates at 20 to 30 rps (revolutions per second). Because each of the color component images is captured individually, in sequence, it takes $\frac{1}{30}$ second (with a 30-rps filter wheel) to capture the three component images that make up a single video image. If there is relative motion between the endoscope and the object being viewed, as often occurs during endoscopy, the three component images may differ slightly with respect to object size and position. When these three RGB images are subsequently superimposed on the video monitor, they are likely to be misaligned. This misalignment is clearly visible if the endoscopist happens to freeze the image while it is moving rapidly. Although the RGB sequential videoscope has difficulty reproducing motion, the color-chip videoscope is excellent at imaging moving tissue because all three color components of the image are captured simultaneously. Because the illumination is continuous and nonstrobed and the frame rate is

consistent with contemporary television standards, reproduction of moving images with a color-chip videoscope is smooth and natural.

Another unique advantage of a color-chip videoscope is a feature that allows its effective shutter speed to be shortened to increase the sharpness of captured images. The color-chip system normally captures a new video image every $\frac{1}{60}$ second. Although this time period is relatively short, quickly moving subjects that are frozen may appear to be slightly blurred (but with no color separation) because of movement during the capture period. To reduce this blur, it is advantageous to shorten the electronic capture period to a fraction of its normal time (e.g., from $\frac{1}{60}$ second to $\frac{1}{250}$ second). As in traditional film photography, the shorter the exposure period, the sharper the subject, but the more brightly the subject must be illuminated to prevent underexposure. The fast-shutter mode found on many color-chip endoscopes may not provide enough light for distant panoramic images, but in situations in which it is truly needed, the fast-shutter capture mode is very effective at producing bright, sharp, frozen images (i.e., close-up still images of quickly moving mucosa).

Advantages of a Color-Chip Videoscope

The color-chip videoscope has several inherent advantages over the RGB sequential system (**Table 3.1**). Advantages

Table 3.1 Advantages and Disadvantages of Videoscope Imaging Systems

Advantages	Disadvantages
COLOR CHIP SYSTEM	
Smooth, natural reproduction of motion	Difficult to adapt to color analysis research
No color separation on captured images	
Fast shutter mode prevents image blur even when subject is moving	
Uses standard (nonstrobing) xenon light source	
Transillumination is possible under normal viewing conditions	
Superior performance during laser therapy	
RGB SEQUENTIAL SYSTEM	
High-resolution image possible	Image slip between RGB component images
Each pixel images all three colors	"Rainbow effect" on rapidly moving objects
Advanced color analysis is possible by changing filters	Requires strobed light source
	Laser therapy is hindered by white aiming beam and image "bloom"
	Transillumination requires removing filter wheel and produces a black and white image

RGB, Red, green, and blue.

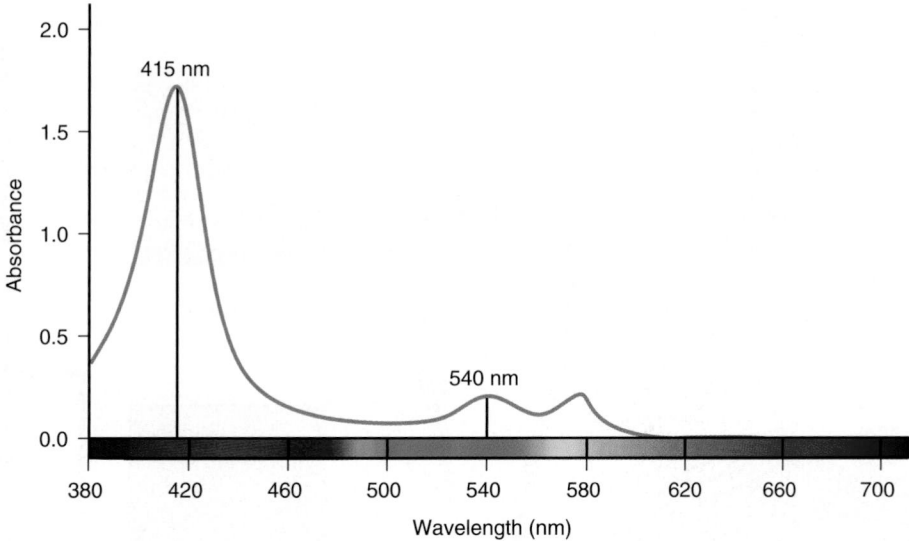

Fig. 3.20   Absorbance spectra of oxyhemoglobin.

discussed previously include (1) a smooth, natural reproduction of motion; (2) the absence of color separation on frozen images; and (3) a fast-shutter mode that prevents image blur of even the fastest moving subjects. Additional advantages include (4) compatibility with standard (nonstrobing) xenon light sources, (5) increased transillumination, and (6) superior performance during laser therapy. With RGB sequential endoscopes, abdominal transillumination is problematic because its strobed light output is substantially weaker than that of nonstrobed systems. Many RGB sequential light sources have a means for temporarily removing the spinning filter wheel from the light path when operating in the "transillumination" mode. A steady, intense white light that is ideal for transillumination is produced. However, once the filter wheel is removed, the image is lost because in most cases the illumination is so intense that it saturates the CCD, producing a largely white image. Even if an image is visible, it is in black and white because the filter wheel must be in its proper position to reproduce color.

Advantages of the Red, Green, and Blue Sequential Videoscope

A major advantage of the RGB sequential videoscope is the opportunity for increased resolution. Image resolution depends heavily on the number of pixels in the original image. The color-chip system requires information from several pixels, which is processed via an algorithm, to obtain the RGB component values for each individual point within the image. In the RGB system, each pixel is illuminated by RGB light sequentially. Each pixel provides information on each of the three color components in turn. The fact that a single pixel can provide all three color components is an advantage for small imaging devices such as endoscopes. In practice, this advantage is not significant for most videoendoscopes, but it is a significant advantage when the thinnest possible endoscope is required (e.g., videocholedochoscope). Because the RGB sequential videoscope uses primary-colored filters and because the color components are isolated, captured, and

processed separately within the videoprocessor, this type of videoscope provides very accurate color information. This potential advantage is not usually apparent with routine endoscopy; however, in image analysis research, the RGB sequential system is better than the color-chip system.

Narrow Band Imaging with a Red, Green, and Blue Sequential Videoscope

In recent years, Olympus (Tokyo, Japan) has introduced videoendoscopy systems with a new observation mode called *narrow band imaging (NBI)*.[6–9] The purpose of this feature is to enhance the observation of mucosal surface detail (e.g., pit patterns) and to increase the contrast between microvascular structures and the surrounding tissue through the selective manipulation of the imaging of hemoglobin. Hemoglobin is a major chromophore in tissue. **Fig. 3.20** shows the relative absorbance of light by oxyhemoglobin over the visible spectrum. Peak absorption occurs at 415 nm (blue light). A secondary peak is observed around 540 nm (green light). It is clear from **Fig. 3.20** that hemoglobin reflects rather than absorbs red light, giving hemoglobin its characteristic color. Using such information regarding the characteristic absorbance of hemoglobin, it is possible to design an imaging system that increases image contrast based on the relative presence or absence of hemoglobin in the tissue being endoscopically studied.

Fig. 3.21 schematically illustrates the implementation of NBI imaging in an RGB sequential videoscope system. The light source has the same xenon lamp and the same rotating RGB filter wheel as the standard endoscopy system illustrated in **Fig. 3.16**. However, for NBI imaging, a special NBI filter has been temporarily placed in front of the xenon lamp. This device filters the broad-spectrum white light produced by the xenon lamp (Spectrum 1 in **Fig. 3.21**) and allows only a very narrow band of blue light with wavelengths centered around 415 nm and a very narrow band of green light with wavelengths centered around 540 nm to pass through the filter (Spectrum 2 in **Fig. 3.21**). It is this use of narrow bands of

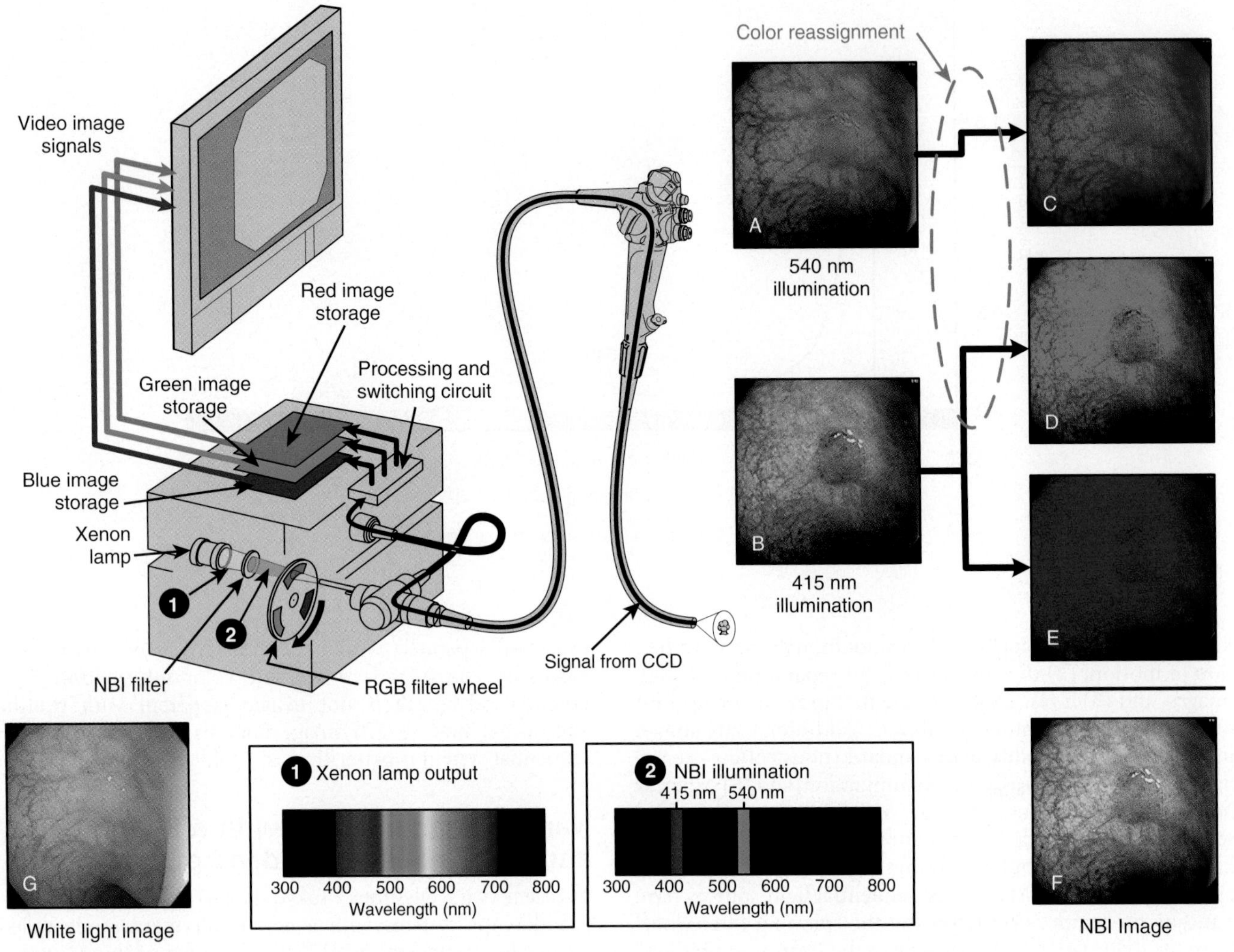

Video image signals

Red image storage

Green image storage

Processing and switching circuit

Blue image storage

Xenon lamp

1

2

NBI filter

RGB filter wheel

Signal from CCD

Color reassignment

A
540 nm illumination

B
415 nm illumination

C

D

E

F
NBI Image

G
White light image

1 Xenon lamp output

300   400   500   600   700   800
Wavelength (nm)

2 NBI illumination
415 nm   540 nm

300   400   500   600   700   800
Wavelength (nm)

Fig. 3.21 Narrow band imaging (NBI) with red, green, and blue (RGB) sequential videoendoscope system. *(Endoscopic images courtesy of Y. Sano and S. Yoshida.)*

light (i.e., very limited wavelengths of light) to illuminate the tissue that gives NBI its name.

The imaging sequence of an RGB sequential NBI system is as follows: When the red filter segment is in the light path, no light enters the endoscope because there is no red light in the NBI-filtered light. No image is created, and no image is stored at this point. The filter wheel rotates to the green filter segment. The green light (540 nm) passing through the NBI filter also passes through the green segment of the rotating filter wheel, passes through the endoscope, and illuminates the tissue. (The 415-nm blue light emitted by the NBI filter is blocked by the green filter in the rotating filter wheel.) A monochromatic (black and white) image of the tissue as it appears under this narrow band of 540-nm green illumination is captured by the CCD (see **Fig. 3.21A**); however, rather than storing this image in the expected green image memory bank, the videoprocessor switching circuit sends the 540-nm image to the empty red image storage bank (see **Fig. 3.21C**). This action is an intentional reassignment of color.

Finally, the filter wheel rotates to the blue filter segment. This filter segment passes the 415-nm blue light from the NBI filter, and the tissue is illuminated by a narrow spectrum of blue light centered at 415 nm. The CCD captures a black

and white image of the mucosa as it appears under 415-nm illumination (see **Fig. 3.21B**), and the videoprocessor stores the image as expected in the blue memory bank (see **Fig. 3.21E**). The videoprocessor also stores an identical copy of this 415-nm image in the green memory bank (see **Fig. 3.21D**), a second intentional reassignment of color. The red component image now consists of an image of the tissue as it appeared under 540-nm narrow band illumination (green light), and the green and blue component images now consist of images of the tissue as it reflected the 415-nm narrow band illuminating light (blue light). After one complete rotation of the RGB filter wheel and the assignment of images to each of the RGB image storage areas, the three RGB component images are sent simultaneously to the video monitor, where the three component images (see **Fig. 3.21C-E**) are superimposed as a final full-color NBI image (see **Fig. 3.21F**). This final NBI image is quite different from the image of the tissue as it would appear under normal white light illumination (see **Fig. 3.21G**). The color reassignment has altered the natural coloration of the tissue, and the selective illumination of the tissue using only the wavelengths that are highly absorbed by oxyhemoglobin has greatly increased the surface pattern of the mucosal lesion.

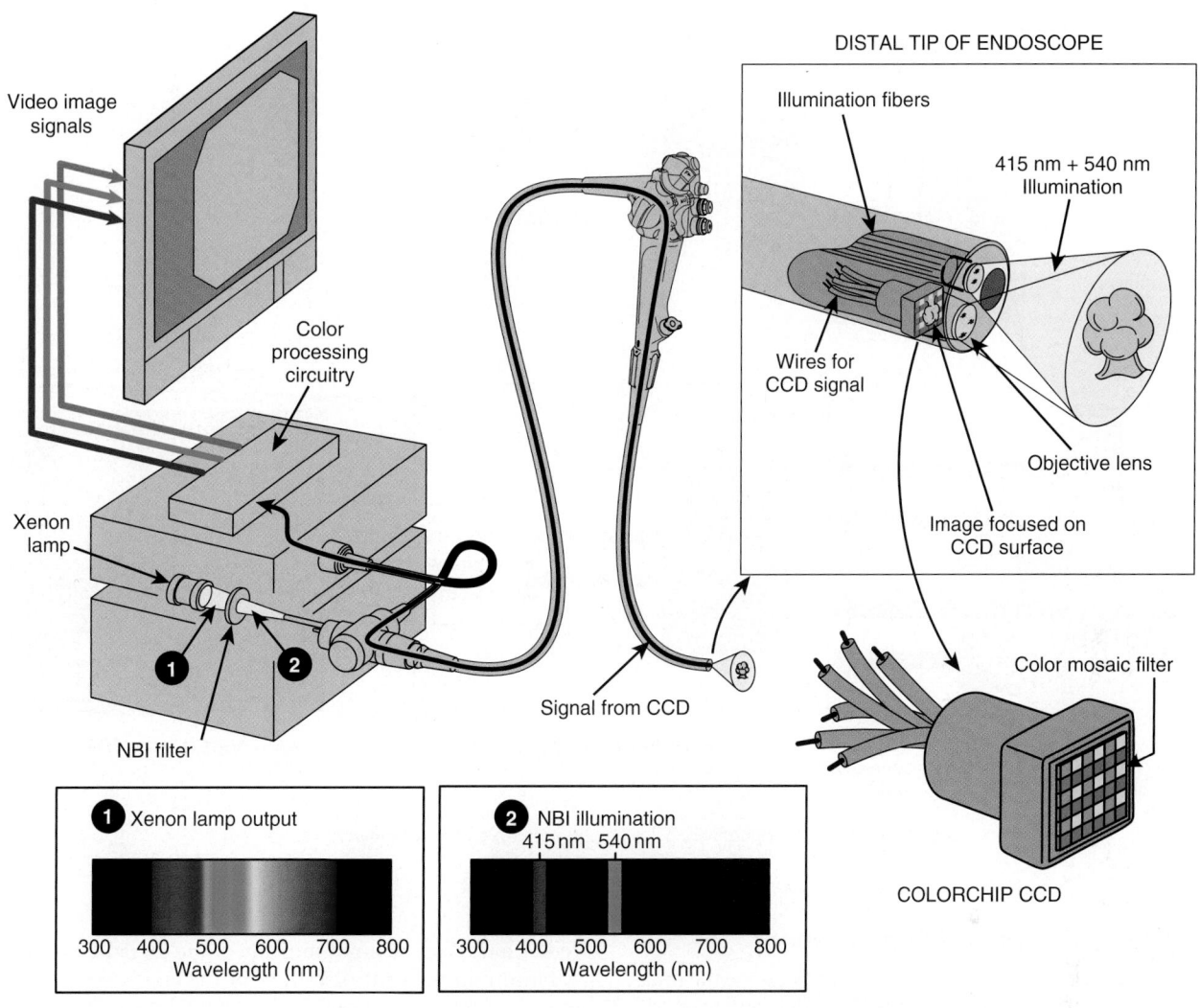

DISTAL TIP OF ENDOSCOPE

Video image signals

Color processing circuitry

Xenon lamp

NBI filter

① Xenon lamp output

③②

300 400 500 600 700 800
Wavelength (nm)

② NBI illumination
415 nm   540 nm

300 400 500 600 700 800
Wavelength (nm)

Signal from CCD

Illumination fibers

415 nm + 540 nm Illumination

Wires for CCD signal

Objective lens

Image focused on CCD surface

Color mosaic filter

COLORCHIP CCD

Fig. 3.22   Narrow band imaging (NBI) with color-chip videoendoscope system.

Narrow Band Imaging with a Color-Chip Videoscope

NBI can also be implemented on color-chip video platforms. **Fig. 3.22** illustrates the insertion of an NBI filter in the light source of a color-chip endoscope. The NBI filter filters the broad-spectrum white light emitted by the xenon lamp (Spectrum 1 in **Fig. 3.22**) to the same NBI spectrum used in the RGB sequential system. Color-chip NBI illumination consists of continuous, simultaneous illumination of the tissue by 415-nm and 540-nm narrow band light. The color-chip CCD in the endoscope captures an image of the tissue reflecting under this special NBI illumination. Following image capture, the image information is processed by the videoprocessor before display. **Fig. 3.23** summarizes the processing of the color-chip NBI image. The color mosaic filter on the CCD filters the image as explained earlier. However, because there are no red wavelengths in the NBI illumination, there is no red image information entering the color processing circuits in the videoprocessor—only blue and green information is available. Similar to the RGB sequential NBI system, the green color information is intentionally reassigned by the videoprocessor for display as a red component image. Also similar to

the RGB sequential system, the blue image information is displayed as a blue component image and is intentionally reassigned as a green component image. When these RGB component images, as defined, are simultaneously displayed on the video monitor, the color-chip videoscope system displays an NBI image that is similar to that of the RGB sequential videoscope system.

The NBI function in both types of systems is easily turned on and off via a switch on the endoscope or via a button on the videoprocessor. The endoscopist can quickly alternate between standard white light and NBI imaging at will.

Image Processing

All videoprocessors convert the endoscopic image to a digital format during processing. When in a digital format, it is very easy to manipulate the image via various algorithms. Some more typically used algorithms are designed to produce various levels of "edge enhancement" or "texture enhancement." These algorithms do not intentionally change the color of the tissue but add image contrast to enhance the delineation of edges or enhance tissue topography. In a sense, they attempt to "sharpen" the image.

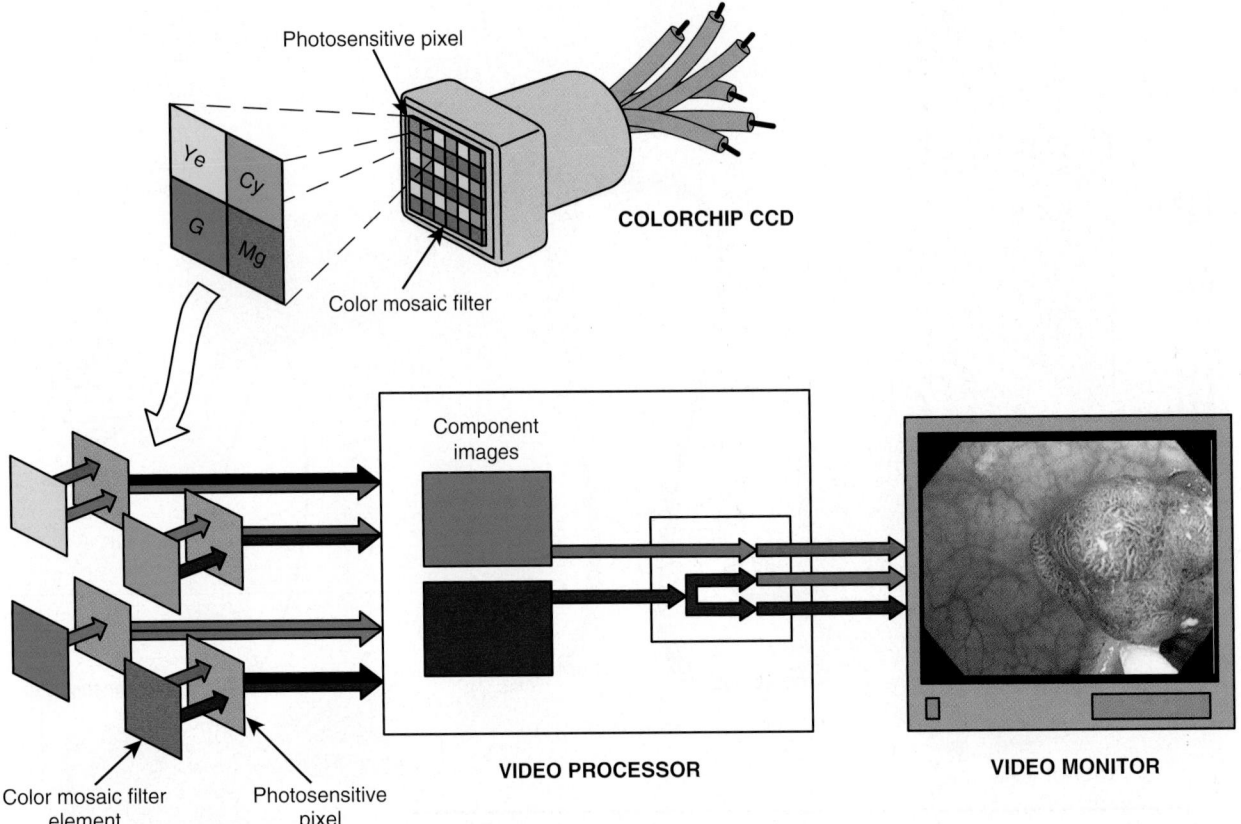

Fig. 3.23 Narrow band imaging (NBI) color processing with color-chip videoendoscope system.

Postprocessing Image Enhancement

Efforts have been made more recently to manipulate the image (postprocessing) to obtain data similar to that obtained with NBI. Fujinon (Saitama, Japan) has introduced a feature called *FICE* (Fuji Intelligent Color Enhancement), and Pentax (Montvale, NJ) has introduced a feature called *i-Scan,* which intentionally manipulate the color of the endoscopic image.[10–13] These postprocessing features are designed to enhance the display of mucosal blood vessels and surface structure. Olympus' NBI feature does this through illuminating the tissue at selected wavelengths corresponding to the natural absorption of hemoglobin. FICE and i-Scan use normal white light illumination, capture a normal white light image, and perform digital manipulations on the resulting normal endoscopic image. This process is variously referred to as "optimal band imaging" or "multiband imaging." When the endoscopic image is in a digital form, it is easy to identify the specific color of each point (pixel) in the captured image and to select only the pixels that fall within a designated color range. These selected colors can be displayed as a new image, manipulated to perform a desired enhancement, or reassigned for display as a different color.

The FICE system allows the user to select from the white light image certain narrow ranges of color that are then used as "optimal band images." Three such optimal band images can be selected by the user and assigned to the RGB monitor inputs. Ten factory-determined optimal band presets are available in FICE configured processors; however, presets can be customized by the user. Any of 60 estimated wavelengths

(color hues) can be input into any of the three RGB channels. A button on the control section of the endoscope allows the operator to switch from conventional white light imaging to real-time multiband imaging.

The optimal multiband imaging presets for tissue diagnosis or differentiation are yet to be determined; however, the concept is easily illustrated. Although endoscopic diagnosis typically consists of interpreting subtle changes in the various hues of red seen in endoscopic images, postprocessing is more easily shown using a photograph containing vivid colors; **Fig. 3.24A** is such an image of a hot-air balloon launch. Once the image is in digital form, it is easy for a software algorithm to select and extract only certain specific hues from the image. In the case of **Fig. 3.24B**, the software (Adobe Photoshop) has selected a specific range of blues and a specific range of greens as colors of interest. This range of colors could be chosen to be very narrow (e.g., a certain shade of dark blue) or could be chosen to be very broad (e.g., ranging from light blue to dark blue). These selected colors can be displayed as they would normally appear or reassigned to a different color to create added emphasis. In **Fig. 3.24C**, the selected blue colors were reassigned to be green, and the selected green colors were reassigned to be blue.

As one can imagine, the ways in which images can be manipulated by digital postprocessing are endless. However, in every case, the colors of the original white light image are being manipulated. NBI manipulates the interaction of the illuminating light with the tissue itself by illuminating the tissue with only specific wavelengths that achieve the desired

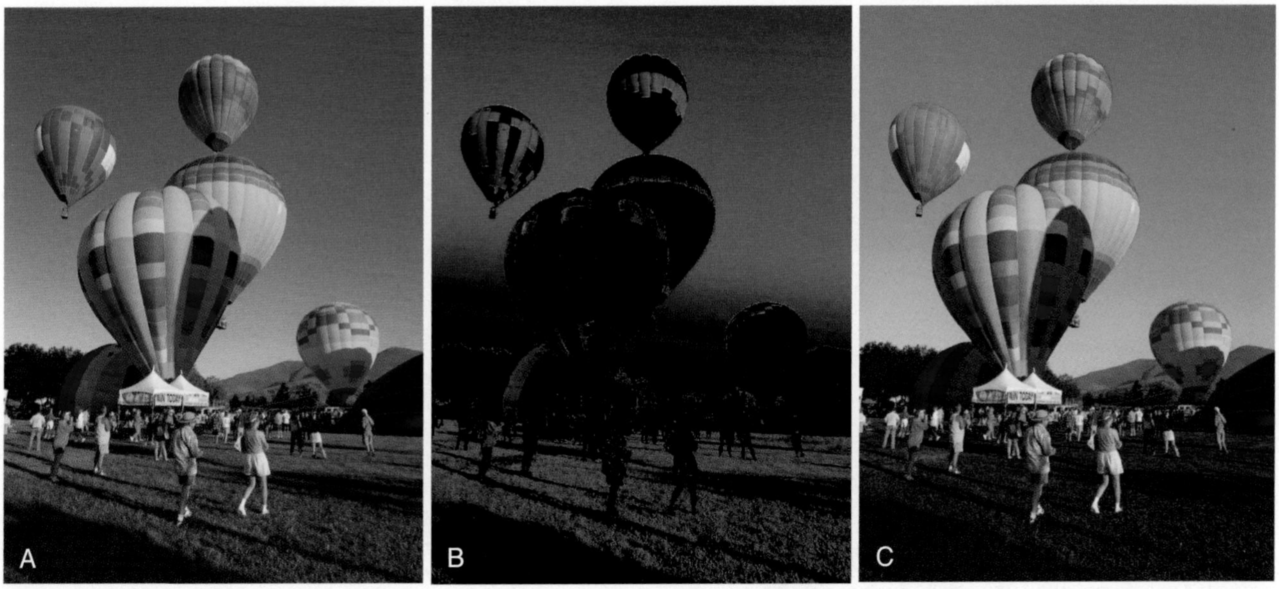

Fig. 3.24   Example of image processing. **A,** Original image. **B,** Selection of colors with blue and green hues. **C,** Color reassignment of selected colors.

contrast change in the tissue. In the postprocessing example shown in **Fig. 3.24C**, although the software effectively exchanged the colors of the sky and the grass, it also changed the colors of other objects in the scene that had similar colors in the white light image (e.g., the blue band on the highest central balloon). If certain endoscopic structures, such as capillaries, glands, and pits, always had a unique characteristic color, it would be possible to design a software algorithm to identify and enhance them. Although no image processing schema has been validated or standardized for routine clinical use, research is ongoing to identify valuable algorithms.

Endoscopic Ultrasound Instrumentation

Olympus introduced the first endoscopic ultrasound (EUS) instruments into general use in 1984. The initial instrument (GF-UM2) was a fiberoptic endoscope with a mechanical scanning piezoelectric transducer at its tip. Although video-based gastroscopes and colonoscopes became available in the mid-1980s, the first video-based EUS instruments were not introduced until 1998. Now video imaging dominates the EUS field as well. The previous discussions about overall instrument construction; insertion tube components; air, water, and suction systems; and video imaging technology generally apply to EUS instruments as well. In addition to these systems, EUS instruments must incorporate extra components for ultrasonic wave generation, coupling, and detection.

To achieve good acoustic coupling, EUS instruments typically have a water-filled latex balloon at their tip. The injection and removal of water from this balloon requires an additional balloon inflation channel running the length of the insertion tube and additional controls (special valves) to fill and empty the balloon. EUS instruments employ either mechanical scanning or electronic scanning technology to create their ultrasound image. The earliest EUS endoscopes used a single

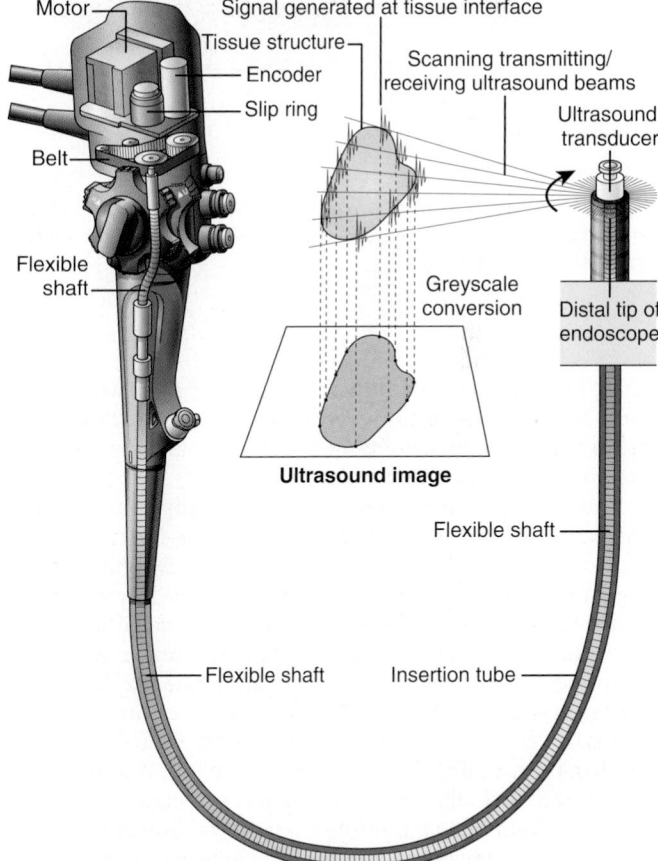

Fig. 3.25   Schematic of mechanical radial scanning endoscopic ultrasound (EUS) instrument.

piezoelectric transducer that was mechanically rotated around an axis parallel to the central axis of the endoscope (**Fig. 3.25**). A 360-degree radial ultrasound image plane was created that was perpendicular to the axis of the endoscope, with the endoscope itself located at the center of the image. Mechanical

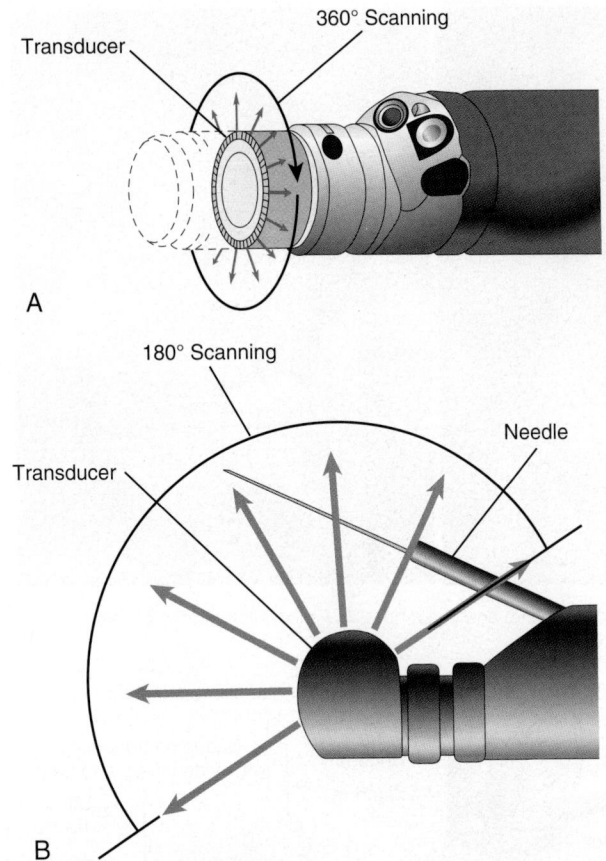

Fig. 3.26 **A,** Distal tip of electronic radial scanning endoscopic ultrasound (EUS) endoscope. **B,** Distal tip of curvilinear EUS fine needle aspiration (FNA) endoscope.

radial EUS endoscopes typically operate at 7.5 to 20 MHz, and for 2 decades these were the primary diagnostic EUS instruments because of their conveniently oriented image plane and their high-resolution EUS image.

In 2003, Pentax introduced an electronic radial image echoendoscope. This was the first radial scanning instrument to provide complex ultrasound features such as Doppler image capability. The image was limited to a 270-degree sector, however. Subsequently, Olympus introduced a radial scanning EUS endoscope that employed a full 360-degree array of piezoelectric transducers in lieu of the single mechanically rotated crystal (**Fig. 3.26A**). Electronic radial scanning instruments by Pentax and Olympus have now supplanted the older mechanical scanning design. In the early 1990s, Pentax introduced the first electronic scanning EUS endoscope that employed a curvilinear transducer array. This instrument produced an image plane aligned with the long axis of the endoscope and for the first time allowed practical fine needle aspiration (FNA) because the entire needle tip lay within the EUS image plane. In contrast to mechanical scanning instruments, electronic scanning endoscopes are capable of color Doppler (a function that shows the direction and the average velocity of blood flow) and power Doppler (a function that has increased sensitivity for measuring the velocity of flow but that provides no information on the direction of flow). Curvilinear array endoscopes typically have a 150-degree to 180-

degree angle of view (ultrasound image) and operate with a transducer frequency of 5 to 10 MHz. The optical direction of view is in a forward oblique direction and aligned in the general direction of the FNA needle (**Fig. 3.26B**). An elevator in the distal tip of the endoscope allows up-and-down movement of the needle, with the elevator being similar to the elevator on a duodenoscope but with a more limited range of motion.

Factors to Consider When Evaluating a Video Image Endoscope

A video image endoscope is a technologically advanced and complex clinical tool. When these instruments first entered the market, published comparison reports of various commercially available models were common.[14–16] Now that the technology of videoendoscopy has matured, such published technical comparisons are rare, but summaries of the specifications of commercially available models are periodically published.[17–19] It is difficult to identify any single design criterion as the deciding factor in selecting the best videoscope for a particular clinical application. When evaluating a videoendoscope, the following criteria should be considered:

1. *Image quality:* Does the instrument have a sufficiently wide angle of view, with good depth of field, high image resolution, good image contrast, accurate color, clear frozen images, and a wide dynamic range (ability to see clearly in light and dark areas of the image)?
2. *Illumination characteristics:* Does the instrument have adequate image brightness under all clinical conditions? Is illumination evenly distributed from image center to image edge? Does the system have responsive automatic brightness adjustment as viewing distances change?
3. *Basic endoscope functions:* Does the instrument have responsive handling and appropriate insertion tube characteristics? Does it have smooth tip angulation; a control section of appropriate shape and weight; conveniently positioned angulation knobs and valves; and good suction, insufflation, and lens washing performance?
4. *Basic specifications:* Does the manufacturer have a full range of instrument models, with a variety of insertion tube diameters and biopsy channel capacities to meet all clinical needs?
5. *Suitability for special therapeutic procedures:* Is the videoendoscope well protected against image noise from electrosurgical generators? Is image quality acceptable when using lasers?
6. *System features:* Are the videoprocessor controls easy to understand? Are the endoscope switches for the control of remote devices easily accessible? Does the size and weight of the equipment allow for easy transportation?
7. *System expansion and integration:* Is the system capable of easily interfacing with hard copy devices, videotape recorders, and computerized image management systems?

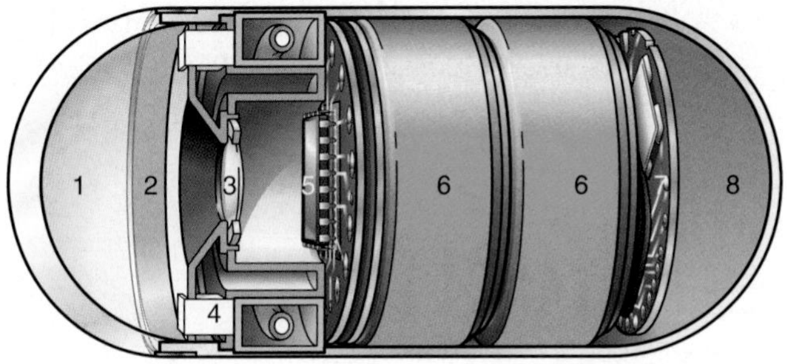

1. Optical dome
2. Lens holder
3. Lens
4. Illuminating LEDs (Light Emitting Diode)
5. CMOS (Complementary Metal Oxide Semiconductor) imager
6. Battery
7. ASIC (Application Specific Integrated Circuit) transmitter
8. Antenna

Fig. 3.27 Schematic of Given Imaging M2A capsule. *(Redrawn from Pillcam, Given Imaging, Yoqneam, Israel.)*

Capsule Endoscopy

The past decade has witnessed the remarkably rapid development and clinical acceptance of capsule endoscopy. The first experiments in animals were published in the journal *Nature* in 2000,[20] and clinical trials for GI bleeding of obscure origin were first reported in the literature in 2001.[21,22] Capsule endoscopy has been a major development in the trend toward minimally invasive examination of the GI tract. Currently, a capsule endoscopy system comprises three distinct components: (1) the capsule, (2) the data receiving and storage system, and (3) a workstation for image review and analysis.

The first capsule cleared by the U.S. Food and Drug Administration (FDA) (August 2001) for small bowel observation was the M2A capsule by Given Imaging, Inc. (Yoqneam, Israel). The capsule was 11 mm in diameter and 26 mm long. The capsule and its component parts are illustrated in **Fig. 3.27**. One end of the capsule has a clear optical dome, behind which sits the imaging system. The capsule is symmetric in shape and small enough to tumble in the intestine; it images the mucosa proximally or distally in a random fashion as it traverses the GI tract. Behind the clear dome is an aspheric lens with four light-emitting diodes (LEDs) arranged around it. The lens focuses the image onto a complementary metal oxide semiconductor (CMOS) imager. Behind this are two

silver oxide batteries, sufficient to power the LEDs, the imager, and the transmitter for at least 8 hours. A transmitter and antenna are located at the back of the capsule. The capsule is packaged adjacent to a magnet. Removal of the capsule from the magnet trips a switch, activating the LEDs and starting the image transmission. Two images are captured and transmitted each second, synchronized with illumination from the flashing LEDs. The small amount of illumination from the LEDs is adequate because the bowel is collapsed (i.e., no air insufflation is added) and the observed tissue is very close to the optical dome.

Given Imaging has launched an updated small bowel capsule called the PillCamSB. Olympus has launched a similar small bowel capsule called the EndoCapsule.[23] All three capsules are exactly the same size. The more recent capsules have improved image resolution, a wider angle of view, six LEDs instead of four, and improved workstation software. Some systems also offer a real-time viewer. The Olympus EndoCapsule uses a CCD image sensor in place of the CMOS image sensor in the Given Imaging capsules. During capsule endoscopy, the patient has a series of eight sensors taped to the anterior abdominal wall. These sensors detect the signal transmitted from the capsule. By measuring the relative strength of the signal from different sensors, the approximate location of the capsule within the abdominal cavity can be determined. The workstation software displays the path taken by the capsule alongside the capsule image. The sensor leads connect to a small data recorder worn on a belt. The belt apparatus is relatively light and does not significantly impede normal nonexertional activities. The patient can ambulate and need not remain in the hospital during the recording phase of the examination. After the examination, the sensors and belt are removed from the patient. The recorded data are downloaded to a computer workstation, which converts the approximately 50,000 images of the study into a video file that is stored on the computer's hard drive. The study is viewed on the workstation screen as a video at speeds determined by the reviewer.

In 2004, Given Imaging received FDA clearance on PillCam ESO, a dual imaging capsule for examining the esophagus. This capsule is currently marketed for diagnosing Barrett's esophagus and esophageal varices. Given Imaging is also developing PillCam COLON, a capsule for examining the colon. Several companies are developing methods to propel capsules actively within the GI tract. Capsule development continues.

References

The complete reference list is available online at www.expertconsult.com.

I

Chapter 4

Cleaning and Disinfecting Gastrointestinal Endoscopic Equipment

Douglas B. Nelson

Introduction

Articles in the lay press suggesting that endoscopes are inadequately reprocessed have raised undue fear regarding the potential for transmission of infection during endoscopy. When current guidelines for endoscope cleaning and disinfection are followed, this risk is virtually eliminated. This topic has largely been taken for granted by many endoscopists, however. Standardized cleaning and disinfection protocols have been available for some time, and, with few exceptions, changes have been gradual. This situation may have engendered some complacency on the part of endoscopists, to the point that many endoscopists were only vaguely aware of what went on "behind the curtain" of the endoscope reprocessing room; instruments were used on patients, taken away by gastrointestinal (GI) nurses or other health care personnel, reprocessed, and returned ready for patient use. As the amount of information available to patients increases via the Internet (often not based on scientific evidence), endoscopists must be able to discuss this subject confidently with their patients.

Since the first report of fiberoptic GI endoscopy in 1961,[1] the endoscope has undergone almost continuous evolution in design. Although most of these developments have been aimed at improving the diagnostic and therapeutic capability of GI endoscopy, the introduction of fully immersible endoscopes in 1983 greatly facilitated cleaning and disinfection of the internal channels of the endoscope.[2,3] The development of video imaging technology, which provided a tremendous increase in the quality and resolution of the endoscopic image, had few implications for endoscope reprocessing. However, some changes have come at the cost of increasing complexity of design, presenting new challenges to cleaning and disinfection. The addition of an elevator lever to the duodenoscope allowed easier cannulation of the papilla during endoscopic retrograde cholangiopancreatography (ERCP), although the new exposed movable part at the distal tip of the instrument and the associated control-wire channel also added new reprocessing steps. A similar type of elevator is present on current endoscopic ultrasound (EUS) endoscopes, or echoendoscopes. Echoendoscopes also possess an additional channel to inflate a balloon at the tip (needed to create the acoustic interface) that must be cleaned and disinfected. The incorporation of a dedicated high-flow water irrigation channel (distinct from the standard air and water channels) in some models of endoscopes adds yet another channel that requires reprocessing (regardless of use) in addition to the external equipment that connect to this channel.

Current reprocessing guidelines are discussed in detail. These guidelines, although applicable to nearly all GI endoscopes, do not apply to sheathed endoscope systems. One endoscopic sheath system that is approved by the U.S. Food and Drug Administration (FDA) is commercially available.[4-8] In contrast to the popular misconception of an "endoscope condom," the sheath is actually a part of the endoscope insertion tube and contains several channels. Because this is a complete endoscope system, the sheaths are not compatible with other endoscopes. Although the sheath itself is disposable and does not need conventional cleaning and disinfection (i.e., a new sheath is used for each procedure), the control dials on the handpiece are not protected and do require reprocessing. These dials are removable and require conventional cleaning and disinfection or sterilization. There are two main disadvantages of the system: (1) The only currently marketed sheathed endoscope for use in the GI tract is a flexible sigmoidoscope; (2) the imaging technology of the instrument uses fiberoptic rather than video-chip technology.[9] Readers should refer to the manufacturer's instructions for reprocessing this type of endoscope.

Principles of Disinfection

Definitions

Cleaning is a term that is both simple to understand and difficult to define precisely in terms of a measurable endpoint. The official definition of cleaning used by the FDA is "the removal, usually with detergent and water, of adherent visible soil, blood, protein substances, and other debris from the surfaces, crevices, serrations, joints, and lumens of instruments, devices, and equipment by a manual or mechanical process that prepares the items for safe handling and/or further decontamination."[10] Although this definition seems straightforward, there is as yet no uniform consensus on how this process is operationally defined or what the endpoint of the process should be. How hot should the water be, and what concentration of detergent should be used? How many times should the cleaning brush be passed down the endoscope channels? What does "visibly clean" mean, and how can this be applied to the internal channels of an endoscope that cannot be examined? Many experimental methods can be used to determine the efficacy of cleaning by the detection of residual protein, carbohydrate, blood, or viral or bacterial RNA or DNA,[11–16] although these are impractical for routine clinical use.

Despite the difficulty in precisely defining the process or the subsequent endpoint, there is ample evidence that endoscope cleaning (as currently performed) is an essential part of the disinfection process. Mechanical cleaning alone reduces microbial counts by approximately 10^3–10^6 (three to six logs), or a 99.9% to 99.9999% reduction.[17–24] Cleaning is an integral part of any endoscope reprocessing regimen because failure to clean endoscopes or their accessories adequately can defeat disinfection or sterilization processes.[25]

Antiseptics are chemicals intended to reduce or destroy microorganisms on living tissue (e.g., skin), as opposed to *disinfectants*, which are used on inanimate objects (e.g., medical devices such as endoscopes). *Disinfection* is defined broadly as the destruction of pathogenic and other types of microorganisms. There are three levels of disinfection, as follows:

1. *High-level disinfection:* The destruction of all mycobacteria, nonlipid or small viruses, fungi, vegetative bacteria, and lipid or medium viruses and most, although not necessarily high numbers of, spores.
2. *Intermediate-level disinfection:* The destruction of all mycobacteria, vegetative bacteria, and fungal spores and some nonlipid viruses but not bacterial spores.
3. *Low-level disinfection:* The destruction of most bacteria (except mycobacteria), most viruses (except some nonlipid viruses), and some fungal spores (and not bacterial spores).[10]

For liquid chemical germicides (LCGs), high-level disinfection is operationally defined as the ability to kill 10^6 mycobacteria

---

Box 4.1 Descending Order of Resistance of Microorganisms to Liquid Chemical Germicides

Prions (transmissible spongiform encephalopathy agents)
  Creutzfeldt-Jakob (CJD)
  Variant Creutzfeldt-Jakob (vCJD)
Bacterial spores
  Bacillus subtilis
  Clostridium sporogenes
Mycobacteria
  Mycobacterium tuberculosis
Nonlipid or small viruses
  Poliovirus
  Coxsackievirus
  Rhinovirus
Fungi
  Trichophyton spp.
  Cryptococcus spp.
  Candida spp.
Vegetative bacteria
  Pseudomonas aeruginosa
  Salmonella choleraesuis
  Enterococci
Lipid or medium-sized viruses
  Herpes simplex virus (HSV)
  Cytomegalovirus (CMV)
  Coronavirus
  Hepatitis B virus (HBV)
  Hepatitis C virus (HCV)
  Human immunodeficiency virus (HIV)
  Ebola virus

Modified from Bond WW, Ott BJ, Franke KA, et al: Effective use of liquid chemical germicides on medical devices: instrument design problems. In Block SS, editor: Disinfection, sterilization, and preservation, ed 4, Philadelphia, 1991, Lea & Febiger, pp 1097–1106.

(a six-log reduction). The FDA defines a high-level disinfectant as a sterilant that is used for a shorter contact time.[26] This difference in the way the same chemical is used to achieve different levels of disinfection and sterilization is important for endoscopy because the contact times for sterilization with any given LCG are generally much longer (hours) than for high-level disinfection (minutes) and may be detrimental to the endoscope. The relative resistance of various microorganisms to LCGs is shown in **Box 4.1**.

Sterilization is the destruction or inactivation of all microorganisms, or the absence of all microbial life. As an endpoint, it is an absolute (sterile or not sterile). The process is operationally defined as a 12-log reduction of bacterial endospores.[27] Not all sterilization processes are alike, however. Steam and dry heat are the most extensively characterized processes; both are thermal methods that do not require the same physical contact as LCGs to achieve sterilization, and the processes are routinely monitored by the use of biologic indicators (e.g., spore test strips) to show that sterilization has been achieved. Although theoretically sterilization could be achieved with LCGs, the FDA and other authorities have stated that these processes do not convey the same sterility assurance as other sterilization methods.[26,28,29]

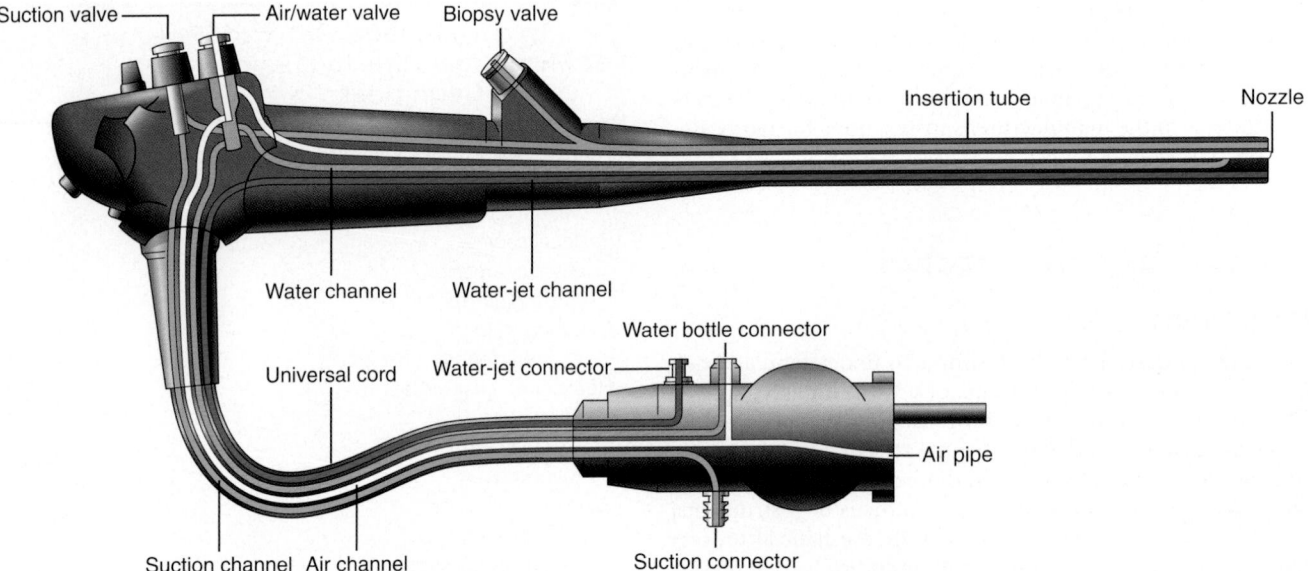

Fig. 4.1 Schematic of internal channels of an endoscope. *(Adapted from Olympus America. Copyright © Olympus America Inc., 2003.)*

The Spaulding classification system divides medical devices into categories based on the risk of infection involved with their use.[30,31] With some modifications, this classification scheme is widely accepted nationally and internationally and has been used by the FDA, the Centers for Disease Control and Prevention (CDC), epidemiologists, microbiologists, and professional medical organizations to determine the degree of disinfection or sterilization needed for various medical instruments. Three categories of medical devices and their associated level of disinfection are recognized, as follows:

1. *Critical:* Devices or instruments that are introduced into the human body and come into contact with normally sterile tissue or the vascular system. Because of the potential for infection if the device is contaminated with microorganisms, these devices require sterilization.
2. *Semicritical:* Devices that contact intact mucous membranes and do not ordinarily penetrate sterile tissue. They should receive at least high-level disinfection.
3. *Noncritical:* Devices that do not ordinarily touch the patient or touch only intact epithelium (e.g., stethoscopes or patient carts). These items may be cleaned by low-level disinfection.

Disinfection and Gastrointestinal Endoscopy

GI endoscopes are considered semicritical devices and should undergo at least high-level disinfection. This standard has been endorsed by the FDA[32]; the CDC[33]; and numerous professional medical organizations, including the American Society for Gastrointestinal Endoscopy (ASGE), the American College of Gastroenterology (ACG), the American Gastroenterology Association (AGA), the Society of Gastroenterology Nurses and Associates (SGNA), the Association of Perioperative Registered Nurses (AORN), the Association for Professionals in Infection Control and Epidemiology (APIC), and the American Society for Testing

and Materials (ASTM).[34–37] Because of design considerations, GI endoscopes can be a challenge to clean and disinfect. Endoscopes are heat-labile instruments and cannot be steam autoclaved. They possess several long, narrow internal channels with bends (**Fig. 4.1**) that require exposure to the LCG to achieve high-level disinfection. Generally, the air and water channels are too narrow to allow the passage of a cleaning brush (although the LCG is routinely circulated through this channel); however, one manufacturer has designed an endoscope with air and water channels that can be brushed.[38] Despite the complex internal design, high-level disinfection is not difficult to achieve with rigorous adherence to currently accepted guidelines. Most accessory instruments used during endoscopy either contact the bloodstream (e.g., biopsy forceps, snares, and sphincterotomes) or enter sterile tissue spaces (e.g., biliary tract) and are classified as critical devices. As such, these devices require sterilization.

Most accessories used during GI endoscopy are labeled by the FDA for single use (i.e., disposable) and are intended to be discarded at the end of the procedure. Because these items are sterilized by the manufacturer, reprocessing is not an issue. However, some accessories are designed to be resterilized and reused and are designated as such by FDA. In this case, cleaning and sterilization is performed by the user according to the manufacturer's instructions. The issue of sterilization of endoscopic accessories becomes considerably more complex when the reuse of single-use devices (SUDs) is considered. Although labeled for single use (disposable), many hospitals safely clean, resterilize, and reuse SUDs, resulting in decreased costs and reduced medical waste generation.[39–42] Despite the absence of evidence suggesting that this practice resulted in patient injury, the FDA issued a guidance document on August 14, 2000, that altered the agency's regulatory policy. The FDA considered the process of reprocessing (i.e., cleaning and sterilizing) a used SUD into a ready-for-patient-use device as "manufacturing," and as a result hospitals or third-party reprocessing companies that reprocessed SUDs were required to follow the same regulations as the original equipment manufacturers: premarket notification and approval requirements,

Table 4.1 Pathogens Reportedly Transmitted during Gastrointestinal Endoscopy

Organism	Probable Cases	Failure in Reprocessing Guideline
Pseudomonas aeruginosa	227	Failure to clean/disinfect between patients Inadequate cleaning Inadequate disinfectant Failure to disinfect all channels (particularly elevator channel) Failure to disinfect/sterilize water bottle Failure to dry with 70% alcohol Faulty/contaminated AER (*n* = 143)
Salmonella spp.	48	Inadequate cleaning Inadequate disinfectant Failure to sterilize forceps
Helicobacter pylori	10	Forceps not cleaned or sterilized between patients Inadequate cleaning Inadequate disinfectant
Klebsiella pneumoniae	5	Failure to dry with 70% alcohol Failure to disinfect elevator channel
Hepatitis C virus	4	Inadequate disinfectant Inadequate exposure to LCG Failure to disinfect all channels with LCG Failure to sterilize forceps
Serratia marcescens	2	Inadequate disinfectant Failure to dry with 70% alcohol Failure to disinfect elevator channel
Enterobacter spp.	2	Inadequate cleaning Inadequate disinfectant
Hepatitis B virus	1	Inadequate cleaning Inadequate disinfectant Failure to disinfect all channels with LCG
Trichosporon spp.	1	Failure to sterilize forceps

AER, automatic endoscope reprocessor; LCG, liquid chemical germicide.
From Nelson DB: Infectious disease complications of GI endoscopy. Part II. Exogenous infections. Gastrointest Endosc 57:695–711, 2003, with permission from the American Society for Gastrointestinal Endoscopy.

including 510(k) and premarket approval application (PMA); registration and listing; submission of adverse event reports; manufacturing and labeling requirements; tracking of devices; and correcting or removing from the market unsafe medical devices. Enforcement of these regulations was phased in over the subsequent 18 months (all aspects taking effect by February 14, 2002). The most onerous requirement was that a 510(k) or PMA was needed for each device that the institution intended to reprocess (both manufacturer and model-specific).[43] The regulatory burden imposed by these requirements essentially eliminated the practice of reprocessing of SUDs by most hospitals.

Risks of Inadequate Disinfection

Before discussing the specifics of current guidelines for endoscope cleaning and disinfection, it is helpful to understand how guidelines evolved over time in response to episodes of infection to minimize or eliminate vulnerabilities in the reprocessing procedure. Initially, endoscopes were simply washed with tap water and detergent, followed by exposure to alcohol.[44] In the 1970s, centers began using various "disinfectants" to reprocess endoscopes.[45–52] The germicides used were generally antiseptic agents. Many of the agents that were considered to be effective at that time (e.g., alcohols, phenolics, iodophors, quaternary ammonium compounds, and chlorhexidine) have

since been shown to be inadequate for high-level disinfection of GI endoscopes (**Table 4.1**).[53]

To standardize the cleaning and disinfection process, the ASGE, the AGA, and the ACG published joint guidelines on endoscope reprocessing in 1988. Key components of these guidelines were the emphasis on thorough manual cleaning of the instrument and all channels, high-level disinfection with an approved LCG (with a 10-minute exposure for glutaraldehyde specified at that time), a water rinse to remove residual sterilant, and a final drying step with forced air. The handles of nonimmersible endoscopes were to be cleaned with alcohol.[54] The British Society of Gastroenterology (BSG) published similar guidelines the same year, although notable differences included a recommended exposure time for glutaraldehyde of 4 minutes, the use of quaternary ammonium detergents as an acceptable second-line disinfectant, and only a brief mention of drying.[55] One of the authors of the BSG guidelines interpreted the guidelines as applying only to the insertion tube (which had direct patient contact) rather than to the entire endoscope (particularly the control handpiece, which was not high-level disinfected) and recommended that if the handpiece was "extensively contaminated," or if the next patient was known to be immunocompromised, only then was high-level disinfection of the entire instrument necessary. If the instrument was not submersible, cleaning with alcohol and chlorhexidine was "practical."[56]

More recent guidelines in the United States from multiple organizations have been uniformly consistent (all endorsing a 20-minute exposure to glutaraldehyde at room temperature).[34–36,57] The importance of close adherence to reprocessing guidelines becomes apparent in the subsequent section. The major difference with formal guidelines originating outside the United States has been the endorsement of a shorter glutaraldehyde exposure time of 10 minutes.[58–60] Actual facility practices in other countries can vary substantially, highlighting the difficulty in generalizing reports of infection to the experience in the United States.[61–65]

It is essential that a record be kept of the instrument used for each procedure so that in the event of a possible endoscope-related transmission the history of that instrument from the index case can be traced. This record is particularly important if a patient were subsequently found to have variant Creutzfeldt-Jakob disease (vCJD).

Specific Agents

The most commonly reported infectious agent transmitted during GI endoscopy is *Pseudomonas aeruginosa*, with 227 cases described in the medical literature (see Table 4.1).[25] *P. aeruginosa* is an opportunistic pathogen that is widely found in the environment, and the organism thrives in a moist environment.[66] Endoscopes and their ancillary equipment are a potential reservoir and may serve as a source of contamination. Early reports of *Pseudomonas* transmission during endoscopy (similar to reports of other organisms at that time) were generally related to inadequate cleaning or the use of inadequate disinfectants; however, later reports have centered around the following major areas: (1) flawed automatic endoscope reprocessor (AER) units (responsible for more than half of the reported cases), (2) failure to disinfect or sterilize the irrigation bottle of the endoscope regularly, (3) failure to recognize and disinfect the elevator channel of duodenoscopes, and (4) failure to dry the endoscope and all channels completely with a 70% alcohol solution followed by forced air.

There have been 48 cases of *Salmonella* species attributed to GI endoscopy.[25] In these reports, failure to clean the internal instrument channels mechanically was a uniform occurrence, and this was usually compounded by the use of an ineffective disinfectant. Because these cases were relatively early in the evolution of endoscope reprocessing (and preceded the guidelines standardizing these protocols), it is not surprising that there have been no reported cases of *Salmonella* transmission since 1987.

The 10 reported cases of endoscopic *Helicobacter pylori* transmission are almost as interesting as the initial confirmatory study by Marshall with self-inoculation. In one case, the author underwent endoscopy immediately after the instrument had been used in a patient known to harbor *H. pylori*. The endoscope was reprocessed by wiping the insertion tube with a paper towel soaked with benzethonium chloride and sucking the "disinfectant" through the instrument channels without cleaning. Perhaps predictably, the author developed acute *H. pylori* infection.[67] Another case was associated with endoscopic research dealing with *H. pylori* and was attributed to failure to clean and sterilize (or even disinfect) the endoscopic biopsy forceps between subjects (although reprocessing of the endoscope or other ancillary study equipment is not

mentioned).[68] The remaining cases were due to inadequate cleaning and the use of inadequate LCGs.

Much greater anxiety is associated with the possibility of transmission of viral infections. This anxiety is surprising because the viruses of greatest concern (i.e., hepatitis B virus [HBV], hepatitis C virus [HCV], and human immunodeficiency virus [HIV]) are among the easiest microorganisms to destroy with standard reprocessing. Before the advent of the reprocessing guidelines in 1988, there were three cases of HBV attributed to endoscopy. Two early reports suggested a temporal relationship between the use of an endoscope in an HBV-positive individual preceding the case and subsequent development of HBV infection, although in both cases no actual investigation was performed, and endoscope cleaning and disinfection were unacceptable by current standards.[69,70] In the third case, subtyping of HBV was used to confirm that transmission was likely. In this instance, the air and water channels were not exposed to glutaraldehyde.[71] Two more recent cases of HBV infection attributed to endoscopy are unlikely.[25,72,73]

There have been four cases of HCV transmission during GI endoscopy, all outside the United States. In three cases, a breach in currently accepted guidelines for endoscope reprocessing was reported.[74,75] In the fourth case, the transmission was believed to be due to contamination of multidose vials used for sedation (and associated with the *procedure* but not the endoscope itself).[76] This type of contamination was also the case in outbreaks of HCV at two endoscopy clinics in 2002 and 2007 in the United States. In the first case, the cause was initially attributed to deficient endoscope reprocessing practices by the lay press, but subsequent investigation by the New York State Department of Health determined that the cause was the improper reuse of needles and contamination of multidose vials.[77] A similar cause was found for the transmission of HCV in at least six patients at a Nevada endoscopy clinic.[78] These cases highlight the importance of general infection control practices, which are discussed later.

No cases of endoscopic transmission of HIV have been reported. Three studies have shown that glutaraldehyde disinfection of endoscopes contaminated with HIV completely eliminates the virus.[79–81]

There have been 317 putative episodes of transmission of infection reported in the medical literature. In the absence of defective equipment (notably the automated endoscope reprocessor), there has been a failure to follow currently accepted guidelines for cleaning and disinfection in each case.[25] These deficient practices can be summarized as follows:

1. Mechanical cleaning of the endoscope and channels before disinfection was inadequate or absent.
2. An inadequate or ineffective disinfectant was used.
3. An appropriate disinfectant was not used for an adequate exposure period.
4. Endoscopic accessory instruments were not sterilized.
5. The endoscope and all channels were not dried.

Liquid Chemical Germicides

The FDA defines a *high-level disinfectant* as a sterilant that is used under the same contact conditions except for a shorter contact time. LCGs were previously classified as sterilants by passing the Association of Official Analytical Chemists

Table 4.2 Disinfectants

FDA-Cleared Sterilants and High-Level Disinfectants for High-Level Disinfection of Endoscopes	Disinfectants Inadequate for High-Level Disinfection of Endoscopes (Examples)
2.4%–3.5% glutaraldehyde	Phenolic solutions
	Hexachlorophene
3.4% glutaraldehyde/26% isopropanol	Iodophor solutions
	Povidone-iodine
1.12% glutaraldehyde/1.93% phenol/phenate	quaternary ammonium solutions
	Benzalkonium chloride
	Benzethonium chloride
	Cetrimide
0.55% ortho-phthalaldehyde	Chlorhexidine
0.60% ortho-phthalaldehyde	
5.75% ortho-phthalaldehyde (diluted)	
0.2% peracetic acid	Chlorhexidine/cetrimide
2.0% hydrogen peroxide	Alkyldiaminoethylglycine hydrochloride
7.5% hydrogen peroxide	
8.3% hydrogen peroxide/7.0% peracetic acid	Ethyl or isopropyl alcohol*
7.35% hydrogen peroxide/0.23% peracetic acid	
1.0% hydrogen peroxide/0.08% peracetic acid	
Hypochlorite/hypochlorous acid 650–675 ppm (active free chlorine)	
Hypochlorite/hypochlorous acid 400–450 ppm (active free chlorine)	

*When used for high-level disinfection; appropriate for terminal drying.
FDA, U.S. Food and Drug Administration.
From Nelson DB: Infectious disease complications of GI endoscopy. Part II. Exogenous infections. Gastrointest Endosc 57:695–711, 2003, with permission from the American Society for Gastrointestinal Endoscopy.

(AOAC) Sporicidal Test.[82] Older LCGs (e.g., ≥2% glutaraldehyde) were approved by the FDA for sterilization and high-level disinfection (although the prolonged exposure time required made this impractical). However, more recently approved LCGs, such as 0.55% ortho-phthalaldehyde (Cidex OPA) and hypochlorite 400–450 ppm (Sterilox), that passed the AOAC Sporicidal Test have not been given an indication for device sterilization (i.e., high-level disinfection only). The FDA has approved many LCGs for use as high-level disinfectants or sterilants in the reprocessing of endoscopes and other reusable medical devices (**Table 4.2**). These include 2.4% to 3.5% glutaraldehyde, 3.4% glutaraldehyde/26% isopropanol, 1.12% glutaraldehyde/1.93% phenol/phenate, 0.55% to 0.60% ortho-phthaldehyde, 0.2% peracetic acid, 2.0% and 7.5% hydrogen peroxide, 8.3% hydrogen peroxide/7.0% peracetic acid, 7.35% hydrogen peroxide/0.23% peracetic acid, 1.0%

hydrogen peroxide/0.08% peracetic acid, and hypochlorite/hypochlorous acid 400 ppm or greater active free chlorine.[82]

Many LCGs are labeled for multiple reprocessing cycles for a specific time period. However, as these sterilants are reused, dilution occurs, which can reduce their effectiveness. Product-specific test strips should be used regularly to monitor these solutions to insure that they are above their minimum effective concentration (MEC). Solutions should be discarded whenever they fall below the MEC or when the use-life expires, whichever comes first. Users should consult with manufacturers of endoscopes and AERs (if used) for compatibility before selecting an LCG. Two agents (0.2% peracetic acid, 5.75% ortho-phthalaldehyde) are used for a single disinfection cycle and are not reusable (i.e., single use—each cycle requires new LCG); the hypochlorite/hypochlorous acid solution is generated from electrolysis of a saline solution for each cycle.[83–85]

Automatic Endoscope Reprocessors

Historically, cleaning and high-level disinfection of endoscopes has been performed manually. The high-level disinfection step involved placing mechanically cleaned endoscopes into a basin or container of LCG (usually glutaraldehyde) that was also circulated through the internal channels of the instrument. Exposure of endoscopy personnel to some LCGs has been reported to cause respiratory, nasal, and skin problems, however.[86,87] AERs were designed to ensure that reprocessing is performed consistently and to replace some manual disinfection steps. In addition, AERs may minimize the exposure of endoscopy personnel to the LCG.[88] It is crucial, however, that users understand that endoscopes must be mechanically cleaned before reprocessing in an AER. Although several devices are labeled by the FDA as "washer-disinfectors," and one device has been approved to bypass the mechanical cleaning step, this has not been endorsed or sanctioned by any of the gastrointestinal societies that represent the end-users (mechanical cleaning is still recommended before the use of all AERs). It is also important to verify that the endoscope and the AER are compatible and use appropriate connectors.[89]

Cleaning and Disinfecting Endoscopes

A guideline for reprocessing GI endoscopes that has been endorsed by numerous gastroenterology, infection control, surgical, nursing, and hospital organizations contains detailed recommendations for this process.[90] A similar guideline (although broader in scope) by the Healthcare Infection Control Practices Advisory Committee (HICPAC) of the CDC has been finalized.[91] The pertinent steps to achieve high-level disinfection of endoscopes from these guidelines are summarized as follows:

1. Perform pressure/leak testing after each use according to the manufacturer's guidelines.
2. Disconnect and disassemble endoscope components (e.g., air/water and suction valves) as far as possible and completely immerse the endoscope and components in the enzymatic detergent.

3. Immediately after use, meticulously clean the entire endoscope, including valves, channels, connectors, and all detachable parts, with an enzymatic detergent compatible with the endoscope according to the manufacturer's instructions. Flush and brush all accessible channels to remove all organic (e.g., blood, tissue) and other residues. Repeatedly actuate the valves during cleaning to facilitate access to all surfaces. Clean the external surfaces and components of the endoscope using a soft cloth, sponge, or brushes.

4. Use brushes appropriate for the size of the endoscope channel, parts, connectors, and orifices (e.g., bristles should contact all surfaces) for cleaning. Cleaning items should be disposable or thoroughly cleaned and disinfected or sterilized between uses.

5. Discard enzymatic detergents after each use because these products are not microbicidal and do not retard microbial growth.

6. Use a high-level disinfectant or sterilant approved by the FDA for high-level disinfection (http://www.fda.gov/cdrh/ode/germlab.html).

7. Exposure time and temperature for disinfecting semicritical patient care equipment vary among the FDA-approved high-level disinfectants. Follow the FDA-approved label claim for high-level disinfection, unless several well-designed experimental scientific studies, endorsed by professional societies, show an alternative exposure time is effective for disinfecting semicritical items. The FDA label claim for high-level disinfection with greater than 2% glutaraldehyde at 25° C ranges from 20 to 90 minutes depending on the product. However, multiple scientific studies and professional organizations support the efficacy of greater than 2% glutaraldehyde for 20 minutes at 20° C.

8. Select a disinfectant or sterilant that is compatible with the endoscope. The use of specific high-level disinfectants or sterilants on an endoscope should be avoided if the endoscope manufacturer warns against use because of functional damage (with or without cosmetic damage).

9. Completely immerse the endoscope and endoscope components in the high-level disinfectant or sterilant and ensure all channels are perfused. Nonimmersible GI endoscopes should be phased out.

10. If an AER is used, ensure that the endoscope and endoscope components can be effectively reprocessed in the AER (e.g., the elevator wire channel of duodenoscopes is not effectively disinfected by most AERs, and this step must be performed manually). Users should obtain and review model-specific reprocessing protocols from both the endoscope and the AER manufacturers and check for compatibility.

11. If an AER is used, place the endoscope and endoscope components in the reprocessor and attach all channel connectors according to the instructions of the AER and endoscope manufacturers to ensure exposure of all internal surfaces to the high-level disinfectant or chemical sterilant.

12. If an AER cycle is interrupted, high-level disinfection or sterilization cannot be ensured and should be repeated.

13. After high-level disinfection, rinse the endoscope and flush the channels with sterile, filtered, or tap water to remove the disinfectant or sterilant. Discard the rinse water after each use or cycle. Flush the channels with 70% to 90% ethyl or isopropyl alcohol and dry using forced air. The final drying steps greatly reduce the possibility of recontamination of the endoscope by waterborne microorganisms.

14. When storing the endoscope, hang it in a vertical position to facilitate drying (with caps, valves, and other detachable components removed as per manufacturer instructions).

15. Endoscopes should be stored in a manner that protects the endoscope from contamination.

16. Perform high-level disinfection or sterilization of the water bottle (used for cleaning the lens and irrigation during the procedure) and its connecting tube at least daily. Sterile water should be used to fill the water bottle.

17. Perform routine testing of the liquid sterilant or high-level disinfectant to ensure MEC of the active ingredient. Check the solution at the beginning of each day of use (or more frequently), and document the results. If the chemical indicator shows that the concentration is less than the MEC, the solution should be discarded.

18. Discard the liquid sterilant or high-level disinfectant at the end of its reuse life (which may be single use) regardless of the MEC. If additional liquid sterilant or high-level disinfectant is added to an AER (or basin, if manually disinfected), the reuse life should be determined by the first use or activation of the original solution (i.e., the practice of "topping off" of a liquid sterilant or high-level disinfectant pool does not extend the reuse life).

Although some authorities have advocated that cleaned and disinfected endoscopes that have been stored should undergo an additional cleaning and disinfection process before the beginning of an endoscopy schedule (i.e., first-case reprocessing), there are no data to support this as a routine practice. When GI endoscope cleaning and disinfection guidelines are strictly followed and endoscopes are stored appropriately, this additional procedure is unnecessary. Generally, however, if there is doubt about a cleaning and disinfection cycle, or the instrument is found to be wet after storage (or otherwise stored improperly), the endoscope should be reprocessed.

Disinfection Procedure Compliance

Adherence to established guidelines for the cleaning and disinfection of endoscopes is imperative. When these guidelines are followed, the risk of transmission of infection is virtually eliminated; however, this is not a reason for complacency because compliance with existing reprocessing guidelines is not uniform. In 1991, Gorse and Messner[92] surveyed 2030 SGNA members and found that compliance with existing guidelines was 67% in some areas. A collaborative study by the FDA and three state health departments published in 1992 investigated endoscope reprocessing at 26 health care facilities and found that 24% of patient-ready endoscopes were contaminated, and these were attributed to fundamental errors in the disinfection process.[93,94]

Although office endoscopy has been shown to be as safe as endoscopy practiced in more regulated settings (e.g., hospitals),[95] the absence of formal infection control programs and personnel may leave the office setting more vulnerable to compliance issues with regard to endoscope reprocessing. In one study of 19 family practice and internal medicine offices performing flexible sigmoidoscopy, all were found to deviate from accepted reprocessing guidelines in at least one area.[96] Although two more recent studies suggest that compliance with reprocessing guidelines has improved,[97,98] there is room for further improvement. The challenge facing practitioners in the field of GI endoscopy is to ensure that compliance with these guidelines is universal, regardless of the practitioner or setting.

Reprocessing Personnel

Only trained personnel who understand the importance of strict adherence to established protocols should perform endoscope reprocessing (as a corollary, untrained personnel should not reprocess endoscopes). This training should include device-specific reprocessing instructions (for both the endoscope and the reprocessing equipment) and education regarding the biologic and chemical hazards associated with the cleaning and disinfection of endoscopes with LCGs. These individuals should meet annual competency standards for endoscope reprocessing. In addition, all health care personnel in the endoscopy suite should be trained in and adhere to standard infection control recommendations (e.g., standard precautions), including recommendations to protect both patients and health care workers.[33] Personal protective equipment, such as gloves, gowns, eyewear, and respiratory protection devices, should be readily available. This equipment should be used, as appropriate, to protect reprocessing personnel from exposure to chemicals, blood, or other potentially infectious material.[99–102]

Novel Infectious Agents

Although Creutzfeldt-Jakob disease (CJD) and vCJD are rare, the impact of these diseases on endoscope reprocessing is addressed. CJD and vCJD are degenerative neurologic disorders transmitted by proteinaceous infectious agents called prions (although this is a simplification). Prions are unusually resistant to disinfection by conventional chemical high-level disinfectants or sterilants.[103,104] The incidence of CJD in the United States is extremely low, with approximately 250 cases per year, or 0.97 cases per 1 million persons per year.[105] Tissues and secretions that come into contact with the endoscope during procedures, such as saliva, gingival tissue, intestinal tissue, feces, and blood, are considered noninfectious by the World Health Organization.[103] A draft statement on CJD and medical device reprocessing from the CDC concluded that current guidelines for cleaning and disinfection of these instruments need not be changed.[35] Other infection control experts have concurred, citing the lack of exposure to high-risk tissue and the importance of mechanical cleaning in removing microbial contamination.[31,104]

The clinical relevance of the more recent finding of abnormal prion proteins in the olfactory (but not respiratory) epithelium of affected patients with regard to infection control or endoscope reprocessing is unclear.[106] To date, there have

been no reported cases in the world literature of transmission of CJD (or any other transmissible spongiform encephalopathy) by endoscopy. vCJD is a more recently recognized and even more rare syndrome that is believed to be due to consumption of beef products containing the bovine spongiform encephalopathy (BSE) agent, possibly requiring a susceptible genotype by the individual.[107] The only case of the disease reported in the United States was found in a 22-year-old patient that had moved from the United Kingdom. Despite active surveillance since 1990, BSE has not been detected in the United States.[108] In contrast to CJD, the prions associated with vCJD can be detected in the lymphoid tissue of affected individuals (e.g., tonsil, appendix, and possibly ileum and rectum).[107,109–112] The prions in these tissues are present in lower concentrations and are approximately 50% less infective than central nervous system tissue when homogenated and injected intracerebrally in mice.[113] The infectivity of intact tissue that might be encountered at endoscopy and the risk of subsequent transmission to another individual via gut inoculation are unknown but would undoubtedly be lower.

Given the virtual absence of vCJD in the United States, rigorous adherence to current guidelines for the cleaning and disinfection of endoscopes would seem to be adequate. There is no evidence that changes to current endoscopic practices or endoscope reprocessing guidelines are warranted, but these should be responsive to new information as it evolves. The European Society for Gastrointestinal Endoscopy (ESGE) stated that because it is impossible to ensure that an instrument used in a patient with vCJD can be cleaned, that instrument should either be destroyed or quarantined for use in other vCJD patients only. The safest option is not to perform endoscopy on these patients or, if absolutely necessary, to use an old instrument and subsequently destroy it. A larger potential problem in Europe is the situation in which a patient who has undergone endoscopy is subsequently found to have vCJD. The instrument should be quarantined (or, ideally, destroyed). How to deal with the group of patients who had subsequently undergone endoscopy with that instrument is a complicated issue that would require input from the hospital administration and government infectious diseases authorities.

General Infection Control Practices

The importance of general infection control practices has been highlighted by the transmission of HCV to at least six individuals at a Nevada endoscopy clinic. The subsequent epidemiologic investigation revealed that the outbreak was due to unsafe injection practices, specifically the reuse of syringes and the use of single-use medical vials on multiple patients.[78] A review of nonhospital health care–associated HBV and HCV transmission outbreaks in the United States over the last decade showed that in each case, failure to follow fundamental principles of infection control and aseptic technique was the cause.[114] Although this problem is not unique to endoscopy, it is imperative that health care workers in endoscopy units understand and adhere to recommended infection control practices.

References

The complete reference list is available online at www.expertconsult.com.

Chapter 5

Tissue Sampling, Specimen Handling, and Chromoendoscopy

Wilfred M. Weinstein

Biopsy

Pinch Biopsy Forceps

Forceps Sizes

The most common pinch biopsy forceps used worldwide is one that fits through a 2.8-mm biopsy channel. Infants and very young children often have biopsy specimens taken with a smaller forceps that fits through a 2.2-mm biopsy channel. Pediatric gastroenterologists generally use narrow-bore instruments for routine diagnostic biopsy if the child weighs less than 10 kg.

The aim with pinch biopsy forceps is to obtain a biopsy specimen that contains the full thickness of the mucosa in disorders not associated with a large increase in mucosal thickness, such as hypertrophic gastropathies. The 2.8-mm channel biopsy forceps can generally obtain a full-thickness mucosal specimen except for the greater curve of the gastric body, where the folds are normally thickest.

Larger Capacity Forceps

The large-cup ("jumbo" or "max capacity") forceps requires a large channel, a so-called therapeutic endoscope (biopsy channel 3.6 to 3.7 mm). Some newer designs are intended to provide larger biopsy specimens with the conventional 2.8-mm channels and intermediate-sized channels such as pediatric colonoscopes.[1] Larger capacity biopsy forceps are highly desirable to optimize the diagnostic yield. Part of the reason that only a few endoscopists have used the large-cup forceps is the reluctance to use larger capacity forceps that require the larger channel. There is also a puzzling antipathy toward the use of a larger forceps that obtains superior sized specimens. Studies have been done to show that a larger forceps is unnecessary, as if the larger forceps represented a serious threat or a "ploy."[2]

Larger capacity forceps biopsies yield two to three times the surface area but are not generally much deeper (**Fig. 5.1**). The main objective with biopsy is *not* to obtain more representative sampling of a *whole organ* but to enable the histotechnologist to see the biopsy specimens to orient them (see **Fig. 5.1**).

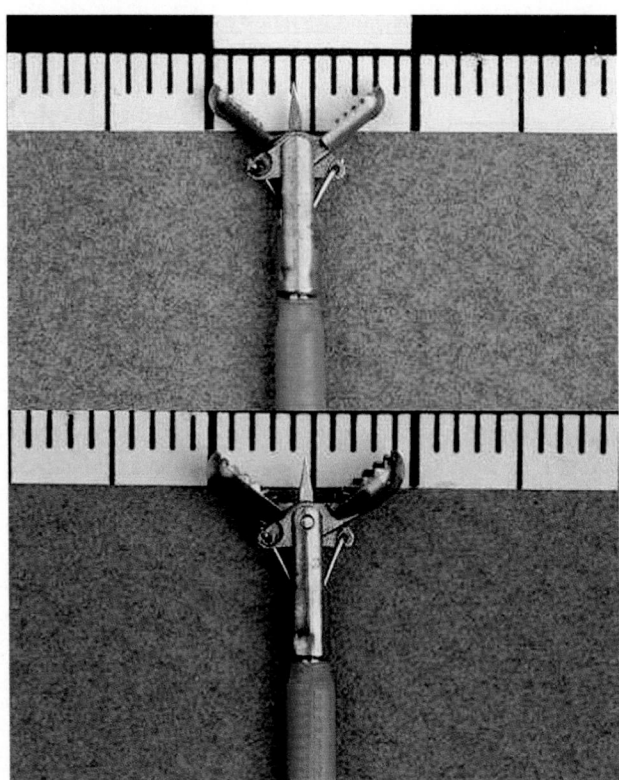

Fig. 5.1 The advantage of a larger capacity forceps is *not* to sample more terrain (e.g., in surveillance in Barrett's esophagus and ulcerative colitis) but to provide larger sized biopsy specimens so that the histotechnologist can orient the specimens for embedding, on edge. That is more difficult with small specimens. With tiny biopsy specimens, it is impossible.

Histotechnologists cannot orient small to tiny specimens. The resultant sections with larger capacity forceps are infinitely superior. Proper orientation during paraffin embedding is impossible with often delivered "fleabite"-sized specimens as part of a group of biopsies in a tissue block.

Orientation for embedding in paraffin is the key to maximizing the diagnostic yield from mucosal biopsies. Orientation with crypts and villi are lined up and not cross cut like a stack of doughnuts. This orientation permits assessment of the amount of lamina propria inflammation, focal lesions such as granulomas, and intraepithelial lymphocytes (especially small bowel). In the colon, oriented sections permit assessment of crypt branching (architectural distortion) for differential diagnosis regarding chronicity and assessment of lesser grades of dysplasia by being able to use crypt architectural disorganization as opposed to only cytologic change in cross-cut sections. Oriented sections are required to maximize the yield for focal lesions.

Biopsy specimens taken with larger capacity forceps usually contain very little submucosa or none at all. It is sometimes difficult to obtain specimens with sufficient submucosa when the objective is to diagnose amyloid or rule out or hunt for vasculitis in submucosal blood vessels.

Multiple Biopsy Specimen Forceps

Multibite forceps are designed to obtain multiple specimens with a single pass. They may be judged as *adequate* by some pathologists, but for what purposes? Biopsy specimens are generally tiny and pale compared with the quality of specimens of other forceps biopsies. The aggregate tissue is considered one advantage, but that does not guarantee any higher yield when the aggregate nets multiple tiny cross-cut sections.

Hot Biopsy Forceps

Hot biopsy forceps are insulated pinch biopsy forceps through which coagulation current is passed. They have been used for removal of diminutive colonic polyps, especially tiny ones in the rectum. They are not commonly used.

Cold Snare Biopsy

Cold snare biopsy is advocated instead of hot biopsy to remove diminutive polyps from the colon and submit them all to the pathology laboratory.[3] A larger capacity biopsy forceps is just as effective for small polyps. In the absence of a cold snare, cold forceps is still preferable to hot biopsy.[3] Fundic gland polyps have a characteristic appearance and location, and cold snare or any kind of snare is not generally required. However, in the case of larger fundic gland polyps, especially in the setting of familial polyposis, removing some may be done to rule out dysplastic change in them. The polyps almost always come off easily without bleeding. If the endoscopist is uncertain that a polyp is fundic gland type, a cautery forceps should be used. The endoscopist should always be prepared to apply a hemostasis technique if bleeding is excessive after a cold snare biopsy. Cold snare biopsy of gastric polyps less than 7 mm to distinguish hyperplastic from adenomatous polyps is useful in the appropriate clinical circumstances.

Suction Biopsy

Suction biopsies are rarely performed.

Grasp Biopsy

Grasp biopsies are performed through a rigid sigmoidoscope using an alligator cutting forceps. These biopsies are rarely performed in clinical gastroenterology practice, but they may be useful for indurated distal rectal tumors that are difficult to grasp with endoscopic biopsy forceps.

Laparoscopic Biopsy

Laparoscopic full-thickness gut biopsies are useful when diagnosis and type classification of intestinal pseudoobstruction is required.[4,5]

Improving the Quality of Forceps Pinch Biopsy Specimens
How Close to the Biopsy Site the Endoscope Should Be Positioned

After biopsy targeting of focal lesions in disorders such as mucosa-associated lymphoid tissue, Barrett's esophagus, and ulcerative colitis, random biopsy specimens can be taken using landmarks or measurements. In these biopsy "mapping" circumstances, it is unnecessary to be close to biopsy sites or to clean each putative biopsy site of mucus or blood that has seeped over from adjacent biopsy sites. The biopsy specimens can in a sense be taken blindly based on measurements or position, after the area has been cleared by biopsy of focal lesions.

Pressure against the Wall

Less tension on the wall helps obtain better-quality biopsy specimens. After the opened forceps is pressed against the wall, it is almost a reflex action to give it a second push into the wall. This unnecessary stretch may result in a shallower or traumatized biopsy specimen. The endoscopist should try to take specimens of folds or valvulae or partially deflate the lumen beforehand or after applying the forceps to the mucosa. Deflation can be achieved very quickly with a few bursts of staccato suction before clamping down on the tissue.

Snapping the Forceps Back Quickly after It Is Closed on the Tissue

There is often an inclination (or urge) to pull back to tent the mucosa surrounding forceps with the trapped biopsy specimen. This urge should be resisted, and the forceps should be snapped back quickly. A delay in snapping the forceps closed and pulling out the forceps quickly may provoke more crush artifact of the tissue.

Double Bites

The term *double bites* refers to taking two specimens with a single pass of the biopsy forceps. With conventional-sized forceps, this double-bite technique often yields a tiny second biopsy specimen, or a "macrocytology" (**Fig. 5.2**). However, the double-bite technique may be used successfully in the colon in ulcerative colitis biopsy surveillance and in the small bowel using a larger capacity forceps. In the esophagus, the double-bite technique is difficult because of the need for angulation and risk of loss of the first biopsy specimen obtained. In the stomach, the size of the specimens is often so generous with the first pass that there is scant room for a second biopsy.

To perform this technique, after the first biopsy specimen is obtained, the closed forceps is placed with slight pressure on the wall where the next specimen is to be taken and is opened against a bit of wall pressure. This pressure helps prevent the first specimen from falling out into the lumen. After opening the forceps poised to biopsy, a few staccato bursts of suction are applied, and then the forceps is closed quickly to obtain the second specimen. One does not always obtain two biopsy specimens. I usually obtain two specimens about once in three to five times.

Turn-in Technique

In areas where one has to perform a biopsy at an oblique angle, as in the esophagus or for gritty lesions, it helps enormously to use the turn-in technique. The opened forceps is first drawn back flush with the endoscope tip. The tip of the endoscope is then deflected 90 degrees against the wall, allowing the forceps to be advanced en face by moving the endoscope in, rather than extending the forceps. It is advanced until resistance is met, then suction is applied briefly, and the forceps is closed. It is not necessary to see what is being biopsied if any targeted areas were cleared with biopsies as in Barrett's esophagus surveillance. In the case of a focal lesion, the endoscope is positioned right over the lesion and turned into it using the large up-down hand control knob on the endoscope. For endoscopists who want experience with the turn-in technique, the best way to obtain it is to try it in more spacious areas, such as the stomach, in the course of performing gastric biopsies.

6 O'clock Position and Biopsies of Gastroesophageal Junction (Cardia) Lesions

When areas are difficult to get at, rotation of the endoscope to the 6 o'clock position makes it infinitely easier to obtain biopsy specimens and to target more accurately (**Fig. 5.3**). This position is especially invaluable in biopsy surveillance of Barrett's esophagus where the 12 o'clock position tends to be ignored for visualization and biopsy targeting. The endoscope is rotated so that what was at 12 o'clock is now at 6 o'clock.

For lesions at the gastroesophageal (GE) junction, it is often invaluable to visualize the area on turnaround in the stomach and target biopsy or endoscopic resection from this

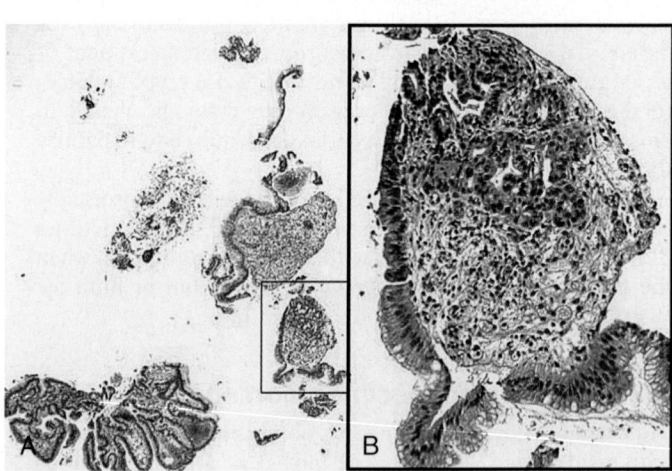

Fig. 5.2 Double-bite inadequate-sized biopsy specimens in Barrett's esophagus. **A,** Specimen at the lower left is the only one that can be oriented, and it is superficial. The others are scrapings. **B,** One of the fragments *(inset in **A** enlarged)* shows high-grade dysplasia.

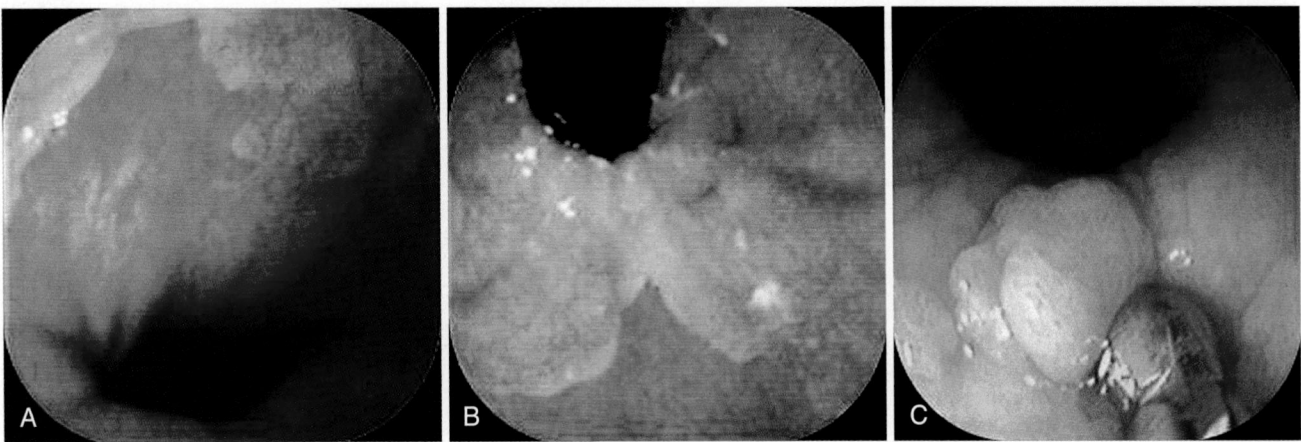

Fig. 5.3 Value of viewing cardia lesions on retroflexion from the gastric side and positioning at 6 o'clock. **A,** End-on view of eccentric Z line. **B,** Retroflexion view in the stomach. Eccentric part is positioned at 6 o'clock. Biopsy, if indicated, is easier from this aspect. **C,** Small gastroesophageal junction mass as viewed from the stomach on retroflexion and rotated to the 6 o'clock position for biopsy.

perspective (see **Fig. 5.3C**). This maneuver works only if the patient has a hiatal hernia. After the turnaround is done in the stomach, air insufflation is set on high. The endoscope is advanced by slowly withdrawing until the endoscope tip advances right to the GE junction. In this way, there is *end-on* visualization of a lesion. Additionally, the endoscope can often be torqued slightly to place the lesion in or near the favored 6 o'clock position (see **Fig. 5.3**). If torque is required for biopsy positioning, the endoscopy assistant maintains it while the biopsy forceps is targeted to the lesion. In the turnaround position from the stomach, some lesions cannot be accessed despite torquing or twisting.

Reducing the Number of Uninterpretable Biopsy Specimens

Independent of which forceps or technique is used, one key way to reduce the uninterpretability rate of biopsy is to have the endoscopy assistant indicate when a biopsy specimen is nearly invisible or when there is only blood or mucus. Such specimens should be discarded. In the process of taking biopsy specimens in our unit, the endoscopy assistant calls out whether a specimen is adequate or otherwise. Apart from size, superficial shallow specimens can be identified by the endoscopy assistant as translucent. Even the most experienced "biopsy veterans" have to go back every five or six biopsies. Unless endoscopists look at the biopsy specimens with the pathologist, they never know how many specimens of a group are interpretable. Histologic diagnoses are sometimes made by piecing together several uninterpretable fragments in the "mind's eye."

Minimizing Biopsy Surveillance Antipathy and Biopsy Exhaustion or Boredom

It is likely nearly impossible to reach a state of "joy of biopsy" even when the reason for the endoscopy is *tissue-is-the-issue.* Examples include surveillance for dysplasia and cancer in ulcerative colitis and Barrett's esophagus. Part of the antipathy to surveillance biopsies is that the "drudgery effect" is eagerly

passed on to fellows from one generation to the next by the endoscopy attending physicians.

When multiple biopsies are required, it helps enormously to have a second assistant in the room to operate the forceps and handle the tissue while the other assistant monitors the patient. For upper endoscopic procedures such as Barrett's esophagus surveillance, a well-sedated patient who does not keep bolting upright helps. The use of an anticholinergic before the procedure may reduce saliva and gastrointestinal secretions, and is routine in some practices.

Tissue Handling
Transferring Biopsy Specimens from Forceps to Fixative

The best way to remove biopsy specimens from the forceps is to use a blunt probe to push the specimen out from the base of the opened forceps cups. If one pushes the specimen out by pressing it from the top of the opened forceps or picking at it, the specimen becomes squashed.

Shaking biopsy specimens off the forceps into a fixative bottle may traumatize the tissue and cause denudation of the epithelium, especially from the gastric body. Endoscopists who use the shake technique should alert the pathologist to look for detached epithelium in biopsy specimens from different parts of the gastrointestinal (GI) tract and give feedback. Most pathologists are so used to seeing detached epithelium that they assume it is a default feature (norm) from the trauma of the scope or the forceps.

When exudative lesions are biopsied for diagnosis, shaking specimens into the fixative may peel off the exudate that contains the evidence for the presence of organisms, especially *Candida* and herpes simplex. These organisms reside in the surface exudate or epithelial slough. Cytomegalovirus does not, and it requires biopsy for diagnosis.

Orientation of biopsy specimens on support materials in the endoscopy unit is not required in clinical practice and in inexperienced hands may lead to more tissue trauma. The key to having well-oriented, high-quality biopsy specimens for histologic examination rests with the pathology histotechnologist's ability and motivation to embed the tissue "on its edge" in paraffin and obtain sections through the central core of the specimens.[6] That depends on providing the histotechnologist with specimens of adequate size.

Number of Biopsy Specimens in a Fixative Bottle

Most histotechnologists cannot line up more than four biopsy specimens in a tissue block during embedding and section them so that all are represented in optimal orientation for interpretation (**Fig. 5.4**). Endoscopists claim that they put 10 or more specimens in a single bottle to reduce the costs. They do not usually get feedback, however, and if they did, they would learn that only half or less of those 10 specimens may be fully interpretable (see **Fig. 5.4**). In one regional community pathology laboratory, the pathologists separate the biopsy specimens themselves for embedding at four or five per cassette.

Polyps: Identifying the Stalk Region

When snare polypectomy is used for the removal of pedunculated or sessile polyps, the key part of the specimen for cancer diagnosis is in the stalk region or the base in the case of sessile polyps (**Fig. 5.5**). Stalks retract right after removal of the polyp and often shrink further and disappear after fixation. The best way to identify the stalk is to impale it with a short (1-inch) 25-gauge needle, right to the hub with the needle point emerging at the most convex part of the tip of the polyp (see **Fig. 5.5**). An alternative is to ink the polyp stalk after removal. After fixation for a few hours, the polyp is bisected with a scalpel or razor blade in the pathology laboratory. The two bisected halves are embedded facedown, and this way the first sections to come off are those that show the stalk region in its best orientation.[6] Larger specimens should go right to the pathology laboratory to be assessed as gross specimens.

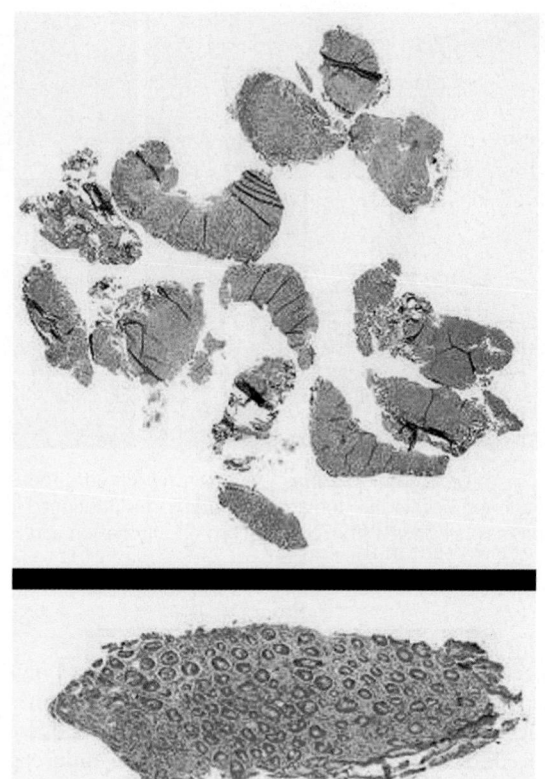

Fig. 5.4 Too many biopsy specimens placed into one fixative bottle and in one tissue block. Fragments of variable sizes cannot be positioned en bloc, and each biopsy specimen is not oriented. Dark lines represent tissue wrinkling in sectioning. The hallmark of grossly misoriented biopsy specimens is shown at the *bottom* as cross-sectioned circles ("doughnut effect") with no clue as to the real architecture.

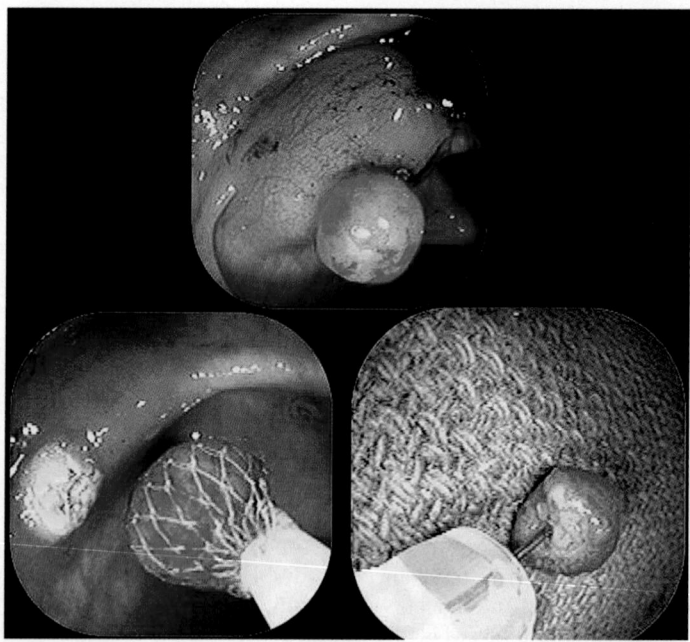

Fig. 5.5 Polypectomy, first preinked. The base of the polyp has a needle inserted through to the tip of the polyp. In the laboratory, the polyp is bisected along the needle path, and the central halves of the polyp are embedded facedown so that the base or stalk zone is represented in the first sections to be collected.

Small Polyps

Small polyps may be retrieved into a suction trap; this does not seem to damage the tissue. One key to using a suction trap without getting the polyp stuck in the suction channel is to have the polyp in a pool of liquid before suctioning. If there is no liquid, saline can be instilled first.

Shave Biopsy

Shave biopsy of larger polyps is to be shunned. The diagnosis of cancer or its exclusion requires that the muscularis mucosae and upper submucosa be visualized. If multiple fragments are submitted with no orientation, the pathologist often cannot provide reassurance that invasion is not present. If there is no choice but to submit two or three pieces of the lesion, each should be marked with ink to show the cut side. This marking permits the pathologist to know where the submucosa is located if present in the specimen. The removal of large specimens requires the same principles that surgeons use in resections.

Endoscopic Mucosal Resection and Endoscopic Resection

Endoscopists and the pathologists who handle specimens from endoscopic resection need to recognize that the specimens should be handled as are any resections for cancer or possible cancer. They are not merely larger biopsy specimens.

It is preferable not to remove the lesions in pieces for the reasons discussed previously. The lesions should be oriented in such a way that there is no doubt about how to handle them. Handling these specimens requires a protocol worked out in advance with the pathologists. The best scheme is to deliver the unfixed specimen to the pathology laboratory so that the pathologist examines it grossly and pins it out before placement in fixative. After fixation, the specimen should be cut into strips and each embedded so that the whole specimen is represented in histologic slides.[7] In this way, the patient and the endoscopist can be reassured that the focal or early lesion was analyzed optimally with respect to maximal invasion.

Brush Cytology

Brush Cytology in the Diagnosis of Infections

Of the three major potential infections of the esophagus, cytomegalovirus, *Candida albicans,* and herpesvirus, the latter two are characterized by having the organisms in surface exudate and surface epithelial slough. Cytomegalovirus is embedded more deeply and is not commonly detected in smears of exudate. Smears of exudates for cytologic examination for herpesvirus may provide a rapid diagnosis. Exudate from the brush is smeared onto slides and placed in Papanicolaou fixative. The brushings may also be used for viral culture for herpesvirus, if desired. For this viral culture, a second brushing is swirled around in a culture medium, or the brush tip is cut off with wire cutters and left in the bottom of the culture

medium container. For *Candida,* in our unit, we cut off the brush tip into a tube with several milliliters of the transport liquid and send for examination for hyphae and pseudohyphae.

One person in the unit should periodically check with the microbiologists to see whether they want to change any transport conditions. With most esophageal infections, it is unnecessary to obtain culture verification. Aspirates of duodenal fluid have been used in the past for the diagnosis of *Giardia lamblia,* but biopsy specimens are at least as sensitive to make the diagnosis.

Brush Cytology for Cancer or Dysplasia Diagnosis

Brush cytology is sometimes the only immediate diagnostic modality available in potentially malignant strictures with marked luminal compromise. One should exercise caution in passing the cytology brush into the lumen of a strictured area to do brushings. Cytologic examinations outside of the setting of endoscopic ultrasound are no longer performed except in the diagnosis of infections (discussed previously). The diagnosis of anal dysplasia, especially in high-risk patients such as patients with human immunodeficiency virus, can be difficult, and anal cytology may be shown to play a diagnostic role in future studies. At the present time, its utility is unknown.

Endoscopist-Pathologist and Pathologist-Endoscopist Communication to Optimize the Diagnostic Yield for Patient Care

A more detailed discussion of the pathologist-endoscopist interaction is available.[8] Dialogue and communication with pathologists and vice versa are a weak and dysfunctional link, virtually unchanged since the advent of flexible endoscopes.[8] The potential consequences of this *dysfunctional relationship* are described subsequently.

False-Positive Diagnoses

False-positive diagnoses may have grave worry consequences for the patients. Three examples follow.

Crohn's Disease

The main question may be to rule out Crohn's disease. That question may virtually seal the diagnosis because almost every mucosal abnormality may be compatible with Crohn's disease. The operative question is *rule out focal inflammation or granulomas or both.* It is the endoscopist's responsibility to integrate the answer to this question with the remainder of the workup. A rush to diagnosis may be premature or erroneous.

Barrett's Esophagus

The endoscopist asks the pathologist if there is Barrett's esophagus in an eccentric Z line. An eccentric Z line *precludes* the diagnosis of Barrett's esophagus. The first criterion for the diagnosis of Barrett's esophagus is endoscopic. There is Barrett's-type mucosa visible in the esophagus above the lower esophageal sphincter (LES). The second criterion is that a biopsy performed above the LES in the esophagus shows intestinal-type goblet cells. An eccentric Z line is not Barrett's esophagus. Up to 30% of patients with gastroesophageal reflux disease (GERD) and no Barrett's esophagus have intestinal metaplasia at the Z line.[9] It is not considered an indication for surveillance. The pathologist may be more circumspect in this example, and instead of calling an eccentric Z line Barrett's esophagus, the pathologist may call it intestinal metaplasia. The endoscopist may recognize the pathologist's circumspection and tell the patient he or she has Barrett's esophagus even if there were no endoscopic criteria for the condition. Commonly, some pathologists compound this in an "enabling" way where no landmarks are given and the biopsy report states "lower esophagus." The enabling report includes a statement that "if the biopsies were from tubular esophagus then this is Barrett's esophagus." This attempt to cover the tracks of the endoscopist results in false-positive diagnoses of Barrett's esophagus with patients worrying about cancer for life and having regular endoscopy assessments for dysplasia.

Celiac Disease

The endoscopist should not ask: *Rule out celiac disease.* That will guarantee that any perceived mild abnormality could be "mild celiac disease." The consequences are predictable: lifelong gluten-free diet, worry, retesting. The operative question should be: *Is there any abnormality, Marsh, or otherwise.* The endoscopist then makes the differential diagnosis. A Marsh 1 lesion (mild) can be seen in numerous conditions.

What Information Should Be Provided to the Pathologist

Tables 5.1 and **5.2** summarize the information that can be incorporated into a standardized biopsy requisition form. **Table 5.1** lists examples of standardized biopsy locations. The endoscopy assistant can prompt the endoscopist if a site given is not "on the list." **Table 5.2** details the other information to be provided to pathologists for them to be able to give more focused diagnoses and differential diagnoses.

Endoscopy Report and History

The endoscopy report is often useless in regard to knowing what was seen. This situation coupled with a lack of any relevant clinical information and a question for the pathologist ensures that the pathologist has to perform a *blind review* of the biopsies. This was discussed previously. The endoscopy report so often tells what the endoscopist believes, not what he or she saw. For example, in an esophagogastroduodenoscopy report, there frequently are two or three diagnoses substituting for what was seen—esophagitis, gastritis, and duodenitis. The history may be brief but relevant. For example, if a patient has diarrhea and has received chemotherapy recently, that should be stated. If radiotherapy has been given, the dates should be indicated so that the pathologist can look

out for the acute mucosal changes that occur soon after radiotherapy is begun or the long-term effects that may occur months or years later. Is the diarrhea bloody or nonbloody? Marked nonbloody diarrhea rules out ulcerative colitis.

Questions for the Pathologist

The Chaucerian attitude of bygone days was to hold back information so it would not "prejudice" the pathologist. This is equivalent to asking a clinician to do a physical examination and make a diagnosis without any history to help guide the examination. So much of modern GI pathology diagnosis is correlative.

Many, if not most, pathologists continue to accept biopsy specimens for examination provided with no history and no questions. Asking the right question presupposes knowledge on the part of the endoscopist regarding what biopsy can do in a given setting and what it cannot accomplish. Frequently, the appropriate question can simply be "what is this lesion?" Endoscopists need to have realistic expectations and not force

Table 5.1 Standardization of Biopsy Locations for Endoscopy Reports and for Pathology Requisition

Esophagus	*LES, Z line, and location of biopsy*—all as centimeters from incisors. If no Barrett's esophagus, LES region and Z line are assumed to be at the same location
Stomach	*Fundus*
	Body, antrum—for each, greater or lesser curvature aspect; proximal, mid, or distal antrum or body
Duodenum and jejunum	*Bulb*
	Second duodenum
	Beyond second duodenum—estimate only, unless enteroscopy done under fluoroscopy
Ileum	As centimeters from ileocecal valve
Colon	*Cecum*
	Ascending colon—cecum and ascending colon normally have more inflammatory cells, so separate them from biopsy specimens from other sites
	Hepatic flexure region
	Transverse colon—if multiple sites here, proximal, mid, and distal
	Splenic flexure region
	Descending and sigmoid colon—if colon straight, as centimeters from anorectal margin; if not straight, site descriptions as descending colon, sigmoid, and rectum
	Rectum—as such or if important focal rectal disease, as centimeters or relationship to valves of Houston

LES, Lower esophageal sphincter.
Modified from Weinstein WM: Mucosal biopsy techniques and interaction with the pathologist. Gastrointest Endosc Clin N Am 10:555–572, 2000.

Table 5.2 Information for the Pathologist to Facilitate More Precise and Relevant Diagnosis

Lesion description	If abnormal, use simple language: *Thick folds* instead of hypertrophic or edematous; *thin* instead of atrophic
	For description of lesion, give what was seen (e.g., erosions, erythema), rather than an interpretation (e.g., gastritis). Erythema is often equated with esophagitis and gastritis—a poor predictor
	Focal lesion: What does it look like? Biopsy it and the adjacent mucosa within a centimeter, and separate the specimens
Biopsy instrument	Detail type of instrument (e.g., hot biopsy forceps, electrocautery snare) if other than a pinch biopsy forceps
Polyps	Give size and whether sessile or pedunculated, and instrument used (e.g., biopsy forceps, hot biopsy forceps, electrocautery snare)
Key drugs	*For all sites:* Immunosuppressives, chemotherapy (if recent) or radiotherapy (current, recent, past), NSAIDs
	Stomach: Proton pump inhibitors, dose and duration; recent or current antibiotics or bismuth compounds
	Colon: Type of preparation, local or oral, and type of oral; 5-ASA compounds or other IBD drugs
History	Brief—one or two lines usually suffices
Questions for the pathologist	*Be as specific as possible:* If biopsy specimens taken from different sites for different questions, indicate the site and the questions associated with it
	What is it? Asking "what is it?" is perfect when the endoscopist does not have any concrete idea

5-ASA, 5-Aminosalicylic acid; IBD, inflammatory bowel disease; NSAIDs, nonsteroidal antiinflammatory drugs.

Modified from Weinstein WM: Mucosal biopsy techniques and interaction with the pathologist. Gastrointest Endosc Clin N Am 10:555–572, 2000.

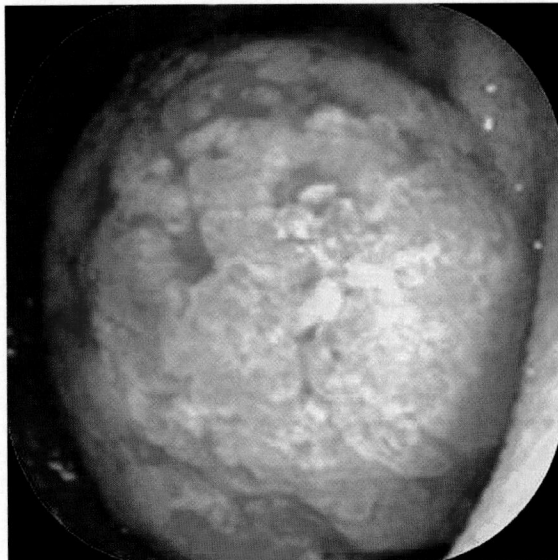

Fig. 5.6 Large tumor of transverse colon seen for the first time. The endoscopist's biopsy specimens were accompanied by the question of "rule out cancer." The pathologist's diagnosis was "adenomatous change, cannot rule out cancer, and recommend rebiopsy." The endoscopist's question should have been "large mass, scheduled for resection, rule out adenomatous change."

pathologists to be apologists. Biopsy of polyps is a good example. Endoscopists biopsy polyps, and the mucosa is frequently normal. Rather than just saying *normal*, the histologic diagnosis is frequently collaborationist: (1) *polypoid fold*, (2) *redundant fold*, or (3) *mucosal tag*. These are meaningless terms. Equating the finding of normal mucosa as a *polypoid fold* may cause worry for patients who see the report and lead to questions every time the individual applies for health, life, and disability insurance. Some pathologists have told me that they are berated or questioned in a hostile manner by endoscopists when a polyp biopsy is signed out as normal. Also, some pathologists have been led to believe that the endoscopist will "get into trouble" if there are too many normal biopsies. That is false. The quality assurance issue with biopsies is whether they are taken according to published guidelines (e.g.,

American Society for Gastrointestinal Endoscopy) for the *indications* for biopsy.

The questions for the pathologist may lead the pathologist astray. For example, the question for sessile polyps that are removed during biopsy should simply be "rule out adenoma," not *rule out complete excision*. In a sessile polyp biopsy, ruling out total excision requires sectioning and examining the whole dome-shaped biopsy specimen from one end to the other.

When an apparent colon cancer mass or large polyp is found, the dialogue should be: *surgical resection is planned; rule out adenomatous change*. Asking to *rule out cancer* may lead to a diagnosis of *adenoma but can't rule out cancer, recommend rebiopsy* (see **Fig. 5.6** to illustrate this point). By alerting the pathologist that surgery is necessary and asking to rule out adenomatous change, the endoscopist may avoid needless repeat biopsy or having the pathologist examine endless numbers of recuts.

Drugs may be responsible for various pathologies that were not imagined previously.[10-12] **Table 5.2** outlines the information regarding drugs or other therapies that can impact any part of the gut and some that are site-specific. Nonsteroidal antiinflammatory drugs should be in the differential diagnosis of unusual lesions anywhere in the gut, although cause and effect in such instances is often difficult to prove. In lymphocytic or collagenous colitis, drugs may trigger symptoms, and the symptoms may be reversed when the offending drugs are removed.[13-16] The importance of some drugs a patient takes may become apparent only after review of the biopsy results. In ischemic colitis in younger people without generalized atherosclerotic disease, the possibility of a wider range of culpable drugs becomes important, including cocaine and oral contraceptives. These can be sought post hoc after the biopsy results are interpreted.

What Pathologists and Endoscopists Can Do to Improve Communication and Biopsy Diagnoses
Feedback

Poor communication between endoscopists and pathologists was discussed previously. For more than 40 years in the flexible endoscopy era, endoscopists have not asked about the quality of their biopsy specimens or the information pathologists need. Pathologists have complied by never spontaneously bringing up these issues. Endoscopists assume that whatever they have submitted is "adequate" and that none of the biopsy specimens in a group defy interpretation because of small size, superficial scrapings, crush to the villi, or crush of the whole specimen. Endoscopists continue taking rapid-fire biopsy specimens and putting 10 or 12 specimens into a bottle for a given site, and virtually all pathologists go along and embed all the specimens into one tissue block (see **Fig. 5.4**).

Radiologists ask in requisitions for a brief overview (two lines), and then what should endoscopists rule out? On many pathology requisitions, there may only be a section for *clinical history*. That may be irritable bowel syndrome or fever of unknown origin. The question on the pathology requisition should be what does the endoscopist want to rule out. Without such information, the pathologist may be left with a rote approach to pathologic diagnosis as opposed to being able to use correlative skills maximally. An example of this inertia is that for some years one of the short courses at the annual meeting of the American Society for Clinical Pathology was "How to Sign out GI Biopsies without Any Clinical Information." This is quintessential *surrender* and *collaboration* of the pathologists to the apathy of endoscopists. This apathy and inertia may compromise patient care.

Modern GI biopsy diagnoses require that the pathologist know the consequences of the diagnoses (e.g., lifelong gluten-free diet for celiac disease; difficulty with life insurance and worry about cancer with ulcerative colitis and Barrett's esophagus). Differential diagnoses should be focused and not just a standard favored group of differential diagnoses.

Improvements in the Quality of Pathology Reporting

The two most needed improvements in the quality of GI pathology reporting are the following:

1. *Avoid calling everything "mild chronic inflammation."* This is a pandemic problem. The pandemic affects nearly all gastric biopsies being signed out as "mild chronic gastritis." The duodenum and colon are also commonly affected by this widespread pandemic in biopsies that are actually normal.
2. *Improve biopsy-processing quality.* Biopsy-processing quality is still lacking in many pathology laboratories with regular production of cross-sectioned specimens. Tearing of tissue and poor staining also compromise the ability to make an accurate diagnosis.

Chromoendoscopy

These are exciting times in GI endoscopy. Novel imaging techniques are being tested.[17-20] They are discussed elsewhere in this book. Optical methods either alone or in combination with chromoendoscopy are likely to hold the key to more targeted biopsies in the search for dysplastic or cancerous mucosa and other mucosal abnormalities. As the technology develops and becomes widely available, chromoendoscopy will become an adjunctive rather than primary tool.

Most endoscopists in the United States do not have access to or use the novel imaging technology. Many do have and use narrow band imaging. In some clinical scenarios, chromoendoscopy with conventional endoscopy may be very useful. With chromoendoscopy, the initial challenge is to learn the difference between normal mucosal variants and the changes that point to the finding of abnormalities such as polyps, cancer in inflammatory bowel disease, early tumors of the stomach and esophagus, and squamous-type or Barrett's-associated esophageal dysplasia.

A Cochrane Collaboration analysis,[21] addressed the question of chromoendoscopy versus conventional endoscopy for detection of polyps in the colon and rectum. Five studies were included. There was strong evidence that *chromocolonoscopy* increased the yield of polyp detection. However, the discussion of the implications for practice correctly cited that the quality of the examination was dependent on complete and careful examination on withdrawal and that training should still focus on this aspect. Speedy withdrawal times have been shown to be one factor contributing to a higher "miss rate."[22,23] There is residual debate about this because of varied study designs and because there are no prospective data from the "fast withdrawal era" (<7 minutes). Some clinicians suggest that "less than 7 minutes" is a factor contributing to a greater miss rate of polyp detection.

Some studies of novel imaging or chromoendoscopy end with enthusiastic conclusions that the studies are ready for routine clinical practice. Chromoendoscopy has never caught on widely in the United States. Spraying a whole colon for a polyp hunt or dysplasia is not a simple undertaking for clinicians who have never done it or plan to do it selectively. The learning curve is related to learning which appearances are normal and which are suspect and, for dysplasia, learning to recognize the patterns. There has been a nearly universal reluctance in the United States to employ even the most useful and simple techniques, such as Lugol's iodine staining of the esophagus to look for dysplastic lesions of the squamous mucosa. Most endoscopy units do not even stock the handful of dyes that can be easily used.

Table 5.3 lists the staining agents and an overview of their staining characteristics and potential utility. There has been a renaissance of research interest in chromoendoscopy worldwide, occurring long after it was developed and first used primarily in Japan. Dyes can help give a landscape view of an area for changes in contour (elevated, depressed) and to define the margins of sessile lesions.

Dyes That Are Most Useful with Conventional Endoscopy

The three dyes that are most useful with conventional endoscopy are discussed subsequently. Following is an overview.

1. *Lugol's iodine:* Lugol's iodine is an important stain in the search for early squamous esophageal cancer or

Table 5.3 Stains for Chromoendoscopy and Most Common Current Uses

Stain Categories and Types	Positive-Staining Color	Potential Utility	Result, Comments
Contrast Stains			
Indigo carmine	Blue-violet (indigo)	Topographic accentuation of lesions, elevated or depressed	Three-dimensional effect; used commonly with other imaging techniques and sometimes with acetic acid
VITAL/ABSORPTIVE			
Lugol's iodine	Dark green-brown to black	Squamous cancer, dysplasia	Negative
		Islands of Barrett's esophagus after ablation	Negative
		Esophagitis or other glycogen-depleting process	Negative, confounding in regard to cancer or dysplasia
Methylene blue (MB)	Blue	IM of stomach	Rarely used in isolation
		Barrett's esophagus—IM component	Positive; in lower esophagus may be heterogeneous
		Adenomatous polyps of duodenum	Negative; *key* with regular imaging
Reactive Stains			
Congo red	Red to blue-black	Stains acid-secreting mucosa	Rarely used
Acetic acid	Bleaches cancer and dysplastic mucosa in stomach	Used with indigo carmine sometimes in various settings. In gastric cancer bleaches, neoplastic or dysplastic edges of cancer and surrounding mucosa remain blue with indigo carmine; not useful in poorly differentiated gastric adenocarcinoma	Not widely used; may lead to detachment of neoplastic or dysplastic epithelium and intramucosal edema
Phenol red	Turns from yellow to red	Map *Helicobacter pylori*–infected epithelium for survey studies	Largely historical interest
TATTOOING AGENTS			
India ink	Black at injection site	For polyps removed and worrisome for cancer (superficial) or lesions for surgical resection (map for surgeon)	Permanent black color

IM, Intestinal metaplasia.

squamous dysplasia, either in isolation or in association with squamous cancer. Other potential uses are described subsequently in relation to Barrett's esophagus.

2. *Indigo carmine:* Indigo carmine is the most widely used dye to highlight subtle changes in terrain, bumpiness, elevations, and depressions. It is a versatile highlighter that can be used throughout the GI tract to give a three-dimensional appearance to visible or suspect lesions and to lesions before endoscopic removal.

3. *Methylene blue(MB):* MB for duodenal polyps in familial adenomatous polyposis (FAP) is discussed subsequently. MB gives a "terrain view" of the duodenum that makes it much easier to see the sizes and numbers of smaller lesions that are often nearly or totally invisible. This application is also discussed subsequently.

Safety of Dyes

Patients who are to receive Lugol's iodine should be questioned regarding iodine sensitivity. Application of the dye to iodine-allergic patients may cause a frightening reaction. In Lugol's staining of the proximal esophagus, it is prudent to have patients intubated so that they do not aspirate the Lugol's irritant. See the section on MB for a discussion of the controversy concerning safety.

Preparation of the Patient and the Mucosa for Chromoendoscopy

As mentioned, if the use of Lugol's iodine is contemplated, it should be ascertained that the patient is not allergic to iodine. For MB staining, the patient should be told that the urine and stool might adopt a blue color for 1 or 2 days.

The enemy of good chromoendoscopy is surface mucus, blood, or retained food material. The surface to be examined after application of dye should be washed. For the vital/absorptive dyes (e.g., Lugol's, MB), it is especially useful to wash with 20 mL or more of 10% N-acetylcysteine. An alternative is to have the patient take a 20,000-U pronase drink before the procedure. This is followed by another wash with water or saline after 1 to 2 minutes, using 100 mL or more of tap water to remove nonabsorbed stain. The washes may also contain a small amount of antifoam solution. Washes may be done using a 60-mL syringe with forceful pressure through the spray catheter or through a syringe without the spray catheter.

The use of an anticholinergic such as glycopyrrolate 0.2 mg intravenously is effective in reducing secretions, and the addition of glucagon (0.25 to 0.50 mg) just before or during the procedure helps to reduce peristalsis and spasm. When taking biopsy specimens from multiple polyps in FAP, after the first few biopsies (e.g., in the third or fourth duodenum), there is often a marked increase in peristalsis. Glucagon (0.25 mg intravenously) stops peristalsis and permits quicker and more biopsy sampling.

Contrast Stains

Contrast stains help most in the delineation of superficial neoplastic lesions, such as in the stomach and of all lesions before endoscopic resection.[7] In the latter instance, the often irregular margins of the lesion to be excised are better defined. One disadvantage of contrast stains is that it requires some experience to recognize what is normal mucosa and what is not if there are no obviously elevated areas. In the stomach, pit openings and areae gastricae may make the field look abnormal.

The most popular dye stain is indigo carmine used as a contrast stain (see **Table 5.3**). Although many experts indicate that it should not be washed off after application, some washing off after application leaves the innate color of the lesion in question still preserved (**Fig. 5.7**). Often all one needs are thin lines of stain in grooves or edges of lesions to define borders and provide a three-dimensional effect (see **Fig. 5.7**).

Other stains can be used for contrast staining. MB is one such dye, provided that there is no intestinal absorptive epithelium because it binds the dye. With ordinary endoscopy, MB as a contrast stain has no advantages over indigo carmine. MB can be used as a contrast stain in a different sense. When saline is being injected before endoscopic resection, a few drops of MB into a 30-mL syringe filled with saline provides a sky blue color to the injected submucosa and provides a better contrast between the lesion to be removed and the uninvolved part of the submucosa below.

Esophagus
Squamous Carcinoma and Dysplasia of the Esophagus

One of the most important potential applications of chromoendoscopy in the clinical arena is in the delineation of squamous carcinoma and dysplasia with Lugol's solution. The iodine in the solution stains the glycogen in normal squamous epithelium. Negative staining indicates a mucosal disorder that also includes inflammatory change and reactive changes with surface glycogen depletion.

The esophagus is sprayed with 10 to 30 mL of the solution (see **Table 5.3**). The esophagus can be sprayed efficiently by beginning at the GE junction and applying the spray as the endoscope is moved cephalad. The lumen can be partially collapsed, and when the upper extent of the sprayed area is reached, it can be totally collapsed to permit apposition of the stained walls for more uniform staining. After 1 to 2 minutes, the lumen is insufflated, and any pale-staining areas can be resprayed. The color ranges from dark green to brown to black in normal squamous epithelium. After 10 to 15 minutes, the stain intensity starts to fade, sometimes dramatically.

Areas of dysplasia and carcinoma are glycogen-depleted, so negative staining occurs; this is also true for areas of eroded mucosa, or mucosa markedly thinned by injury or regeneration.[24] Examples of mucosa thinned by regeneration are after healing of erosive esophagitis and after restoration of neosquamous epithelium following ablation of Barrett's esophagus.

With negative staining, Lugol's highlights areas of dysplasia or early carcinoma that can be missed or poorly visualized in terms of margins (**Fig. 5.8A and B**). In a study in Linxian, China, which has among the highest rates of esophageal cancer, the rate of dysplasia and cancer detection increased from 62% to 96% with a specificity of 63% with the use of Lugol's stain.[25] The technique is very useful to detect recurrent or metachronous squamous cell esophageal carcinoma.[26] It is also useful in patients with head and neck cancers where there is an increased risk of squamous cell esophageal cancer.[24]

Residual Islands of Nonsquamous Mucosa after Ablation of Barrett's Esophagus

Lugol's makes it simple to do "final checks" for nonsquamous islands after ablation. These islands may be invisible in the

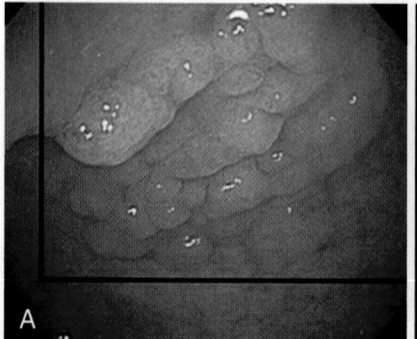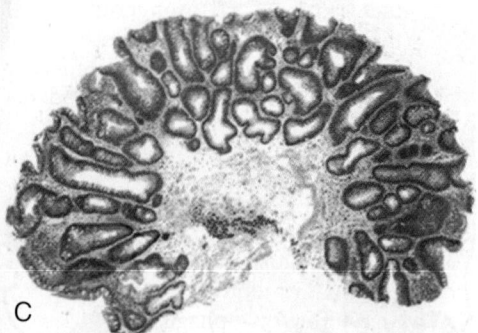

Fig. 5.7 **A** and **B,** Cluster of confluent colonic bumps. With indigo carmine top right (much of it intentionally washed off), the margins of the lesion are crisp. **C,** Adenomatous change. This "spreading lesion" needs to be endoscopically removed en bloc.

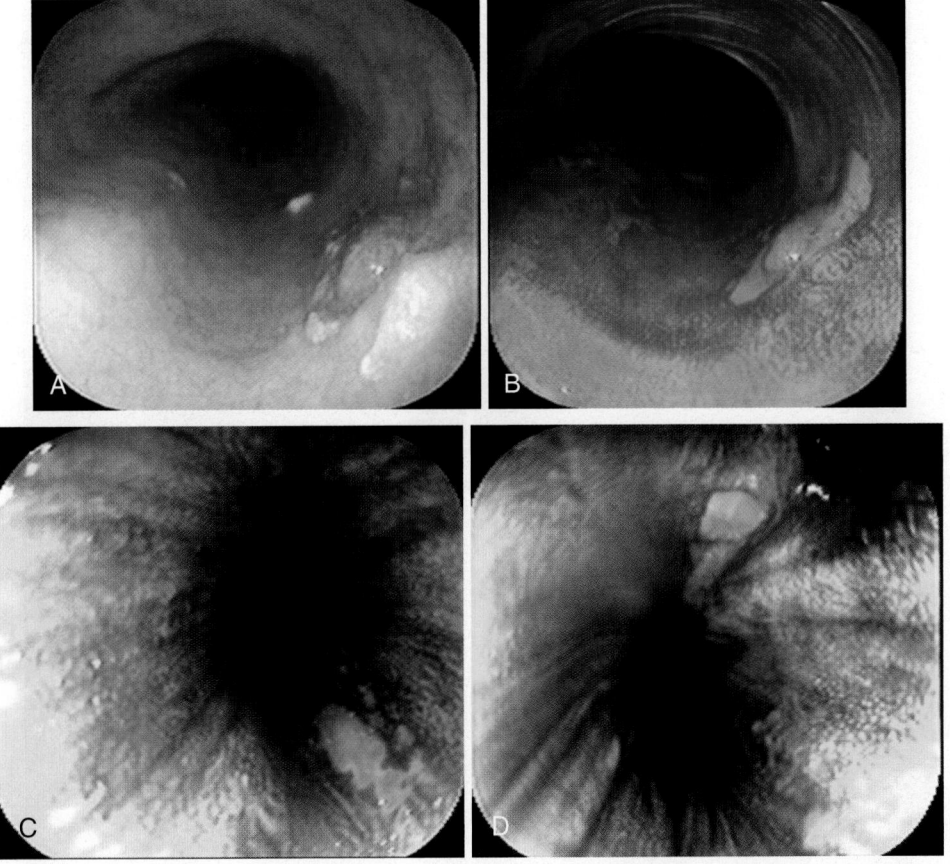

Fig. 5.8   **A** and **B,** Comparison of the appearance of squamous cancer before **(A)** and after **(B)** Lugol's staining. Lugol's-stained mucosa provides crisp definition of the margins of the lesion and its extent. **C** and **D,** Two small nonstaining areas after ablation for Barrett's esophagus. At this stage, they do not require biopsy, just "touchup" ablation.

unstained state (**Fig. 5.8C and D**). Neosquamous postablation mucosa is thinner initially, with less glycogen. It may be paler than usual with Lugol's staining but not completely negative. I use Lugol's iodine as the final "gold standard" for complete return of neosquamous epithelium after ablation of Barrett's esophagus.

Methylene Blue

Sprayed MB induces oxidative damage of DNA when it is photosensitized by white light.[27-29] The concern in Barrett's esophagus is that the stain may further the promutagenic DNA damage that may already exist, and this raises the question about increased rate of carcinogenesis. This situation is controversial with vigorous arguments[28] that the studies of cellular damage used higher doses for longer than the conventional spray at endoscopy and other variables. To resolve this controversy, cellular damage or lack of it needs to be studied in a fashion that is comparable in dose and duration to MB as used in chromoendoscopy.

MB staining is and will be used even more as an adjunct to novel imaging techniques. It has been used alone in research studies of Barrett's esophagus with conventional endoscopy (**Fig. 5.9**). Canto and colleagues[30] did much of the seminal work with MB. MB binds to intestinal absorptive epithelium, be it normal small intestine or the intestinal metaplasia that

is characteristic of Barrett's esophagus and intestinal metaplasia of the stomach.

METHYLENE BLUE PROCEDURE

First, a mucolytic is given (*N*-acetylcysteine or pronase, the latter more commonly in Japan). Next, 0.5% MB is sprayed with a spray catheter, and 2 minutes later the mucosa is washed off. One should avoid staining clothing, and patients should be told not to be concerned by the passage of blue or green urine in the next 1 or 2 days. There is an acknowledged learning curve, and the staining procedure adds 2 to 12 minutes to the procedure and on the order of 10 to 15 minutes if one includes setup and postprocedure cleanup times and learning curves. Canto advised that beginners in chromoendoscopy take multiple photographs and compare staining characteristics with pathologic diagnoses of biopsy specimens of stained areas.[34]

In Barrett's esophagus, there are two areas of interest in studies with MB. One is to identify intestinal epithelium (positive staining) in apparent or possible short-segment Barrett's esophagus, and the second is to detect dysplasia by negative staining. With conventional endoscopy, a meta-analysis failed to show superiority of MB (to provide targeting of areas for biopsy) over random four-quadrant biopsy.[31] In a prospective randomized crossover trial, the dysplasia detection rate was

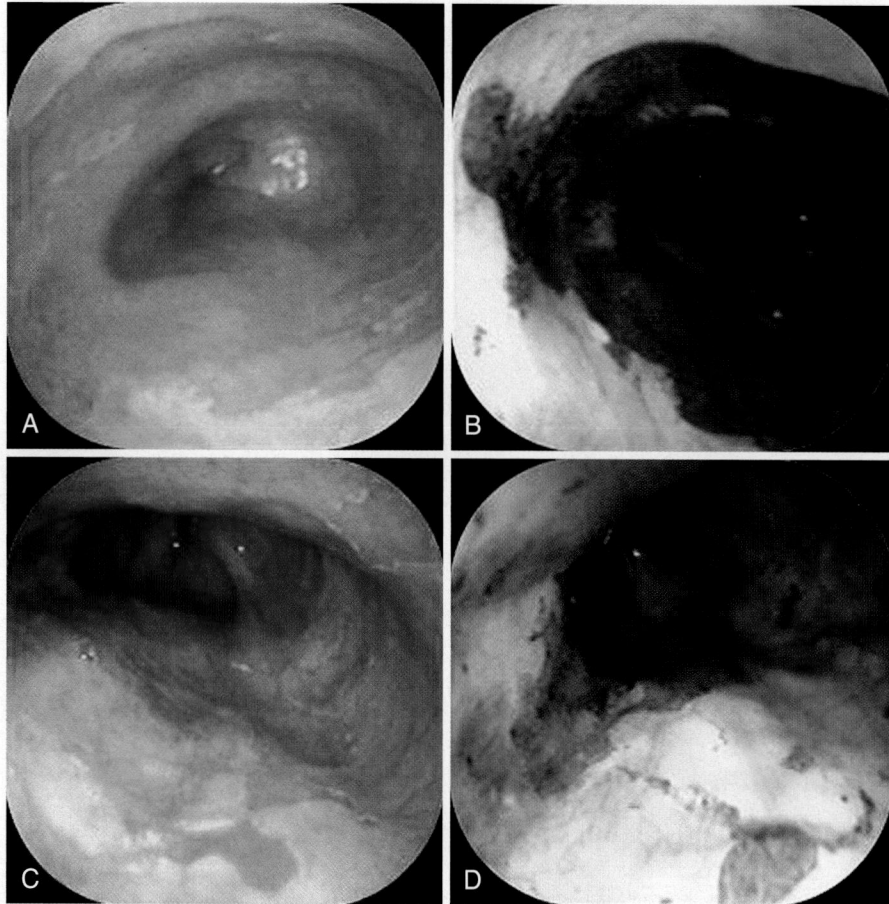

Fig. 5.9 **A** and **B,** Long-segment Barrett's esophagus before and after methylene blue staining. Staining intensity is dark and uniform. **C** and **D,** Short-segment Barrett's esophagus before and after methylene blue staining. Staining intensity is lighter and more patchily distributed.

similar with MB versus four-quadrant biopsy.[32] The miss fraction for dysplasia was 5/21 with MB and 3/21 with four-quadrant random biopsy. Fewer biopsy specimens were taken in the MB group (for targeting), however. MB may be useful in trying to define the region around the LES to determine whether there are short tongues of Barrett's esophagus above a normally positioned Z line.

SHORT-SEGMENT BARRETT'S ESOPHAGUS AND INTESTINAL METAPLASIA OF THE CARDIA

If biopsy specimens of apparent 2-cm tongues of Barrett's esophagus at endoscopy are found histologically to have intestinal-type goblet cells, the diagnosis of short-segment Barrett's esophagus is made. If intestinal-type goblet cells are absent, Barrett's esophagus should not be diagnosed. Staining with MB in suspected short-segment Barrett's esophagus is intended to help increase the yield in biopsies of areas with intestinal metaplasia (blue staining) to clinch the diagnosis.

When used for the detection of short-segment Barrett's esophagus (≤3 cm in length), the staining pattern is less diffuse and patchier than cephalad than in longer segments of Barrett's esophagus (see **Fig. 5.9**). The reason is that in short-segment Barrett's esophagus there is a greater mix of intestinal and nonintestinal columnar cells present than in the more diffuse intestinal change of long-segment Barrett's esopha-

gus.[33,34] In the final analysis, the finding rate of intestinal-type goblet cells in short-segment Barrett's esophagus of the tongue variety is no greater than targeted biopsies without chromo-endoscopy. Fewer biopsies may be needed, so the main value is for clinicians who like it because it is a "biopsy aversion technique."

MB staining has also been used to identify intestinal metaplasia of the cardia right at the GE junction in patients without endoscopically visible Barrett's esophagus. In practice, there is no reason to biopsy a normal-appearing Z line. Intestinal metaplasia may occur in 30% of individuals with GERD and no Barrett's esophagus. It is also common in individuals with no GERD.[9] Its presence is not an indication for biopsy surveillance.

HIGH-GRADE DYSPLASIA AND ENDOSCOPICALLY INVISIBLE ADENOCARCINOMA

Studies with MB (with or without acetic acid) for detecting dysplasia or early cancer in Barrett's esophagus generally have an adjunctive role coupled with novel imaging methods.[35-38] Acetic acid (1.5%) blanches the esophagus white and leaves Barrett's esophagus and gastric mucosa looking red. The objective is to target the areas most likely to contain neoplastic change and to reduce the numbers of random biopsies.

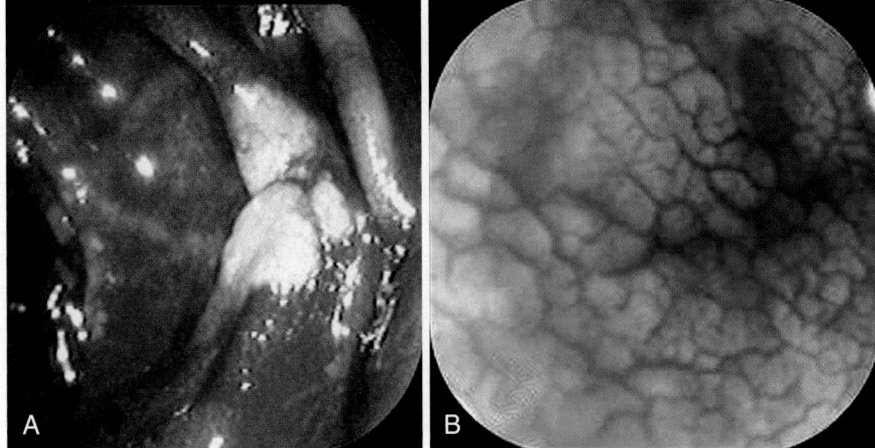

Fig. 5.10 Small intestinal chromoendoscopy. **A** and **B,** Typical flat to minimally raised adenomas in duodenum typical of adenomas seen in familial polyposis coli. They are easily highlighted and more readily recognized with methylene blue staining. Methylene blue stains intestinal mucosa and leaves adenomas negatively stained.

Well-designed larger prospective studies are needed to settle whether these dyes with novel imaging have any advantage over dyes with conventional endoscopy.

SUMMARY: DYE STAINING IN BARRETT'S ESOPHAGUS

Given the available data and the extra time involved, MB or other dye techniques for detecting intestinal metaplasia and dysplasia are not likely to be incorporated into routine clinical practice in the United States.

Stomach

Apart from the use of contrast stains to detect subtle lesions or to define the margins of lesions[39] with or without novel imaging, there is no type of chromoendoscopy that has widespread applications in the stomach. MB stains intestinal metaplasia of the stomach a dark blue, and it has been combined with magnification endoscopy to examine its utility in more precise characterization of intestinal metaplasia and gastric dysplasia.[40,41]

Small Intestine
Celiac Disease

The endoscopic signs of celiac disease include decreased numbers of valvulae, scalloped valvulae, a mosaic pattern, and visualization of underlying blood vessels. A host of new imaging technologies are being examined in celiac disease, including some with dyes such as MB or a contrast stain.[42]

If the objective is to rule out celiac disease, biopsy specimens from three sites in the duodenum should be taken to rule out patchy involvement with lesions of lesser severity: mid–second duodenum, third duodenum, and fourth duodenum or proximal jejunum. Dye stains are generally not helpful nor worth the extra time. *Biopsy specimens should be taken even if the mucosa looks normal.*

Other Small Bowel Lesions

Nowhere is MB more useful than in the assessment of the duodenal sweep in patients with FAP or more atypical polyposis

syndromes. Some lesions are easily visible; however, most duodenal adenomas in FAP are flat, often along valvulae, and barely raised if at all. MB stains the nondysplastic mucosa deep blue and leaves dysplastic areas unstained. Spraying of the whole duodenum permits a sweeping view of the terrain for targeting biopsy (**Fig. 5.10**). This stain or a contrast stain, such as indigo carmine, may be very useful before endoscopic resection of one or more of these lesions.

Colon
Polyps of the Colon

Chromoendoscopy has been directed toward two aspects of polyps of the colon. One is to determine the difference between hyperplastic and adenomatous polyps on gross examination. The second is to increase the detection rate, especially of adenomas. The favorite stain has been indigo carmine spray, with or without magnifying endoscopy or high-resolution endoscopy. Other creative approaches to dye staining have put the dye into the electrolyte purging solution or into capsules.[43,44]

HYPERPLASTIC VERSUS ADENOMATOUS POLYPS

A pit or pitted pattern denotes a hyperplastic polyp, and a grooved or sulcus appearance denotes adenoma. Most of the pioneering work in this area was done in Japan.[45] Among numerous studies examining the potential of chromoendoscopy has been a U.S. prospective multicenter study, in which 92.3% of the polyps could be classified according to the dye staining pattern. For adenomatous polyps, the sensitivity, specificity, and negative predictive values were 82%, 82%, and 88%.[46]

INCREASED DETECTION RATE OF ADENOMAS

Flat and depressed adenomas refer to adenomas that are raised but pancakelike (with or without depressed centers) and not generally dome-shaped. One endoscopic definition that has been used is that they are either flat or depressed lesions with a height less than half of the diameter of the lesion.[47] To prove that they were not just a Japanese phenomenon, a Japanese endoscopist, Saitoh, who was experienced in the detection of these lesions, was recruited to the United States to perform a study using indigo carmine and conventional endoscopy. He did left-sided colonic indigo carmine staining from splenic flexure to rectum for colonoscopies in 211 patients.[47] Flat and depressed lesions were found in 22.7%. These were more likely adenomas than hyperplastic polyps (87% vs. 67%), and the advanced lesions with high-grade dysplasia or cancer were significantly smaller than comparable conventional polypoid lesions (10.75 mm vs. 20 mm). In a randomized controlled trial of 259 patients using total colonic dye spray, more diminutive adenomas were detected proximal to the sigmoid colon, and more patients were identified with three or more adenomas.[48] Increased detection rates with indigo carmine staining were also found in a study in Korea, a country with a lower incidence of colorectal neoplasia compared with Western countries.[49]

APPLICATION IN PRACTICE

The distinction of hyperplastic from adenomatous polyps holds some appeal, especially proximal to the rectum and distal sigmoid colon. In the latter distal locations, hyperplastic polyps may be numerous and easy to identify as such because of their whitish or neutral appearance. Colon dye spray adds time to the colonoscopy procedure; it requires a motivated endoscopist and gaining of a certain amount of experience. It remains to be seen whether their use in prospective studies will find carcinomas at an earlier stage or whether optical techniques alone that can scan the mucosa will be the answer for easier detection (e.g., narrow band imaging). The greatest theoretical potential for any optical aid is in finding flat adenomas in the 8- to 10-mm range that contain carcinoma. It is unknown how many of these would be missed by experienced endoscopists with conventional colonoscopy; also, the temporal biologic behavior of these lesions is unknown.

Chromoendoscopy and Inflammatory Bowel Disease

Chromoendoscopy was studied in a randomized controlled trial of 174 patients with long-standing ulcerative colitis comparing conventional surveillance biopsy with total spray of the colon with MB.[50] Investigators compared 32 lesions with intraepithelial neoplasia (24 of 32 low grade; 24 of 32 in flat mucosa) in the dye group with 10 lesions (8 of 10 low grade; 4 of 10 in flat mucosa) in the conventional endoscopy group. The dye spray group also predicted the degree of histologic inflammation better than the conventional group, but that is not the primary message.[51]

References

The complete reference list is available online at www.expertconsult.com

Chapter 6

Electrosurgery in Therapeutic Endoscopy

Marcia L. Morris and Ian D. Norton

Introduction

Endoscopic electrosurgery involves the use of electrical current to achieve a desired tissue effect (cutting, tissue ablation, desiccation, or a combination of these). Electrical energy to produce heating and tissue effect has been a part of endoscopy since the early 1970s.[1,2] Common indications include biliary sphincterotomy, polypectomy, hemostasis and ablation of vascular lesions such as arteriovenous malformations, radiation proctopathy, and other forms of vascular ectasia. Other forms of nonelectrosurgical thermal effect may be achieved without the direct use of electrical current, such as laser photoablation and heater probe. Incorrect use of electrical equipment may contribute to poor patient outcomes, such as postpolypectomy serositis; colonic perforation; and biliary sphincterotomy–associated complications such as acute pancreatitis, hemorrhage, and duodenal perforation.

From the clinician's point of view, this field has been hampered by problems with nomenclature (**Table 6.1**). First, there is often lack of uniformity in terms used by different manufacturers (e.g., *blend* may have quite different characteristics from one manufacturer's generator to another). Second, the terms themselves may be misleading (e.g., a low duty-cycle waveform may be called *pure coag* but be capable of cutting tissue; this situation leads to statements such as "I only cut with coag") Lastly, some terms in common usage are manufacturer specific (e.g., *Endocut* refers specifically to an ERBE [Marietta, GA] generator output). Usually a clinician becomes adept with the particular generator that he or she uses, and most modern generators have storable or preset parameters

for common scenarios such as polypectomy and sphincterotomy. Problems may occur, however, when the clinician is confronted with a different generator (most likely to happen in an unusual and stressful environment, such as an emergency procedure in the operating room or emergency department or first list at a new appointment).

A clinician with no electrosurgical "conscious competence" would be unable to troubleshoot generator problems or be flexible in unusual situations. Understanding the basic type of current delivery (bipolar vs. monopolar) has important implications for patients with implanted devices, such as pacemakers, defibrillators, and deep brain stimulators. For these reasons, the clinician should have a basic knowledge of electrosurgical generator principles. This chapter outlines the basic principles of electrosurgery pertaining to flexible endoscopy. As far as possible, the use of proprietary-specific terms is minimized.

Electricity and Tissue

Early pioneers of electrosurgical devices discovered that applying an electrical current to biologic tissue might produce different effects. The first effect was electrolytic. Charged molecules in the tissue flowed toward the opposite poles of an electrode if the current applied was direct or alternated slowly. Alternating the current more rapidly eliminated the electrolytic effect and produced heating at a cellular level. However, a current alternating at less than 100 kHz resulted in undesired neuromuscular effects (the result of applying household

Table 6.1 Monopolar Output Names with Corresponding Duty Cycle*

Duty Cycle (%)	Meditron UGI 3000B	Microvasive Endostat	ValleyLab SSE2	ValleyLab Force2	ValleyLab ForceFX	ValleyLab ForceEZ	ERBE ICC 200E/A
100	Cut	Cut	Cut	Cut	Cut low (voltage limited) and cut pure	Cut pure and coag low 2 (330 Vp) and coag low 3 (550 Vp)	Autocut (Vp >200) and soft coag (Vp <200)
50	Blend 1	Blend	Blend	Blend 1	Cut blend	Cut blend	NA
37	NA	NA	NA	Blend 2	NA	NA	NA
25	Blend 2	NA	NA	Blend 3	NA	NA	NA
12	Blend 3	Coag	Coag	NA	NA	NA	NA
8	NA	NA	NA	NA	Desiccate	Coag low 1	NA
4–6	Coag	NA	NA	Coag	NA	NA	Forced coag

*Endostat is a trademark of Microvasive Corp; Operator's manual, 1992. SSE2, Force2, ForceEZ, and ForceFX are trademarks of ValleyLab, Inc., a division of Tyco Healthcare; SSE2 and Force2 user's guides, 1994; ForceFX user's guide, 1997, EZ-20 user's guide, 1999. ICC 200 E/A is a trademark of ERBE, USA, Inc; Operator's manual V 2.X, 2001. Meditron is a division of Cooper Surgical, Inc; UGI 3000 and UGI 3000B operator's manuals, 1995–1999.
Coag, coagulation; NA, not applicable; Vp, peak velocity.

current of 60 Hz is well known). Alternating at very high frequency (300 kHz) eliminates neuromuscular effects but retains the desired cellular heating effects. This thermal effect is the basis for all electrosurgery.[3]

Endoscopic Thermal Modalities

Monopolar Electrosurgery

Monopolar output involves use of an electrode at the luminal site and a return electrode at a remote site (usually an adhesive pad placed on the thigh). The current flows from the electrode site, through the patient's tissue to an electrode on the skin, and back to the generator, completing an electrical circuit. Monopolar is the most common form of endoscopic electrosurgery and is commonly used in hot biopsy forceps (HBF), polypectomy snares, sphincterotomes, needle-knives, and endoscopic mucosal dissection devices. As discussed subsequently, variables in current flow and current density result in different tissue effects, ranging from desiccation to cutting.

Bipolar (Multipolar) Electrosurgery

Bipolar (multipolar) electrosurgery uses technology similar to the monopolar circuit, but both electrodes are on the tip of the instrument. Current flows through a relatively small area of tissue, and there is no need for a return electrode on the patient's skin. The common uses for this technology are coagulation of arteriovenous malformations and ulcer hemostasis. Bipolar (or multipolar) probes have been shown to be effective devices for hemostasis for bleeding peptic ulcers. Optimal results seem to be obtained by using forceful tamponade, large probes, low power settings (15 to 25 W) and prolonged contact times (10 seconds).[4,5] This technique uses relatively low power outputs (approximately 16 W) with limited depth of injury.[6] Bipolar snares, biopsy forceps, and sphincterotomes have been developed but are not widely used. A new, important use of bipolar current is radiofrequency ablation catheters employed

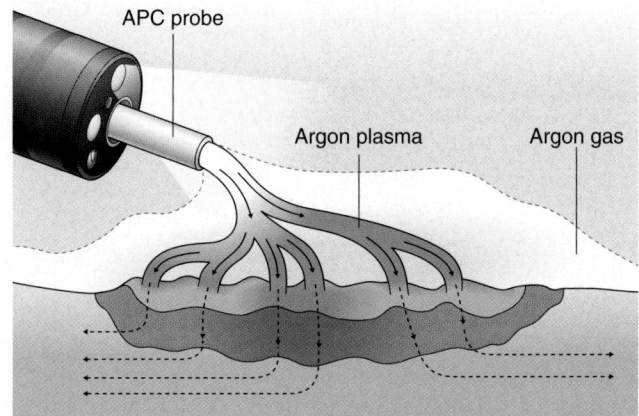

Fig. 6.1 Argon plasma coagulation.

to ablate Barrett's esophagus. In this situation, the current moves from one adjacent electrode on a balloon catheter to another. This energy passes via the mucosa and is sufficient to obliterate the mucosa, while being superficial enough to prevent significant submucosal damage, minimizing stricture formation.

Argon Plasma Coagulation

Argon plasma coagulation (APC) is a newer technique in flexible endoscopy with many potential applications, including tumor debulking,[7] ablation of vascular malformations,[8] and coagulation of peptic ulcer bleeding sites.[9] It also has a role in "tidying up" residual adenoma after piecemeal polypectomy, although overuse in this setting suggests poor polypectomy technique. APC is a unique means of energy delivery (**Fig. 6.1**). Argon gas flows from the catheter tip and provides a medium for current flow from the catheter tip to an adjacent mucosal surface (and via the patient to a remote return pad). APC is a form of monopolar electrocoagulation, unique in its noncontact nature. It can be used effectively either tangential or perpendicular to the mucosal surface. Side-firing catheters are available, but the standard end-firing catheter can be used for tangential and perpendicular applications.

High current density at the mucosal surface leads to tissue effect. At high power output (e.g., 75 to 90 W), APC results in tissue debulking. At lower energy levels (e.g., 30 to 45 W), tissue desiccates with limited depth of injury.[10] It has been theorized that as tissue desiccates, its electrical resistance increases, resulting in electrical arcing to adjacent, nondesiccated tissue. This mechanism could act to limit depth of injury. It has been shown, however, that APC can cause transmural injury at high power outputs,[10] and there have been reports of perforation using this device.[11,12] Nonetheless, the relative ease of use, nontouch technique, and relatively shallow depth of injury make this a versatile and useful instrument, especially in thin parts of the bowel such as small intestine and right colon.

Heater Probe

The heater probe unit (Olympus Corporation, Melville, NY) comprises a power source, catheter, and irrigation system. At the tip of the catheter is a heating coil within a polytef (Teflon) cap. This energy delivery is unique because it supplies a predetermined amount of energy (e.g., 30 J) to the cap without an electrical circuit flowing through tissue. Because this is a direct transfer of heat, it is an example of *electrocautery,* not electrosurgery. The main indications are ulcer hemostasis and coagulation of angiodysplastic lesions. Heater probe results in ulcer hemostasis in 80% to 90% of bleeding lesions.[13] The energy and probe size are inadequate for tumor ablation indications, and this method cannot produce any electrosurgical cutting effect.

Principles of Electrosurgery

Electrical output from generators used in endoscopy are at high frequencies (300 to 950 kHz). The output is beyond the frequency range that causes neuromuscular stimulation, generally preventing muscular side effects and always preventing "electrocution."

Tissue effect is determined by the rapidity of tissue heating. Rapid heating causes intracellular boiling and explosion of cells resulting in a cleavage plane (incision).[14] In contrast, slow heating results in protein denaturization and desiccation or "coagulation" of tissue.[15] Understanding the different characteristics of tissue heating under different circumstances is essential to understanding electrosurgery.

Variables in Electrosurgery

Many variables in electrosurgery can influence tissue effect.

Power Output

Power output is the amount of energy flowing through the circuit per unit of time (i.e., power = joules per second) measured in watts. The higher the power, the greater the tissue heating.

Two formulas, including Ohm's law, elegantly relate all of the electrosurgical variables:

1. $V = IR$, where V is voltage, I is current, and R is resistance
2. $P = I^2R$, where P is power, I is current, and R is resistance

Power and voltage are also directly related (e.g., $P = V^2/I$).

These formulas illustrate that there is a relationship between power output and tissue resistance. As the resistance (or *impedance*) in the tissue increases (as it desiccates), power falls off unless either current or voltage is increased. Manufacturers addressed this problem by developing microprocessor-controlled generators that could measure resistance in the circuit and adjust output automatically (within certain set parameters) to maintain the desired tissue effect.[16] Some power outputs are constant over a wide range of resistance; when this is graphically represented, it results in the so-called flat or wide power curve (**Fig. 6.2**). The initiation of an incision is problematic for generators, especially if the electrode is pressed firmly against the tissue surface because this presents a large surface area with low current density and low tissue impedance. The generator must supply particularly high power output to initiate the formation of microelectric arcs and commencement of the cutting effect. This initial power output is often greater than the output needed to continue the incision. Microprocessors can recognize this situation and transiently provide a high power output to initiate cutting.

Voltage

Voltage refers to the potential difference between the two electrodes and defines the force making electrons move from one point in the circuit to another. Using the analogy of a waterfall, with current being the water flowing, voltage is analogous to the height of the waterfall. As one can see from the aforementioned formulas, voltage is an integral determinant of circuit behavior (and tissue effect). To complete a circuit, sufficient voltage must exist across the device-patient interface for microelectric arcs to occur between patient and tissue. Generally, a peak of at least 200 V is required. At greater than 500 V, tissue tends to char. Manufacturers have manipulated voltage in an attempt to create specific effects. In particular, increasing the voltage for a given continuous sinusoidal output (i.e., pure cut) varies the depth of coagulation adjacent to the cut; this has been termed *cut effect 1, cut effect 2,* and so forth (**Figs. 6.3 and 6.4**).

Duty Cycle

Current flows for only a fraction of each second that the activating pedal is depressed. This fraction or percentage of time current flows is the *duty cycle.* A *pure-cut* mode delivers current during most or all of the activation period, whereas *blended* mode delivers current in an interrupted fashion (e.g., 25% to 50%). A *pure coag* mode may have a duty cycle of 6% to 10% (see **Fig. 6.4**). This mode gives tissue time to dehydrate (rather than rapid heating causing an explosive tissue cleavage seen in cutting mode). Some new generators have an alternating cut and coagulation mode (e.g., 50 msec of pure cut followed by 700 msec of coagulation). This mode results in a characteristic "staccato" type of incision. The aim of this type of output is to slow the rate of incision and prevent uncontrolled ("zipper")

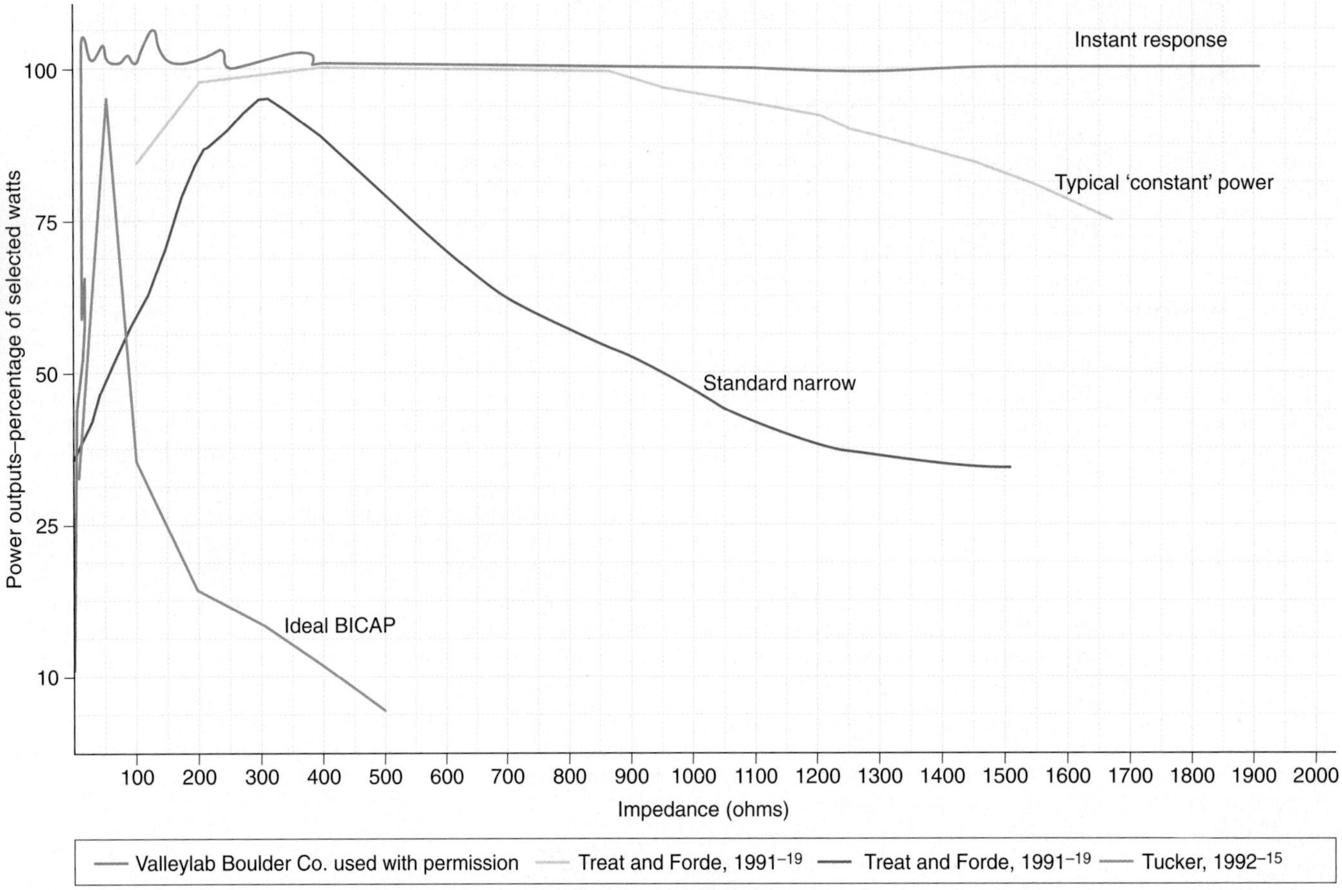

Fig. 6.2   Typical power curves.

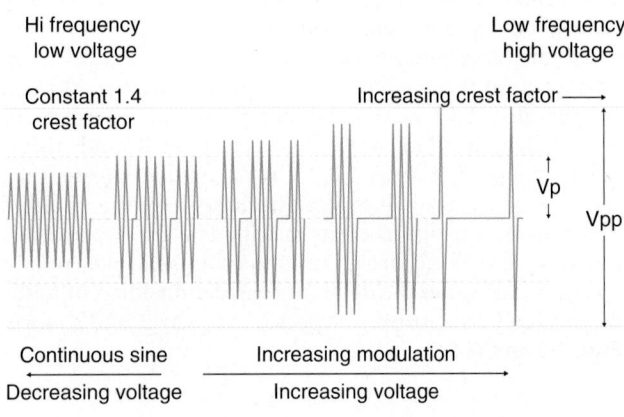

Fig. 6.3   Electrosurgical waveform patterns.

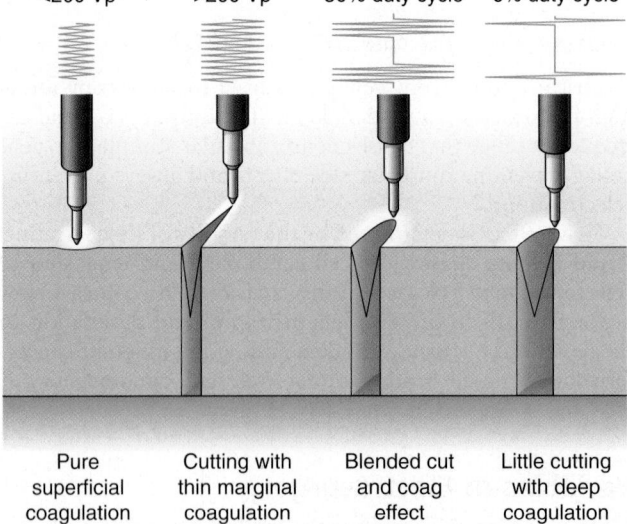

| Pure superficial coagulation | Cutting with thin marginal coagulation | Blended cut and coag effect | Little cutting with deep coagulation |

Fig. 6.4   Tissue effect changes with changing waveform.

cut[17]; whether this translates to improved patient outcome is yet to be determined.

Current Density

Current density relates to the ratio between current and the volume of tissue through which it passes. Heat generation is proportional to the square of the current density. The smaller the area of electrode in contact with tissue, the greater the effect. Practical aspects of cutting effect and current density include the following:

1. Sphincterotomy progresses much better when a small amount of wire is in contact with the tissue.
2. Polypectomy may be difficult to initiate if the polyp has a very thick stalk (i.e., large circumference of tissue is in contact, or the snare is squeezed too tightly so that more of it is surrounded by tissue).

3. Return electrode burn is prevented by having a large surface area of conductive surface in contact with the patient skin (i.e., low current density). The corollary is that reduced contact with skin could result in a skin burn at the return electrode site. Modern generators avoid this danger by having a feedback mechanism that automatically switches off the circuit if the return pad becomes partially disconnected. This feedback mechanism is achieved using a split pad system.[18]

Tissue Tension

Some degree of tissue tension is necessary for progression of an incision (e.g., polypectomy or sphincterotomy). However, overzealous tension may result in poor control of cutting, leading to a rapid incision with inadequate vessel coagulation and increased risk of hemorrhage.

Tissue Resistance

Tissue resistance varies during the incision as tissue characteristics vary (e.g., fibrosis and water content). Resistance increases substantially as tissue becomes desiccated; this can reduce energy flow sufficiently to "stall" the cut unless another variable is adjusted (tissue tension, voltage, or power). Tissue resistance is a dynamic variable that alters as tissue desiccates during the incision. There is a fixed interrelationship between power, voltage, and resistance such that as resistance increases, power or voltage or both also must change. New-generation generators detect alteration in circuit (tissue) resistance and automatically adjust output to maintain cutting effect over a wide range of tissue resistance (a so-called flat or wide power curve).

Blood Flow

Blood flow may help dissipate heat at the site of the tissue. Similarly, submucosal saline injection may act as a "heat sink" and help dissipate energy and prevent transmural injury during polypectomy.[19] Saline is widely used in clinical practice to reduce the risk of transmural injury, but it has not been proven to increase safety.

Electrical Hazards
Electrical Shock

As mentioned previously, generator output is at a high frequency, which does not cause neuromuscular stimulation, but conduction of main power from faulty equipment via the patient could cause electrical shock. Leakage of faulty current can flow along any conductive pathway from an electrical instrument that is connected to a power line. This problem is prevented by grounding the external conducting surfaces and by isolating conductors in contact with the patient. There are strict standards relating to the use of electrical equipment with patients, and equipment should be checked at regular intervals.

High-Frequency Burn

The most common electrical complications associated with monopolar electrosurgery are burns to the patient and surgeon caused by the following:

- Defective patient return electrodes
- Insufficient patient contact with the return electrode
- Poor technique.

In old machines, the return electrode was no more than a large flat metal plate on which the patient was positioned. Contact could easily become partial (resulting in increased current density and the risk of a skin burn). New return pads minimize the possibility of a burn at the return site by ensuring adequate patient contact (reducing the amount of energy passing through each square centimeter of skin—i.e., ensuring low current density). First, these are flexible adhesive pads, preventing the patient from partially rolling off the electrode during the procedure. Second, new pads comprise two electrically isolated pads. A small current flows from one side of the pad to the other. If this small circuit is lost (indicating poor skin contact), a return electrode fault registers, and the generator does not activate. Rarely, an alternating current in one appliance can induce a "capacitance" current in an adjacent conductive wire without there being an actual physical contact between the two wires. This occurrence is made possible by the flux of positive and negative charge in one circuit inducing an opposite electron flow in the other (e.g., if a nonshielded wire was used to maintain access to the biliary tree during sphincterotomy). An induced current in the access wire could cause a burn within the liver. This risk highlights the importance of using only guidewires approved for access during sphincterotomy. It is also important not to lay active cords, such as cords attaching a polypectomy snare to the generator, closely along the wire leads from patient monitor patch electrodes. Current can concentrate under the patch electrode causing a burn.

Cardiac Pacemakers and Implanted Defibrillators

Guidelines for endoscopic electrosurgery in the presence of cardiac pacemakers and implanted defibrillators have been published by the American Society for Gastrointestinal Endoscopy (ASGE).[20] Electrosurgical units should be used with caution in patients with these devices. Although there have been no reports of serious adverse events in endoscopic applications, monopolar electrosurgical energy in urology and general surgery has been reported to cause pacemaker dysfunction, especially in older pacemakers. In short, the electrical current flowing through the body could be misinterpreted by an implanted defibrillator as a tachyarrhythmia, leading to an unnecessary shock, or could interfere with pacemaker sensing. General principles for the use of electrosurgery in the presence of a permanent pacemaker are as follows:

1. Power delivery should be kept to short bursts (<1 second) with at least 5 seconds between each activation.
2. Try to keep the path from active electrode to return pad distant from the permanent pacemaker and its leads.
3. If possible, consider using bipolar circuitry or a heater probe.
4. Permanent pacemakers can be put into a safe default mode by placing a strong magnet over the pacemaker box for the duration of the procedure.

5. The patient should have continuous electrocardiogram (ECG) monitoring during the procedure.

Implanted defibrillators should be turned off for the duration of the procedure, and the patient should have continuous ECG monitoring during the procedure.

Deep brain electrode stimulation is increasingly used for refractory Parkinson's disease. Although no adverse effects with electrosurgery have been reported, manufacturers and neurologists are very reluctant to allow patients to have any monopolar electrosurgery. There is a single case report of severe lancinating pain experienced by a patient with one of these devices while undergoing dermatologic surgery with a monopolar instrument.[21]

Endoscopic Electrosurgical Techniques

Biliary and Pancreatic Sphincterotomy

Transpapillary division of the biliary sphincter has become a routine part of endoscopic retrograde cholangiopancreatography (ERCP) to facilitate biliary access, remove calculi, improve drainage in biliary dyskinesia, prevent biliary stenosis after ampullectomy, and aid in stent placement. Sphincterotomies are done using monopolar current. Most sphincterotomies are performed using a "pull" type of sphincterotome. The tip of the instrument has an exposed wire (20 to 30 mm) that forms a bow with the catheter when a handle is tightened; this puts tension between the cutting wire and the roof of the papilla. Only the tip of the exposed wire is used for cutting (to increase current density and improve operator control of the incision). Most procedures are wire guided, that is, with a shielded guidewire in the bile duct to ensure that the pancreatic duct is not inadvertently incised.

Cutting may be performed with either pure-cut (100% duty cycle) or blended (approximately 50% duty cycle) current. Use of pure-cut current results in a more rapid incision with less edema of surrounding tissues but less hemostasis. Several studies have shown reduced risk of pancreatitis in patients having pure-cut sphincterotomy compared with coag current.[22,23] As would be expected with less coagulation, increased mild hemorrhage is seen, but this does not translate into clinically significant bleeding.[22,23] However, because of the potential for less control of a rapid incision with pure-cut current, great care must be taken with this current output. As mentioned earlier, new generators automatically switch between cut and coag settings or interrupted pulses of cut current alone during the course of the incision. As with colonic polypectomy, excessive tissue desiccation should be avoided because this may lead to stalling of the incision.

Needle-Knife Sphincterotomy

Needle-knife sphincterotomy employs a fine, stiff wire projecting approximately 5 mm beyond the tip of a catheter. This type of sphincterotomy is used to cut a pathway into the bile duct and is usually reserved for cases of failed cannulation in which biliary access is of particular importance.

Complications of Sphincterotomy—Link with Electrosurgery

Common complications of endoscopic sphincterotomy include pancreatitis, hemorrhage, and perforation. Each complication may be influenced by the type of current used.

PANCREATITIS

Acute pancreatitis is the most common complication of endoscopic sphincterotomy, occurring in at least 5% of cases.[24,25] Development of pancreatitis may be partly a function of iatrogenic trauma to the periampullary region. This trauma results in edema and obstruction to pancreatic flow. Post-ERCP pancreatitis may be reduced by the use of pure-cut current instead of the usual blended current.[22]

HEMORRHAGE

Hemorrhage during endoscopic sphincterotomy is due in part to inadequate coagulation effect of tissue during the incision. Mild oozing at the sphincterotomy site at the time of endoscopic sphincterotomy is common, settles spontaneously, and is of no clinical significance. Minor bleeding at the time of sphincterotomy may be more common with pure-cut technique.[22] Significant hemorrhage occurs in 1% to 3% of patients[26] with an associated mortality of less than 1%.[26–28] This hemorrhage is due to incision of a significant vessel, which is partly "bad luck" and sometimes due to poor orientation of the incision, cutting into a diverticulum or overcutting the incision. Arterial bleeding is not prevented by one electrosurgical output versus another. It is believed, however, that a half-incised vessel (the ends of which cannot retract) bleeds much more than a fully cut one, implying that cutting a little more may be useful in this situation.

PERFORATION

Duodenal perforation during endoscopic sphincterotomy is usually the result of a poorly aligned or too long incision beyond the boundaries of the intramural common bile duct. Clinically significant perforation occurs in less than 1% of sphincterotomies.[24,29] The risk of perforation may be 8% in patients with a small papilla and patients with papillary stenosis.[30] Asymptomatic perforation may be more common, possibly occurring in 15% of sphincterotomies.[31] Duodenal perforation may occur during a rapid, uncontrolled cut of the sphincter ("zipper cut"). The occurrence of this type of rapid incision is a function of current delivery to the tissue and operator experience.

Polypectomy

Polypectomy is most commonly used to remove colonic polyps, either in one piece or piecemeal. Polypectomy and other thermal ablative techniques such as hot biopsy and ablation have the potential to cause transmural damage, resulting in either serosal inflammation (postpolypectomy syndrome) or perforation. Perforation occurs in 0.1% to 0.8% of colonoscopic polypectomies.[32,33] Serositis without perforation occurs in 1% of polypectomies[32]; it manifests 6 hours to 5 days after the procedure with pain, fever, and leukocytosis. The right side of the colon is particularly at risk because of its thinner wall.

Immediate hemorrhage occurs in about 1% of polypectomies, and delayed bleeding may occur in 2% of polypectomies.[34] Significant hemorrhage is much more likely when cutting through a thick stalk. Delayed bleeding may occur any time up to 2 weeks after the procedure. From the preceding discussion, it can be seen that sphincterotomy and polypectomy complications may be related partly to either an overrapid, poorly controlled incision or an overdesiccated, poorly progressed incision. Modern generators use bursts of cut alternating with coagulation to progress the incision in a predictable fashion. Microprocessor-controlled feedback varies generator output in response to changes in tissue resistance (i.e., increasing desiccation) to prevent stalling of the incision.

Osmotic sugar preparations (e.g., mannitol) should be avoided because gut fermentation generating hydrogen could cause explosion during colonic electrosurgery. This risk has been greatly reduced with the introduction of nonfermentable preparations. Nonetheless, to reduce risk of explosion further, preparation should be optimized to reduce fecal residue and colonic gas (i.e., hydrogen and methane). Explosion has also been reported with the use of APC of the rectum after enema preparation.[35–37] If cautery must be performed on an unprepared colon, effort to exchange the gas in the colon with repeated insufflation and suction should be undertaken. Carbon dioxide (CO_2) insufflation, mainly used for patient comfort, may reduce the risk of gas ignition further.

Hot Biopsy Forceps

HBF have been a popular means of removing diminutive polyps for many years.[38] HBF employs monopolar circuitry.

Blended or coagulation current should be used, at a relatively low setting and applied only until blanching of the tissue occurs (1 to 2 seconds). The bowel should be deflated before power application, and care must be taken not to touch other parts of the bowel wall with the cups while coagulating. Postpolypectomy syndrome, perforation, and significant bleeding all have been reported after removal of diminutive polyps using HBF.[38] This technique is relatively poor at removing all polyp tissue.[39]

Cold Snare Technique

Chopping polyps off without using any thermal energy has been advocated for polyps less than 5 mm.[40,41] The technique is fast, but, more importantly, it does not leave a significant thermal ulcer, which may take 2 weeks to heal. This technique has particular appeal for patients requiring anticoagulation after the procedure.

Summary

There are a variety of indications for electrosurgery throughout the gastrointestinal tract for cutting or ablating tissue. All of these techniques involve manageable risks of perforation or hemorrhage. New devices, techniques, and generators intended to reduce these risks do not replace the responsibility of the clinician to have a working knowledge of the principles underlying the tools in use.

References

The complete reference list is available online at www.expertconsult.com.

Chapter 7

Sedation and Monitoring in Endoscopy

Matthew R. Banks, George J. M. Webster, and Liang H. Wee

Introduction

Sedative and analgesic drugs are frequently used to facilitate endoscopic procedures. The principal aim of sedation is to maintain a cooperative patient so that the endoscopic procedure can be completed effectively and safely. The potential benefits of sedation can be realized in terms of patient satisfaction and the efficiency of the procedure. Sedation is associated with potential problems, however. Sedation-related complications have been implicated in more than 50% of all reported endoscopic complications and include aspiration, oversedation, hypoventilation, and airway obstruction.[1,2] Sedation has time, cost, and staffing implications in terms of additional monitoring and recovery. With these issues in mind, there have been studies and expressed opinion in favor of unsedated endoscopy, with attempts at selecting tolerant patients (see Chapter 10).[3-6] The practice of unsedated endoscopy varies greatly geographically and culturally; rates are particularly low in the United States.[7]

When using sedation, several factors may influence the class of sedative, the depth of sedation, and the necessary level of anesthetic expertise present during the procedure. These factors include the length and complexity of the procedure, the degree of discomfort expected or experienced, and patient comorbidity. Patients vary in their sensitivity to sedation and their tolerance of endoscopy. The level of sedation may be broadly considered on a spectrum from no sedation to general anesthesia (Table 7.1). The most frequently used level in endoscopic procedures is conscious sedation, whereby the patient is able to make purposeful responses to verbal or tactile stimuli and with ventilatory and cardiovascular functions maintained. This level of sedation is normally achieved with a benzodiazepine alone or combined with an opiate. There has been an increase in the use of deep sedation, most commonly with propofol.

This chapter discusses all aspects of sedation and patient safety. Patient evaluation and risk assessment, presedation preparation, and issues of consent are discussed. The attributes of sedative drugs are discussed in the context of level of sedation and monitoring required.

Patient Evaluation and Preparation

Appropriate preprocedural evaluation of the patient's history and physical findings reduces the risk of adverse outcomes (see

Table 7.1 **Levels of Sedation**	
Level 1: Minimal sedation	Drug-induced state, during which patient responds normally to verbal commands. Cognitive function and coordination may be impaired. Ventilatory and cardiovascular function are unaffected
Level 2: Conscious sedation	Drug-induced depression of consciousness, during which patient responds purposefully to verbal commands, either alone or accompanied by light tactile stimulation. Patent airway is maintained without help. Spontaneous ventilation is adequate, and cardiovascular function is usually maintained
Level 3: Deep sedation	Drug-induced depression of consciousness, during which patient cannot be easily aroused but responds purposefully to repeated or painful stimulation. Patient may require assistance maintaining an airway. Spontaneous ventilation may be inadequate, and cardiovascular function is maintained
Level 4: General anesthesia	Patient is not able to be aroused even by painful stimuli. Patient often requires assistance in maintaining patent airway. Positive-pressure ventilation may be required owing to respiratory depression or neuromuscular blockade. Cardiovascular function may be impaired

From Bryson HM, Fulton BR, Faulds D: Propofol: an update of its use in anesthesia and conscious sedation. Drugs 50:513–559, 1995.

Table 7.2 **Definition of American Society of Anesthesiologists Status**	
Class 1	Patient has no organic, physiologic, biochemical, or psychiatric disturbance. Pathologic process for which operation is to be performed is localized and does not entail systemic disturbance
Class 2	Mild to moderate systemic disturbance caused either by the condition to be treated surgically or by other pathophysiologic processes
Class 3	Severe systemic disturbance or disease from whatever cause; it may be impossible to define degree of disability with finality
Class 4	Severe systemic disorders that are already life-threatening, not always correctable by operation
Class 5	Moribund patient who has little chance of survival but is submitted to operation in desperation

Chapter 8).[8] The clinicians responsible for sedation should familiarize themselves with specific and relevant aspects of the medical history, including abnormalities of major organ systems, previous adverse experience with sedation and analgesia, current medications and drug allergies, time of the last oral intake, and history of alcohol or recreational drug use. A thorough physical examination is required particularly to assess the heart and lungs in addition to the airway. It may be useful to consider the patient in terms of the American Society of Anesthesiologists (ASA) status classification (**Table 7.2**). There is usually no indication to perform laboratory tests, unless particular concern is raised during assessment.

Although there are no data to support the provision of information about sedatives to patients, counseling may improve patient satisfaction. Patients undergoing sedation should be informed of the benefits, risks, and limitations associated with sedation and possible alternatives. This process should be part of the patient consent. Patients' expectations regarding the discomfort they are likely to experience while sedated during the procedure should be realistic and as accurate as possible.

Procedural Monitoring

Patients undergoing endoscopic procedures should have continuous monitoring before, during, and after the administration of sedatives.[9] Monitoring should be discontinued only when the patient is fully awake. The literature and medical opinion suggest that continuous recording of the patient's level of consciousness, respiratory function, and hemodynamics reduces the risk of sedation-related adverse outcomes.[8] Early detection of adverse events induced by sedatives, such as hypoxemia and cardiovascular compromise, allows intervention to prevent life-threatening complications. Each of the parameters monitored is addressed.

Level of Consciousness

Decreasing level of consciousness is associated with loss of reflexes that normally protect the airway and prevent hypoventilation. The response of patients to commands during sedation serves as a guide to their level of consciousness (see **Table 7.1**). Spoken responses also provide an indication that the patient is breathing. During procedures in which verbal responses are impossible, such as upper gastrointestinal (GI) endoscopy, other responses should be sought, including hand movements or a nod of the head. Lack of response to verbal or tactile stimuli suggests a greater level of sedation and should be treated accordingly.

Pulmonary Ventilation

Respiratory depression is probably the central event in sedation-related complications, and monitoring of ventilatory function reduces the risk of adverse outcomes. Ventilatory function can be monitored by observation of respiratory movement or by direct pulmonary auscultation. If ventilatory function cannot be observed, transcutaneous carbon dioxide (CO_2) and end-tidal CO_2 can be measured by capnography. Capnography measures CO_2 indirectly by light absorption in the infrared region of the electromagnetic spectrum. If a patient's ventilation is compromised, CO_2 retention occurs, which is identified as an early event on capnography often before oxygen desaturation.[10] Unless the breathing system is a closed circuit, the exact measurement of CO_2 is inaccurate. The presence of a CO_2 trace on capnography is reassuring that the patient is still breathing, however. Alternatively, respiratory activity can be continuously measured graphically using expired air CO_2 detectors.[11] This method can detect the early phases of respiratory depression. No studies have addressed whether capnography improves outcome in patients with conscious sedation.

Pulse Oximetry

Pulse oximetry is a noninvasive method of measuring oxygen saturation from a light signal transmitted through tissue, taking into account the pulsatile volume changes that occur. The probes differentiate the absorption of incidental light by the pulsatile arterial component from the static component—hence the term pulse oximeters. The pulse oximeter estimates the oxygen saturation by measuring the pulsatile signals across perfused tissue at two distinct wavelengths, which allows the differentiation of reduced hemoglobin and oxyhemoglobin. Oxyhemoglobin absorbs light in the infrared band, whereas reduced hemoglobin absorbs light in the red band. The functional oxygen saturation is defined as the ratio of oxyhemoglobin to all functional hemoglobins. The oxyhemoglobin dissociation curve is sigmoid, which limits the degree of desaturation that can be tolerated. Between 90% and 100% saturation, the partial pressure of arterial oxygen is maintained at a high level; however, at less than 90%, the curve becomes steeper, and small decreases in the oxygen saturation correspond to large decreases in partial pressure.

Various probes are available; however, the most commonly used probe is a reusable one for use on fingers or toes. Pulse oximetry in sedated patients has been shown to improve assessment of respiratory status.[12] The routine use of pulse oximetry in unsedated endoscopy is not always indicated, however.[13] Although oximetry is not a substitute for monitoring ventilatory function, hypoxemia is more likely to be detected using oximetry in addition to clinical assessment. Pulse oximeter probes occasionally detect peripheral oxygen saturation poorly, however, resulting in a falsely low or absent oxygen saturation reading. Failure rates have been shown to be 7%,[14] although the accepted error is 3% when compared with arterial blood gases.[15] Failure is more common in patients who are ASA class 3 and higher, patients with hypertension or hypotension, patients with hypothermia, patients with pigmented skin, elderly patients, and patients with renal failure. Pulse oximeters require adequate pulsations to distinguish arterial blood light absorption from venous blood and tissue light absorption. The reading may be unreliable or absent if there is loss or diminution of the peripheral pulse; this may occur with blood pressure cuff inflation, improper positioning, hypothermia, hypotension, and peripheral vascular disease. Although the response time of the pulse oximeter is fast, there may be a significant delay in the alveolar oxygen tension and change in oximeter reading.[16]

Some shades of nail polish may cause significantly lower saturation readings. This problem can be overcome by placing the probe across the finger rather than from nail to finger dorsum. False alarms frequently occur during continuous monitoring and are usually due to motion artifact. Poor signal quality and sensor displacement are also common and can be avoided by changing position of the probe or warming a limb to improve circulation. Other maneuvers to reduce false alarms include delaying the time between detection of a low oxygen saturation and alarm activation, although this may lead to a delay in resuscitation in the event of a true alarm. Pulse oximetry is a valuable monitor because endoscopic procedures are performed with dim ambient light, which makes clinical assessment of a patient's oxygenation difficult. Most patients undergoing an endoscopic procedure under sedation have supplemental oxygen administered. Their saturations remain at a normal level despite having profound respiratory depression, and this needs to be borne in mind.

Hemodynamic Measurements

Sedative agents and analgesics may have mild direct effects on hemodynamic control, such as hypotension and cardiovascular response to stress. These changes can be detected by regular measurement of pulse and blood pressure. Changes in blood pressure and pulse may represent responses to hypoxemia, oversedation, or possibly patient distress to procedure-induced pain. Although no evidence shows that blood pressure monitoring during endoscopy influences morbidity and mortality, it has been suggested that both regular blood pressure measurements and pulse be measured throughout procedures performed under sedation.[17] There is wide geographic variation in this practice, however. Continuous electrocardiogram (ECG) monitoring should be considered in high-risk patients, such as patients with disturbances in cardiac rhythm or ischemic heart disease. The necessity for ECG monitoring has not been shown in clinical trials.

Supplemental Oxygen

Oxygen given via nasal cannulas or via a mask has been shown to reduce oxygen desaturation during endoscopy performed under sedation[18,19] and should be given to all patients receiving sedation. However, because supplemental oxygen delays the onset of hypoxemia in sedated patients who are hypoventilating, it is important not to rely solely on oximetry to monitor ventilation but to employ additional techniques, including assessment of respiratory rate.

Intravenous Access

In patients receiving intravenous sedatives, intravascular access should be maintained throughout the procedure until the patient is no longer at risk from cardiopulmonary or respiratory depression. Immediate access is available for administration of reversal agents in the event of oversedation or emergency drugs in the event of arrhythmias. In patients who are receiving sedatives via nonintravascular routes (e.g., pediatric patients undergoing endoscopic procedures), intravenous access should also be obtained if the patient is likely to have any cardiopulmonary depression.

Sedation and Consent

There are two issues surrounding consent and sedation. The first is that the patient should be fully informed of the indications, risks, and alternatives to sedation. The second is whether the patient while under sedation is able to withdraw consent. If a sedated patient indicates during endoscopy that he or she wishes the procedure to be terminated, should the clinician complete the procedure or stop, given it may be in the patient's best interests to complete it? In a study, 88% of colonoscopists stated that they would stop only after repeated requests by the sedated patient, and only 45% of colonoscopists thought patients were capable of making rational decisions while under sedation.[20] From the patient's perspective, opinion is evenly divided into terminating the examination immediately or completing.

Staffing Levels and Training

A clinician performing a procedure is unable to observe and assess fully the patient under sedation. Another individual should be available to monitor the patient's status in terms of conscious level, ventilatory function, and hemodynamic parameters. The presence of another individual is likely to improve patient comfort and satisfaction. Several areas of expertise are required while managing sedated patients, including knowledge of administered drugs and management of adverse events. All staff members administering sedative drugs should be familiar with the pharmacology of all drugs used. In particular, staff members should be aware of the time to onset of action, elimination half-life, interactions, adverse reactions, contraindications, and pharmacology of appropriate antagonists.

Specific areas of concern include the potentiation of sedative-induced respiratory depression by concomitantly administered opioids and benzodiazepines and inadequate time intervals between doses of sedatives. Individuals monitoring sedated patients should be able to recognize complications associated with the sedative drugs. Given that most complications associated with sedatives are cardiopulmonary, at least one individual should be familiar with advanced airway and ventilation management. Failing this, guidelines recommend an advanced resuscitation provider be immediately available in the event of an emergency.[8] Resuscitation equipment must be readily available and should include a cardiac defibrillator, advanced airway and positive-pressure ventilation equipment, and all the appropriate drugs including sedative antagonists (**Box 7.1**).[8]

Postprocedural Monitoring

After completion of the procedure, the patient is still at risk of sedative-related complications. The risk of upper airway obstruction and hypoxemia after significant conscious sedation for endoscopic retrograde cholangiopancreatography (ERCP) seems to be greatest immediately after removal of the endoscope. Monitoring should continue until the patient has reached an acceptable level of consciousness, with normal ventilation, oxygenation, and hemodynamic parameters. Before discharge of the patient, although the patient's conscious level seems normal, it should be recognized that there may be a prolonged period of amnesia with impairment of cognition and judgment. Patients may also be mildly dehydrated, especially after colonoscopy, and fluid replacement should be addressed. After an outpatient procedure, the following instructions apply for 24 hours after discharge:

- Patients should not drive.
- Patients should not operate heavy or dangerous machinery.

> **Box 7.1 Appropriate Emergency Equipment to Have Available When Using Sedative or Analgesic Drugs Capable of Causing Cardiorespiratory Depression**
>
> **Intravenous Equipment**
> - Gloves
> - Tourniquets
> - Alcohol wipes
> - Sterile gauze
> - Intravenous cannulas
> - Intravenous tubing
> - Intravenous fluids
> - Needles and syringes
>
> **Basic Airway Management Equipment**
> - Source of oxygen
> - Suction
> - Suction catheters (Yankauer catheters)
> - Face masks
> - Self-inflating breathing bag valve mask set
> - Oral and nasal airways (Guedel)
>
> **Advanced Airway Management Equipment**
> - Laryngoscope handles and blades
> - Endotracheal tubes
> - Stylet
>
> **Pharmacologic Antagonists**
> - Flumazenil
> - Naloxone
>
> **Emergency Medications**
> - Epinephrine
> - Ephedrine
> - Atropine
> - Lidocaine
> - Glucose (50%)
> - Diphenhydramine
> - Hydrocortisone and methylprednisolone
> - Diazepam or midazolam
>
> *From Practice guidelines for sedation and analgesia by non-anesthesiologists: A report by the American Society of Anesthesiologists Task Force on sedation and analgesia by non-anesthesiologists. Anesthesiology 84:459–471, 1996.*

- Patients should not sign any legally binding documents.
- Patients should arrange escort home with an able companion.
- Patients should be given written instructions regarding the signs and symptoms of any adverse outcomes of the procedure and contact numbers for 24-hour advice.

In a placebo-controlled study, the benzodiazepine antagonist flumazenil was shown to enhance recovery from sedation and amnesia without any risk of resedation.[21] Use of flumazenil increases the expense of the procedure, but it may be preferable to patients. Use of flumazenil does not preclude the need for postprocedural monitoring, and the advantages of routine use may be negligible and are as yet unproven.

Drugs for Sedation

Characteristics of an ideal sedative agent include the following:

- Rapid onset of action
- Practical means of delivery
- Short half-life with rapid recovery
- Safe with predictable sedative response (pharmacodynamics)
- Minimal or no cardiovascular or respiratory effects
- Effective, producing a calm, pain-free, cooperative patient

The most commonly used drugs are benzodiazepines used alone or in combination with an opiate. It is vital that clinicians become familiar with some specific sedatives (e.g., either pethidine or fentanyl). More recently, propofol has been used as an agent to induce deep sedation. The benzodiazepines midazolam and diazepam are frequently used and have been found to have similar efficacy.[22,23] Midazolam is a more attractive agent because of its rapid onset of action, short half-life, and amnestic properties. Fentanyl, meperidine, and pethidine are the most commonly used opiates, with fentanyl preferred because of its rapid action and absence of nausea.

A combination of a benzodiazepine and an opiate is frequently used in endoscopy, although this may lead to a greater incidence of sedation-related complications.[24] In colonoscopy, opiates combined with benzodiazepines are frequently used, but their combined use has not been shown to be more efficacious than benzodiazepines alone. Combination therapy in colonoscopy and upper GI endoscopy does not seem to improve pain and tolerance compared with individual agents.[24–26] The literature generally suggests that administration of intravenous sedatives or analgesics is achieved safely by giving small incremental doses until the desired level of sedation is attained, rather than giving a single dose based on patient weight. The drug should be titrated with sufficient time elapsed between doses to allow for the full effect of each dose to be assessed before subsequent drug administration. Although not based on evidence, it has been suggested that opiate drugs are administered before benzodiazepines to titrate the latter carefully because of their greater sedative effects.

Droperidol has been used in the sedation of agitated patients. However, it is associated with hypotension and a prolonged recovery period. The U.S. Food and Drug Administration (FDA) has issued a warning following droperidol-induced cardiac arrhythmias. Nitrous oxide has been used as a form of patient-controlled analgesia in several studies involving colonoscopy.[27,28] Potential benefits include an absence of sedation-related risks and a rapid recovery. In terms of patient tolerance, the studies were inconsistent showing no or reduced benefit compared with traditional sedation.

Propofol and Deep Sedation

In certain circumstances, standard conscious sedation is inadequate, and patients may require deep sedation. These circumstances include patients who are not tolerant of endoscopy under conscious sedation and procedures that are painful, prolonged, or complex, such as ERCP and endoscopic ultrasound. Deep sedation can be achieved with benzodiazepine and narcotic combinations. Droperidol, diphenhydramine, and promethazine all have been combined with benzodiazepines and narcotics to potentiate the sedative effects to achieve deep sedation.

Propofol is increasingly used for GI endoscopy because of its rapid onset, rapid recovery, and attainable depth of sedation. Propofol is an anesthetic agent with a rapid onset of action, amnestic properties, and a very short context-sensitive half-life of 2 to 8 minutes, rendering it an attractive agent for endoscopic procedures. Patients who regularly use sedatives and narcotics are often insensitive to standard benzodiazepine sedation and may benefit from propofol sedation. There are disadvantages associated with propofol use, however. Because of its short context-sensitive half-life, propofol must be continuously titrated to maintain sedation. The narrow therapeutic window between conscious sedation, deep sedation, and anesthesia necessitates close monitoring. Compared with midazolam, the amnestic properties of propofol are inferior.[29] As a result of peripheral vasodilation and impairment of cardiac contractility, propofol may cause profound hypotension. Propofol causes apnea more readily than midazolam, so managing the airway and breathing is more critical if propofol is used.

Propofol Use in Standard Endoscopic Procedures

Propofol has been compared with midazolam in several trials during standard endoscopic procedures.[30,31] Although the results are inconsistent, propofol seems to improve patient cooperation and reduces recovery time. There does not seem to be any consistent difference in patient tolerance or safety. Because propofol has no analgesic properties, its use in combination with fentanyl has been investigated and compared with standard benzodiazepine and narcotic combinations.[32,33] The results were inconsistent in terms of sedation, analgesia, recovery, and incidence of side effects, suggesting propofol confers no additional benefit over standard sedation regimens.

Propofol Use in Complex Endoscopic Procedures

The use of propofol in complex and prolonged procedures has also been investigated. In a randomized trial, Wehrmann and colleagues[34] compared propofol with midazolam for ERCP and found patient cooperation to be superior and recovery times to be less in the propofol group; however, patient tolerance was the same. A patient in the propofol group required ventilatory support. The benefit of propofol over midazolam was replicated in two other studies for ERCP with endoscopic ultrasound and ERCP with sphincter of Oddi manometry.[35,36]

Nurse-Administered Propofol Sedation

Given the narrow therapeutic window and potential for cardiopulmonary adverse events, many endoscopists favor the expertise of an anesthetist to administer and monitor propofol sedation. Using an anesthetist incurs additional costs, which offsets any cost advantage gained by a more rapid sedation induction and recovery time. There is growing evidence, however, to support the practice of nurse-administered propofol sedation (NAPS). In a study involving a series of 9152 patients given NAPS under the supervision of an endoscopist, NAPS was found to be safe and effective. The nurses were trained and registered to administer and monitor propofol sedation and were not nurse anesthetists. There were seven cases of respiratory compromise (three prolonged apnea, three laryngospasm, one aspiration) associated with upper endoscopy, which required mask ventilation only. The greater frequency of respiratory adverse events with upper endoscopy is probably related to the deeper level of sedation required to prevent reflex gagging. The ideal procedures for administration of NAPS are lower endoscopic procedures, in which adverse complications are particularly low. The colonic perforation rate was less than 1:1000, and patients preferred NAPS over previous experiences with benzodiazepines.[37] In a randomized study comparing NAPS and nurse-administered midazolam for colonoscopy, time to sedation was more rapid with propofol, recovery was faster, and patient satisfaction was improved.[33] NAPS is also cost-effective compared with anesthetist-administered propofol.[35]

Propofol Patient-Controlled Analgesia

Patient-controlled analgesia and sedation (PCS) with propofol has been assessed in several studies. PCS using propofol and alfentanil was compared with diazepam (Diazemuls) and pethidine given as a bolus during colonoscopy in 66 randomly assigned patients. PCS provided lighter sedation, less analgesia, faster recovery, with similar patient satisfaction.[38] In a more recent study, Kulling and associates[39] compared PCS using propofol and alfentanil, continuous infusion, or NAPS and found PCS to exhibit a higher degree of patient satisfaction with faster recovery. Similar results were generated when comparing propofol PCS with midazolam.[40]

Propofol and Patient Monitoring

Patients receiving propofol for procedures probably require more monitoring than patients undergoing conscious sedation, although there is as yet no evidence to support additional monitoring. Preprocedural assessment should include a full history of sedation-related risk factors and airway assessment. Risk factors include conditions such as age extremes, cardiopulmonary disease, hepatic or renal impairment, narcotic or sedative use, and a potentially difficult airway for intubation (**Box 7.2**). Trials of NAPS have selected only patients with ASA status class 1 or 2 for propofol.[37] The ASA Task Force stated that if the patient has one or more sedation-related risk factors, coupled with the potential for deep sedation (with propofol), the incidence of adverse sedation-related events is likely to be high. In these circumstances, an anesthetist should be consulted before the procedure. Vargo and coworkers[11] used capnography to guide propofol titration, allowing respiratory depression to be identified early, although this was not shown to have an impact on outcome.

Pharyngeal Anesthesia in Sedation

Topical anesthetic agents are often used in addition to sedation to suppress the gag reflex and facilitate upper endoscopy. The most frequently use agent is lidocaine, administered as an aerosol spray to the pharynx. Other, less commonly used

---

Box 7.2 American Society of Anesthesiologists Task Force Situations Associated with Difficult Airway Intubation

Patients with previous problems with anesthesia or sedation

Patients with a history of stridor, snoring, or sleep apnea

Patients with dysmorphic facial features, such as Pierre-Robin syndrome or trisomy 21

Patients with oral abnormalities, such as small opening (<3 cm in an adult), edentulous, protruding incisors, loose or capped teeth, high arched palate, macroglossia, tonsillar hypertrophy, or invisible uvula

Patients with neck abnormalities, such as obesity involving the neck and facial structures, short neck, limited neck extension, decreased hyoid-mental distance (<3 cm in an adult), neck mass, cervical spine disease or trauma, tracheal deviation, or advanced rheumatoid arthritis

Patients with jaw abnormalities such as micrognathia, retrognathia, trismus, significant malocclusion

---

agents include tetracaine, cetacaine, and benzocaine. All topical agents induce anesthesia for up to 1 hour with some evidence of impaired pharyngeal coordination. Patients should be advised not to eat or drink until sensation has returned to minimize the potential risk of bronchial aspiration. Data regarding the benefit of pharyngeal anesthesia in addition to sedation are conflicting. Because topical anesthetics have been associated with adverse reactions such as methemoglobinemia, their use should be limited to minimally sedated or unsedated patients.

Management of Oversedation

Sedatives have been implicated in more than 50% of all endoscopy-related complications; the most common adverse reactions are oversedation and respiratory depression. The expected mean desaturation during all sedated endoscopic procedures is about 3% from baseline.[41] The availability of reversal agents for sedative drugs is associated with a decreased risk of sedation-related adverse events. The specific antagonists available include flumazenil for benzodiazepines and naloxone for opioids. No antagonists exist for propofol, although the short context-sensitive half-life lends to a rapid reversal of sedation when the infusion is ceased. The literature supports the use of flumazenil and naloxone individually to reverse benzodiazepine-induced and opioid-induced sedation and ventilatory depression. In patients who have received both a benzodiazepine and an opioid, flumazenil reverses sedation but not respiratory depression. Similarly, naloxone monotherapy has not been shown to reverse respiratory depression induced by opioid and benzodiazepine combinations. In the setting of combination therapy–induced respiratory depression, it is recommended that naloxone is given in addition to flumazenil. At the time of reversal or before reversal, the following should be done:

- Perform basic airway management
  - Clear airway including suction (if appropriate)
  - Jaw thrust maneuver
  - Guedel airway if necessary

- Administer supplemental oxygen or increased oxygen
- Encourage or stimulate deep breaths
- Administer positive-pressure ventilation if spontaneous ventilation is inadequate

Flumazenil and naloxone previously were reserved for the treatment of oversedation and respiratory depression. However, prolonged recovery times associated with the use of benzodiazepines have prompted research into the feasibility of using flumazenil routinely to reduce recovery times with potential cost savings.[21,42]

Unsedated Endoscopy

Because of the risks and additional costs associated with the use of sedative drugs in endoscopy, unsedated endoscopy is increasingly being considered. In particular, the availability of ultrathin endoscopes (5 to 6 mm) has rendered unsedated endoscopy far more attractive. Several studies have shown comparable and improved tolerance using the ultrathin compared with standard endoscopes.[43] The transnasal approach does not seem to be different from the peroral route.[44,45] The benefits of unsedated endoscopy include a reduction in morbidity associated with sedative drugs, reduced patient monitoring, more rapid recovery, less time off work, and reduced cost. The potential disadvantages include poor patient satisfaction, with refusal to undergo repeat procedures; incomplete examination because of patient intolerance; and the inability to perform therapeutic procedures. The refusal rate for upper GI endoscopy remains high.[46]

Patient selection is of paramount importance before unsedated upper endoscopy. Several studies suggested older age, low anxiety scores, tolerance of pharyngeal anesthesia, and tolerance of prior endoscopy were associated with tolerance of unsedated upper endoscopy.[47] The data regarding the benefit of pharyngeal anesthesia in unsedated endoscopy are inconsistent, although the larger studies suggest improvement in patient tolerance and ease of performance.[48] Several studies have shown colonoscopy can be completed successfully without sedation in up to 95% of patients in one series.[49,50] The refusal rate for unsedated colonoscopy can be 83%.[51]

Review of Specific Drugs

Benzodiazepines

Benzodiazepines are central nervous system (CNS) depressants that induce sedation, hypnosis, amnesia, and anesthesia. The mechanism of action seems to intensify the physiologic inhibitory mechanisms mediated by γ-aminobutyric acid (GABA).

Midazolam
PHARMACOLOGY

Midazolam is a short-acting benzodiazepine with an intravenous peak onset of action of 2 to 5 minutes depending on the dose given and level of consciousness attained. If given with an opioid, the onset of action is more rapid (1.5 minutes)

and sedation is deeper, and a dose reduction of 30% is recommended. At doses sufficient to induce sedation, midazolam decreases the ventilatory response to increased CO_2 in normal patients and in specific patients with chronic airway limitation. The pharmacokinetic profile of midazolam is linear over 0.05 to 0.4 mg/kg lending predictable dosage titration. The elimination half-life is 1 to 2.8 hours with a large volume of distribution. The drug is metabolized rapidly to 1-hydroxymethyl midazolam in the liver, conjugated, and secreted in the urine. The elimination half-life is increased in elderly patients and patients with renal failure.

ADMINISTRATION

Midazolam should be titrated in doses of 0.5 to 2 mg at intervals of 2 to 3 minutes to a total dose of 5 mg. Higher doses may be required but should be used with caution.

PRECAUTIONS AND ADVERSE REACTIONS

When given with an opioid analgesic, there is an increased sedative effect necessitating administration in small incremental steps and a usual requirement of a 30% reduction in dose. Sensitivity increases with age. Caution is required when using midazolam in elderly patients, patients with hepatic or renal impairment, and patients with airflow limitation. Owing to a reduced rate of plasma clearance, patients with heart failure eliminate midazolam more slowly. Paradoxic reactions may occur with restlessness, agitation, and disinhibition. Hypotension is a recognized association of midazolam, particularly if given with an opioid.

CONTRAINDICATIONS

Midazolam should not be given to patients with myasthenia gravis, alcohol intoxication, or narrow-angle glaucoma.

INTERACTIONS

The sedative effects of midazolam are enhanced by other CNS depressants, including neuroleptics, alcohol, tranquilizers, antidepressants, analgesics, antiepileptics, and anxiolytics. The effects of midazolam are attenuated by drugs that induce cytochrome P450 (rifampicin, carbamazepine, and phenytoin) and enhanced by inhibitors (erythromycin, diltiazem, antiviral agents, and fluconazole). In particular, midazolam should be given with care in patients receiving combination antiretroviral therapy.

Diazepam
PHARMACOLOGY

Diazepam is metabolized in the liver to the active metabolites temazepam, nordiazepam, and oxazepam, all of which are renally excreted. Plasma concentrations of diazepam and its active metabolites exhibit considerable interpatient variation. The intravenous plasma time curve is biphasic, with an initial rapid increase with a half-life of up to 3 hours and a second elimination phase with a half-life of 20 to 70 hours. The elimination half-life is increased in elderly patients and in patients with renal and hepatic impairment.

ADMINISTRATION

Diazepam should be titrated in doses of 2 to 4 mg to a total of 10 to 20 mg in some circumstances.

PRECAUTIONS AND ADVERSE REACTIONS

Caution is required in patients with renal, hepatic, and cardiopulmonary impairment. Hypotension occurs rarely. Other precautions, contraindications, and drug interactions are similar to midazolam.

Opioid Analgesics
Fentanyl
PHARMACOLOGY

Fentanyl is a synthetic opioid with an estimated 80-fold greater potency than morphine. In contrast to other opioids, fentanyl does not induce histamine release. After intravenous injection, fentanyl reaches peak analgesic effects within 1 to 2 minutes, with a duration of 30 to 60 minutes. Serum concentrations decrease rapidly within 5 minutes to 20% of peak concentrations, followed by a slow decrease over 30 minutes. The drug is metabolized in the liver to active metabolites, all of which are excreted in the urine.

ADMINISTRATION

A dose of 50 to 100 μg should be given before benzodiazepine, to enable accurate sedative dose titration.

PRECAUTIONS AND ADVERSE REACTIONS

Fentanyl causes respiratory depression for periods extending beyond the analgesic effect. In light of the elimination, a reduced dose should be used in hepatic and renal impairment. In view of the marked respiratory depression, caution is required in patients with pulmonary disease.

CONTRAINDICATIONS

Fentanyl may cause severe bronchospasm and is contraindicated in asthma. Fentanyl may cause severe muscle rigidity and is contraindicated in patients with myasthenia gravis.

INTERACTIONS

The sedative effect of fentanyl is enhanced by other CNS depressants, such as other opioids, benzodiazepines, alcohol, neuroleptics, and tranquilizers. In particular, fentanyl has been associated with hypotensive adverse events with monoamine oxidase inhibitors and neuroleptics.

Pethidine
PHARMACOLOGY

Pethidine is a synthetic opioid with sedative and analgesic properties. Similar to other narcotics, pethidine causes respiratory depression and suppresses the cough reflex. The sedative and analgesic effects of pethidine after intravenous dosing occur within 2 to 4 minutes, and the analgesic effects can last

4 hours. The elimination half-life is 3.2 hours, and metabolism is predominantly hepatic conjugation. Pethidine elimination is prolonged in patients with hepatic impairment.

PRECAUTIONS AND ADVERSE REACTIONS

Care should be taken when giving pethidine concurrently with other neurodepressants. The most common adverse reaction is respiratory depression. Pethidine may also result in profound hypotension. One active pethidine metabolite, norpethidine, has convulsant properties, and elimination is prolonged in patients with renal impairment and elderly patients. In these patients, high doses of pethidine may lead to convulsions, agitation, irritability, and tremors.

ADMINISTRATION

Pethidine should be given at an intravenous dose of 25 to 50 mg. Higher doses are more likely to result in adverse events.

DRUG INTERACTIONS

The sedative effects of neurodepressants all are potentiated by pethidine. In addition, when given with phenothiazines, CNS toxicity and hypotension may occur. Interactions with monoamine oxidase inhibitors may be fatal and result in excitation, sweating, rigidity, hypertension or hypotension, and coma.

Propofol
PHARMACOLOGY

Propofol is distributed rapidly and induces sedation within 30 to 60 seconds. The context-sensitive half-life is only 2 to 8 minutes. Metabolism is by hepatic conjugation with renal excretion of inactive metabolites. Propofol is a centrally acting neural depressant without any analgesic properties and rapidly crosses the blood-brain barrier to potentiate GABA activity.

CONTRAINDICATIONS

Propofol is contraindicated in patients with known allergy to propofol.

PRECAUTIONS AND ADVERSE REACTIONS

The most important effect to be monitored with propofol is respiratory depression and apnea, occurring frequently with deep sedation. Hypotension is also common. Patients with ASA class 3 or higher, elderly patients, and patients using sedatives or opioid agents are at particular high risk for developing these cardiorespiratory complications. Apnea and hypotension can occur in 75% of patients. In endoscopic trials using propofol, ventilatory support was necessary in 10% of patients, although incidence of respiratory depression necessitating support was far greater in complex procedures requiring a cooperative patient.[34] Excitatory phenomena such as tremors, twitches, hypertonus, and hiccups can occur in 14%. Rarely, pulmonary edema, hypertension, cardiac arrhythmias, bronchospasm, and laryngospasm have occurred. Pain at the injection site is the most frequent local complication and occurs in 5% to 50% or more of patients.[52]

ADMINISTRATION

Propofol has been given in endoscopic studies by repeated bolus injections or as an infusion. Propofol is usually administered as an initial bolus dose of 20 to 40 mg followed by maintenance doses of 10 to 20 mg to attain the required level of sedation. Alternatively, propofol can be infused at a dose of 0.5 to 1.0 mg/kg over 1 to 5 minutes to induce deep sedation, followed by maintenance infusion at a dose of 1.5 to 3 mg/kg/hr. For anything other than very short procedures, administration of propofol as an infusion is preferable because this produces better steady-state levels and more stable operating conditions.

INTERACTIONS

The sedative effect of propofol is enhanced by other sedative agents and analgesics, when dose requirements are reduced.

Flumazenil
PHARMACOLOGY

Flumazenil is an imidazobenzodiazepine and antagonizes benzodiazepines through competitively inhibiting central receptors. Its effects are rapid within 30 to 60 seconds, and it has an elimination half-life of 53 minutes. Clearance is entirely hepatic, where it is conjugated to form inactive metabolites.

CONTRAINDICATIONS

Flumazenil should not be given to patients with known sensitivity to flumazenil.

PRECAUTIONS AND ADVERSE REACTIONS

Care should be taken when administering flumazenil to patients with known benzodiazepine dependence because this may precipitate withdrawal or convulsions. Consideration should be given to the possibility of resedation and respiratory depression following the use of flumazenil. Patients should be monitored for an appropriate period based on the dose and duration of effect of the benzodiazepine used. Despite the use of reversal agents, patients should still be given postprocedural warnings as previously described. Flumazenil is not recommended in epileptic patients taking benzodiazepines because this may give rise to convulsions. Seizures have been reported in patients with epilepsy and hepatic impairment.

INTERACTIONS

Flumazenil also blocks the effects of nonbenzodiazepines acting on benzodiazepine receptors such as zopiclone.

ADMINISTRATION

The recommended initial dose is 0.2 mg administered intravenously over 15 seconds. This dose can be repeated using 0.1-mg doses every 60 seconds to achieve reversal to a total dose of 2 mg.

Naloxone
PHARMACOLOGY

Naloxone is a competitive antagonist at opiate receptor sites and can reverse the sedative and respiratory effects of opiates. The effects of intravenous naloxone are apparent within 2 minutes, and a single dose from an ampule of 0.2 mg lasts 20 to 30 minutes. The effects of pethidine and other opioids last longer than this, so repeated doses of naloxone may need to be given. Naloxone is conjugated in the liver with renal excretion of the metabolites. Elimination half-life is 60 to 90 minutes.

CONTRAINDICATIONS

Naloxone should not be administered to patients with known hypersensitivity.

PRECAUTIONS AND ADVERSE REACTIONS

Care is required in patients who are dependent on opiates because naloxone can precipitate withdrawal syndrome. A rapid reversal of opioids can induce catecholamine release and cause excitation, ventricular arrhythmias, hypotension, pulmonary edema, convulsions, and death. Care should be used in patients with preexisting cardiac abnormalities.

ADMINISTRATION

Naloxone can be given intravenously or intramuscularly at an initial dose of 0.4 to 2 mg. Doses can be repeated at 2- to 3-minute intervals until a total dose of 10 mg is reached.

References

The complete reference list is available online at www.expertconsult.com.

Chapter 8

Patient Preparation and Pharmacotherapeutic Considerations

Mark Schoeman and Nam Q. Nguyen

Introduction

Correct patient preparation is essential for all endoscopic procedures because it contributes significantly to the safety and success of the procedure. Many requirements must be considered during the preparatory phase; patient preparation is not limited to statements regarding fasting or how to complete a bowel preparation. The clinician must consider issues such as timing and patient-specific factors that must be taken into account when preparing for an endoscopic procedure. If the patient has had this type of information explained, he or she is more likely to comply with preparation instructions in a safe manner. As part of this phase and as part of the explanation about what the procedure involves, it is also necessary to explain potential risks and complications. All of this communication with the patient contributes to the process of obtaining informed consent, which is a crucial part of the preparation process.

Informed Consent

The process of informed consent varies from country to country. In many parts of Europe, a formal consent is not required before endoscopic examinations. If the patient comes to have the procedure performed, these systems assume an implied consent. In other parts of the world, such as the United States and Australia, the consent process is a very detailed and potentially complex process that requires considerable attention by the endoscopist (see Chapter 9).

General Information about Patient Preparation

Numerous aspects must be considered when preparing patients for endoscopic examinations, including the following:

- Understanding of the patient's particular clinical problem
- Awareness of the patient's clinical history
- Knowledge of the patient's recent (and past) medication history
- Requirements of procedure-specific preparation
- Requirements of patient-specific preparation
- Informed consent
- Postprocedure observation and discharge planning

The endoscopist must have knowledge of the indication for the procedure because this determines not only what procedure is performed but also what interventions or treatment might be required during the procedure. Implicit also is an understanding of the patient's clinical history and the results of any recent investigations. The preprocedure assessment must extend to the patient's past medical and surgical history, previous endoscopy results, current medical therapy (including over-the-counter and intermittent medications), and drug allergies. Specific clinical history such as diabetes, a personal or family history of bleeding disorder, anesthetic reactions, or previous adverse reactions to other medical interventions (including reactions to radiologic contrast agents) should also be considered. Armed with this information, the endoscopist is able to determine the proper preparation and any specific modifications that might be required for the individual patient (see Chapter 7).

After the procedure preparation, risks, and potential complications have been discussed, the next phase of the explanatory process is to discuss discharge guidelines. Most endoscopic examinations are performed as day procedures, and frequently patient sedation is administered. Most institutions require that sedated patients are discharged in the care of a responsible person who not only can supervise transportation of the patient home but who also is able to respond to any delayed complications or difficulties. The level of postprocedure supervision depends on the type of intervention and sedation, specific patient factors such as mobility and age, and such things as geographic isolation. These issues must be brought to the patient's attention before the procedure so that proper planning can occur. Difficulties with discharge arrangements should always be resolved before the endoscopic procedure and never left to be discussed after the procedure has been performed. Although the previous process may seem cumbersome, there are significant advantages for the patient and the endoscopist, such as the following:

- Ability to obtain informed consent
- Proper patient preparation
- Greater patient confidence with preparation
- Decreased failure of patient to attend endoscopic examination
- Correct procedure being performed
- Improved diagnostic yield
- Decreased patient anxiety and potentially improved patient tolerance of the procedure
- Improved discharge outcome

Preparation for Endoscopy and Enteroscopy

Patients should not eat solid food for 6 hours or drink fluids for at least 4 hours before an elective endoscopy.[1] If a delay in gastric emptying is known or suspected, longer fasting or a period of a fluid-only diet should be considered. Many centers use prokinetic agents to speed gastric emptying in patients when fasting time is inadequate (see subsequent section on special circumstances). In situations in which there is a delay in gastric emptying or in which there is inadequate fasting time, there is a significant risk of pulmonary aspiration, and airway protection with airway intubation should be considered. Normally, it is acceptable for patients to take their usual medicines with a sip of water before endoscopy. Special consideration must be given to patients taking anticoagulant medication or medication to treat diabetes (see separate section).

No data support routine blood tests before diagnostic endoscopy, and screening tests are not required. If a bleeding disorder is suspected or known, tests to evaluate this and direct therapy are indicated. Similarly, if the patient's clinical condition is unstable or indicates that an abnormality in the blood tests is likely to be present, appropriate testing and correction of relevant abnormalities is indicated. Preparation for antegrade enteroscopy is the same as described earlier. If retrograde enteroscopy is to be performed, preparation requirements are the same as for colonoscopy.

Preparation for Endoscopic Retrograde Cholangiopancreatography

The preparation of patients for endoscopic retrograde cholangiopancreatography (ERCP) is similar to the preparation for endoscopy.[1] Generally, patients undergoing ERCP almost always require sedation, and the duration of the procedure is longer; this should be taken into account for purposes of discharge planning. Patients with suspected or proven biliary or pancreatic duct obstruction generally are given prophylactic intravenous antibiotics if there is a clinical suspicion of inadequate duct drainage. Antibiotics may also be given in patients with sclerosing cholangitis and in patients after liver transplantation. Before ERCP, it is important to determine if the patient has a known history of reaction to iodinated contrast agents. Although reaction to the contrast agent in allergic patients during ERCP is rare, it is generally considered appropriate to administer prophylactic steroids, often in combination with an intravenous antihistamine agent. In severe cases, enlisting support of an anesthetist in case of a reaction is a prudent precaution. The use of a noniodinated contrast agent is an alternative strategy.

Because ERCP is performed with radiologic imaging of the abdomen, patients who have had recent barium studies or other oral contrast agents should be checked to ensure that the field of view is clear for the ERCP to be successfully completed. If there is residual contrast material in the gut, a formal bowel preparation may be required. Women of childbearing age must be asked if they are pregnant. If there is uncertainty, the ERCP may need to be deferred until a pregnancy test can be done. If ERCP is considered necessary in a pregnant woman, appropriate lead shielding of the lower abdomen is recommended to protect the fetus. Similarly, pelvic shielding is appropriate for any premenopausal woman.

No data support routine blood tests before diagnostic ERCP, and screening tests are generally not required. If a bleeding disorder is suspected or known, tests to evaluate this and direct therapy are indicated. Similarly, if the patient's clinical condition is unstable or indicates that an abnormality in the blood tests is likely to be present, appropriate testing and correction of relevant abnormalities is indicated. In patients presenting for ERCP with a history or signs of biliary obstruction, the possibility of disordered coagulation exists. Correction of this type of abnormality before the procedure is appropriate.

Preparation for Colonoscopy

Of all endoscopic procedures, the quality of the preparation before colonoscopy has the greatest effect on the outcome of the procedure.[1] The preparation is often regarded as the most unpleasant part of colonoscopy, and many patients are more concerned about this aspect than having the procedure performed. It is vital that the patient be given detailed verbal and written instructions to complete the preparation safely. If the correct preparation is not followed, the procedure usually has to be deferred. The American Society for Gastrointestinal Endoscopy (ASGE) published a technology status evaluation report on colonoscopy preparation that reviews the various bowel preparations in detail.[2] Good bowel preparation is essential to provide an optimal view for colonic examination and to minimize the risk of colonic trauma during the procedure resulting from poor view.

To determine the correct preparation, the clinician requires a careful patient assessment to determine which bowel cleansing agent should be used and what modifications to the patient's diet and regular medications are required. The addition of simethicone to the bowel preparation does not improve cleansing but does reduce bubbles, which may improve the endoscopic view.[3] As part of the preparation, most patients are advised to have only a clear liquid diet for 24 hours before the examination.[1] Routine blood testing before colonoscopy is not required. Management of patients taking antiplatelet and anticoagulation medications should be carefully considered before the examination to minimize the risk of procedure-related bleeding (see later guidelines). In addition, any medication that might be associated with constipation should be temporarily stopped to facilitate the bowel cleansing process. In particular, oral iron can make the stool black and viscous, and iron should be stopped at least 5 days before the colonoscopy.[1] Lastly, specific instructions should be given to diabetic patients who are taking oral hypoglycemic medications or insulin to avoid periprocedural hypoglycemia.

Intravenous sedation is administered to most patients who undergo colonoscopy. It is necessary for the patient to fast before the procedure to reduce the potential for aspiration. The duration of fasting can be comparatively brief because the patient will have been on clear fluids only for 24 hours before the procedure while undergoing bowel preparation. A fasting time of 2 to 4 hours is generally considered adequate.

There are many independent predictors for a potential inadequate bowel preparation, such as a late colonoscopy start time; failure to follow preparation instructions; inpatient status; procedural indication of constipation; use of drugs that impair gut motility (e.g., tricyclic antidepressants, calcium channel blockers, iron); male gender; and a history of cirrhosis, stroke, dementia, obesity, or diabetes mellitus.[4-7] A prior history of failed colonoscopy preparation is also highly predictive of a failed second or subsequent attempt at preparation.[8] In these various patient groups, a more prolonged bowel preparation may be required. Many studies have shown an improved effect of the preparation if half is given the day before the procedure and half is given on the day of the examination. This approach also improves patient adherence and tolerance and is a useful strategy if difficulties with the preparation are anticipated. Other options include abstinence from dietary fat for 1 week and a morning procedure time. In patients who develop nausea, vomiting, or excessive bloating and patients who do not tolerate the preparation, one of the following measures can be used:

- Stop the preparation early if a clear fecal fluid output is achieved.
- Interrupt the preparation temporarily for 1 to 2 hours and then resume.
- Use a trial dose of metoclopramide or another prokinetic agent.
- Chill the bowel preparation solution (very cold solution is not recommended).
- Add clear, sugar-free flavor enhancers or lemon juice.
- Slow the rate of consumption of the solution.

Currently, the three widely accepted bowel preparations for colonoscopy are polyethylene glycol (PEG)–based solutions, sodium phosphate–based solutions, and sulfate-based preparations. Stimulant and hyperosmotic laxatives, such as castor oil, senna, mannitol, sorbitol, and lactulose, are no longer used because they are ineffective. Nonabsorbable sugars may be metabolized by colonic bacteria, generating hydrogen, and carry the risk of explosion during electrosurgical procedures.[9]

Polyethylene Glycol–Based Preparations

Golytely, developed in 1980, was the first osmotically balanced electrolyte purge solution. Since then, several modifications of the solution have been made to improve tolerability. An oral purge using 4 L of a PEG-based solution, given the day before colonoscopy at the rate of approximately 1 L/hr, is associated with a good cleansing efficacy and reasonable patient tolerance.[10-12] Adding a flavor to the preparation is often preferred by patients. Approximately 19% of patients are unable to complete the preparation because of its large volume and unpalatable taste.[13] Newer PEG-based solutions such as MoviPrep (supplied by Norgine in Europe and Australia and Salix Pharmaceuticals in the United States) are better tolerated because the ingested volume has been reduced (2 L), and the taste has been significantly improved.[14] The efficacy of the lower volume preparation is similar to the standard 4-L products, and the side-effect profile is similar. Metoclopramide may be helpful in selected patients to decrease nausea and vomiting, although routine use of metoclopramide did not confer any significant benefit in a small, randomized trial.[15] PEG-based oral lavage (or any form of bowel preparation) is contraindicated in patients with an ileus, significant gastric retention, suspected or established mechanical bowel obstruction, severe colitis, or neurologic impairment that prevents safe swallowing.[1] For patients with swallowing difficulties, a nasogastric tube can be used to administer the solution.

Sodium Phosphate–Based Preparations

The sodium phosphate–based bowel preparation is a smaller volume and can be safely given to most healthy individuals. Traditionally, sodium phosphate preparations have been available in liquid form, but more recently Diacol (Pharmatel Fresenius Kabi, Australia, and Dr Falk Pharma, Europe) and Visicol and OsmoPrep (Salix Pharmaceuticals, United States) have been released with sodium phosphate in a tablet form. Less taste than the liquid formulations may improve tolerance, and efficacy seems comparable. Sodium phosphate preparations are administered in split doses before colonoscopy with the exact timing depending on the time that the colonoscopy is to be performed. The preparation acts by exerting a hyperosmotic effect and by indirectly stimulating stretch receptors to increase peristalsis.[13] Sodium phosphate–based preparations have been shown to be superior in tolerance and at least as effective as PEG-based preparation.[13,16–19]

Because of its rapid osmotic effect and the possibility of significant hyperphosphatemia, it is recommended that sodium phosphate–based bowel preparation be avoided in patients sensitive to sudden volume shifts, such as patients with congestive heart failure and renal impairment. Caution is also required in patients with the potential for disordered sodium or phosphate balance, such as patients with decompensated cirrhosis, small or large bowel dysmotility, and other preexisting electrolyte imbalances.[1,16,17,19] In addition, this preparation is not recommended in patients with proven or suspected inflammatory bowel disease because it can cause colonic inflammation and aphthous ulceration in 25% of cases compared with 2% to 3% in PEG-prepared patients.[20] Patients in whom this preparation is prescribed must be advised to drink as much clear fluids as can be tolerated to reduce the risk of dehydration and to facilitate the cleansing effect of the medication. For this reason, it has been suggested that sodium phosphate–based preparations are inappropriate for elderly patients, but Thomson and coworkers[21] found that this preparation was safe, effective, and well tolerated in most elderly patients (mean age 72 years). Caution is nonetheless advised because a more recent study has shown sodium phosphate–based solutions are associated with a decline in glomerular filtration rate in elderly patients with creatinine levels in the normal range.[22]

Other Preparations

Colocap Balance was released more recently; this is a capsule that contains magnesium sulfate. The capsules have no taste and may be easier for patients who are unable to tolerate the taste of the liquid bowel preparation regimens. This product is currently undergoing clinical trials. Oral sulfate solutions are also available. A randomized controlled trial showed that these agents are as effective as low-volume PEG-based regimens.[23] There seemed to be an advantage if the preparation was split with half administered the day before colonoscopy and half administered on the day of the procedure.

Preparation for Flexible Sigmoidoscopy

Preparation before flexible sigmoidoscopy generally requires cleansing of only the left colon.[1] In most cases, this cleansing can be achieved by administering one or two enemas 1 hour before the procedure. Several types of enemas are available:

- Microlax enema
- Fleet enema (sodium phosphate)
- Tap water enema
- G&O enema (3 parts glycerin, 3 parts olive oil, and 3 parts water)

A more extensive bowel preparation may be required in severely constipated patients or in patients in whom a therapeutic procedure is required, such as polypectomy or argon plasma coagulation therapy. In these cases, 2 L of PEG-based bowel preparation with 24 hours of clear fluid may be adequate. In contrast, bowel preparation may be unnecessary in patients with active colitis or watery diarrhea. Generally, patients undergoing flexible sigmoidoscopy do not require intravenous sedation. If sedation is required, the patient should be advised to fast for 2 to 4 hours before the procedure.

Preparation for Endoscopic Ultrasound

Patient preparation for endoscopic ultrasound is similar to preparation for upper gastrointestinal (GI) endoscopy.[1] Patients must fast for at least 4 hours before the procedure. In patients in whom a biopsy or therapeutic intervention is considered necessary, a platelet count and coagulation studies may be appropriate before the procedure if a bleeding disorder is suspected. In addition, antiplatelet and anticoagulation therapies must be reviewed, and where appropriate modification or cessation of this therapy may be required. Antibiotic prophylaxis generally is not required unless fine needle aspiration (FNA) of a cystic lesion is being performed. FNA of cystic lesions is considered high risk for infection, and antibiotics are recommended. FNA of solid lesions in the upper GI tract[24,25] or in the lower GI tract[26] has been shown to be a low-risk procedure and does not warrant antibiotic prophylaxis.

Preparation for Capsule Endoscopy

Optimizing conditions for capsule endoscopy continues to be an area of interest. Most centers prefer a slightly longer fasting time than for routine endoscopy. Generally, clear fluids are given after lunch on the day before the examination, and the patient fasts for 12 hours before the examination is scheduled to begin. No medication should be taken within 2 hours of ingestion of the capsule. In some centers, 2 L of a PEG-based bowel preparation regimen is given before the patient begins the 12-hour fast.[27,28] This additional step might be particularly important if the patient has had a recent barium study or has had some other form of oral radiologic contrast agent. Some units ask the patient to ingest a small amount of simethicone preparation before the procedure,[29] and some units use a prokinetic such as metoclopramide. The use of a purgative preparation improves the quality of the small bowel images obtained during the capsule endoscopy study and diagnostic yield.[30] The purgative preparation does not seem to influence completion rate of the study, however. The optimal preparation regimen is not yet established, so instructions may be individualized for the patient. It is prudent to review the patient's medications and consider holding any medication that might slow GI motility. Iron supplements should be stopped at least 3 days before the examination.

Preparation for Endoscopic Procedures in Patients with Diabetes

There are no controlled trials to guide preparation for endoscopic procedures in diabetic patients.[1] The approach to these patients must be individualized, and factors such as usual glycemic control and the patient's ability to manage his or her diabetes are important considerations. There are no specific requirements in diabetic patients who are controlled on diet alone. In patients taking oral hypoglycemic agents, medications are generally withheld during preparation for the procedure. During this time, the patient must monitor his or her serum glucose and be able to manage or get assistance if there is evidence of progressive hyperglycemia. Hypoglycemia is managed with sugar-containing clear fluids or candy. In patients taking insulin, dose reduction while undergoing the preparation is normal. For upper GI procedures, the usual dose may be given the evening before the procedure, but only half the dose is given on the morning of the examination. The remaining dose can be given if appropriate after the procedure has been completed.

Insulin-dependent diabetics undergoing preparation for colonoscopy should have their diabetic treatment individually modified with clear instructions provided as to how hypoglycemia and hyperglycemia should be managed. Diabetic patients should preferentially be scheduled for a morning procedure and ideally be the first case for the day. During the preparation, the patient must be advised to monitor serum glucose regularly. Patients with brittle diabetic control, patients unable to manage hypoglycemia or hyperglycemia, and patients with significant other comorbidity may need medical or nursing supervision during bowel preparation.

Special Circumstances

Preparation for Endoscopy in Case of Ingestion of a Foreign Body or for Food Bolus Obstruction

Ingestion of foreign bodies occurs mainly in children and mentally disabled patients. Food bolus obstruction is relatively common in adults.[31,32] Endoscopic assessment and removal is the main modality of treatment for objects below the level of the cricopharyngeal muscle. The nature of the patient's symptoms determines the urgency of the procedure. Emergency procedures should be performed for patients who

are unable to swallow their saliva, patients with sharp objects (e.g., fish bones, pins, dentures, razor blades), and patients with impacted disk batteries.[32,33] The procedure is probably technically easier if performed early. Plain x-rays of the chest and neck may be advisable before the endoscopic procedure if the nature of the object or the site of obstruction is unclear from the history. The x-ray film may also show ectopic gas patterns to indicate a silent perforation. Oral radiologic contrast material generally is best avoided because of the risk of aspiration and because it may obscure the endoscopic field.[34,35]

With regard to food bolus impaction, glucagon or another prokinetic can be given while the patient is waiting for endoscopy, but this is usually unsuccessful and should not delay endoscopy.[36,37] Special attention should be given to airway protection to avoid the risk of airway obstruction during the procedure. Continuous oral suction and the availability of a laryngoscope are also important. General anesthesia with endotracheal intubation is usually required if airway protection is needed, but this is required in less than 25% of cases.[38] An alternative strategy to protect the airway is the use of an esophageal overtube. General anesthesia with muscle relaxation often facilitates removal of difficult or large items, particularly as they pass through the upper esophageal sphincter; this is particularly true for swallowed dentures (see Chapter 19).

Preparation for Endoscopy in Patients with Upper Gastrointestinal Bleeding

Preparation of an acutely bleeding patient for endoscopy requires additional precautions and care. The first step is to ensure that the patient is adequately resuscitated because any subsequent endoscopy is best performed when the patient is hemodynamically stable. Volume replacement and correction of any coagulation or platelet function disturbance are important. If there is evidence of ongoing bleeding, urgent endoscopy with airway protection, even in an unstable patient, may be the best way of getting better clinical control of the situation. If time permits, a 6-hour fast is desirable because this would improve the endoscopic view. However, a fast is often not practical, particularly if there is evidence of active bleeding. Sometimes gastric lavage can be used to empty the stomach of blood before endoscopy is performed. Care must be taken not to suck too aggressively with the gastric lavage tube because significant mucosal trauma can occur, and this can make interpretation of the subsequent endoscopic findings difficult. One randomized, placebo-controlled study showed improved endoscopic view with intravenous erythromycin administered 2 hours before endoscopy.[39]

Endoscopy in patients with upper GI bleeding is usually performed after the patient has received intravenous sedation.[40] Endotracheal intubation should be considered in patients with active hematemesis or other perceived increased risk of aspiration. If the patient is suspected to have a bleeding peptic ulcer, an intravenous proton pump inhibitor before the endoscopy should be considered. Studies have suggested that a proton pump inhibitor can significantly improve outcome in these patients.[41-44] Similarly, patients suspected to have variceal bleeding may benefit from an octreotide infusion (see Chapter 13).[45-47]

Preparation for Colonoscopy in Patients with Lower Gastrointestinal Bleeding

In patients with lower GI bleeding, colonoscopy is the procedure of choice to identify the site of bleeding and in some circumstances allows therapeutic intervention (see Chapter 14).[48] Before the procedure, patients should be resuscitated, and their general condition should be stabilized. Routine blood tests and coagulation profile are generally performed in patients with GI bleeding, and these should be corrected if abnormal. Generally, most colonoscopies in patients with lower GI bleeding are performed on a semiurgent basis to allow time for some form of bowel preparation. The view at colonoscopy is often a problem in procedures performed urgently, although some studies suggest that urgent colonoscopy is not only technically possible and safe but also effective in controlling bleeding.[49,50] Blood itself is a cathartic; many clinicians perform the procedure in an unprepared bowel.[51] Other clinicians preferring a bowel preparation generally give 4 L of PEG over 4 hours before the procedure.[49,52–54] This solution can be given orally or via a nasogastric tube. In elective procedures, the colon can be prepared in a standard fashion. Because these patients are at higher risk of a disturbance of intravascular volume, it is generally advisable to avoid sodium phosphate–based preparations. A prokinetic agent may facilitate the bowel preparation. In general, patients should not have barium studies before colonoscopy because it would interfere with the view and may obscure flat mucosal lesions such as angiodysplasia. If an obstructive lesion is suspected, a clear water-soluble contrast agent such as Gastrografin should be used.

Antiplatelet and Anticoagulation Therapy

The decision to discontinue antiplatelet or anticoagulation therapy depends on two important factors: the risk of bleeding related to an endoscopic intervention and the risk of a thromboembolic event related to interruption of these medications. The risk stratification of these two factors is summarized in **Table 8.1**.[55] If anticoagulation therapy is temporary, elective procedures should be delayed until the anticoagulation has been stopped. For patients receiving warfarin who undergo a low-risk procedure, no adjustment to the anticoagulation therapy is needed, regardless of the underlying condition. In contrast, anticoagulation therapy should be discontinued 3 to 5 days before the procedure in patients who undergo high-risk procedures, and anticoagulation therapy generally can be resumed the night of the procedure. The decision to obtain a preprocedure international normalized ratio (INR) should be individualized.

Increasingly, patients who require anticoagulation therapy are being managed with low-molecular-weight heparin (LMWH) because therapy is more reliable and easier to manage. The ASGE has published a guideline on management of LMWH and nonaspirin antiplatelet agents before endoscopic procedures.[56] For elective procedures, no specific modification is required for low-risk procedures. For high-risk procedures, LMWH should not be given for at least 8 hours before the procedure and then restarted when deemed safe for the individual patient. LMWH is often used as a bridge in patients taking warfarin for high-risk cardiovascular or thrombotic conditions before an endoscopic procedure. In

Table 8.1 Risk Stratification of Bleeding from Endoscopic Procedures and the Condition Risk for Thrombosis and Embolism

High-Risk Procedures	Low-Risk Procedures
PROCEDURE RISK FOR BLEEDING	
Polypectomy	Diagnostic endoscopy ± biopsy
Biliary sphincterotomy	Diagnostic flexible sigmoidoscopy ± biopsy
Pneumatic or bougie dilation	Diagnostic colonoscopy ± biopsy
PEG or PEJ placement	Enteroscopy ± biopsy
EUS-guided fine needle biopsy	ERCP without sphincterotomy
Laser ablation and coagulation	Biliary/pancreatic stenting without sphincterotomy
Variceal treatment	EUS without fine needle biopsy
CONDITION RISK FOR THROMBOSIS OR EMBOLISM	
Atrial fibrillation with valvular heart disease	Deep venous thrombosis
Mechanical valve in mitral position	Uncomplicated nonvalvular atrial fibrillation
Mechanical valve with prior thromboembolic event	Bioprosthetic heart valve
	Mechanical valve in aortic position

ERCP, endoscopic retrograde cholangiopancreatography; EUS, endoscopic ultrasound; PEG, percutaneous endoscopic gastrostomy; PEJ, percutaneous endoscopic jejunostomy.

Adapted from Eisen GM, Baron TH, Dominitz JA, et al; American Society for Gastrointestinal Endoscopy: Guideline on management of anticoagulation and antiplatelet therapy for endoscopic procedures. Gastrointest Endosc 55:775–779, 2002, with permission from the American Society for Gastrointestinal Endoscopy.

these patients, LMWH is started 3 to 5 days before the endoscopic procedure when the warfarin is stopped. LMWH is then stopped at least 8 hours before the procedure. The decision when to restart therapy should be individualized.

Generally, endoscopic procedures may be performed in patients taking aspirin or other nonsteroidal antiinflammatory drugs (NSAIDs) in standard doses, provided that they do not have a preexisting bleeding disorder.[55] This recommendation is based on limited published studies suggesting that aspirin and NSAIDs in standard doses do not increase the risk of significant bleeding after gastroscopy or colonoscopy with biopsy, polypectomy, and biliary sphincterotomy.[57,58]

For newer antiplatelet agents, such as clopidogrel, ticlopidine, and glycoprotein (GP) IIb/IIIa inhibitors, limited data are available to make firm recommendations. As mentioned, the ASGE has published a guideline on management of LMWH and nonaspirin antiplatelet agents before endoscopic procedures.[56] Decision making should be individualized. These agents generally should be stopped in patients who present with acute GI hemorrhage. The risks of this decision should be balanced against the risk of an ischemic or thrombotic event, especially if the patient has recently had implantation of a drug-eluting coronary stent. If rapid reversal is required, a platelet transfusion may be appropriate. For low-risk procedures, adjustment to clopidogrel and ticlopidine therapy is not required. For high-risk procedures, one approach is to stop the agent for 7 to 10 days before the procedure.

In patients who take clopidogrel or ticlopidine in combination with aspirin, it may be appropriate to revert to a single agent (aspirin) before an elective endoscopic procedure. Dipyridamole may be used alone or in combination with aspirin for low-risk procedures. The risk of dipyridamole in high-risk procedures is unclear, but cessation may be prudent if the risk of thrombosis or ischemia is low. Patients undergoing elective endoscopic procedures generally are not exposed to GP IIb/IIIa inhibitors. For patients requiring emergency endoscopy for acute GI hemorrhage, GP IIb/IIIa inhibitors should be discontinued. Eptifibatide and tirofiban have a relatively short duration of action (4 hours), whereas abciximab may last 24 hours. Platelet transfusion or desmopressin (DDAVP) may be useful for major bleeding.

Particular care needs to be taken in patients with coronary artery stents, in whom a high risk of stent occlusion exists if antiplatelet therapy is stopped. This risk is of particular concern in patients with a drug-eluting coronary artery stent. Antiplatelet therapy should not be modified within 1 month of insertion of a bare metal coronary stent and within 12 months of a drug-eluting coronary stent. Consideration should be given to deferring elective endoscopic procedures during these times. Consultation with the patient's cardiologist is advised before stopping antiplatelet agents in this setting.

Management of Disorders of Hemostasis before Endoscopic Examinations

Management of patients with hemostasis disorders should be individualized and when possible should be in close collaboration with an experienced hematologist in a specialized center with a specialist coagulation laboratory. The endoscopist must assess the risk of bleeding based on the procedural risk and the severity of the underlying disorder of hemostasis and plan the endoscopic procedure accordingly.[59]

Von Willebrand's Disease

von Willebrand's disease (vWD) is the most common inherited disorder of hemostasis; therapy before endoscopic procedures depends on the type of vWD. For less severe type I disease, treatment with DDAVP starting 1 hour before the procedure and once daily thereafter for 2 to 3 days is adequate for patients undergoing diagnostic procedures and mucosal biopsies. However, for therapeutic procedures, infusion of factor VIII 1 hour before the procedure to achieve a factor VIII activity of 0.80 to 1.20 U/mL is required. After the procedure, factor VIII activity of at least 0.30 to 0.50 U/mL must be maintained for up to 2 weeks to minimize the risk of rebleeding.[46] For more severe type II and type III disease, the same factor VIII replacement regimen is required for diagnostic (maintenance duration of 2 to 3 days) and therapeutic procedures (up to 2 weeks).[59]

Hemophilia A and B

Preprocedural assay of factor VIII or IX activity is essential to determine the dosage of replacement therapy in patients with hemophilia. Before the procedure, factor VIII infusion is required to achieve an activity of 0.80 to 1.20 U/mL. Postinfusion factor assay should be obtained to determine the patient's response to the infusion. For purely diagnostic procedures, no further infusion is required. If mucosal biopsies are performed, 75% of the initial dose should be given every 24 hours for an additional 2 to 3 days. If therapeutic procedures are performed, twice-daily factor VIII infusion is required to achieve a maintenance activity of 0.30 to 0.50 U/mL for up to 2 weeks. Adequate factor VIII maintenance activity must be confirmed by at least daily factor VIII assay. Indications for factor IX replacement are identical to the indications for factor VIII infusion except that the maintenance dose is administered at intervals of 24 hours because the half-life of factor IX is longer.[59]

Liver Disease

The possible hemostatic defects in patients with liver disease are coagulopathy and thrombocytopenia. Correction is usually not required for diagnostic endoscopic procedures, but most centers would consider correction if the INR is greater than 2.5. Correction is necessary if therapeutic maneuvers are needed. These recommendations are based on limited data. If high-risk procedures are done, correction of an INR to less than 1.4 to 1.7 is advisable[59]; this can be accomplished by a combination of fresh frozen plasma and vitamin K replacement. Correction of significant thrombocytopenia is discussed later.

Renal Failure

The main hemostatic defect in patients with renal failure is an acquired qualitative platelet defect secondary to uremia. Bleeding complications in these patients undergoing renal biopsy, abdominal surgery, liver and bone biopsies, or tooth extraction are rare.[60] In addition, measurement of preprocedural bleeding time is not helpful because it does not predict outcome.[60] Platelet infusion is not routinely recommended, unless concurrent significant thrombocytopenia exists.[59] Because uremia is thought to be the cause of platelet dysfunction, dialysis with limited heparin shortly before high-risk procedures is recommended to reduce serum urea nitrogen to less than 50 to 75 mg/dL.[59,61]

Thrombocytopenia

There are no prospective data on the need for prophylactic platelet transfusion, and the following guidelines have been based on decision analysis.[59,62,63] Platelet transfusion to increase the platelet count to greater than 20×10^9 platelets/L is required for low-risk procedures, and a count greater than 50×10^9 platelets/L is required for high-risk therapeutic procedures. For patients with immune thrombocytopenia, elective procedures should be postponed until an appropriate improvement in platelet count (20 to 30×10^9 platelets/L) is observed with standard therapy. If endoscopic procedures cannot be postponed and immediate intervention is necessary, a platelet transfusion should be given just before the procedure.[59] If bleeding occurs after the procedure, further platelet transfusion should be given. Input from a hematologist is recommended if response to platelet transfusion is poor.[59]

Antibiotic Prophylaxis

GI procedures are commonly associated with bacteremia. The complications of these endogenous bacteria are rare. There are, however, specific high-risk procedures and high-risk patient conditions for which it is considered appropriate to use prophylactic antibiotics. High-risk procedures include PEG insertion, ERCP in patients with obstructed biliary or pancreatic ducts, or ERCP in patients with inadequate duct drainage on completion of the procedure. High-risk patient factors that warrant specific consideration for antibiotic prophylaxis include patients with cirrhosis and ascites and patients with primary sclerosing cholangitis.

The British Society of Gastroenterology more recently released guidelines for antibiotic prophylaxis in GI endoscopy.[64] The executive summary includes the following recommendations:

- Patients undergoing ERCP for treatment of cholangitis should be established on antibiotics before the procedure, and an additional single dose of antibiotic is not recommended (the collection of a bile sample for culture to guide subsequent therapy should be considered).
- Routine prophylactic antibiotics for ERCP is no longer considered appropriate. If biliary duct decompression cannot be achieved, full antibiotic therapy should be instituted until this goal can be achieved either by repeat procedure or by alternative means.
- Specific circumstances in which antibiotic therapy should be used to cover ERCP include:
  - Patients with biliary disorders such as primary sclerosing cholangitis or hilar cholangiocarcinoma in whom complete biliary drainage would be difficult or impossible to achieve during one procedure
  - Patients with a history of liver transplantation
  - Patients with a pancreatic pseudocyst
  - Patients with severe neutropenia or advanced hematologic malignancy
- Patients having a percutaneous endoscopic gastrostomy or jejunostomy should receive prophylactic antibiotics, unless they are already receiving broad-spectrum antibiotics.
- Patients with suspected variceal bleeding or patients with decompensated liver disease who develop acute GI bleeding should receive antibiotics before endoscopy.
- Antibiotic prophylaxis is recommended before FNA of cystic lesions in or adjacent to the pancreas and for endoscopic drainage of pseudocysts and postpancreatitis collections.
- Patients with severe neutropenia or advanced hematologic malignancy or patients with a profound immunocompromised state should receive antibiotics if they undergo procedures that are known to be associated with a high risk of bacteremia.

The choice of antibiotic to be used in the above-listed circumstances is beyond the scope of this chapter. Local guidelines should be followed, and microbiologic advice should be sought if necessary. Recent positive cultures if available should be taken into account when deciding on antibiotic regimens. In addition, many institutions modify recommendations depending on whether the patient is an existing inpatient or presents to the hospital from the community.

Antibiotic Prophylaxis for Prevention of Infective Endocarditis

The practice of antibiotic prophylaxis in GI endoscopy to prevent infective endocarditis has previously been common. Antibiotic guidelines have previously recommended antibiotic prophylaxis for the prevention of infective endocarditis.[65] For more than 50 years, patients and physicians have been accustomed to this practice. However, the data on which this practice has been based have been scanty. In addition, the risk of infective endocarditis as a result of a GI procedure is extremely low, and true causality is usually lacking in the few case reports that do exist.

A consensus document has been published looking at the role of antibiotic prophylaxis for the prevention of infective endocarditis.[66] These guidelines were prepared in collaboration with many learned societies and advisory groups and have been broadly adopted internationally. The guidelines conclude that:

- Only an extremely small number of cases of infective endocarditis might be prevented by antibiotic prophylaxis.
- Antibiotic prophylaxis is not recommended based solely on an increased lifetime risk of acquisition of infective endocarditis.
- Administration of antibiotics solely to prevent endocarditis is not recommended for patients who undergo GI tract procedures.
- Antibiotic prophylaxis is reasonable only for patients with an underlying cardiac condition associated with the highest risk of an adverse outcome from infective endocarditis.

Antibiotic prophylaxis may be considered in very-high-risk cardiac conditions. The cardiac conditions that are considered the highest risk for adverse outcome from endocarditis include the following:

- Prosthetic cardiac valve or prosthetic material used for cardiac valve repair
- Previous history of infective endocarditis
- Congenital heart disease
  - Unrepaired cyanotic congenital heart disease, including palliative shunts and conduits
  - Completely repaired congenital heart defect with prosthetic material or device during 6 months after the procedure
  - Repaired congenital heart disease with residual defects at the site or adjacent to the site of a prosthetic patch or prosthetic device
- Cardiac transplant recipients who develop cardiac valvulopathy

The major challenge that exists with the introduction of these new guidelines is patient education. Many patients remain very anxious and require reassurance that their expected administration of antibiotics is no longer required.

If antibiotics are required, it is recommended that a single dose be given before the procedure. If the antibiotic inadvertently is not administered before the procedure, it may be given up to 2 hours after the procedure. The gut contains a wide variety of bacteria, but of these enterococci are the most likely to cause infective endocarditis. If an antibiotic is required for a high-risk patient, amoxicillin and ampicillin are the preferred agents for enterococcal cover. Vancomycin may be used in patients who are allergic to penicillin. Vancomycin administration should be slow (10 mg/min) to avoid complications. If patients are already receiving antibiotics, a different class of agent should be chosen rather than increasing the dose of the existing treatment. Antibiotic prophylaxis is generally given intravenously. Intramuscular injections should be avoided in patients who are anticoagulated.

Antibiotic Prophylaxis for Patients with Vascular Grafts and Other Implanted Devices

It has been suggested that some delayed infections of orthopedic, neurosurgical, and other prostheses may be due to bacteremia associated with endoscopic procedures.[64] However, the risk from endoscopic procedures is negligible compared with other daily activities associated with bacteremia, such as chewing or oral hygiene measures such as tooth brushing. Any benefit of antibiotics to cover these activities would be outweighed by the adverse effects. The British Society of Gastroenterology, the ASGE, and the American Society of Colon and Rectal Surgeons do not recommend the use of antibiotics before endoscopy in patients with orthopedic prostheses, central nervous system vascular shunts, vascular grafts or stents, penile prostheses, intraocular lenses, pacemakers, or local tissue augmentation materials.

Antibiotic Prophylaxis for Percutaneous Endoscopic Gastrostomy or Percutaneous Endoscopic Jejunostomy

A single dose of an appropriate antibiotic given 30 minutes before percutaneous endoscopic gastrostomy or jejunostomy insertion is routinely recommended for all patients who are not already receiving antibiotics because the risk of peristomal wound infection is significantly reduced.[64] However, for patients who are already receiving appropriate antibiotics, no additional prophylaxis may be required. Patients known to be colonized with multiple resistant organisms or patients who have been hospitalized for some time before percutaneous endoscopic gastrostomy or jejunostomy insertion and who are likely to be colonized with resistant organisms should receive antibiotic prophylaxis appropriate to cover multiple resistant organisms. Local guidelines should be followed when choosing the antibiotic before percutaneous endoscopic gastrostomy or jejunostomy insertion. The choice of drug should be carefully considered in patients who are allergic to penicillin.

Antibiotic Prophylaxis for Patients with Variceal Bleeding or Patients with Decompensated Liver Disease Who Develop Acute Gastrointestinal Bleeding

Prophylactic antibiotics in patients with variceal bleeding or in patients with decompensated liver disease who develop acute GI bleeding improves short-term survival and may be associated with a reduced risk of rebleeding.[64] It is recommended that patients receive antibiotics before endoscopy. The choice of antibiotics is determined by local guidelines, but ceftriaxone is frequently used.

Antibiotic Prophylaxis for Patients with Neutropenia or Who Are Immunocompromised

Neutropenia ($<0.5 \times 10^9$/L) predisposes to sepsis after procedures such as endoscopy, but the level of risk is unclear.[64] Patients who are febrile should already be treated with empiric antibiotics according to local hematology guidelines. In afebrile patients, antibiotic prophylaxis should be offered for high-risk procedures such as sclerotherapy, esophageal dilation, or ERCP with duct obstruction. Gram-negative aerobic and, less frequently, anaerobic organisms are likely pathogens, and the choice of antibiotic should reflect local sensitivities. No data support the use of prophylactic antibiotics in patients who have a normal neutrophil count but who are nonetheless immunocompromised (e.g., organ transplants). Routine antibiotic prophylaxis is not recommended in patients with human immunodeficiency virus (HIV) infection.

References

The complete reference list is available online at www.expertconsult.com.

Reporting, Documentation, and Risk Management

Ian D. Norton and Kenneth Schroeder

Introduction

Endoscopic services have developed rapidly over the past 30 years such that the practice of gastroenterology is a procedural specialty for most practitioners. Procedural activities carry specific risks to the patient and expose the gastroenterologist to more potential for litigation than many other physicians; this is particularly the case because most procedures are performed on "the walking well"—patients without a defined major illness who have little expectation of a poor outcome (e.g., compared with cardiologists performing infarct angioplasty). Despite this increased potential for litigation, a review of medical claims in the United States ranked gastroenterologists 23rd of 28 specialties in number of claims.[1]

It is a reality of practice for gastroenterologists in many societies that malpractice litigation is a real possibility (or even probability) during their career. Nothing can eliminate this risk, but sound medical practice, good documentation, and appropriate informed consent processes reduce the chance of poor outcomes and litigation when adverse events occur. These all are elements of good practice, and the principles outlined in this chapter are as relevant to gastroenterologists practicing in highly litigious environments (e.g., the United States and Australia) as they are to practitioners in areas where litigation is almost nonexistent (e.g., New Zealand and parts of Western Europe). These regional differences are partly due to patient (consumer) expectation and the local legal compensation framework.

Relationship of Medical Practice to Litigation

Several large studies have examined the impact of medical error on patient care.[2–5] Up to 36% of hospital admissions are associated with some form of error during the admission, usually trivial and of no clinical impact. However, a study of 20,000 surgical admissions noted an iatrogenic disability rate of 4.6%. Most of these disabilities were attributable to "acceptable risk," but the authors concluded that 17% of these injuries would have probably been successfully litigated. In other words, almost 1% of surgical admissions could result in a successful lawsuit against the surgeon. In the Harvard Medical Practice Study,[4] less than 2% of patients with an iatrogenic injury filed a claim. Other factors in addition to injury determine whether a claim is filed. Several studies have addressed this issue and found that major determinants of a patient's decision whether to sue are patient dissatisfaction and the physician's communicative and interpersonal skills.[6–9]

Communication with the patient and family is of utmost importance, particularly when mishaps occur. Patients experiencing a significant complication often have their care transferred to an appropriate specialist for correction of the problem (e.g., intensivist or surgeon). It is an important risk management strategy for a physician to be available to the patient and family even if no longer participating in the direct care of the patient. This availability shows empathy and prevents anger arising from the perception of being "abandoned" by the physician.

Claims against Gastroenterologists

Data regarding claims against gastroenterologists are difficult to assess because not all insurers are equally forthcoming with their data, and some major U.S. institutions self-insure and do not release their data for review. The Physician Insurers Association of America pools information from 20 member insurers and periodically publishes their data.[1] These data have also been reviewed and published in the gastrointestinal (GI) literature.[10,11] The claims fall into the following groups:

1. *Iatrogenic injury:* Nearly 30% of claims are related to improper endoscopic practice causing injury. Of these cases, 95% were perforation or laceration of the gut and its sequelae. Other injuries such as pancreatitis, hemorrhage, dental injury, and falling from the bed while sedated also constituted claims.
2. *Errors in diagnosis:* About 25% of claims are related to errors in diagnosis, two-thirds of which were missed malignancies, particularly of the right colon and stomach. Missed colon cancer accounted for more than 50% of colonoscopy claims and more than 75% of claims relating to sigmoidoscopy. Another relatively frequent scenario was delay in diagnosis of malignancy through failure to perform endoscopic examinations. When claims against gastroenterologists were examined, another frequent scenario was delayed diagnosis of non–GI tract neoplasia, especially gynecologic and pulmonary. Gastroenterologists must be diligent in investigating the GI tract and must ensure that their endoscopic examination is adequate (both in terms of bowel preparation and ensuring that the cecum is reached or, if not, that further steps are taken to complete the evaluation). Gastroenterologists must be clear where their duty of care to the patient ends. Consider a scenario in which a 60-year-old woman with new-onset abdominal bloating is referred to a gastroenterologist. It is inadequate merely to examine the bowel, find no abnormality, and reassure the patient. In this scenario, the physician must either investigate further or make it clear to the referring physician and patient that although the GI tract is normal, other possibilities (e.g., ovarian cancer) should be considered.
3. *Medication error:* Medication error was uncommon, accounting for less than 10% of gastroenterology claims. However, two notable areas are endoscopist-supervised sedation and prescription of corticosteroids and immunosuppressive agents. Overall, approximately two-thirds of claims against gastroenterologists could be considered "cognitive," and one-third could be considered "procedural mishap." Problems with informed consent were mentioned in about half of the cases.

Specific Endoscopic Procedures

In the study by Gerstenberger[10,12] of 610 endoscopic claims, the relative risk of litigation arising from various procedures (relative to sigmoidoscopy) varied by less than a factor of 2, as follows: sigmoidoscopy, 1.0; gastroscopy, 1.2; colonoscopy, 1.7; and endoscopic retrograde cholangiopancreatography (ERCP), 1.6. This small variation occurred despite the fact that ERCP and colonoscopy result in far more complications than sigmoidoscopy and gastroscopy. This seeming paradox is probably explained by the use of more intensive informed consent processes for ERCP and colonoscopy compared with the technically less challenging procedures. This study illustrates the important principle of informed consent as a risk management strategy (see later).

Legal Principles in Medical Practice

Principles of Tort Law

Claims for medical negligence fall under the principles of tort law. A knowledge of the principles of tort law is germane to the physician's understanding of his or her responsibilities. Torts are "civil wrongs," where one private citizen has brought legal proceedings against another (in this case, the physician). Tort law does not involve criminal behavior and is usually settled with financial compensation to the injured party (the award of "damages").

Tort law (with respect to medical negligence) involves four steps, as follows:

1. *A duty:* The physician has a responsibility to the patient to comply with professional standards of practice.
2. *A breach of duty:* The physician did not fulfill that responsibility.
3. *Causation:* The physician's failure was a proximate cause of the patient's suffering.
4. *Injury:* The patient suffered a defined injury (be it physical, financial, or psychological).

Duty

The physician's duty to the patient comes from the physician-patient relationship. The physician enters into a contract with the patient to provide the patient with medical services to a reasonable standard; this does not mean a consultation. For example, a complication may arise from a preparation suggested for a patient undergoing an open-access procedure. One way to reduce liability to the patient is to demarcate clearly where duty of care begins and ends. If a physician diagnoses colon cancer, it is prudent to document clearly a management plan with subsequent specialists and to document that the patient understands the condition and how it is being managed and that both the patient and his or her primary care physician are aware of this plan and how to take this management further. This communication and documentation prevent complications from delay in definitive management and might help to reduce subsequent vicarious liability (e.g., the physician's level of responsibility for subsequent malpractice by other health care professionals).

Breach of Duty

In a breach of duty, the physician failed to provide a reasonable standard of care after entering into the physician-patient

Box 9.1 **Professional Gastroenterology Societies**	
American Gastroenterology Association	www.gastro.org
American Society for Gastrointestinal Endoscopy	www.asge.org
American College of Gastroenterology	www.acg.org
British Society of Gastroenterology	www.bsg.org.uk
Gastroenterology Society of Australia	www.gesa.org.au
World Gastroenterology Organization	www.worldgastroenterology.org

relationship. This reasonable standard is often difficult to define and usually is established with the aid of expert witnesses—not to the level of an emeritus professor in that field but to a level acceptable to the physician's peers (i.e., sound medical practice; published guidelines can be useful in this context but ironically are more often used for the plaintiff's case). Many societies (e.g., American Society for Gastrointestinal Endoscopy [ASGE], British Society of Gastroenterology, and Gastroenterology Society of Australia) publish guidelines for endoscopic practice. The set of guidelines published by the ASGE, in particular, is an excellent resource that is available on the Internet (**Box 9.1**). Medical practice often varies depending on many variables, such as comorbidities, patient wishes, physician expertise, and available resources. If one deviates substantially from common practice, it is essential to note the reasons for this in the medical record.

Causation

The plaintiff must prove that the physician's breach of duty caused the injury. The breach must be a "proximate cause" or a substantial (vs. remote) factor in bringing about the injury. For example, a patient with weight loss, back pain, and diabetes undergoes endoscopic ultrasound, and the endoscopist fails to diagnose a pancreatic cancer. The patient is diagnosed with metastatic disease to the liver 2 months later. Even though the endoscopist missed the lesion, it is unlikely that finding it would have altered the eventual outcome. This example also highlights the fact that no procedure is 100% sensitive, and the endoscopist's report and subsequent communication with the referring physician should reflect this fact, perhaps with suggestions for further assessment if the clinical suspicion is high.

Injury

The patient must be able to show some form of suffering; this is usually physical, including the steps necessary to correct the initial injury (e.g., colonic perforation followed by surgery). In some circumstances, the injury could be psychological, although this is harder to prove and quantify. Monetary losses as a result of the injury (e.g., medical costs, lost earnings, and future lost earnings) are also a relevant factor. Intangibles, such as pain and suffering and emotional distress, are also compensable in the United States.

Damages

As mentioned earlier, the outcome of a successful malpractice suit is usually a monetary assessment of damages. The total payout may comprise three types of damages, as follows:

1. *General damages:* This includes payment for pain and suffering.
2. *Special damages:* This includes compensation for medical expenses, lost earnings, and future earning capacity.
3. *Punitive damages:* This is a payment as a punishment for gross negligence, which usually means conscious indifference, fraud, or intentional harm. Punitive damages are rarely part of medical malpractice awards and may not be covered by malpractice insurance.

Standards of Care

Standards of care is a legal concept that attempts to determine the duty physicians must fulfill in their care of a patient. Failure to practice to this standard constitutes a breach of duty. The court usually determines this standard by hearing expert testimony and relying on published data, such as peer-reviewed journal articles and practice guidelines.[13,14] The standard is tailored to the specific case under review and should reflect current practice at the time of the injury. Although society practice guidelines and publications may be an important part of the evidence used to help determine this standard, they do not replace the court's or jury's determination in a particular case. Similarly, a case's judgment is not designed to dictate future clinical practice (although this often is the case). The standard of care is best described as good patient care. It is not defined as best medical practice (e.g., that provided by a world leader in a field) but rather what would be expected from a peer under the same circumstances.

Majority and Minority Standards

There are often many ways to manage a clinical problem. Generally, it is easier to defend the approach taken by most peers (the *majority standard*). Less common approaches, or a *minority standard*, may be valid, but if used such approaches should ideally be accompanied by good documentation explaining why the usual clinical pathway was not followed and clear documentation that alternative strategies and their relative risks and benefits were discussed with the patient. Many societies (e.g., the ASGE) publish excellent guidelines for endoscopic practice. Generally adhering to guidelines such as these is a good risk management strategy. Conversely, physicians who practice in ignorance of the majority standard do so at their peril.

Defining Responsibility
Joint Liability and Comparative Fault

The concept of joint liability and comparative fault recognizes that many health care workers may be involved in the circumstances leading to an adverse outcome. The blame may be appropriately shared over many physicians, nurses, and institutions. For example, a colonic perforation is not, of itself, negligent; however, if it occurred with inadequate consent, liability may be shared by the endoscopist, the referring physician, and the nurse who obtained consent.

Respondeat Superior and Vicarious Liability

Respondeat superior is a legal term referring to the concept that a master is responsible for the mistakes of his servant. *Vicarious liability* means a corporation is responsible for the acts of its employees and agents. In this sense, a consultant supervising a fellow doing an ERCP may be liable for a proportion of the damages arising from a duodenal perforation. The degree of liability varies depending on factors such as whether the patient had consented that the procedure would be performed by a trainee, the degree of seniority and supervision of the trainee, and whether the trainee was performing appropriately. Similarly, a physician may be held responsible for an adverse outcome resulting from incompetency by office staff, and hospitals may be held partly responsible for the mistakes of a physician in the employ of the institution.

Informed Consent

It is a basic legal principle that a competent individual has the right to determine what shall happen to his or her body. The physician must obtain the consent of the patient (or his or her legal guardian) before performing any procedure, with certain exceptions (see later). Historically, touching a patient without the patient's consent constituted a battery (a criminal offense). Over time, however, negligence theory has tended to replace battery where cases of inadequate consent are tried. Inadequate consent issues are likely to be heard in civil rather than criminal proceedings. It is crucial to understand that informed consent is a process, not a signed piece of paper. Although most institutions use a signed consent form, it is usually a generic document and may not reflect that the patient was aware of all the elements necessary for informed consent for that particular procedure in that particular patient. Nonetheless, a signed consent form is very useful in court as tangible evidence that a defendant did go through some process of consent and provided the opportunity to ask questions.

Informed consent comprises several elements, as follows:

1. *Risks:* All procedures have some risk, and patients must be made aware of any risk that, in the view of a reasonable person, might have played a role in that specific patient's decision to proceed. Discussion of risks typically includes the most severe complications (e.g., death, hemorrhage, disability) and common side effects.
2. *Benefits:* The patient must understand why he or she is undergoing the procedure.
3. *Alternatives:* The patient must understand the relative risks and benefits of alternative investigations. The patient should also understand the alternative of not performing any procedure. The courts have struggled with what constitutes reasonable disclosure of alternatives. It should be a discussion of alternatives relevant to the patient concerned and not a recitation of medical casebook history.[15]
4. *Opportunity to ask questions.*

The standard of disclosure presents difficulty with regard to all these elements. Traditionally, the *professional standard of disclosure* has been used. This standard may be defined as "as much information as would have been provided by a physician's peers in the same situation"[16] and was defined by a landmark case in 1960. It assumes that the physician is acting in the best interest of the patient. However, it was noted in the 1970s that this standard implies a paternalistic physician-patient relationship, which impinges on the patient's right to self-determination. The *lay* or *patient-oriented standard* subsequently evolved. This standard was first enunciated in 1972, when a judge commented that "... a risk is thus material when a reasonable person, *in what the physician knows or should know to be the patient's position,* would be likely to attach significance to the risk or cluster of risks in deciding whether or not to forego the proposed therapy."[17]

In other words, the lay standard dictates that the physician must supply any information to which *that particular patient* would attach significance (e.g., a 1:10,000 risk of pharyngeal perforation might hold different significance to an opera singer compared with the average person). This standard is potentially much more difficult for the physician to defend because it requires a subjective assessment of what that *specific* patient would want to know.

It is important for the physician to avoid coercion of any sort. The physician should not be judgmental or emotive when explaining the procedure or the consequences of not following medical advice. It has been proposed by some authorities that obtaining informed consent in the endoscopy room immediately before the procedure could be perceived as being coercive because the patient, having taken time off work and being prepared, gowned, and possibly with an intravenous line in situ, is unlikely to refuse the procedure. Also, the endoscopy suite environment is unlikely to provide the patient with an adequate opportunity to ask questions. These issues are especially important in the setting of open-access endoscopy. Informed consent must be obtained in the language suitable to the patient's comprehension. If the patient speaks only a foreign language, consent should be obtained though a health care professional fluent in the language or interpreter service. A friend or relative of the patient should not act as interpreter because this may constitute a breach of confidentiality, and the patient may be misled by the friend or relative's own biases about what he or she wishes the patient to hear. In one study, a videotape discussing the proposed procedure was shown to patients and was found to be as useful as discussion with the physician without the tape. If information tapes are used, there must be the opportunity for the patient to ask questions that might arise from the viewing.[18]

Exceptions to Informed Consent
Emergency

To satisfy the requirements for emergency, the patient must be incapacitated such that he or she cannot provide consent, and delay in obtaining consent from other sources would put the patient at risk of permanent disability or death. It occasionally may be appropriate to perform additional procedures during the patient's consented procedure that could not have been reasonably foreseen and for which allowing the patient to recover only to submit to another procedure would be unreasonable. It would be reasonable to obtain a biopsy specimen of a suspected early esophageal malignancy during gastroscopy performed to assess peptic ulcer disease. Another example is that a patient may require an intervention to correct a mishap that occurred during the procedure.

Waiver

A patient may occasionally assign his or her right to determination to the physician for the management of a specific condition. This waiver must be well documented, ideally with a document signed by the patient.

Therapeutic Privilege

Therapeutic privilege refers to an unusual situation in which the physician believes that fully informing the patient would be detrimental to the patient. This situation usually refers to emotional issues. There is a danger here that mental health patients could be denied a basic right of self-determination. The physician must fully document why he or she has withheld information and should provide as much information to the patient as possible.

Legal Mandate

In some circumstances, the court may order that a patient undergo a medical procedure without requiring the patient's consent. Obtaining concealed contraband and forensic pathology specimens are examples. A more difficult situation is performing a procedure on a minor against the wishes of the parent.

Incompetency

If the patient is incompetent to make decisions, the patient's legal guardian has the responsibility of providing informed consent.

Informed Refusal

The inverse of informed consent is informed refusal. If a patient refuses specific medical treatment, there is a duty of care for the physician to ensure that the refusal is informed. It is negligent to allow a patient to leave the hospital against medical advice without informing the patient of the risks of doing so.

Documentation

Sound documentation is an important risk management tool and a component of good medical practice. Nothing in a patient's management plan should be left to the memory of the physician. A case may come to trial years after the event. It is highly unlikely that the physician would be able to remember details of a consultation with the clarity of the plaintiff (on whom this brief physician-patient interaction has had a major impact). The plaintiff would appear to be a much more credible witness unless the physician has comprehensive notes. Generally, a court would accept that something was discussed or did occur if it was documented in the notes at the time.

Conversely, a court or jury may decide that a conversation did not occur if the plaintiff denies it and the physician only "remembers" the conversation or states that it is always his or her practice to discuss a certain aspect of care. Videotaping the consent process has been mentioned as a method of documenting exactly what occurred.[19]

Medical record retention laws vary, and the physician should be acquainted with how long records of adults and minors need to be retained. The physician owns the record, but the patient has the right to control access to the information. The patient has a right to see the medical record and copy it for an appropriate fee. Documents should be concise, logical, and legible. All entries must be dated. The physician should never make demeaning or insulting comments about the patient. If an error occurs, it should be struck through once (still legible), and a correction should be made, signed, and dated. *Notations must never be altered.* Forensic techniques are available to determine whether numbers have been changed subsequently. Notations can be corrected or supplemented if the changes are clearly identified and dated.

Electronic Media

The gist of telephone conversations should be recorded in the notes. E-mail is increasingly used to communicate with other health care professionals and patients. A physician using e-mail should consider using encryption software to protect confidentiality. All communications should be printed, and a hardcopy should be kept with the notes. Patients communicating with their physician via e-mail must understand that sending an e-mail does not mean that the physician has received and read it. (An automatic reply message can be sent warning patients of a delay and urging them to call or go to the nearest hospital if their concern is urgent.) Patients should also be aware that in many circumstances e-mail is a poor substitute for a standard consultation. Care must be taken to ensure the security of data kept on computers and personal data assistants (PDAs). PDAs are of particular concern because they may be lost easily and may have inadequate password protection to prevent data retrieval of sensitive patient information.

Procedure Documentation

Procedures may be documented by dictated or handwritten notes, or documentation may be generated by databases. Regardless of the method of documentation, all procedural reports should contain the following information:

Date
Patient identification (at least name and medical record number)
Proceduralist
Assistants present
Instrument used
Sedation
Monitoring
Use of topical anesthesia
Indication
Findings
Interventions performed
Impediments to the study (e.g., preparation)

Complications
Recommendations
Follow-up

It is wise to include postprocedure documentation because many patients have persistent amnesia attributable to the effects of sedation at the time of discussion before leaving the endoscopy unit (despite appearing to be alert). This documentation should include advice regarding driving, important decision making, or dangerous activities following sedation; follow-up arrangements; and a plan in case of emergency after the procedure. Depending on the findings of the procedure and the level of relationship between the endoscopist and the patient, it may or may not be appropriate to include a summary of the findings of the procedure. Several software reporting systems incorporate many of the necessary elements of the report, including embedding of photographs that may be used to document pathology and the adequacy of the examination (e.g., documentation of visualization of the ileocecal valve).

Risk Management

Risk management is an evolving process that aims to identify potential sources of poor outcome and undergo steps to correct these issues. Risk management has the following objectives:

1. To define instances that place the endoscopist at risk
2. To determine the frequency and significance of these instances
3. To apply risk management to individual cases
4. To develop preventive measures

Many of the issues already discussed constitute important aspects of risk management:

1. *Sound medical practice:* The best defense against poor outcomes and possible litigation is good medical practice. Efforts on the part of the individual and the institution to remain current with the medical literature and practice in line with government statutes and societal guidelines is an important aspect of sound medical practice. Courts have been reluctant to accept financial constraint as a mitigating factor when assessing a poor outcome (although this may shift some blame from the individual to the institution).
2. *Good documentation: See previous discussion.*
3. *Informed consent: See previous discussion.*
4. *Peer review:* Peer review is a vital mechanism to identify endemic problems and to recognize and discuss problems to prevent their recurrence. Peer review must always be done in a nonthreatening manner to maintain a true reflection of the unit's complication profile. It should be a formal process, usually involving a meeting of all senior staff on a regular basis with recording of minutes. Physicians should be aware of their own complication profiles and where they stand relative to their peers. Some very experienced proceduralists may have high complication rates because of the complexity of work they perform, and in this circumstance, they should have some way of illustrating their work mix. Patients have a right to know, in general terms, a physician's complication and outcome profile.

5. *Adequate indemnity insurance:* Some large institutions may self-insure their employees, but it is the responsibility of every physician to ensure that he or she has adequate indemnity cover both for claims occurring now and for claims that may occur years into the future (although many states have a statute of limitation on medical malpractice claims).

Quality Agenda in Endoscopy

As previously stated, the best defense against poor outcomes and litigation is good medical practice. In recent years, a great deal of attention has focused on issues regarding quality assurance in endoscopy units. There are several reasons for this interest, as follows:

1. *The rollout of colorectal cancer screening programs:* Regardless of type of screening program, healthy, asymptomatic individuals are being advised to undergo colonoscopy. Most of these people will not have a significant colonic lesion. It is imperative that colonoscopy under these circumstances is as safe as possible. A healthy person with no colonic pathology who is advised to undergo a colonoscopy is much more likely to be upset over a complication than a patient presenting with symptoms.
2. *Recognition of limitations in current clinical practice:* Prominent publications have suggested that the quality of screening colonoscopies may be inferior to that previously supposed. A large review of colonoscopy in England under the auspices of the National Health Service reported surprisingly poor quality indices, such as an adjusted cecal intubation rate of 56%.[20]
3. *Increasing sophistication of the "consumer":* The consumer of endoscopic services in this context includes not only the patient but also government health authorities, health insurance providers, and indemnity providers. Patients are increasingly likely to query the experience of a proceduralist, including Internet searches of the proceduralist and the procedure. In some areas of medicine, the concept of a publicly available "report card" is gaining acceptance, although there is concern that this concept may act as a disincentive to perform high-risk procedures.
4. *Appropriateness of endoscopic procedures:* Concerns over appropriateness of endoscopic procedures are increasing. Such concern is especially relevant with regard to ERCP because competing noninvasive imaging technologies are making "diagnostic" ERCP increasingly difficult to justify in many circumstances. This issue was highlighted in a review of 59 medicolegal opinions offered by a single experienced endoscopist; in more than half of these cases, the main basis for litigation was that the procedure was not indicated.[21] As major endoscopy societies expand their roles, they are developing clinical guidelines for appropriate use of endoscopic procedures.[22]

Knowledge of these quality assurance issues can assist referring primary physicians and may be used by other groups, such as insurers, to ensure proper endoscopic practice.

Specific Quality Indicators in Endoscopy

National and international endoscopy bodies, such as the American Society of Gastrointestinal Endoscopy, American College of Gastroenterology, World Gastroenterology Organization, British Society of Gastroenterology, and Gastroenterology Society of Australia, have published guidelines on quality indicators related to various aspects of endoscopy (see **Box 9.1**). Objective procedural quality indicators have been suggested by ASGE[21] for colonoscopy and for ERCP:

- Colonoscopy
  - Cecal intubation rates of greater than 90% and greater than 95% for screening colonoscopy
  - Withdrawal times from cecum of 6 minutes or longer when no biopsies or other maneuvers are performed
  - Adenoma detection rate of greater than 25% for men and 15% for women older than age 50
  - Perforation rates of less than 1:1000 for screening colonoscopy and less than 1:500 for all colonoscopy procedures
- ERCP
  - Desired duct cannulation rate of greater than 85%
  - With regard to choledocholithiasis, bile duct clearance rate of greater than 85%

Such guidelines are designed to help ensure appropriate, safe, and cost-effective endoscopic practice and should help assist endoscopists and endoscopy units in establishing quality criteria in monitoring their activities. The increasing use of computerized reporting systems should make data capture for the purposes of quality audits (individual and institutional) easier in the future. Photographic documentation, especially of colon landmarks, is increasingly recommended. Sedation-related issues are also being recognized as an important aspect of quality endoscopic practice.[23] As risks associated with sedation are being recognized and guidelines regarding appropriate care are disseminated, endoscopists and endoscopy units will need to monitor their experience in this aspect of endoscopic practice.

Medicolegal Consultation

A detailed discussion of medicolegal consultation is beyond the scope of this textbook. An expert medical witness provides an important service to the community, provided that the opinion is unbiased. The American College of Physicians has developed guidelines to assist physicians engaged in this activity. These guidelines state that expert witnesses should be appropriately licensed and board certified and should have been practicing in the area for at least 3 of the previous 5 years. Reasonable compensation should be provided, but contingency fees (i.e., fee structure based on the outcome of the case) are unethical. Some states cap the proportion of income that a physician can derive from this type of activity; this is an effort to prevent "hired guns" who provide opinions clouded by a perception of what the client would like them to say. The opinion should be unbiased, such that it should be irrelevant to the expert whether he or she is retained by the plaintiff or defendant. The opinion must be nonemotive.

In most cases, being an expert witness requires a review of a medical record and summarizing an opinion regarding the patient's care. Because most cases are resolved long before trial, usually this is all that is needed. If the case does proceed to trial, the witness may be required to supply an affidavit, give a deposition, or, less commonly, testify in court. When in court, witnesses should have detailed notes and not rely on their memory of the case. Answers should be succinct and respond directly to the question. It is crucial to answer only the question posed and fight the tendency to embellish an answer. If a physician witness does not know the answer to a question, he or she should say so. The physician should be nonemotive and recognize that it may be the aim of one of the teams to discredit his or her answers and position as an expert.

References

The complete reference list is available online at www.expertconsult.com.

Chapter 10

Small-Caliber Endoscopy

Christopher J. Gostout

Video related to this chapter's topics can be found online at expertconsult.com.

Introduction

Small-caliber endoscopy has selective appeal. Sedation may be responsible for a substantial proportion of the morbidity and mortality of endoscopic procedures. The opportunity to perform diagnostic endoscopy without sedation can overcome the issues relative to sedation, especially in high-risk patients. The administration of sedatives increases the preprocedure preparation, total procedure, and postprocedure recovery times. Finally, the "sedationless" argument gains strength with regard to lifestyle impact, allowing the patient to minimize time away from work or family and eliminating the need for an accompanying responsible person. Despite its potential safety and cost-effectiveness, however, the practice of unsedated endoscopy with small-caliber endoscopes has not gained wide acceptance. Many factors may be responsible, including inadequate evidence for efficacy, poor patient acceptance, lack of physician incentives, and limited opportunities for training.

Small-caliber endoscopy has other practical uses. Patients who may be predictably intolerant of endoscopy with sedation, such as young patients, are potential candidates for this option. Small-caliber endoscopy offers a dramatically reduced procedure stress for patients who have fragile cardiopulmonary disease. The small-caliber endoscope provides an effective and well-tolerated option for the placement of transnasal feeding tubes and the placement of jejunal extensions via an existing percutaneous feeding gastroscopy site.[1-3] Patients with high-grade esophageal strictures with existing percutaneous feeding gastrostomy may have primary or rendezvous attempts at dilation with placement of guidewires using a small-caliber endoscope via the gastrostomy site.[4,5]

Small-Caliber Endoscopy Insertion Techniques

Small-caliber upper endoscopy can be performed either transnasally or perorally (**Fig. 10.1**). Transnasal endoscopy is feasible with endoscopes measuring 6 mm or less in outside diameter. **Table 10.1** summarizes specifications of small-caliber endoscopes used in the reviewed studies and other endoscopes that are commercially available. Both videoesophagogastroduodenoscopes and esophagoscopes are currently available. Videoesophagogastroduodenoscopes have a working length of 1030 to 1330 mm, and esophagoscopes have a working length of only 600 mm. The outer diameter of videoesophagogastroduodenoscopes is between 5.1 mm and 6 mm. Esophagoscopes have an outside diameter between 3.1 mm and 4 mm. The relative outside diameters of small-caliber pediatric and conventional esophagogastroduodenoscopes are shown in **Fig. 10.2A**. Some esophagogastroduodenoscopes allow right and left and up and down angulation, whereas others provide only up and down angulation (**Fig. 10.2B**).

Careful patient selection and preparation are of utmost importance. Uncooperative patients and young patients with a high preprocedure anxiety level are not well suited for unsedated procedures. Elderly patients tolerate the examination extremely well—so well that in our institution we contemplated offering this exclusively for patients 80 years or older undergoing diagnostic endoscopy. Because the tolerability of the procedure is related to preprocedure anxiety, the procedure must be explained clearly before intubation.

Topical anesthesia in the form of a spray or jelly is useful before endoscope insertion. The application of 2% lidocaine

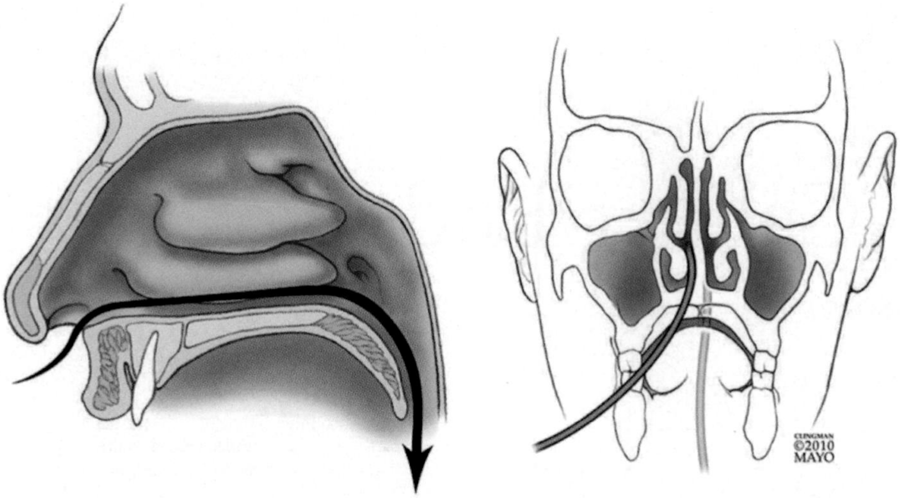

Fig. 10.1   Nasal passage anatomy. Small-caliber endoscope is passed directly back along the floor of the nasal passage, along the medial septum, avoiding the turbinates, with flexion of the tip down into the posterior pharynx *(line arrow)*.

Table 10.1 Fiberoptic and Video Small-Caliber Endoscopes Available for Unsedated Upper Endoscopy

Company/Model	Imaging	Outer Diameter* (mm)	Working Length (mm)	Instrument Channel (mm)	Angulation Up/Down–Right/Left
Pentax					
EG-1540	Video	5.1	1050	2.0	210/120–0/0
EG-1840	Video	6.0	1050	2.0	210/120–120/120
OLYMPUS					
GIF-XP N180	Video/NBI	5.5	1100	2.0	210/90–100/100
GIF-N180	Video	4.9	1100	2.0	210/90†
XGIF-N160Y1	Video	5.3	1330	2.0	180/180†
GIF-N30	Fiberoptic	5.3	930	2.0	180/180–160/160
GIF-XP20	Fiberoptic	7.9	1030	2.0	210/90–100/100
XEF-DP‡	Fiberoptic	3.1	600	—	90/90†
LF-GP‡	Fiberoptic	4	600	—	90/90†
XEF 140I	Video	4	600	—	90/90†
FUJINON					
EG-470 N/EG-270 N	Video	6.0	1100	2.0	210/90–100/100

Note: Endoscopes with a working length of 600 mm are used for esophagoscopy only. Some esophagoscopes are battery-operated.
*Values correspond to the outside diameter of the insertion tube.
†Two-way deflection only.
‡Battery-operated esophagoscope.
NBI, Narrow band imaging.

jelly into the more patent nostril as determined by visual inspection is recommended for this approach to topical anesthesia. Pharyngeal anesthesia is also recommended. Local vasoconstrictors may also be beneficial, especially when a 6-mm diameter instrument is inserted transnasally. If a 4-mm or smaller caliber endoscope is used, a local vasoconstrictor may be of marginal value to aid insertion, but it may minimize epistaxis.

The procedure can be performed either in the standard left lateral decubitus position for conventional endoscopy or in the upright position (**Fig. 10.3**). Whether the upright position decreases the aspiration risk is unknown. The transnasal procedure should be performed with minimal air insufflation. The endoscope should be inserted slowly and gently, keeping the insertion tube of the endoscope straight such that it passes along the floor and septum of the nasal cavity and it does not migrate upward and laterally into turbinates interrupting passage, causing pain, and inducing bleeding. Slow progressive insertion with flexion of the endoscope tip over the base of the tongue is recommended for unsedated peroral

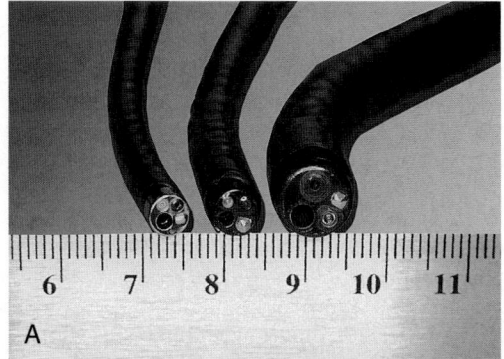

Fig. 10.2   Small-caliber upper endoscopes. Distal ends of a small-caliber, pediatric, and conventional esophagogastroduodenoscope are shown **(A)** along with the handle of a small-caliber endoscope with only one ratchet for up and down control **(B)**.

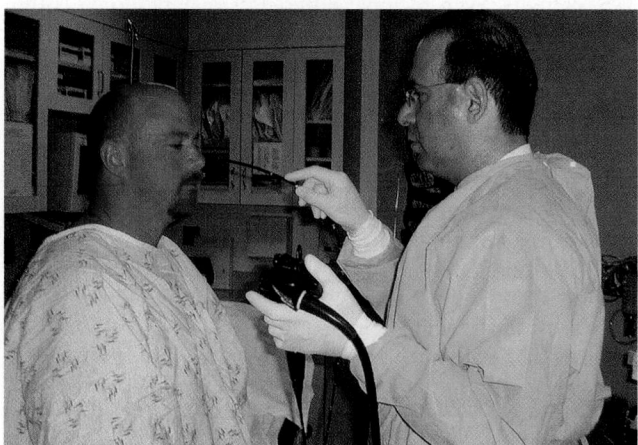

Fig. 10.3   Patient is shown undergoing transnasal small-caliber esophagogastroduodenoscopy in the upright position.

examinations. Vigorous movements of the endoscope cause greater nasal discomfort with the transnasal route and more gagging with the peroral approach. During the procedure, conversing with the patient and pointing out findings on the video monitor reassure patients and may improve tolerability and reduce discomfort.

Unsedated Small-Caliber Upper Endoscopy

The impact of unsedated small-caliber endoscopy on the everyday practice of esophagogastroduodenoscopy (EGD) is complex. There are no data from large randomized controlled trials. Although lower procedure cost and complication rate favor unsedated EGD, poor patient tolerance, suboptimal visualization, and failure to complete the procedure could increase the cost of upper endoscopy secondary to repeated examination by sedated EGD. Analyses of the few existing randomized controlled studies provide sufficient evidence that unsedated small-caliber upper endoscopy is feasible and tolerable in select patient groups. Most evidence suggests, however, that small-caliber endoscopy is slightly less sensitive.

There are conflicting reports regarding the transnasal approach and whether or not it is preferred over the peroral route. Based on a questionnaire provided to patients undergoing endoscopy at our outpatient units, patient preference is actually for peroral intubation. This preference has been well appreciated within our motility practice, which for decades has performed esophagogastroduodenal motility via a peroral catheter approach. Data are insufficient regarding the safety of unsedated small-caliber endoscopy compared with sedated conventional endoscopy. Finally, the cost-effectiveness of unsedated small-caliber endoscopy is yet to be determined. With that in mind, the following sections summarize the literature addressing the various aspects of unsedated small-caliber endoscopy.

Technical Feasibility of Unsedated Small-Caliber Endoscopy

Feasibility of unsedated small-caliber endoscopy is mainly a subjective measure defined by the endoscopist. It can be affected by many factors, including the diameter of the small-caliber endoscope, endoscope maneuverability, image quality, patient tolerability, and the skills of the endoscopist. Feasibility of unsedated endoscopy is particularly linked to tolerance, which is discussed in the next section. In the crudest sense, technical feasibility represents the successful completion of the intended procedure by intubating the duodenum if an EGD is being performed or intubating the stomach if esophagoscopy is being done. Several investigators have reported the feasibility of transoral or transnasal unsedated EGD.[6–18] Most of these studies have not been prospective randomized controlled trials. The patient populations have been either small in size or not representative of the general U.S. population. Studies addressing the feasibility of EGD that warrant attention are described next.

Wilkins and coworkers[6] randomly assigned 72 patients to undergo either unsedated small-caliber EGD or sedated conventional EGD. Despite a highly selected and motivated U.S. Air Force community population, only 29 of the 33 patients (88%) had a complete unsedated small-caliber EGD. In another controlled study, Mulcahy and coworkers[7] compared the feasibility of unsedated small-caliber EGD with unsedated conventional EGD in 322 patients. EGD was completed in 160 of the 163 patients (98%) undergoing unsedated EGD with a 6-mm gastroscope compared with 145 of the 159 patients (91%) undergoing unsedated EGD with a 9.8-mm gastroscope. These investigators subsequently reported 39 (8%) failures in a prospective study of 508 patients undergoing routine unsedated gastroscopy.[8] Failure was associated with larger scope diameter (>9 mm), higher preprocedure anxiety, and younger age.

Ristikankare and colleagues[9] randomly assigned 180 patients undergoing EGD to receive intravenous (IV) midazolam, IV saline, or no IV access. Although the procedure was perceived "less difficult" in the IV midazolam group compared with the IV saline group, the difference was not statistically significant. The power to detect differences between the three groups was not determined in this study. The small patient population and the lack of validated criteria to assess the difficulty of an EGD limit the utility of the evidence.

The feasibility of unsedated small-caliber EGD was also assessed as part of the multiphase Mayo Clinic Rochester study of a select group of highly motivated patients and volunteers.[10] The second portion of the duodenum was reached in 20 sedated and 20 unsedated volunteers in this prospective, nonrandomized study. Among the patients, 50 subjects successfully underwent sedated small-caliber EGD followed by sedated conventional EGD, and 38 of 40 patients underwent successful unsedated small-caliber EGD followed by sedated conventional EGD. Overall, the technical feasibility was not significantly affected by sedation in this study. A type II error (failure to detect a significant difference when there is a difference) cannot be ruled out, however, because the sample size to detect a significant difference was not calculated.

Investigators have also studied the feasibility of unsedated transnasal small-caliber EGD. Saeian and coworkers[11] showed that unsedated transnasal esophagoscopy with a 5.3-mm gastroscope was feasible in 15 cirrhotic patients. The study was uncontrolled, and the population was very small. Zaman and colleagues[13] compared peroral and transnasal approaches for EGD with the same small-caliber instrument using a prospective randomized crossover study design. Of 105 patients, 60 (57%) agreed to undergo unsedated small-caliber EGD. Peroral unsedated EGD was feasible in 34 of 35 (97%) patients, including 4 who failed transnasal EGD and were crossed over. Unsedated transnasal EGD was feasible in only 25 of 29 (86%) patients. The statistics were not reported, and a sample size based on a study hypothesis was also not calculated before study initiation.

Campo and coworkers[14] randomly assigned 181 Spanish patients to undergo transnasal small-caliber EGD or peroral conventional EGD. Insertion failed in six (3.3%) patients; four had been randomly assigned to the transnasal route and two to the peroral route. In a prospective randomized trial in Australia, Craig and colleagues[17] compared the feasibility of unsedated transnasal with unsedated peroral small-caliber EGD. A complete examination was feasible in 74 of the 84 (88%) transnasal and 85 of the 86 (99%) transoral procedures ($P = .004$).

Dumortier and coworkers[18] reported that unsedated transnasal EGD was feasible in 1033 of 1100 (94%) patients studied prospectively at three French medical centers. Failures were mainly due to the inability to insert the small-caliber endoscope (62.7%). Other reasons for failure included patient refusal and nasal pain. In their prior study published in 1999, the same investigators showed that unsedated transnasal EGD was feasible in 82% of the study population and was associated with less nausea and choking.[19] The feasibility of transnasal small-caliber EGD was initially assessed in 100 patients in this two-phase study; 150 patients were then randomly assigned to undergo peroral conventional EGD with a 9.8-mm videoendoscope, peroral small-caliber EGD with a 6-mm videoendoscope, or transnasal small-caliber EGD with a 6-mm videoendoscope.

The evidence that supports the feasibility of unsedated upper endoscopy compared with sedated endoscopy is limited. The randomized studies that have been reviewed failed to specify the study hypothesis and to calculate a sample size before study initiation. These studies may have failed to detect a difference because of a type II error. The studies have also used different caliber instruments, and there is some evidence suggesting that the feasibility of an unsedated examination may be better with smaller diameter instruments. None of the studies had sufficient power to examine whether unsedated endoscopy is feasible for all indications. Comparative studies comparing transnasal and peroral approaches have given variable results. However, the weight of the evidence suggests that transnasal intubation may not be feasible in all patients.

Tolerability of Unsedated Small-Caliber Endoscopy

The tolerability of unsedated small-caliber esophagoscopy or EGD is of utmost importance. It directly affects patient or physician acceptance, examination adequacy, and technical feasibility. Many studies have measured the tolerability of unsedated upper endoscopy by evaluating specific symptoms, such as gagging, choking, pain, and discomfort, on a Likert scale. Tolerability of unsedated endoscopy varies considerably across countries and patient populations. Although unsedated upper endoscopy may be considered the norm in some countries, the idea may not be appealing to U.S. endoscopists and U.S. patients. Even regional differences may be noted within the United States.

Tolerability is a complex variable, which is likely affected by numerous patient-related and operator-related factors, including patient education, prior endoscopic experience, preprocedure anxiety, patient age, patient gender, endoscopist skill, and technical performance of the endoscope. A prohibitively large and diverse patient population would be required to determine how all of these factors affect the tolerability and acceptance of unsedated endoscopy. Catanzaro and coworkers[20] evaluated patient tolerability of unsedated endoscopy with a 4-mm esophagoscope. This study enrolled 51 patients; 30 patients underwent an unsedated procedure. Of these patients, 18 preferred the peroral route, and 12 preferred the transnasal route. Patient tolerability and acceptability of unsedated esophagoscopy with the 4-mm esophagoscope compared favorably with a historical group of patients examined with a 3-mm esophagoscope.

In an earlier study, Catanzaro and colleagues[21] assessed the use of a 3.1-mm, battery-operated esophagoscope in an unsedated procedure. Examination with the battery-operated esophagoscope was performed in 98 patients. Of the 56 patients undergoing an unsedated examination, 43 preferred the peroral approach. Although the endoscopist's perception of patient discomfort was not significantly different, the patients undergoing unsedated small-caliber esophagoscopy reported significantly more choking, pain, and overall discomfort with the 3.1-mm, battery-operated esophagoscope.

Faulx and coworkers[22] approached 98 patients to undergo unsedated esophagoscopy with a 3.1-mm esophagoscope before conventional EGD. Only 46% of the 52 patients participating in the study preferred unsedated 3.1-mm esophagoscopy over conventional EGD in the future. Of patients, 16 chose the peroral approach, and 36 chose the transnasal approach. Patients who chose the peroral route were more likely to prefer unsedated small-caliber endoscopy with the 3.1-mm esophagoscope compared with the transnasal approach (58% vs. 23%).

Saeian and colleagues[11] performed sedated conventional EGD following unsedated small-caliber EGD and reported no significant difference in choking, discomfort, and sore throat in a population of 15 cirrhotic patients. In contrast, Wilkins and coworkers[6] reported increased gagging and choking in the 33 patients randomly assigned to undergo unsedated small-caliber EGD compared with the 39 patients who underwent sedated conventional EGD. However, most patients tolerated unsedated small-caliber EGD.

A prospective study in the United States found that only 52 of 98 patients (53%) approached agreed to undergo unsedated esophagoscopy with a 3.1-mm esophagoscope followed by sedated EGD.[22] Although one may argue that the willingness to undergo unsedated endoscopy may be hampered by undergoing tandem endoscopies, this is one of the few well-designed studies to address the impact of unsedated endoscopy on the practice of EGD. Of the 52 patients who underwent both procedures, only 46% preferred unsedated EGD. Patients who had transnasal esophagoscopy were less likely to prefer an unsedated procedure in the future compared with patients who underwent peroral esophagoscopy (23% vs. 58%). Similarly, Zaman and colleagues[23] reported that 19 (31%) of 62 patients asked to undergo unsedated 6-mm transoral EGD followed by sedated transoral conventional EGD refused. Of the 43 patients who agreed to undergo unsedated small-caliber EGD, 30 (70%) were willing to have unsedated small-caliber EGD in the future.

A prospective randomized controlled trial from a center in the United Kingdom that routinely performs unsedated endoscopies concluded that endoscopists found unsedated examinations easier, but patients reported significantly greater comfort with sedation.[24] Another trial from the United Kingdom that studied 62 elderly patients reported that an equal number of patients undergoing sedated or unsedated EGD described the procedure as "mildly unpleasant."[25] Of the patients who underwent unsedated EGD, 73% did not wish to be sedated for future EGD. Froehlich and colleagues[26] randomly assigned 200 European patients to receive IV midazolam with lidocaine spray, IV placebo with lidocaine spray, IV midazolam with placebo spray, or IV placebo with placebo spray and showed that tolerability, assessed on a visual analogue scale, was significantly improved in patients who received IV sedation.

One major difficulty with the interpretation of the studies comparing the tolerability of unsedated endoscopy with sedated procedures is that benzodiazepines affect recall. The timing of when the patient is questioned may affect the response to the questions. The only prospective controlled trial that compared two unsedated procedures found that patients reported less discomfort when peroral EGD was performed with a 6-mm endoscope compared with a 9.8-mm instrument.[7] Sedation during future examination was requested by 14% of subjects who underwent examination with a 6-mm endoscope compared with 31% of patients examined with a 9.8-mm endoscope.

A few studies have compared the tolerability and acceptance of unsedated transnasal and peroral approaches. In a randomized U.S. trial of unsedated peroral versus transnasal small-caliber EGD, Zaman and coworkers[13] determined that 89% of the patients undergoing peroral EGD and 69% of the patients undergoing transnasal EGD were willing to have unsedated small-caliber EGD in the future. A smaller U.S. study of 24 patients who had undergone transnasal unsedated EGD followed by conventional EGD concluded that transnasal EGD was more acceptable.[15] However, a randomized Australian study of 170 patients found no significant difference in tolerability of unsedated small-caliber EGD with either route.[17] Dumortier and colleagues[18] reported that 95% of 1033 French patients who successfully underwent unsedated small-caliber transnasal EGD were willing to repeat the procedure. Of the 377 patients who had previously undergone unsedated transoral EGD, 91% preferred the transnasal route.

Most of the literature suggests that unsedated endoscopy is not as tolerable as sedated endoscopies. The evidence in support of a transnasal approach to improve procedure tolerability is inconclusive because various studies have reported contradictory results. Patients who have successfully completed unsedated endoscopy seem to have moderate acceptance of the procedure. For reasons not completely understood, U.S. patients may be particularly unwilling to undergo unsedated endoscopy.

Safety of Unsedated Small-Caliber Endoscopy

One of the arguments for advocating unsedated procedures is that the morbidity and mortality of endoscopic procedures are largely related to sedation. The evidence to support this allegation is limited, however. The practice of sedated endoscopy is very safe, and complications are uncommon. The incidence of serious cardiorespiratory complications in an American Society for Gastrointestinal Endoscopy (ASGE)/U.S. Food and Drug Administration (FDA) collaborative study of 21,011 procedures was 5.4 per 1000 cases, and the incidence of death was 0.3 per 1000 cases.[27] A large retrospective German study found that the overall complication rate associated with sedated EGD was 0.009%.[28]

Because of the low complication rate of sedated EGD, any study to determine whether unsedated EGD is safer would require an extremely large patient population. The safety of unsedated EGD has been addressed in several small studies. Limited studies have reported no serious complications in 60 patients[5] and 170 patients[17] who underwent unsedated procedures. Epistaxis is unique to transnasal EGD and can occur in one of five patients[29]; this is not surprising given that insertion of a soft small-bore nasogastric tube may result in epistaxis. The largest prospective study of unsedated transnasal EGD revealed epistaxis in 2.3%, nasal pain in 1.6%, and vasovagal reactions in 0.3% of 1100 consecutive patients participating in the study at three French centers. Much larger studies of unsedated EGD are needed to determine a true cardiorespiratory complication rate of the procedure. Cost prohibits the performance of such a large prospective randomized comparative study on the safety of unsedated and sedated EGD. Although it seems that transnasal unsedated EGD is associated with an increased rate of minor complications (epistaxis) compared with peroral EGD, larger comparative studies with ultrathin endoscopes are required. In the absence of data from large prospective studies, the currently available safety data originate from small prospective or retrospective studies.

Adequacy of Unsedated Small-Caliber Endoscopy and Biopsy

The data on the adequacy of examinations performed using small-caliber endoscopes are even more limited. Image quality, suctioning ability, adequacy of tissue sampling, and ability to perform therapeutic maneuvers are among the main determinants of "adequacy." The specifications of several small-caliber upper endoscopes are listed in Table 10.1. Most commercially available small-caliber endoscopes incorporate video charge-coupled devices technology, although some studies have been performed with fiberoptic instruments. The outside diameter of these endoscopes is 5 to 6 mm, approximately half the diameter of a conventional upper endoscope (see **Fig. 10.2A**). The esophagoscopes have a working length of 600 mm to allow intubation of the stomach. Some are battery-operated, and none allow biopsies. A thinner insertion tube may be too flexible, limiting passage through the pylorus and intubation of the second portion of the duodenum. Some manufacturers have marketed small-caliber endoscopes that have only unidirectional up-and-down tip deflection (see **Fig. 10.2B**), whereas others have bidirectional up-and-down and right-and-left tip deflection similar to conventional instruments. The accessory channel of small-caliber esophagogastroduodenoscopes is generally 2 mm; this limits the size of the biopsy specimens that can be obtained and the ability to perform therapeutic interventions. The smaller diameter of the channels could also impair the ability to aspirate blood, secretions, and debris and the ability to wash the lens. A sample image of the gastroesophageal junction as viewed by a small-caliber endoscope is shown in **Fig. 10.4**, and a brief normal transnasal examination is presented as a video clip.

Wildi and coworkers[30] and Catanzaro and colleagues[20,21] addressed the accuracy of small-caliber esophagoscopes. Wildi and coworkers[30] assessed the diagnostic accuracy of sedated esophagoscopy performed by a nurse practitioner using a 4-mm esophagoscope compared with sedated conventional EGD performed by an experienced gastroenterologist. There were 40 patients who underwent tandem procedures in a blinded fashion. For all esophageal lesions, the sensitivity and specificity of the examination by the nurse practitioner were 75% and 98%. All four Schatzki rings were missed.[30] In their study of 51 patients undergoing esophagoscopy using the 4-mm esophagoscope, Catanzaro and colleagues[20] reported sensitivity, accuracy, and specificity of 91%, 98%, and 99% for

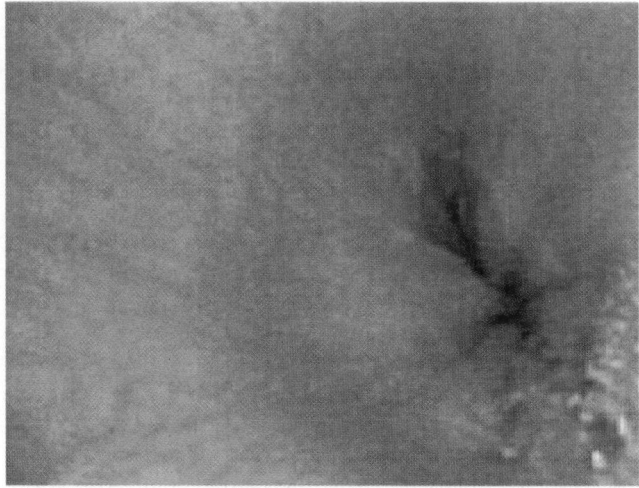

Fig. 10.4 Endoscopic image of a normal squamocolumnar junction as viewed by a videoesophagogastroduodenoscope.

detecting all esophageal lesions. The first 24 patients underwent endoscopy using the battery-operated fiberoptic esophagoscope, and 27 patients were examined with the 4-mm videoesophagoscope. In an earlier study, Catanzaro and coworkers[21] reported that the accuracy of esophageal examination with a 3.1-mm endoscope is substantially inferior to conventional EGD. The sensitivity for detecting Barrett's esophagus, esophageal tumors, and esophageal varices was 54.5%, 66.7%, and 80%. Optical quality was reported as less than 4 on a scale of 1 to 5 in 42% of the cases.

In the study of Dumortier and colleagues,[18] endoscopic biopsy specimens, obtained in 457 subjects undergoing a transnasal examination, were considered "sufficient." Four esophageal cancers and one gastric cancer were correctly diagnosed by biopsy. Although this is the largest study addressing the adequacy of samples obtained at the time of unsedated transnasal EGD, this outcome was not the primary or even secondary goal of the study. Criteria for determining sample adequacy were not defined. Zaman and coworkers[18] reported that unsedated peroral small-caliber EGD with a video instrument missed 5 of 59 lesions identified by conventional EGD in 62 patients, yielding an accuracy of 92%. The optical quality of the images was rated as good in 84%, 65%, and 78% of the subjects when examining the esophagus, stomach, and duodenum. In a similar study of unsedated transnasal EGD, Dean and colleagues[15] found a sensitivity of 89% and a specificity of 97% using a fiberoptic instrument.

In the only study examining the effect of sedation and endoscope caliber, Sorbi and coworkers[10] showed that the accuracy for major endoscopic findings was 96% for the 50 patients who underwent sedated transoral small-caliber EGD and 97% for the 40 patients who underwent unsedated transoral small-caliber EGD. The view was particularly limited because of the inability to aspirate secretions and clear bubbles rapidly. These results suggest that caliber, and not sedation, may be the primary factor determining the accuracy of unsedated small-caliber endoscopy. The 4-mm diameter may be the lower limit for upper endoscopes to maintain adequate image quality.

Regardless of whether a videoendoscope or a fiberoptic endoscope is used, studies comparing small-caliber upper endoscopy with conventional upper endoscopy have uniformly reported that the smaller caliber instruments have a slightly lower accuracy. Lesions missed by small-caliber instruments tend to be mild esophageal stenoses or lesions located in the second portion of the duodenum. Although small-caliber endoscopes apparently are accurate for detecting common lesions, the studies have not addressed the accuracy of small-caliber endoscopy for detecting subtle rare mucosal abnormalities such as early malignancies. There is also insufficient evidence whether biopsy specimens obtained by small-caliber endoscopes are adequate for detecting dysplasia in Barrett's esophagus.

Cost-Effectiveness of Unsedated Small-Caliber Endoscopy

Cost may be the major impetus behind the practice of unsedated endoscopy. Elimination of sedation may significantly reduce the cost of endoscopy. However, the total expense of unsedated endoscopy must be studied in view of its impact on the everyday practice of EGD. Unsedated small-caliber endoscopy can result in savings only if the general population finds it acceptable and if most unsedated examinations are adequate and a repeat examination under sedation is not required. The impact of unsedated endoscopy on the cost of EGD has been evaluated only in a few studies. In a case-control study, Gorelick and colleagues[31] assessed the potential cost savings associated with unsedated small-caliber EGD in 16 patients undergoing unsedated transoral small-caliber EGD matched for age, gender, indication, and procedure day with a control group of 16 patients who underwent sedated conventional EGD. The mean procedure room time was 16.3 minutes for unsedated small-caliber EGD and 34.9 minutes for sedated conventional EGD ($P < .0005$). The mean recovery room time was 9.0 minutes for unsedated small-caliber EGD and 41.3 minutes for sedated conventional EGD ($P < .00001$). The mean cost for unsedated small-caliber EGD was $462 and was considerably lower than the mean cost of sedated conventional EGD, which was reported as $587 ($P < .0006$).

In a controlled study, Wilkins and coworkers[6] randomly assigned 72 patients to undergo either unsedated small-caliber EGD or sedated conventional EGD. The procedure time (mean ± standard error of the mean) for the 33 patients who underwent unsedated small-caliber EGD was 21.5 ± 2.3 minutes, whereas the procedure time for the 39 patients who underwent sedated conventional EGD was 55.4 ± 2.3 minutes. Without performing a formal cost analysis, the investigators suggested that unsedated small-caliber EGD performed by primary care physicians could increase access while decreasing the cost of upper endoscopy. Bampton and colleagues[32] compared unsedated transnasal EGD with sedated transoral EGD. The mean procedure times of 15 minutes for the unsedated procedure and 20 minutes for the sedated procedure were not significantly different. However, the mean recovery time was 7 minutes for the unsedated transnasal examination compared with 37 minutes for the transoral sedated EGD, emphasizing the shorter recovery time when no sedation is administered. A formal cost-effectiveness analysis of unsedated versus sedated endoscopy that accounts for variations in the patient population, patient acceptance, completion rates, and diagnostic accuracy is yet to be performed to determine the utility of this approach in the daily practice of upper endoscopy.

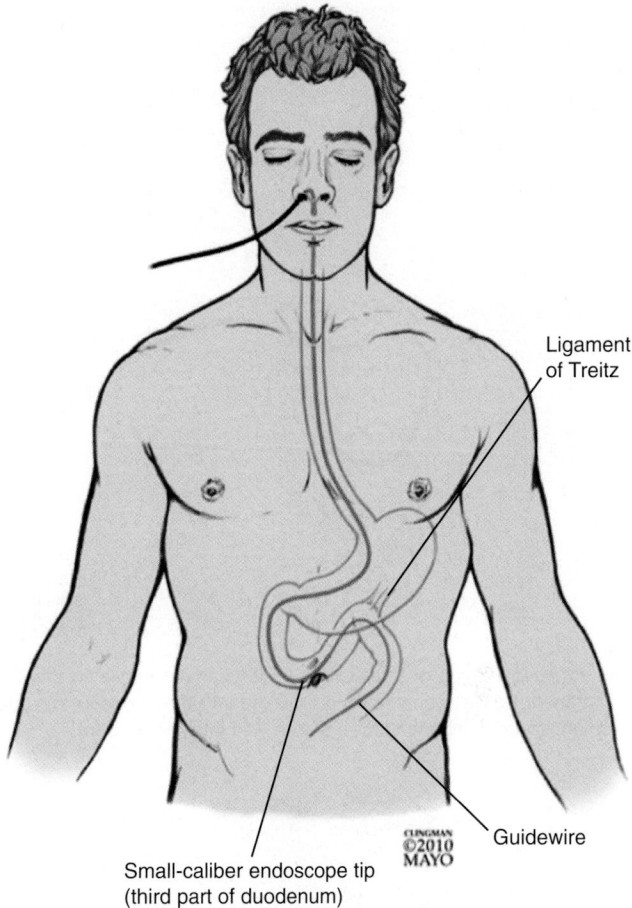

Ligament of Treitz

Guidewire

Small-caliber endoscope tip (third part of duodenum)

CLINGMAN ©2010 MAYO

Fig. 10.5 Illustration of small-caliber endoscope passed transnasally into postbulbar duodenum with guidewire placement beyond the ligament of Treitz (using supplemental fluoroscopy).

Therapeutic Applications for Small-Caliber Endoscopy

The following are common and practical applications:

1. Guidewire placement and dilation of pharyngeal and cervical esophagus in patients who have undergone cancer surgeries with and without radiation
2. Guidewire placement and dilation of high-grade esophageal strictures
3. Transnasal guidewire and nasogastric or nasojejunal tube feeding tube placement (**Fig. 10.5**)
4. Percutaneous transgastric conversion of a gastric feeding tube to a jejunal extension (**Fig. 10.6**)
5. Retrograde percutaneous transgastric intubation of a feeding gastrostomy for access to the esophagus in the setting of a high-grade stricture at any level with placement of a guidewire to enable dilation
6. Retrograde percutaneous transgastric intubation of a feeding gastrostomy for rendezvous access to near-total esophageal stricture using simultaneous peroral endoscopy (**Fig. 10.7**)
7. Percutaneous evaluation of persistent long-standing fistulas with closure using injected fibrin sealants or cyanoacrylate glues

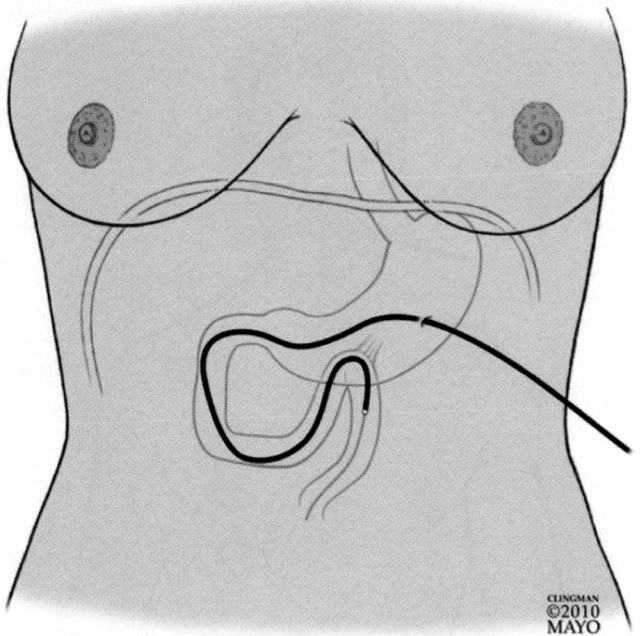

Fig. 10.6   Illustration of small-caliber endoscope passed via an existing percutaneous gastrostomy feeding tube site into the duodenum to the ligament of Treitz with guidewire placed well into the jejunum.

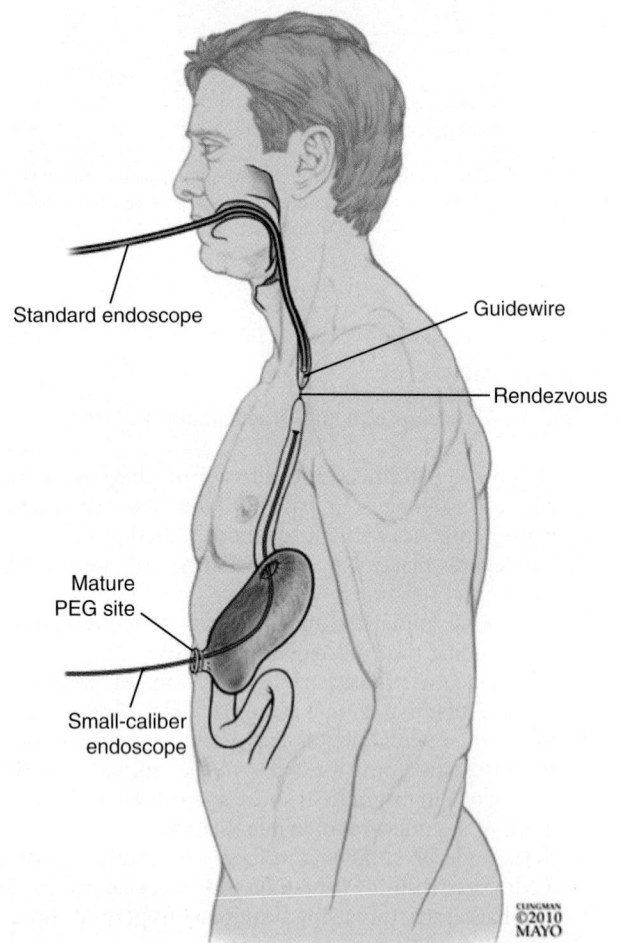

Fig. 10.7   Illustration of small-caliber endoscope passed via an existing percutaneous gastrostomy feeding tube site into the esophagus. There is simultaneous placement of a standard endoscope perorally down to the level of esophageal obstruction with a guidewire extended beyond the endoscope to probe a potential lumen site.

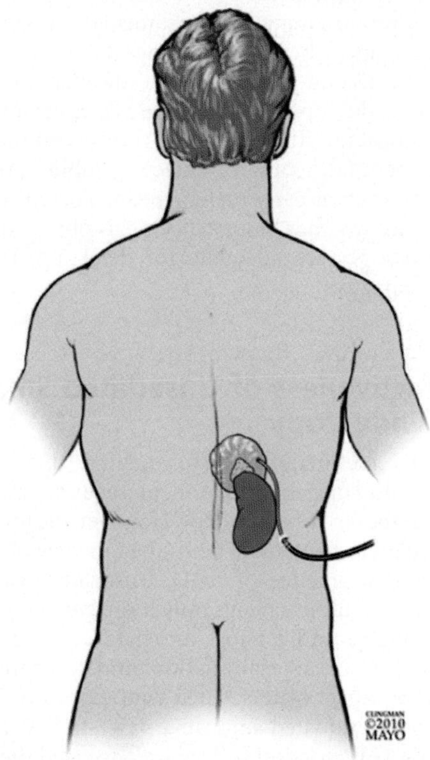

Fig. 10.8   Illustration of small-caliber endoscope passed via a right flank percutaneous tract into the right perinephric space exploring residual necrotic material and eventually directing more accurate catheter drainage. Necrotic material is the result of extensive organized necrosis, loculated contiguous to the kidney, subsequent to acute pancreatitis.

8. Percutaneous entry via cholecystostomy tract or transhepatic tract for stone clearance[33]
9. Percutaneous evaluation and initiation of drainage procedures for abdominal and retroperitoneal abscesses (**Fig. 10.8**).

Small-caliber endoscopes nearly uniformly provide 2.0-mm working channels. These do not prevent the use of standard 0.035-inch guidewires. The longer small-caliber endoscopes (e.g., Olympus N180 series 100 cm) are perhaps more advantageous for placement of jejunal feeding tubes. These instruments offer only up-and-down tip deflection. The insertion tube is soft enough to enable torquing movements that conveniently replace the left-and-right tip deflection options. Small-caliber endoscopy via an existing percutaneous gastrostomy site can be performed without sedation.

As noted earlier, patients with persistent well-organized abscesses and collections of necrotic material, in either the peritoneal or the retroperitoneal spaces, who have had percutaneous catheter efforts performed for the purpose of drainage and resolution typically have well-established fistulas into the persistent cavity and collection. The small-caliber endoscope can provide useful identification of unaccessed collections and facilitate their drainage by visually directing catheter placement for drainage or dilating the percutaneous fistulas via guidewire placement, allowing larger endoscopes to be passed for débridement. This is a very unique application that can provide a successful outcome for difficult management situations. Passage of small-caliber endoscopes percutaneously via established fistula tracts into either the liver or the gallbladder for stone clearance has been well established.

Conclusion

The practice of gastrointestinal endoscopy is constantly evolving. Unsedated small-caliber upper endoscopy is intuitively appealing, and sufficient data exist to support the feasibility of unsedated small-caliber endoscopy in selected patients. Adequate data suggest that the sensitivity of small-caliber endoscopes may be slightly less than conventional EGD.

Current literature lacks sufficient evidence, however, to provide guidelines on how to select the suitable patient population and whether or not unsedated endoscopy results in cost savings without significantly compromising comfort. There are more useful applications of the small-caliber endoscope, to enable sedated examinations in poorly tolerant or fragile patients and, even more so, to facilitate feeding tube placement, resolve complex strictures, and resolve abdominal abscesses and necrosis collections.

References

The complete reference list is available online at www.expertconsult.com.

Chapter 11

Postsurgical Endoscopic Anatomy

Arnaldo B. Feitoza

Video related to this chapter's topics can be found online at expertconsult.com.

CHAPTER OUTLINE

Introduction

Patients who have undergone surgical procedures that alter the anatomy of the upper gastrointestinal (GI) tract are often referred for endoscopic evaluation.[1] If meaningful and accurate diagnostic information is to be obtained in these patients, it is important that the endoscopist fully understand the anatomic changes resulting from the surgical procedures.[2] Knowledge of the new anatomy is essential to define the type of endoscope and accessories and to determine the need for supplementary studies during or before the endoscopic procedure.[3,4] In addition, accurate interpretation of endoscopic findings may permit the endoscopist to identify an unknown previous surgical procedure. This chapter discusses the most common operations in the upper GI tract that are relevant to the endoscopist. Technical details and common variations are described for each surgical procedure and correlated to the findings and to the anatomic alterations observed endoscopically. Surgical terms are also presented to assist the endoscopist in the interpretation of the surgical reports, which should always be reviewed before the endoscopic examination.

Antireflux Procedures

Nissen Fundoplication

Fundoplications to treat gastroesophageal reflux disease (GERD) are performed without gut resection to restore the competency of the cardia (**Fig. 11.1**). The plication has to be created over the distal esophagus just proximal to the cardioesophageal junction to be effective.[5] Modifications to the original fundoplication described by Nissen decreased the incidence of postoperative gas-bloat syndrome and dysphagia at the same time that the laparoscopic approach proved to be safe and reliable.[6–10] Shortening from 5 cm to 2 cm and loosening of the fundoplication resulted in the so-called floppy Nissen, which was performed laparoscopically and became the surgical "gold standard" treatment for GERD.[11]

The distal esophagus, the cardioesophageal junction, the gastric fundus, and the right and left crura are dissected in the same way for the open or laparoscopic procedure. Careful dissection is required to avoid transection of the nerve of Latarjet on the right side of the stomach. After reduction of the hernia, the left and right crura are approximated by sutures, gently snuggling the hiatus around the esophagus, which accommodates a previously inserted 60-Fr dilator (**Fig. 11.1A**). Division of the short gastric vessels may be required to mobilize the fundus.[12,13] The gastric fundus is passed behind the esophagus from left to right creating a 360-degree wrap by the placement of two or three sutures involving stomach-esophagus-stomach in the anterior portion of the wrap. The anterior and posterior vagus nervus are usually contained into the wrap, attached to the esophagus. At the end of the procedure, the wrap must lie below the diaphragm without tension (**Fig. 11.1B-1**).[14,15]

An intact Nissen fundoplication appears to the endoscopist as a narrow, easily transposable distal esophagus, with noninflamed mucosa and reduced distention to air insufflation. An

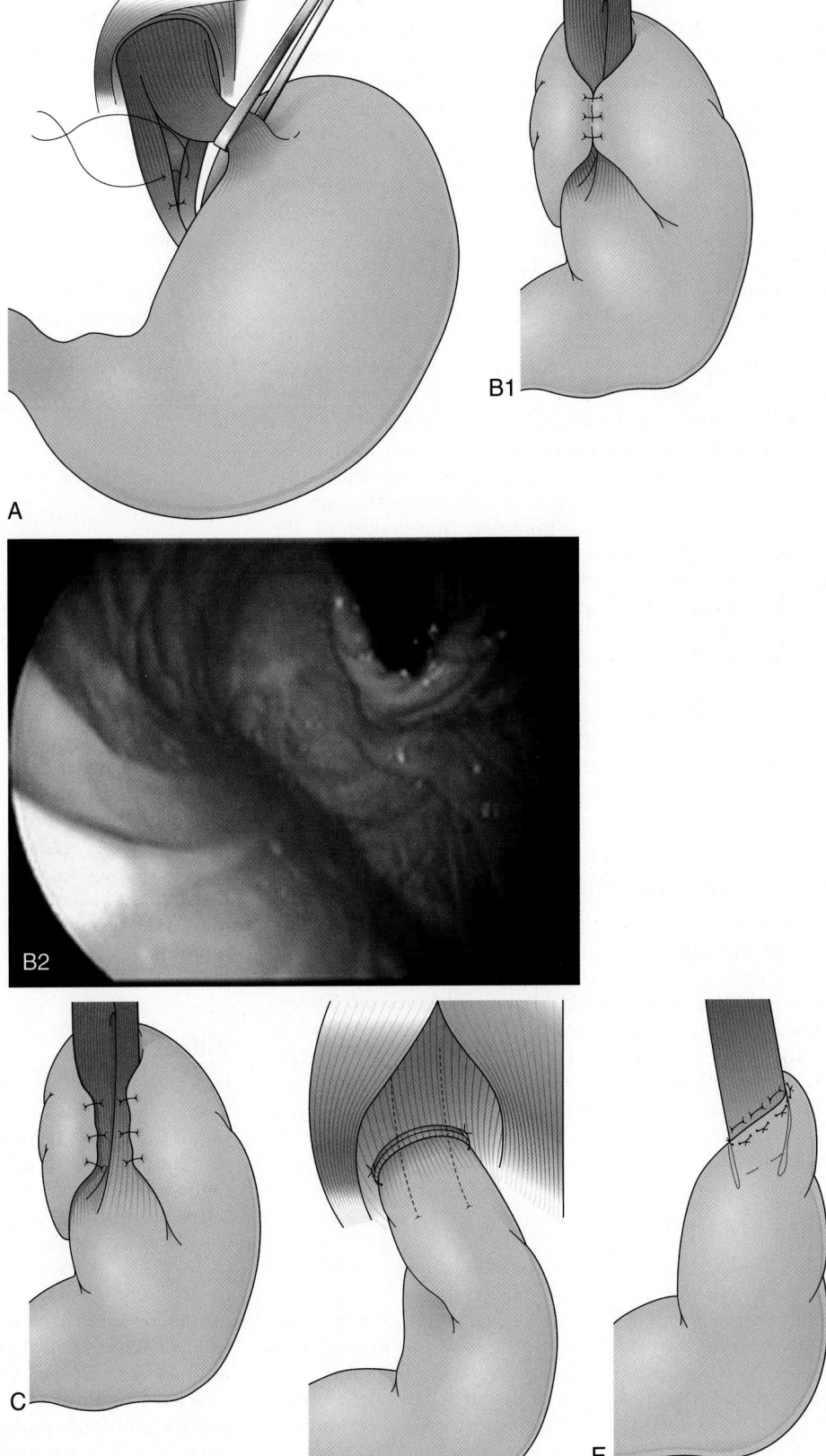

Fig. 11.1 Antireflux procedures. **A,** Esophageal hiatus is narrowed by sutures that approximate the crura of the diaphragm. **B-1,** Nissen fundoplication: A short and loose 360-degree wrap is created around the distal esophagus; **B-2,** parallel rugal folds encircle the cardia and the insertion tube of the endoscope. The cardia is below the diaphragm, and there is no hiatal enlargement. **C,** Toupet fundoplication: A posterior partial wrap is created by suturing the edges of the stomach to the anterior esophagus, leaving a space in between. **D,** Dor procedure: A partial anterior fundoplication usually performed following a Heller myotomy. **E,** Belsey-Mark IV procedure: A partial wrap is created through a thoracotomy by progressive invagination of the esophagus into the stomach.

encircling redundant fold overlies the cardia on a retroflexed view and snuggles the endoscope. Edema accentuates the prominent cardia in the early postoperative setting, and the area of the fundus becomes less capacious than normal. Late evaluation of the wrap may reveal several rugal folds parallel to each other and to the markings on the insertion tube of the endoscope (**Fig. 11.1B-2**). Although this is a 360-degreee wrap, endoscopically the redundant fold appears as a 270-degree free cuff margin because the border continuous with the lesser curvature is not evident.[16] The crural closure should maintain the cardia below the diaphragm with the stomach completely insufflated with air. Occasionally, sutures in the distal esophagus may be observed, indicating migration through the wall or inappropriate penetration depth of the stitches during the procedure; this may or may not be associated with symptoms.[17]

Findings that could be associated with failure of the fundoplication include esophagitis, lack of the encircling fold on a retroflexed view, patulous gap between the endoscope tube and the wrap, migration of the wrap through an enlarged esophageal hiatus, hourglass appearance of the proximal stomach indicating slippage through the valve, and irregularity in the dome shape of the fundus indicating parahiatal hernia. The squamocolumnar junction located more than 1 cm proximal to the margin of the wrap has been reported to be a major endoscopic clue in diagnosis of postfundoplication problems.[18] Gastric food retention may be related to damage to the vagus nerves during the procedure.[19] Some patients with persistent dysphagia have a tight wrap that causes resistance to the advance of the endoscope, and these patients may benefit from endoscopic dilation.[20]

Partial Fundoplications (Dor and Toupet)

Partial fundoplications are created with the fundus involving partially the distal esophagus. A Dor fundoplication is performed anteriorly, and a Toupet fundoplication is performed posteriorly (**Fig. 11.1C and D**). Both procedures can be performed to treat GERD; however, they are best indicated in patients who underwent a Heller myotomy (Dor) or with impaired esophageal body motility (Toupet).[21–23] Partial fundoplications also have a prominent fold overlying the cardia, which is not less evident than 360-degree wraps when observed endoscopically.[24]

Belsey Mark IV

With the advent of laparoscopy, the Belsey Mark IV fundoplication is performed only occasionally because it requires a thoracotomy. A circumferential invagination of the distal esophagus into the proximal stomach is performed with two layers of stitches, including anchoring to the diaphragma in the last one. The crura are also sutured to narrow the esophageal hiatus. The final result is a 270-degree wrap around the distal esophagus, placed in the abdomen, and a hiatal repair (**Fig. 11.1E**). Endoscopically, Belsey Mark IV and Nissen fundoplications are similar, with folds encircling the endoscope at the level of the cardia. However, coils of gastric rugae as seen after Nissen repair are not evident, and there is an anterior compression that corresponds to the attachment of the esophagus to the diaphragm.[16]

Collis Gastroplasty

A short esophagus, usually caused by chronic scarring resulting from GERD, can be repaired surgically through a Collis gastroplasty. This gastroplasty creates a tubular segment of stomach in continuity to the esophagus, long enough to be encircled by a 360-degree fundoplication placed below the diaphragm. The fundoplication around this tubular segment within the positive pressure of the abdomen prevents the gastroesophageal reflux.[25] Short esophagus is declining possibly because patients with GERD are medically diagnosed and treated earlier.[26] Endoscopically, the squamocolumnar junction is observed above a short tubular segment of stomach, which may not distend properly because of the wrap. The Collis gastroplasty resembles the Nissen fundoplication on a retroflexed view with a less capacious fundus.

Operations without Alteration of the Pancreaticobiliary Anatomy

Billroth I

Billroth I is a type of reconstruction after a partial gastrectomy in which the stomach is anastomosed to the duodenum (**Fig. 11.2A**).[27] The stomach resection is usually restricted to the antrum, and a truncal vagotomy is often associated. A considerable amount of remaining stomach with refluxed bile is observed endoscopically. The gastroduodenostomy is found toward the greater curvature. A prominent fold representing the closed part of the stomach is often observed along the lesser curvature ending at the gastroduodenostomy. A mucosal pattern change from gastric folds to flat duodenal surface indicates the anastomosis site. The duodenum is rectified, and the circular folds of the second portion are close to the anastomosis because of the partial resection of the bulb. Major and minor papillae appear to be more proximal in the duodenum than in a patient with intact anatomy.

Billroth II

In a Billroth II reconstruction after a partial gastrectomy, the duodenal stump is closed and a gastrojejunostomy is created (**Fig. 11.2B**). This type of reconstruction, commonly used for complicated ulcer disease in the past, is now used more often in the treatment of gastric neoplasia in which extensive resections are required. The remaining stomach is variable in length allowing the retroflexion maneuver if a long segment is present. The gastric remnant usually contains frothy bile and mucosal erythema from the alkaline reflux.[28] The gastrojejunostomy is located at the distal end of the stomach where two stomal openings corresponding to an end-to-side anastomosis can be identified (**Fig. 11.2C**).

Several surgical techniques are employed to perform the gastrojejunostomy leading to distinct endoscopic presentations. The chosen technique depends on surgeon preference, and there is no consensus for the ideal one. The gastrojejunostomy can vary in the size of the anastomosis, in the orientation of the jejunal loop to the stomach, and in the position of the anastomosis to the transverse colon. If the whole length of the transected stomach is anastomosed to the jejunum (oralis totalis or Polya), several rows of jejunal folds are observed

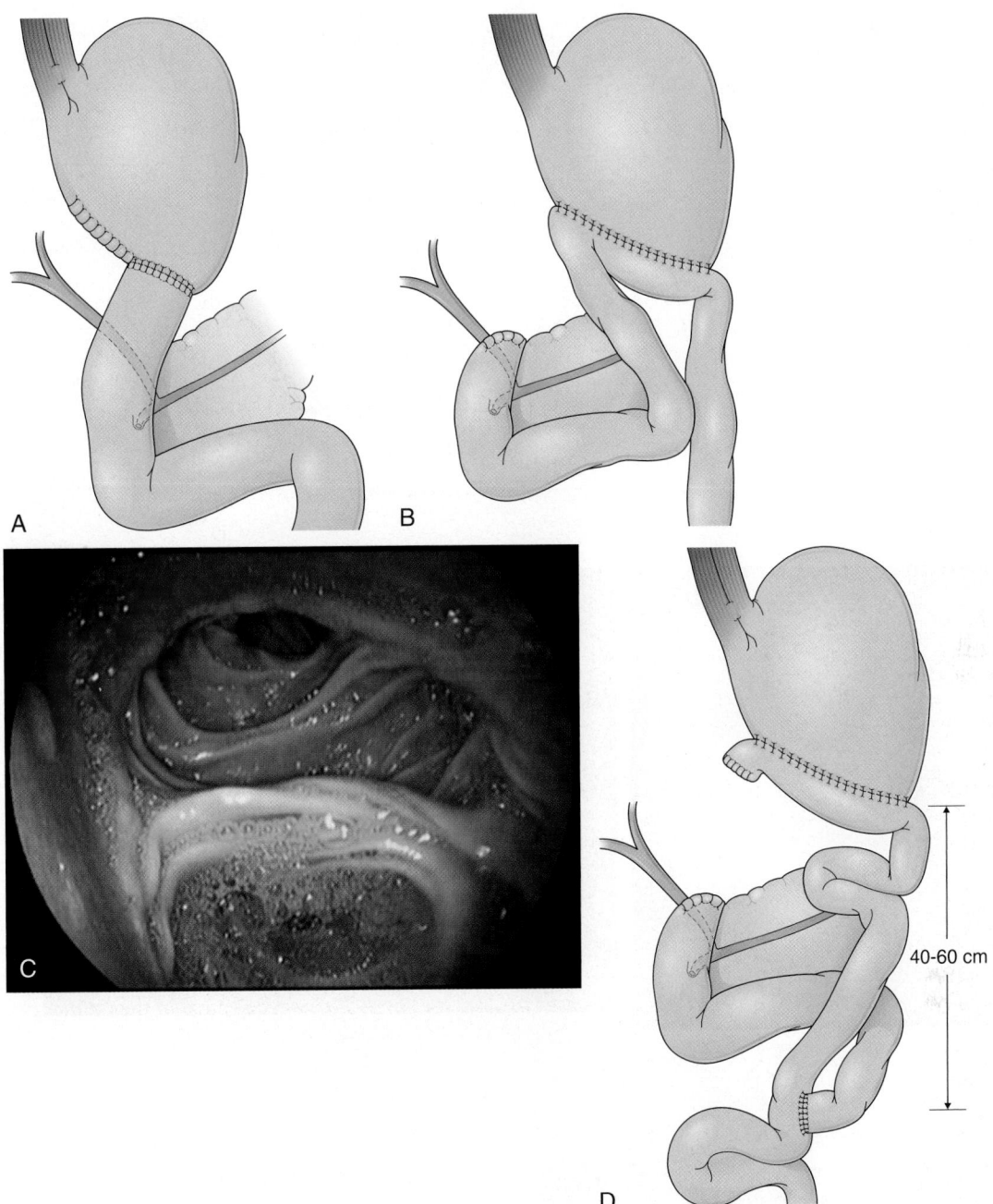

Fig. 11.2 Three types of reconstruction after partial gastrectomy. **A,** Billroth I: A gastroduodenostomy is performed toward the greater curvature. **B,** Billroth II: A gastrojejunostomy is created to reestablish the alimentary transit. Several variations may be observed in this type of reconstruction. **C,** Frothy bile coming from the anastomotic opening linked to the lesser curvature indicates the afferent limb (anisoperistaltic anastomosis). **D,** Roux-en-Y: A gastrojejunostomy only is created with the efferent limb to prevent biliopancreatic reflux into the stomach. A 40-cm to 60-cm efferent limb leads to the jejunojejunostomy and afferent limb.

between the two stomal openings (**Fig. 11.3A**). Conversely, if only a segment of the transected stomach is anastomosed to the jejunum (oralis partialis or Hoffmeister), few or no folds are evident. In this case, the stomach is partially closed, always from the lesser curvature, to reduce the diameter of the anastomosis, which is observed toward the greater curvature. Some surgeons attach the jejunal limb to the suture line that is closing the stomach to prevent dehiscence when performing an oralis partialis anastomosis (**Fig. 11.3B**).[29] In this case, a sharp angulation might be negotiated to enter the correspond-

ing jejunal limb, and a prominent fold may be seen emanating from the lesser curvature to the anastomosis. The small anastomosis diameter in association with the sharp angulation of this type of reconstruction may make the anatomy difficult to define endoscopically.

Gastrojejunostomies performed with staplers are usually oralis partialis. In some cases, the stomach is completely closed at the distal end, and the gastrojejunal anastomosis is performed with a linear or a circular stapler in a side-to-side fashion at the posterior wall, 2 cm proximal to the end of the

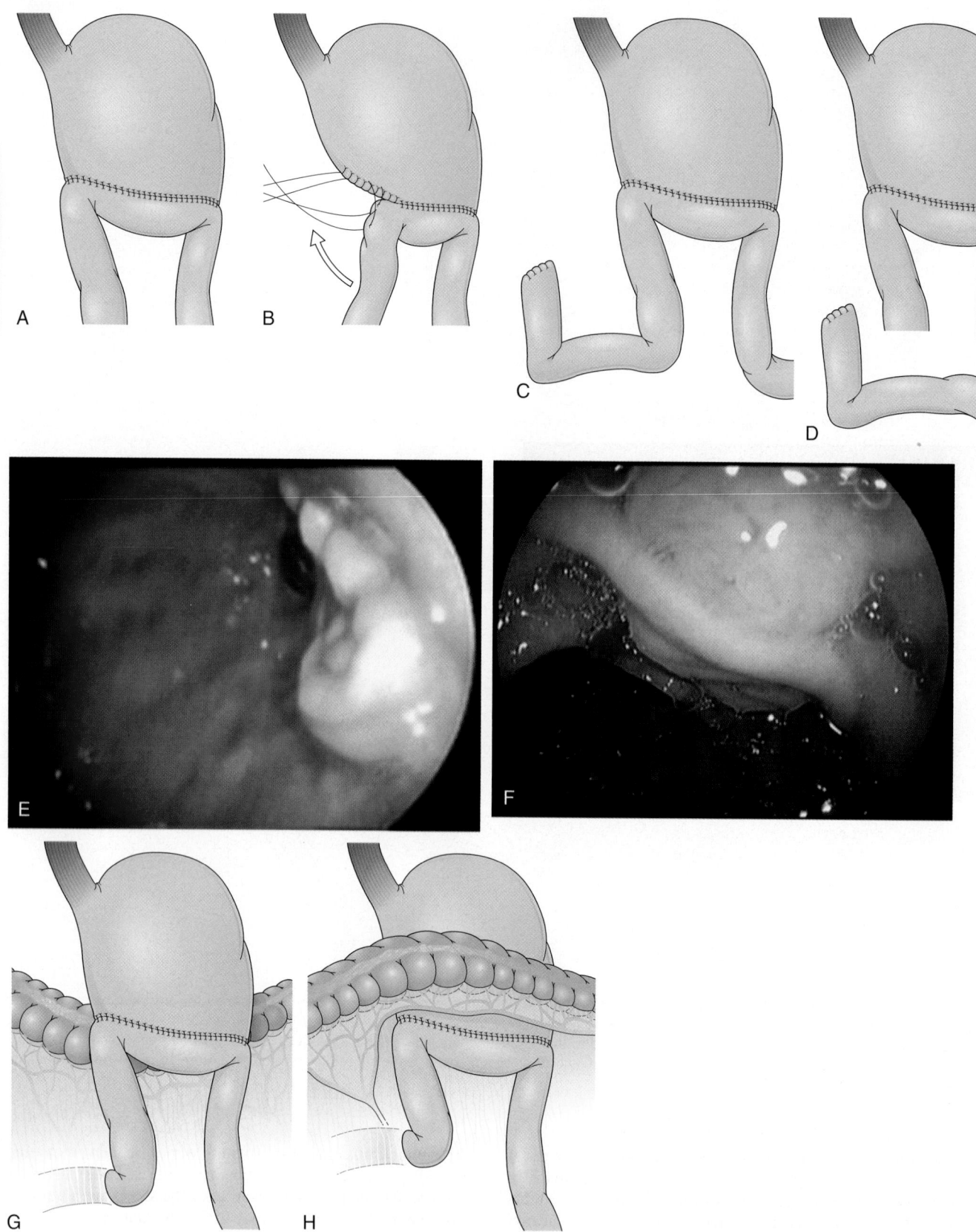

Fig. 11.3   Variations of Billroth II reconstruction. **A,** Oralis totalis (Polya): The anastomosis occupies the entire length of the distal stomach. **B,** Oralis partialis (Hoffmeister): The anastomosis occupies only part of the distal stomach. In some cases, the jejunal limb is sutured to the lesser curvature to protect the suture line of the stomach from disruption. In this scenario, a sharp angulation must be negotiated to advance the endoscope through the stomal opening linked to the lesser curvature. **C,** Antiperistaltic anastomosis: The afferent limb is attached to the lesser curvature. **D,** Isoperistaltic anastomosis: The afferent limb is attached to greater curvature. **E,** Sharp verticalization of the gastroenteroanastomosis impairs advance of the endoscope to this afferent limb. **F,** Retrograde view of the major papilla through the afferent limb. **G,** Antecolic reconstruction: The anastomosis is anterior to the transverse colon leading to a longer afferent limb. **H,** Retrocolic reconstruction: The anastomosis passes through the mesocolon creating a shorter afferent limb.

stomach.[30] When observed endoscopically, however, this side-to-side anastomosis is almost indistinguishable from a short end-to-side anastomosis. The jejunum can be anastomosed to the stomach with the afferent limb attached to the greater curvature (isoperistaltic) or to the lesser curvature (antiperistaltic). The afferent limb refers to the jejunal limb that is in continuity with the duodenum, whereas the efferent limb refers to the one that leaves the stomach toward the distal jejunum. The two stomal openings observed endoscopically may represent the afferent or efferent limb depending on how the reconstruction was performed (**Fig. 11.3C and D**). If the reconstruction is isoperistaltic, the opening linked to the greater curvature corresponds to the afferent limb. If the reconstruction is antiperistaltic, the opening linked to the greater curvature corresponds to the efferent limb. Usually the stomal opening linked to the lesser curvature is more difficult to access with the endoscope because of the relative verticalization of the anastomosis (**Fig. 11.3E**).[31]

Gastrectomies usually include the lesser more than the greater curvature in the resection. In addition, the information from surgical notes about the type of reconstruction, peristalsis, and bile flow might help to define the limbs endoscopically. On careful observation of the anastomosis, bile may be seen coming predominantly from the afferent limb. Introducing the endoscope through this opening should reveal an increasing volume of bile as the endoscope advances toward the bulb, although bile may also be observed in the efferent limb. Visible peristaltic waves advancing away from the endoscope suggest that the instrument is in the efferent limb. When the duodenal stump is reached, the flat mucosa of the residual bulb with a scarlike deformity in a cul-de-sac can be identified. A careful withdrawal of the endoscope exposes the major papilla, usually located at the right upper quadrant on the monitor screen (**Fig. 11.3F**).

In patients with Billroth II anatomy, the papilla is rotated 180 degrees in the endoscopic visual field. This "upside down" position requires distinct techniques to perform endoscopic retrograde cholangiopancreatography (ERCP), including dedicated sphincterotomes, needle-knife cut technique over the stent, or balloon dilation of the papilla.[32–36] If the duodenal stump cannot be identified, the endoscope should be withdrawn, and the other limb should be intubated as far as possible. Fluoroscopic guidance may indicate that the efferent limb has been entered when the instrument is seen to pass deep into the pelvis. Conversely, passage of the endoscope into the right upper quadrant toward the liver or previous cholecystectomy clips suggests entry into the afferent limb.[37]

The length of the afferent limb also varies depending on the surgical technique. The afferent limb naturally fixed at the ligament of Treitz and surgically fixed to the stomach should be tensionless but not redundant. There are two ways to position the afferent limb in relation to the transverse colon during a Billroth II reconstruction. If an antecolic anastomosis is performed, the gastrojejunostomy is placed anterior to the transverse colon (**Fig. 11.3G**). Antecolic reconstructions frequently have long afferent limbs because of the distance between the ligament of Treitz and the remaining stomach, over the mesocolon, omentum, and transverse colon. Conversely, retrocolic reconstructions are performed through an opening in the transverse mesocolon, shortening the distance between the ligament of Treitz and the remaining stomach

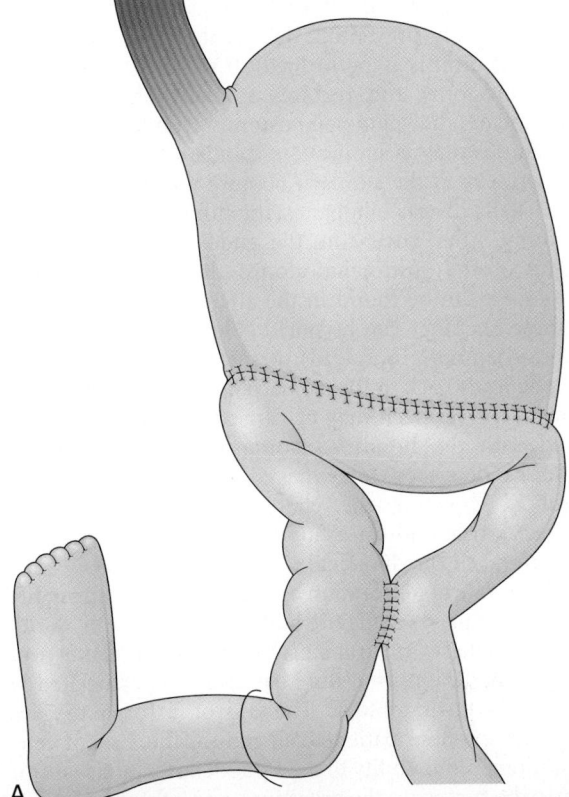

A

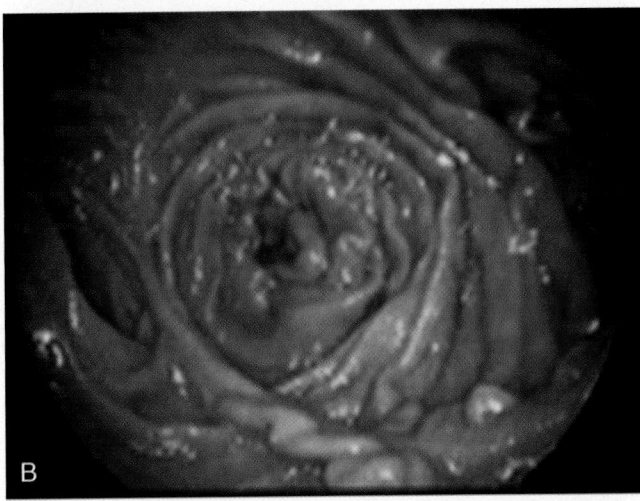

B

Fig. 11.4 **A,** Braun procedure after a Billroth II gastrectomy: An anastomosis between the afferent and efferent limb is created to prevent biliopancreatic reflux to the stomach or alleviate pressure in the afferent limb. **B,** Braun jejunojejunostomy: Three openings resulting from a side-to-side enteroanastomosis.

(**Fig. 11.3H**).[38,39] Antecolic and retrocolic anastomoses are similar endoscopically except for the unspecific observation obtained from the length of the limbs. Caution should be taken if a percutaneous endoscopic gastrostomy is indicated for a patient with a previous partial gastrectomy and retrocolic reconstruction.

Billroth II reconstruction can be associated with a side-to-side jejunojejunostomy, referred to as the Braun procedure (**Fig. 11.4A**).[40] This procedure creates an anastomosis between the afferent and the efferent limb to divert bile from the gastric remnant and to release the pressure of the afferent limb, supposedly preventing duodenal stump fistula.[41] The Braun anastomosis is performed 10 to 15 cm distal to the gastrojejunostomy and requires a longer afferent limb to accommodate the jejunojejunostomy.[42] Endoscopically, the gastrojejunostomy is similar to a standard Billroth II. Frothy bile is present in the stomach because the Braun procedure only partially diverts biliopancreatic fluids from the gastrojejunostomy. After advancing the endoscope through either opening of the gastrojejunostomy, the side-to-side Braun anastomosis can be found in the afferent and efferent limb, and three openings can be noted (**Fig. 11.4B**). One leads to the distal jejunum, one leads to the afferent limb, and the third one leads back to the stomach. A complete reverse intubation of the stomach may be carried out through the loop created with the Braun anastomosis. The same anatomic landmarks described for other Billroth II procedures are helpful in directing the endoscope through the limbs. However, a trial-and-error approach may be necessary ultimately to reach the duodenal stump.

A higher rate of perforation has been reported during ERCP while traversing the afferent limb compared with standard ERCP, particularly when a stiff therapeutic duodenoscope is used.[43,44] The Braun procedure has also been associated with perforations during ERCP. The use of a forward-viewing endoscope in these patients can reduce the risk of jejunal perforations.[45] The ability to use a duodenoscope elevator may increase the success of the procedure, and a flexible diagnostic duodenoscope may be safer than a stiff therapeutic instrument. If the papilla cannot be located with a side-viewing endoscope, a forward-viewing endoscope should be attempted and vice versa. Patients with an excessively long afferent limb may require longer endoscopes to reach the papilla.

Roux-en-Y Gastrectomy

In a Roux-en-Y reconstruction, the jejunum is transected close to the ligament of Treitz, creating two distinct segments. The distal segment is sutured to the gastric remnant (gastrojejunostomy) becoming the efferent limb. The proximal segment is sutured to this efferent limb (jejunojejunostomy) approximately 40 cm below the gastrojejunostomy (see **Fig. 11.2D**). The proximal segment is called the afferent limb, which connects the duodenum to the efferent limb instead of the stomach as in Billroth II reconstructions. The Roux-en-Y prevents biliopancreatic fluids from refluxing into the stomach in patients who have undergone gastric resection. It can be performed as the initial reconstruction after a gastrectomy or as the treatment for postgastrectomy syndrome resulting from a previous Billroth II reconstruction.[46–48] Truncal vagotomy is commonly performed in association with Roux-en-Y to prevent peptic ulcers in the efferent limb, which is no longer washed by the alkaline contents of the biliopancreatic fluid.[49]

The gastrojejunal anastomosis is end-to-side, and two stomal openings are seen. The reconstruction can be isoperistaltic or antiperistaltic, antecolic or retrocolic, and oralis totalis or partialis, as described for Billroth II. In contrast to the Billroth II, one of the two limbs is extremely short and ends blindly almost immediately. On entering a long limb with a patent lumen, it is almost certain that the endoscope is within the efferent limb. If the Roux-en-Y was performed after an initial Billroth II reconstruction, the endoscopist

should be aware that the blind limb might be patent for several centimeters before ending in a cul-de-sac. This short segment of patent limb occurs because conversion from a Billroth II to a Roux-en-Y sometimes has to be performed farther from the gastrojejunostomy to avoid adhesions from the initial surgery.

In effective Roux-en-Y reconstructions (**Fig. 11.5**), the remnant stomach is completely clean of bile (see **Figs. 11.3A and B and 11.5A and B**). However, because Roux-en-Y gastrojejunostomy increases the risk for delayed gastric emptying, residual contents in the stomach, including bezoars, and in the efferent limb may impair visualization of these segments or progression of the endoscope. The absence of bile in an operated stomach should always alert the endoscopist for a Roux-en-Y reconstruction, and the presence of residual food in this case should not lead to an erroneous conclusion of efferent limb obstruction. Total obstruction of the afferent limb in a Billroth II reconstruction could also prevent bile to reflux to the stomach, mimicking a Roux-en-Y, but this is uncommon.[50] Conversely, presence of bile does not exclude a Roux-en-Y reconstruction. In this case, a short-length efferent limb may be responsible for the reflux. To be effective, the efferent limb has to measure at least 40 cm from the gastrojejunal anastomosis to the jejunojejunal anastomosis.[51] Longer limbs (up to 60 cm) may also be encountered.[52]

Intubation through the efferent limb usually follows a straight route with variable looping. The enteroenteric anastomosis is usually end-to-side, but it may be side-to-side with a blind end. In either case, the endoscope has to leave the efferent limb and enter the afferent limb to reach the major papilla in the duodenum (see **Fig. 11.5C**). If a side-to-side anastomosis is present, three openings can be observed. The opening in continuity with the efferent limb leads to the distal jejunum, the second opening leads to a blind distal end of the afferent limb, and the third one leads to the duodenum through the afferent limb (see **Fig. 11.5D**). An end-to-side anastomosis has two openings. One is a continuation of the efferent limb and leads to the distal jejunum; the other opening leads to the afferent limb. Different degrees of angulation have to be negotiated to enter the afferent limb depending on the anastomosis configuration. Once the afferent limb is entered, progressively more bile should be seen until the duodenal stump is reached.

A complete visualization of the Roux-en-Y gastrojejunostomy during a routine esophagogastroduodenoscopy (EGD) can be performed with a forward-viewing gastroscope, including the jejunojejunostomy. In contrast, when patients with Roux-en-Y gastrectomy require ERCP, endoscopes with a longer insertion tube are usually needed (pediatric and adult colonoscopes, push-enteroscopes). In addition to the difficulties to reach the papilla, the small diameter of the working channel of these endoscopes and the short length of the endoscopic accessories contribute to the high rate of ERCP failures in these patients (compared with Billroth II patients).[53]

Gastrojejunostomy without Gastric Resection

Gastrojejunostomy without gastric resection is performed to bypass the distal stomach or the duodenum mostly in cases of malignant obstruction that cannot be resected. In major

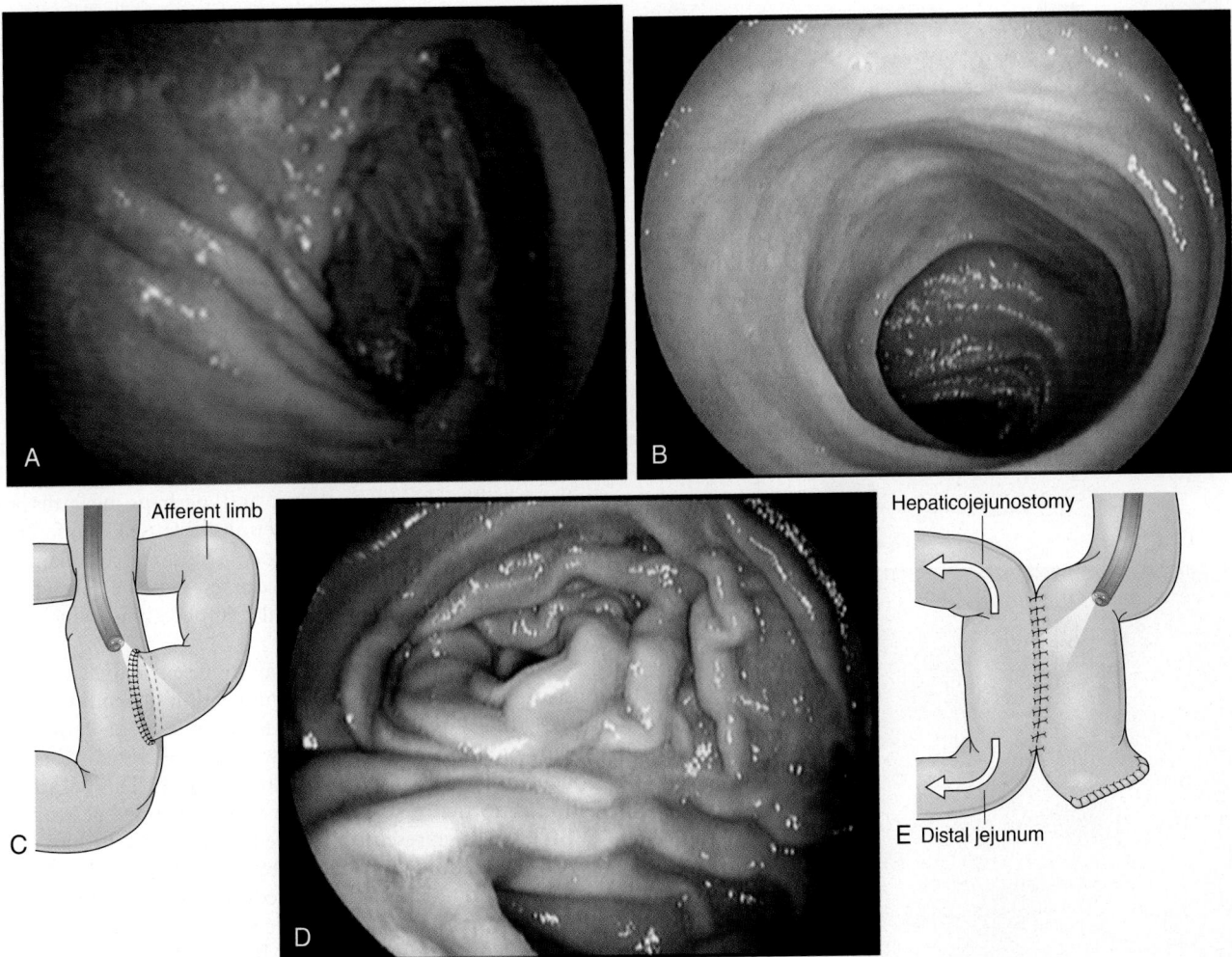

Fig. 11.5 Roux-en-Y gastrectomy. **A,** Gastrojejunostomy clean of bile with two openings (one is short and ends blindly). **B,** Lack of bile in typical Roux-en-Y efferent limb. **C,** Terminolateral anastomosis in a Roux-en-Y gastrectomy: Two openings are observed at this level; one leads to the distal jejunum, and the other leads to the ampulla via the afferent limb. **D,** Two openings are at the level of a side-to-side jejunojejunostomy. The third opening is located proximally and out of the field. Bile is usual at this level where the efferent limb connects to the afferent limb. **E,** Laterolateral anastomosis in a hepaticojejunostomy: The endoscope has passed through the stomach, duodenum, and proximal jejunum reaching the jejunojejunal anastomosis. Three openings are noted, including a blind one. In contrast to a Roux-en-Y gastrectomy **(A),** the loop in which the endoscope is located ends blindly.

duodenopancreatic trauma with a high risk for fistulas, a gastrojejunostomy may also be performed in association with a temporary closure of the pylorus as part of the duodenal exclusion.[54] Occasionally, the gastrojejunostomy is created prophylactically during the surgical exploration of a patient with unresectable adenocarcinoma of the head of the pancreas to prevent subsequent gastric outlet obstruction.[55] The gastrojejunostomy is usually performed along the greater curvature of the distal body or the proximal antrum of the stomach (**Fig. 11.6A**). It may involve the anterior or the posterior wall at the surgeon's discretion. In all cases, a side-to-side anastomosis is performed with the first jejunal loop that can be sutured without tension to the stomach. The anastomosis can be isoperistaltic or antiperistaltic, retrocolic or antecolic, as described for a Billroth II gastroenteroanastomosis. The definition for the length of the anastomosis does not apply (oralis totalis or oralis partialis) because this is a side-to-side anastomosis. However, this anastomosis usually resembles an oralis partialis in length.

The gastrojejunostomy appears endoscopically as a vertical anastomosis with two stomal openings that correspond to the afferent and efferent limbs. Either one of the limbs may be in a superior (upper) or inferior (lower) position, depending on the technique used during the surgery. If an isoperistaltic gastrojejunostomy has been created, the opening of the afferent limb should be expected in the upper position. The endoscopist should look carefully for a gastrojejunostomy in a patient with an upper tract obstruction who had undergone surgery. This anastomosis may become easily overlooked because it is typically not large, usually located among edematous gastric folds, and associated with gastric contents resulting from outlet obstruction (**Fig. 11.6B**). Ulcerations are also common and may impair intubation of the jejunal openings resulting from tissue retraction.[56] Access to the papilla can be achieved by passing the endoscope retrograde through the afferent limb when a gastric outlet obstruction has been established. The Braun procedure may be added to the gastrojejunostomy as previously described for Billroth II reconstruction (**Fig. 11.6C**).

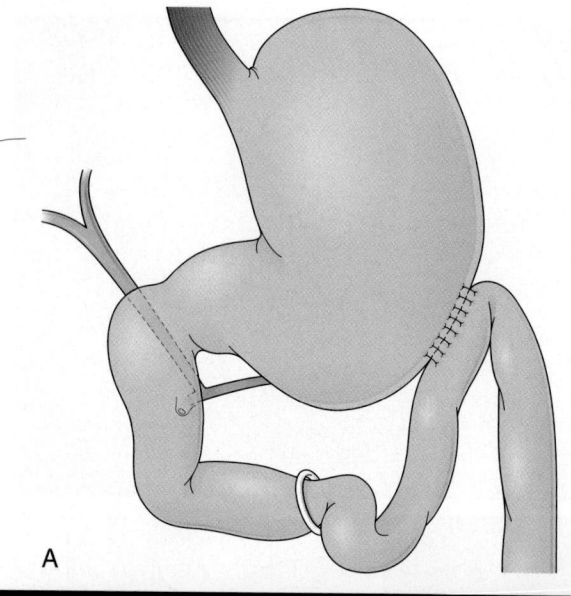

A

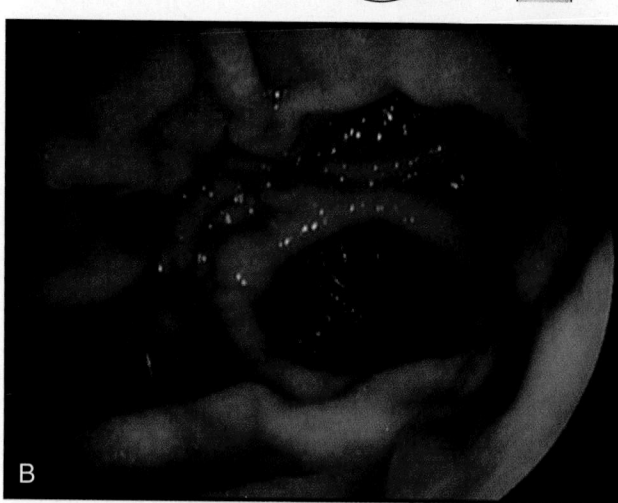

B

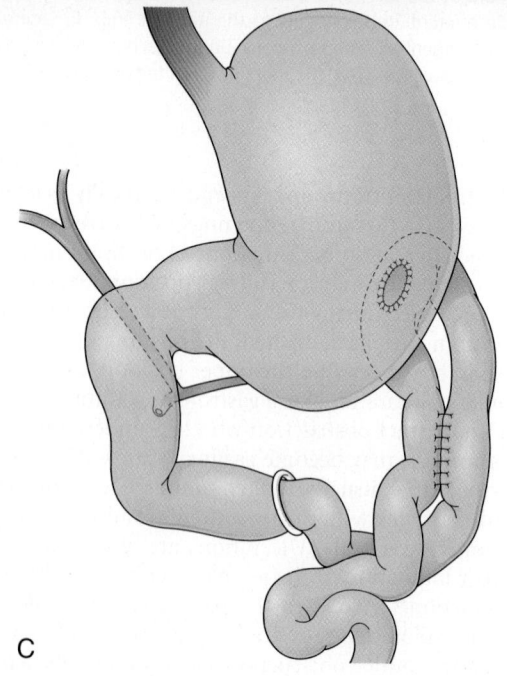

C

Fig. 11.6 Gastroenteroanastomoses. **A,** Antiperistaltic gastroentero-anastomosis is created along greater curvature. **B,** Gastrojejunostomy without gastric resection: Residual contents, enlarged gastric folds, and suboptimal air insufflation may obscure this anastomosis. **C,** Isoperistaltic gastroenteroanastomosis is created on the posterior wall of the stomach in association with Braun procedure.

Bariatric Surgery

The National Institutes of Health (NIH) Consensus Conference in 1985 recognized obesity as a health risk, acknowledged the importance of treating this condition, and recommended the body mass index (BMI) to classify patients.[57,58] Indications for bariatric procedures are increasing because of the increase in prevalence of obesity, including childhood obesity, and the lack of effective nonsurgical treatments. A growing number of patients with altered anatomy and perhaps new diseases should be expected in endoscopy units because GI complaints are frequent after bariatric surgery. The same complaints in uncomplicated postoperative courses can be present in patients with important surgical complications, which may require surgical revision.[59-61]

Some endoscopic findings may represent either a normal postsurgical appearance or a complication depending on the surgery that was performed.[62] An example is the endoscopic finding of a communication between a short proximal gastric pouch with a normal-size remnant stomach. This communication is normally expected in a vertical banded gastroplasty (VBG), but it represents a failure (gastrogastric fistula) if the surgical procedure was a gastric bypass (GB). Familiarity with the most common bariatric procedures is essential for optimal endoscopic assistance to bariatric patients and surgeons. Surgical procedures to treat obesity have evolved during the last 5 decades. They can be simplified in two types, restrictive and malabsortive.[63] Selection of a procedure is based on individual patient characteristics and surgeon preference.[64-66]

Jejunoileal Bypass

Jejunoileal bypass (JIB) was the first procedure proposed to induce malabsorption in 1954.[67] It is technically simple and safe because it involves only enteroanastomosis, and the surgical steps are performed in the middle abdomen. In JIB, the proximal jejunum and the distal ileum are transected. The long jejunoileal segment in between these two transections is excluded from the intestinal transit by suturing the proximal margin in a close end and the distal margin to the sigmoid. An enteroanastomosis is performed between the proximal jejunum and the distal ileum, leaving a short segment of small bowel to absorption (**Fig. 11.7**). This procedure does not alter the endoscopic anatomy of the upper GI tract. JIB is no longer performed because of severe hepatic complications.[68] Patients with intact JIB should be considered to revert the operation.

Gastric Bypass

GB includes partition of the stomach creating a small-volume pouch (15 to 50 mL) in the proximal stomach.[69,70] With the distal stomach completely disconnected, the proximal gastric pouch is anastomosed with a Roux-en-Y limb that ranges from 50 to 200 cm to reestablish the alimentary transit (**Fig. 11.8A**).[71]

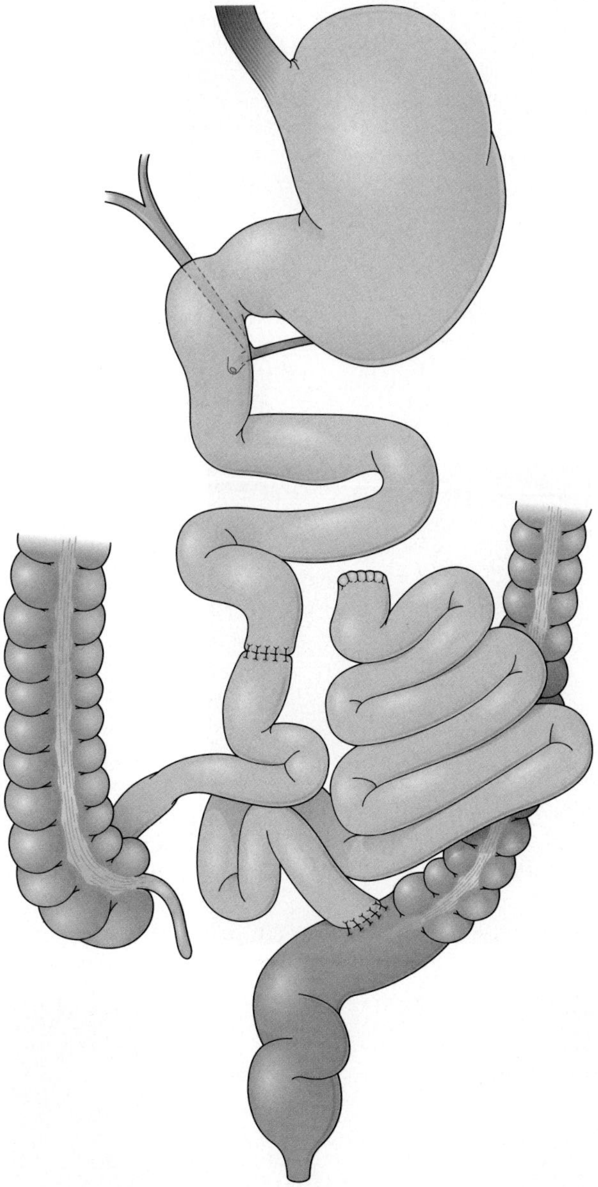

Fig. 11.7   Jejunoileal bypass. This operation reduces the small bowel absorptive surface and leaves a long nonfunctional segment of small bowel. Endoscopically, there is no change in the anatomy for upper endoscopy and endoscopic retrograde cholangiopancreatography (ERCP).

For the endoscopist, GB may be compared with a Roux-en-Y gastrectomy. The differences are the size of the proximal gastric pouch, the length of the Roux-en-Y limb, and the fact that the distal stomach is not resected. Surgical technical variations can be observed in GB in regard to the orientation of the pouch (horizontal vs. vertical), partition of the stomach (transection vs. no transection), use of a Silastic ring around the gastrojejunal stoma, length of the Roux-en-Y limbs, and surgical access (laparoscopy vs. open surgery), among others.[72–74]

The procedure proposed by Capella and Capella[75] incorporates a Silastic ring in the upper gastric pouch to prevent late stretching and the suture of the Roux-en-Y limb to the staple line of the pouch to prevent late gastrogastric fistulas (**Fig. 11.8B-D**). GB is a restrictive and malabsorptive procedure.[76] Upper endoscopy in a patient with GB shows a small proximal pouch immediately after the esophagogastric junction with a

narrow stoma leading to the small bowel and a long limb before reaching the jejunojejunal anastomosis, which may be inaccessible depending on the length of the limb (**Fig. 11.8E**). The gastric partition may include only the staple line, without division of the stomach (undivided bypass), or a complete transection of the stomach (divided bypass) (**Fig. 11.8F**). Undivided bypass presents a higher rate of fistulas between the pouch and the distal stomach compared with divided bypass. A gastrogastric fistula leads to a failure in weight loss and to a higher incidence of peptic ulcers beyond the gastro-jejunal anastomosis.

The gastrojejunostomy may be to the side or to the end of the jejunum or stomach. The small gastric pouch makes lateral and terminal gastric anastomoses indistinguishable. However, lateral and terminal anastomoses are different in the jejunal side. Lateral jejunal anastomosis has two openings. One ends blindly shortly after the anastomosis; the other leads to the distal jejunum (efferent limb) (**Fig. 11.8G**). Terminal anastomosis has one opening that should be readily accessible endoscopically. The blind end of a lateral anastomosis should not be confused with stenosis of the efferent limb, particularly when scarring alters the anatomy. Abnormal endoscopic findings include esophagitis, pouch or esophagus dilation, stomal stenosis, stomal ulceration, prosthesis erosion at the stoma, and breakdown of the partition staple line. Stomal ulceration has been related to staple line dehiscence in which a gastrogastric fistula occurs, although other factors may be involved.[77,78]

Access to the major papilla and to the disconnected part of the stomach is often impossible per os in patients with GB using regular endoscopes.[79–81] A gastrostomy tract created in the distal stomach is used as an alternative to access these areas with the endoscope.[82,83] Double-balloon enteroscopy has emerged as an alternative to access the biliopancreatic ducts and the disconnected part of the stomach in these patients.[84–87]

Biliopancreatic Diversion

Biliopancreatic diversion (BPD) is a malabsorptive procedure to delay the involvement of bile and pancreatic juice in digestion.[88] BPD was first reported in 1979 by Scopinaro and colleagues[89] and is also known as the Scopinaro procedure. In BPD, the small bowel is divided creating two limbs. The distal limb is anastomosed to the stomach, and the proximal limb is anastomosed to the ileum. After completion, the small bowel has a new anatomic configuration with three distinct channels: common, alimentary, and biliopancreatic (**Fig. 11.9A**). BPD requires no small bowel resection and does not leave a nonfunctional small bowel segment. The results of the procedure depend on the length of the channels, which are variable because of the individual patient characteristics and surgeon preferences. Typically, a 50-cm to 100-cm common channel and a 150-cm to 200-cm alimentary channel are created. The remaining small bowel constitutes the biliopancreatic channel.

The common channel length is the determinant for long-term weight maintenance and steatorrhea, and the total common alimentary channel is for the temporary mild short-gut syndrome. In addition, the stomach is altered via a partial resection or a GB to prevent peptic ulcer and to limit food intake. The gastric component of the BPD is easily accessible endoscopically, and the findings vary according to the procedure performed. Nevertheless, bile should never be observed, and peptic ulceration at the gastroenteroanastomosis and

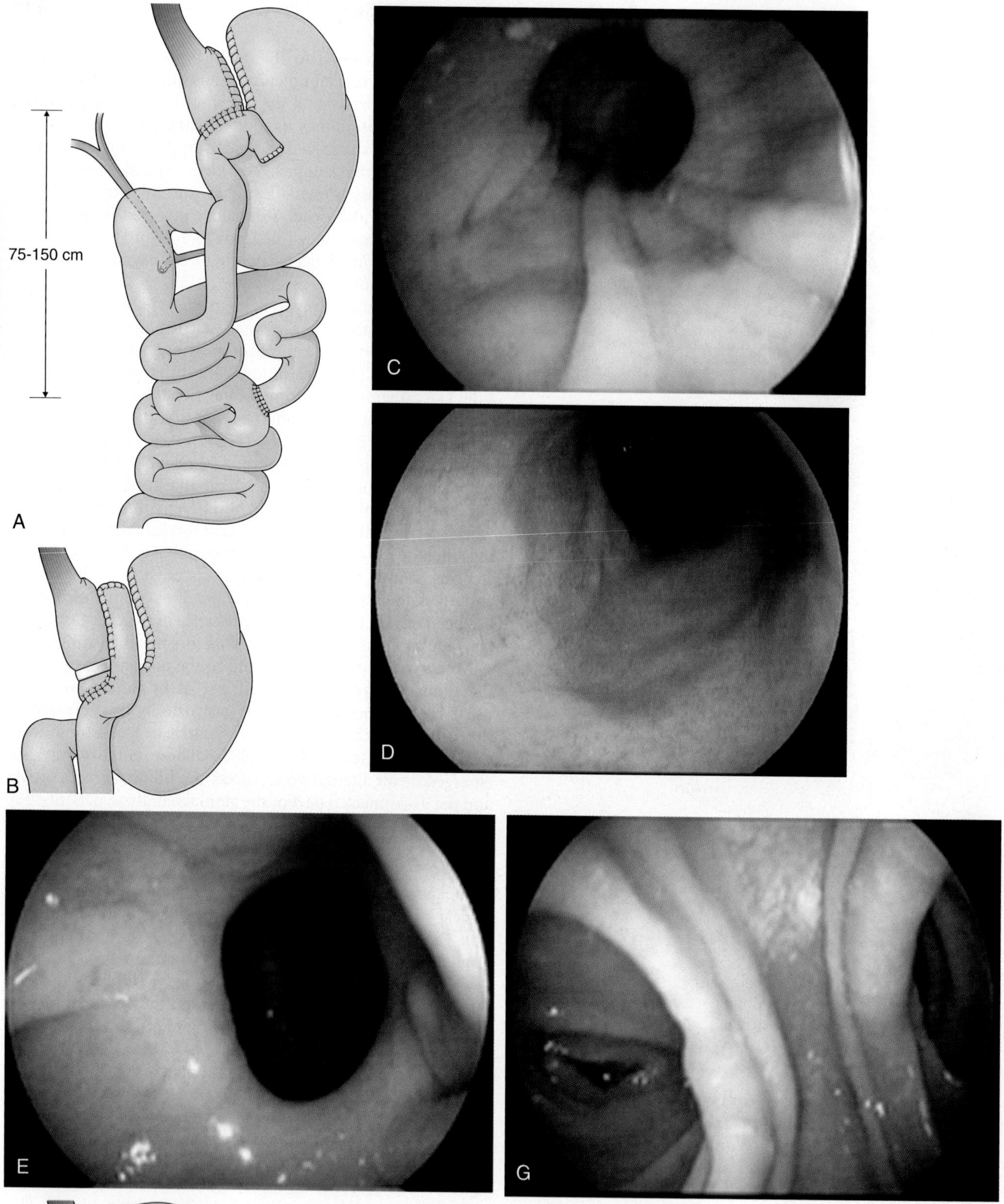

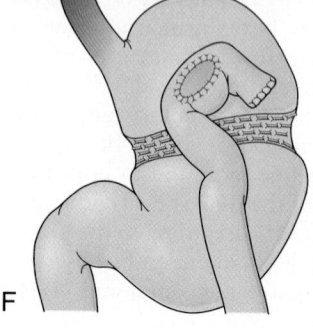

Fig. 11.8 Gastric bypass. **A,** Small-volume pouch (15 to 50 mL) is created just beyond the gastroesophageal junction and is anastomosed to a jejunal loop in a Roux-en-Y fashion. The efferent limb ranges from 75 to 150 cm. The distal stomach is not resected and may be used to create a gastrostomy through which the endoscope can be advanced to perform endoscopic retrograde cholangiopancreatography (ERCP) or gastroduodenoscopy. **B,** A technical variation includes the attachment of the jejunal limb to the gastric partitioning to prevent gastrogastric fistulas and the placement of a Silastic ring in the distal portion of the pouch to prevent dilation. **C,** Small gastric pouch with a subtle circumferential compression proximal to the anastomosis indicating an external ring. **D,** Intact stapler line at the gastric pouch. **E,** Small-diameter gastrojejunostomy. **F,** Undivided gastric bypass: The staple line is not transected, and the pouch is horizontal. This type of gastric bypass has been associated with failures in weight loss because of dilation of the pouch and disruption of the staple line. **G,** End-to-side gastrojejunostomy with two openings. The right one is the efferent limb. The left one ends blindly.

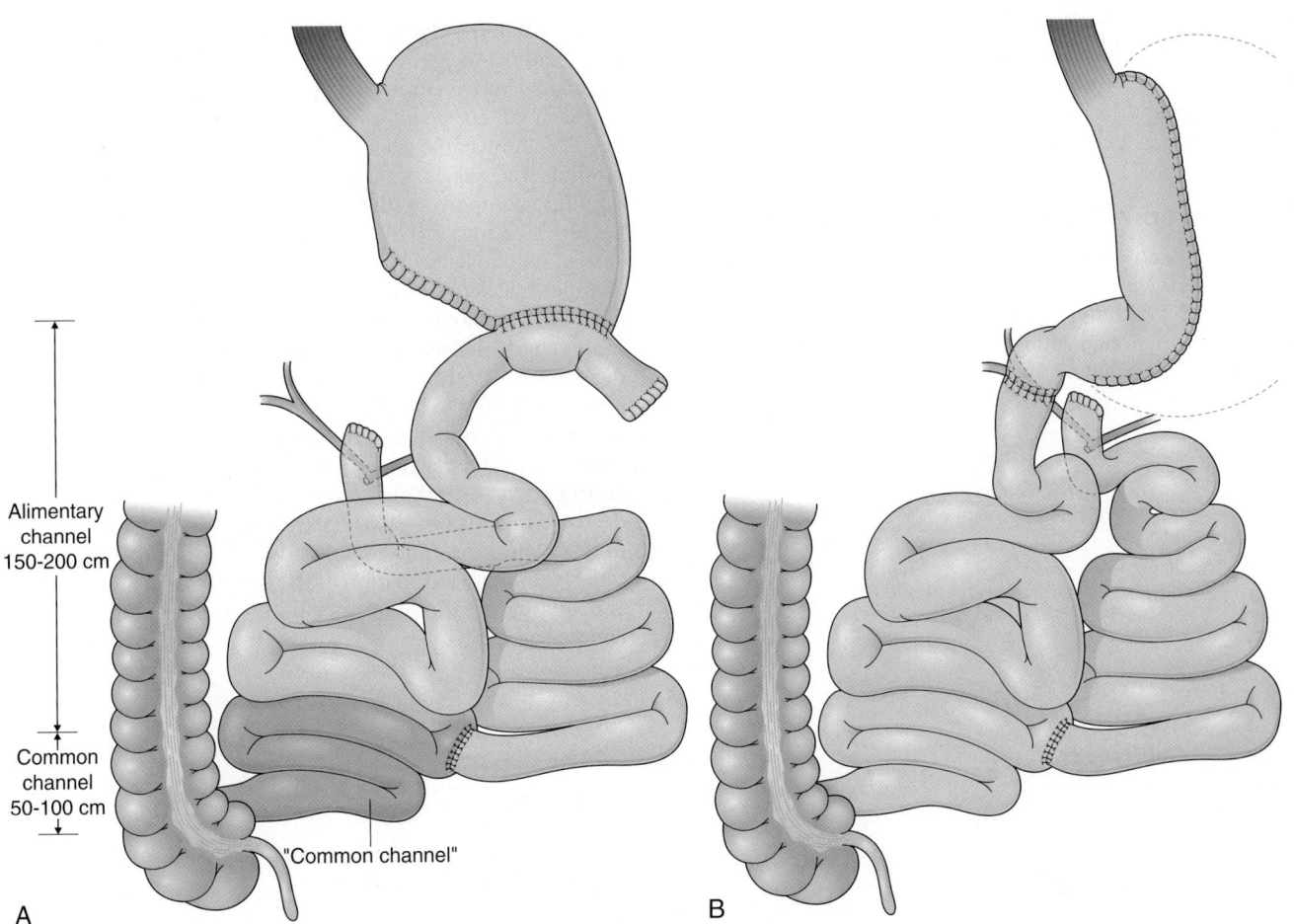

Fig. 11.9 Malabsorptive bariatric surgeries. **A,** Biliopancreatic diversion: A partial gastrectomy is reconstructed in a Roux-en-Y fashion with long afferent and efferent limbs (biliopancreatic and alimentary channels). *Shadowed area* represents the short length common channel (50 to 100 cm). **B,** Duodenal switch: A sleeve gastrectomy with preservation of the pylorus leads to a duodenojejunostomy rather than a gastrojejunostomy. Jejunal limbs are reconstructed as in a biliopancreatic diversion.

small bowel always should be carefully investigated. If a partial gastrectomy was chosen, the stomach resembles a Roux-en-Y gastrectomy with a short proximal gastric pouch. A GB may appear as a vertical small gastric pouch or a horizontal pouch that includes the fundus. In a horizontal pouch, the anastomosis with the jejunum should be observed toward the greater curvature. A GB does not include stomach resection, leaving a nonfunctional distal gastric segment, and it can be divided or undivided.

Performing ERCP in a patient with BPD is nearly impossible per os because the endoscope has to be advanced all the way through the small bowel except for the common channel to reach the major papilla. Alternatives to access the major papilla are through a gastrostomy (surgical or radiologic) or through a disrupted staple line between the pouch and the stomach. These alternatives apply only for patients who had a GB because gastric resection precludes both options. Double-balloon enteroscopy has the potential to advance through the altered BPD anatomy and reach the major papilla.

Duodenal Switch

The duodenal switch (DS) procedure is a variation of BPD. This procedure includes a sleeve gastrectomy preserving the pylorus and anastomosis of the enteric limb end-to-end with the postpyloric duodenum (**Fig. 11.9B**).[88] A lower prevalence

of side effects has been reported for DS compared with BPD. The same principles described in regard to BPD apply to DS during the endoscopic evaluation except that a duodenojejunostomy rather than a gastrojejunostomy is present.

Vertical Banded Gastroplasty

Initial gastroplasty configurations proved inadequate in terms of weight loss, and the procedure was refined by Mason into VBG. VBG, a pure restrictive procedure, is the result of a search for a simpler operation compared with GB.[90] VBG involves the creation of a small pouch in the proximal stomach and the encirclement of the outlet channel to prevent dilation. The pouch is created along the lesser curvature with a stapled partition precisely at the angle of His to accommodate a volume of 15 mL or less. The outlet channel of the pouch is stabilized by the encirclement of a 5-cm circumference band or a Silastic ring (**Fig. 11.10A**). A technical variation includes dividing the stapled partition (**Fig. 11.10B**).

Upper endoscopy in patients with intact VBG shows a small tubular pouch immediately after the esophagogastric junction with a narrow outlet channel that once transposed leads to the remaining distal stomach. Abnormal endoscopic findings include esophagitis, staple line dehiscence, food impaction, stenosis of the pouch outlet, and erosion of the gastric wall by the material used to encircle the outlet channel.[91,92] The remaining stomach, duodenal bulb, and biliopancreatic ducts are readily accessible for endoscopy if the outlet channel permits passage of the endoscope. The outlet channel is ideally 11 mm wide and 15 mm long, and it can be dilated endoscopically in cases of stenosis.

Laparoscopic Adjustable Gastric Banding

Laparoscopic adjustable gastric banding (LAGB) is a restrictive procedure largely used in European countries and Australia.[93] LAGB involves placing a band around the proximal stomach to create a 15-mL pouch without the need of resecting or stapling the stomach (**Fig. 11.11A**). LAGB is now performed using a

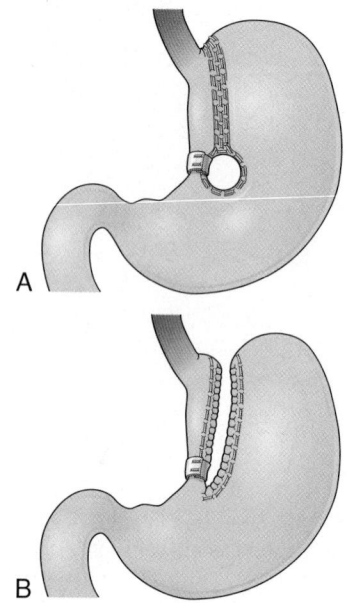

Fig. 11.10   Vertical banded gastroplasty. A 15-mL pouch is created at the angle of His, and the outlet channel is encircled by a circumferential band. **A,** Circular and linear staplers are used to create this uncut gastroplasty. **B,** The staple line may be divided separating the two gastric parts to prevent gastrogastric fistula.

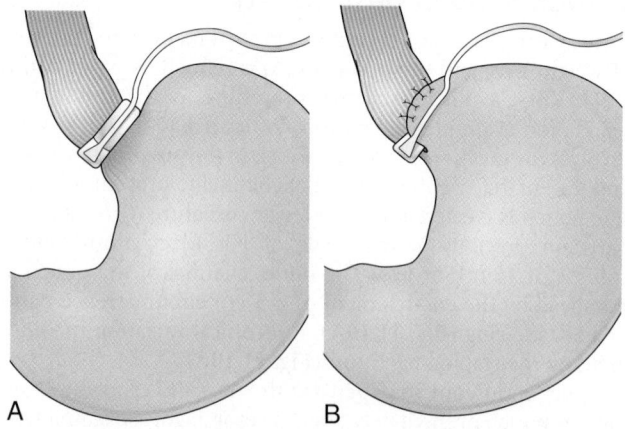

Fig. 11.11   Laparoscopic adjustable gastric banding. **A,** A 15-mL pouch is created in the proximal stomach with a banding device. The device can be adjusted to narrow the opening to the distal stomach by percutaneous injection of fluids. **B,** A gastrogastric suture is placed anteriorly over the band to prevent gastric herniation.

silicone material device that can be inflated with saline solution to adjust the gastric-pouch outflow. The inflatable part of the band device is connected by tubing to a reservoir implanted and secured to the abdominal fascia that can be accessed via a needle.[94] Adjustable silicone gastric bands reduce the risks of eroding the gastric wall and the incidence of uncontrolled vomiting compared with former types of gastric banding.

Upper endoscopy in a patient with LAGB shows a small gastric pouch at the level of the cardia with a narrow outlet channel that leads to the distal normal stomach. Esophageal dilation, esophagitis, gastric pouch dilation, gastric slippage, outlet channel stenosis, and gastric wall erosion by the band device are the most common abnormal findings observed after LAGB.[95,96] Occasionally, a marked gastric fold surrounding the pouch outlet channel can be observed in a retroflexed view within the distal stomach. This fold corresponds to the gastrogastric sutures placed anteriorly over the band device to decrease the risks of gastric herniation (**Fig. 11.11B**). Similar to VBG, once the endoscope is advanced through the pouch-outlet channel, examination of the distal stomach, duodenum, and biliopancreatic ducts can be performed as in a regular endoscopy.

Operations with Alteration of the Pancreaticobiliary Anatomy

Pancreaticoduodenectomy (Whipple Procedure)

The Whipple procedure is performed to resect malignant or benign lesions in the head of the pancreas or in the second portion of the duodenum.[97] The extent of the resection classifies this procedure as classic or pylorus-preserving.

Classic Whipple Procedure

In the classic Whipple procedure, the gastric antrum, duodenum, head of the pancreas, and distal bile duct are resected. This extensive resection has led to the proposal of at least 68 techniques for reconstruction of the alimentary and pancreaticobiliary tract during the evolution of this operation.[98] Currently, one well-accepted technique is to create all necessary anastomoses with a single limb of small bowel (**Fig. 11.12**).[99,100] In this case (**Fig. 11.12A**), a side-to-side gastroenteroanastomosis is encountered endoscopically, usually oralis partialis and with the resection limited to the antrum. All the variations regarding orientation, position to the transverse colon, and stoma size described for the Billroth II gastroenteroanastomosis apply here. On entering the afferent limb, which may range from 40 to 60 cm and include a Braun procedure, the anastomosis with the biliary and pancreatic ducts can be identified. Sharp angulations resulting from fixation to adjacent organs may be encountered before reaching the blind end of the most proximal portion of the afferent limb, where the pancreaticojejunostomy is found.

The pancreaticojejunostomy may be end-to-end or end-to-side. In either case, the pancreaticojejunostomy may also be a mucosa-to-mucosa or a "dunking" anastomosis (**Fig. 11.13**).[101] A mucosa-to-mucosa anastomosis creates a small opening by suturing the pancreatic duct to the jejunal mucosa. The

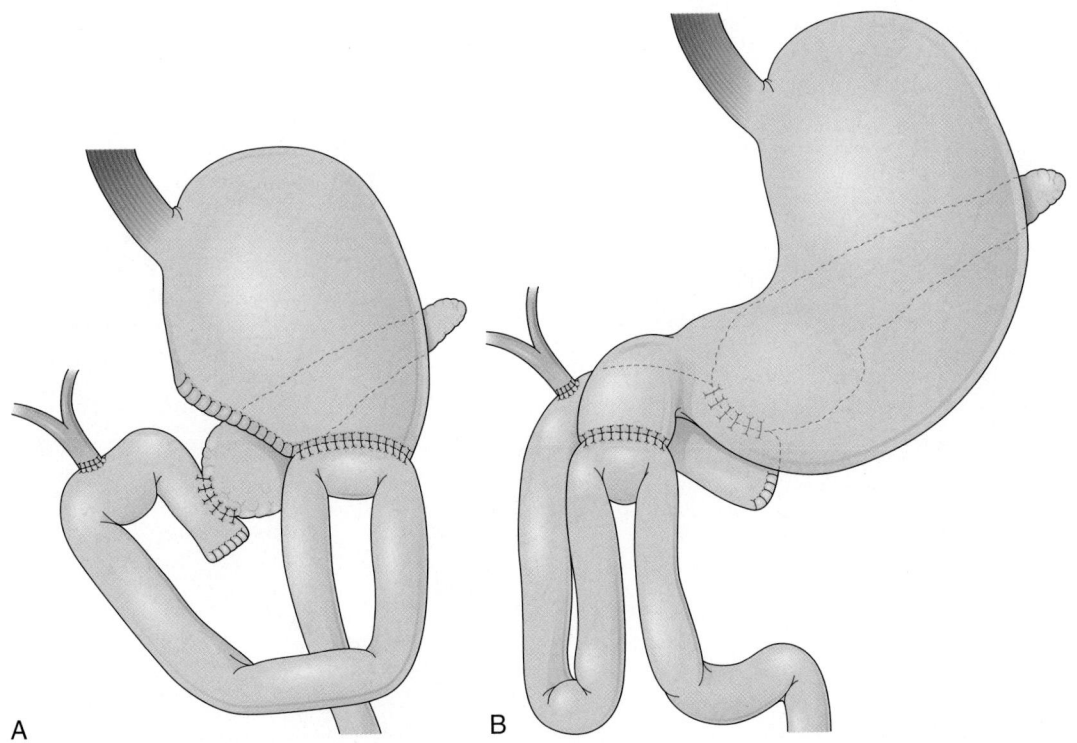

Fig. 11.12 Whipple operations. **A,** Classic Whipple: The distal stomach, head of the pancreas, distal biliary duct, and duodenum are resected. A single loop of jejunum is used to the anastomoses with the stomach and biliary and pancreatic ducts. A partial isoperistaltic gastroenteroanastomosis is shown. **B,** Pylorus-preserving Whipple: A duodenojejunostomy rather than a gastrojejunostomy is created in this procedure.

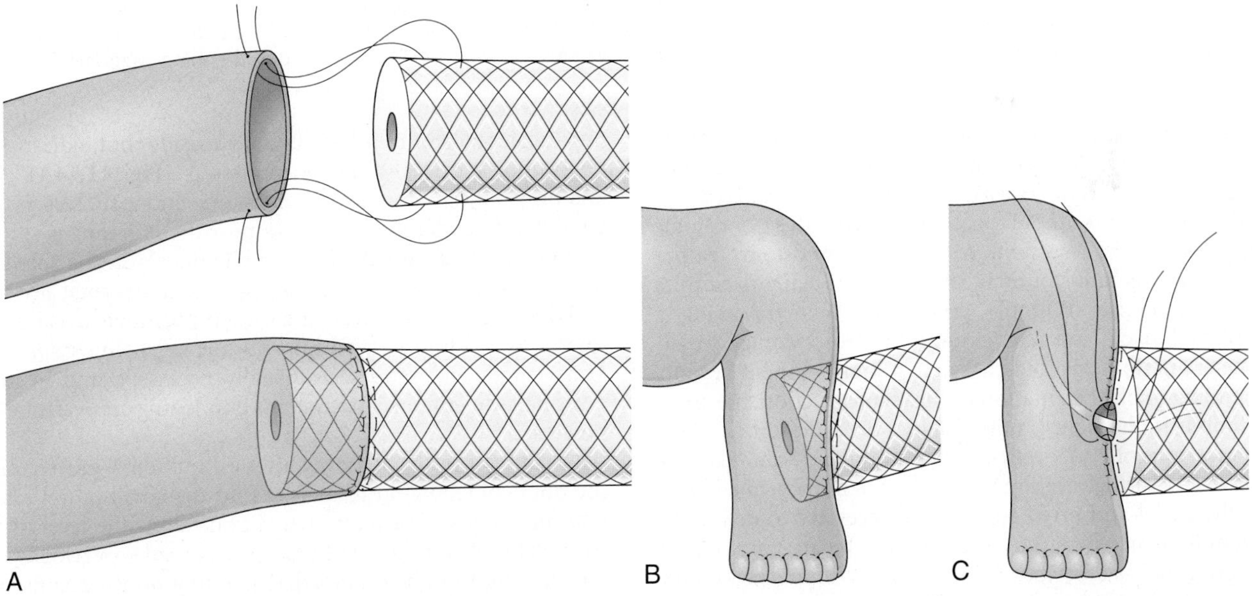

Fig. 11.13 Pancreaticojejunostomies. **A,** Terminoterminal dunking anastomosis in which the pancreas is invaginated into the jejunum. **B,** Terminolateral dunking anastomosis. **C,** Mucosa-to-mucosa pancreaticojejunostomy.

dunking anastomosis differs from the mucosa-to-mucosa anastomosis in that the pancreas is invaginated into the jejunum. The opening of the pancreatic duct varies from a flat, small-diameter anastomosis (mucosa-to-mucosa) to a protuberant, sometimes downward-oriented anastomosis (lateral dunking), making the identification and cannulation of this duct technically challenging. The hepaticojejunostomy is located approximately 10 cm proximal (endoscopically) to the

pancreaticojejunostomy. It is always an end-to-side anastomosis located in the antimesenteric border of the limb, occasionally subtle or hidden by a fold.

Pylorus-Preserving Whipple Procedure

The pylorus-preserving Whipple procedure differs from the classic Whipple operation in that the stomach is not resected

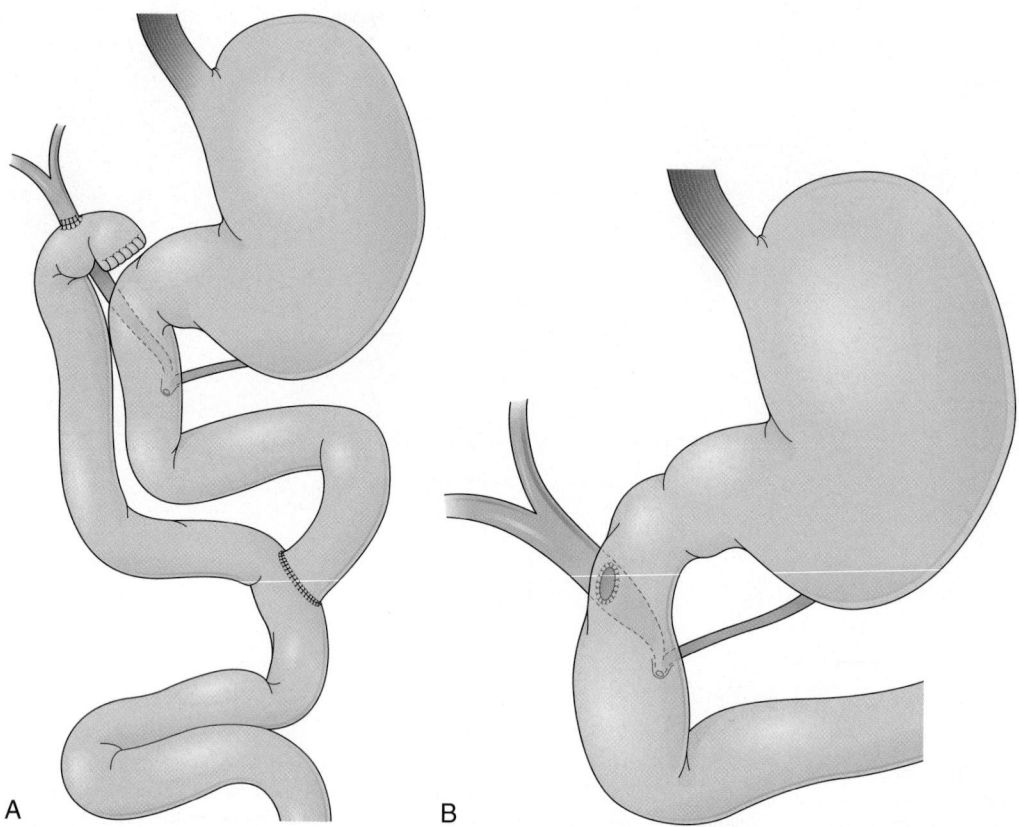

A   B

Fig. 11.14   Bilioenteric anastomoses. **A,** Roux-en-Y hepaticojejunostomy: The bile duct is anastomosed to a limb of jejunum in a lateral or terminal fashion. A side-to-side anastomosis preserves cannulation of the intrahepatic ducts through the papilla if no obstruction is present. The pancreatic duct remains accessible through the second portion of the duodenum. **B,** Choledochoduodenostomy: Usually a side-to-side anastomosis is accessible on the second portion of the duodenum. The distal bile duct may be filled with residual enteric contents leading to the sump syndrome.

and a short segment of the proximal bulb remains to be anastomosed with the jejunum (see **Fig. 11.12B**).[102] This modification has proved to decrease the morbidity of pancreatico-duodenectomies without compromising the oncologic principles of the resection. A duodenojejunostomy rather than a gastrojejunostomy is observed in patients with a pylorus-preserving Whipple procedure. After traversing a normal stomach and the pylorus, a two-opening, small-diameter anastomosis is identified in a short segment of bulb. Depending on the orientation of the reconstruction, the afferent limb is to the right (antiperistaltic) or to the left (isoperistaltic). Antecolic or retrocolic anastomosis can also be observed, creating variations on the length of the jejunal limb. Usually, a trial-and-error approach is necessary to define the afferent limb, in which the pancreatic and biliary anastomosis are performed as described for the classic Whipple procedure. In patients who have undergone either Whipple operation, the biliary and pancreatic anastomosis may be reached with a side-viewing or a forward-viewing endoscope, owing to the relatively short afferent limb.

Roux-en-Y Hepaticojejunostomy

Anastomosis of the hepatic duct to a loop of jejunum without disturbing the gastroduodenal anatomy is usually performed for biliary disease or during liver transplantation when the native bile duct cannot be used to create a duct-to-duct anastomosis (e.g., in the setting of sclerosing cholangitis).[103] The hepaticojejunostomy is usually end-to-side, but side-to-side anastomosis can also be encountered (**Fig. 11.14A**). The anatomy of the stomach, duodenum, and pancreas is not altered, and endoscopic evaluation of these organs is similar to a nonoperated stomach. If the bile duct must be accessed, the endoscope has to be advanced through a normal stomach and duodenum before reaching the jejunojejunal anastomosis that leads to a Roux-en-Y limb with the hepaticojejunostomy. Long-length endoscopes are usually necessary, and in most cases balloon enteroscopy systems employing an overtube are now used.[104–106]

In contrast to the anatomy after a Roux-en-Y gastrectomy, the duodenojejunal limb merges into the small bowel rather than merging with a loop of small bowel. At the level of the jejunojejunostomy, three lumens (side-to-side) or two lumens (end-to-side) can be observed, depending on the reconstruction (see **Fig. 11.5E**). One lumen leads to the distal jejunum, and the other leads to the limb that contains the hepaticojejunostomy. The third lumen (only if side-to-side) observed along the initial limb occupied by the endoscope ends blindly just beyond the anastomosis. A trial-and-error approach to the first two limbs reveals the one with the hepaticojejunostomy. The end-to-side hepaticojejunostomy is similar to the one described in the Whipple procedure except that here the location is closer to the blind end of the limb. In contrast to the end-to-side hepaticojejunostomy, the side-to-side hepaticojejunostomy preserves the access to the biliary ducts through the major papilla if the distal common bile duct is not obstructed. In this case, a cholangiogram can be obtained with the aid of an occlusion balloon inflated proximal to the hepaticojejunostomy, avoiding the demanding insertion of the endoscope through the Roux-en-Y limb. Air within the intrahepatic ducts is common in bilioenteric anastomosis and may be useful to evaluate patients in whom the hepaticojejunostomy is not reachable with the endoscope (air cholangiogram).[4,107]

Choledochoduodenostomy

Choledochoduodenostomy is the anastomosis of the bile duct to the second portion of the duodenum, usually performed in a side-to-side fashion (see **Fig. 11.14B**). Endoscopically, after traversing the pylorus, the choledochoduodenostomy is found at the level of the major papilla on the opposite wall of the duodenum. The anastomosis may be sufficiently wide to allow visualization and partial intubation of the extrahepatic ducts. A side-to-side anastomosis has two lumens. One lumen leads to the proximal biliary tree, and the other leads to the distal common bile duct. Because there is no alimentary diversion from the anastomosis, food impaction may occur in the distal common bile duct causing the sump syndrome, which may be the indication for ERCP in these patients.[108] Because the biliary duct can be accessed through the major papilla and through the choledochoduodenostomy, a combination of accesses can be used to manipulate the different portions of the ducts, including anterograde cannulation of the papilla. The approach to the pancreatic duct is the same as for standard ERCP.

References

The complete reference list is available online at www.expertconsult.com.

Section II

Luminal Gastrointestinal Disorders

Christopher J. Gostout and Michael L. Kochman

Benign Disorders

Neoplastic Disorders

Esophagus

Gastroduodenum

Colorectum

Chapter 12

Nonvariceal Upper Gastrointestinal Bleeding

Yakub I. Khan and Naresh T. Gunaratnam

Video related to this chapter's topics can be found online at expertconsult.com.

Introduction

Upper gastrointestinal (GI) bleeding is a common GI emergency. Frequency of occurrence is 40 to 150 cases per 100,000 in the Western population, and it accounts for a total expenditure of $2.5 billion annually in the United States.[1,2] Significant advances have been made not only in decreasing the overall incidence, but also in treatment (medical treatment and endoscopic hemostasis), prevention of complications, and recurrence of bleeding.[3] These advances have resulted in an overall decrease in the rate of hospitalizations and mortality associated with upper GI hemorrhage in the Western world.[4] However, more recent data suggest that although hospital admission rates may have decreased, patients being admitted are older and have more comorbid illnesses. These patients are known to carry a worse prognosis.[3] Acute nonvariceal upper GI bleeding is still associated with significant morbidity and mortality despite significant development in the understand-

ing of the pathophysiology of the disease and the armamentarium available to the endoscopist for endoscopic therapy to treat these lesions. This chapter discusses the approach, assessment, and management strategies in patients presenting with nonvariceal upper GI bleeding.

Clinical Presentation

The presentation of GI bleeding depends on the volume and site of bleeding. *Hematemesis* is vomiting of blood and is the most common presentation of an upper GI bleed. The source is almost always proximal to the ligament of Treitz. Blood may be bright red, indicating a recent bleed, or resemble "coffee grounds," representing older blood reduced by acid in the stomach. *Melena* is black, tarry, and sticky stool with a specific foul odor caused by degradation of blood in the intestines and colon. This presentation most commonly indicates an upper

Table 12.1 Hypovolemic Shock: Manifestations and Fluid Resuscitation

Blood loss (mL)	<750	750–1500	1500–2000	>2000
Blood loss (% body weight)	<15%	15%-30%	30%–40%	>40%
Pulse (beats/min)	<100	100–120	120–140	>140
Blood pressure (mm Hg)	>100	>100	<100	<100
Pulse volume	Normal	Decreased	Decreased	Decreased
Respiration rate (breaths/min)	14–20	20–30	30–35	>35
Hourly urine output (mL)	>30	20–30	<20	<20
Mental status	Marked anxiety	Mild anxiety	Anxiety, confusion	Confusion, drowsiness
Fluid therapy	Crystalloids	Crystalloids	Crystalloids, colloids, blood	Crystalloids, colloids, blood

From Celinski K, Cichoz-Lach H, Madro A, et al: Non-variceal upper gastrointestinal bleeding—guidelines on management. J Physiol Pharmacol 59(Suppl 2):215–229, 2008.

GI source; however, blood from the right colon may also manifest as melena. A massive upper GI bleed can manifest as *hematochezia* (bright red blood per rectum) in 15% of cases and carries a worse prognosis.[5]

Initial Evaluation

The initial assessment of a patient suspected to have an acute GI bleed must focus on hemodynamic stability so that resuscitative measures can be started without delay. Good clinical assessment determines the fluid requirement for hemodynamic stabilization.[6] A focused history and physical examination provides vital information on the severity of bleeding and other confounding medical problems (e.g., coronary disease, chronic obstructive pulmonary disease, malignancy) that may affect medical management and therapeutic intervention. The initial evaluation should focus on vital signs and orthostatic changes because postural hypotension represents a significant volume loss (>15%) and is predictive of a poor outcome (**Table 12.1**).[7,8]

Peripheral intravenous (IV) access with two large-bore (at least 18-gauge) catheters or central venous access must be achieved in patients with an acute bleed, especially if the patient is hemodynamically unstable. Crystalloids (normal saline or lactated Ringer's solution) are the initial fluids of choice and are administered rapidly to restore intravascular volume to ensure adequate tissue perfusion and oxygen delivery. Continuous monitoring is required, especially for fragile patients with comorbid cardiopulmonary disease.

Nasogastric Aspirate

Nasogastric tubes can be helpful in the localization of bleeding because a positive nasogastric aspirate (coffee ground or bright red blood) confirms the source to be from the upper GI tract. However, the localization of bleeding can be determined by a careful history and physical examination. A reliable history of hematemesis confirms the source to be proximal to the ligament of Treitz. Use of a nasogastric tube to stratify patients with high-risk lesions is controversial.[9] In the national survey of the American Society of Gastrointestinal Endoscopy (ASGE), about 16% of patients with clear nasogastric aspirates

were found to have active bleeding at the time of endoscopy.[10] The bleeding sources in these patients also included esophagitis (10.7%) and varices (5.1%).

Aljebreen and colleagues[11] performed a retrospective analysis on 1869 patients with upper GI bleeding. A bloody nasogastric aspirate was significantly associated with high-risk lesions (active bleeding, nonbleeding visible vessel, adherent clot). A bloody aspirate had a specificity of 75.8% and negative predictive value of 77.9% for high-risk lesions. Although nasogastric lavage provides no information about the etiology of bleeding, it can be valuable in localizing the source in a hemodynamically unstable patient because it is a quick and easy test that is performed at bedside. A negative or bilious aspirate does not rule out upper GI bleeding. Nasogastric suction often is not needed with the availability of large-channel therapeutic endoscopes, with forward water jets built into the endoscope and the ability to suction directly from the endoscopic channel port, bypassing the internal suction channeling that passes through the handle of the endoscope and through the umbilicord, which can contain a stepdown in channel size.

Laboratory Data

Laboratory tests appropriate at initial presentation include hemoglobin level, hematocrit, platelet count, prothrombin time, and partial thromboplastin time. Initial hemoglobin level may not depict the degree of bleeding, and initial decision making must be based on clinical grounds. An increased blood urea nitrogen (BUN)-to-creatinine ratio (>36) has been suggestive of an upper GI source of bleeding with a sensitivity of 90% and specificity of 27%.[12] BUN levels can weakly predict severity of bleeding but are not helpful in predicting high-risk lesions.[13] BUN values can be helpful in the diagnosis; however, the clinical picture is often complicated by other medical illnesses (e.g., renal insufficiency, congestive heart failure) and polypharmacy. Other important laboratory data include liver function tests and cardiac enzyme analysis.

Risk Stratification

Most GI bleeds stop spontaneously without any recurrence. Approximately 20% of bleeds can continue or recur leading

Table 12.2 Statistically Significant Predictors of Persistent or Recurrent Bleeding

Risk Factor	Odds Ratio for Increased Risk
Age	
>65 yr	1.3
>70 yr	2.3
Shock (systolic blood pressure <100 mm Hg)	1.2–3.65
Comorbid illness	1.6–7.63
Transfusion requirements	NA
Initial hemoglobin <10 g/dL	0.8–2.99
Coagulopathy (prolonged prothrombin time)	1.96 (1.46–2.64)
Melena	1.6
Blood in nasogastric tube or stomach	1.1–11.5
Hematemesis	1.2–5.7
Continued bleeding	3.14 (2.4–4.12)
Need for emergency surgery	NA

NA, Not available.
Modified from Barkun A, Bardou M, Marshall JK; Nonvariceal Upper GI Bleeding Consensus Conference Group: Consensus recommendations for managing patients with non-variceal upper gastrointestinal bleeding. Ann Intern Med 139:843–859, 2003.

Table 12.3 Modified Forrest Criteria

Forrest Class	Type of Lesion
IA	Arterial spurting
IB	Active oozing
IIA	Ulcer with nonbleeding visible vessel
IIB	Ulcer with adherent clot on surface
IIC	Ulcer with red or dark blue flat spot
III	Ulcer with clean base

to patient morbidity and mortality.[14] Numerous clinical factors have been identified that predict a high rate of recurrent bleeding or poor outcome. Old age (>65 years), shock, comorbid illnesses, low hemoglobin on evaluation, melena, multiple transfusions (more than five), hematochezia, fresh blood emesis or nasogastric aspirate, and need for emergency surgery are clinical predictors of increased risk of rebleeding.[15,16] A history of alcoholism, a history of cancer, and an Acute Physiology, Age, and Chronic Health Evaluation (APACHE) II score of 11 or greater have also been associated with poor outcomes.[17,18]

Chiu and colleagues[19] prospectively studied 3220 patients with bleeding peptic ulcers from 1993 to 2003 and identified risk factors for mortality. Among patients with bleeding peptic ulcers after endoscopic hemostasis, advanced age, multiple comorbidities, hypovolemic shock, in-hospital bleeding, rebleeding, and need for surgery were significant factors predicting in-hospital mortality (**Table 12.2**). Based on these individual clinical criteria and endoscopic findings, numerous scoring systems have been formulated to try to stratify high-risk patients for appropriate intervention.

Blatchford and associates[20] devised a scoring system based on admission hemoglobin, BUN, pulse, systolic blood pressure, presentation with syncope and melena, and evidence of hepatic disease and cardiac failure. Their criteria could identify 20% of patients with very low risk of needing treatment to control bleeding, who could be offered outpatient treatment. The Blatchford scoring system has been validated by other investigators.[21] In 1974, Forrest and colleagues[23] first classified stigmata of active or recent bleeding based on visualization at the time of endoscopy (**Table 12.3**). *Visible vessel*

is the term used for an elevated area within the ulcer base. It is thought to be a coagulum over a small-caliber arterial vessel in the ulcer base.[24] The color of the lesion can also be predictive of rebleeding: Nonpigmented lesions (white-pale) have a higher risk (71%) than pigmented lesions (38%).[25] The frequency with which a visible vessel can be found also depends on the timing of endoscopy and how aggressively the clot is washed to expose the ulcer base. Chung and coworkers[26] reported disappearance of visible vessels in 62 patients who underwent endoscopy for 3 consecutive days.

Rockall and colleagues[27] developed a scoring system involving clinical and endoscopic criteria. The main aim is to predict risk of rebleeding and mortality. An initial calculation is based on clinical parameters, and further categorization of the bleeding lesion and the stigmata of hemorrhage at the time of endoscopy enables the complete score to be calculated. A total score of less than 3 was associated with excellent prognosis, whereas a score greater than 8 carried a high mortality. For cases with a score less than 3, rebleeding occurred in less than 5%, and mortality was 0%. Multiple studies have been performed to validate the Rockall scoring system.[28,29] It has been validated in other studies to be predictive and cost-effective (**Table 12.4**).[30]

Hay and coworkers[31] derived a scoring system by using hemodynamics, time from bleeding, comorbidity, and endoscopy findings. Use of the practice guidelines reduced hospital stay in low-risk patients from 4.6 to 2.9 days ($P < .001$). Saeed and associates[32] proposed another scoring system based on endoscopy findings. In a retrospective analysis, Chuan and colleagues compared the Blatchford score with the Rockall score in 354 patients. The Blatchford score identified 92.1% of patients, whereas the Rockall score identified 70.1%. Blatchford scoring based on clinical and laboratory parameters was concluded to have a higher sensitivity to identify high-risk patients ($P < .0001$).[33,34]

Kim and associates[35] conducted a prospective study to compare the clinical utility of five scoring systems for the prediction of rebleeding and death in patients with nonvariceal upper GI bleeding. Using five scoring systems (Forrest classification, Rockall scoring system, Cedars-Sinai Medical Center Predict Index, Blatchford scoring system, and Baylor College scoring system), 239 consecutive patients were investigated. All patients underwent endoscopy for nonvariceal bleed. There were 35 patients (14.6%) who experienced rebleeding and 20 patients (8.4%) who died. Forrest classification was superior to the others in predicting rebleeding and death. The Cedars-Sinai Medical Center Predict Index and the Rockall scoring system showed high positive predictive values for predicting rebleeding (Cedars-Sinai Medical Center Predict

Table 12.4 Rockall Scoring System for Risk of Rebleeding and Death after Admission to the Hospital for Acute Gastrointestinal Bleeding

Variable	Score			
	0	*1*	*2*	*3*
Age (yr)	<60	60–79	>80	
Shock	No shock (systolic BP >100 mm Hg, pulse <100 beats/min)	Tachycardia (BP >100 mm Hg, pulse >100 beats/min)	Hypotension (systolic BP <100 mm Hg, pulse >100 beats/min)	
Comorbidity	Nil	Nil	Cardiac failure, ischemic heart disease, any major comorbidity	Renal failure, liver failure, disseminated malignancy
Diagnosis	Mallory-Weiss tear, no lesion or no SRH	All other diagnoses	Malignancy of upper GI tract	
Major SRH	None or dark spot		Blood in upper GI tract, adherent clot, visible or spurting vessel	

BP, Blood pressure; GI, gastrointestinal; SRH, stigmata of recent hemorrhage (blood in upper GI tract, adherent clot, visible vessel, spurting vessel, dark spot).
From Rockall TA, Logan RF, Devlin HB, et al: Risk assessment after acute gastrointestinal haemorrhage. Gut 38:316–321, 1996.

Index) and death (Rockall scoring system). Forrest classification was thought to be the most useful scoring system for the prediction of rebleeding and death in patients with nonvariceal upper GI bleeding. The development of clinical scoring systems is very encouraging because these can be used by emergency department physicians, general practitioners, and junior house staff to triage patients effectively. These scoring systems have been validated in large cohorts in diverse populations and have been shown to be effective in risk stratification and cost-effectiveness.

Timing of Endoscopy

Endoscopy primarily is used to determine the cause of bleeding, prognosticate, and administer appropriate endoscopic therapy to control bleeding and prevent rebleeding.[36,37] The timing of endoscopy has been a subject of debate, especially in patients who are clinically stable with no evidence of further bleeding. It is now evident that early endoscopy provides essential data affecting patient triage.

Lee and associates[38] showed that early "endoscopy triage" leads to early discharge of patients with low risk of rebleeding, without increasing morbidity and mortality. Median cost savings were $2068. Cipolletta and coworkers[39] used endoscopic and clinical criteria to identify patients at low risk for recurrent bleeding. Patients were randomly assigned to outpatient care versus hospital admission. No patients underwent surgery or died. Rates of recurrent bleeding were comparable (2.1% and 2.2%) in both groups. Median costs were $340 for outpatients and $3940 for inpatients. Based on multiple studies confirming the beneficial effects of endoscopic therapy, urgent endoscopy has been recommended by the National Institutes of Health[40] and ASGE[41] for patients who have active bleeding or who are at high risk for rebleeding. The definition of *urgent endoscopy* ranges in various studies from 2 to 24 hours after presentation to the hospital. It has been determined that 76% to 78% of patients with acute GI bleeding undergo endoscopy within the first 24 hours.[42,43] Even if discharge is not always the best option,

triage results might help choose the correct level of care within the hospital.

Preparation and Place for Endoscopy

Endoscopy is best performed in a fully equipped endoscopy suite where staff members are trained to take care of the patient and in the use and maintenance of endoscopes and their accessories (**Fig. 12.1**). A general recommendation is that patients with mild to moderate bleeding can have endoscopy the next day in the endoscopy unit. Patients whose presentation suggests a major or severe bleeding event (e.g., hemodynamic compromise) can undergo endoscopy at the bedside in the intensive care unit after initial resuscitation. Endotracheal intubation to protect the airway and prevent aspiration should be considered in high-risk patients who are experiencing active hematemesis, marked agitation, lethargy, and persistent shock. In the United States, there is increasing use of propofol for routine and even emergency endoscopy; use of propofol not administered by an anesthetist has also been studied but is not widely employed in current practice.[44]

In patients with active or recent hemorrhage, residual blood in the stomach, especially in the fundus, can limit the quality of the examination, and residual clots must be removed or flushed away. Poor visualization at the time of endoscopy has been associated with worse outcomes.[45] Multiple methods have been proposed to overcome this problem. Vigorous gastric lavage using a large-bore nasogastric tube at the time of endoscopy and instillation of 3% hydrogen peroxide[46] to dissolve small clots have been proposed. Use of an endoscope with a large device channel may offer a convenient and effective method to remove clots and blood from the stomach.[47,48] Connecting a suction line directly to the endoscope device channel, bypassing the internal system, provides rapid and impressive clearing of blood and clot. Randomized controlled trials have looked into using erythromycin as a promotility agent to improve quality and yield of endoscopy.[49-52] Patients with acute GI bleeding were randomly assigned to receive

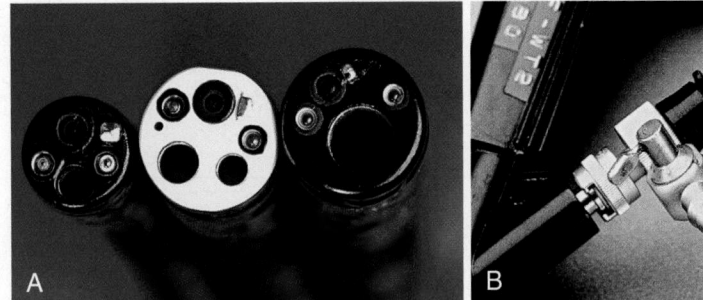

Fig. 12.1   A, Comparison of the tips of endoscopes: diagnostic (tip diameter approximately 10 mm, channel size 2.8 mm); dual-channel therapeutic (tip diameter approximately 12 mm, channel sizes 3.4 mm and 2.8 mm); jumbo-channel therapeutic (tip diameter approximately 13 mm, channel size 6.0 mm). **B,** Jumbo-channel endoscope uses the biopsy channel port as the site for a separate suction line. A specialized toggle-type switch allows the suction to be controlled as desired and maintain use of the channel for devices. Use of the biopsy port with a second suction line is a practical method to deal with quick evacuation of blood and clot with any type of endoscope.

Table 12.5   American Society of Gastrointestinal Endoscopy Bleeding Survey: Endoscopic Diagnosis for Upper Gastrointestinal Bleeding in 2225 Patients

Diagnosis	Frequency (%)
Duodenal ulcer	24.3
Gastric erosions	23.4
Gastric ulcer	21.3
Varices	10.3
Mallory-Weiss tear	7.2
Esophagitis	6.3
Erosive duodenitis	5.8
Neoplasm	2.9
Stomal ulcer	1.8
Esophageal ulcer	1.7
Miscellaneous	6.8

erythromycin (3 mg/kg intravenously) and were compared with a no treatment arm. The treatment group (erythromycin 3 mg/kg intravenously 20 to 60 minutes or 120 minutes before endoscopy) had an improved quality of endoscopic examination and reduced need for second-look endoscopy, and erythromycin was deemed a cost-effective strategy.

Etiology of Nonvariceal Upper Gastrointestinal Bleeding

Causes of nonvariceal upper GI bleeding are presented in **Table 12.5.**

Gastric and Duodenal Ulcers

Gastroduodenal ulcer disease is the most common cause of acute GI bleeding in the Western world despite an overall decline in the disease incidence in the last 3 decades.[53–56] Ulcer disease is responsible for 50% of patients presenting with upper GI bleeding.[57] With better understanding of the risk factors and better treatment protocols, overall prevalence and

hospital admissions for peptic ulcer disease have decreased. The hospitalization rate for ulcer-related GI bleeding has not changed significantly, however.[56] More elderly patients (>65 years old) are being hospitalized with bleeding ulcers.[54,58–60] Mortality associated with peptic ulcer disease is still about 14% and is known to increase progressively with age.[14,61] Previously, all peptic ulcers were considered idiopathic; in the 1980s and 1990s, most ulcer disease was attributed to *Helicobacter pylori* and nonsteroidal antiinflammatory drugs (NSAIDs). *H. pylori* was associated with 90% of duodenal ulcers and 70% of gastric ulcers.[62] With awareness and aggressive therapy, there has been a decline in the prevalence of *H. pylori* in the Western world. The epidemiology of peptic ulcer disease has changed with a much higher percentage of *H. pylori*–negative ulcer disease now being reported.[63,64]

Mamdani and colleagues[65] reported an increase in admission rate from upper GI bleeding in patients older than 65 years with greater use of cyclooxygenase-2 (COX-2) and NSAIDs. *H. pylori* infection and NSAID use both increase risk of peptic ulcer disease and upper GI bleeding.[14,66–68] In a meta-analysis by Huang and colleagues,[66] NSAID use was significantly greater in patients with peptic ulcer disease than in matched controls. *H. pylori* infection marginally increased the risk of ulcer bleeding. Risk of bleeding was much greater when both risk factors coexisted, having an additive effect. COX-2 inhibitors increase the risk modestly—less than NSAID use but higher than no use at all.[69] Cardiovascular risks associated with some COX-2 inhibitors must also be taken into consideration. Patients seen with GI bleeding with ulcers with high-risk features (active bleeding, nonbleeding visible vessel) commonly have continued or recurrent bleeding, and up to 35% require urgent surgery.[70] Over the last 15 to 20 years, endoscopic therapy has been shown to benefit this population of patients. Endoscopic therapy has been associated with reduction in the rates of rebleeding, blood transfusion, length of hospital stay, need for other therapeutic interventions, costs, and mortality.[71–73]

Indications for Endoscopic Therapy for Gastroduodenal Ulcers

After initial resuscitation of patients with severe upper GI bleeding and initiation of medical therapy for patients with suspected ulcer hemorrhage, urgent endoscopy is integral to the initial care, permitting effective triage of patients into low-risk and high-risk categories. Endoscopic treatment directed at major stigmata for ulcer hemorrhage should be intentionally planned because it has shown to improve outcome. A multicenter U.S. trial of 4090 patients hospitalized for non-variceal GI bleeding showed 10.3% had active bleeding (arterial or oozing), 12.2% had nonbleeding visible vessel, 8.3% had adherent clot, 9.9% had flat spot, and 58.4% had an ulcer with clean base.[74] Endoscopic treatment is not recommended for patients with low-risk endoscopic stigmata, including an ulcer with a clean base or a dark nonprotuberant pigmented spot in the ulcer base. Patients who have active bleeding, spurting or oozing from the ulcer, or a nonbleeding visible vessel in the ulcer base should receive endoscopic therapy.[75,76] In a meta-analysis by Bardou and colleagues,[77] endoscopic treatment was associated with statistically significant absolute decrease in rates of rebleeding, surgery, and mortality.

Nonbleeding Adherent Clot

Endoscopic therapy for ulcers with an adherent clot is also recommended. A high rate of rebleeding has been documented in these patients (33% to 40%) caused by an underlying visible vessel. Earlier studies did not show any benefit of endoscopic monotherapy in ulcers with adherent clots.[78,79] Severe bleeding may be induced from removal of the clot.[76] This observation has often been a deterrent to intervention and has led to confusion regarding whether or not to intervene. Later studies have shown combination therapy to be superior to medical therapy.

In a multicenter study organized by the Mayo Clinic GI Bleeding Team, Bleau and colleagues[80] randomly assigned patients with adherent clots to receive medical therapy or endoscopic therapy. In the treatment arm, 1:10,000 epinephrine was injected in four quadrants around the ulcer before removing the overlying clot aggressively (cold snare, suction, manipulation with biopsy forceps and tip of the endoscope). Underlying stigmata were treated with heater probe coagulation. Rates of rebleeding were 34.3% in the medical treatment arm and 4.8% in the endoscopic treatment arm. Jensen and coworkers[81] randomly assigned 32 patients with severe bleeding and adherent clots to combination endoscopic therapy or medical management. In their study, after epinephrine injection in four quadrants, cold guillotining was used to shave off the clot to 3 to 4 mm above the ulcer base. The residual clot was treated with coaptive coagulation. Rebleeding rate in the medical treatment group was 35.3% and in the endoscopic therapy group was 0%.

A meta-analysis by Kahi and associates[82] of six studies comprising 240 patients showed significant reduction in rebleeding rates (relative risk 0.35, 95% confidence interval [CI] 0.14 to 0.83) in patients who received endoscopic treatment versus medical treatment alone (8.2% vs. 24.7%). Other outcomes, such as length of hospital stay, need for surgery, transfusion requirements, and surgery, were not significant. The underlying mechanism of rebleeding in the case of an adherent clot is thought to be stigmata underlying the clot, which are the major determinants of rebleeding. Evaluation of the ulcer base is vital. Injection of 1:10,000 epinephrine seems to reduce the risk of bleeding and allows for the safe removal of the overlying clot.

Although these studies are promising, aggressive removal of clot and endoscopic therapy have their own risks. Adherent

clot removal is advisable in the appropriate clinical setting (high-risk patients) in the hands of expert endoscopists. It is important for the endoscopist to maintain the entire clinical picture in focus, including the appearance and location of the ulcer, before removing a clot. Large ulcers (>2 cm) and especially deep ulcers may contain exposed serosally based arteries that are expectedly large. Ulcers with these features in the posterior duodenal bulb and along the lesser curvature of the stomach may be particularly vulnerable to containing large compromised arteries—the gastroduodenal in the posterior duodenal bulb and the left gastric along the lesser curve. The caliber of these arteries may exceed the capabilities of standard endoscopic therapies. If there is question regarding the size of a potential artery underlying a dense adherent clot, endoscopic ultrasound (EUS) may be performed to screen the lesion. Preliminary data suggest that EUS-guided therapy may have an important role in delivering more effective treatment.[83]

Available Modalities for Endoscopic Therapy

Endoscopic therapy is now an accepted community standard of care in patients with acute GI bleeding, with earlier defined risk factors and stigmata for rebleeding. Endoscopic therapy can be broadly divided into four categories: injection therapy, thermal coaptive therapy, mechanical devices, and combination methods. Combination therapies are more popular with data supporting this method of therapy in specific situations. Data are also supportive of thermal or mechanical therapy over injection therapy alone. For this reason, monotherapy with injection cannot be supported.

Injection Therapy

Injection therapy is used as an adjunct with other modalities for ulcer hemostasis. Epinephrine is the most established injection agent used for peptic ulcer injection therapy. Epinephrine diluted to 1:10,000 or 1:20,000 in normal saline is found to be most effective and safest.[84,85] The mechanism of action is thought to be vasoconstriction, platelet activation, and stimulation of the coagulation cascade.[86] In addition, a tamponade effect resulting from the volume of fluid injected into the ulcer base is thought to be therapeutic.[87]

Technique

A disposable injection needle with a retractable tip is used. Injection is undertaken in 0.5- to 1.0-mL increments in all four quadrants around the nonbleeding stigmata because the path of the exposed artery is unknown. A total volume of 20 to 45 mL may be injected to achieve the desired results.[88,89] No cardiac side effects have been reported as a result of larger volume of epinephrine being injected. In the setting of active bleeding, if the initial injection results in noticeable slowing and, more so, cessation of bleeding, a single injection site may suffice. Additional volume may be injected via a single site as long as any lifting effect does not impair access to the bleeding vessel for second-line therapy with coaptive coagulation or mechanical closure.

Thermal Coaptive Therapy

Thermal methods formerly included the neodymium:yttrium-aluminum-garnet (Nd:YAG) laser and presently include heater probe and electrocoagulation (**Fig. 12.2**). Laser therapy and monopolar coagulation are no longer popular because of the lack of portability to bedside, high cost, and perforation risks. Multipolar electrocoagulation and heater probe are the most widely used thermal modalities. The advantages of these devices are their excellent efficacy; safety; portability; and ability to combine irrigation, tamponade, and coagulation.

In coaptive coagulation, the probe is used to compress physically and tamponade the bleeding vessel, followed by thermal energy sealing the walls of the vessel. In an animal model, arteries with a diameter of 2.5 mm can be coagulated with a heater probe using this technique.[93]

Technique
BIPOLAR ELECTROCAUTERY (MULTIPOLAR PROBE)

The technique for applying bipolar electrocoagulating energy has not been standardized and varies among reported clinical trials. In canine models, a large (3.2-mm) multipolar probe produced better hemostasis than a smaller (2.3-mm) probe.[94,95] Laine[96] recommends forcefully applying a large (3.2-mm) bipolar circumactive probe (BICAP) on a power setting of 3 to 5 for a prolonged duration, such as 14 seconds, or seven pulses of 2 seconds each. Jensen and Hirabayashi[94] used a setting of 3 to 4 with 10-second pulses on a BICAP II generator. The Gold Probe (Boston Scientific, Microvasive Endoscopy, Natick, MA), which contains a gold foil–wrapped tip, has been shown in clinical trials to be effective at low power settings with longer pulse duration.[97]

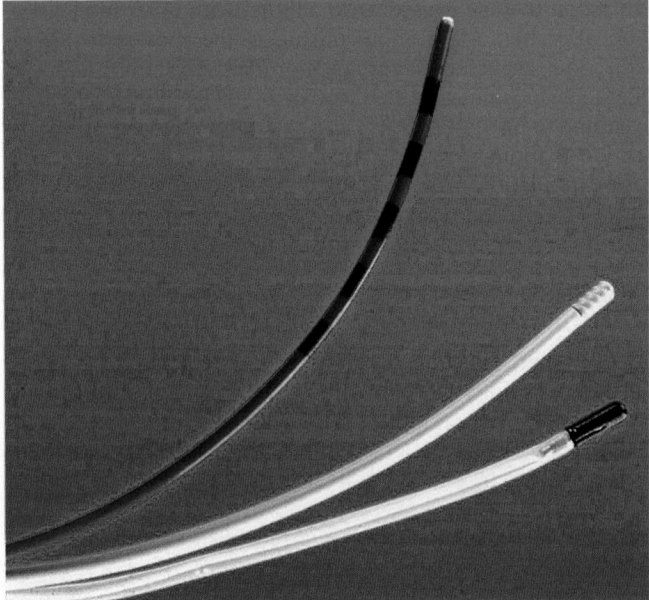

Fig. 12.2 Coagulation probes *(from top down)*: argon plasma coagulation end-firing probe, Gold Probe (Boston Scientific, Microvasive Endoscopy, Natick, MA), and heater probe (Olympus America, Center Valley, PA).

HEATER PROBE

The present technique for bleeding peptic ulcers involves using the larger heater probe, firm tamponade directly on the bleeding point or visible vessel, and coagulation with at least 120 J (four pulses of 30 J each) before moving the probe.[98] An additional application of energy when using the heater probe or multipolar (bipolar) probes as the probe is removed from the treatment site can reduce unwanted tissue adhesion and the inadvertent tearing of the coagulated sealant with resultant rebleeding. In a prospective study by Bianco and colleagues,[99] combined therapy with epinephrine injection with bipolar probe showed better results than epinephrine alone.

Mechanical Devices

Numerous mechanical devices, including hemoclip, endoloop, and rubber band, are now available for endoscopic treatment of GI bleeding. Although endoloop and rubber band ligation have little role in treating peptic ulcer bleeding, use of hemoclips has become very popular for emergency nonvariceal hemostasis. The underlying mechanism of action is mechanical clamping of the bleeding vessel. Various clips are available (**Table 12.6**). Multiple randomized trials have compared use of clips alone or in combination with other therapies. Most studies have been performed on first-generation clips. Jensen and associates[100] studied hemostasis capability of three presently available clips in a canine model; initial hemostasis was 100% for all types with longer retention times reported for the largest of the available clips, which can also be opened and closed on demand before deployment (see **Table 12.6**).

Clips are easier to apply with the scope in straight position. Tangential access makes application a challenge because of the simple mechanics allowing the clip to be extruded from the catheter, opened, and finally closed. Similarly, it is difficult to place a clip in the fundic region with the scope retroflexed. All currently available clips are not designed for use through a side-viewing duodenoscope. The angle of entry of the clipping device and the elevator function challenge current clip designs. Various maneuvers and modifications of the actual device have been identified to allow use of the device in conjunction with a duodenoscope.

Among trials comparing hemoclip with other endoscopic therapy, Cipolletta and colleagues[101] randomly assigned 112 patients with major stigmata to heater probe or hemoclip therapy (**Fig. 12-3**). Rates of recurrent bleeding (21% vs. 1.8%) and need for surgery (7% vs. 3.6%) were significantly lower in the hemoclip group. The investigators concluded that hemoclip therapy was safe and superior to heater probe therapy. In a randomized study by Chou and coworkers,[102] hemoclip therapy was found to be superior to distilled water injection therapy in patients with major stigmata (active bleeding vessel, nonbleeding visible vessel). In their study comparing hemoclip versus heater probe, Lin and associates[103] reported 85% initial hemostasis in the hemoclip group compared with 100% in the heater probe group. Rebleeding rate was 8.8% in the hemoclip group and 5% in the heater probe group. In trials comparing combination therapy, Chung and colleagues[104] prospectively assigned 124 patients to hemoclip, hypertonic saline–epinephrine (HSE), and combined treatment groups. Initial hemostasis was comparable in all groups.

Table 12.6 Single-Use, Disposable Clipping Devices

Manufacturer	Brand Name	Working Length (cm)	Minimum Working Channel (mm)	Opened Clip Width Span (mm)	Features	Price*
Olympus America Inc (Center Valley, PA)	QuickClip2	165 or 230	2.8	9.0	Rotatable	$1800 per box of 20; $475 per box of 5
	QuickClip2Long	165 or 230	2.8	11.0	Rotatable	
Boston Scientific Corp (Natick, MA)	Resolution	155 or 235	2.8	11.0	Reopening and closing capability for clip repositioning	$155 per clip (boxes of 1, 10, or 20)
Wilson-Cook Medical Inc (Winston-Salem, NC)	TriClip (7-Fr)	205	2.8	12.0	Three-prong design	$316 per box of 3
	TriClip (8-Fr)	205	3.2	12.0	Three-prong design; integrated flush port	$316 per box of 3

From Anastassiades CP, Baron TH, Wong Kee Song LM: Endoscopic clipping for the management of gastrointestinal bleeding. Nat Clin Pract Gastroenterol Hepatol 5:559–568, 2008.

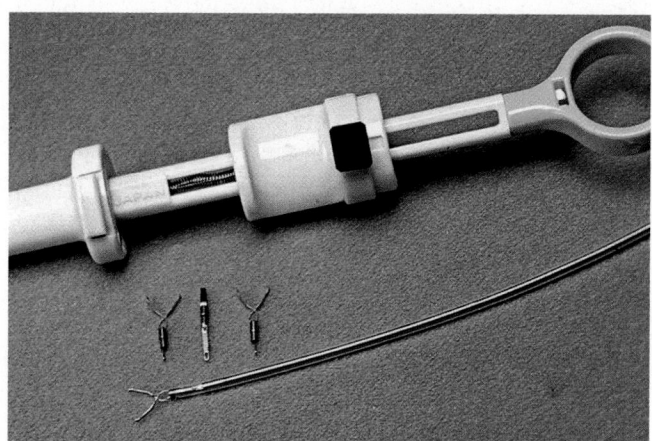

Fig. 12.3 Original manually loaded hemoclip (Olympus America, Center Valley, PA).

Rates of recurrent bleed in hemoclip, HSE, and combination therapy groups were 2.4%, 14.6%, and 9.5%. Buffoli and colleagues[105] did not find an additional advantage of hemoclip therapy when used in combination with epinephrine injection therapy. A favored trend toward reducing surgery was seen in the combination therapy group (0% vs. 7.4%).

Several randomized controlled trials investigating the use of endoscopic clips alone or in combination with other endoscopic modalities have reported variable success (**Table 12.7**).[106] The most important factor seems to be difficulty in appropriate placement of the clip for effective hemostasis, especially for ulcers in difficult-to-approach sites such as high on the lesser curvature and posterior duodenal wall.[103] Improvements in endoscopic clip devices have included single-use, rotatable, and reopening features. Present data suggest clips to be as effective as thermal therapy. The choice between the two modalities is at the discretion of the endoscopist depending on his or her comfort level with the device and the location of the lesion (see **Table 12.7**).[106]

Combination Therapy

There is a theoretical advantage of combining therapies because hemostasis is achieved by different mechanisms. The most popular combination therapy used is injection therapy and thermal coagulation (**Fig. 12.4**); epinephrine causes vasoconstriction, reduced blood flow, and platelet activation, which potentiates the coaptive coagulation by thermal energy. Another advantage may be improved visualization of the target area for thermal coagulation after initial injection therapy in an actively bleeding ulcer. Combination therapy with injection and coaptive therapy has consistently shown superiority over medical therapy.[115]

In a randomized controlled trial, Chung and colleagues[116] compared epinephrine injection with epinephrine injection plus heater probe in actively bleeding ulcers. Patients with major, active arterial bleeding had a better outcome regarding need for surgery (29.6% vs. 6.5%) and length of hospital stay (6 days vs. 4 days) after combination therapy. Combination therapy did not improve outcomes of patients with lesions with oozing only. Lin and coworkers[117] compared epinephrine injection alone, bipolar electrocoagulation alone, and combined treatment. Combination therapy was associated with reduced rate of rebleeding, reduced treatment failure, and reduced transfusion requirements. In contrast, Marmo and associates[118] showed single endoscopic therapy with thermal probes or clips is as effective as combination therapy and may be safer than combination therapy including injection therapy in high-risk ulcers.

A meta-analysis performed by Calvet and colleagues[119] looked at trials comparing epinephrine injection alone versus epinephrine plus a second method (thermal, mechanical, sclerosant) for patients with upper GI hemorrhage from peptic ulcer disease. The analysis included 16 studies with 1673 patients; only studies with major stigmata of bleeding defined by Forrest criteria IA, IIA, and IIB were included. Addition of a second endoscopic method reduced rate of rebleeding (18.4% vs. 10.6%), need for surgery (11.3% vs. 7.6%), and mortality (5.1% vs. 2.6%) compared with epinephrine

Table 12.7 Randomized Controlled Trials of Clipping for Bleeding Peptic Ulcers

Authors	Treatment Modalities	No. Patients	Primary Hemostasis (%)	Rebleeding (%)	Rescue Therapy* (%)	Mortality (%)
Chou et al (2003)[102]	Clipping	39	100	10†	5	3
	Injection (distilled water)	40	98	28†	13	5
Chung et al (1999)[104]	Clipping	41	98	2	5	2
	Injection (HSE)	41	95	15	15	2
	Clipping plus injection	42	98	10	2	2
Gevers et al (2002)[107]	Clipping	35	86	20	0	0
	Injection (epinephrine-polidocanol)	34	97	15	0	0
	Clipping plus injection	32	91	16	0	9
Shimoda et al (2003)[108]	Clipping	42	100	10	0	7
	Injection (ethanol)	42	100	14	0	2
	Clipping plus injection	42	100	7	0	2
Ljubicic et al (2004)[109]	Clipping	31	97	6	3	3
	Injection (polidocanol)	30	97	13	3	0
Park et al (2004)[110]	Clipping plus injection	23	87	9	4	0
	Injection (epinephrine)	45	98	20	4	2
Lo et al (2006)[111]	Clipping plus injection	52	98	4†	0†	2
	Injection (epinephrine)	53	92	21†	9†	0
Cipolletta et al (2001)[101]	Clipping	56	89	2†	4	4
	Heater probe coagulation	57	86	21†	7	4
Lin et al (2002)[103]	Clipping	40	85†	8	5	5
	Heater probe coagulation	40	100†	5	3	3
Lin et al (2003)[112]	Clipping	46	85†	9	0	4
	Injection (HSE) plus heater probe coagulation	47	100†	6	4	2
Saltzman et al (2005)[113]	Clipping	26	100	15	12	0
	Injection (epinephrine) plus bipolar coagulation	21	95	24	5	10
Lin et al (2007)[114]	TriClip	50	76	22	4	4
	Olympus clip	50	94	14	2	0

*Surgery or angiographic embolization.
†$P < .05$.
HSE, Hypertonic saline-epinephrine.
From Anastassiades CP, Baron TH, Wong Kee Song LM: Endoscopic clipping for the management of gastrointestinal bleeding. Nat Clin Pract Gastroenterol Hepatol 5:559–568, 2008.

injection alone. Risk of further bleeding decreased regardless of the type of second method used. Risk of significant complications, including massive bleeding, gastric wall necrosis, and perforation, was the same in both groups (1.1%).

A meta-analysis by Yuan and associates[120] comparing clips with other modalities showed that initial hemostasis was 92% for clips versus 96% for other modalities (CI 0.19 to 1.75); however, rate of rebleeding was 8.5% for clips versus 15.5% for other modalities (CI 0.30 to 1.05). Both values did not reach statistical significance. Hemoclips are equivalent to other endoscopic modalities in terms of initial hemostasis, rebleeding rates, emergency surgery, and mortality rates for treatment of peptic ulcer bleed. Sung and colleagues[121] reached a similar conclusion that hemoclips improved hemostasis

compared with injection alone but were comparable to thermal coagulation. In a Cochrane review meta-analysis in 2007 that included 1763 patients, adding a second procedure reduced further bleeding rate from 18.8% to 10.4% (odds ratio [OR] 0.51), emergency surgery from 10.8% to 7.1% (OR 0.63), and mortality from 5% to 2.5% (OR 0.50). Subanalysis showed that risk decreased regardless of which modality was used as second therapy. Risk was reduced in all groups.[122]

Role of Argon Plasma Coagulator

Argon plasma coagulation (APC) is a noncoaptive method that allows controlled noncontact electrocoagulation via high-frequency monopolar energy delivered to the tissue through

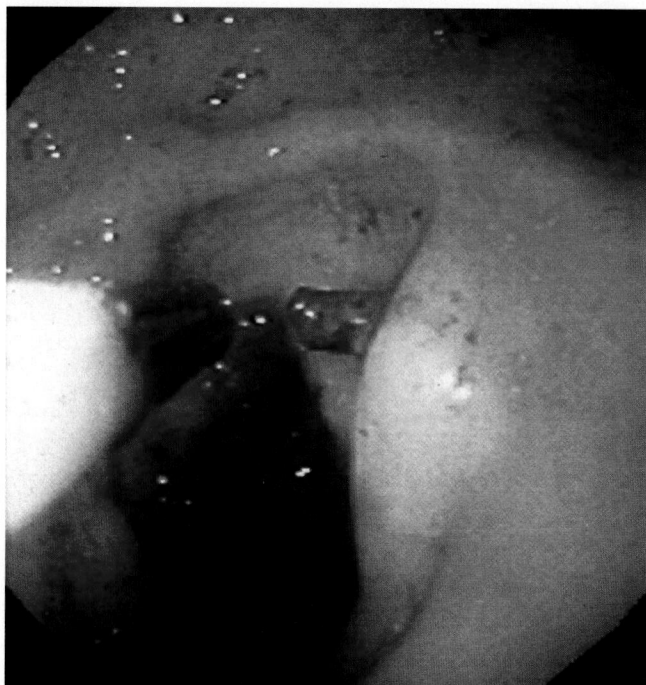

Fig. 12.4 Large-sized heater probe and large-sized visible vessel protruding from an antral ulcer (not seen). Note the surrounding mucosal pallor from prior injection with 1 : 10,000 epinephrine.

ionized gas (argon plasma). It has been used instead of standard electrocoagulation, and preliminary data show some promise. In a prospective trial of 41 patients, Cipolletta and colleagues[123] compared APC with heater probe therapy; rates of initial hemostasis, recurrent bleeding, emergency surgery, and 30-day mortality were comparable in both groups. Chau and coworkers[124] reported similar results in a large (185 cases) randomized trial comparing epinephrine plus heater probe with epinephrine plus APC. A Cochrane review concluded that APC was similar to other endoscopic therapies for nonvariceal upper GI bleeding.[125] These data suggest that APC therapy is safe and effective for treatment of ulcer bleeding.

Other Options

Various agents have been used for injection therapy with variable results, including agents causing tamponade (hypertonic saline, distilled water),[87] sclerosing agents (ethanolamine, cyanoacrylate, polidocanol),[126–128] tissue-fixating (desiccating) agent (alcohol),[129] and agents stimulating clot formation (thrombin, fibrin).[88,130] There is little evidence that addition of other agents significantly reduces the rate of rebleeding. Some of these agents (e.g., alcohol) have been associated with tissue necrosis of injected areas, clinical perforation, and death. Current data do not show superiority of these agents to currently available therapeutic options, including the settings of rebleeding alternative therapy and therapy in patients with coagulopathies.

Recommendations for Endoscopic Stigmata

Arterial spurting: Combination therapy—epinephrine injection, followed by thermal coagulation and hemoclips

Nonbleeding visible vessel: Monotherapy, hemoclips, or thermal coagulation
Active oozing from ulcer base: Monotherapy, thermal therapy favored
Adherent clot: Combination therapy—injection, removal of clot followed by thermal coagulation and hemoclips
Pigmented flat spot or ulcer with clean base: No therapy needed

Injection therapy only is insufficient but may be performed as an adjunctive treatment when access to the bleeding site is suboptimal.

Role of Medical Therapy

Medical management targets reduction in morbidity, risk of rebleeding, need for transfusions, hospitalization duration, need for endoscopic or surgical intervention, and mortality. Testing and eradication for *H. pylori* is important in all patients with peptic ulcer bleeds. Several randomized controlled trials have shown that eradication of *H. pylori* in patients with bleeding peptic ulcers significantly decreases recurrent bleeding compared with nontreated patients.[131,132] In addition to endoscopic therapy, acid suppression therapy has been shown to benefit patients with bleeding peptic ulcers.[133] The role of gastric acid inhibition in stopping bleeding or preventing recurrent bleeding is related to sealant clot stability, which is favored at a higher gastric pH.[134,135] A pH greater than 6 is required for platelet aggregation, whereas clot lysis occurs at pH less than 6. IV and oral H_2 antagonists have previously been used to prevent recurrent bleeding in these patients. Two meta-analyses showed that H_2-receptor inhibitors provide no additional benefit in patients with bleeding duodenal ulcers, but statistically significant absolute risk reductions in rebleeding, surgery, and death were seen in patients with bleeding gastric ulcers.[133,136] Proton pump inhibitors (PPIs) have been found to be more effective than H_2-receptor antagonists in decreasing the rate of recurrent bleeding.[137,138]

Lau and colleagues[139] reported results of a large double-blind randomized trial in which omeprazole was compared with placebo in patients receiving endoscopic therapy for bleeding ulcers (**Table 12.8**). After receiving endoscopic therapy (active bleeding, nonbleeding visible vessel, stigmata under adherent clot), patients were randomly assigned to IV omeprazole (8 mg/hr continuous infusion) versus placebo for 72 hours. Recurrent bleeding at 30 days, the primary endpoint of the study, occurred in 6.7% of the patients in the omeprazole group compared with 22.5% of the patients in the placebo group (relative risk reduction 70%, $P < .001$). Most cases of rebleeding occurred within 72 hours of endoscopic therapy. A Cochrane meta-analysis by Leontiadis and colleagues[146] on the role of PPI therapy in peptic ulcer bleeding included 24 trials with 4373 patients. Reductions in rebleeding, the need of surgery, and repeat endoscopic therapy were statistically significant with PPI use. Other meta-analyses reached similar conclusions.[147–150] Post hoc analysis of the Cochrane data by Leontiadis and colleagues[150] showed important differences between Asian and non-Asian patients. The effects of PPI therapy on rebleeding and need for surgery were more marked in the Asian trials, and PPI therapy was associated with significant reduction in 30-day mortality in Asian patients.

Table 12.8 Effectiveness of Omeprazole in Peptic Ulcer Bleeding

Study	No.	Endoscopic Therapy	Bleeding Rate Control	Omeprazole	P Value
Hasselgren et al (1997)[140]	322	Yes	26/163 (17%)	12/159 (8%)	NS
Schaffalitzky de Muckadell et al (1997)[141]	229	Yes	37/118 (25%)	20/111(18%)	NS
Khuroo et al (1997)[142]	220	No	40/110 (36%)	12/110(11%)	<.001
Lin et al (1998)[143]	100	Yes	8/50 (16%)	0/50 (0%)	.01
Lau et al (2000)[139]	240	Yes	24/120 (23%)	5/120 (7%)	<.001
Javid et al (2001)[144]	166	Yes	18/84 (21%)	6/82 (7%)	.02
Sung et al (2003)[145]	156	Yes	7/78 (7%)	0/78 (0%)	.01

NS, Not significant.

Lau and coworkers[151] prospectively showed that IV bolus followed by infusion of PPI started before endoscopy decreased the need for endoscopic therapy, number of actively bleeding ulcers, and duration of hospitalization. A retrospective study from Keyvani and colleagues[152] showed that PPI (oral and IV) started before endoscopy significantly reduced rebleeding, surgery, duration of hospital stay, and mortality in patients presenting with ulcer hemorrhage. In a meta-analysis, Laine and McQuaid[153] studied the role of PPI therapy as an adjunct to endoscopic therapy. Three groups were analyzed: (1) IV PPI (bolus followed by infusion) versus placebo, (2) IV PPI (bolus followed by infusion) versus H_2 blockers, and (3) oral or intermittent IV PPI versus placebo. Their conclusions were that PPI therapy after endoscopic therapy reduced rebleeding, need for surgery, need for urgent intervention, and mortality. The results were most consistent for bolus followed by continuous IV PPI for 72 hours.

Based on randomized clinical trials, the recommended dose of PPI is equivalent to omeprazole 80 mg IV bolus followed by 8 mg/hr infusion for 72 hours. The U.S. Food and Drug Administration (FDA) has not approved PPIs for the indication of upper GI bleed. In view of their known benefits and very good side-effect profile, starting PPI therapy seems to be a reasonable approach. Increasing data indicate that perhaps it is safe to switch the patient to oral PPI early in the course of management.[154,155] Somatostatin, octreotide, and tranexamic acid may have a theoretical advantage by their different mechanism of action of helping hemostasis, but there is no firm evidence to recommend them over PPI therapy for nonvariceal upper GI bleeding.

Second-Look Endoscopy

Routine repeat (second-look) endoscopy is done 24 hours after the initial procedure with the intent of repeat endoscopic treatment of residual high-risk lesions and has been advocated to be beneficial in some clinical situations. Few randomized trials have addressed the issue, and these trials show conflicting results. Messmann and colleagues[156] reported no improvements in outcomes when scheduled repeat endoscopy was compared with second-look endoscopy performed at recurrent bleeding. Villanueva and associates[157] noted a nonsignificant trend toward better outcomes in the group that received routine second-look endoscopy within 24 hours. Saeed and colleagues[158] adopted an approach of scheduled retreatment in high-risk patients based on a composite clinical and endoscopic score and showed significant benefit in the prevention of rebleeding.

Pooled data on second-look endoscopy showed that routine second-look endoscopy with retreatment significantly reduced the risk of recurrent bleeding compared with expectant management (absolute risk reduction 6.2%, $P < .01$, number needed to treat 16).[159] The risk of surgery and death were not significantly influenced by second-look endoscopy. Cost-effectiveness of repeat endoscopy has been verified in a hypothetical model,[160] but no prospective studies are available to date. Routine second-look endoscopy in all patients is not recommended. It may be justified in selected high-risk patients. Second-look endoscopy may be needed in patients with an incomplete initial endoscopy because of poor visualization or other technical difficulties.

Recurrent Bleeding

The size and the depth of ulcer influence the bleeding rate. Increased ulcer size (>1 cm) is associated with an increased risk of rebleeding and mortality. The failure rate of therapeutic endoscopy is much greater in ulcers larger than 2 cm.[161] Ulcers located high on the lesser curvature of the stomach and on the posteroinferior wall of the duodenum also seem to have a higher rate of rebleeding.[24] Primary hemostasis is achieved in greater than 95% of patients with bleeding peptic ulcers and ulcers with a nonbleeding visible vessel. Rebleeding can occur in 10% to 20% of these patients with mortality of 4% to 10%. In a prospective study, Manguso and colleagues[162] recruited patients admitted for nonvariceal upper GI bleeding with Forrest I lesions (active bleeding) at time of endoscopy. All patients received standard endoscopic therapy and IV PPI. The investigators reported a rebleeding rate of 12%, 2.8% of patients required surgery, and there was an overall mortality of 5.6% in a 24-day period.

Rebleeding occurs within 48 to 72 hours and is highly infrequent after 96 hours. In most patients, repeat endoscopy for diagnosis of the bleeding site and a renewed effort at endoscopic hemostasis is the next intervention. The number of repeated efforts at endoscopic therapy depends on various individualized factors. Repeat endoscopic intervention should include an evaluation for the selection of endoscope and therapy. The original presentation of the bleeding site, access to it, and the tissue response to the original therapy are important considerations. Angiography and surgery should be considered for patients with refractory recurrent bleeding and massive recurrent bleeding associated with hypotension, patients receiving transfusion of 4 or more units of blood for a resuscitative event, and patients receiving transfusion of 8 or more units of blood.

In a retrospective trial of patients with nonvariceal upper GI bleeding, rate of recurrent bleed was 20% after endoscopic therapy. The authors developed a score to predict rate of rebleeding in patients after endoscopic therapy. The score was based on six factors: failure to use a PPI after the procedure, endoscopically shown active bleeding, treatment with epinephrine monotherapy, peptic ulcer as a source of bleeding, IV heparin or low-molecular-weight heparin after procedure, and moderate or severe cirrhosis.[163]

In a prospective randomized trial, Lau and coworkers[164] randomly assigned 92 patients with recurrent bleeding after endoscopic hemostasis; 48 patients were assigned to repeat endoscopic therapy, and 44 patients were assigned to emergency ulcer surgery. Of patients in the repeat endoscopic therapy group, 73% (35 of 48) had long-term control of bleeding by repeat endoscopic therapy; 27% (13 of 48) required surgery because of 11 endoscopic failures and 2 perforations secondary to thermal coagulation. Overall, a lower complication rate (14.6% vs. 36.4%) was seen in the repeat endoscopy group. This study suggests that repeat endoscopy is effective in reducing the need for surgical intervention and its associated complications.

During endoscopic retreatment with coagulation therapy, a large thermal probe (3.2-mm) is desirable. Repeat thermal therapy at the same location increases the risk of clinical perforation and should be used with caution in therapy of acute lesions, such as a Mallory-Weiss tear, stress ulcer, and Dieulafoy's lesion in the gastric fundus, and in severely ill immunocompromised patients with poor tissue healing capability.[164] Injection therapies may be ineffective because of increased fibrosis, especially of chronic and penetrating ulcers. Injection therapy is reasonable to attempt during active spurting. If there is no immediate response, alternative therapy is needed. Refractory rebleeding in patients who are not candidates for surgical intervention or who have also failed angiographic intervention may be candidates for EUS-guided therapy by direct vascular injection of embolic material or glue. Fine needle application of tissue glues and even alcohol can be performed into specific types of lesions (e.g., gastrointestinal stromal tumors, pseudoaneurysms).[165]

Complications of Endoscopic Therapy

The most feared complications of endoscopic hemostatic therapy are perforation and induction of uncontrollable bleeding. Both of these complications are relatively rare, however. One must be prepared for the possibility of inducing massive bleeding when a deeply penetrating ulcer is encountered with focally pulsating stigmata of a large visible vessel,

especially when there is a fresh dense adherent clot attached to the stigmata. These are unique circumstances for which careful planning is required to ensure that blood products are readily available, endotracheal intubation is performed, and surgical backup has been readied.

Perforations are typically small (probe-sized), and efforts should be directed at closing the perforation with hemostatic clips. For larger perforations in the stomach, except posteriorly, and in the anterior duodenum, omental fat can be grasped and pulled into the defect, then clipped into place (omental patch). Laine and Peterson[14] reported induction of uncontrollable bleeding requiring urgent surgery in 0.3% of cases and perforation in 0.5% of patients who underwent endoscopic therapy for peptic ulcer hemorrhage. In a meta-analysis by Cook and associates,[71] endoscopic hemostasis induced bleeding requiring surgery in 0.39% and 0.4% of cases for contact thermal devices and injection therapy, and perforation rates of 0.7% and 0% were reported.

Failure of Endoscopic Therapy

Surgery for bleeding peptic ulcer has declined in the past 2 decades secondary to improvements in endoscopic hemostasis techniques and acid suppression therapy. However, active nonvariceal GI hemorrhage that cannot be controlled by endoscopic intervention and especially hemorrhage that overwhelms the ability to visualize any bleeding site requires an urgent operation. It is imperative to obtain surgical consultation in all patients presenting with the aforementioned clinical situation. Accurate prediction of patients likely to do poorly after endoscopic therapy is desirable. Wong and colleagues[166] analyzed risk factors associated with treatment failure with combined injection therapy and heater probe thermal coagulation. Hypotension, hemoglobin less than 10 g/dL, fresh blood in the stomach, ulcer with active bleeding, and ulcers larger than 2 cm were independent risk factors predicting poor outcome. In a prospective study by Chung and coworkers,[167] presence of spurting and ulcers larger than 2 cm were significantly related to failure of endoscopic therapy. Few data support elective surgery in these patients after their first endoscopic intervention, although it sounds appealing in theory because elective surgery carries a much lower mortality than emergency surgery. Maximal acid suppression therapy, close monitoring for signs of rebleeding, and surgical team on standby may be the best treatment strategy.

Therapeutic Angiography

Therapeutic angiography is an alternative option for patients who have failed endoscopic therapy and have a high surgical risk. Therapeutic options include selective intraarterial vasopressin infusion or embolization with microcoils, gelatin, or polyvinyl alcohol particles. Embolization has been shown to stop bleeding in massive gastroduodenal ulcers. Detection of bleeding site at the time of endoscopy provides vital information to the interventional radiologist to select the target area for catheterization. Technical success rates have been reported to be 50% to 90%.[168–170] Known complications of embolization are bowel ischemia, necrosis with perforation, abscess formation, and hepatic infarction especially in patients with poor hepatic reserve.

Prevention of Recurrent Bleed

Prevention of recurrent ulcer disease and bleeding is very important in patients with ulcer hemorrhage. Convincing data indicate that treatment with PPIs prevents ulcer rebleeding. Follow-up endoscopy is warranted to exclude malignancy in certain patients with gastric ulcer. The data linking persistent *H. pylori* with recurrent ulcer hemorrhage are compelling, making eradication of infection the best approach for these patients.[171–174] Most tests of active infection may exhibit increased false-negative rates in the context of acute bleeding.[175–178] The optimal diagnostic approach may include testing for *H. pylori* by antral biopsy at the time of endoscopy, with reconfirmation of negative results by repeat testing outside the acute setting of bleeding. Oral therapy can be started immediately or during follow-up in patients found to have *H. pylori*. Patients with peptic ulcer bleeding should be encouraged to discontinue use of NSAIDs. If stopping NSAID usage is impossible, therapy with misoprostol (200 µg four times daily) or omeprazole seems to be effective in prevention of gastroduodenal ulcers and erosions.[171,179] Switching to COX-2 inhibitors would still require concurrent prophylaxis therapy.

Dieulafoy's Lesion

Dieulafoy's lesion is an uncommon cause of acute nonvariceal GI bleeding, but it can be associated with massive, life-threatening hemorrhage. Originally described by Gallard in 1884 and designated "exulceratio simplex" by the French surgeon Dieulafoy 14 years later, Dieulafoy's lesion consists of an abnormal, submucosal "caliber persistent artery" (1 to 3 mm diameter) that retains the large caliber and typically protrudes through a small mucosal defect without any surrounding ulceration.[180] The underlying mechanism is poorly understood but thought to be due to mechanical compression of overlying mucosa by the large artery resulting in small erosion with rupture of the vessel into the lumen.[181] Dieulafoy's lesion accounts for 1.2% to 1.9% of cases of acute nonvariceal upper GI bleeding,[182,183] but an incidence of 5.8% has been reported.[184] Although reported in all age groups, Dieulafoy's lesion predominantly manifests in old men with multiple comorbid conditions.[181,184] Typically, a Dieulafoy lesion is located in the stomach usually within 6 cm of the gastroesophageal junction, the classic site, in 60% to 64% of cases and in the duodenum in another 14% to 18%.[184,185]

Diagnosis

The endoscopic criteria for the diagnosis of Dieulafoy's lesion are (1) active arterial spurting or micropulsatile streaming; (2) visualization of a protruding vessel with or without active bleeding; or (3) fresh, densely adherent clot with a narrow point of attachment, from a minute (<3 mm) mucosal defect or through normal surrounding mucosa (**Fig. 12.5**).[186] Diagnosis at the time of endoscopy can be difficult because there is no identifying lesion (ulcer) to indicate the source. The diagnosis rates for initial endoscopy range from 49% to 63%, and repeat endoscopy is often required.[182,187] In view of the intermittent nature of bleeding from Dieulafoy's lesion, which can span years, the sensitivity of endoscopic diagnosis is increased through early endoscopy in patients with acute GI bleeding.

Dieulafoy's lesion should be suspected in specific clinical situations. One clinical scenario involves a patient with repeated unexplained acute upper GI tract bleeding with repeatedly negative endoscopy. Another clinical scenario involves a patient who presents with a major acute bleed with the finding only of blood, fresh or altered in the stomach or duodenum. Repeat endoscopy timed as close as possible to a rebleeding event is crucial for the diagnosis. In a hospitalized patient in whom a gastric site of bleeding is suspected, a nasogastric tube can be useful to identify a rebleeding event promptly. EUS has been reported to identify Dieulafoy lesions successfully in this patient group and to guide therapy.

Endoscopic Therapy

Hemostasis and long-term ablation of the caliber persistent artery of Dieulafoy's lesion can be achieved by endoscopic treatment in more than 90% of patients.[183,184] Endoscopic therapy can be effective with most methods—injection or thermal probe monotherapy, mechanical devices, or

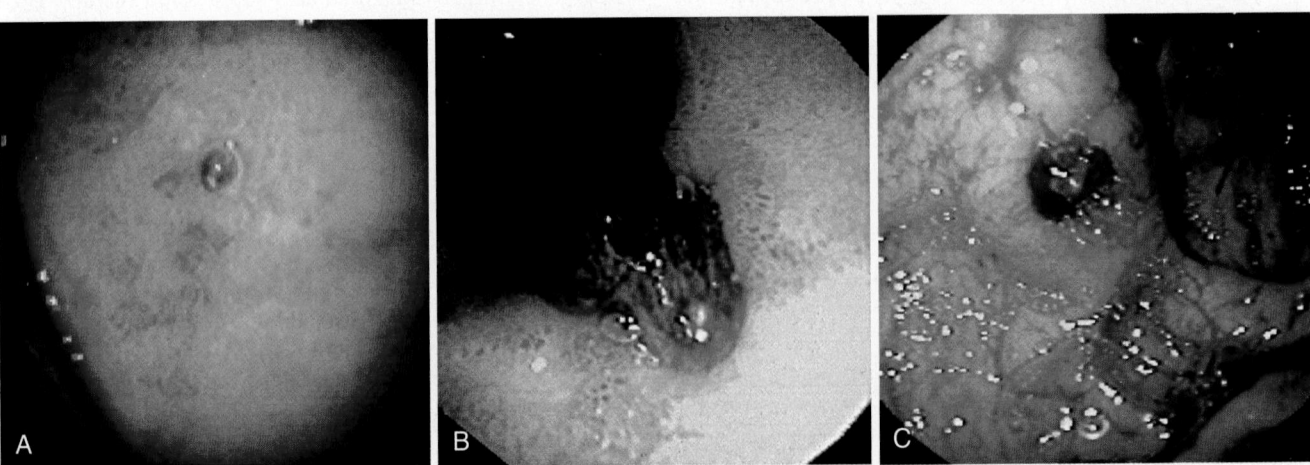

Fig. 12.5 Dieulafoy's gastric lesions. **A,** Lesion with thin rim of surrounding ulceration. **B,** Pale protruding artery with surrounding blood. **C,** Pale centrally protruding artery with surrounding mucosal defect.

combination treatment. Most data are from case series because randomized trials are difficult to perform secondary to the rarity of the condition. Therapy is directed at controlling bleeding and preventing rebleeding over the long-term. To accomplish this goal, the underlying caliber persistent artery must have its path altered. Although mechanical devices (clips) have been successful for controlling bleeding from acute events, it is uncertain that they would provide long-term benefit because this form of therapy is very superficial (mucosal).

Injection and Thermal Monotherapy

Multiple agents, including epinephrine, sclerosant, alcohol, hypertonic glucose, and cyanoacrylate glue, have been reported for successful injection therapy. Although there is a high initial success rate, there seems to be a high rate of rebleeding with injection monotherapy. Baettig and colleagues[184] treated 19 patients using injection therapy with epinephrine or polidocanol and had a rebleeding rate of 21%, whereas Kasapidis and colleagues[188] in their retrospective analysis reported a rebleeding rate of 55% in patients with Dieulafoy lesions treated with injection therapy using epinephrine, ethanolamine oleate (5%), or combination of the two.

Thermal probe monotherapy has been found to be effective, but variable success rates have been reported. Lin and coworkers[189] had 100% success in their six patients. Parra-Blanco and associates[190] had two of six patients with recurrent bleed after treatment with heater probe.

Combination Therapy

Combination therapy with injection followed by thermal probe coagulation seems to offer more secure hemostasis compared with monotherapy. Prior injection therapy with epinephrine may be a useful adjunct to slow or stop bleeding before targeted ablative therapy or before clot guillotine.

Stark and colleagues[191] presented the Mayo Clinic GI Bleeding Team data of 10 years on management of Dieulafoy's lesion. Dieulafoy's lesion was found in 19 of 1124 consecutive patients with upper GI bleeding. Patients (18 of 19) treated with combination therapy with epinephrine injection and thermal therapy (17 heater probe, 1 BICAP) had a 100% success rate of initial hemostasis, and only 1 patient had rebleeding in the follow-up period. In a review of 6 years of experience at a tertiary care center, 40 cases of Dieulafoy's lesion were identified with a 90% success rate of hemostasis with endoscopic therapy. Combination therapy with epinephrine injection and heater probe was used in most (28 of 40) patients. Rates of rebleeding were not specified, but only two patients required surgical intervention in the combined treatment group.[180] Kasapidis and colleagues[188] retrospectively compared injection therapy (epinephrine, ethanolamine) with thermal therapy alone or in combination with epinephrine injection. Initial hemostasis was achieved in all 18 patients. Five of nine patients had recurrent bleeding, whereas none of the patients in the other group (eight of nine had combined therapy; one of nine had heater probe only) had rebleeding.

Mechanical Devices

Among mechanical devices, hemoclip application and endoscopic rubber band ligation have been successfully used to

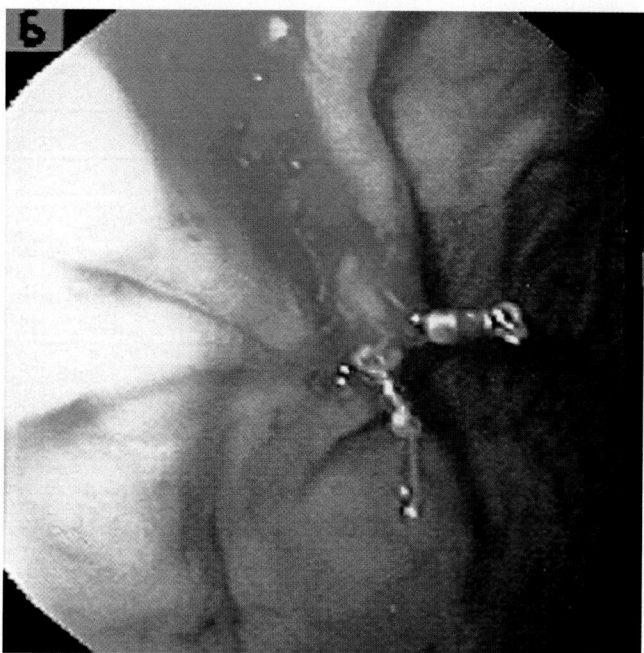

Fig. 12.6 Fundal Dieulafoy's lesion treated by clipping.

treat bleeding from Dieulafoy's lesion. The rationale of using mechanical devices is the small size of the lesion with normal surrounding tissue, which can be compressed along with the caliber persistent artery.

Hemoclip Application

Hemoclip application hemostasis has been used for Dieulafoy's lesion (**Fig. 12.6**) similar to other lesions. Yamaguchi and coworkers[192] used hemoclip application as first-choice hemostatic treatment for bleeding from Dieulafoy's lesion. Initial hemostasis was achieved in 94.1% of patients requiring 3.1 (mean, range 1 to 6) clips per patient. Rate of recurrent bleeding was 9.4%, which was successfully treated with repeat endoscopic therapy. None of the patients required surgery. Parra-Blanco and associates[190] used hemoclip application to control bleeding from Dieulafoy's lesion in 69% of their patients. Initial success rate was 97% (17 of 18) with a mean of 2.7 clips per patient.

In a randomized prospective trial, Chung and colleagues[193] compared mechanical methods (hemoclip and band ligation) with injection therapy with HSE (**Table 12.9**). Of 24 patients, 12 were assigned to mechanical therapy (9 hemoclip, 3 rubber band ligation), and 12 were assigned to the injection therapy group. Mechanical therapy was more effective than injection therapy in terms of initial hemostasis (91.7% vs. 75%), recurrent bleeding (8.3% vs. 33.3%, $P < .05$), and need for surgery (0% vs. 17%).

Endoscopic Rubber Band Ligation

Matsui and coworkers[196] compared endoscopic rubber band ligation with bipolar electrocoagulation in patients with acute GI hemorrhage exclusive of chronic gastroduodenal disease (**Fig. 12.7**). Endoscopic therapy was provided to 27 patients with Dieulafoy's lesion. Success rate of hemostasis was 100%

Table 12.9 Randomized Controlled Trials of Clipping for Dieulafoy Lesions						
Authors	**Treatment Modalities**	**No. Patients**	**Primary Hemostasis (%)**	**Rebleeding (%)**	**Rescue Therapy* (%)**	**Mortality (%)**
Chung et al (2000)[193]	Clipping	9	89	11	0	0
	Injection (HSE)	12	75	33	17	0
Park et al (2003)[194]	Clipping	16	94	0†	0	0
	Injection (epinephrine)	16	88	36†	13	0
Park et al. (2004)[195]	Clipping	13	100	8	0	0
	Band ligation	13	100	8	0	0

*Surgery or angiographic embolization.
†$P < .05$.
HSE, Hypertonic saline-epinephrine.
From Anastassiades CP, Baron TH, Wong Kee Song LM: Endoscopic clipping for the management of gastrointestinal bleeding. Nat Clin Pract Gastroenterol Hepatol 5:559–568, 2008.

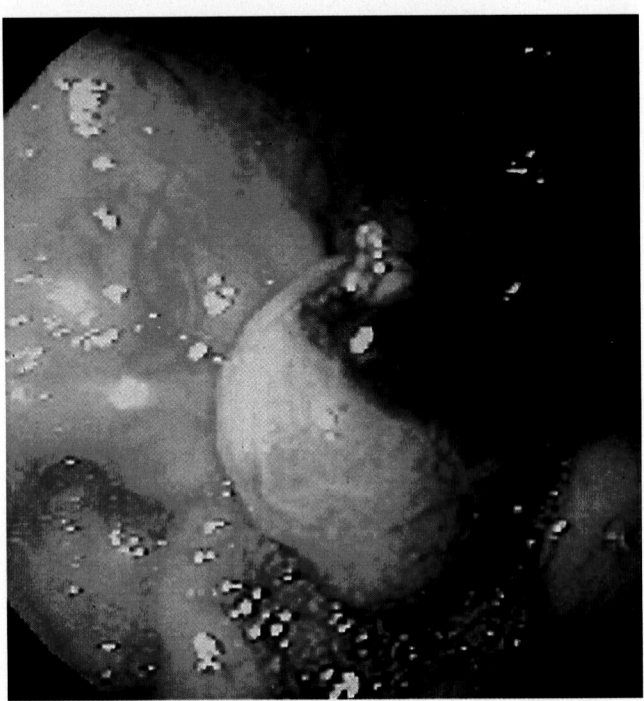

Fig. 12.7 Gastric Dieulafoy's lesion (from Fig. 12.5C) treated by band ligation. Note very prominent translucent protruding artery.

(13 of 13) for endoscopic band ligation versus 85.7% (12 of 14) for bipolar electrocoagulation. In a retrospective Veterans Affairs study, Mumtaz and colleagues[197] presented data of 23 patients with Dieulafoy's lesion treated with endoscopic band ligation (14 of 23) and injection with or without thermal therapy. Initial hemostasis was achieved in all patients in both groups, and only one patient had early rebleeding (within 72 hours) in both groups. Nikolaidis and associates[198] retrospectively reviewed the results of endoscopic band ligation in 23 patients with Dieulafoy's lesion. Initial hemostasis success rate was 96% (22 of 23). One patient with jejunal Dieulafoy's lesion required surgery for rebleeding.

Recurrent Bleeding

There is little evidence to support acid suppression therapy to prevent rebleeding from Dieulafoy's lesions. Because the underlying pathophysiology that causes the aberrantly located artery to bleed is unknown, long-term use cannot be justified. It is often administered either as empiric therapy for acute GI bleeding or to treat concurrent GI pathology. Short-term recurrent bleeding is common, occurring in 9% to 22% of cases.[182,184,186,187,189,199] In case of rebleeding, repeat endoscopic therapy is recommended to destroy the aberrant artery effectively because it is successful in most patients. The long-term rate of recurrent bleeding is low once Dieulafoy's lesion is completely treated. Studies have reported no recurrent bleeding with follow-up of up to 3 years after treatment[188,190]; however, repeat bleeding from the same site has been known to occur 6 years after the initial episode.[186]

Salvage Therapy

Despite a high success rate of endoscopic therapy, surgery may be required as salvage therapy in 3% to 16% of patients. Endoscopy is extremely important for localizing the lesion. Surgical oversewing of the vessel is associated with a higher risk of recurrent bleeding for reasons mentioned earlier. Wedge resection is more intuitive and is a better surgical procedure for these patients with refractory bleeding.[185,187] Angiography can be used not only to localize but also to embolize the bleeding vessel selectively. Variable success has been reported, and angiography should be reserved for patients who have failed endoscopic therapy and are poor candidates for surgical intervention. After the vessel site has been identified and bleeding has become refractory, EUS-guided ablative therapy may become the next and more ideal choice over angiography and surgery.

Mallory-Weiss Tear

Mallory-Weiss tears are a common cause of nonvariceal upper GI bleeding and account for 3% to 10% of cases.[200,201] A Mallory-Weiss tear was found by endoscopy in 7% of patients in the ASGE survey.[10] Mallory-Weiss tear is a mucosal laceration at the gastroesophageal junction or gastric cardia usually caused by retching or forceful vomiting. The underlying mechanism is thought to be rapid propulsion of gastric cardia into the thoracic cavity through the hiatus from retching or vomiting. If this is forceful enough, a longitudinal laceration can follow. Most patients with Mallory-Weiss tears are in their third to fifth decade, and there is a male preponderance in most case series.[200,201] Alcohol use is a common factor and is found in 40% to 70% of patients with Mallory-Weiss tear.[202–204] Many other factors have been associated with the development of Mallory-Weiss tears, including severe coughing, pregnancy, heavy lifting, straining, and colonic lavage using polyethylene glycol. Mallory-Weiss tears are well known, although uncommon complications of upper endoscopy.[205]

Risk Assessment

Few prospective data exist about clinical or endoscopic stigmata of recent hemorrhage and benefits of endoscopic hemostasis for bleeding Mallory-Weiss tears. Bharucha and colleagues[200] did a retrospective review of 56 patients presenting with acute GI bleeding to the Mayo Clinic GI Bleeding Team over a 4-year period. Clinical features and endoscopic findings were compared to determine prognostic factors for rebleeding and outcomes. Rebleeding, although unusual (7%), was significantly greater in patients with bleeding diathesis ($P = .02$); only active bleeding (not other stigmata) was associated with a higher transfusion requirement. The investigators concluded that GI bleed from a Mallory-Weiss tear without (1) clinical features of severe bleeding (hematochezia, hemodynamic instability), (2) coagulopathy or other major systemic disease, or (3) active bleeding at endoscopy can be managed with a brief period of observation.

Kortas and colleagues[202] did a retrospective analysis of 73 cases of Mallory-Weiss tear. The most common risk factor was alcohol use (40%). A complicated course was present in 17 (23%) patients. Among the factors studied, a complicated course was associated with a low hematocrit ($P = .009$) and active bleeding on initial endoscopy ($P = .013$).

Endoscopic Stigmata

Present data suggest that endoscopic stigmata that predict a high risk of rebleeding in peptic ulcer disease do not apply to Mallory-Weiss tears. Jensen and colleagues showed that less than 20% of patients with Mallory-Weiss tears with nonbleeding visible vessels or adherent clots had rebleeding with medical management. In the study by Chung and associates,[206] no recurrent bleed (0 of 40) was reported with medical management in patients with Mallory-Weiss bleed with a protruding vessel (23 patients) and adherent clot (17 patients). Bataller and coworkers[207] reported similar results where none (0 of 18) of the patients with an adherent clot had rebleeding in the medical management group. In view of current data, endoscopic therapy is recommended for active spurting and active oozing. Data do not show any benefit of endoscopic treatment of a visible vessel or an adherent clot in patients with Mallory-Weiss tear with an acute GI hemorrhage. Despite the above-described general experience, a Mallory-Weiss tear, if sufficiently deep, can compromise an esophageal branch from the left gastric artery, which would result in massive life-threatening bleeding. This is a very infrequent occurrence for which awareness is appropriate.

Endoscopic Therapy

Similar to other etiologies of GI bleeding, different endoscopic methods have been used to achieve hemostasis, including injection. Laine[208] showed that, compared with medical treatment, multipolar electrocoagulation is beneficial in achieving hemostasis, reducing emergency interventions and transfusion requirements in patients with major GI bleeding from a Mallory-Weiss tear.

Peng and colleagues[209] retrospectively compared data of 76 patients with Mallory-Weiss bleeding. Patients with visible vessel or fresh blood coating the tear were included. Isotonic saline–epinephrine injection (15 of 36) was compared with conservative management (21 of 36). The initial hemostasis rates (93% vs. 95%) and rebleeding rates (7% vs. 5%) were similar in the two groups. Llach and colleagues[210] showed injection sclerotherapy (epinephrine and polidocanol) to be superior to conservative management (rebleeding; 25.8% vs. 6.2%, $P < .05$) in patients with active bleeding or nonbleeding visible vessel with Mallory-Weiss tear.

Chung and associates[206] studied 76 patients with Mallory-Weiss tear in whom there was active bleeding, who contained a protruding vessel, or who had an adherent clot. The first 30 patients were randomly assigned to injection therapy with HSE ($n = 14$), hemoclipping, or band ligation. In the remaining 46 patients, lesions were irrigated with a 1 : 100,000 epinephrine solution until hemostasis occurred (medical management group). All patients received IV H_2 blockers. Rebleeding occurred in 1 of 6 patients with oozing in the medical management group and 3 of 15 patients in the endoscopic therapy group. All of these patients received injection therapy; no bleeding occurred with mechanical hemostasis (hemoclip, band ligation). The authors concluded that endoscopic therapy for Mallory-Weiss tear is unnecessary in patients without active bleeding, and mechanical hemostatic method is more effective than HSE injection.

Huang and colleagues[211] prospectively compared epinephrine injection therapy ($n = 17$ of 35) with endoscopic hemoclip application ($n = 18$ of 35) in patients with spurting vessels or active oozing from Mallory-Weiss tears (**Table 12.10**).[106] In each group, there was one case of recurrent bleeding that was successfully controlled by repeat endoscopic therapy. There were no procedure-related complications, and none of the patients required surgery. Cho and colleagues[212] found hemoclip placement and band ligation to be equally effective and safe for the management of active bleeding even in patients with shock or comorbid diseases.

Future Directions for Endoscopic Therapy

Doppler ultrasound may provide objective findings in patients with ulcer hemorrhage. Doppler signal correlates with rebleeding suggesting that it may be useful to continue endoscopic treatment until underlying signal of blood flow stops.[213,214] Interobserver disagreement in interpretation and its availability preclude wide use of Doppler ultrasound at present.

Table 12.10 Randomized Controlled Trials of Clipping for Mallory-Weiss Tears

Authors	Treatment Modalities	No. Patients	Primary Hemostasis (%)	Rebleeding (%)	Rescue Therapy* (%)	Mortality (%)
Huang et al (2002)[211]	Clipping	18	100	6	0	6
	Injection (epinephrine)	17	100	6	0	0
Chung et al (2002)[206]	Clipping or banding	16	100	0†	0	0
	Injection (HSE)	14	71	29†	0	0
Cho et al (2008)[212]	Clipping	21	100	4.9	0	0
	Banding	20	100	10	0	0

*Surgery or angiographic embolization.
†$P < .05$.
HSE, Hypertonic saline-epinephrine.
From Anastassiades CP, Baron TH, Wong Kee Song LM: Endoscopic clipping for the management of gastrointestinal bleeding. Nat Clin Pract Gastroenterol Hepatol 5:559–568, 2008.

EUS-guided therapy has been used in sporadic cases to control refractory bleeding.[165] EUS-guided therapy has the advantage because therapy is delivered under ultrasound guidance, and direct visualization may not be needed. Hemoclips are the only mechanical device available for widespread clinical use, but it is expected that development of natural orifice transendoscopic surgery will offer additional endoscopic suturing devices that eventually will be applicable to endoscopic therapy of nonvariceal bleeding.[215]

References

The complete reference list is available online at www.expertconsult.com.

Portal Hypertensive Bleeding

Charanjit Virk, Nayantara Coelho-Prabhu, and Navtej S. Buttar

Video related to this chapter's topics can
be found online at expertconsult.com.

Introduction

Portal hypertension is a clinical syndrome defined as an increase in portal venous pressure greater than 5 mm Hg.[1,2] It can arise from any condition interfering with the blood flow within the portal system. Among several complications of portal hypertension, including ascites, hepatic encephalopathy, and renal insufficiency, variceal hemorrhage is the most dramatic with a high mortality. Under physiologic conditions, collaterals exist between the portal venous system and the systemic venous circulation; in portal hypertension, these collaterals enlarge in an attempt to decompress the portal circulation and form varices. This chapter focuses on the gastrointestinal (GI) bleeding that results from portal hypertension; other complications of portal hypertension are reviewed separately.

Etiopathogenesis

The portal vein supplies about 1050 mL of blood into the liver sinusoids every minute. An additional 300 mL of blood is supplied by the hepatic artery with the total averaging around 1350 mL/min, which amounts to about 27% of the cardiac output. The liver receives fresh oxygenated blood from the hepatic artery and nutrient-rich blood from the stomach, spleen, and small and large intestine via the portal vein. Measuring approximately 8 cm in length, the portal vein is formed by the union of the superior mesenteric vein and splenic vein behind the neck of the pancreas. Immediately before reaching the liver, the portal vein divides into right and left branches. The right branch receives the cystic vein and enters the right lobe of the liver. The left branch receives the umbilical and paraumbilical veins, which can dilate to form caput medusae in cirrhosis. Blood from the hepatic artery and blood from the portal vein mix for the first time in the hepatic sinusoids. After mixing, the blood is drained from the lobule by the central vein, a branch of the hepatic vein. With this understanding, the portal system can be divided anatomically into presinusoidal, sinusoidal, and postsinusoidal. Portal hypertension can arise from any condition interfering with blood flow at any level within the portal venous system (**Table 13.1**).

Cirrhosis is the most common cause of portal hypertension in the Western world,[3,4] accounting for about 90% of cases; schistosomiasis is the leading cause in many developing countries. Other causes of portal hypertension include portal vein thrombosis, polycystic liver disease, nodular regenerative

Table 13.1 **Common Causes of Portal Hypertension**		
Prehepatic	**Hepatic**	**Posthepatic**
Portal vein thrombosis	Presinusoidal	Inferior vena cava obstruction
	NCPF	
	IPH	
	Sarcoidosis	
	Schistosomiasis	
	Nodular regenerative hyperplasia	
	Myeloproliferative disorders	
Splenic vein thrombosis	Sinusoidal	Cardiac failure
	Cirrhosis	
Hepatoportal arteriovenous fistula	Postsinusoidal	Constrictive pericarditis
	Budd-Chiari syndrome	
	Venoocclusive disease	
Splenomegaly		

IPH, Idiopathic portal hypertension; NCPF, noncirrhotic portal fibrosis.

hyperplasia of the liver, congenital hepatic fibrosis, myeloproliferative disorders, hepatic sarcoidosis, and hereditary hemorrhagic telangiectasia. The primary factors influencing increased pressure in the portal hepatic system are resistance and flow. In cirrhosis, both resistance and flow are altered. Increased portal venous resistance is central to the development of portal hypertension in cirrhosis. This increased resistance can be attributed to two specific factors. The first is mechanical obstruction to flow secondary to fibrotic disruption of the liver architecture and regenerative nodules. The second factor is a dynamic component produced by active contraction of vascular smooth muscles and activated stellate cells, believed to be due to a relative deficiency of nitric oxide (vasodilator),[5,6] and high levels of endothelin-1 (vasoconstrictor) leading to increased sinusoidal resistance.[7-9] Also, cirrhosis results in a hyperdynamic circulatory state that is characterized by peripheral and splanchnic vasodilation, reduced mean arterial pressure, and increased cardiac output. Nitric oxide–mediated splanchnic vasodilation[8-16] produces an increase in inflow of systemic blood into the portal circulation, which causes an increase in portal pressure.[10,11]

The correlation between collateral blood flow and the transmural pressure gradient in the varix is expressed as: $P1 - P2 = Q \times R$, where $P1$ and $P2$ are the pressures within and outside the varix, Q is the blood flow per unit of time, and R is the resistance to flow through the varix. Poiseuille's formula states that the resistance to flow may be expressed as follows: $R = 8 \; nl/p \; r4$, where n is blood viscosity, l is length, and r is radius of the vessel. The transmural pressure and radius of the varix along with the mural thickness of the varix (w) determines the wall tension of the varix according to the law of Laplace: Wall tension = $Q \times (8 \; nl/p \; r4) \times r/w$. The propensity for a varix to bleed is directly linked to its wall tension. Theoretically, large long varices with thin walls and high rates of flow are most prone to bleed. Decreasing collateral flow (by decreasing portal pressure) should decrease the risk of variceal rupture.[12,13]

Clinical Presentation

Portal hypertension should be suspected in all patients with GI bleeding in conjunction with signs of liver disease, such as ascites, jaundice, spider angiomata, gynecomastia, palmar erythema, testicular atrophy, and splenomegaly. Variceal bleeding classically manifests as effortless and recurrent hematemesis with or without dark red stools (melena). In the stomach, portal hypertension may manifest as portal hypertensive gastropathy (PHG)[14,15] or gastric antral vascular ectasia (GAVE).[16,17] Bleeding from either of these two conditions is usually more indolent and chronic (**Fig. 13.1**).

Variceal bleeding is usually associated with systemic effects including hypotension, shock, new onset of spontaneous bacterial peritonitis, or worsening encephalopathy. Spontaneous bacterial peritonitis after variceal bleeding is believed to be secondary to translocation of bacteria across the compromised mucosae.[18,19] Patients with spontaneous bacterial peritonitis who were not given antibiotics had a high failure to control bleeding and higher rates of rebleeding.[20] Also, in patients with ascites, infections may induce acute impairment in systemic circulatory function and hepatorenal syndrome. It is proposed that endotoxins released during bacterial infection result in an increase in portal pressure through the introduction of endothelin (a potent substance for contraction of the stellate cells), vasoconstrictive cyclooxygenase products, and contraction of hepatic stellate cells. Endotoxin-induced nitric oxide and endothelin-induced prostacyclin could inhibit platelet aggregation and reduce hemostasis at the level of the varix. Hepatic encephalopathy, which is a serious and potentially reversible disorder and known to be associated with advanced liver failure, can also be exacerbated by portal hypertension–associated GI bleeding. GI bleeding and consequent cerebral adaptation to gut-derived neurotoxins is one possible explanation. Increased levels of ammonia and mercaptans by the intestinal bacteria lead to impaired neural function secondary to cellular swelling and depletion of glutamate.

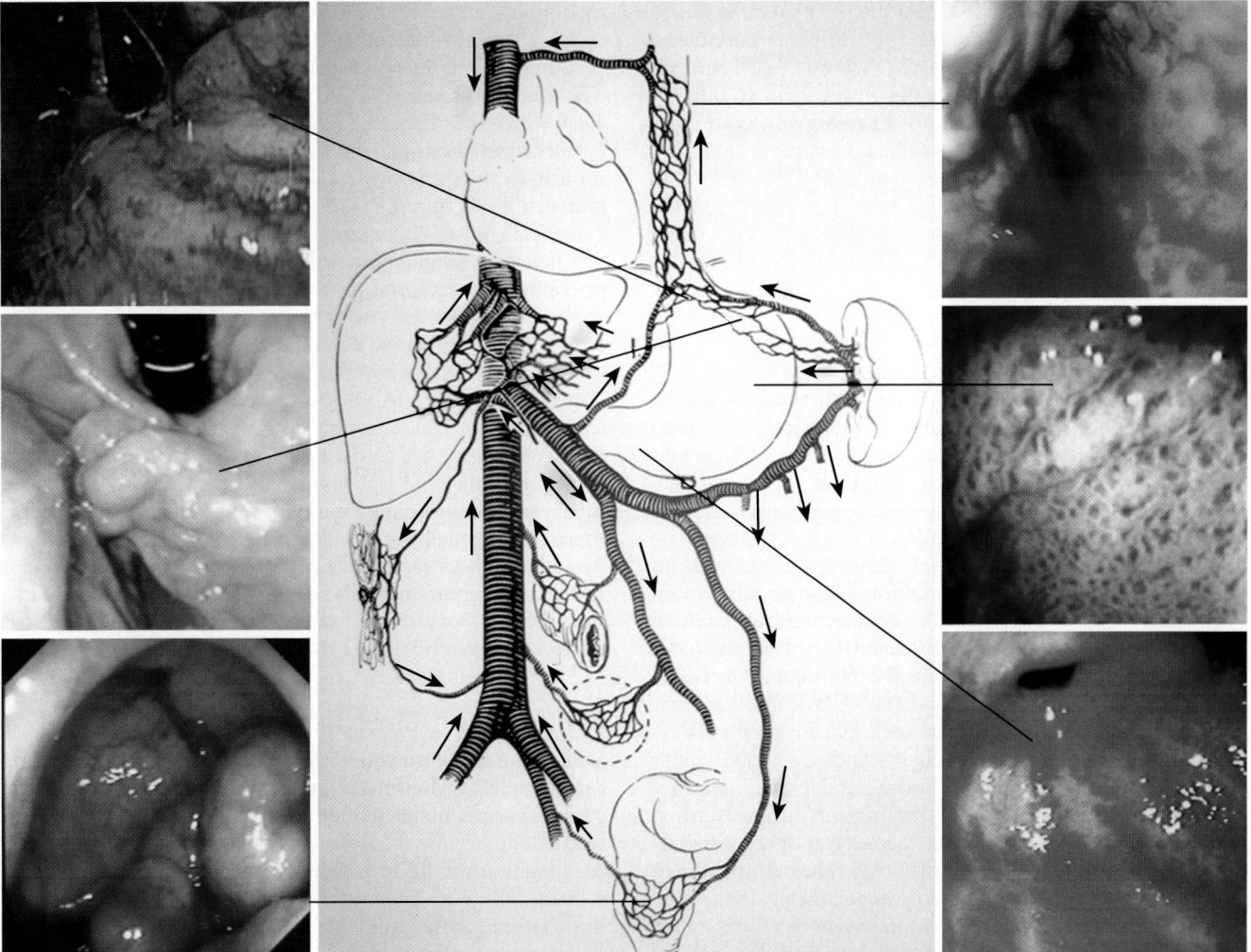

Fig. 13.1 Anatomic localization of portal hypertension–related gastrointestinal bleeding: Esophageal varices *(right upper panel)*, cardia varices *(left upper panel)*, fundic varix *(left middle panel)*, colonic varix *(left lower panel)*, portal hypertensive gastropathy and gastric antral vascular ectasia *(right middle and lower panels)*.

Diagnosis

The mainstay of diagnosis for varices is esophago-gastroduodenoscopy (EGD); however, several invasive and noninvasive methods can help predict the risk of bleeding from varices.

Endoscopy

EGD is the most effective method for screening and surveillance of portal hypertension in patients with cirrhosis.[21] The distal esophagus is the most common location for varices; however, varices can also develop in the stomach and small and large intestine.[2,22] Esophageal varices occur in about 50% of all patients with cirrhosis. Gastric varices are found in approximately one of five patients with portal hypertension. About 5% to 10% of patients with gastric varices may not have esophageal varices.[23] Although endoscopic evaluation of small or large bowel is not recommended in patients who are suspected to have portal hypertension (unless symptoms warrant), varices could be encountered in the small or large intestine (see **Fig. 13.1**).

Although EGD is recommended for all patients with a new diagnosis of cirrhosis to screen for varices, the procedure is costly, may be unpleasant, and has potential risk for complications. EGD is often performed under sedation,[24–26] which includes its own cost and complications that may be more severe in patients with cirrhosis. Unsedated EGD performed with small-diameter endoscopes is being evaluated as an alternative to conventional endoscopy to avoid the direct and indirect costs of conscious sedation.[27,28]

Hepatic Vein Pressure Gradient

The hepatic vein pressure gradient (HVPG) is more invasive but is an accurate tool to measure portal hypertension. Portal venous pressure can be measured either directly by portal venography or indirectly by HVPG. HVPG is the difference between the wedged hepatic venous pressure (a measure of portal venous pressure) and the free hepatic vein pressure.[29,30] In acute variceal bleeding, the measurement of HVPG provides prognostic information and identifies difficult-to-treat patients. In patients with acute variceal bleeding, HVPG of 20 mm Hg or greater measured soon after admission was associated with a significantly longer intensive care unit (ICU) stay, longer hospital stay, greater transfusion requirements, and worse short-term and long-term survival (1-year mortality 64% vs. 20%; $P > .002$).[31] HVPG greater than 10 mm Hg is a good predictor of the development of varices. A threshold value of 12 mm Hg has been identified for variceal rupture.[32] In cirrhotic patients with portal hypertension, the reduction of HVPG to less than 12 mm Hg or by 20% or more of the baseline value significantly reduces the risk of bleeding. Most importantly, a reduction of HVPG 20% or greater of baseline reduces the risk of death.[33,34]

Other Methods

Several methods have been proposed as alternatives to conventional EGD or HVPG for noninvasive diagnosis of esophageal varices,[35] including platelet count-to-spleen diameter ratio, Fibrotest, and Fibroscan. Multidetector computed tomography (CT) esophagography and esophageal capsule endoscopy are considered minimally invasive. Transient elastography (Fibroscan) is a novel noninvasive method for assessing liver stiffness and is useful for diagnosis of advanced fibrosis and portal hypertension. Transient elastography is painless, rapid, and easy to perform at the bedside or in the outpatient setting. Results are expressed in kilopascals (kPa), and values range from 2.5 to 75 kPa.[36] A study assessed the correlation between liver stiffness with Fibroscan and HVPG in diagnosing significant portal hypertension in 150 patients who underwent a liver biopsy and hemodynamic measurements.[37] In patients with significant portal hypertension (HVPG >10 mm Hg), area under the receiver operating characteristic curves for Fibroscan was 0.945. The cutoff value of 21 kPa accurately predicted significant portal hypertension in 92% of patients for whom measurements were successful. Larger studies are needed to define precisely the role of Fibroscan in the diagnosis of portal hypertension.

Esophageal capsule endoscopy is a practical, safe, well-tolerated, and accurate method for the diagnosis of esophageal varices.[38] However, interpretation of esophageal capsule endoscopy can be compromised by the presence of secretions or bubbles, and it does not detect gastric varices. An unpredictable transit time and poor interobserver agreement could account for a significant rate of failure (6% in some studies). The use of multidetector CT esophagography to grade esophageal varices has been evaluated more recently.[39,40] The esophagus is insufflated with air via a catheter passed through the mouth. In the study by Kim and associates[39] that included 90 patients with cirrhosis, 30 patients had large esophageal varices. CT scan performance for the diagnosis of large varices was 0.931 to 0.958 (estimated by the area under the receiver operating characteristic). Perri and colleagues[40] prospectively evaluated 102 patients who underwent both CT and endoscopic screening for gastroesophageal varices. CT was found to have approximately 90% sensitivity for the identification of large esophageal varices but only about 50% specificity. The sensitivity of CT in detecting gastric varices was 87%.

Gastric varices are harder to detect by endoscopy, especially if they are small and isolated. Small varices in the fundus are often mistaken for a mucosal fold. Their identity as varices is based on their shape (grapelike clusters) and their bluish tinge. At endoscopic ultrasound (EUS), they can be seen as circular or linear anechoic channels within the gastric wall. The addition of color Doppler or through the scope Doppler probe can differentiate gastric varices from mucosal folds.[41]

Grading and Classification of Varices

Varices are easily diagnosed by upper GI endoscopy and are categorized by their location into esophageal and gastric varices. Varices are most often seen in the distal esophagus and may extend beyond the Z line into the gastric cardia. The distal esophagus must be insufflated with air while assessing the variceal size. The most recent guidelines by the American Association for the Study of Liver Diseases (AASLD) recommend classifying esophageal varices as either small (<5 mm) or large (>5 mm) (**Fig. 13.2**).[42]

Esophageal varices can also be graded using several classifications for documentation and research purposes.[43–45] According to Conn,[43] the number of varices is graded as follows: 1+, a single varix; 2+, two to three varices; 3+, four to

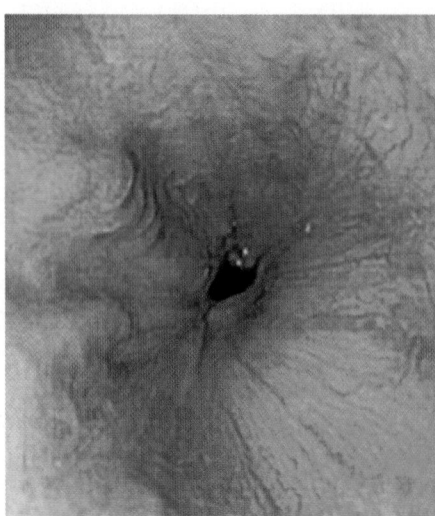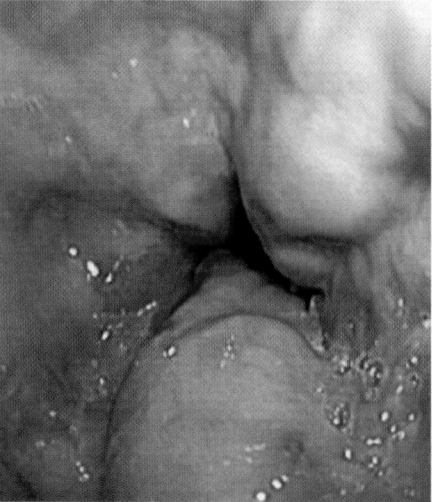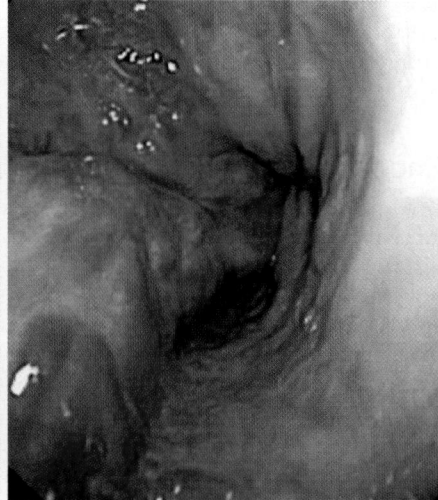

Fig. 13.2 Classification of esophageal varices: Small esophageal varices without red signs *(left panel)*, large varices without red signs *(middle panel)*, and large varices with red signs *(right panel)*.

Classification of GV

Based on location

Gastroesophageal varices (GOV)

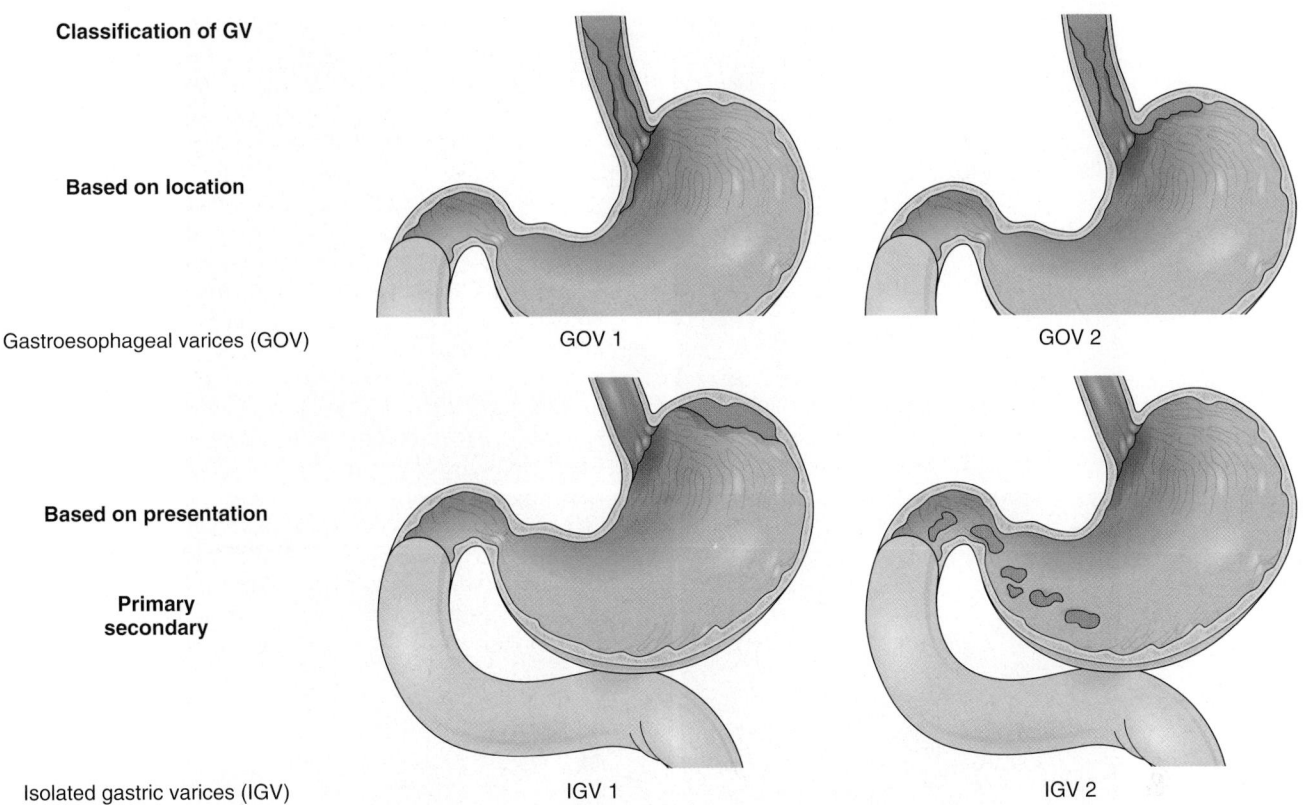

GOV 1   GOV 2

Based on presentation

Primary
secondary

Isolated gastric varices (IGV)

IGV 1   IGV 2

Fig. 13.3 Gastric varices are classified based on location and presentation.

six varices; and 4+, more than six varices. The size of the varices is graded as follows: 1+, small varices detectable only on performing Valsalva maneuver; 2+, small varices (approximately 1 to 3 mm in diameter) visible without Valsalva maneuver; 3+, varices of moderate size (3 to 6 mm in diameter); and 4+, large varices (>6 mm). Extent of esophageal involvement is graded as follows: 1+, terminal 3 cm; 2+, terminal 6 cm; 3+, terminal 9 cm; and 4+, involving more than the terminal 9 cm.

The Japanese Research Society for Portal Hypertension criteria evaluate the following endoscopic signs:

1. *Fundamental color of varices:* Divided into white (Cw) and blue (Cb) color
2. *Red color signs:* Dilated small vessels or microtelangiectasia on the variceal surface subdivided into cherry red spot, red wale marking, and hematocystic spot; depending on the number and the extent of distribution, each of these three red color signs is graded as absent (−), 1+, or 2+
3. *Form of varices:* Small straight varices (F1), enlarged tortuous varices occupying less than one-third of the esophageal lumen (F2), and largest sized coil-shaped varices occupying more than one-third of the esophageal lumen (F3)
4. *Location:* Longitudinal extent of varices—located in the lower third of the esophagus, locus inferior (Li); varices extending up to the tracheal bifurcation, locus medialis (Lm); and varices that extend beyond the tracheal bifurcation, locus superior (Ls).

Certain types of varices are more likely to appear depending on the cause of portal hypertension. Isolated gastric varices

located on the fundus (IGV1) classically occur in association with splenic vein thrombosis. Duodenal and biliary varices can occur more often with extrahepatic causes of portal hypertension.[46] A simple classification of gastric varices depending on their anatomic location in the stomach can also help in understanding their natural history and approach to management.[47] Gastroesophageal varices are located in the esophagus and extend in continuity to the lesser curve (GOV1) or greater curve (GOV2) of the stomach. Isolated gastric varices are located usually on the fundus (IGV1) or greater curve or other sites in the stomach or first part of duodenum (IGV2) (**Fig. 13.3**). In more recent publications as well as in our own experience, the use of a through the scope Doppler probe not only facilitates the diagnosis, but it also confirms successful therapy of gastric varices (**Fig. 13.4**).[41]

Predictors of Variceal Bleed

The North Italian Endoscopic Club uses the extent of liver disease, large variceal size, and the presence of red color signs on endoscopy as an index for the likelihood of first variceal bleeding.[48] Of the above-mentioned indicators, variceal size seems to be the most important predictor of first variceal bleeding. The probability of variceal bleeding is significantly greater in patients with larger esophageal varices ($P = .0001$), with more severe red wale marks ($P = .0001$), or with more severe liver dysfunction according to the Child-Pugh classification ($P = .007$).[49] However, because only one-third of patients who present with variceal hemorrhage have the previously mentioned risk factors, a better definition of predictive factors is needed.

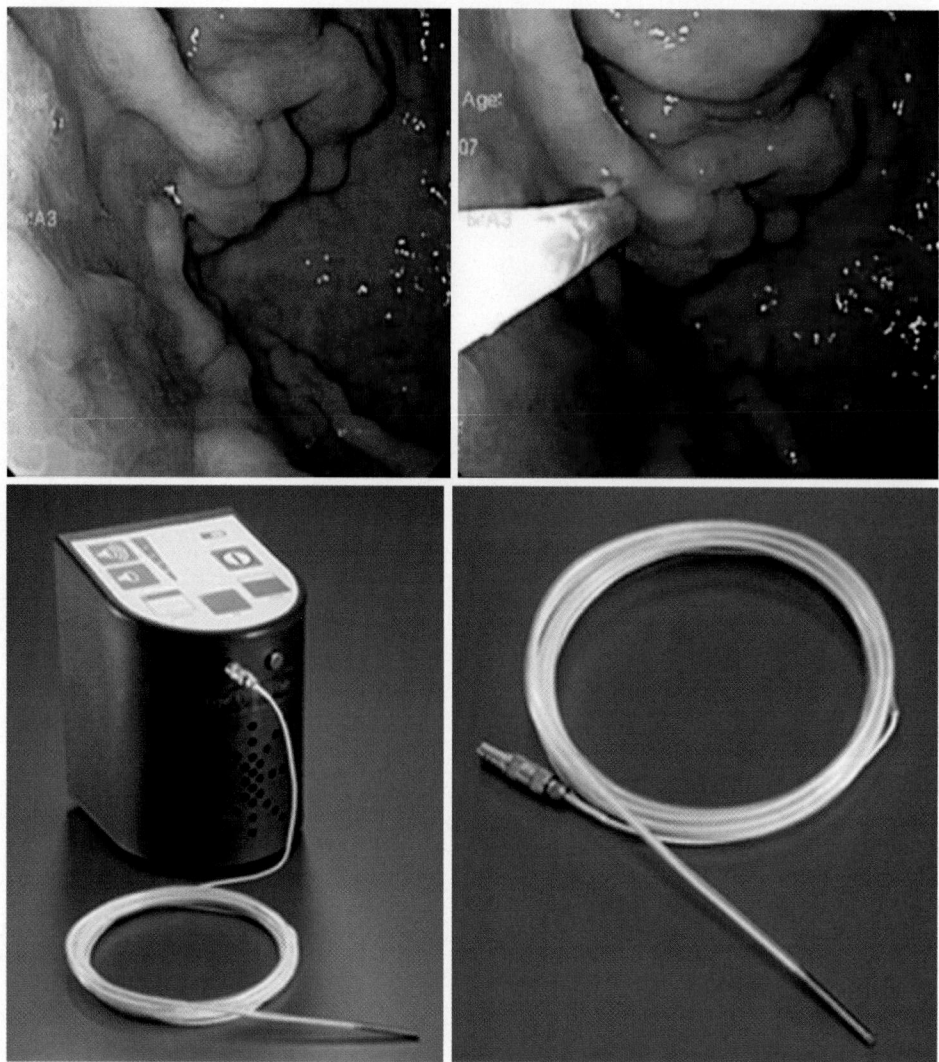

Fig. 13.4 Differentiation between gastric folds and varices. Using a VTI Doppler (Vascular Technology, Nashua, NH) that has a through the scope disposable probe, gastric varices can be differentiated from a gastric fold. Blood flow in the gastric varices gives a distinct sound that resembles high-speed wind.

Sarin and Kumar[47] examined 12 clinical, endoscopic, and hemodynamic variables in 126 patients with portal hypertension (72 bleeders and 54 nonbleeders). The variceal size and intravariceal pressures were the most important predictors of hemorrhage. In another study, the risk of bleeding was 0% when the variceal pressure was 13 mm Hg or less, 9% when the variceal pressure was 13 to 14 mm Hg, 17% when the variceal pressure was 14 to 15 mm Hg, 50% when the variceal pressure was 15 to 16 mm Hg, and 72% when the variceal pressure was greater than 16 mm Hg.[50]

HVPG is a measure of portal pressure and intravariceal pressure in patients with cirrhosis. Garcia-Tsao and colleagues[32] found that HVPG was significantly greater in 49 patients who had bled from esophageal varices than in 44 patients with cirrhosis who did not bleed (20.4 ± 5.1 mm Hg vs. 16.0 ± 5.2 mm Hg). They also found that none of the patients who had bled had HVPG less than 12 mm Hg. In one study, the portocaval pressure gradient decreased after transjugular intrahepatic portosystemic shunt (TIPS) procedure (from 19.7 ± 4.6 mm Hg to 8.6 ± 2.7 mm Hg), and a subsequent increase in pressure greater than 12 mm Hg (18.4 ± 7.46 mm Hg) was associated with rebleeding.[51] Moitinho and coworkers[31] reported that patients admitted because of variceal bleeding who had HVPG greater than 20 mm Hg measured within 48 hours had a fivefold increased risk of (1) failure to control bleeding with the emergency treatment or (2) experiencing early rebleeding. Dynamic measurements of HVPG are more valuable to assess the influence of therapeutic interventions or alcohol abstinence. Active bleeding at endoscopy was statistically shown to be an independent risk factor in predicting failure to control variceal bleeding.[52]

Natural History of Varices

Gastroesophageal varices are the most significant portosystemic collaterals because their rupture results in variceal hemorrhage, the most common lethal complication of cirrhosis.[53] The prevalence and rate of growth of varices in cirrhotics are often related to the severity of liver disease. All patients should be screened for varices at the time of diagnosis of cirrhosis.

Patients who have no varices on screening endoscopy should be rescreened every 2 to 3 years if their liver function is stable or earlier if there are signs of hepatic decompensation. Patients who have small varices on screening endoscopy should be rescreened every 1 to 2 years because the development of large varices is greater in patients with small varices on initial endoscopy compared with patients with no varices.[42]

About one-third of patients with varices experience a variceal hemorrhage. The 2-year bleeding risk in patients with cirrhosis and moderate to large varices is 25% to 30%. Lifelong risk of variceal bleeding is almost 50%.[54] In portal vein obstruction, the bleeding rate is even higher. After varices start bleeding, hemorrhage spontaneously stops in only 50% of cases. Patient's with Child C cirrhosis and actively spurting varices are particularly likely to continue to bleed without active intervention. After cessation of active bleeding, the risk of rebleeding is higher for approximately 6 weeks. The risk of early rebleeding is greatest within the first 48 hours, and about half of all early rebleeding episodes occur during this time. Risk factors for early rebleeding include large varices, age older than 60 years, severity of initial bleed, renal failure, ascites, active bleeding on endoscopy, and red wale marks (defined as longitudinal dilated venules resembling whip marks on the variceal surface). Aggressive volume replacement may exacerbate portal hypertension and precipitate early rebleeding.

Of patients who bleed from esophageal varices, the variceal hemorrhage is fatal in roughly 20% of patients. The incidence of new varices is approximately 5% to 15% per year, depending on the Child-Turcotte-Pugh class[1] and the etiology of the liver disease.[2,22] The risk of gastric variceal bleeding is lower than the risk of esophageal variceal bleeding, but gastric variceal bleeding, especially fundal varices, tends to be more severe, to require more transfusions, and to have a higher rate of mortality.[23] Gastric variceal bleeding has been reported to account for 3% to 30% of all acute variceal bleeding episodes. The risk of bleeding from gastric varices depends on the location. Although GOV1 constitute more than 70% of gastric varices, only 11% of GOV1 ever bleed. In contrast, although IGV1 constitute less than 8% of all gastric varices, 80% of IGV1 bleed.[19] IGV1 are often fed by spontaneous large collaterals that partly decompress the portal vein, and IGV1 are associated with lower portal pressures than esophageal varices. IGV2 are rare (4.7% of all gastric varices); commonly seen in antrum (53%), duodenum (32%), or at both sites (11%); and rarely in body and fundus (4%). Overall, gastric varices bleed less often but more severely than esophageal varices.[55]

Management

Major progress has occurred in endoscopic, surgical, radiologic, and pharmacologic treatments for GI bleeding resulting from portal hypertension. Management varies depending on the presentation of the patient and the disease stage.

Endoscopic and Pharmacologic Therapy

Endoscopic or pharmacologic interventions can be used to prevent the first variceal bleeding (primary prophylaxis), to manage the acute episode of bleeding, or to prevent recurrent bleeding (secondary prophylaxis). Although endoscopic

variceal ligation (EVL) is the most commonly used endoscopic approach, sclerotherapy and thermal and mechanical modalities are also reported as management options. Pharmacotherapy is mainly directed toward the reduction of portal pressure.

Primary Prophylaxis to Prevent Esophageal Variceal Bleeding

Primary prophylaxis of variceal bleeding or prevention of the first episode of variceal hemorrhage is the most logical approach to decrease morbidity and mortality after a variceal bleed. Because only about 10% to 20% of patients bleed, it is essential to select carefully patients who are at a high risk of variceal hemorrhage. In patients without varices, nonselective β blockers were proposed with the aim of preventing the development of varices.[56] In a large multicenter study, 213 cirrhotic patients with portal hypertension (HVPG >5 mm Hg) but without varices were randomly assigned to receive timolol or placebo in double-blind conditions for a median of 55 months.[57] The rate of the development of esophageal varices did not differ between the two groups, and the timolol group reported more adverse events. These results do not support the universal use of β blockers in cirrhotics without varices. In patients with no varices on endoscopy, there is no indication for treatment to prevent the formation of varices.

Patients who have varices may benefit from the interventions directed toward prevention of first bleeding. Endoscopic sclerotherapy, which is not commonly used at the present time, was compared with no treatment in 20 randomized trials that included 1756 patients, most of whom had medium-sized or large-sized varices. In the sclerotherapy group, there was a significant reduction in bleeding in 5 trials, increase in bleeding in 2 trials, and no difference in 13 trials.[58] Because of significant heterogeneity in the results with regard to bleeding and mortality among the different trials, prophylactic sclerotherapy is not recommended for primary prophylaxis.[59,60] In patients who have small varices that have not bled, β blockers can be used to prevent the progression of varices and bleeding. A meta-analysis evaluating nonselective β blockers in the prevention of first variceal bleed investigated the results of three trials that included patients with small varices.[61] The group receiving β blockers showed a reduction in the incidence of first variceal hemorrhage (2% over 2 years) compared with the nontreated group (7% over 2 years), but the reduction was not statistically significant.

Prophylaxis is important in patients who are considered at high risk for bleeding because of advanced liver disease and the presence of red wale marks on varices.[21] Regarding patients with medium to large varices, a meta-analysis of 11 trials comprising 1189 patients evaluated nonselective β blockers (i.e., propranolol, nadolol) versus placebo in the prevention of first variceal bleeding and showed that the risk of bleeding was significantly reduced by β blockers (30% in control vs. 14% in β blocker group). This meta-analysis indicates that one bleeding episode is avoided for every 10 patients treated. More importantly, mortality was lower in the β blocker group compared with the control group, and this difference has been shown to be statistically significant.[62] β blockers might not be tolerated by all patients, and there might be some contraindications, such as in patients with asthma, insulin-dependent diabetes, and peripheral vascular disease. The most common

Table 13.2 Endoscopic Variceal Ligation (EVL) versus No Treatment for Prevention of First Bleeding from Esophageal Varices

Reference	Therapy	No.	Eradication (%)	Variceal Bleeding (%)	Recurrence (%)	Mortality (%)
Sarin et al (1996)[63]	Control	33	—	39.4	—	24.2
	EVL	35	96	8.6	29	11.4
Lay et al (1997)[64]	Control	64	—	60	—	58
	EVL	62	60	19	42	28
Triantos et al (2005)[65]	Control	27	—	7	—	40
	EVL	25	—	20	—	28

Table 13.3 Primary Prophylaxis of Bleeding from Esophageal Varices

Reference	Therapy	No.	Variceal Bleeding (%)	Mortality (%)
Sarin et al (1999)[66]	Propranolol	44	43	11
	EVL	45	15	11.1
Lui et al (2002)[62]	Propranolol	66	9	21
	ISMN	62	19	19
	EVL	44	6.8	25
Lo et al (2000)[107]	EVL + propranolol + sucralfate	60	12	16
	EVL	62	29	32
Sarin et al (2005)[68]	EVL + propranolol	72	7	8
	EVL	72	11	15
Tripathi et al (2009)[67]	Carvedilol	77	10	35
	EVL	75	23	37

EVL, Endoscopic variceal ligation; ISMN, isosorbide mononitrate.

side effects in cirrhotics are lightheadedness, fatigue, and shortness of breath.

In the last 2 decades, EVL has essentially replaced sclerotherapy as a mode of variceal eradication, and it has been evaluated for preventing the first bleed from esophageal varices. In a series of 68 patients, Sarin and coworkers[63] showed the superiority of EVL compared with no therapy to prevent first variceal bleed (**Table 13.2**). Their results were subsequently confirmed by Lay and colleagues,[64] who found significant reduction in the incidence (19% vs. 60%) and mortality (28% vs. 58%) of first bleed when EVL was compared with no therapy. In contrast to these reports, a more recent study showed no benefit of EVL; however, the patients included in this study were either intolerant to or had contraindication for the use of β blockers.[65]

After the initial encouraging reports, it was logical to assess whether EVL is comparable to the current therapy for primary prophylaxis—β blocker therapy. Sarin and coworkers[66] randomly assigned 89 patients with high-risk varices to receive EVL or propranolol. The actuarial probability of bleeding at 18 months was significantly lower in the EVL group (15.8%) compared with the propranolol group (43%). There was no survival benefit with EVL, however. Lui and colleagues[62] assigned 172 patients to EVL (*n* = 44), propranolol (*n* = 66), or isosorbide mononitrate (ISMN) (*n* = 62) therapy (**Table 13.3**). On intention-to-treat analysis, variceal bleeding was

observed in 7% of patients randomly assigned to EVL, 14% of patients randomly assigned to propranolol, and 23% of patients randomly assigned to ISMN; the difference between EVL and nitrates was significant. A significant number of patients reported side effects with drug treatments (45% propranolol and 42% ISMN vs. 2% EVL), resulting in withdrawal from treatment in 30% of patients receiving propranolol and 21% of patients receiving ISMN. There was no significant difference in mortality rates in the three groups.

A more recent randomized controlled trial found carvedilol to be more effective in preventing first variceal bleed than EVL in patients with high-risk esophageal varices.[67] Sarin and coworkers[68] noted that although addition of propranolol to EVL does not decrease the probability of first bleed or death, the recurrence of varices is lower if propranolol is added to EVL. Several meta-analyses have been performed comparing EVL with β blockers.[69-71] The meta-analysis performed by Imperiale and Chalasani[69] included five trials with 601 patients. Khuroo and associates[70] included eight trials comprising 596 patients. More recently, Gluud and coworkers[71] performed a meta-analysis of 15 randomized controlled trials comprising 1174 patients. Imperiale and Chalasani[69] and Khuroo and associates[70] concluded that in patients with large varices that are high risk for bleeding, EVL decreases bleeding episodes; however, there was no reduction effect on mortality. Gluud and coworkers[71] noted that the positive effects associated with the EVL group were more commonly seen in the trials that had shorter follow-up.

There are several distinct advantages of EVL over β blockers, as follows:

1. There are no contraindications (unless endoscopy is contraindicated).
2. The required therapy of 3 to 4 weeks is of short duration, so there is improved compliance.
3. There is no need to measure hemodynamic parameters to assess 25% reduction in HVPG after drug therapy; in EVL, the achievable endpoint, the variceal eradication, is visible endoscopically.
4. There is no need for indefinite therapy. It has been shown that patients who are on long-term propranolol therapy do not fare well on stopping the drug; the rebleeding rate becomes the same as before starting the drug with higher mortality.

Teran and colleagues[72] examined the cost-effectiveness of various treatments in primary prophylaxis of variceal bleeding. They found that β blockers were more cost-effective than sclerotherapy or shunt surgery in patients with cirrhosis with a cost savings between $440 and $1460. The other treatments were not cost-effective. Spiegel and coworkers found empiric β blocker therapy for primary prophylaxis of variceal hemorrhage to be a cost-effective measure because the use of screening endoscopy to guide therapy adds significant cost with only marginal increase in effectiveness.

The Baveno IV consensus recommended that nonselective β blockers should be considered as first-choice treatment to prevent first variceal bleeding in patients with high-risk varices, and EVL should be offered to patients with contraindications or intolerance to β blockers.[21] HVPG can also be monitored while receiving treatment with a β blocker. If HVPG is reduced by 25% or more or the gradient is less than 12 mm Hg after 4 to 6 weeks of therapy, the drug should be continued. A more noninvasive method of measuring efficacy of β blockers is by noting a decrease in the patient's pulse rate. AASLD and American College of Gastroenterology also consider β blockers as first choice in patients with medium to large varices that have not bled and are not high risk. In patients with high-risk varices, the combination of EVL and β blockers is considered first-choice therapy.

Management of Active Esophageal Variceal Bleeding

Active bleeding has been defined by the Baveno II Consensus Workshop as oozing or spurting at the time of endoscopy. Clinically significant bleeding is defined as bleeding with a transfusion requirement of 2 or more units of blood within 24 hours of time zero, together with a systolic blood pressure less than 100 mm Hg or a postural change of greater than 20 mm Hg or pulse rate greater than 100 beats/min at time zero.[73]

RESUSCITATION

The mortality rate from active variceal bleeding has declined because of improved diagnosis and treatment. Patients with bleeding esophageal varices should be admitted to the ICU for

resuscitation and management. Airway protection should be provided without delay to prevent aspiration of blood before endoscopy. The patient should receive prompt blood volume restitution using crystalloids and blood transfusion with the goals of maintaining hemodynamic stability. Conversely, vigorous resuscitation should be avoided because it can precipitate recurrent variceal hemorrhage. Packed red blood cells should be used to keep the target hemoglobin at approximately 8 g/dL.

PHARMACOTHERAPY

The advantage of pharmacotherapy is that it is generally applicable and can be administered as soon as the diagnosis of variceal hemorrhage is suspected. Vasoactive therapy should be initiated before diagnostic EGD. Several vasoactive agents have been evaluated extensively. Vasopressin and its analogue terlipressin and somatostatin and its analogues octreotide, lanreotide, and vapreotide have been studied. β blockers should not be used in the acute setting because they decrease blood pressure and blunt a physiologic increase in heart rate associated with bleeding. The use of vasoactive drugs alone in acute variceal bleeding has not proved to be more effective than endoscopic treatment. Adding octreotide to EVL in patients with acute variceal bleeding was beneficial in one study but not in another.[74,75] A meta-analysis of 15 trials comparing emergency sclerotherapy and pharmacologic treatment (vasopressin with or without nitroglycerin, terlipressin, somatostatin, or octreotide) showed similar efficacy but with fewer side effects in the pharmacologic therapy group.[76]

The use of somatostatin and analogues such as octreotide and vapreotide also produces splanchnic vasoconstriction, which is thought to be indirect via the inhibition of the release of vasodilatory peptides, primarily glucagon. More recent studies imply that octreotide has local vasoconstrictive effects. Somatostatin and its analogues have the advantage of being safe and can be used continuously for 5 days or longer. Terlipressin is a synthetic analogue of vasopressin and has the benefit of longer biologic activity with significantly fewer side effects. Terlipressin should be the first choice because it is the only drug that has been shown to improve survival; however, it is unavailable in the United States. Terlipressin is also the only pharmacologic treatment that has been shown to improve prognosis of variceal bleeding in placebo-controlled randomized controlled trials and meta-analysis. The most common side effect is abdominal pain; more serious side effects such as peripheral or myocardial ischemia may occur in less than 3% of patients.[77] Of the somatostatin analogues, only octreotide is available in the United States; it may be used as an adjunct to endoscopic therapy. The combination of pharmacologic and endoscopic therapy is considered to be the most effective treatment for acute variceal bleeding at the present time.

ACID SUPPRESSION

Many uncontrolled studies suggest a beneficial effect of acid suppression as an adjunct to sclerotherapy. In three controlled studies, the effect of sucralfate on healing of sclerotherapy-induced ulcers or preventing ulcer bleeding was found to be controversial. In one controlled study, ranitidine had a significant effect on ulcer healing, whereas omeprazole had no effect in another study.[78]

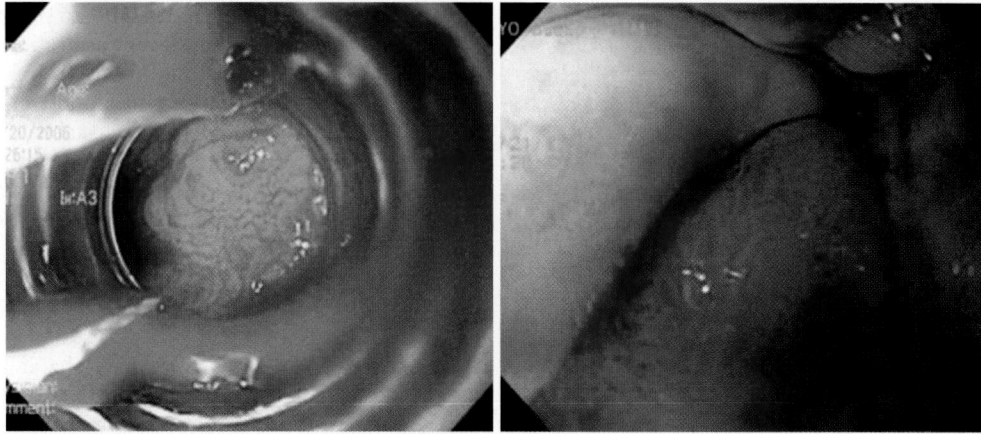

Fig. 13.5 Endoscopic band ligation is commonly used to treat active esophageal varices (*left panel* shows band ligation of gastroesophageal junction varix with a fibrin plug); however, active bleeding occasionally requires injection of sclerosing agents (*right panel* shows bluish discoloration of esophageal varix after sclerotherapy).

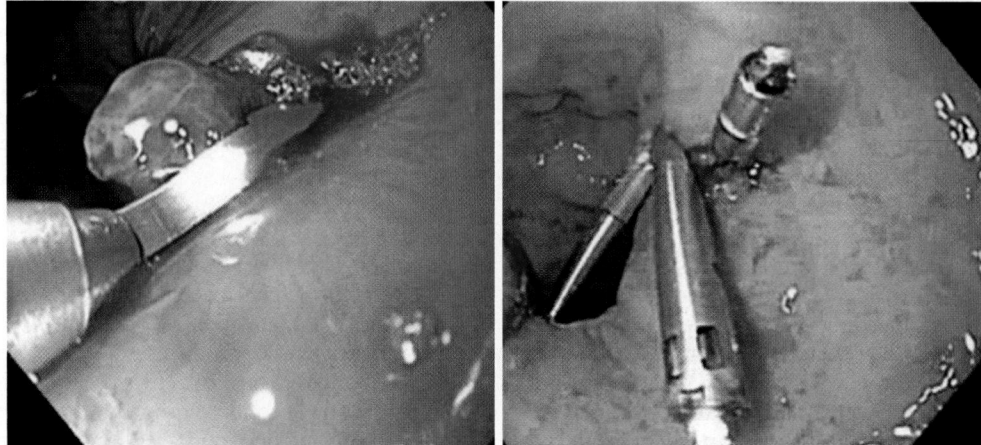

Fig. 13.6 Bleeding after band ligation can be managed by repeat band ligation or sclerotherapy or as shown here with hemoclips.

ANTIBIOTICS

Patients with cirrhosis are prone to developing spontaneous bacterial peritonitis among other infections. Consequently, antibody prophylaxis is an integral part of therapy for patients with variceal bleeding and should be started at admission.[21] Patients with Child class B and C cirrhosis are at the highest risk for developing bacterial infections. The use of prophylactic antibiotics is associated with a decrease in the rate of infections and improved survival. The improved survival is considered to be related to a decrease in the incidence of early rebleeding in patients who receive prophylactic antibiotics. Oral norfloxacin (400 mg twice daily) or intravenous ciprofloxacin (in patients in whom oral administration is not feasible) is the recommended antibiotic.[79,80] Antibiotics must be started on admission even if there is no apparent ascites.

ENDOSCOPIC VARICEAL LIGATION THERAPY

The current recommendation is to perform EVL after initial resuscitation when the patient is stable and the bleeding has ceased or slowed. Endoscopic sclerotherapy has largely been replaced by EVL. Sclerotherapy can be used when poor visualization prevents effective band ligation for bleeding varices (**Fig. 13.5**). Rarely, in cases with failed band ligation, our group and others have attempted mechanical closure of the bleeding site with hemoclips (**Fig. 13.6**).[81]

EVL was initially introduced in 1986 and is now established as standard therapy for the management of bleeding esophageal varices. Rubber bands are placed with the help of an endoscope to strangulate a varix, resulting in thrombosis and necrosis of the varix. The mucosa sloughs, and a mural scar is formed. A banding device consists of a cylinder preloaded with elastic rubber bands that is attached to the tip of the endoscope; the varix is suctioned into the cylinder, and a trigger device allows the deployment of a band around the varix. The optimal technique for ligation of esophageal varices involves initial application of bands distally at the gastroesophageal junction, followed by placement of bands proximally until all protruding varices are captured, which is usually accomplished in the distal 5 cm of the esophagus. Varices in the middle or proximal esophagus usually do not need to be banded because these varices have a lower propensity to bleed as they are compressed via perforating veins. The advantage of starting distally is that it allows for complete visualization and avoids the potential risk of dislodging a band during advancement of the endoscope past a previously captured varix. During variceal band ligation, transient bleeding can occur because of rupture of the varix. Single or multiple bands can be applied using different devices.

Generally, five to eight bands are deployed circumferentially in one session. Band ligation is ideally repeated at 2- to 4-week intervals until the varices are obliterated.

Endoloops

Endoloops have been used as an alternative to rubber bands. They can be placed during the same endoscopy without taking the endoscope out. Although they may exert more effective compressive force on tissue than bands, endoloops may cause tearing if tightened excessively. Endoloops also need repeated loading.

Endoscopic Sclerotherapy

Endoscopic sclerotherapy consists of injection of a sclerosing agent into the lumen of a varix (intravariceal) or immediately adjacent to the vessel to tamponade flow (paravariceal).[82] The injected sclerosant achieves its immediate hemostatic effect by coagulation necrosis, and variceal thrombosis and subsequently the inflammation of the surrounding tissue and scarring lead to variceal obliteration. The most commonly used sclerosants, with nearly comparable efficacy, are ethanolamine oleate, polidocanol, absolute alcohol, sodium tetradecyl sulfate, and sodium morrhuate.[22,82-84] Absolute alcohol is a potent, aqueous, readily available low-cost agent and is comparable to 5% ethanolamine oleate and 3% sodium tetradecyl sulfate.[82,84] Endoscopic sclerotherapy is performed using freehand technique. An injector with a retractile needle is passed through the operating channel of the endoscope, and the sclerosant is injected into the varix. During an acute bleed, injections are directed at the bleeding site. Endoscopic sclerotherapy can effectively arrest active esophageal variceal bleeding in about 95% of cases. Sclerotherapy is associated with significant complications, which have led to infrequent use of this modality in present-day practice. Its use is mainly limited to actively bleeding cases in which banding is not feasible or has failed.

Endoscopic Variceal Ligation versus Sclerotherapy

EVL and sclerotherapy have been compared and shown to be effective in the control of acute variceal bleeding. Two randomized trials compared EVL versus sclerotherapy in acute variceal bleeding.[85,86] In the first trial, 71 cirrhotics with active variceal bleeding were randomly assigned to receive EVL (37 patients) or sclerotherapy (34 patients) immediately after endoscopic examinations. Treatment failure within 1 month was 8% in the EVL group versus 30% in the sclerotherapy group ($P = .02$). Blood transfusion requirements were significantly lower in the EVL group than in the sclerotherapy group (3.2 ± 1.2 U vs. 4.5 ± 1.8 U, $P < .01$). There were significant complications in 5% in the EVL group and 30% in the sclerotherapy group ($P = .007$). In the second trial, patients admitted with acute GI bleeding and with suspected cirrhosis received somatostatin infusion for 5 days. Patients underwent endoscopy within 6 hours, and patients with esophageal variceal bleeding were randomly assigned to receive either sclerotherapy ($n = 89$) or EVL ($n = 90$). Therapeutic failure occurred in 21 patients treated with sclerotherapy (24%) and in 9 patients treated with EVL (10%) (relative risk 2.4, 95% confidence interval 1.1 to 4.9). Failure to control bleeding occurred in 15% versus 4% ($P = .02$). Side effects occurred in 28% of patients receiving sclerotherapy versus 14% receiving EVL (relative risk 1.9, 95% confidence interval 1.1 to 3.5); the side

effects were serious in 13% versus 4% ($P = .04$). The 6-week survival probability without therapeutic failure was better with EVL ($P = .01$).

The efficacy of EVL for the control of acute bleeding has been debated technically because it may be difficult to visualize and band a bleeding varix. This technical difficulty could be overcome by placing four bands, one in each quadrant, just above the gastroesophageal junction and a second set 3 to 4 cm proximal. Stiegmann and coworkers[87] randomly assigned patients who bled from esophageal varices to sclerotherapy or EVL. The control of active bleeding was comparable—77% in the sclerotherapy group and 86% in the EVL group. Mortality was higher in the sclerotherapy group (45%) compared with the EVL group (28%). Avgerinos and colleagues[88] randomly assigned 71 patients with cirrhosis and active variceal bleeding to EVL or sclerotherapy. The bleeding was controlled in 97% of patients in the EVL group and 76% of patients in the sclerotherapy group.

Meta-analyses show that EVL is better than sclerotherapy in the initial control of bleeding and is associated with fewer adverse events and improved mortality. HVPG increases significantly immediately after both EVL and sclerotherapy. However, HVPG decreases to baseline within 48 hours in patients who underwent EVL but not in patients who received sclerotherapy. EVL is the preferred method, and sclerotherapy is recommended in patients in whom EVL is not feasible.

ADJUVANT AND ALTERNATIVE TREATMENTS TO ENDOSCOPIC MODALITIES IN THE TREATMENT OF ACUTE VARICEAL BLEEDING

Balloon tamponade using a triple-lumen Sengstaken-Blakemore tube or a four-lumen Minnesota tube stops acute variceal bleeding effectively. The Zimmon tube allows endoscopy through the inflated rim of the balloon that abuts against the gastroesophageal junction and compresses the bleeding varices. Balloon tamponade is not routinely used before therapeutic endoscopy because it has a high rate of complications.[54,89-91]

Secondary Prophylaxis to Prevent Recurrent Esophageal Variceal Bleeding

All patients who survive an episode of acute variceal bleeding should undergo secondary prophylaxis. The rebleeding rate in untreated patients is around 60% within 1 to 2 years of the index hemorrhage. The risk of rebleeding is greatest within the first 6 weeks, with more than half of rebleeding episodes occurring within 3 to 4 days. Several risk factors have been recognized and include severe initial bleeding as defined by a hemoglobin less than 8 mg/dL, gastric variceal bleeding, active bleeding at endoscopy, and elevated HVPG.[92,93] It is vital that preventive therapy should be initiated before discharge from the hospital in patients who have recovered from an episode of hemorrhage for at least 24 hours.

Pharmacologic Therapy

Pharmacologic therapy using nonselective β blockers with ISMN has been proposed as a modality to prevent recurrent variceal bleeding. The combination therapy has synergistic

Table 13.4 Endoscopic Sclerotherapy versus Band Ligation for Prevention of Rebleeding from Esophageal Varices

Reference	Therapy	No.	Eradication (%)	Rebleeding (%)	Variceal Recurrence (%)	Follow-up
Hou et al (1995)[95]	EST	67	79	42	30	9.7 ± 6.4 mo
	EVL	67	86	19	48	10.5 ± 6.3 mo
Baroncini et al (1997)[96]	EST	54	92.5	19	13	53.4 ± 42 days
	EVL	57	93	16	30	496 ± 40 days
Sarin et al (1997)[97]	EST	48	93.8	21	7	8.3 ± 4.2 mo
	EVL	47	93.6	6	29	8.6 ± 4.6 mo
de la Pena et al (1999)[98]	EST	46	71	50	28	16 mo
	EVL	42	79	31	45	18 mo
Zargar et al (2005)[100]	EST	36	92	19	9	28 mo
	EVL	36	95	3	11	30 mo

EST, Endoscopic sclerotherapy; EVL, endoscopic variceal ligation.

effects on reducing portal pressures. Gournay and colleagues[94] tested the effectiveness of ISMN as an adjunct to propranolol for the prevention of variceal rebleeding. The study included 95 patients randomly assigned to combination treatment (46 patients) or propranolol alone (49 patients). The group receiving combination therapy had less rebleeding (33% vs. 41%); however, it was not statistically significant.

Endoscopic Variceal Ligation

EVL has essentially replaced sclerotherapy owing to faster reduction and obliteration of varices and by requiring fewer procedures with lower rates of complications (**Table 13.4**).[95–99] EVL was compared with sclerotherapy for the prevention of recurrent bleeding in 18 studies (n = 1509 patients). Meta-analyses have shown that the number of sessions, the time for obliteration, and the rebleeding rates are significantly lower with EVL compared with sclerotherapy. Sarin and associates[97] observed a faster variceal eradication with EVL requiring fewer sessions but with a higher recurrence rate compared with sclerotherapy group over a follow-up period of 8.5 ± 4.4 months. The higher recurrence with EVL is probably because ligation does not occlude the perforators as is done by injecting a sclerosant. The incidence of PHG was greater after sclerotherapy than after EVL (20.5% vs. 2.3%). The infrequent occurrence of PHG after EVL may be due to the fact that band ligation does not occlude the esophageal perforators, which allow blood to be drained away to paraesophageal collaterals, resulting in less congestion of gastric microcirculation but a higher rate of recurrence of esophageal varices. EVL has also been found effective in extrahepatic portal venous obstruction.[100]

Endoscopic Variceal Ligation and Sclerotherapy

EVL and sclerotherapy together during the same session (synchronous combination) for obliteration of esophageal varices has been proposed as a more effective management option compared with their individual use. Two meta-analyses, one comprising seven trials and a more recent one comprising eight trials, showed no differences in rebleeding, death, or number of sessions to variceal obliteration between groups and a higher incidence of esophageal strictures in the combination therapy group.[101,102] Consequently, EVL should not be combined with sclerotherapy.

Endoscopic Variceal Ligation and Pharmacotherapy

Combined EVL and pharmacotherapy using β blockers have also been proposed for secondary prophylaxis of variceal hemorrhage. The results of four trials are presented in **Table 13.5**.[103–106] EVL was also compared with the combination of EVL, β blockers, and sucralfate; 62 patients received EVL alone, and 60 received combination therapy.[107] After a median follow-up of 21 months, rebleeding and variceal recurrence occurred in 30% and 50% of patients in the EVL group and in 11.6% and 26% of patients in the combination group (P < .05). In addition, a large meta-analysis from Spain, which included 1860 patients in 23 trials, showed that combination therapy reduced overall and variceal rebleeding in cirrhotics more than either therapy alone,[108] supporting that this is a better approach for secondary prophylaxis.

Argon Plasma Coagulation and Microwave Coagulation

Argon plasma coagulation and microwave coagulation are other approaches to improve the rate of long-term eradication of esophageal varices after EVL by causing fibrosis of the esophageal wall. The techniques of argon plasma coagulation, low-power diode laser treatment, and microwave are still experimental.[109–113]

Gastric Varices

Bleeding from gastric varices is less frequent than bleeding from esophageal varices, but it is usually more severe and is

Table 13.5 Randomized Controlled Trials Comparing Combination Pharmacotherapy with Endoscopic Therapy for Prevention of Variceal Rebleeding

Reference	Therapy	No.	Rebleeding (%)	Deaths (%)	Follow-up (mo)
Villanueva et al (1996)[103]	Nadolol + ISMN	43	26	9	18
	Sclerotherapy	43	53	21	18
Villanueva et al (2001)[104]	Nadolol + ISMN	72	33	32	20
	Band ligation	72	49	42	22
Lo et al (2002)[105]	Nadolol + ISMN	61	57	13	24
	Band ligation	60	38	25	25
Patch et al (2002)[106]	Propranolol + ISMN	44	37	33	8
	Band ligation	47	53	33	12

ISMN, Isosorbide mononitrate.

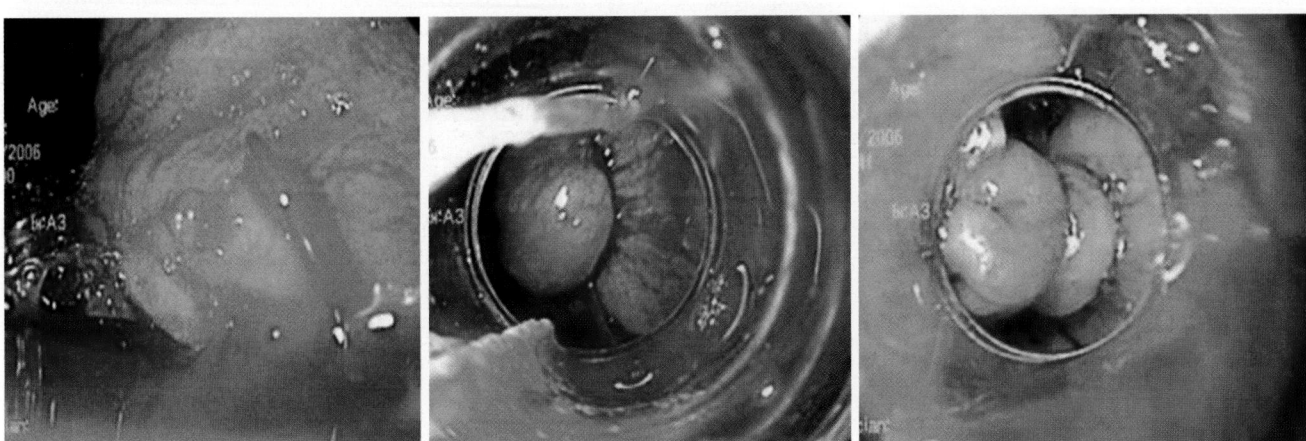

Fig. 13.7 Active bleeding from gastric cardia varix (gastroesophageal varix extending to lesser curve [GOV1]) treated with band ligation. Gastric cardia varices are amenable to band ligation in antegrade or retrograde fashion.

associated with a higher mortality rate. Gastric varices develop in approximately 20% of patients with portal hypertension.[55] The management of bleeding gastric varices depends on the natural history of different types of gastric varices. Although GOV1 disappear with the obliteration of esophageal varices in nearly 60% of patients, GOV2 and IGV1 require specific therapy.[114] GOV1 can also be managed with EVL in either an antegrade or retrograde fashion (**Fig. 13.7**). The risk of bleeding from IGV1 was shown to correlate with variceal size (>10 mm), Child class, and the presence of red color signs on varices.[22] IGV2 are uncommon varices, rarely bleed, and can be managed similar to IGV1.

At the present time, endoscopic therapy of isolated gastric varices is indicated in the presence of active bleeding (spurting or oozing) and the presence of a clot or other stigmata of a recent bleed on the varix. Several issues related to gastric varices have not been well studied, including the risk of bleeding from gastric varices after an episode of bleeding from esophageal varices, whether eradication of esophageal varices increases the risk of bleeding from gastric varices, and whether nonbleeding gastric varices that accompany bleeding esophageal varices should be treated prophylactically. At the present time, empirically, the decision to treat gastric varices prophylactically could be made on the basis of location and size of gastric varices, presence of red color signs, Child score, and

the patient's access to cyanoacrylate treatment in the event of sudden hemorrhage.

Endoscopic Sclerotherapy

Endoscopic sclerotherapy has not been highly successful in the treatment of gastric varices. The reason has been the high incidence of complications associated with sclerotherapy, which include gastric ulceration and perforation and recurrent bleeding rates of 37% to 53%.[115] Endoscopic sclerotherapy does not achieve thrombosis of the entire varix, and the necrosis caused by it may induce massive bleeding from the nonthrombosed high-flow gastric varix, leading to high mortality.[60]

Endoscopic Variceal Ligation

EVL and detachable snares have also been used by some groups to control acute gastric variceal bleeding and reduce the risk of rebleeding. Limited efficacy data are available, however.[116,117]

Tissue Adhesive Agents

Tissue adhesive agents have been reported to be effective in treating bleeding gastric varices. Compared with endoscopic

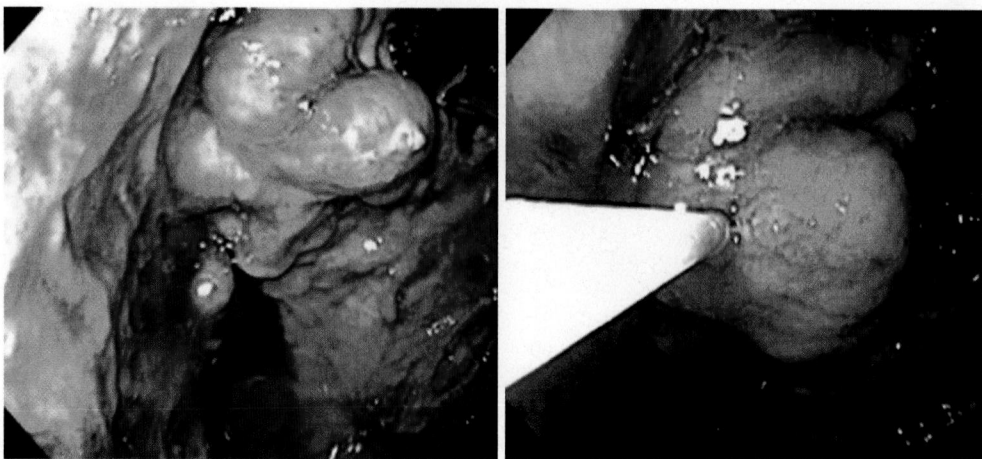

Fig. 13.8 Gastric varix with fibrin plug *(left panel)* treated with 3 mL of cyanoacrylate using Marcon-Haber needle (Cook Endoscopy, Winston-Salem, NC).

Table 13.6 Endoscopic Glue Injection for Treatment of Gastric Varices

References	No.	Hemostasis (%)	Rebleeding (%)	Mortality (%)	Follow-up (mo)
Lee et al (2000)[125]	47	95.7	12.8*/44.7†	17	24
Kind et al (2000)[123]	174	97.1	15.5	19.5	36
Battaglia et al (2002)[126]	32	96.8	34.4	18.7	45.4
Huang et al (2000)[124]	90	93.3	23.3	2.2	13
Sarin et al (2002)[118]	11	100	27	9	—
Greenwald et al (2003)[127]	44	95	18	22	12
Fry et al (2008)[128]	33	88	15	3	60

*≤48 hr.
†>48 hr.

sclerotherapy or EVL, endoscopic variceal obturation with tissue adhesive such as *N*-butyl-cyanoacrylate, isobutyl-2-cyanoacrylate, or thrombin is more effective for acute gastric variceal bleeding, especially fundal varices, with better control of initial hemorrhage and lower rates of rebleeding (**Fig. 13.8**). Native cyanoacrylate (*N*-butyl-2-cyanoacrylate [Histoacryl]) is a liquid with a consistency similar to water and lends itself to intravariceal injection. On contact with a physiologic medium such as blood, it rapidly polymerizes, forming a hard substance that plugs the bleeding varix and serves as a useful treatment option. However, the rapid polymerization can block the needle or damage the endoscope. Histoacryl must be diluted with lipiodol (0.5:0.8 mL) to delay the polymerization reaction to complete the injection and remove the needle. The individual dosage of Histoacryl per injection should be limited to 2 mL for fundal varices. Obliteration is tested by palpating the varix with the needle retracted. If soft, the varix is injected with additional aliquots of Histoacryl; after 3 to 4 days of injection, necrosis occurs on the variceal walls, and the cast is slowly extruded. The extrusion process may last several weeks and sometimes even months.

With Histoacryl, control of active bleeding from gastric varices has been reported to range from 93% to 100% of patients, and rate of rebleeding is generally less than 30%.[118-125] Huang and coworkers[124] reported 94% hemostasis in 90

patients with active or recent variceal bleeding from fundal varices. Tumorous gastric varices had a higher rebleeding rate than the tortuous and nodular type (34.4% vs. 17.2%). Kind and associates[123] reported their 12-year experience with the use of Histoacryl in 174 patients with bleeding gastric varices. The hemostasis rate was 97.1% with an early rebleeding rate of 15.5% and a hospital mortality rate of 19.5%. Complications including chest pain and treatment-related, ulcer-induced bleeding occurred in 2.9% of patients. However, these investigators reported high rebleeding rates in patients with prehepatic block with IGV1-type varices. **Table 13.6** summarizes other studies that have used Histoacryl.[118,123-128]

The use of glue has also been compared with other modalities.[121] A large prospective, randomized trial comparing gastric variceal obturation with Histoacryl versus EVL in patients with acute gastric variceal hemorrhage showed that control of active bleeding was similar in both groups but that rebleeding over a follow-up period of 1.6 to 1.8 years occurred significantly less frequently in the GVO group (23% vs. 47%), with an average of only 1.5 sessions (range 1 to 3).[129] Sarin and coworkers[118] found Histoacryl to be more effective than absolute alcohol for controlling acute bleeding (89% vs. 62%) and obliteration of gastric varices (100% vs. 44%) (**Table 13.7**). Histoacryl has also been shown to be superior to ethanolamine.[119] Combination of a sclerosing agent (ethanolamine

Table 13.7 Endoscopic Sclerotherapy versus Histoacryl Injection for Active Gastric Variceal Bleeding

Reference	Agent	No.	Hemostasis (%)	Rebleeding (%)	Ulcer (%)	Mortality (%)
Oho et al (1995)[121]	EO	24	67	12.5	25	67
	Histoacryl	29	93	10	30	38
Ogawa et al (1999)[119]	EO	21	81	35	—	23.8
	Histoacryl	17	100	0	—	0
Sarin et al (2002)[118]	AA	9	44	33	—	33
	Histoacryl	11	100	27	—	9

AA, Absolute alcohol; EO, ethanolamine oleate.

oleate) and Histoacryl has not been found to be of added advantage.[120,130] Glue injection has also been found superior to EVL of gastric varices.[122] Repeat glue injection into the gastric varix to obliterate it completely may be better than injection on demand (or response to recurrent bleed).[125]

Histoacryl injection has some adverse effects. Although uncommon, embolization of the adhesive into the lung, spleen, portal vein, renal vein, inferior vena cava, or brain poses a serious problem. The incidence varies from 2% to 5%; most often, the embolization is small. Because of the fear of embolization, some operators prefer to inject undiluted Histoacryl. However, the disadvantage of using undiluted adhesive is that the device channel of the endoscope may get blocked, or the injector needle may get glued into the varix.[130,131] Modifications of the injection technique, such as applying a silicone coating of the injection needle and sheath and new cyanoacrylate compounds such as acrylic glue (2-octyl-cyanoacrylate), can reduce the risk of such complications. Cases of visceral fistula have also been described after glue injection.[132] EUS with or without Doppler probe could be used to guide the injection of glue into gastric varices and to assess adequate obliteration. EUS could also help in assessing the paraesophageal collaterals and obliteration of perforators in esophageal variceal sclerotherapy or ligation.[133]

The hemostatic efficacy of glue injection coupled with the high mortality associated with nonendoscopic methods strongly favors glue injection as initial treatment in patients with active bleeding from GOV2 and IGV1. The treatment of GOV1 persisting after obliteration of esophageal varices must be separately planned. Modifications of the injection technique and new cyanoacrylate compounds such as acrylic glue (2-octyl-cyanoacrylate) may reduce or eliminate the risk of embolization.

Other agents, including thrombin alone or in combination with fibrinogen ("fibrin glue"), are useful to stop excessive surface bleeding.[134] Poly-N-acetyl glucosamine (P-GLc NAc) isolated from marine microalgae is a polysaccharide polymer that was shown to stop variceal hemorrhage quickly in dogs. An open trial of endoscopic gastric intravariceal injection treatment with Beriplast (fibrin sealant) enrolled 15 patients presenting with gastric variceal bleeding and followed them up to 1 month after endoscopic treatment. There was failure to control bleeding in one patient. Four patients had rebleeding after the index bleed. All patients were followed for 30 days. There were 14 patients who were discharged from the hospital after the first episode of gastric variceal bleeding.

None of the patients had injection-induced complications. Beriplast injection seems to be a safe, simple, and effective endoscopic treatment in acute gastric variceal bleeding. It is undergoing further evaluation.[135]

Ectopic Nongastroesophageal Varices

Ectopic varices occur at sites other than the gastroesophageal junction and account for a small percentage of variceal bleeding.

Anorectal Varices

Anorectal varices result from collaterals between the superior hemorrhoidal vein (portal) and the middle and inferior hemorrhoidal veins (systemic). Hemorrhoids must be differentiated from anal varices; the former appear as purple, well-vascularized mucosa in the lower 4 cm of the anal canal. Varices in the anal canal appear as either discrete veins or saccular blue or slate gray swellings. Rectal varices start above the dentate line and are easy to diagnose. Anorectal varices are more common in patients with extrahepatic portal venous obstruction and noncirrhotic portal fibrosis (89%) compared with cirrhosis (56%) and are more common in patients who are bleeders than in nonbleeders.[136]

In contrast to esophageal varices, anorectal varices rarely bleed, but if they bleed, they often bleed massively. The incidence of bleeding from rectal varices was 1.4%, 6.7%, and 18% in three studies, with more bleeding in patients with noncirrhotic portal hypertension.[136-138] For bleeding anorectal varices, endoscopic injection sclerotherapy, EVL, embolization, cryosurgery, and underrunning of the varices with sutures all have been tried but often with limited success. EVL seems to be a safe and effective therapy, but this requires further study to become the standard of care. Portosystemic shunt or TIPS is the other option if EVL fails to decompress and prevent rectal variceal bleeding.[46,82]

Duodenal, Jejunal, Ileal, and Colonic Varices

Duodenal, jejunal, ileal, and colonic varices are rare and are usually found incidentally at the time of endoscopy, more often in patients with extrahepatic portal vein obstruction or in cirrhotics with portal vein thrombosis. Usually the afferent vessel of the duodenal varices is the superior or inferior pancreaticoduodenal vein originating in the portal vein trunk or superior mesenteric vein. The efferent vein drains into the inferior vena cava. In a review of 169 cases of bleeding ectopic varices, 17% occurred in the duodenum, 17% in the jejunum or ileum, 14% in the colon, 8% in the rectum, and 9% in the peritoneum.[139]

Duodenal varices more often are secondary; that is, they appear after obliteration of esophageal varices. When a patient with portal hypertension has melena without hematemesis, the possibility of a bleeding duodenal varix should be considered. Sometimes these patients present with active upper GI bleed. Successful control of bleeding after injection of cyanoacrylate, sclerosant, or thrombin and sclerosant combination has been reported.[46,139] Data regarding EVL of duodenal varices and other ectopic varices are limited. Even in patients with reasonable liver function, surgical mortality rates for treating actively bleeding duodenal varices range from 30% to 40%. Radiologic procedures such as selective embolization and TIPS may be effective but have not been extensively studied. Jejunal and ileal varices involving the small intestine are rare. They are commonly found at the anastomotic sites and in adhesions.

Patients who present with bleeding jejunal or ileal varices typically have a history of portal hypertension, prior abdominal surgery, and hematochezia without hematemesis. Small bowel varices can occur in the absence of cirrhosis when there is mesenteric or splenic vein thrombosis and even with concomitant nonbleeding esophageal varices. The common locations are ileum (47%) and jejunum (39%). Push enteroscopy and venous phase of angiography may reveal the bleeding source. Small bowel varices can also be identified by wireless capsule endoscopy and retrograde ileoscopy. Successful sclerotherapy and glue injection to treat bleeding jejunal varices have been reported.[140]

Stomal Varices

Stomal varices may form in and around the stoma in a patient who has had a colectomy for ulcerative colitis who develops portal hypertension resulting from sclerosing cholangitis or in a cirrhotic with ileostomy. Bleeding is usually recurrent and problematic, with an estimated 3% to 4% risk of death at each episode. The time frame for development of these varices and hemorrhage from them is unclear but ranges from 1.5 to 348 months with an average of 28 months for colostomy and 48 months for ileostomy. Local compression with gauze soaked in dilute epinephrine, sclerotherapy, and surgical variceal ligation are useful in temporarily controlling the bleed. Transcatheter embolization, disconnection of the stoma or portosystemic shunting, and TIPS placement have been used with variable success.

Biliary Varices

Biliary varices have been reported in the gallbladder and the bile ducts, more often in patients with portal vein thrombosis. Usually varices of the biliary tree are found incidentally during ultrasound, Doppler, CT scan, or endoscopic retrograde cholangiopancreatography (ERCP) imaging. Bile duct varices may produce narrowing, irregularity, and nodular extrinsic defects termed *portal biliopathy* on ERCP.[141] Spontaneous bleeding from biliary varices is rare. Portal decompressive measures should relieve venous dilation and consequent obstructive jaundice, if present.

Portal Hypertensive Gastropathy

PHG, known earlier as congestive gastropathy, relates to gastric mucosal changes seen endoscopically in patients with portal hypertension. Mild PHG manifests as a mosaiclike pattern without discrete red spots and is unlikely to cause significant blood loss. In severe PHG, mucosal red spots become confluent and give rise to deeply erythematous areas that are susceptible to bleeding. PHG can also be seen in patients without portal hypertension and in healthy subjects.[142] PHG is a dynamic condition that can progress from mild to severe and vice versa or even disappear completely. Acute bleeding from PHG is relatively rare, and bleeding from PHG is less severe than bleeding from gastroesophageal varices. After the first bleed from PHG, rebleeding seems to be very common, with reported figures of 62% and 75%. Effective treatment of PHG requires a reduction in the increased portal pressure, which can be accomplished pharmacologically by β blockers with or without nitrates, radiologically by TIPS, by surgical shunts, or by liver transplantation. Argon plasma coagulation through endoscopy was found to be effective in two of nine patients when performed every 2 to 3 weeks in one small series, but this is not an established therapy.[143]

Gastric Antral Vascular Ectasia

Two endoscopic manifestations of GAVE are currently recognized: (1) watermelon stomach and (2) diffuse antral vascular ectasia. The endoscopic description of watermelon stomach is diagnostic and includes the presence of longitudinal rugal folds traversing the antrum and converging on the pylorus; overlying these folds are myriad angioectasias linearly arrayed, the aggregate resembling the stripes of a watermelon. Some workers have described a more diffuse endoscopic form of GAVE (**Figs. 13.9 and 13.10**) that sometimes is difficult to differentiate from PHG.[144] **Table 13.8** outlines the differences and the management options for PHG and GAVE. Patients with GAVE present with significant occult or overt blood loss. Severe anemia is one of the most common presentations, and about 25 mL of blood is estimated to be lost per day by these lesions.[145]

The etiology of GAVE is uncertain, but it has been proposed that gastric peristalsis causes prolapse of the loose antral mucosa into the duodenum with consequent elongation and ectasia of the mucosal vessels.[146,147] GAVE is more prevalent among patients with chronic liver disease but not infrequently occurs in patients without hepatic pathology. When associated with cirrhosis, the evolution to portal hypertension does not seem to be a prerequisite. Reduction in portal pressure does not improve the endoscopic appearance or bleeding propensity of GAVE. However, liver transplantation leads to rapid regression of the lesions. These features indicate that portal hypertension per se is not the sole pathogenetic mechanisms for GAVE. At the present time, treatment of GAVE is unsatisfactory because reduction of portal pressure by β blockers is of limited help. Drugs such as tranexamic acid, glucocorticoids, and estrogen-progesterone combination may help in reducing transfusion requirements, but their true efficacy remains equivocal.

Our group had reported the use of endoscopic neodymium:yttrium-aluminium-garnet (Nd:YAG) laser coagulation to be effective in 12 of 13 patients after a median

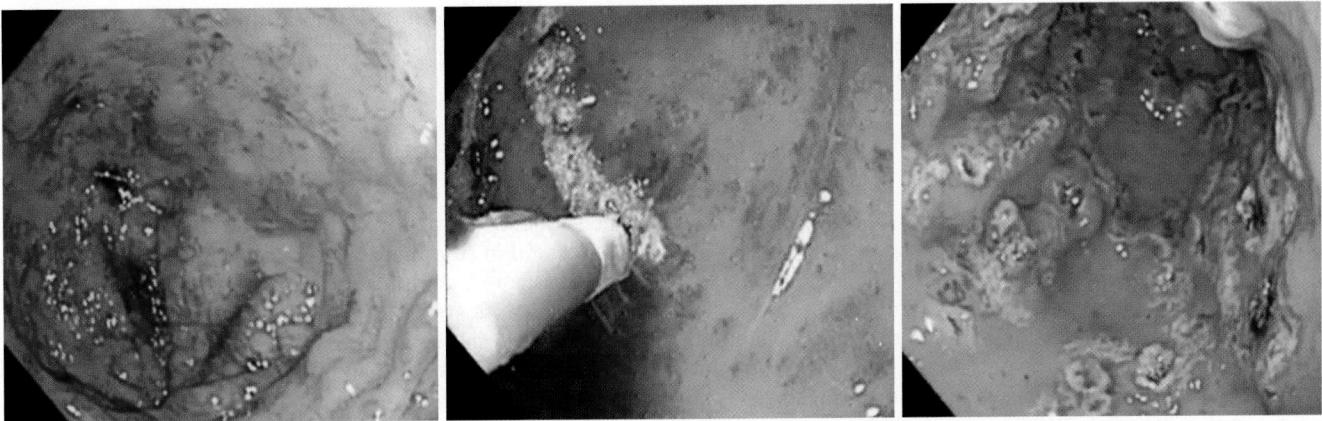

Fig. 13.9 Paintbrush technique to treat gastric antral vascular ectasia using argon plasma coagulator.

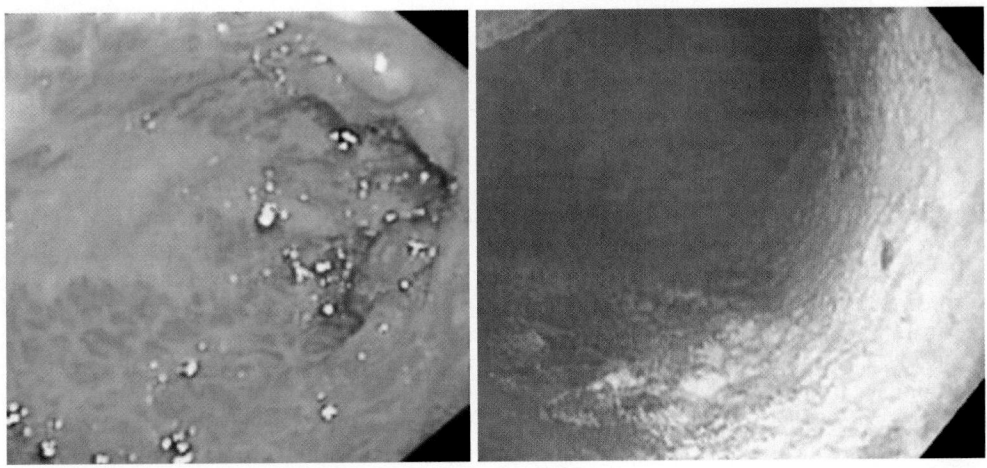

Fig. 13.10 Diffuse gastric antral vascular ectasia treated with cryotherapy. *Right panel* shows immediate postprocedure frosting of mucosa.

Table 13.8 Portal Hypertensive Gastropathy (PHG) versus Gastric Antral Vascular Ectasia (GAVE)

	PHG	GAVE
Distribution in stomach	Proximal	Distal
Mosaic pattern	Present	Absent
Red signs	Present	Present
Biopsy		
Thrombi	—	+++
Spindle cell proliferation	+	++
Fibrohyalinosis	+	+++
Treatment	β blockers	APC
	TIPS	Transplant

APC, Argon plasma coagulation; TIPS, transjugular intrahepatic portosystemic shunt.
Courtesy of Patrick Kamath.

period of 6 months, eliminating the need for transfusion.[145] Similar experience was reported by others without complications.[148] However, success in the diffuse form of GAVE is limited. Cryotherapy is used as an experimental technique, but experience is limited.[149,150] Although surgical antrectomy can cure GAVE, liver transplantation is the best option.

Portal Hypertensive Enteropathy and Colonopathy

Portal hypertension–related mucosal abnormalities affecting the small intestine are less frequent with low bleeding propensity.[151] Diarrhea and protein-losing enteropathy, which improved after TIPS placement, could be other manifestations of portal hypertensive enteropathy. Kozarek and coworkers[152] reported that 14 (70%) of 20 cirrhotics had multiple vascular-appearing lesions (10 with cherry red spots, 6 with spider telangiectasias), 4 of whom also had endoscopic features suggesting a mild, chronic colitis, most commonly involving the right colon. Other investigators have observed colonopathy in 52% of patients with portal hypertension, more often in bleeders (52%) than in nonbleeders (12.5%).[137] Portal hypertensive colonopathy is rarely a cause of significant portal hypertension–related bleeding. Colonopathy is usually diagnosed endoscopically and not histologically. Endoscopic lesions of portal hypertensive colonopathy include colonic angioectasias, mucosal abnormalities such as erythema, friability, and edema.[153,154]

Transjugular Intrahepatic Portosystemic Shunt in the Management of Bleeding Related to Portal Hypertension

TIPS creates a communication between the hepatic vein and an intrahepatic branch of the portal vein using an expandable metallic stent and decompresses high portal pressures. The shunt is placed by an interventional radiologist via a transjugular approach and dilated as needed to reduce the portacaval pressure gradient to less than 12 mm Hg. At the present time, coated stents are used more often to reduce the frequency of shunt stenosis. Immediate complications of TIPS placement include intraperitoneal hemorrhage, sepsis, and cardiopulmonary failure from excessive blood flow into the right heart. Early complications include shunt thrombosis or migration, hepatic encephalopathy, progressive hepatic failure, and pulmonary artery hypertension. Late complications include shunt stenosis, progressive hepatic encephalopathy, portal vein thrombosis, and heart failure. The best indicator of failure of TIPS is recurrence of GI bleeding. TIPS should be avoided in patients with a Model for End-Stage Liver Disease (MELD) score greater than 24 because these patients have a reduced survival.[155,156] In patients with a MELD score of 14 or less, survival is excellent. Severe hepatic encephalopathy is a relative contraindication for TIPS.

The best method to evaluate the patency of TIPS is by hepatic venogram and measurement of the portacaval pressure gradient. TIPS has been compared with sclerotherapy in two meta-analyses, involving 811 patients and 750 patients.[157,158] The median follow-up period ranged from 10 to 32 months in various trials. Both meta-analyses concluded that TIPS is more effective in preventing variceal rebleeding than endoscopic sclerotherapy (19% vs. 47%). However, because of the increased risk of posttreatment encephalopathy and the lack of improvement in survival, TIPS is not recommended as first-line treatment for preventing variceal rebleeding. A high rate of stent dysfunction requiring revision is another limitation of TIPS.

TIPS is better than the combination of ISMN and propranolol and better than endoscopic therapy in the prevention of variceal rebleeding, although at the expense of an increased risk of encephalopathy.[63,64] Also, there is no increased survival benefit. A more recent trial showed that although pharmacologic (propranolol plus nitrates) therapy was less effective than TIPS in preventing rebleeding, it was associated with less encephalopathy, identical survival, and more frequent improvement in Child-Pugh class with lower costs than TIPS.[159] These findings are supported further by a meta-analysis of 11 published randomized controlled trials.[158] TIPS is considered a salvage therapy for patients who bleed despite adequate medical and endoscopic treatment. TIPS is very effective in the treatment of bleeding gastric varices. It has a success rate of greater than 90% for initial hemostasis and a very low rebleeding rate.[160,161] A more recent trial has shown that TIPS is more effective than cyanoacrylate glue injection

in preventing rebleeding; however, the rate of complications and survival was not different.[162]

Surgical Management of Portal Hypertensive Bleeding

When endoscopic, pharmacologic, and radiologic options are unsuccessful in stopping acute or recurrent variceal bleeding, portal system decompression created by a shunt between the portal and systemic venous circulation is considered. Portosystemic shunts can be classified as selective, nonselective, or partial depending on how much hepatic portal flow is preserved. Selective shunt—chiefly, the distal splenorenal shunt (DSRS)—involves an anastomosis between the distal splenic vein and the renal vein and interruption of all collaterals connecting the superior mesenteric and the gastrosplenic components of the portal system. Although DSRS can decrease portal pressure, it may worsen ascites from continuous mesenteric venous hypertension. It is relatively contraindicated in patients with a splenic vein diameter less than 7 mm because of a high incidence of shunt thrombosis. DSRS has been compared with nonselective shunts in several controlled trials, none of which have shown a survival advantage for either procedure.[163] Encephalopathy seems to be less with DSRS compared with nonselective shunts, and DSRS can be recommended even for alcoholic patients. Survival after DSRS is higher among patients with nonalcoholic cirrhosis, however, possibly because of better preservation of hepatic portal perfusion.

Partial shunt using polytetrafluoroethylene (PTFE) is a small-diameter shunt that attempts to decompress varices while preserving hepatic portal flow. When partial PTFE shunt is combined with coronary vein ligation and division of collaterals, it offers a fixed resistance and is more likely to maintain hepatopetal portal flow.[164] Nonselective shunts divert all portal blood flow and in doing so decompress the entire portal venous system. Examples of nonselective surgical shunts include end-to-side shunt, side-to-side shunt, and conventional splenorenal shunt. The end-to-side shunt, also known as Eck fistula, was compared with medical therapy in four randomized clinical trials, none of which showed a survival advantage. Patients in the shunted group had excellent control of bleeding but at the expense of increased encephalopathy. Bleeding was the most common cause of death in the medically treated group, whereas accelerated hepatic failure was the leading cause of death in the surgical group.[89]

Surgical options also have been proposed as secondary prophylaxis. Orozco and coworkers[165] compared elective treatment of variceal hemorrhage with β blockers (propranolol), endoscopic sclerotherapy, and portal blood flow–preserving surgical procedures (selective shunts and the Sugiura-Futagawa operation). The investigators found that rebleeding rate was significantly lower in the surgical group compared with the other two groups. Survival was better for low-risk patients (Child A) in the three groups, but when the three options were compared, no significant difference was found. A randomized controlled trial compared distal splenorenal shunt with TIPS and found similar efficacy in the control of refractory variceal bleeding in Child-Pugh class A and B patients. Reintervention was significantly greater for TIPS compared with the shunt.[166]

Summary

Management of esophageal and gastric varices poses considerable challenges and requires a team approach and a dedicated ICU. The combination of EVL with vasoactive drugs or with β blockers to reduce portal pressure is effective in controlling active bleeding and preventing rebleeding. In patients who do not respond to these measures, TIPS or rescue surgery must be offered. Although prevention of infection and hepatic encephalopathy can help improve survival, HVPG determines the outcome in such patients. A first variceal bleed from high-risk varices can be prevented by reduction in HVPG by β blockers with or without adding nitrates. In patients who do not achieve 20% or greater reduction in HVPG or who have contraindications or side effects to β blockers, EVL offers an equally effective and safe alternative. Effective strategies are needed to prevent development of varices or delay the increase in size of small varices. Reduction in portal pressure also helps to reduce bleeding from PHG and ectopic varices but not from GAVE. Liver transplantation offers a lasting cure because it treats the cirrhosis and the portal hypertension.

References

The complete reference list is available online at www.expertconsult.com.

Chapter 14

Lower Gastrointestinal Bleeding

Thomas J. Savides

 Video related to this chapter's topics can be found online at expertconsult.com.

Introduction

Acute severe lower gastrointestinal (GI) bleeding is a common problem. Colonoscopy is often performed for diagnosis and sometimes treatment. It is often mild and self-limited. For purposes of this discussion, only moderately severe hematochezia, which results in decreased hematocrit greater than 8%, hospitalization, and possible blood transfusion, is considered. In addition, this chapter focuses only on colonic sources of lower GI bleeding, which is the most common site for severe hematochezia.

Epidemiology

Acute severe lower GI bleeding occurs with an annual hospitalization rate of 22 per 100,000 adult population; this is based on a retrospective study of middle-class Americans who were members of Kaiser Permanente Health Care system in San Diego, California.[1] Assuming that an average full-time clinical gastroenterologist is responsible for 50,000 adult lives, he or she would see more than 10 cases per year. Most cases occur in elderly patients, given the increased frequency and risk for diverticulosis, vascular disease, and colonic malignancy.[1] Risk of lower GI bleeding is also associated with the use of aspirin and nonsteroidal antiinflammatory drugs (NSAIDs).[2,3]

Initial Approach to a Patient with Severe Hematochezia

Initial patient assessment includes history, vital signs with orthostatic blood pressure determination, and physical and rectal examinations. Patients should be asked about whether they saw red blood or dark maroon blood, duration of symptoms, abdominal pain, prior history of lower GI bleeding, prior pelvic radiation, history of diverticulosis, and prior colon imaging studies. Patients should also be asked about use of medications associated with GI bleeding (e.g., aspirin, NSAIDs, anticoagulants, and *Ginkgo biloba*). Weight loss or a change in bowel habits suggests possible colon cancer. Abdominal pain usually suggests ischemic colitis, although abdominal pain can be present in other colitides and malignancy.

The most important parts of the physical examination are the vital signs and the stool examination. The presence of bright red blood on rectal examination strongly suggests the possibility of colonic bleeding. Bright red blood per rectum is always a colonic source, unless it is accompanied by hypotension, which can occur during a severe upper GI or small bowel bleed with rapid transit of blood.[4] In the setting of hematochezia without hypotension, placement of a diagnostic nasogastric (NG) tube is usually unnecessary because it is unlikely that there is a severe upper GI bleed without hypotension.

If there is hypotension and hematochezia, a severe upper GI bleed is possible, and an NG tube should be placed. A clear NG tube lavage does not always imply a lower GI source because 16% of patients with duodenal ulcer bleeds have negative NG lavage.[5] If bile is seen in the NG tube lavage, it is unlikely to be an upper GI bleed. Physical examination should also focus on abdominal tenderness, surgical scars, and stigmata of liver disease. Most patients with severe hematochezia do not need placement of an NG tube for diagnostic lavage, unless there is a strong suspicion for an upper GI source. At least one large-bore (14-gauge or 16-gauge) intravenous catheter should be placed, with two placed in the setting of ongoing bleeding.

Blood should be sent for hematocrit, platelets, prothrombin time, partial thromboplastin time, chemistry panel, and type and crossmatch for packed red blood cells. Resuscitation should be initiated simultaneously with assessment. Normal saline is infused as fast as needed to keep systolic blood pressure greater than 100 mm Hg and pulse lower than 100 beats/min. Patients are transfused with packed red blood cells, platelets, and fresh frozen plasma as necessary to maintain hematocrit greater than 24%, platelet count greater than 50,000/mm[3], and prothrombin time less than 15 seconds. A GI endoscopist should be notified as soon as possible to expedite patient diagnosis and possible therapy; this is especially important in terms of coordinating timing of the bowel purge and procedure.

Most patients with lower GI bleeding can be admitted to internal medicine or gastroenterology services rather than to the general surgery services because these patients rarely require emergency surgical intervention, and given their elderly age, they usually require management of comorbid diseases by an internist. Patients should be admitted to an intensive care unit (ICU) or monitored intermediate care unit. Patients should have automatic blood pressure monitoring every 5 minutes if unstable and hourly if stable. Each patient should receive cardiac rhythm monitoring to observe for arrhythmias and to follow the heart rate as a sign of continued or recurrent bleeding. Laboratory-determined hematocrits (not finger-stick hematocrits, which are less reliable) should be obtained every 4 to 6 hours until the patient has a stable hematocrit. In cases of active bleeding, an indwelling bladder catheter should be placed to help monitor fluid status. Swan-Ganz catheter monitoring is unnecessary except for patients with a history of congestive heart failure or unstable cardiac disease. Patients older than age 60 or with risk factors for coronary artery disease should also have serial electrocardiograms and cardiac enzyme evaluation to determine whether there is any cardiac ischemia.

Endoscopy of any sort should be done only when it can be performed safely and when the information may influence patient care. Patients should be medically resuscitated with fluids and transfusions before endoscopy. Ideally, patients should be hemodynamically stable, with a heart rate of less than 100 beats/min and systolic blood pressure greater than 100 mm Hg. Hematocrit, especially in elderly patients, ideally should be greater than 28%. Severe thrombocytopenia (platelet count <50,000/mm[3]) should be corrected with transfusions before emergency endoscopy, and prolonged prothrombin time (>15 seconds) should be corrected with fresh frozen plasma. Performance of endoscopy in the middle of the night should be avoided unless well-trained endoscopy nurses, appropriate endoscopy equipment, and surgical backup are available.

Early Predictors of Severity in Acute Lower Gastrointestinal Bleeding

Early predictors (within 4 hours of admission) of severity for continued or recurrent bleeding after 24 hours of hospitalization include heart rate greater than 100 beats/min, systolic blood pressure less than 115 mm Hg, syncope, nontender abdominal examination, observed rectal bleeding during the first 4 hours of hospital evaluation, aspirin ingestion, and the presence of more than two comorbid conditions (**Box 14.1**).[6,7] This prediction model has been prospectively validated; the low-risk group had 0% rebleeding, the moderate-risk group had 45% rebleeding, and the high-risk group had 77% risk of rebleeding.[7] It is possible that factors such as these can be used to help triage patients to the appropriate level of care, such as ICU, hospital ward, or outpatient evaluation and urgent versus elective endoscopic evaluation.

Mortality in Severe Lower Gastrointestinal Bleeding

A large U.S. database study comprising 227,000 patients with discharge diagnoses of lower GI bleed in 2002 reported an overall mortality rate from lower GI bleeding of 3.9%.[8] Multivariate analysis found that independent predictors of in-hospital mortality were age (>70 years), intestinal ischemia, presence of two or more comorbid illnesses, bleeding while hospitalized for a separate process, coagulopathies, hypovolemia, transfusion of packed red blood cells, and male gender. Colorectal polyps and hemorrhoids were associated with a lower mortality risk. Patients who develop severe lower GI bleeding while hospitalized for other lesions have a much higher mortality rate than patients admitted with lower GI bleeding. In a large Kaiser Permanente San Diego retrospective study, the in-hospital mortality rate for patients with lower GI bleeding who began as outpatients was 2.4% compared

---

Box 14.1 Early Predictors of Severity of Continued or Recurrent Lower Gastrointestinal Bleeding

Heart rate >100 beats/min
Systolic blood pressure <115 mm Hg
Syncope
Nontender abdominal examination
Observed rectal bleeding during first 4 hours of hospital evaluation
Aspirin
More than two comorbid conditions

From Strate LL, Orav EJ, Syngal S: Early predictors of severity in acute lower intestinal tract bleeding. Arch Intern Med 163:838–843, 2003; and Strate LL, Saltzman JR, Ookubo R, et al: Validation of a clinical prediction rule for severe acute lower intestinal bleeding. Am J Gastroenterol 100:1821–1827, 2005.

with 23% for patients with in-hospital lower GI bleeding ($P < .001$).[1]

Diagnostic Options

Most patients undergo initial evaluation with colonoscopy after bowel preparation, although in selected cases flexible sigmoidoscopy without bowel preparation or with enema preparation may be performed. Other diagnostic tests may be used in selected cases or when colonoscopy is unsuccessful.

Anoscopy

Anoscopy can be useful if actively bleeding hemorrhoids are suspected. However, nearly every patient requires additional visualization of the more proximal colon using colonoscopy or possibly sigmoidoscopy.

Flexible Sigmoidoscopy

Occasionally, flexible sigmoidoscopy may be performed to evaluate the left side of the colon quickly for any bleeding site stigmata rather than waiting for a full colonoscopy bowel preparation, and this results in a diagnosis in approximately 9% of cases.[9] Flexible sigmoidoscopy may be especially useful in patients with strongly suspected diverticular bleeding or ischemic colitis.

Barium Enema

There is no role for emergency barium enema in a patient with severe lower GI bleeding. This test is rarely diagnostic because it cannot show vascular lesions and may be misleading if only diverticula are present. It also fails to detect 50% of polyps greater than 10 mm in size.[10] Subsequent colonoscopy is needed for any suspicious lesions seen on barium enema, and no therapy can be performed.

Nuclear Medicine Scintigraphy

Nuclear medicine scintigraphy involves injecting a radio-labeled substance in the patient's bloodstream and then performing serial scintigraphy to detect focal collections of radiolabeled material. It has been reported to detect bleeding at a rate of 0.1 mL/min.[11] The overall positive diagnostic rate is approximately 45%, with a 78% accuracy in the localization of the true bleeding site.[12] The most common false-positive result occurs when there is rapid transit of luminal blood such that labeled blood is detected in the colon, although it originated in the upper GI tract.

Angiography

Angiography is positive when the arterial bleeding rate is at least 0.5 mL/min.[13] The diagnostic yield depends on patient selection, timing of the procedure, and the skill of the angiographer, with positive yields in 12% to 69% of cases. An advantage of angiography is that embolization can be performed to control some bleeding lesions. There is also a 3% rate of major complications, however, including hematoma formation, femoral artery thrombosis, contrast dye reactions, renal failure, and transient ischemic attacks.[14]

Computed Tomography Colonography

Computed tomography (CT) visualization of the colon is increasingly used to evaluate the colon for polyps and masses and may be of some benefit in lower GI bleeding. Faster scanners allow CT angiography, CT colonography, and CT evaluation of the small bowel to be performed. Use of CT potentially could allow diagnosis of mass lesions and vascular lesions, which would be an advantage compared with other radiologic imaging studies. One study from France reported that CT accurately diagnosed 17 of 19 lower GI bleeding sites, including diverticula, tumors, angiomas, and varices.[15]

Colonoscopy

Urgent colonoscopy using a rapid sulfate purge has been shown to be safe, to provide important diagnostic information, and sometimes to allow therapeutic intervention.[16] Patients usually ingest 4 to 8 L of polyethylene glycol either orally or via NG tube over 3 to 5 hours until the rectal effluent is clear of stool, blood, and clots. Metoclopramide may be given intravenously before the purge and repeated every 3 to 4 hours to facilitate gastric emptying and reduce nausea.

Most "urgent" colonoscopy for lower GI bleeds is performed 6 to 36 hours after the patient is admitted to the hospital. Because most bleeding stops spontaneously, cases are often performed more electively the day after initial hospitalization to allow the patient to receive blood transfusions and to have the bowel preparation during the 1st day of hospitalization.

The overall diagnostic yield of a presumed or definite etiology using colonoscopy in lower GI bleeding ranges from 48% to 90%, with an average of 68%, based on a review of 13 studies.[12] The problem with interpreting these data is that it is often impossible to determine a definite diagnosis of the cause of the bleeding, unless bleeding stigmata are identified such as active bleeding, a visible vessel, an adherent clot, mucosal friability or ulceration, or the presence of fresh blood limited to a specific part of the colon. A presumptive diagnosis often is made, especially in the case of diverticulosis, in which no blood is seen but there is a potential bleeding site present.

The optimal time for performing urgent bowel preparation and colonoscopy is unknown. Theoretically, the sooner the endoscopy is performed, the higher the likelihood of finding a lesion that might be amenable to endoscopic hemostasis, such as a bleeding diverticulum or polyp stalk. However, a retrospective study from the Mayo Clinic suggested that there was no significant association between the time of endoscopy (0 to 12 hours, 12 to 24 hours, >24 hours) and the findings of active bleeding or other stigmata that would prompt colonoscopic hemostasis in patients with diverticular bleeding.[17] Early colonoscopy has been associated with fewer hospitalization days.[18] Active bleeding or lesions at risk for rebleeding can be treated with colonoscopic hemostasis; this mostly applies to postpolypectomy bleeding and diverticula and is discussed later.

Surgery

Surgical management is rarely needed for lower GI bleeding because most bleeding is either self-limited or easily managed

Table 14.1 Etiology of Severe Lower Gastrointestinal Bleeding*

Cause	Cases (%)
Diverticulosis	33
Cancer/polyps	19
Colitis	18
Unknown	16
Angiodysplasia	8
Other	8
Postpolypectomy	6
Anorectal	4

*Summary of 1333 patients in seven published studies.
From Zuckerman GR, Prakash C: Acute lower intestinal bleeding. Part II. Etiology, therapy, and outcomes. Gastrointest Endosc 49:228–238, 1999.

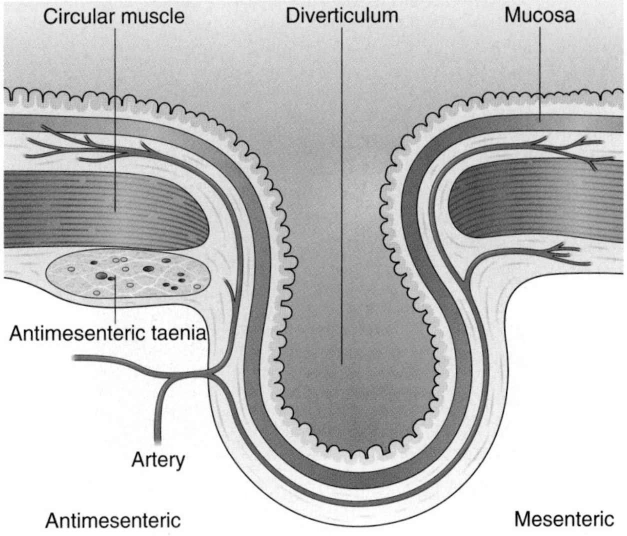

Fig. 14.1 Vascular anatomy of colonic diverticulum.

with medical or endoscopic therapy. The main indications for surgery are malignant lesions and recurrent bleeding from diverticula. For this reason, it seems prudent that most stable patients be managed by an internist or gastroenterologist rather than a surgeon.

Etiology and Pathogenesis of Severe Lower Gastrointestinal Bleeding

It is not always possible to visualize active bleeding during colonoscopy. The timing of endoscopy may influence visualization: Earlier colonoscopy should increase the chances of detecting an actively bleeding lesion. A definite diagnosis of a bleeding lesion can usually be made if active bleeding is seen or there is an obvious stigma, such as clot or visible vessel. A presumptive diagnosis can be made if there is a suspicious lesion and no other possible sources. **Table 14.1** lists the frequency of various presumed or definite sites of acute colonic bleeding.[19] Potential colonic lesions amenable to endoscopic hemostasis include diverticula, postpolypectomy sites, angiomas, hemorrhoids, Dieulafoy's lesions, tumors, ulcers, and radiation proctitis.

Diverticular Bleeding

Colonic diverticula are herniations of colonic mucosa and submucosa through the muscular layers of the colon. Diverticula in the colon are actually pathologic pseudodiverticula because true diverticula contain all layers of the intestinal wall. Colonic diverticula seem to form when colonic tissue is pushed out by intraluminal pressure. Diverticula occur at the point of entry of the small arteries that supply the colon, the vasa recta, as they penetrate the circular muscle layer of the colonic wall. The entry points of the vasa recta are areas of relative weakness through which the mucosa and submucosa can herniate when under increased intraluminal pressure. They vary in diameter from a few milliliters to several centimeters. The most common location is the left colon.

Most colonic diverticula are asymptomatic and remain uncomplicated. Bleeding may occur from vessels at the neck or base of the diverticulum (**Fig 14.1**).[20] Diverticula are common in Western countries, with a prevalence of 50% in older adults.[21] In contrast, less than 1% of people living in continental Africa and Asia have diverticula.[22] This finding has led to the hypothesis that regional differences in prevalence can be explained by the low amounts of dietary fiber in Western diets. Presumably, a low-fiber diet results in less stool content, longer fecal transit time, increased colonic muscle contraction, and, ultimately, increased intraluminal pressure that results in the formation of propulsion diverticula. In addition, diverticula occur with increasing frequency with advanced age, which could be a result of weakening of the colonic wall and muscle tone.

It has been estimated that 3% to 5% of patients with diverticulosis develop diverticular bleeding.[23] Although most diverticula are in the left colon, several series suggest that bleeding diverticula occur more often in the right colon.[20,23-25] Patients with diverticular bleeding are typically elderly and present with painless hematochezia. They often have been taking aspirin or NSAIDs.[2] In at least 75% of patients with diverticular bleeding, the bleeding stops spontaneously.[24] Patients in whom bleeding stops usually require less than 4 U of blood. In one surgical series, surgical resection was needed in 60% of patients, most of whom had continued bleeding despite transfusion of 4 U of blood.[24] Patients with successful resection of a bleeding diverticulum had a rebleed rate of 4%.[24] Among patients in whom bleeding stopped spontaneously, the rebleeding rate from colonic diverticulosis was 25% to 38% over the next 4 years.[1,24] Urgent colonoscopy after rapid bowel preparation often reveals that bleeding has stopped by the time of colonoscopy, and only nonbleeding diverticula are detected. These patients are given the diagnosis of "presumptive diverticular bleed" because the diverticula are the only likely source of bleeding, although no stigmata were identified.

Occasionally, urgent colonoscopy reveals stigmata of recent bleeding, such as active bleeding, a visible vessel, clot, or blood limited to one segment of the colon (**Fig. 14.2**). It seems

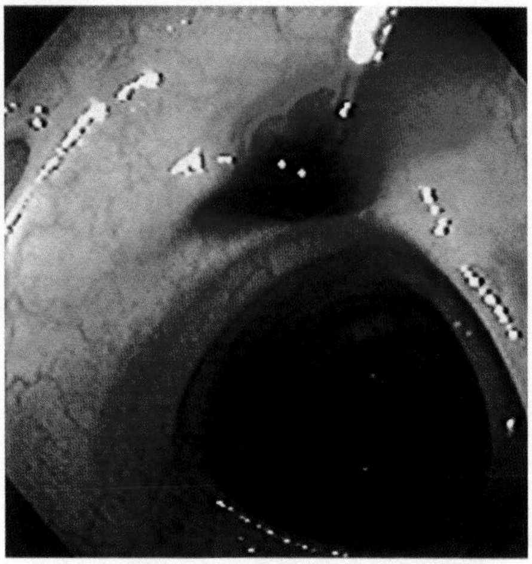

Fig. 14.2 Active diverticular bleeding.

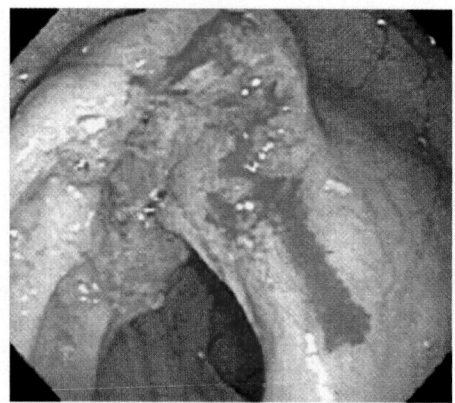

Fig. 14.3 Colon cancer as a cause of severe hematochezia.

possible that earlier colonoscopy in lower GI bleeding would result in a greater frequency of finding stigmata of recent diverticular bleeding, although a small case series study from the Mayo Clinic did not find any difference if colonoscopy was performed between 0 and 12 hours, between 12 and 24 hours, or more than 24 hours from the time of hospital admission.[17] There have been attempts to stratify patients with diverticular bleeding at increased risk for rebleeding employing the same endoscopic stigmata used in high-risk peptic ulcer bleeding (active bleeding, visible vessel, and clot), although the natural history for each of these untreated stigmata is unknown. The "pigmented protuberance" found on the edge of some diverticula at histopathology is usually clot at the edge of a ruptured blood vessel.[26]

The UCLA/CURE group[17] found that among patients with stigmata of recent diverticular hemorrhage (six active bleeding, four visible vessels, and seven adherent clots), there was a very high rebleed rate of 53% and emergency surgery rate of 35%.[27] Colonoscopic hemostasis of actively bleeding diverticula has been reported using bipolar probe coagulation, epinephrine injection, metallic clips, rubber band ligation, and fibrin glue.[26–33] If fresh red blood is seen in a focal segment of colon, we try to examine this segment of bowel carefully to detect the exact bleeding site. If the bleeding is coming from the edge of the diverticulum or there is a pigmented protuberance on the edge, we initially inject 1:10,000 epinephrine in 1-mL aliquots using a sclerotherapy needle into four quadrants around the bleeding site. Then we use either an endoscopic clip or a bipolar probe at a low power setting (10 to 15 W) and light pressure for a 1-second pulse duration to cauterize the diverticular edge and stop bleeding or flatten the visible vessel. If there is a nonbleeding adherent clot, we inject around the clot with 1:10,000 epinephrine in four quadrants with 1 mL per quadrant and remove the clot in piecemeal fashion using a cold polyp snare. The clot is shaved down until it is 3 mm above the diverticulum, and then the underlying stigma is treated with either endoscopic clip or bipolar probe coagulation as discussed previously. After performing endoscopic hemostasis of a bleeding diverticulum, a permanent submucosal tattoo and a metal clip (if not previously placed) should be placed in the adjacent mucosa to identify the site in case colonoscopy, angiographic embolization, or surgery is required for recurrent bleeding. For long-term management

after colonoscopic hemostasis, patients are told to avoid aspirin (if approved by their cardiologist) and NSAIDs and to take a daily fiber supplement.

In 2000, Jensen and colleagues in the UCLA/CURE group[27] published their results on urgent colonoscopy for diagnosis and treatment of severe diverticular hemorrhage. The investigators found that 20% of patients with severe hematochezia had endoscopic stigmata suggesting a definite diverticular bleed. Compared with a historical control group with high-risk stigmata but no colonoscopic hemostasis, the group receiving colonoscopic hemostasis had a rebleed rate of 0% versus 53% and an emergency hemicolectomy rate of 0% versus 35%. After 3 years of follow-up, there were no rebleeding episodes in the patients who underwent colonoscopic hemostasis. In contrast to the UCLA experience, a smaller, retrospective review of the Duke University Medical Center Endoscopic Database revealed 13 patients with active bleeding or stigmata who received endoscopic treatment with epinephrine or bipolar coagulation or both.[34] The 30-day rebleed rate was 38%; four of these patients underwent surgery. The long-term rebleed rate was 23% with a mean follow-up of 3 years.

Angiographic embolization can also be performed in selected cases of diverticular bleeding, but there is a risk of bowel infarction, contrast reactions, and renal failure. Angiography can be helpful before surgical resection. Surgical resection for diverticular bleeding is usually reserved for recurrent bleeding episodes. Resection should be guided by colonoscopic, angiographic, or nuclear medicine studies showing the likely bleeding site. The need for surgery is often guided by certainty regarding the bleeding site and medical comorbidity because diverticular bleeding is often mild, and the risks of surgical complications are increased in elderly patients.

Colon Cancer

Most patients with colon cancer present with occult GI blood loss rather than hematochezia. For adult patients with hematochezia, determining the presence or absence of a colon cancer is imperative because early diagnosis improves survival. Because a cancer must ulcerate for overt bleeding to occur, most bleeding cancers are at a relatively advanced tumor stage (**Fig. 14.3**). Colon cancer can occur anywhere in the colon or rectum, but there is increased prevalence of right-sided tumors in elderly patients.

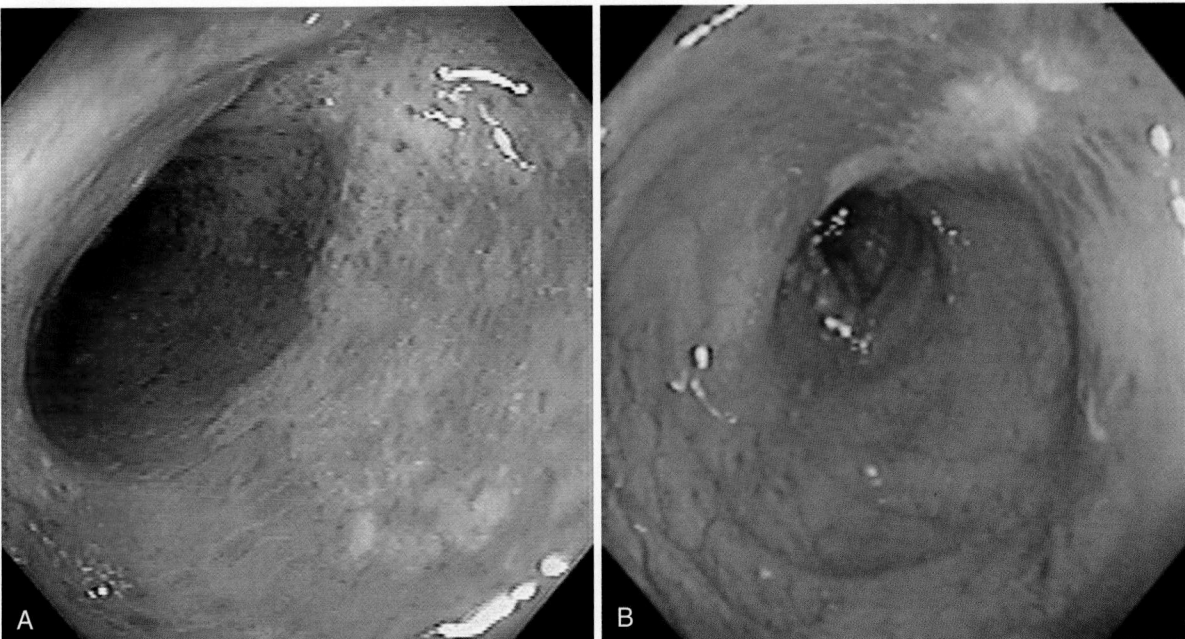

Fig. 14.4   Ischemic colitis.

Colitis

The term *colitis* refers to any form of inflammation of the colon. With regard to severe lower GI bleeding, this is usually ischemic colitis, inflammatory bowel disease, or possibly infectious colitis. Ischemic colitis generally manifests as hematochezia with mild left-sided abdominal discomfort. It results from mucosal hypoxia and is thought to be caused by hypoperfusion of the intramural vessels of the intestinal wall rather than by large vessel occlusion. Most cases do not have a recognizable cause, but associated conditions include recent aortic or cardiac surgery, vasculitis, and medications.[35,36] Because of collateral circulation, ischemic involvement is usually segmental and primarily affects the mucosal aspect of the intestine. The colon is mostly affected in the watershed areas, such as the splenic flexure or rectosigmoid junction in which there is reduced collateral circulation, although ischemia can occur anywhere.

The diagnosis is usually confirmed by colonoscopy but can be suspected by "thumbprinting" on plain film radiographs or colonic wall thickening on CT scan. The colonoscopic appearance includes erythema, friability, and exudate (**Fig. 14.4**). Biopsy specimens may be suggestive of ischemic changes but more importantly are used to exclude infectious changes or Crohn's disease. Ischemic colitis generally resolves in a few days and does not require colonoscopic hemostasis. In a large retrospective series from Kaiser Permanente San Diego, there were no episodes of rebleeding from ischemic colitis over a 4-year period.[1] Inflammatory bowel disease affecting the colon can rarely cause severe acute lower GI bleeding. In a case series from the Mayo Clinic, most patients had Crohn's disease.[37] Most patients were successfully treated medically. Three of the 31 patients in the series received endoscopic therapy with epinephrine injection alone or with bipolar coagulation for adherent clots or oozing ulcers in Crohn's disease. These patients had no rebleeding. Rebleeding occurred in 23% of patients a median of 3 days after the initial bleed

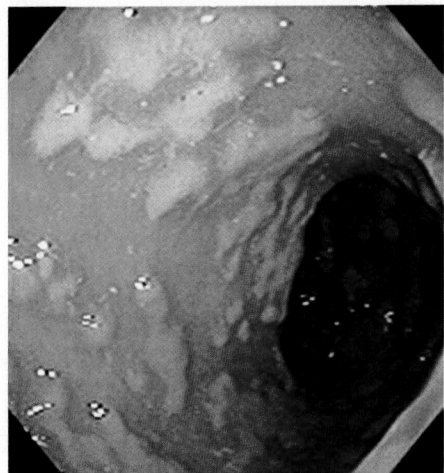

Fig. 14.5   *Clostridium difficile* colitis.

(range 1 to 75 days). Of the patients with Crohn's disease with severe bleeding, 39% required surgical management.

Infectious colitis should always be excluded in any patient with severe lower GI bleeding and colitis. Lower GI bleeding can occur with infection by *Campylobacter jejuni, Salmonella, Shigella,* invasive *Escherichia coli, E. coli* 0157, or *Clostridium difficile* (**Fig. 14.5**). Significant blood loss is rare. Diagnosis is made by stool cultures and flexible sigmoidoscopy.

Angiodysplasia

Colonic angiomas are also referred to as angiodysplasia, arteriovenous malformations, or vascular ectasias. They are generally uncommon: Less than 1% of asymptomatic patients undergoing screening colonoscopy were found to have angiodysplasia.[38] The lesion seems to increase with age and may represent degeneration of previously normal blood vessels in

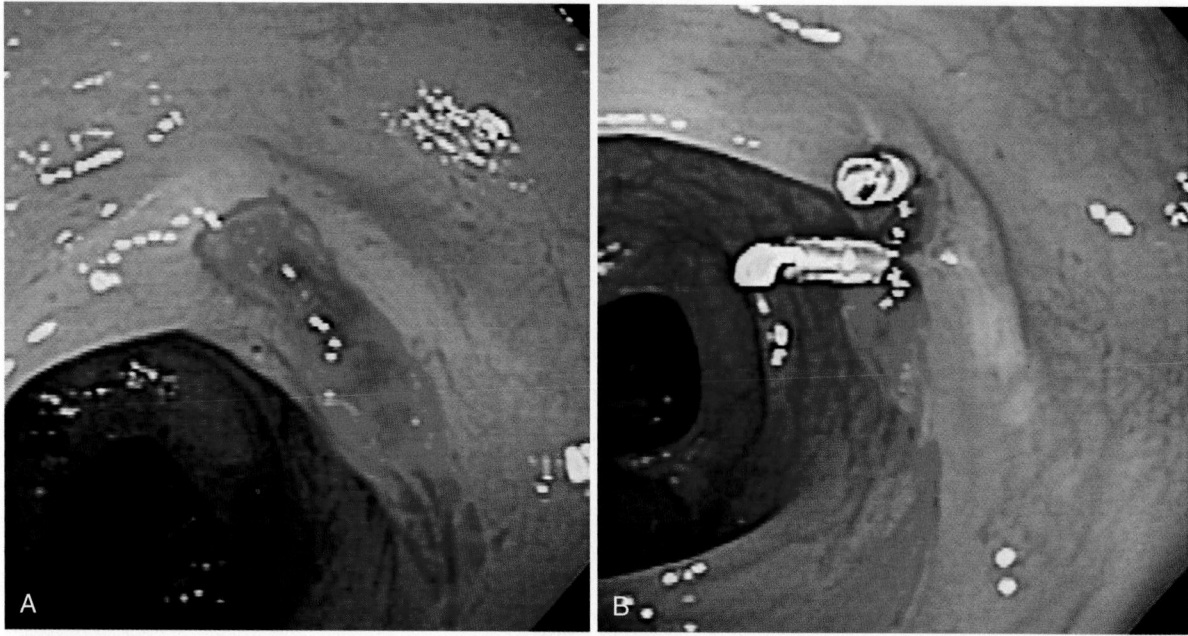

Fig. 14.6 A, Postpolypectomy bleeding. **B,** Polypectomy site after placement of clips.

the cecum and proximal ascending colon. Histopathology reveals a large, dilated, submucosal vein and, in advanced cases, dilated mucosal veins with small arteriovenous communications. Proposed explanations for angioma formation include the partial obstruction of submucosal veins passing through the colonic muscle layers, with eventual dilation of the submucosal and mucosal veins, and local mucosal ischemia.

Medical conditions associated with angiomas include chronic renal failure and hereditary hemorrhagic telangiectasia (Osler-Weber-Rendu syndrome). There have been reports suggesting that aortic stenosis is associated with lower GI bleeding, presumably from colonic angiomas.[39] The potential biologic explanation is that aortic stenosis causes defects in von Willebrand factor, which causes the patient to have decreased platelet adhesion and increased bleeding tendency, especially if there were preexisting mucosal GI lesions such as angiomas.[40,41] Clinical studies do not support the association between aortic stenosis and the presence of angiomas, however.[42,43] Bleeding from angiodysplasia is usually painless. The bleeding usually occurs from the right colon or cecum.

In the past 2 decades, it seems that the reported frequency of angiomas as the source of lower GI bleeding has decreased.[16,27] This may be because of better recognition of angiomas with improved endoscope technology and increased attribution to presumed diverticular bleeding as the cause of hematochezia. Endoscopic hemostasis has been successfully reported using thermal modalities (e.g., bipolar probe, heater probe, laser) and injection therapy.[44] Hormonal therapy has been reported as useful for decreasing bleeding from angiodysplasia, but a more recent randomized controlled trial found no benefit.[45]

Postpolypectomy Bleeding

Postpolypectomy bleeding occurs after 1% to 6% of polypectomies, usually within the first 7 days.[46] It is generally mild and self-limited. Reported risk factors for postpolypectomy bleed-

ing include large polyps (>2 cm), thick stalks, sessile polyps, and right colon polyps.[46] Endoscopic management techniques include resnaring the stalk (without cautery), epinephrine injection, thermal coagulation, hemoclips, and endoloops (**Fig. 14.6**).[46–49] In a case series from the Mayo Clinic, the median time to bleeding after polypectomy was 5 days (range 0 to 17 days).[48] Of patients, 65% received aspirin, NSAIDs, warfarin (Coumadin), heparin, or steroids after polypectomy; 76% required transfusions; and 96% were managed endoscopically with coagulation or epinephrine injection or both. The routine use of placing hemoclips after colonic polypectomy or endoscopic mucosal resection does not decrease the subsequent postpolypectomy bleeding rate.[50] However, in selected patients who have had polypectomies and who were believed to be at increased risk for bleeding, prophylactic hemoclip placement or other endoscopic hemostasis may be considered.

Radiation Proctitis

Radiation proctitis usually causes mild chronic hematochezia but occasionally can cause acute severe lower GI bleeding. Ionizing radiation can cause acute and chronic damage to the normal colon and rectum after radiation treatment for gynecologic, prostatic, bladder, or rectal tumors. Approximately 75% of patients who receive 4000 rad develop acute, self-limited diarrhea, tenesmus, abdominal cramping, and rarely bleeding during the first few weeks. Chronic radiation effects occur 6 to 18 months after completion of treatment. Bowel injury resulting from chronic radiation is related to vascular damage, with subsequent mucosal ischemia, thickening, and ulceration. Much of this damage is believed to be due to chronic hypoxic ischemia and oxidative stress. Flexible sigmoidoscopy reveals telangiectasia, friability, and ulceration in the rectum.

Patients should be instructed to avoid all aspirin and NSAIDs and should be put on a high-fiber diet. Medical

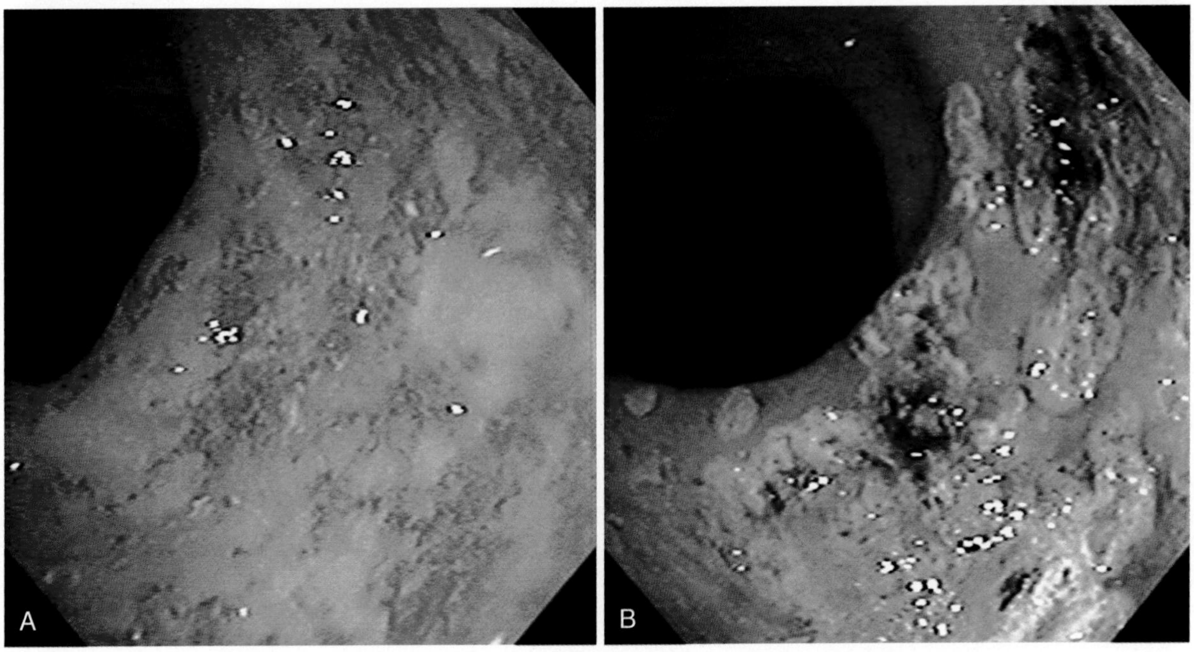

Fig. 14.7 **A,** Radiation proctitis. **B,** Radiation proctitis after argon plasma coagulation.

therapies with topical or oral 5-aminosalicylic acid, sucralfate, or steroids can be tried but are usually unsuccessful.[51] Thermal therapy can be quite successful, including argon plasma coagulation, bipolar probe coagulation, radiofrequency ablation, and cryotherapy (**Fig. 14.7**).[52–54] Topical formalin applied directly to the rectal mucosa can reduce bleeding.[55] In refractory cases, hyperbaric oxygen can also be used successfully.[56,57] A few pilot studies suggest that antioxidant vitamins, such as vitamins A, C, and E, can also decrease bleeding resulting from chronic radiation proctitis.[58]

Hemorrhoids

Hemorrhoids are a plexus of veins just above the rectal squamocolumnar junction. Internal hemorrhoids are located above the dentate line, and external hemorrhoids are located below the dentate line. Symptomatic hemorrhoids are common in adults, mostly associated with prolonged straining during bowel movements, chronic constipation, pregnancy, obesity, and low-fiber diet. Bleeding is characterized by bright red blood per rectum that can coat the outside of the stool, may drip into the toilet bowel, and is present when wiping with tissue. Usually this is mild bleeding, but occasionally severe bleeding may occur from hemorrhoids. Treatment of hemorrhoids usually starts with medical therapy consisting of fiber supplementation to soften stool, lubricant rectal suppositories (with or without steroids), and warm sitz baths. Anoscopic therapy can also be used, including injection sclerotherapy, rubber band ligation, cryosurgery, infrared photocoagulation, and bipolar and direct current electrocoagulation. The use of a flexible endoscope and esophageal band ligation devices has also been described (**Fig. 14.8**).[59] Surgery is reserved for refractory bleeding not controlled with other mechanisms. Most patients respond to medical management.

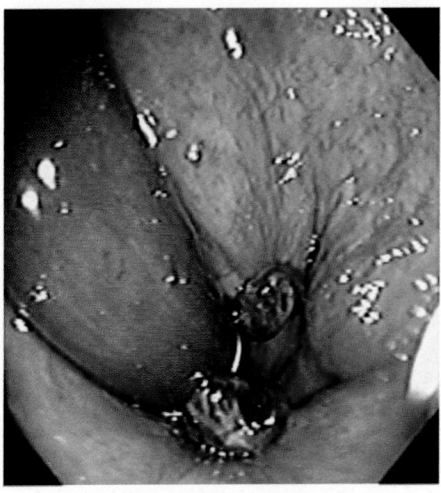

Fig. 14.8 Hemorrhoid banding.

Rectal Varices

In response to portal hypertension, varices can develop in the rectal mucosa between the superior hemorrhoidal veins (portal circulation) and the middle and inferior hemorrhoidal veins (systemic circulation). With anoscopy or sigmoidoscopy, rectal varices are seen as vascular structures located several centimeters above the dentate line. The incidence of rectal varices increases with the degree of portal hypertension. About 60% of patients with a history of bleeding esophageal varices have rectal varices. Rectal varices can be treated similarly to esophageal varices, with sclerotherapy, rubber band ligation, or portosystemic shunts.[60,61]

Rectal Dieulafoy's Lesion

Dieulafoy's lesions are large submucosal arteries without overlying mucosal ulceration, which can cause massive bleeding from anywhere in the GI tract, although bleeding is usually from the stomach. There have been reports of bleeding Dieulafoy's lesions in the rectum that were treated successfully with endoscopic hemostasis.[62,63]

Summary

The source of severe lower GI bleeding usually can be diagnosed by urgent colonoscopy. The differential diagnosis of lower GI bleeding includes diverticulosis, cancer, colitis, angiomas, postpolypectomy sites, radiation proctitis, internal hemorrhoids, and rectal varices. Patients should be stabilized with medical resuscitation and transfusion before urgent colonoscopy. Urgent colonic purge allows for earlier colonoscopy and the increased possibility for colonoscopic hemostasis. Bleeding diverticula and postpolypectomy bleeding can be treated with epinephrine injection, bipolar coagulation, or clipping. Radiation proctitis and angiomas can be treated with thermal coagulation. Most patients who have successful colonoscopic hemostasis do not experience rebleeding. After endoscopic hemostasis, medical management can often help reduce the chances of rebleeding. Urgent colonoscopy should be performed in all patients with severe hematochezia who are suspected to have a lower GI bleed.

References

The complete reference list is available online at www.expertconsult.com.

Obscure Gastrointestinal Bleeding

Itay Maza and Ian M. Gralnek

Video related to this chapter's topics can be found online at expertconsult.com.

Introduction

Obscure gastrointestinal (GI) bleeding accounts for approximately 5% of all GI bleeding and is defined as bleeding from an unknown source that persists or recurs after negative endoscopic diagnostic evaluation.[1] A negative diagnostic evaluation is commonly agreed on as consisting of negative upper endoscopy (esophagogastroduodenoscopy [EGD]) and colonoscopy with careful evaluation of the terminal ileum. Obscure GI bleeding is subcategorized as overt or occult. *Obscure-overt* GI bleeding is persistent or recurrent visible evidence of bleeding (hematemesis, hematochezia, or melena), whereas *obscure-occult* GI bleeding is persistent or recurrent positive fecal occult blood, iron deficiency anemia, or both, when there is no evidence of visible blood loss to the patient or health care provider.[2]

Etiology of Obscure Gastrointestinal Bleeding

Obscure GI bleeding has numerous possible causes and may originate from the upper GI tract (proximal to the ligament of Treitz), the mid-GI tract (ligament of Treitz to the terminal ileum), or the colon. Most causes (approximately 75%) of obscure GI bleeding are found between the ligament of Treitz and the ileocecal valve—in other words, in the small bowel.[3] Arteriovenous malformations (AVMs) of the small bowel

account for 30% to 40% of obscure GI bleeding and are the most common source of obscure GI bleeding in older patients (**Fig. 15.1**).[4] In persons 30 to 50 years of age, tumors such as GI stromal tumors, leiomyomas, leiomyosarcomas, schwannomas, carcinoids, lymphomas, and adenocarcinomas predominate (**Fig. 15.2**). Younger individuals most commonly have obscure bleeding from Crohn's disease or Meckel's diverticula–associated ulceration (**Fig. 15.3**).[5] Nonsteroidal antiinflammatory drug (NSAID) enteropathy has been associated with erosions, ulcers, and strictures of the small bowel and can also be a potential cause of obscure GI bleeding.[6] Less common causes of obscure GI bleeding include Dieulafoy's lesions, hemosuccus pancreaticus, *Strongyloides stercoralis* infection, radiation-induced enteritis, and pseudoxanthoma elasticum (**Table 15.1**).[7-11]

Investigating Obscure Gastrointestinal Bleeding

Medical history, patient age, symptoms, physical examination findings, and laboratory data all may provide clues and help guide diagnostic investigations. Several elements of the medical history and physical examination can provide important information about the etiology of obscure bleeding and help define the intensity with which a bleeding site should be sought. Recurrent hematemesis indicates bleeding proximal to the ligament of Treitz, whereas recurrent passage of

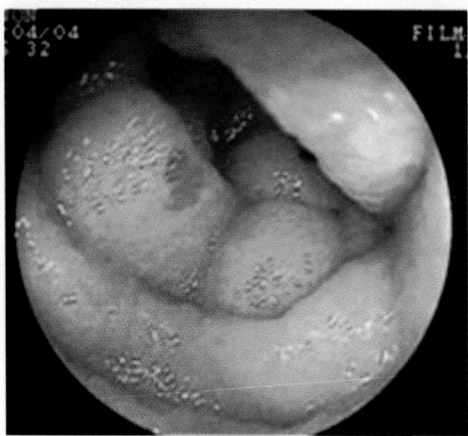

Fig. 15.1 Arteriovenous malformation of the small bowel as seen by capsule endoscopy.

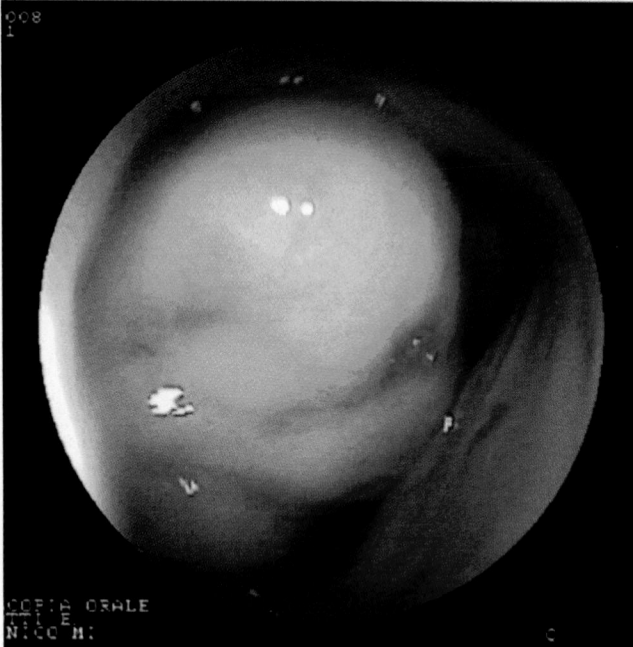

Fig. 15.2 Gastrointestinal stromal tumor as seen by double-balloon enteroscopy. *(Courtesy of Professor Roberto De Franchis.)*

PillCam® SB

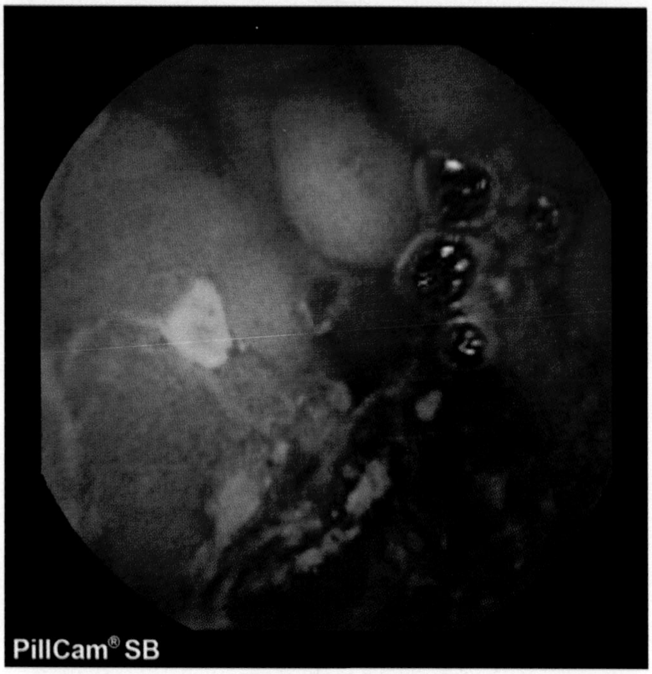

Fig. 15.3 Small bowel ulceration in Crohn's disease as seen by capsule endoscopy.

Table 15.1 Etiology of Obscure Gastrointestinal (GI) Bleeding

UPPER GI LESIONS	Older than 40 Years of Age
Cameron's erosions	
Fundic varices	Angiectasis
Peptic ulcer	NSAID enteropathy
Angiectasis	Celiac disease
Dieulafoy's lesion	Hemobilia
Gastric antral vascular ectasia	Hemosuccus pancreaticus
	Aortoenteric fistula
MID–GI TRACT LESIONS	
	LOWER GI LESIONS
Younger than 40 Years of Age	
	Angiectasis
Meckel's diverticulum	Neoplasms
Crohn's disease	
Celiac disease	
Tumors	
Dieulafoy's lesion	

NSAID, Nonsteroidal antiinflammatory drug.

hematochezia suggests a colonic source. Melena can originate from bleeding anywhere from proximal to the ligament of Treitz to the right colon. As a result, a history of melena provides only limited value in terms of localization of obscure GI bleeding.

A review of medications (including over-the-counter medications) may reveal inadvertent use of NSAIDs or products containing acetylsalicylic acid (ASA) and NSAIDs. A family history of cancer occurring at an early age, particularly colorectal or endometrial, may suggest the presence of hereditary nonpolyposis colorectal cancer. Skin, nail, and oral mucosal changes may suggest the presence of several disorders associated with obscure GI bleeding or iron deficiency anemia, including telangiectasias, which may reflect hereditary hemorrhagic telangiectasia (Osler-Weber-Rendu syndrome); dermatitis herpetiformis, which may reflect celiac disease; or other conditions with cutaneous and GI manifestations (e.g.,

Kaposi's sarcoma, Peutz-Jeghers syndrome, tylosis, pseudoxanthoma elasticum, Ehlers-Danlos syndrome, blue rubber bleb nevus syndrome, Henoch-Schönlein purpura, neurofibromatosis, malignant atrophic papulosis, and Klippel-Trenaunay-Weber syndrome).[2]

Diagnostic Investigations

Numerous diagnostic investigations may be performed to identify the etiology of obscure GI bleeding. Endoscopic investigations include repeat EGD and colonoscopy, push enteroscopy, capsule endoscopy (CE), deep enteroscopy using

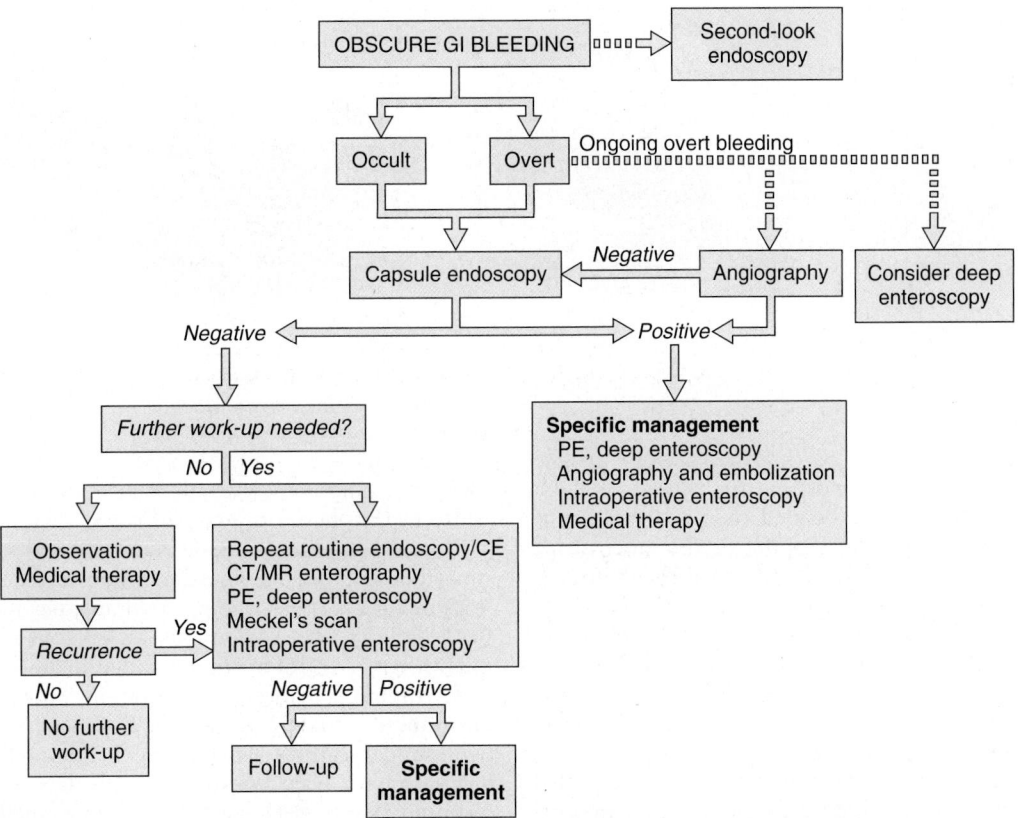

Fig. 15.4 Proposed algorithm for diagnosis and management of obscure gastrointestinal bleeding. CE, Capsule endoscopy; PE, push enteroscopy. *(Adapted from Pennazio M, Eisen G, Goldfarb N: ICCE consensus for obscure gastrointestinal bleeding. Endoscopy 37:1046–1050, 2005.)*

balloon-assisted or non–balloon-assisted techniques, and intraoperative enteroscopy (IOE). Radiologic testing includes barium studies such as small bowel follow-through and enteroclysis, nuclear medicine studies such as tagged red blood cell (RBC) scan and Meckel's scan, computed tomography (CT) and magnetic resonance (MR) imaging in combination with enteroclysis (CT and MR enterography), and angiography (**Fig. 15.4**).

Endoscopic Investigations

Repeat Upper Endoscopy (Esophagogastroduodenoscopy) and Colonoscopy

Second-look upper endoscopy may be helpful in identifying lesions potentially overlooked or unrecognized at the time of the initial endoscopic evaluation.[12] Data suggest that 20% of lesions leading to obscure GI bleeding may be overlooked and are within reach of a standard upper endoscope.[13] Commonly overlooked lesions in the upper GI tract include Cameron's erosions or ulcerations in large hiatal hernias, isolated gastric fundal varices, peptic ulcers, AVMs including gastric antral vascular ectasia (watermelon stomach), and Dieulafoy's lesion (**Fig. 15.5**).[14-16] An aortoenteric fistula should be considered in patients with prior abdominal aortic aneurysm repair. Although the reported yield of repeat colonoscopy is low (3% to 6%), it may be helpful in selected patients when the original colonoscopy examination was documented to have had a mediocre or poor preparation, the extent of the examination

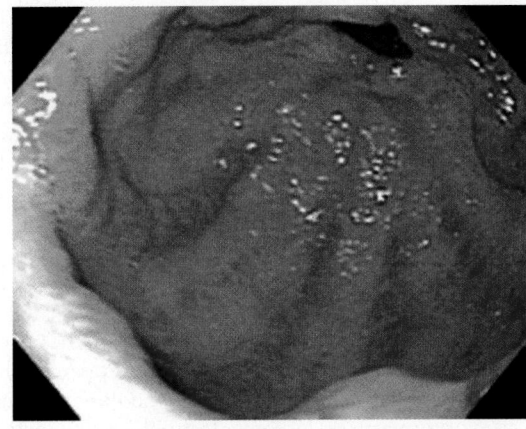

Fig. 15.5 Gastric antral vascular ectasia, also referred to as watermelon stomach.

was not to the cecum, or the terminal ileum was not evaluated.[17] Lesions missed or unrecognized during colonoscopy may include AVMs, polyps, solitary rectal ulcers, rectal varices, and neoplasms.

Push Enteroscopy

Push enteroscopy permits evaluation of the proximal small intestine to a distance that is approximately 50 to 100 cm beyond the ligament of Treitz. Dedicated videoenteroscopes (160 to 250 cm in length) are commercially available, but if these instruments are not available at the endoscopy site, a

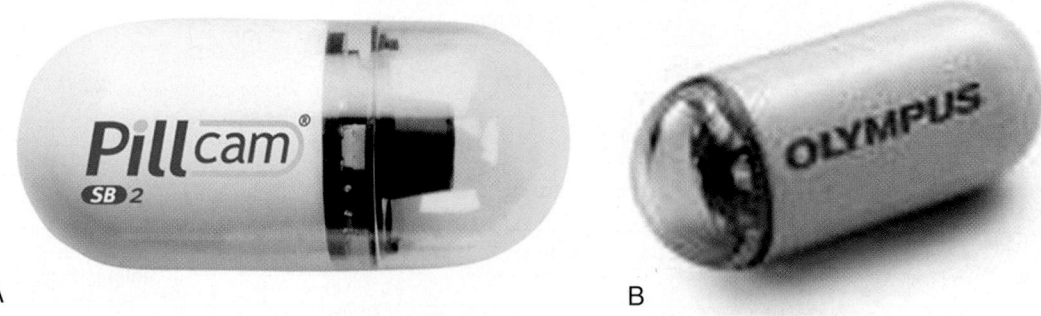

Fig. 15.6 **A,** Capsule endoscope (Pillcam SB 2). **B,** Capsule endoscope (Olympus EndoCapsule). (*A, Courtesy of Given Imaging Ltd, Yoqneam, Israel; B, courtesy of Olympus Corporation, Tokyo, Japan.*)

pediatric or standard adult colonoscope can be used instead.[18] The use of an overtube, back-loaded onto the endoscope insertion tube, may help limit looping of the enteroscope within the stomach and facilitate deeper small bowel intubation.[19] The diagnostic yield of push enteroscopy is reported to increase with greater depth of scope insertion. When using a pediatric or adult colonoscope, the reported diagnostic yield in the evaluation of obscure GI bleeding ranges from 13% to 38%. With the use of a dedicated videoenteroscope, reported diagnostic yield rates increase to 26% to 80%.[13,20,21]

With the development of endoscopic devices for dedicated videoenteroscopes, such as biopsy forceps, snares, thermal probes (contact and noncontact), and injection needles, push enteroscopy is preferred over radiologic diagnostic modalities because of the ability to obtain tissue, perform polypectomy or hemostasis if necessary, and mark lesion sites with India ink tattoo.[13] However, push enteroscopy does not allow for the visualization of the entire small bowel, and complications, including perforation and mucosal laceration, have been reported with the use of an overtube. With the advent of CE and "deep" enteroscopy, diagnostic push enteroscopy is less commonly used.

Capsule Endoscopy

CE is an endoscopic technology that is capable of obtaining endoscopic images from the entire small bowel.[22,23] CE is safe, easy, minimally invasive, and patient-friendly and has become a first-line tool in imaging small bowel pathologies. With this realization, there has been rapid uptake and wide acceptance of this revolutionary endoscopic technology for detecting small bowel abnormalities.[24]

The Pillcam SB video capsule endoscope (Given Imaging Ltd, Yoqneam, Israel) is a wireless capsule (11 mm × 26 mm) composed of a light source, lens, complementary metal oxide semiconductor imager, battery, and wireless transmitter. The Pillcam SB has a battery life of approximately 7 to 8 hours in which time the capsule captures two images per second (approximately 60,000 total images per examination) in a 140-degree field of view and 8:1 magnification.[25] The smooth outer coating of the capsule allows easy ingestion and prevents adhesion of intestinal contents, whereas the capsule moves via natural peristalsis from the mouth to the anus. Endoscopic images are transmitted via sensor arrays to a recording device worn as a belt by the patient. The recorded images are downloaded into a Reporting and Processing of Images and Data (RAPID) computer workstation and reviewed as a continuous video by the physician. The PillCam SB 2 video capsule offers advanced optics and a wider field of view for imaging the small bowel. It has the same dimensions as the PillCam SB and captures nearly twice the mucosal area per image compared with the PillCam SB. The PillCam SB 2 also provides Automatic Light Control for optimal illumination of each image.

Olympus (Olympus Corporation, Tokyo, Japan) has introduced a wireless capsule endoscope (EndoCapsule) with similar features. The Pillcam SB, Pillcam SB 2, and Endo-Capsule have been approved by the U.S. Food and Drug Administration (FDA) (**Fig. 15.6**). Other small bowel capsule endoscopes available in the marketplace but not yet approved by the FDA are the OMOM pill (Jinshan Science & Technology, Chongqing, China) and the MiroCam (Intromedic, Seoul, Korea).

Compared with other diagnostic modalities for evaluating obscure GI bleeding (e.g., small bowel series and enteroclysis, push enteroscopy, IOE), CE has been shown to have very good test characteristics and diagnostic yields in the range of 63% to 74%.[2] Patient selection is important and seems to influence the diagnostic yield of CE. CE performed close to the time of the bleeding event, hemoglobin less than 10 g/dL, recurrent episodes of bleeding, or persistent bleeding (>6 months) may increase CE diagnostic yield.[2] Limitations of CE include that at the present time biopsy, therapy, and endoscopic marking (e.g., India ink tattooing) are impossible. In addition, not all CE examinations reach the cecum (complete small bowel examination occurs approximately 80% to 85% of the time), and in some patients, luminal debris and bubbles interfere with viewing. Some physicians use polyethylene glycol–based preparations, prokinetic agents, simethicone, or a combination of these products before capsule ingestion.[26] Other limitations are that the imaging cannot be controlled or localized, and images are not viewed in real time.

Some patients may be unsuitable candidates for CE, including patients with cardiac pacemakers, patients with defibrillators, and patients with suspected small bowel obstruction. However, small case series suggest that CE, when performed with careful patient monitoring, is safe in patients with pacemakers and cardiac defibrillators.[2] Patients with swallowing disorders may have the capsule placed endoscopically into the duodenum using a capsule delivery device. Capsule retention is the major, and for all practical purposes, the only complication of CE. The reported incidence of capsule retention ranges from 0% in healthy volunteers, to 1.4% in patients with

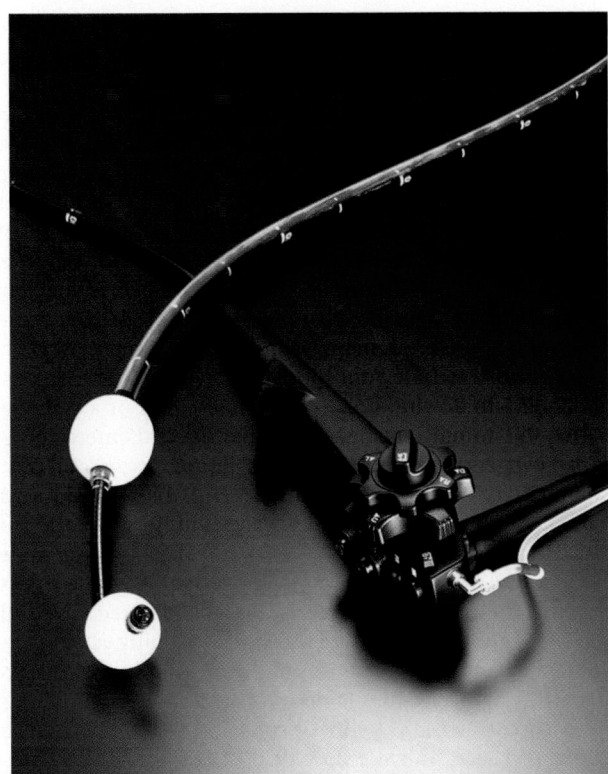

Fig. 15.7 Double-balloon enteroscope. *(Courtesy of Fujinon Inc, Saitama, Japan.)*

obscure GI hemorrhage, to 21% in patients with suspected small bowel obstruction.[27]

Double-Balloon Enteroscopy

Double-balloon enteroscopy (DBE), initially described and reported by Yamamoto and colleagues,[28] is a novel endoscopic insertion technique that attempts to improve on currently available endoscopic insertion methods to evaluate the entire length of the small bowel. The DBE system (Fujinon Inc, Saitama, Japan), uses a high-resolution, dedicated videoendoscope that has a working length of 200 cm and two soft, latex balloons: One balloon is attached to the tip of the endoscope, and the other is attached to the distal end of a soft, flexible overtube (**Fig. 15.7**). The balloons can be inflated and deflated using an air pump that is controlled by the endoscopist while monitoring air pressure.[29] The balloons grip the wall of the bowel, allowing the endoscope to be advanced without looping.

The procedure can be performed via an oral or anal approach with or without fluoroscopic guidance. Choice of oral or transanal approach may be dictated by suspicion for the location of a possible lesion as determined by preceding small bowel CE or other nonendoscopic small bowel imaging technique.[30,31] In a peroral approach, when the two balloons reach the duodenum, the overtube balloon is inflated to fix the overtube to the small bowel wall. The overtube is held in place as the endoscope is inserted further. Once the tip of the endoscope is maximally inserted, the balloon on the tip of the endoscope is inflated, the balloon on the overtube is deflated, and the overtube is advanced over the shaft of the endoscope. When the distal end of the overtube reaches the tip of the endoscope, the overtube balloon is reinflated, again fixing the

overtube to a second point on the small bowel wall. This sequence is repeated until the entire small bowel is evaluated or further advancement of the endoscope is difficult.[32]

Two types of double-balloon enteroscopes are available: one for general diagnostic use (EN-450P5) and one for therapeutic use (EN-450T5). The EN-450P5 is a thinner endoscope with an external diameter of 8.5 mm and maximum working channel diameter of 2.2 mm. The EN450T5 has an external diameter of 9.4 mm and working channel of 2.8 mm.[29] DBE has been shown to be able to visualize the entire length of the small bowel and allows for biopsy, marking of lesions for subsequent surgical resection (e.g., India ink tattoo), and therapeutics.

Published studies evaluating DBE for obscure GI bleeding have reported diagnostic yields ranging from 40% to 80% and diagnostic or treatment success in 43% to 76% of cases.[2] Limitations of DBE include concerns about the endoscopic learning curve, common need for endoscopy on two separate days (peroral followed by transanal approach), limitations in visualization of the entire small bowel, miss rates for submucosal lesions owing to insufflation issues, time-consuming procedure that also requires a high level of ancillary staffing, increased sedation requirements (including possible anesthesiology support), and patient tolerance and preferences. Although initial reports of complete evaluation of the small bowel using DBE were encouraging, subsequent studies have failed to show similar results.[2] In addition, although uncommon, the reported incidence of severe complications associated with DBE has ranged from 0% to 2.5% and has included pancreatitis, perforations, bleeding, abdominal pain, and fever.[29]

Single-Balloon Enteroscopy

A novel balloon enteroscope system has been developed more recently using only a single balloon (single-balloon enteroscopy [SBE]) (**Fig. 15.8**). The endoscopist needs to manipulate only one balloon, and time and complexity for preparation of the system and for the examination itself may be reduced.[33] Data for the SBE system to compare its performance and safety profile with DBE are sparse.[34] In the limited literature available, SBE seems to provide similar diagnostic and therapeutic yield compared with DBE.[35,36] SBE is performed using the SBE endoscope system (SIF-Q180, Olympus Optical Co, Ltd, Tokyo, Japan). The SBE endoscope consists of a 200-cm long videoendoscope with an outer diameter of 9.2 mm and a flexible overtube with a length of 140 cm and an outer diameter of 13.2 mm. One single silicone balloon is attached to the tip of the overtube. The insertion process follows the method used for DBE, but instead of inflation of the endoscope balloon, the tip of the endoscope may be optionally angulated during the pullback or straightening of the enteroscope and balloon-inflated overtube.[37] Similar to DBE, SBE can be performed via an oral or transanal approach, according to suspicion for the location of a possible small bowel lesion.

Spiral Enteroscopy

Spiral enteroscopy is an alternative technique for accomplishing deep small bowel intubation that uses a special overtube (Endo-Ease, Discovery Small Bowel (DSB), Spirus Medical) to pleat the small bowel onto itself (**Fig. 15.9**).[38] The DSB overtube can be paired with existing enteroscopes or colonoscopes.

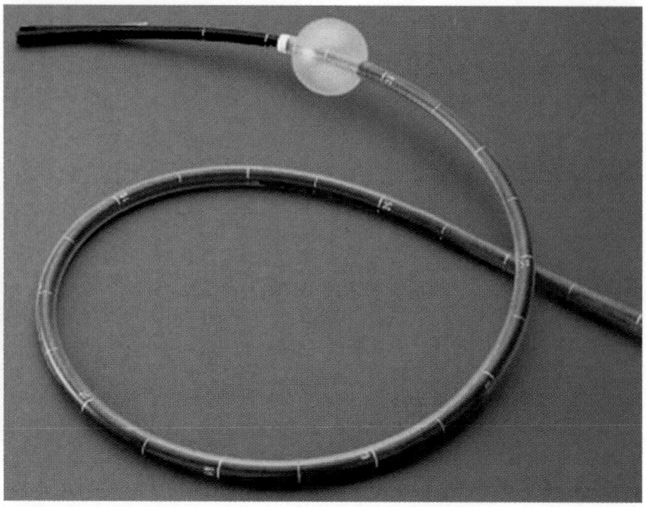

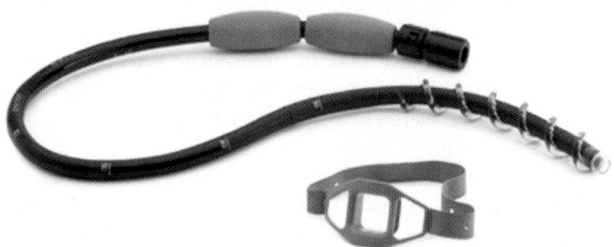

Fig. 15.8 Single-balloon enteroscope. *(Courtesy of Olympus Optical Co, Ltd, Tokyo, Japan.)*

Fig. 15.9 Spiral enteroscope. *(Courtesy of Spirus Medical.)*

Rotation of the DSB beyond the ligament of Treitz allows the manually rotating overtube with an outer fixed spiral coil to pleat the small bowel onto the overtube. Preliminary data suggest that use of the Endo-Ease DSB overtube for enteroscopy is a safe and effective technique for visualization of the small bowel.[39] Studies of spiral enteroscopy have shown diagnostic yield, total time of procedure, and depth of small bowel insertion to compare favorably with DBE and SBE.[40] The strengths of spiral enteroscopy are rapid advancement in the small bowel and controlled, stable withdrawal that facilitates endoscopic therapy.

Intraoperative Enteroscopy

Exploratory laparotomy with IOE has been used since the 1980s and is a diagnostic and potentially therapeutic endoscopic modality in suspected small bowel disease.[41,42] IOE is considered to be the ultimate endoscopic evaluation of the small bowel. In addition to being able to diagnose small bowel sources of obscure bleeding, IOE allows for identification of lesions for definitive surgical resection. Using an orally passed colonoscope or, more optimally, a dedicated small bowel videoenteroscope, the endoscope is either advanced beyond the ligament of Treitz into the proximal jejunum or advanced into a mid–small bowel enterotomy. The latter technique expedites the examination, especially of the distal small bowel, and minimizes the potential for iatrogenic trauma to the small bowel arising from excessive manipulation that can arise from

peroral passage. At that point, the surgeon gently telescopes the small bowel over the shaft of the endoscope, allowing for the careful inspection of the mucosa.

Inspection of the small bowel mucosa should be performed in an anterograde manner. When using a mid–small bowel enterotomy, the endoscope is first advanced toward the cecum and then redirected toward the stomach. Dimming the operating room lights facilitates endoscopic visualization and extrinsic inspection of the bowel by the surgeons. Lesions identified endoscopically can be marked for resection by the surgeon with a suture placed on the serosal aspect of the bowel. After completion of the enteroscopy and withdrawal of the endoscope, the marked sites can be surgically resected. An alternative approach to IOE involves insertion of a sterilized endoscope through multiple, surgically created enterotomies, rectal insertion, or laparoscopy-assisted enteroscopy.

Reported complications associated with IOE include mucosal lacerations, perforations, prolonged ileus, abdominal abscess, and bowel ischemia.[41,42] Because of its invasive nature and potential for complications, the decision to perform IOE must not be made lightly. All risks and benefits need to be fully considered and explained well to the patient; only experienced endoscopists and surgeons should perform this procedure. Currently, this technique is reserved as a last option if deep enteroscopy using DBE, SBE, or spiral enteroscopy cannot be performed successfully because of the presence of abdominal adhesions, obesity, or other technical factors.

Small Bowel Contrast Radiography

A small bowel series (upper GI series with small bowel follow-through) involves the oral ingestion of a dilute barium solution with serial abdominal images obtained of the small bowel. Enteroclysis is a double-contrast study performed by passing a tube into the proximal small bowel and injecting barium, methylcellulose, and air.[43] This technique is considered to be superior to standard small bowel follow-through.[44] An upper GI series with small bowel follow-through is sometimes used to evaluate obscure GI bleeding either before performing push enteroscopy or after a negative push enteroscopy examination.

The role of small bowel series and enteroclysis in the evaluation of obscure GI bleeding has declined substantially because of low diagnostic yield (0% to 6% for small bowel follow-through and 10% to 25% for enteroclysis) and the advent of improved endoscopic diagnostic techniques for the small bowel.[45,46] In addition to limited diagnostic sensitivity in obscure GI bleeding, enteroclysis can be uncomfortable for the patient and involves more radiation exposure than small bowel follow-through. Generally, the role of enteroclysis in the evaluation of obscure GI bleeding is limited to settings in which CE and enteroscopy are unavailable or contraindicated, such as clinical situations that suggest small bowel obstruction secondary to malignancy, Crohn's disease, or prior significant NSAID use. Otherwise, there is little or no role today for either small bowel series or enteroclysis in the evaluation of obscure GI bleeding.

Cross-Sectional Imaging

Novel cross-sectional imaging techniques for evaluation of the small bowel include helical CT enteroclysis, helical CT angiography, and MR enteroclysis.[2] Helical CT enteroclysis combines standard enteroclysis to distend the small bowel followed by helical CT.[47] More recent reports suggest the utility of helical CT in identifying small and large intestinal bleeding angiectasias.[48,49] Further research and clinical experience should define the precise role of CT enteroclysis in the investigation of small bowel disease.

CT angiography involves catheterization of the abdominal aorta followed by helical CT angiography before and after intraarterial injections of a contrast medium. The site of hemorrhage is recognized as a hyperdense area owing to the extravasation of contrast medium into the intestinal lumen. In a prospective study of 18 patients with bleeding colonic angiectasis, the sensitivity, specificity, and positive predictive value of helical CT angiography were 70%, 100%, and 100% compared with a "gold standard" of colonoscopy and mesenteric angiography.[50] In a report of 22 patients with obscure GI bleeding, CT enteroclysis was found to be inferior to CE in the detection of potential bleeding lesions such as angiectasis in the small bowel.[51]

Nuclear Medicine Scans

Tagged RBC scans are noninvasive, safe, and readily available. Most commonly performed with technetium-labeled RBCs, a radionuclide bleeding scan detects bleeding that is occurring at a rate of 0.1 to 0.5 mL/min. It is of little or no value in patients with obscure-occult bleeding who appear to have a low rate of blood loss because the rate of bleeding is too slow to be detected. Bleeding scans may be more sensitive than angiography but less specific than either a positive endoscopic or angiographic examination.[52,53] Early scans (up to 4 hours after initial injection) may be helpful in gross localization of bleeding when the rate of blood loss exceeds 0.1 to 0.5 mL/min. Tagged RBC scans can identify only a general area of bleeding, however, and assessment with other diagnostic modalities such as angiography is often necessary after nuclear scans. The role of nuclear scans continues to be limited in patients with obscure GI bleeding, and the ability to localize the source of bleeding accurately is poor.[54]

Angiography

The data on the clinical utility of angiography in the setting of obscure GI bleeding are very limited.[55] Compared with tagged RBC scans, mesenteric angiography is more likely to document the specific site of bleeding, yet the rate of bleeding must be greater than 0.5 mL/min. Angiography can also identify lesions that are not actively bleeding because of demonstration of typical vascular features seen in vascular ectasia (e.g., slow-emptying veins, vascular tuft, and early-filling veins) and tumors. It is possible to administer embolization therapy if an amenable lesion is detected.

Provocation angiography using anticoagulation, vasodilators, or thrombolytic agents may increase the likelihood that

a source of bleeding can be identified and has been advocated by some investigators.[56,57] However, the risk of inducing uncontrolled bleeding limits the use of this technique. As noted with tagged RBC scans, the utility of mesenteric angiography in the evaluation of patients with obscure GI bleeding is limited, and it is not commonly recommended.

Proposed Diagnostic Strategy

In a patient with obscure GI bleeding, defined as careful, quality endoscopic examinations (EGD plus ileocolonoscopy) being negative, the small bowel should be assumed to be the source of blood loss. Unless contraindicated, CE should be the next method of small bowel evaluation (see **Fig. 15.4**).[2,58] In patients with obscure overt bleeding, data support the role of expedited CE.[12,59] CE performed closer to the episode of obscure overt bleeding has a higher likelihood of finding the site of small bowel bleeding.[12,59] If CE defines a small bowel source of obscure bleeding, appropriate specific therapy may be instituted (e.g., endoscopic, surgical, or pharmacologic). If no small bowel source is identified, a decision must be made as to whether additional diagnostic evaluations are immediately indicated (e.g., repeat EGD with or without ileocolonoscopy, repeat CE, Meckel's scan in pediatric and young adult patients) or a period of "watchful waiting" may be warranted.

Pharmacologic Therapy

Pharmacotherapy should be considered whenever endoscopic therapy, surgical intervention, or angiographic therapy is impractical or ineffective, such as in patients in whom the source and the etiology of bleeding remains undefined or the underlying bleeding pathology is too diffuse to be amenable to ablative therapies. The role of hormonal therapy continues to be most debated.[60,61] Somatostatin and its analogue octreotide have been anecdotally reported to be beneficial in patients with obscure GI bleeding from angiectasis and blue rubber bleb nevus syndrome, possibly secondary to their inhibitory effect on angiogenesis and splanchnic blood flow.[62–64] A beneficial effect of thalidomide and its antiangiogenic effects in patients with obscure GI bleeding secondary to angiectasis and hereditary hemorrhagic telangiectasia has also been reported.[65,66] In a case report, erythropoietin was believed to stop chronic diffuse hemorrhage from the GI mucosa. The exact mechanism of erythropoietin is unknown but may be related to the complex effect of erythropoietin on the platelet-subendothelial interactions and on protein C, protein S, and anti–thrombin III levels.[67]

References

The complete reference list is available online at www.expertconsult.com.

Chapter 16

Chronic Gastrointestinal Bleeding

Miguel Muñoz-Navas and Maite Betés Ibáñez

Introduction

Chronic gastrointestinal (GI) hemorrhage may be overt or occult. Overt bleeding is defined as chronic if it is persistent but not severe enough to cause circulatory compromise. It may be seen in the form of melena or red rectal bleeding. If bleeding is occult, the clinical presentation is anemia, and evidence of occult bleeding is found on testing of the stools. In some patients, chronic hemorrhage may be clinically interspersed with acute episodes.[1] Acute GI bleeding is discussed in detail in other chapters.

Chronic GI bleeding includes common clinical scenarios, yet the meaning and diagnostic criteria for the different terms are not well delineated.[2] Chronic bleeding from the gut is always significant; in particular, malignant tumors of the gut that are curable may be present. There is no universal agreement regarding the nomenclature of GI lesions that can cause chronic bleeding. Development of new technology, mainly wireless video capsule endoscopy and balloon-assisted enter-

oscopy has provided an opportunity to revisit the traditional classifications of the source of GI bleeding into upper or lower GI bleeding based on the location of the bleeding either proximal or distal to the ligament of Treitz.[3]

Some authors propose reclassifying GI bleeding into three categories: upper GI, mid-GI, and lower GI bleeding. Bleeding above the ampulla of Vater, within the reach of esophagogastroduodenoscopy (EGD), is defined as upper GI bleeding; small intestinal bleeding from the ampulla of Vater to the terminal ileum, best investigated by capsule endoscopy and balloon-assisted enteroscopy, is defined as mid-GI bleeding; and colonic bleeding, which can be evaluated by colonoscopy, is defined as lower GI bleeding. A simple classification is presented in **Table 16.1**. This chapter discusses some of the most frequent causes of chronic GI bleeding. Vascular lesions are an important cause of chronic GI bleeding. They may be solitary, multiple, or diffuse and may exist as isolated abnormalities or be part of a syndrome or a systemic disorder. The internationally accepted term for the endoscopic finding of a mucosally

Table 16.1 Causes of Chronic Gastrointestinal Bleeding

Gastrointestinal Lesions	
Within Reach of Upper Endoscope	**May Be beyond Reach of Upper Endoscope**
Esophagitis	Celiac sprue
Cameron's erosions	Crohn's disease
Peptic ulcer disease	Intestinal lymphoma
Gastritis and erosions	Small bowel angiodysplasia
Duodenitis and erosions	Small bowel tumors
Angiodysplasia	Small bowel ulcers and erosions, including NSAID- and other drug-induced lesions
Portal hypertensive gastropathy	Small bowel diverticulosis
Gastroesophageal cancer	Small bowel varices
Gastric or duodenal polyps	Lymphangioma
Gastroduodenal lymphoma	Radiation enteritis
Partial gastrectomy	Blue rubber bleb nevus syndrome
GAVE	Osler-Weber-Rendu syndrome
Dieulafoy's lesion	Small bowel polyposis syndromes
	Gardner's syndrome
	Amyloidosis
	Meckel's diverticulum
	Hemosuccus pancreaticus, hemobilia
	Klippel-Trénaunay-Weber syndrome
Colonic Lesions	
Colon polyps Colon cancer Angiodysplasia Colonic ulcers Colitis and IBD Parasitic infestation Hemorrhoids Diverticular bleeding	

GAVE, Gastric antral vascular ectasia; IBD, inflammatory bowel disease; NSAID, nonsteroidal antiinflammatory drug.

based vascular malformation is *angiectasis*. The categorization of vascular abnormalities in the GI tract has been inconsistent and a source of confusion.[4,5] It can be based on histologic characteristics, gross appearance, or association with systemic diseases. These considerations permit categorization into three broad groups, as follows:

1. *Vascular tumors,* which can be benign (e.g., hemangiomas) or malignant (e.g., Kaposi's sarcoma or angiosarcoma)
2. *Vascular anomalies* associated with congenital or systemic diseases, such as blue rubber bleb nevus syndrome, Klippel-Trénaunay-Weber syndrome, Ehlers-

Danlos syndrome, pseudoxanthoma elasticum, the CREST (*c*alcinosis, *R*aynaud's phenomenon, *e*sophageal dysmotility, *s*cleroderma, and *t*elangiectases) variant of scleroderma, and hereditary hemorrhagic telangiectasia
3. *Acquired or sporadic lesions,* such as angiodysplasias, gastric antral vascular ectasia (GAVE), radiation-induced vascular ectasias, and Dieulafoy's lesions.

Angiodysplasia of the Gastrointestinal Tract

Vascular ectasia of the GI tract, also referred to as angiodysplasia or less accurately as arteriovenous malformation, is a distinct clinical and pathologic entity.[6–8] It is the most common vascular abnormality of the GI tract and probably the most frequent cause of lower intestinal bleeding in patients older than 60 years. Although the terms *angiodysplasia* and *arteriovenous malformation* have been used synonymously, the term *angiodysplasia* (Greek *angeion*, "vessel"; *dys*, "bad" or "difficult"; *plasis*, "a molding"), means a poorly formed vessel but with a lesser connotation of congenital origin than with the word *malformation*. Angiodysplasias are usually distinguished from telangiectasias, which, although anatomically similar, are usually referred to in the context of systemic or hereditary diseases. Because most vascular abnormalities are detected during endoscopy, a classification based on endoscopic appearance has been proposed.[9] The classification system recognizes the location, size, and number of angiodysplasias.

Pathogenesis

Angiodysplasias are composed of ectatic, dilated, thin-walled vessels that are lined by endothelium alone or by only small amounts of smooth muscle. Their anatomy has been best shown by studies in which casts of the vessels were made by injecting a silicone material.[10] These studies showed that dilated tortuous submucosal veins are the most prominent feature in angiodysplasias. Small arteriovenous communications are present because of incompetence of the precapillary sphincter. Enlarged arteries are also present in bigger angiodysplasias and may be associated with arteriovenous fistulas, which explains why bleeding can be a risk in some patients.

Histologic examination shows dilated vessels in the mucosa and submucosa, sometimes covered by a single layer of surface epithelium. These features are shared by angiodysplasias in the colon and stomach.[11] Increased expression of angiogenic factors has been found in human colonic angiodysplasias.[12] The pathogenesis of angiodysplasias is not well understood. Four theories have been proposed, as follows:

1. Angiodysplasias may develop in response to chronic partial, intermittent, low-grade obstruction of the submucosal veins at the point where they penetrate the muscle layers of the colon.[10] Following this logic, the prevalence of vascular ectasias in the right colon can be attributed to a greater tension in the cecal wall compared with other parts of the colon, according to LaPlace's principle. Over many years, repeated contraction and distention of the cecum results in dilation and tortuosity of the submucosal vein and, later, the venules

and capillaries draining into it. Finally, the capillary rings dilate, the precapillary sphincters become incompetent, and a tiny arteriovenous fistula develops.

2. Angiodysplasias may be a complication of chronic mucosal ischemia, which can occur during episodes of bowel obstruction or straining stools.[13]
3. Angiodysplasias may be a complication of local ischemia associated with cardiac, vascular, or pulmonary disease.[14]
4. Angiodysplasias may be congenital, which is probably more likely in young patients or patients who have angiodysplasias associated with congenital diseases.

Epidemiology and Natural History

The prevalence of GI angiodysplasias in the overall population is not well known because asymptomatic individuals usually do not undergo endoscopic evaluation. Angiectases have been seen in 0.2% to 2.9% of "nonbleeding persons"[15,16] and in 2.6% to 6.2% of patients evaluated specifically for occult blood in the stool, anemia, or hemorrhage.[15–17] Angiodysplasias occur most often in the colon, where they are an important cause of lower GI bleeding, particularly in patients older than 60,[18–20] although presentation in patients in their 30s has been described.[21] There is no gender predilection.

Clinical Manifestations

Angiodysplasias can remain clinically silent or cause bleeding. The estimated incidence of active GI bleed in patients with angiodysplasia is less than 10%. These lesions may be located throughout the GI tract with a variable rate of bleeding associated with them and presentation ranging from hematemesis or hematochezia to occult anemia.[3,22] Bleeding is usually chronic or recurrent and, in most cases, low grade and painless.

GI bleeding from small bowel lesions has occurred in 22% of patients in whom angiodysplasia of the colon was the presumed index source of bleeding. In 40% to 60% of patients with gastric and duodenal angiodysplasia, multiple lesions are observed at endoscopy. Colonic lesions are associated in 15% to 20% of these patients. In addition, angiodysplastic lesions in the colon are frequently multiple. To diagnose and treat patients with suspected angiodysplasia, the propensity for multiplicity at different levels within the gut must be considered. Hematemesis can rarely be observed in patients with angiodysplasia of the upper GI tract. Presentation with hemodynamically well-compensated, chronic bleeding is more typical. Bleeding from colonic lesions most often is chronic, intermittent, and low grade, with 15% of patients presenting with acute hemorrhage.

Patients with colonic angiodysplasia may present with hematochezia (0% to 60%), melena (0% to 26%), Hemoccult-positive stool (4% to 47%), or iron deficiency anemia (0% to 51%). Melena occurs in at least one-fourth of patients with colonic bleeding. The nature and degree of bleeding frequently vary in the same patient with different episodes, and patients may have bright red blood, maroon-colored stools, and melena on separate occasions. In 20% to 25% of episodes, only tarry stools are passed, and in 10% to 15% of patients, bleeding is evidenced only by iron deficiency anemia, with stools that are intermittently positive for occult blood.[23] With effective diag-

nostic and therapeutic endoscopy, the percentage of patients who have had operations has decreased because most lesions are being identified and treated at the time of the first episode.[24] Angiodysplasia can be confidently considered to be a source of GI bleeding in an anemic patient only if it is seen to be actively bleeding. The risk of bleeding in patients who are incidentally found to have nonbleeding colonic angiodysplasia is unknown. The number of lesions and the presence of coexisting coagulopathy or platelet dysfunction may increase the risk for bleeding. Patients who have bled from colonic angiodysplasias are at increased risk for subsequent bleeding.[10]

Stomach and Duodenum

Angiodysplasias of the stomach have been found to be the cause of blood loss in 4% to 7% of patients with GI bleeding.[18,25] Angiodysplasias in the stomach or duodenum are found incidentally in approximately 50% of cases.[26]

The risk that an incidentally found gastric or duodenal angiodysplasia will subsequently bleed is uncertain. Patients who have bled from gastric or duodenal angiodysplasias do rebleed. This rebleeding was illustrated in a series of 30 patients with gastric or duodenal angiodysplasias; 77% had experienced at least one episode of overt bleeding before diagnosis.[18]

Small Intestine

Approximately 5% of patients presenting with GI hemorrhage have no source found by upper endoscopy and colonoscopy. In approximately 75% of these patients, responsible lesions can be detected in the small bowel. In patients presenting with obscure overt bleeding (defined as the presence of recurrent melena or hematochezia with normal evaluation by upper endoscopy and colonoscopy), small bowel angiectases are detected in 30% to 60% of examinations.[3,27]

Colon

The colon is the most common site of angiodysplasias in the GI tract; colonic lesions are most often found in the cecum and ascending colon. In some reported experiences, angiodysplasias of the colon account for approximately 20% to 30% of cases of acute lower GI bleeding, approaching the frequency of acute colonic diverticular bleeding.[28] Foutch and colleagues[29] noted the prevalence of angiodysplasia to be 0.93% from three prospective studies in which screening colonoscopies were performed in 964 asymptomatic individuals (mean age 61 years).

Conditions with Increased Prevalence
End-Stage Renal Disease

Angiodysplasia is the second most common cause of GI bleeding in patients with end-stage renal disease.[30] These lesions account for about 20% of upper GI bleeds and 30% of lower GI bleeds[30] and approximately 50% of recurrent upper GI bleeds.[31] In a prospective study of upper GI hemorrhage over a 50-month period, vascular ectasia was the etiology of upper GI hemorrhage in 13% of patients with renal insufficiency and was the etiology of bleeding more often in patients with renal insufficiency than in patients with normal renal function.[32] The prevalence of vascular ectasia as a cause of upper GI bleeding was related to the duration of renal failure and the requirement of hemodialysis. The lesions can occur anywhere along the GI tract and are usually multiple.[31] The reason for the increased prevalence among patients with end-stage renal disease is unknown. One possible explanation is that the lesions are detected more frequently because of the increased risk of bleeding associated with uremia-induced platelet dysfunction.

von Willebrand's Disease

The association of abnormal von Willebrand's factor (vWF) is receiving increasing attention in the management of patients with bleeding GI angiectasias. von Willebrand's disease is a bleeding disorder that results from a qualitative or quantitative defect in vWF. vWF is a complex multimeric glycoprotein present in platelets, plasma, and subendothelium. vWF is essential to platelet adhesion and aggregation at the site of vascular injury. In a study of patients with both bleeding and nonbleeding angiectasias of the GI tract and control patients with colonic diverticular hemorrhage, Veyradier and associates[33] showed that most patients with bleeding angiectasias of the GI tract lack the largest multimers of vWF induced by a latent acquired form of von Willebrand's disease. Because these specific multimers are the most effective in inducing platelet aggregation in high shear stress that is commonly present in the microcirculation of angiectasias, it was concluded their deficiency contributes to active bleeding.

An association between angiodysplasias and congenital or acquired von Willebrand's disease had been reported previously.[34,35] Patients with angiodysplasia found on endoscopy were prospectively tested for von Willebrand's disease at the Mayo Clinic, but no associations were identified.

Aortic Stenosis

Approximately 50% of patients with bleeding vascular ectasias have evidence of cardiac disease, and 25% have been reported to have aortic stenosis. Bleeding from angiodysplasias in patients with aortic stenosis (Heyde's syndrome) has been repeatedly reported but is highly controversial.[36] In support of this relationship is the observation that bleeding may be improved after aortic valve replacement.[37–39] Two possible explanations have been proposed to explain this observation. Patients with aortic stenosis may develop an acquired form of von Willebrand's disease, which can be reversed after aortic valve replacement.[33,40,41] The mechanism is thought to involve mechanical disruption of vWF multimers during turbulent passage through the narrowed valve.[42] Patients with aortic stenosis may be more likely to bleed from existing angiodysplasias. The observation that angiodysplasias persist after aortic valve replacement despite the fact that bleeding stops supports this hypothesis.[11,43] Another explanation is that existing angiodysplasias may bleed as a result of ischemic necrosis in patients who have a low cardiac output.[13,43] However, this explanation is inconsistent with the observations that bleeding angiodysplasias have not been observed with other forms of heart disease associated with a low cardiac output and that a low cardiac output is a late complication of aortic stenosis.

Several retrospective, uncontrolled studies[44,45] and a prospective, controlled investigation[46] do not substantiate a causative role or association of aortic valve diseases with colonic angiectases. Replacement of the aortic valve for control of bleeding secondary to these vascular lesions is not universally accepted.[24] A logical approach to patients with both lesions is to treat the colonic lesion first endoscopically, regardless of whether the patient's cardiac status warrants surgery. If valve replacement is necessary and endoscopic therapy is unsuccessful, further endoscopic or surgical treatment of the colonic angiodysplasia should be delayed until after cardiac surgery. Further attempts at endoscopic treatment or surgical resection are indicated if bleeding recurs.[47] The association between chronic GI bleeding in elderly patients and aortic stenosis becomes more relevant with the advent of transcatheter aortic valve implantation that can be offered even to elderly patients with comorbidities, which could make conventional surgery impossible.[48]

Progressive Systemic Sclerosis

Vascular lesions are a prominent feature of progressive systemic sclerosis, especially in the CREST variant.[49] Angiodysplasias are usually distinguished from telangiectases, which, although anatomically similar, are usually referred to in the context of systemic or hereditary diseases. In patients with progressive systemic sclerosis, sites most frequently involved by telangiectases are the hands, lips, tongue, and face, but gastric, intestinal, and colorectal lesions have been reported. These lesions may be the source of occult or clinically significant bleeding and are best treated by endoscopic coagulation.[50]

Diagnosis

Angiectases have a characteristic appearance of a cherry-red, fernlike pattern of arborizing, ectatic blood vessels radiating from a central vessel (**Fig. 16.1**). This pattern should be specifically looked for because angiectases may be confused with other erythematous mucosal lesions or with normal vessels (**Table 16.2**).[24,51] Because traumatic and endoscopic suction artifacts may resemble vascular lesions, all lesions must be evaluated immediately on insertion of the colonoscope, rather than during withdrawal. "Anemic halos" are often seen surrounding angiectases of the bowel. Although these "halos" do not differentiate the various types of vascular lesions, they distinguish true vascular lesions from artifacts.[47] Newer alternative imaging options, such as narrow band imaging, allow precise discrimination of vascular structures from artifactual mucosal hemorrhage. Punch biopsy samples of vascular lesions obtained during endoscopy are usually nonspecific; the bleeding induced by performing biopsies of these abnormalities is not justified.

Angiectases may be difficult to visualize during colonoscopy in patients who do not have an optimal bowel cleaning. Because the appearance of angiectases is influenced by blood pressure, blood volume, and state of hydration, these lesions may not be evident in patients with severely reduced blood volumes or who are in shock until red blood cell and volume deficits are corrected. Cold water lavage of the colon, as is sometimes done to clean the luminal surface from debris during colonoscopy, reportedly may mask these lesions.[52]

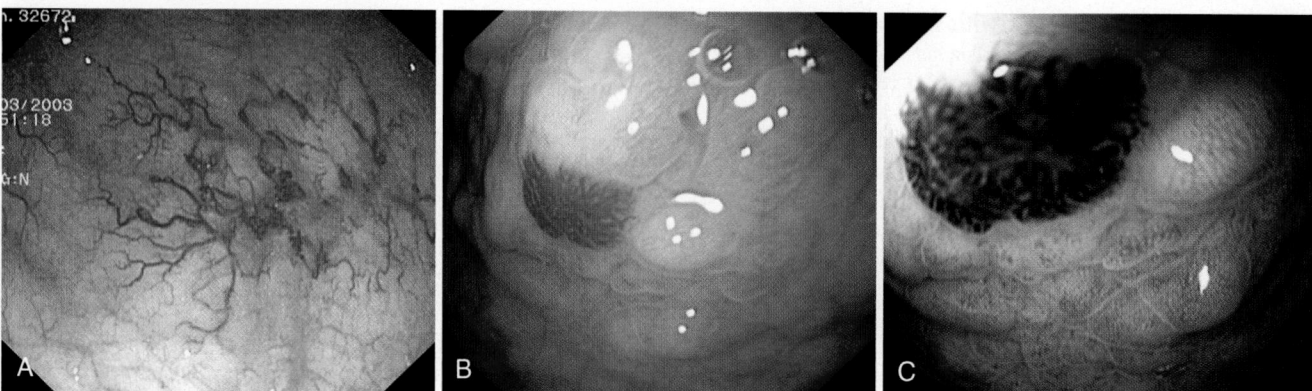

Fig. 16.1 A, Typical angiodysplasia in right colon. Angiodysplastic lesions are seen as slightly dilated tortuous vessels. **B,** Angiodysplasia in the stomach. **C,** Narrow band imaging of same lesion.

Table 16.2 **Lesions Confused with Angiectasias on Endoscopy**

Vascular	Nonvascular	Colitis
Arteriovenous malformations	Trauma	Ischemic
Angiomas	Polyps	Infectious
Phlebectasia	Adenomatous	Radiation (acute)
Varices	Hyperplastic	Inflammatory bowel disease
Venous stars	Lymphoid	

Meperidine also has been implicated in masking lesions because of a transient decrease in mucosal blood flow. Minimizing use of meperidine and reversal with naloxone to increase the yield of detection have been advocated by some clinicians. Naloxone has been reported to enhance the appearance of normal vasculature in about 10% of patients and to cause angiectases to appear (2.7%) or increase in size (5.4%).[53] Reversal of narcotic analgesia may affect the comfort of an examination, particularly if therapeutics are performed.

Some patients presenting with GI bleeding have no source found by upper endoscopy and colonoscopy.[3] In these cases of obscure chronic GI bleeding, endoscopic examination of the small bowel has been limited by several factors. The length of the small intestine, in addition to its free intraperitoneal location, vigorous contractility, and overlying loops, confounds the usual diagnostic techniques, including barium studies, endoscopic intubation, and identification of specific sites by special imaging techniques of nuclear medicine scans and angiography. The bleeding rate may be slow or intermittent, not allowing identification by either angiography or radionuclide bleeding scan. Because of the inability to localize a bleeding site in the small bowel, patients with obscure GI bleeding from a small bowel source typically presented with prolonged occult blood loss or recurrent episodes of melena or maroon stool without a specific diagnosis. In this group of patients, previous noninvasive tests, such as small bowel follow-through, radioisotope-labeled red blood cell scan, and push enteroscopy, have had suboptimal diagnostic yields of 20% to 40%. Invasive methods, such as laparotomy or intraoperative enteroscopy, may improve the yield up to 70%.[54]

For patients with obscure chronic GI bleeding, an early diagnosis of the bleeding site was the exception rather than the norm until more recently with the development of capsule endoscopy and balloon-assisted enteroscopy. The last American Gastroenterological Association Institute medical position statement on obscure GI bleeding considered that for patients with obscure GI bleeding and associated anemia or overt bleeding, repeat endoscopic examinations can be worthwhile.[55] Useful adjunctive diagnostic maneuvers include use of a cap-fitted endoscope to examine blind areas, such as the high lesser curve, under the incisura angularis, and the posterior wall of the duodenal bulb; use of a side-viewing endoscope to examine the ampulla in patients with suspected pancreaticobiliary pathology; and use of a push enteroscope to examine the C-loop of duodenum carefully after injection of glucagons. Although the yield is low (6%), repeat colonoscopy may be useful in the setting of prior poor bowel preparation. Use of naloxone may improve the detection of colonic angiectases that were not obvious at the index examination.[3]

When all the findings on standard examinations (EGD and colonoscopy) are negative, the small bowel may be assumed to be the source of blood loss. Capsule endoscopy should be the third test in the evaluation of patients with GI bleeding.

Capsule Endoscopy

The first capsule endoscope, referred to as the M2A ("mouth to anus"), was approved for clinical use late in 2001. The capsule endoscope is a wireless miniature camera that can be swallowed to obtain images of the GI mucosa; the camera contains a light source, batteries, and a radio transmitter. Video images are transmitted via radiotelemetry to a skin surface patterned antenna that allows images to be captured and localizes the relative position of each image in the abdomen.[56] In July 2003, the capsule endoscope was approved by the U.S. Food and Drug Administration (FDA) as a first-line tool for the detection of abnormalities of the small bowel, based on evidence provided by a meta-analysis (**Fig. 16.2**). M2A was renamed PillCam SB (SB means "small bowel").[57]

Obscure GI bleeding is the main clinical indication for capsule endoscopy; approximately 70% to 80% of patients undergo capsule endoscopy for this indication. The American Society for Gastrointestinal Endoscopy (ASGE) Technology Assessment Committee concluded that capsule endoscopy provided superior yield compared with radiographic contrast

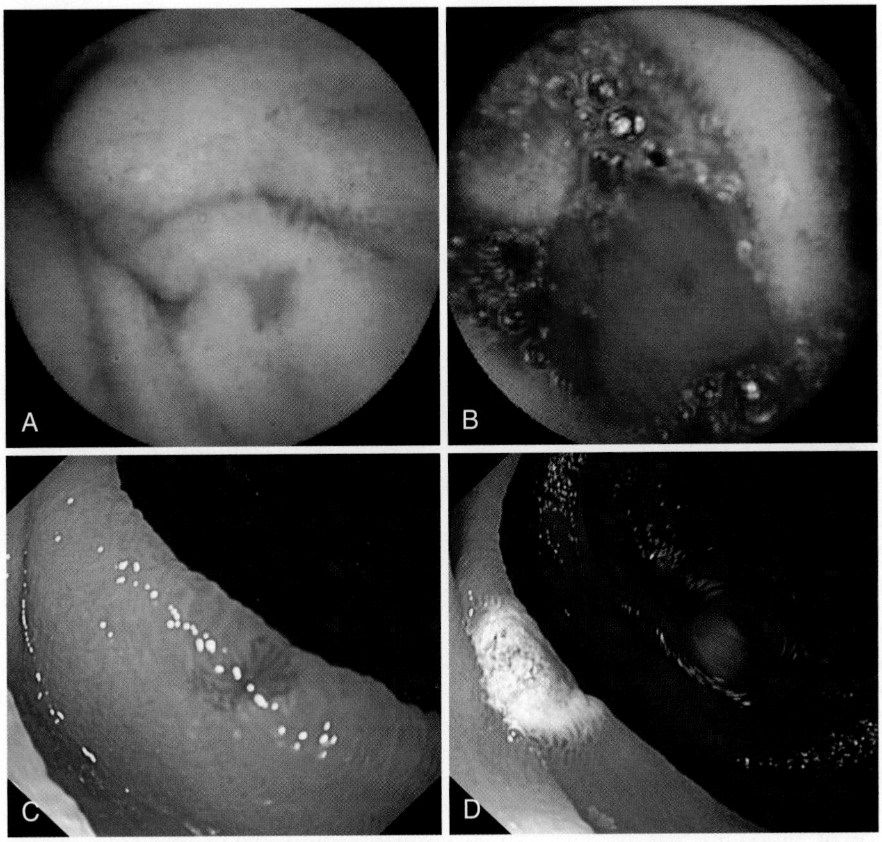

Fig. 16.2 Small bowel angiodysplasias in patients with obscure gastrointestinal bleeding. **A,** Nonbleeding angiodysplasia diagnosed by wireless capsule endoscopy. **B,** Active bleeding angiodysplasia visualized by capsule endoscopy. **C,** Small bowel angiodysplasia seen with balloon enteroscopy. **D,** Same lesion treated with argon plasma coagulation.

studies and push enteroscopy.[58] Two published meta-analyses support the utility of capsule endoscopy in obscure GI bleeding.[59,60] The ASGE Technology Assessment Committee also concluded that capsule endoscopy is indicated not only for evaluating obscure GI bleeding, but also for evaluating unexplained iron deficiency anemia.[58]

The EndoCapsule EC type 1 is another small bowel capsule endoscope, developed by Olympus America (Center Valley, PA). This capsule uses a high-resolution CCD and an external real-time image viewer (External Viewer) monitor.[61] A randomized study comparing these two types of capsule endoscope reported a statistically nonsignificant trend for the EndoCapsule to detect more bleeding sources in patients with suspected small bowel bleeding than the PillCam SB.[62] Future capsule designs may emerge with expanded capabilities that include fluid sampling, mucosal biopsy, targeted labeling, and controlled movement. With future innovation and study, the indications for capsule endoscopy are likely to expand and become more focused.

Balloon-Assisted Enteroscopy

Push-and-pull enteroscopy with the double-balloon technique (double-balloon enteroscopy [DBE]) for inspection of the entire small bowel was first performed in the Western world in 2003.[63] The earliest case report documenting the success of this method was published by Yamamoto and colleagues in 2001.[63a]

DOUBLE-BALLOON TECHNIQUE

The endoscope is introduced into the small bowel within a soft overtube. The balloon at the tip of the endoscope is inflated to hold it in place while the overtube, with deflated balloon, is passed distally until it reaches the tip of the endoscope. Both balloons are inflated, and the entire system is slowly pulled back; this results in an accordionlike sleeving of the small bowel onto the overtube. In the next step, the overtube balloon is kept inflated while the endoscope balloon is deflated and the endoscope is pushed 40 cm deeper into the small bowel. This method is repeated until the enteroscope has been passed as far as technically possible. In approximately 10% of cases, the entire small bowel can be visualized in a single session, typically via an antegrade approach. Carbon dioxide insufflation improves depth of insertion especially during antegrade approaches.[64] In most cases, however, antegrade and retrograde examinations are required for the entire small bowel to be visualized. In this setting, the distalmost point in the small bowel that is reached after antegrade passage is tattooed to provide an endpoint during the retrograde examination.

The push-and-pull technique is used in reverse to withdraw the endoscope from the small bowel; while the endoscope is being withdrawn, the small bowel can be carefully reinspected. The enteroscope is 2 m long and has an outer diameter of either 8.5 mm (standard size channel) or 9.5 mm (therapeutic size channel). The endoscope is outfitted with capabilities similar to a conventional endoscope: The endoscope optics or the bowel itself can be rinsed by the instillation of fluid through the device port, biopsy samples can be taken, and a full range of therapeutic interventions can be performed.

SINGLE-BALLOON ENTEROSCOPY

Antegrade DBE can examine three times the length of small bowel as push enteroscopy, with a corresponding increase in diagnostic yield.[65] More recently, single-balloon enteroscopy (SBE) was introduced in the United States (Olympus America, Center Valley, PA).[66] The single-balloon and double-balloon systems share many features, including scope length, diameter, accessory channel size, and overtube design. The most important design difference between the two systems is that the single-balloon enteroscope does not have a distal balloon on the scope; the only balloon is on the tip of the overtube. As a result, the sequence of steps to advance the scope through the small bowel is simplified in SBE.

Although there are some minor differences between the systems, use of either scope requires a technician to assist with handling of the overtube and balloon inflation and deflation. In addition, both systems require fluoroscopy to monitor scope position and sedation appropriate for prolonged procedures. Early clinical experience using SBE on average reported a depth of insertion (270 cm) and diagnostic yield (54%) similar to DBE with a shorter procedure time.[67] Comparison studies between DBE and SBE are inherently difficult to design and carry out. For this reason, accurate comparisons are impossible. Choice of procedure has become a user preference.

COMPLICATIONS

Abdominal pain is common after DBE and can be lessened by the use of carbon dioxide insufflation. Diagnostic DBE has an overall complication rate of 1.7% (perforation 0.3%, bleeding 0.8%, pancreatitis 0.3%).[68] The cause of pancreatitis is uncertain. Advancing the overtube and enteroscope into the jejunum before inflating balloons and avoiding excessive tension on the mesentery during push-pull cycles may limit this risk. Therapeutic DBE has a relatively high complication rate of 4.3% (polypectomy bleeding 3.3%, argon plasma coagulation [APC] perforation 1.2%, dilation perforation 2.9%). DBE evaluation of the entire small bowel is possible in 45% to 84% of patients in whom it is attempted, although it can rarely be achieved with antegrade DBE alone. In the evaluation of obscure GI bleeding, DBE has been reported to identify a bleeding source in 53% to 80% of cases.[69,70]

Three prospective studies compared capsule endoscopy with DBE. Combining the results of the three studies, capsule endoscopy and DBE agreed in 68% of all cases and in 63% of positive cases. A meta-analysis that included these three prospective studies and results published only in abstract form compared diagnostic outcomes between capsule endoscopy and DBE. There was no difference in diagnostic yield between capsule endoscopy and DBE.[71] Another meta-analysis reached the same conclusion.[72] A new enteroscopy technology consists of a 48-Fr rotating overtube with spiral threads (Discovery SB; Spirus Medical, Inc, Stoughton, MA). The overtube is backloaded on any enteroscope[73] or on a pediatric colonoscope.[74] After intubation of the stomach with the endoscope, the overtube is rotated clockwise through the upper GI tract until the spiral threads engage in the jejunum; once free in the abdominal cavity, clockwise spinning of the overtube results in rapid pleating of small bowel onto the overtube. In a preliminary report,[75] average procedure time for spiral enteroscopy was shorter (32 minutes) than times reported for DBE and SBE. The diagnostic yield is lower (32%) compared with balloon-assisted enteroscopy. The depth of insertion into the small bowel and the overall safety of the large twisting overtube have not been shown.

Summary

Balloon-assisted enteroscopy seems to have superior diagnostic capability compared with push enteroscopy and equivalent yield compared with intraoperative enteroscopy without the associated morbidity of the latter procedure. Although balloon-assisted enteroscopy does not allow visualization of the entire small bowel in one examination, compared with capsule endoscopy, it has been shown to be associated with an equivalent detection rate, has the capability to detect lesions missed by capsule endoscopy, and offers the advantages of therapeutic treatment. In patients with a positive finding on capsule endoscopy, balloon-assisted enteroscopy provides a safe method to achieve a favorable clinical outcome, including significant reduction in recurrent bleeding and transfusion requirements.[76] With the advent of balloon-assisted enteroscopy, intraoperative enteroscopy can be relegated to cases in which the success of balloon-assisted enteroscopy is limited by body habitus, the presence of adhesions, or other anatomic factors.[3] Most existing trials have focused on the diagnostic value of capsule endoscopy, with few examining the impact on the long-term outcome of obscure GI bleeding. In a 1-year study based on telephone interviews, the negative predictive value of capsule endoscopy for clinical rebleeding was 87%.[77] In another more recent report, the negative predictive value was 89%.[78] Capsule endoscopy can guide the management of these small bowel lesions.

Similar to other authors,[57,80] we[79] recommend capsule endoscopy as a first-line investigation over balloon-assisted enteroscopy in view of its convenience, higher chance to visualize the entire small intestine, and similar diagnostic yield. A proposed algorithm for capsule endoscopy in cases of obscure GI bleeding is shown in **Fig. 16.3**. No test substitutes for good clinical judgment, however, and all small bowel diagnostic studies must be considered in difficult cases of obscure GI bleeding, particularly in a young patient.[81]

In the setting of obscure overt bleeding, capsule endoscopy should be performed close to the bleeding episode. We recommend that a second endoscopist reread the capsule endoscopy study. We also recommend a second-look EGD with special attention to areas less optimally examined by capsule endoscopy, especially the duodenum, before concluding with a final diagnosis of obscure GI bleeding. Second-look capsule endoscopy has also been suggested for patients with a prior nondiagnostic capsule endoscopy. Bar-Meir and associates[82] reported that 7 of 20 patients (35%) who underwent second-look capsule endoscopy had positive or suspicious findings. Another study showed that patients with a nondiagnostic capsule endoscopy test would benefit from a second-look capsule endoscopy if the bleeding presentation changed from occult to overt or if the hemoglobin value decreased 4 g/dL or more.[83]

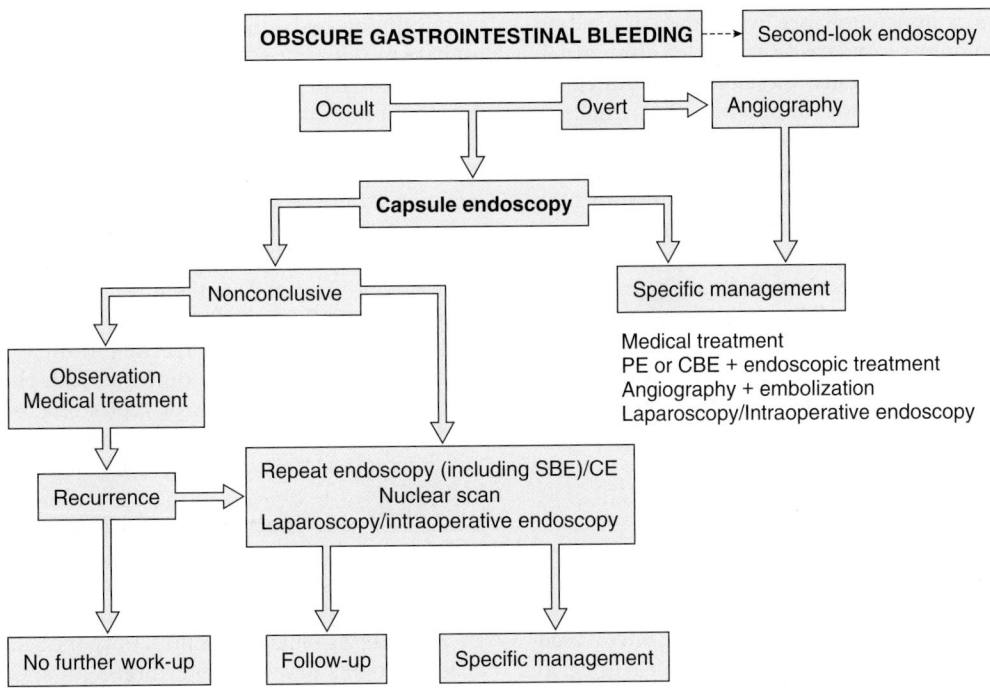

Fig. 16.3 Diagnostic algorithm for obscure gastrointestinal bleeding. *(Adapted from Nakamura T, Terano A: Capsule endoscopy: Past, present, and future. J Gastroenterol 43:93–99, 2008.)*

Angiography is used to determine the site and nature of lesions during bleeding. It may permit therapy in patients who are bleeding and can identify some vascular lesions even when bleeding has ceased. The three reliable angiographic signs that help diagnose angiectases are a densely opacified, slowly emptying, dilated, tortuous vein; a vascular tuft, and an early-filling vein.[84] A fourth sign, extravasation of contrast material, identifies the site of bleeding when bleeding volume is at least 0.5 mL/min but does not contribute to the diagnosis of an angiectasis. Nuclear scan is another diagnostic technique that can be used in selected patients.[85,86] Provocative scintigraphy with heparin can enhance diagnosis with further localization of bleeding.[87]

Helical computed tomography (CT) angiography may provide another method to help diagnose angiectases. Accuracy may be high,[88] although studies are needed to understand the role of this technique better in the management of patients with GI bleeding. In a report of 22 patients with obscure GI bleeding, CT enteroclysis was found to be inferior to capsule endoscopy in the detection of potential bleeding lesions such as angiectases in the small bowel.[89] In another more recent study performed in 28 patients with obscure GI bleeding, capsule endoscopy detected more lesions (72%) than CT angiography (24%) or standard mesenteric angiography (56%).[90] The aggressiveness of the approach should be individualized depending on the clinical circumstances. Evaluation of the small bowel may be deferred in patients with negative upper and lower endoscopy until or unless the patient is bleeding severely enough to require a transfusion.[55]

Management

Management of bleeding angiectases consists of three phases[24]: (1) diagnosis; (2) conversion of acute bleeding manifesting as

an emergency to elective care by control of the acute hemorrhage; and (3) definitive treatment of the lesions by endoscopic ablation, angiography, or surgical removal. The natural history of colonic angiectases is benign in healthy, asymptomatic individuals, and the risk of bleeding is small.[29] It is estimated that only about 50% of colonic lesions ever bleed. There is a risk of bleeding and perforation following attempts at endoscopic obliteration. For all these reasons, in incidentally found angiectases at all levels of the gut, endoscopic therapy is not warranted.[91]

Pharmacologic Treatment

IRON FORMULATIONS

Nonbleeding angiodysplasia detected during evaluation of occult bleeding or iron deficiency anemia should be considered to be causative. In patients with occult bleeding, bleeding from angiodysplasia may be more likely in patients who have multiple lesions and a bleeding diathesis (e.g., anticoagulation). As a result, a graduated approach with primary or adjunctive iron replacement therapy may be initiated, with pursuit of more aggressive therapeutic options guided by the clinical circumstances.[91–93] The aims of iron replacement therapy should be to restore hemoglobin levels and mean corpuscular volume to normal and to replenish body stores.

Laboratory measurements of body iron stores such as serum ferritin are helpful to assess the effectiveness of iron supplementation. Iron supplementation is achieved most easily with oral iron supplementation. Numerous oral iron preparations are available, although ferrous sulfate and ferrous gluconate are preferred forms of oral iron because of low cost and high bioavailability. A liquid preparation often is tolerated better. Ascorbic acid enhances iron absorption. Parenteral iron should be used when there is intolerance to at least two oral iron preparations or noncompliance, when there is a suboptimal clinical response secondary to suspected iron malabsorption, and when blood transfusion becomes difficult to achieve because of excessive antibodies that challenge crossmatching.

Some patients with obscure GI bleeding are managed clinically with intermittent blood transfusions along with other nonspecific supportive measures, such as avoidance of aspirin, avoidance of anticoagulants, and oral iron supplementation. These patients often do not have a definite diagnosis despite extensive work-up, have diffuse GI angiectases often in inaccessible locations, have failed endoscopic or surgical or other specific therapies, or are elderly with many comorbid conditions and the risk of further diagnostic evaluation is considered to be greater than the risk of nonspecific management.

HORMONAL THERAPY

Estrogen-progesterone combination hormonal therapy has been used to treat patients with angiectases of the GI tract.[94,95] The effect, which is not immediate, seems to be estrogen dose–dependent. Hormonal therapy acts by enhancing microvascular circulation, coagulation, and vascular endothelial integrity. The most common combination schedule has been ethinyl estradiol 0.01 to 0.05 mg and norethisterone 1 to 3 mg. This therapy should be used in 6-month courses with pauses to reduce the incidence of adverse effects, mostly secondary to the estrogen component. The results of several prospective, controlled trials examining hormonal therapy have been divergent.[96–99] In a long-term observational study, combination hormonal therapy was shown to stop bleeding in patients with occult GI bleeding of obscure origin, likely to have resulted from small bowel angiodysplasias.[98] Although uncontrolled studies suggest that combination estrogen-progesterone therapy prevents bleeding episodes secondary to angiodysplasia, the evidence from the largest placebo-controlled trial to date suggests that this therapy is ineffective.[100] These authors considered that efficacy of hormonal therapy in these patients remains to be proven by a large, randomized, placebo-controlled trial with long-term follow-up.

This pharmacologic therapy is not without complications. The main side effects include fluid retention, uterine bleeding, increased plasma triglycerides, pancreatitis, hypercoagulability, breast tenderness or enlargement, headache, and increased incidence of gallbladder disease. Contraindications for hormonal therapy include thromboembolic disease, cholestatic jaundice, endometrial hyperplasia, known or suspected breast cancer or estrogen-dependent neoplasia, vaginal bleeding, and gynecomastia. In clinical practice, estrogen-progesterone therapy should be used for patients with symptomatic recurrent episodic bleeding in which other therapies have failed.

OCTREOTIDE

Reports of efficacy of octreotide in the treatment of angiodysplasia have been limited to case reports and small series in which a response has been reported in some patients.[95,101–103] Octreotide produces vasoconstriction secondary to inhibitory effects on growth hormone and multiple GI vasodilator hormones and markedly reduces splanchnic blood flow. Its antiangiogenic properties have been shown in different tissues (eye, placenta, liver, and GI neuroendocrine tumors); however,

applicability and utility in obscure GI bleeding remain unknown.

The dosage of octreotide can be tapered to the lowest quantity that prevents rebleeding. Response is immediate, and the drug can be administered intravenously (50 µg/hr) or subcutaneously (50 to 100 µg two or three times a day).[95] Its subcutaneous administration and its longer half-life (90 to 100 minutes) make octreotide superior to somatostatin and allow use in the outpatient setting. A 6-month course of therapy has been used to treat most patients. The first comparative cohort study showing the benefit of long-term octreotide compared with placebo in preventing bleeding from angiodysplasia was reported more recently.[104] Compared with placebo, octreotide markedly reduced the risk of rebleeding with a significant decrease in iron requirements, but there were no differences in hemoglobin levels or transfusion requirements between the two groups.

Mild GI side effects have been reported with octreotide. Inflammation at the injection site has been noted. Mild steatorrhea and mild hyperglycemia may result from the inhibition of pancreatic exocrine and endocrine secretion. Octreotide therapy alters gallbladder contractility, inducing biliary sludge. A few patients develop acute cholecystitis. Cost-effectiveness of this treatment has not been shown to date.

Sandostatin LAR Depot is a depot formulation of octreotide for long-term maintenance therapy currently approved for acromegaly and GI and pancreatic neuroendocrine tumors. Compared with conventional octreotide, Sandostatin LAR Depot is administered intramuscularly once a month with a similar efficacy and safety profile and does not require hospital admission, which makes it an attractive outpatient option for long-term therapy in patients with chronic GI bleeding. The effectiveness of Sandostatin LAR Depot at a dose of 20 mg intramuscularly once a month for obscure GI bleeding has been described in several small series.[95,102,105–107] The main disadvantage of this drug formulation may be its cost compared with conventional octreotide. However, in very specific cases, it may prove to be cost-effective. The appropriate dose and schedule required for long-term therapy are unknown.

NONSELECTIVE β BLOCKERS

Nonselective β blockers aim to control hemorrhage by reducing GI blood flow secondary to splanchnic vasoconstriction and reduction of cardiac output. The benefit of nonselective β blockers in primary and secondary prophylaxis of variceal bleeding in portal hypertension has been shown in many studies, sometimes for portal hypertensive gastropathy (PHG) and colopathy; however, its use in obscure GI bleeding is anecdotal.

THALIDOMIDE

Thalidomide is a drug with powerful immunomodulatory, antiinflammatory, and antiangiogenic effects that was withdrawn from the market in the 1960s because of its teratogenicity; it has been reintroduced more recently for the treatment of leprosy, multiple myeloma, and various tumors. Vascular endothelial growth factor (VEGF) has been identified as the key mediator for endothelial vessel formation in early phases of angiogenesis. High concentrations of VEGF result in aberrant angiogenesis with formation of angiectasias that lack a smooth muscle cell layer and are more susceptible to rupture and bleeding. VEGF-dependent angiogenesis is inhibited by thalidomide. Thalidomide is an innovative and promising therapeutic option for GI bleeding associated with angiodysplasia and can be used in refractory cases or when other drugs or therapies are contraindicated.[95]

Thalidomide is administered orally at a variable dose of 100 to 300 mg/day.[95] No significant adverse effects have been reported except transient fatigue; however, thalidomide is contraindicated in patients with peripheral neuropathy and pregnant women and women with childbearing potential because of its teratogenic effects, and it should be used cautiously in patients with cardiovascular or neurologic disorders and hepatic or renal impairment. Owing to its immunosuppressant activity by blocking tumor necrosis factor, use of thalidomide may be also discouraged in patients at risk for infection or chronic infectious disease, especially patients with human immunodeficiency virus (HIV) infection. In all these clinical settings, Sandostatin LAR Depot may be safer than thalidomide.

There are few reports in the literature about the effectiveness of thalidomide for chronic GI bleeding. It was successfully used in a patient with von Willebrand's disease and life-threatening bleeding caused by small bowel angiodysplasia refractory to other pharmacologic treatments and endoscopic cauterization with argon beam laser.[108] It has also been proven effective in controlling bleeding from diffuse idiopathic angiodysplastic lesions in the small bowel.[109,110] Bauditz and coworkers[111] studied the effect of thalidomide at a dose of 100 mg daily for 3 months in three patients with chronic bleeding from small bowel angiodysplasia as evidenced by wireless capsule endoscopy. Bleeding was controlled in all cases for a median follow-up of 34 months despite drug discontinuation. Repeat capsule endoscopy after therapy revealed a substantial reduction in lesion numbers, size, and color intensity.

MISCELLANEOUS AGENTS
Antifibrinolytics

Tranexamic acid is a synthetic lysine analogue that inhibits the conversion of plasmin to fibrinogen. It has been used successfully for chronic bleeding from angiodysplasia in patients with end-stage renal failure at doses of 10 to 20 mg/kg every 48 hours; it remains unclear whether long-term therapy or as-needed therapy is preferable during hemorrhagic crises.[95,112] The main risk derived from the use of antifibrinolytics is thrombosis, so thrombophilia should be ruled out before prescribing them. Adverse events associated with tranexamic acid may be frequent, and use of these drugs is not supported by randomized controlled trials, which makes antifibrinolytics a last option for chronic GI bleeding. Because of their mechanism of action, antifibrinolytics may have a more important role in the treatment of patients with hematologic disorders.

Danazol

Danazol is an antigonadotropin drug with weak androgenic activity that blocks pituitary secretion of follicle-stimulating hormone and luteinizing hormone, leading to ectopic and normal endometrial tissue atrophy. It has been used for endometriosis and uterine bleeding disorders. Anecdotal reports suggest a partial improvement in patients with GI bleeding and hereditary hemorrhagic telangiectasia.[44,45] Cosmetic stigmata (acne, hair loss, mild hirsutism) and uncommon but severe adverse effects (intracranial hypertension, peliosis hepatis, thrombosis, seizures) consign danazol to a secondary role in chronic GI bleeding, to be used when other therapies have failed.

Desmopressin

Desmopressin is a synthetic analogue of the antidiuretic hormone vasopressin that lacks vasopressor activity. It increases vWF and factor VIII levels and enhances hemostasis in patients with defective platelet function. It is indicated as a hemostatic agent for patients with hemophilia A and von Willebrand's disease, and it can be administered intravenously, subcutaneously, or by intranasal spray. An isolated report showed a benefit of intravenous desmopressin for life-threatening GI bleeding in a patient with hereditary hemorrhagic telangiectasia and vWF deficiency, allowing elective colectomy and bleeding resolution.[113]

Recombinant Activated Factor VII

Recombinant activated human factor VII is a novel drug that strongly promotes hemostasis and is currently indicated for patients with hemophilia A and hemophilia B with antibody inhibitors to coagulation factors VIII or IX, congenital deficiency of factor VII, and Glanzmann's thrombasthenia. This drug has been used for controlling hemorrhage, with or without hematologic disorders, in massive or uncontrollable bleeding at any location. Its short half-life of 2 hours requires frequent boluses or continuous infusion to achieve hemostasis, and it can induce definitive control of bleeding or be a bridge until a causal therapy can be instituted.

Recombinant activated human factor VII has been used mainly in upper GI hemorrhage related to cirrhosis or acute liver failure,[114,115] although it has been used in other settings, including refractory bleeding after endoscopic sphincterotomy in patients with preexisting coagulopathy.[116] Sporadic reports have shown the effectiveness of factor VIIa in patients with von Willebrand's disease for chronic GI bleeding secondary to small bowel angiodysplasia or of unknown origin.[117] Secondary myocardial and cerebrovascular infarctions have been described while using factor VIIa owing to its marked prothrombotic activity,[118] so particular care should be taken in patients with a high-risk cardiovascular profile, and the indication should be assessed for each individual case.

SUMMARY

Pharmacotherapy should be considered whenever endoscopic therapy, surgical intervention, or angiographic therapy is impractical or ineffective, such as in patients in whom the source and the etiology of bleeding are unknown or the pathology is too diffuse to be amenable to ablative therapies. Combined hormonal therapy and other miscellaneous treatments (antifibrinolytics, desmopressin, danazol, recombinant activated factor VIIa) should be considered currently useful for chronic GI bleeding in patients with hereditary hemorrhagic telangiectasia, von Willebrand's disease, and end-stage renal disease. In patients with bleeding from small bowel angiodysplasia or of unknown origin without the abovementioned diseases, octreotide is effective and safe, but it requires administration several times a day. In the future, Sandostatin LAR Depot, oral thalidomide, and nonselective β blockers are likely to become the pharmacologic cornerstone replacing hormonal therapy and conventional octreotide, owing to easy administration, good tolerability, and absence of major adverse effects. Further studies are needed to confirm this hypothesis and to elucidate the adequate dose and schedule needed for these novel and promising drugs.

Endoscopic Treatment

The goal of endoscopic therapy is thrombosis of the bleeding vessel. Studies directly comparing the effectiveness of the different approaches have not been performed. The approach depends on the location of the lesion, the experience of the endoscopist, and the availability of equipment.

BIPOLAR OR HEATER PROBE COAGULATION

Bipolar or heater probe coagulation is said to be effective for treatment of angiodysplasia,[119,120] and these modalities have replaced monopolar coagulation.[14,121]

SCLEROSANT

Injection of a sclerosant, such as ethanolamine, has been used to obliterate lesions.[122] Epinephrine injection works by volume tamponade of the bleeding vessel and transient vasoconstriction.[123] Sclerosants should probably be avoided, however, because of the risk for bleeding from injection site ulceration and perforation.[47]

BAND LIGATION

Band ligation has been used to treat angiectasia of the stomach.[124,125] The relatively small surface area incorporated into the ligation site (e.g., in GAVE or "watermelon stomach") and, more so, the expense of the therapy outweigh any perceived benefits. The walls of the small and large intestine above the rectum (especially the right colon) are thinner than the stomach. For this reason, band ligation therapy cannot be advocated owing to the recognized risk for perforation.[126,127]

LASERS

Argon and neodymium:yttrium-aluminum-garnet (Nd:YAG) lasers have been used in the past.[128–130] These techniques require expensive equipment and specific training. More convenient and safer coagulation options have replaced laser therapy except for treatment of "watermelon stomach" (GAVE). APC has become the dominant therapy for GAVE. A few patients are refractory to this therapy. These patients most often respond to treatment with Nd:YAG laser.

ARGON PLASMA COAGULATION

APC is a monopolar electrosurgical procedure in which electrical energy is transferred to the target tissue using ionized and conductive argon gas (argon plasma).[131] The plasma beam follows the path of least electrical resistance. This phenomenon permits the argon plasma to be applied both en face and tangentially, allowing treatment of regions that are normally

difficult to access. A second-generation APC (VIO APC; Erbe Elektromedizin, Tuebingen, Germany; and Beamer, Con Med, Utica, NY) offering a broader bandwith of APC modes compared with the earlier generators has been introduced more recently to GI endoscopy. The optional coagulation modes (e.g., "forced," "pulsed," and "precise") of second-generation devices provide different coagulation tissue effects. These effects include a continuous energy output, pulsed energy (with high energy per pulse with longer pauses per pulse or a greater number of pulses with a lower energy per pulse with a constant voltage maintained for each pulse option).

The newer power applications such as "forced" and "pulsed" of second-generation APC devices have been reported to be 30% to 50% higher compared with the ICC/APC300 system. Another power delivery mode ("precise") uses an integrated regulation system that adjusts the argon plasma regardless of impedance and is characterized by continuous application of energy and by an increase of plasma intensity. In this application, the tissue effect becomes independent of the distance between the APC probe and the target tissue (within 5 mm). The three most important factors influencing the thermal impact of APC are the duration of application, the power setting, and the probe-to-tissue distance. The lowest power settings and the shortest duration of coagulation energy applied to a focal point have the lowest risk of deep tissue injury.

APC has been used for various bleeding lesions, including angiectases.[132,133] Its great advantage over laser or photodynamic therapy is the limited depth of tissue injury and lower cost. Shallow tissue injury is due to the fact that the argon stream always seeks electrically conductive areas of tissue, avoiding the coagulated zones, which have lost their electrical conductivity as a result of desiccation. Perforation of the cecum has been reported.[132] APC seems to be most effective[131] in the treatment of vascular lesions (GAVE, angiodysplasias, and Dieulafoy's lesions).

The utility of obtaining a submucosal saline solution cushion before APC therapy to prevent deep tissue injury has been shown in a porcine model.[134] Before APC, it is recommended to collapse the lumen partially while maintaining the treatment site in view. It is important to avoid thinning of the colonic wall with excessive air insufflation because this increases the risk for perforation during therapy, especially in the cecum.[123]

CRYOTHERAPY

Safety and efficacy of cryotherapy have been reported for treatment of diffuse mucosal lesions of the GI tract.[135] The effectiveness of endoscopic treatment of angiectases is difficult to assess owing to the absence of prospective controlled trials. Recurrent bleeding from cecal angiodysplasia seems to be reduced after laser photocoagulation or thermal ablation via heater probe or bipolar electrocoagulation, with long-term control of bleeding requiring more than one treatment.[136] Aside from perforation, the main risks of thermal therapy for colonic angiectases are bleeding in 5% of patients and postcoagulation syndrome in 1.7% of cases.[120] Endoscopic treatment of vascular lesions in patients known to have coagulation disorders carries an increased risk of procedure-induced hemorrhage.

When treating large lesions, some experienced endoscopists recommend[47] to ablate first the periphery of the lesion to create a collar of edema that theoretically reduces the vascular supply to the lesion and diminishes the potential for immediate or delayed hemorrhage. Some clinicians have placed mechanical clips around the margins of large lesions also to reduce the blood supply and facilitate effective coagulation. Others typically target the central portion of the angiodysplasia because ensuing coagulation and edema obstruct the peripheral branches and limit the extent of coagulation needed. Also, for a very large angiodysplasia, epinephrine injection may contract the lesion and reduce the amount and area of coagulation needed for eradication.[123] Recurrent bleeding can be expected in approximately 20% of patients with colonic angiectases and in a greater percentage of patients with associated coagulopathies, renal failure, portal hypertension, or additional upper GI vascular lesions.[47] It is reasonable to attempt endoscopic therapy in patients with accessible lesions despite various coexisting morbidities that may allow only short-term success. Patients with multiple lesions or an underlying bleeding diathesis are less likely to benefit long-term from endoscopic therapy and are at increased risk of complications, especially delayed bleeding from treatment site thermally induced ulceration. Such patients benefit from any attempts to improve their underlying bleeding tendency.

In preparation for endoscopic ablation of vascular lesions, aspirin, nonsteroidal antiinflammatory drugs, anticoagulants, and antiplatelet agents should be withdrawn at least 1 week to 10 days before the procedure. Care should be taken not to distend the cecum fully because the wall would be thinned further, and the risk of perforation would be increased.[24,123] After therapy, patients must be cautioned not to resume full doses of anticoagulants or antiplatelet agents for at least 1 week. Coagulated tissues are at their maximum of thermal injury by 5 to 10 days, and the onset of hemorrhage may be delayed.

Angiography

Localization of active bleeding permits embolization or infusion of vasopressin. Because angiography occasionally causes serious complications, such as arterial thrombosis, contrast reactions, and acute renal failure, its use before definitive surgical therapy has been questioned.[137] Angiography should be reserved for patients with life-threatening bleeding, patients who are not surgical candidates, and patients in whom localization of lesions is desired before surgical resection. Intravenous or intraarterial vasopressin infusions through the angiographic catheter successfully arrest hemorrhage from vascular ectasias in more than 80% of patients in whom extravasation is demonstrated.[16] The intravenous route seems to be as effective as the intraarterial route when the bleeding is in the left colon, but intraarterial administration is more successful when the bleeding is from the right colon or small bowel. Infarction of the sigmoid colon and severe arterial spasm and lower extremity ischemia have resulted from vasopressin infusions into the inferior mesenteric artery given at the same rate as used in the superior mesenteric artery. These complications may be avoided by infusing less than 0.4 U/min (the dose of superior mesenteric artery infusions), recognizing the lesser blood flow of the inferior mesenteric artery.

Surgery

Surgical resection is definitive for lesions that have been clearly identified as the source of bleeding. Recurrent bleeding may

occur, however, from lesions elsewhere in the GI tract. Preoperative or intraoperative enteroscopy and wireless capsule endoscopy are helpful for localizing lesions. Right hemicolectomy remains the treatment of choice for a patient who has bled and whose right colonic angiectases have been identified by either colonoscopy or angiography if:

1. The bleeding is refractory (especially with redevelopment of recurrent lesions).
2. Endoscopic ablation is unavailable.
3. Endoscopic ablation has been unsuccessful or is not feasible for technical reasons.

In the latter two situations, right hemicolectomy is done as an elective procedure after active bleeding is controlled. The entire right half of the colon needs to be removed to ensure that no angiectases are left behind. Recurrent bleeding can be expected in 20% of patients. Subtotal colectomy should be performed only as a last resort in circumstances in which colonic bleeding is strongly suspected but the site and cause are unknown.[24] Richter and colleagues[16] studied the course of 101 patients with angiodysplasias to determine the natural history and compare the efficacy of medical therapy, endoscopic electrocoagulation, and surgery (right hemicolectomy). Similar rates of recurrent bleeding were observed for medically and endoscopically treated groups during a mean follow-up of 22 months. Surgically treated patients had a frequency of recurrent bleeding less than half that of the other groups.

Hereditary Hemorrhagic Telangiectasia

Hereditary hemorrhagic telangiectasia, or Rendu-Osler-Weber disease, is an uncommon, autosomal dominant disorder characterized by telangiectases and arteriovenous malformations that affect many organs, including the skin, periungual areas, lips, oral and nasopharyngeal membranes, tongue (**Fig. 16.4A**), lungs, GI tract (**Fig. 16.4B**), liver, and brain,[138,139] and can result in bleeding. Lesions consist of irregular, ectatic, tortuous blood spaces lined by a single layer of endothelial cells and supported by a fine layer of fibrous connective tissue. In these vessels, no elastic lamina or muscular tissue is present, so they cannot contract; this property may explain why these lesions tend to bleed.[24]

Clinical Manifestations

Manifestations of hereditary hemorrhagic telangiectasia are not generally present at birth but develop with increasing age. Epistaxis is usually the earliest sign of disease, often occurring in childhood; pulmonary arteriovenous malformations become apparent from puberty; mucocutaneous and GI telangiectases develop progressively with age; and, finally, GI bleeding occurs well into adulthood.[140] A family history has been reported in approximately 80% of patients with this disease[141] but is less common in patients who manifest bleeding after age 50 years.[47] Severe GI bleeding is unusual before the 5th or 6th decade[142]; occurs in 25% to 33% of patients with hereditary hemorrhagic telangiectasia; is challenging to treat; and can cause significant morbidity, resulting in severe anemia and high blood transfusion requirements.[143,144]

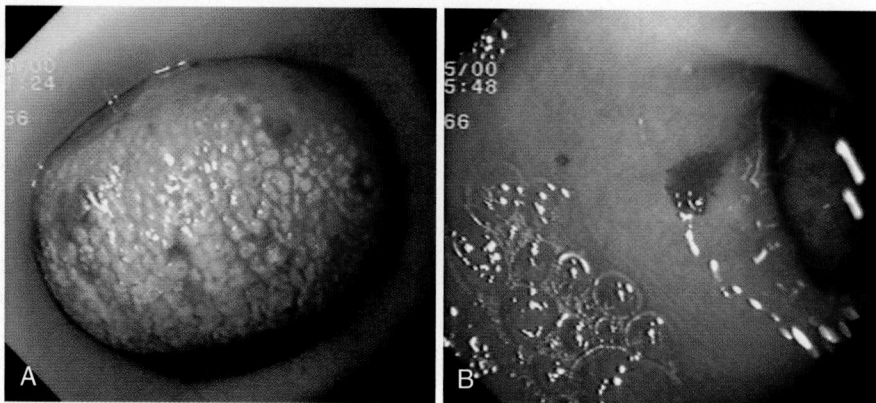

Fig. 16.4 Hereditary hemorrhagic telangiectasia, or Rendu-Osler-Weber syndrome. Patient with multiple telangiectases involving the tongue **(A)** and the stomach **(B)**.

Endoscopy may reveal telangiectases in the stomach (see **Fig. 16.4B**), duodenum, small bowel, or colon that are punctiform, discrete, red spots or with a classic fernlike border similar to all other angiectases. Lesions are usually flat, although they may be slightly raised 1 to 3 mm, similar in size and appearance to angiectases of the nasal and oral mucosa.[142] Telangiectases are more common in the stomach, duodenum, or jejunum than in the colon.[140] They also may have a characteristic pale mucosal halo. Capsule endoscopy contributes significantly to defining the extent of small intestinal telangiectases and can be used to stage the disease to decide on the extent and form of endoscopic therapy.[139] Selective mesenteric arteriography may localize the precise bleeding site, but in most cases this is unnecessary.[145]

Management

Therapies for GI bleeding range from various pharmacologic agents to endoscopic and surgical treatment. Drug therapies include ethinyl estradiol and norethisterone,[96] danazol,[146] and aminocaproic acid.[147] Endoscopic therapy is the most effective form of treatment in stopping hemorrhage from actively bleeding lesions. Because of the multiplicity of lesions and the redevelopment of lesions, sometimes within weeks, bleeding recurs at varying intervals after therapy, depending on the extent and thoroughness of ablative therapies.[141] There are several reports of endoscopic therapy, including sclerotherapy with sodium morrhuate,[148] ethanol, and polidocanol[149]; monopolar and bipolar coagulation and heater probe[150,151]; APC[149]; YAG laser[152]; and clip application.[153] Surgical therapy with resection of involved bowel has limited success because of recurrent disease[140] but may be useful for emergency control of hemorrhage from discrete lesions identified as the source of the bleeding that do not respond to medical or endoscopic therapy.[141] Surgical intervention has otherwise been more common owing to excessive bleeding from thermally induced ulcerations after endoscopic therapy and perforation.

Gastric Vascular Lesions in Patients with Cirrhosis

After variceal bleeding, hemorrhagic gastritis is the most frequent cause of upper GI bleeding in cirrhotic patients with portal hypertension.[154] The term *hemorrhagic gastritis* has included bleeding from various nonvariceal mucosal lesions, such as multiple ulcerations, PHG, and GAVE.[154–156] PHG and GAVE can cause acute and chronic upper GI blood loss.[157] These conditions frequently, but not invariably, are diagnosed by upper endoscopy. Although they are fairly prevalent, only 15% to 20% of affected individuals experience symptomatic GI blood loss.

Portal Hypertensive Gastropathy

PHG describes the endoscopic appearance of gastric mucosa, with a characteristic mosaiclike pattern with or without red spots, seen in patients with cirrhotic or noncirrhotic portal hypertension. The mosaiclike pattern appears as a white reticular network separating areas of raised red or pink mucosa, resembling the skin of a snake ("snakeskin appearance"). PHG is seen mainly in the body and the fundus of the stomach but is also seen rarely in the gastric antrum (**Fig. 16.5**). These changes are not unique to gastric mucosa. Similar changes are rarely seen in the small intestine and colon, especially in the presence of extrahepatic portal hypertension. With the broad use of capsule endoscopy, different manifestations of portal hypertension have been reported, although their clinical implications are uncertain to date.[158,159] When PHG is severe, it can include discrete cherry-red spots, fine pink speckling, or scarlatina-type rash, collectively called *red marks*.[160] The characteristic histologic finding of PHG is dilated capillaries and venules in the mucosa and submucosa without erosion, inflammation, or fibrinous thrombi.[161]

Classification

There is no general consensus on the endoscopic classification of PHG. The most widely used classification is the one recommended by McCormack and colleagues,[161] who classified PHG into mild and severe (**Table 16.3**). Mild PHG is defined by the presence of only a mosaiclike pattern, whereas severe PHG is diagnosed when red point lesions, cherry-red spots, or black-brown spots are present. The popularity of this classification relates in part to its simplicity and its ability to predict the risk of bleeding, with an increased risk of gastric hemorrhage in severe cases (38% to 62%) compared with mild cases (3.5% to 31%).[155,156] Observed endoscopic findings often are of an intermediate severity, however, and are not well represented as being either mild or severe. Tanoue and colleagues[162] and

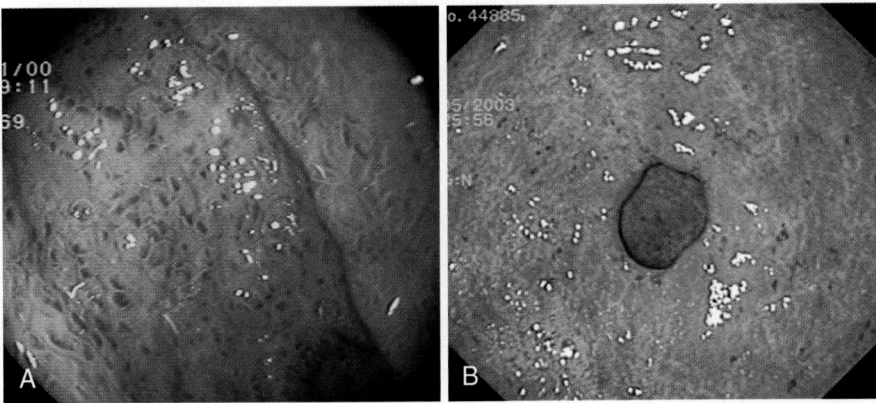

Fig. 16.5 Portal hypertensive gastropathy with mosaic pattern and cherry-red spots in the body of the stomach **(A)** and localized in the antrum of a cirrhotic patient **(B)**.

Table 16.3 Classification of Portal Hypertensive Gastropathy

McCormack et al[161]	Tanoue et al[162]	Primignani et al (NIEC)[163]
Mild	**Grade I**	**Mosaic pattern**
Fine pink speckling (scarlatina-type rash)	Mild reddening	Mild—diffuse pink areola
Superficial reddening	Congestive mucosa	Moderate—flat red spot
Mosaic pattern		Severe—diffuse red areola
Severe	**Grade II**	**Red mark lesion**
Discrete red spots	Severe redness and fine reticular pattern separating areas of raised edematous mucosa	Discrete
Diffuse hemorrhagic lesion		Confluent (diffuse)
	Grade III	**Black brown spot**
	Point bleeding + grade II	

NIEC, New Italian Endoscopic Club.

the New Italian Endoscopy Club[162,163] have described a more detailed scoring system. Tanoue and colleagues[162] classified PHG into four grades (grade 0 = none, grade 1 = mild, grade 2 = moderate, grade 3 = severe). This grading permits more informative description of the observed endoscopic findings. A simpler classification system such as recommended by McCormack and colleagues[161] has a better intraobserver and interobserver agreement and reproducibility.[164] Further work needs to be done to improve the currently available grading system.

Prevalence

Prospective studies have reported that PHG is present in more than 50% of patients with cirrhosis.[165,166] The reported preva-

lence varies widely because of patient selection, absence of uniform criteria and classification, and, more importantly, the differences in interobserver and intraobserver variation.[167] Although PHG is usually seen in association with either esophageal or gastric varices, there is no direct linear correlation between portal pressure and the presence or severity of PHG.[168] The cause of portal hypertension is unlikely to be a significant factor.[169–171] The prevalence of PHG does not seem to have a linear relationship with the severity of liver disease, as reported by one study that showed the lowest prevalence of severe PHG in Child C patients.[163] This finding may suggest that other, hitherto unidentified factors may play a role in the pathogenesis of PHG. There is general agreement, however, that the prevalence of PHG increases with variceal obliteration.[170]

Pathogenesis

Portal hypertension, and not liver disease, seems to be the key factor for the development of PHG because PHG is equally common in patients with portal hypertension with or without liver disease.[172,173] The improvement or disappearance of PHG in many patients after transjugular intrahepatic portosystemic shunt (TIPS) and shunt surgery suggests that there is a significant association between PHG and portal hypertension. However, the severity and the presence of PHG do not have a linear correlation with the severity of portal hypertension.[168] Chronic elevation in portal pressure and increased splenic circulation may increase gastric mucosal blood flow; this may be one explanation for the development of PHG, but actual measurement of gastric blood flow using Doppler has shown variable results, suggesting that there may be other explanations for the pathogenesis of PHG.[174,175]

The severity of PHG may increase with more advanced liver disease as shown in some studies, but the results are inconsistent.[163,168,169] Many other explanations have been offered for the pathogenesis of PHG. Experimental evidence suggests that gastric mucosal defense mechanisms are impaired in the presence of portal hypertension.[176–178] Aggravation of PHG after variceal banding or sclerotherapy might be caused by alterations in local hemodynamics after obliteration of the esophageal varices.[179,180] Hepatofugal flow velocity is increased in the left gastric vein in direct relationship with the enlarging size of esophageal varices. Gastric mucosal blood flow is higher in cirrhotic patients whose extrahepatic collaterals are predominantly via esophageal varices. Obliteration of the esophageal collateral venous network may cause higher flow velocity in the gastric vascular bed. It has been speculated that the extravasation of sclerosant into the mediastinum during sclerotherapy may result in chemical vagotomy, and this may cause esophageal dysmotility and delayed gastric emptying, leading to the development of PHG.[181] However, there is no direct evidence to suggest that delayed gastric emptying causes PHG.

Natural History and Complications

The overall incidence of acute bleeding from PHG is low, and acute bleeding is seen mostly in patients with more severe PHG. Bleeding is often mild, and transfusion requirement is usually limited to 1 to 2 U of blood. The prevalence of chronic bleeding cannot be reliably estimated because of the uncertainty of making a firm diagnosis. Major determinants of bleeding from PHG are length of time the patient had PHG and the extent and severity of lesions. The mortality associated with bleeding from PHG is very low because most bleeds are minor compared with variceal bleeding. Death caused by PHG is unusual, and PHG is not an independent risk factor for survival.

The presence and severity of PHG seem to change with time. Although some authors believe that PHG is a progressive lesion,[166,182] others have observed that it may regress in a fair proportion of patients. In one study, during a follow-up of 2 years, the severity of PHG fluctuated with time in 25%, improved in 23%, remained stable in 29%, and deteriorated in 23%.[163] The variability in results can be due to differences in the patient population, the time when the lesions appear, or the influence of endoscopic intervention for varices. Endoscopic sclerotherapy and banding seems to worsen the severity of PHG and increases the risk of bleeding.[161,162,179,180] In one study, 44% of patients developed PHG after variceal eradication by sclerotherapy compared with only 9% before sclerotherapy.[170] The results in this prospective study suggested that if gastropathy persists for more than 3 months, it is likely to persist for longer periods. In a few patients, PHG lesions may still regress within 6 months but are unlikely to regress beyond this period; when PHG was present before endoscopic therapy for varices, the lesions often persisted or progressed after obliteration of esophageal varices. The frequency of bleeding from PHG in these circumstances was high. For these reasons, the study investigators recommended that such patients be followed with serial endoscopies and that the benefits of β blocker therapy be evaluated as prophylaxis against PHG bleeding.[170] However, the efficacy of serial endoscopies simply for monitoring of the progression of PHG remains to be proven.[183]

Management

Clinically significant bleeding is seen only in association with severe PHG. Effective treatment requires a reduction in the portal pressure.

PHARMACOLOGIC TREATMENT

The aim of pharmacologic treatment is (1) to control hemorrhage in patients with actively bleeding PHG and (2) to prevent rebleeding in patients with known PHG.

Nonselective β Blockers

Nonselective β blockers, such as propranolol and nadolol, have been shown to reduce portal pressure and gastric mucosal blood flow. In small studies, propranolol has been shown to reduce bleeding related to PHG.[184,185] In a randomized, controlled trial of 56 patients with PHG, multivariate analysis showed that absence of propranolol treatment was the only predictive variable for rebleeding.[165] The use of propranolol in PHG leads to endoscopic improvement, a cessation of bleeding in acutely hemorrhaging patients, and a decreased incidence of rebleeding from severe PHG. Pharmacologic therapy is typically long-term because of evidence that discontinuation of therapy can lead to rebleeding from PHG. Other medications, such as prednisone, estrogen, and progesterone, are ineffective for bleeding-related PHG.

Vasoactive Agents

Given the proven beneficial effects of vasoactive agents such as somatostatin, octreotide, and terlipressin in variceal bleeding, their role in the management of PHG has also been evaluated. Somatostatin has been shown to reduce gastric mucosal blood flow by decreasing splanchnic blood flow.[186] Similar effects are seen with vasopressin and terlipressin. In patients with acute bleeding, an uncontrolled study showed efficacy with somatostatin and octreotide.[187] A more recent study showed that the decrease in portal pressure is only transient, however, and use of somatostatin or octreotide is unlikely to benefit patients with chronic PHG bleeding.[188] Use of these agents should be limited to patients with acute bleeding. There are no clinical trials directly comparing the efficacy of propranolol versus octreotide for active hemorrhage related to PHG. Some authors use octreotide first in patients with acute bleeding because it is better tolerated than propranolol in this setting.[189]

ENDOSCOPIC TREATMENT

Endoscopic treatment does not have a significant role in the management of PHG bleeding because the bleeding is often mild and diffuse. If an active bleeding site is identified, it could be managed by injection of sclerosant or cauterization using the heater or bipolar probe. Although laser therapy has been shown to be safe and effective in reducing GAVE-associated bleeding, it is unknown whether laser therapy is effective or safe in patients with severe PHG when the predominant lesion is in the gastric antrum.[190]

NONINVASIVE AND INVASIVE SURGERY

Both TIPS and shunt surgery have been shown to be effective for PHG bleeding in anecdotal reports. In a study by Orloff and coworkers,[191] portacaval shunting successfully controlled bleeding, and the gastric mucosa had reverted to normal on follow-up gastroscopies in all 12 patients with repeated bleeding unresponsive to propranolol. TIPS was shown to improve PHG in 9 of 10 patients.[192] TIPS successfully stopped recurrent bleeding refractory to medical therapy in one of these patients. TIPS offers another therapeutic option for patients who have bleeding refractory to medical therapy, especially if they are poor candidates for surgical shunts.[193] Despite these encouraging anecdotal reports, most authors believe[189] that TIPS or shunt surgery should be used only as the last resort in these patients because the risks outweigh the benefits. Currently, the only treatment that could be recommended for prophylaxis of PHG bleeding is nonselective β blockers such as propranolol or nadolol. Pharmacologic therapy is typically long-term because of evidence that discontinuation of therapy can lead to rebleeding from PHG.[193] Efficacy of therapy can be followed clinically and endoscopically; efficacy is evidenced by improved mucosal appearance and diminished portal hypertension.

Gastric Antral Vascular Ectasia

GAVE was first described in 1984 by Jabbari and colleagues.[194] These authors coined "watermelon stomach" to describe GAVE because of its resemblance to the skin of a watermelon. GAVE describes vascular lesions of the antrum organized in a linear array on top of raised convoluted folds radiating outward from the pylorus, similar to spokes from a wheel, and resembling the dark stripes on the surface of a watermelon (**Fig. 16.6A**). The typical histologic appearance of GAVE includes marked dilation of capillaries and collecting venules in the gastric mucosa and submucosa with areas of intimal thickening characterized by fibromuscular hyperplasia, fibrohyalinosis, and thrombi.[155,156,194] An increasing number of reports of GAVE have included some cases in which the endoscopic appearance showed spotty erythemas diffusely scattered in the antral area and coalesced (diffuse antral vascular ectasia or "honeycomb stomach").[4,25] Diffuse antral vascular ectasia is now recognized as the same entity as "watermelon stomach," and both are regarded as GAVE (**Fig. 16.6B**).[26]

The diffuse form is the predominant pattern in patients with cirrhosis. Noncirrhotic patients with GAVE are typically middle-aged or older women; in these patients, GAVE is associated with achlorhydria, atrophic gastritis, CREST syndrome, and post–bone marrow transplantation.[26,49,195]

Pathogenesis

The pathogenesis of GAVE is poorly understood, and there is no single unifying hypothesis. Possible mechanisms include humoral factors and mechanical causes.[155,156,196] Spahr and coworkers[197] observed that GAVE was not improved by successful portal decompression after TIPS (one patient) or by endoscopic laser therapy (one patient), whereas the antral mucosal lesions disappeared completely after liver transplan-

tation. GAVE could be related to increased secretion of yet unidentified vasoactive substances in the presence of liver disease; for example, glucagon and nitric oxide were found to be increased in cirrhotic patients. Local disturbances in vascular tone must be involved to explain that vascular ectasias develop specifically in the antrum. The proponents of a "mechanical" theory have suggested that chronic intermittent venous obstruction associated with powerful muscular contractions of the antrum and pylorus or repeated trauma associated with a loosely attached antral mucosa and prolapse of the antral mucosa through the pylorus may cause GAVE.[194,198,199] The fibromuscular hyperplasia seen at histology in GAVE supports the hypothesis of repeated mechanical stress induced by gastric peristalsis.

Relationship between Portal Hypertensive Gastropathy and Gastric Antral Vascular Ectasia

Some researchers believe that GAVE and PHG are different manifestations of the same pathogenetic process, whereas others view them as separate entities.[156] These lesions can be differentiated by endoscopic and histologic findings. PHG is always associated with cirrhosis and is observed mostly in the fundus and corpus of the stomach; mucosal red spots and the so-called mosaic pattern are present, and the histologic examination shows only microvascular ectasia in the mucosa without signs of inflammation. By contrast, GAVE can occur in cirrhotic and noncirrhotic patients. Lesions are found almost exclusively in the antrum, and the mucosal microvascular ectasias are either aggregated in linear stripes (as in "watermelon stomach") or diffusely spread. Histologically, true ectasia of the mucosal microvasculature is present and associated with fibrin thrombi, fibrohyalinosis, and spindle cell proliferation. This constellation of findings can be identified within the body of the stomach in a patient with PHG but not a patient with GAVE.

In severe PHG, the mucosal vascular ectasias are linearly arrayed in the antrum and resemble GAVE. A GAVE-like appearance is commonly seen in patients with portal hypertension.[164] The dilemma is whether this appearance is GAVE or severe PHG. As mentioned earlier, the histologic appearance of GAVE is confined to the antrum. Similar histologic examination of random biopsy specimens in the body of the

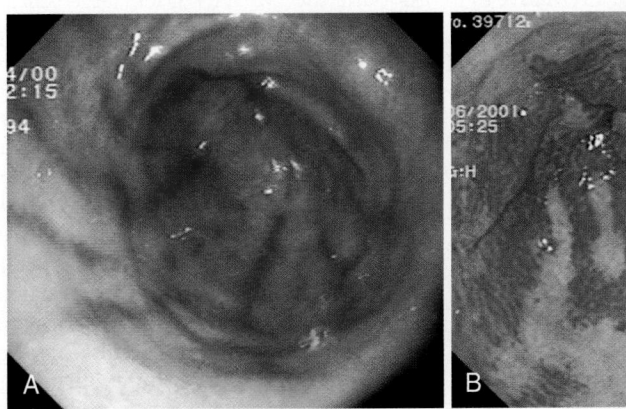

Fig. 16.6 Two different forms of gastric vascular antral ectasia: "watermelon stomach" **(A)** and diffuse vascular antral ectasia **(B)**.

stomach in patients with severe PHG can serve to discriminate between the two. In contrast to PHG, bleeding from GAVE is not known to respond to nonselective β blockers.[156,200] However, a therapeutic challenge is not clinically useful to differentiate these two entities because the response to β blockers is variable in patients with PHG. Kamath and associates[201] showed that compared with patients with PHG, patients with GAVE, in the absence of background mosaic appearance, did not respond to TIPS.

It has been suggested that the same gastric vascular alteration related to portal hypertension may appear grossly and histologically different depending on the anatomic location in the stomach.[166] The hemodynamics of venous drainage of the antrum are different from the body or the fundus of the stomach. It can be argued that the "typical" histologic changes, fibrosis and thrombosis, seen in GAVE are also seen with more chronic and severe PHG confined to the antrum. The variable response to β blockers and TIPS may be a reflection of the advanced histologic changes.[156] Some authors believe that the diagnosis of GAVE should be reserved for patients with the presence of typical, linear red lesions in the gastric antrum without the mosaiclike appearance of mucosal background in the rest of the stomach. When there is evidence of a mosaiclike pattern or evidence of more severe PHG in the body and fundus, some authors favor classifying it as a spectrum of PHG.[164]

Management

Bleeding from gastric mucosal lesions in patients with portal hypertension is a serious complication, although bleeding is usually slow and insidious and rarely massive and life-threatening. However, multiple transfusions may be required during follow-up. Endoscopic therapy generally is preferred because of its efficacy, but pharmacologic treatment may be used as adjunct therapy or in patients with persistent bleeding from mucosal areas not amenable to endoscopic therapy.

PHARMACOLOGIC TREATMENT
Combination Hormonal Therapy

Combination hormonal therapy has been shown to be effective in controlling bleeding from GAVE in some case reports and small trials.[202–205] Hormonal therapy does not improve the endoscopic appearance of this lesion. As with other pharmacologic therapies, hormonal therapy provides an alternative to endoscopic therapy when extensive vascular abnormalities are present. It also eliminates the risk of circumferential scarring and stenosis, which can occur with the endoscopic modalities discussed.

Tranexamic Acid

One case report described the use of tranexamic acid for GAVE.[206] Given the limited experience with antifibrinolytics for GI bleeding, the use of this agent should be reserved for refractory patients who have failed other measures.[189]

Octreotide

Octreotide was used in one trial with successful results.[101] However, at least one case report failed to show a response of GAVE to octreotide.[207]

β Blockers

Treatment with β blockers has been reported to be successful in controlling bleeding from gastric mucosal lesions in cirrhotic patients. However, it is unclear in these reports whether patients bled from PHG or from GAVE.[165,185] In the study from Spahr and coworkers,[197] treatment with the nonselective β blocker nadolol did not control chronic bleeding from GAVE. In addition, the results of this study clearly showed that the decrease in portal hypertension after TIPS or shunt surgery was not effective in controlling chronic blood loss related to GAVE.[197]

ENDOSCOPIC TREATMENT

The current first-line therapy for GAVE consists of endoscopic coagulative ablation. The aim of endoscopic therapy is to eliminate completely or reduce significantly the blood transfusion requirements of a patient with bleeding.

Neodymium:Yttrium-Aluminum-Garnet Laser Coagulation

In a trial by Bourke and associates,[208] Nd:YAG laser coagulation was used in 11 consecutive patients with GAVE. Transfusion dependence was eliminated in two-thirds of the patients and decreased in the remaining patients. In this trial, an average of three sessions per patient was required; sucralfate was used to prevent iatrogenic ulceration. Endoscopic laser therapy is repeated every 8 to 12 weeks until most of the lesions disappear and the hemoglobin remains stable. Sufficient time must be allowed after laser photocoagulation therapy for healing of the thermally induced ulcers to occur and to maximize the assessment of residual vascular lesions. One study indicated that the mean number of treatments needed to obliterate the vascular lesions and eliminate the need for transfusions was less for Nd:YAG laser compared with APC (2.33 ± 0.27 vs. 5.75 ± 0.89).[209]

Heater Probe

The heater probe uses a thermal element that heats the device tip and results in tissue coagulation. Petrini and Johnston[210] described the successful use of a heater probe for management of GAVE. An average of four sessions was required to eliminate the transfusion requirements and improve endoscopic appearance in 8 of 10 patients.

Argon Plasma Coagulation

As with the Nd:YAG laser, large surface areas of involved mucosa can be adequately treated with APC during a single endoscopic session. Several case reports have described the successful use of APC for the management of GAVE.[211,212]

Compared with Nd:YAG laser, APC is more convenient to use. The tangential approach to the vascular lesions, especially along the posterior wall of the antrum, makes APC an attractive tool for use compared with the laser device, which requires a more perpendicular approach. Among noncontact thermal endoscopic treatments for GAVE, APC has gained popularity in recent years and is now widely available in endoscopy units. The results from several small series and case reports so far have been similar to the results achieved with the Nd:YAG laser but with a superior safety profile.[213] Long-term efficacy remains suboptimal, however, with a 22% incidence of recurrent bleeding and with up to 31% of patients requiring ongoing transfusions.[156,214,215] Long-term sequelae of ablation include antral scarring and hyperplastic polyps.[216] Most rebleeding episodes respond to repeated treatment, but these patients may require multiple sessions and commitment to ongoing endoscopic treatments.[213]

Higher power settings should be used for patients with GAVE to provide ablation of the mucosal and submucosal vascular abnormalities. Nd:YAG laser therapy provides a viable option for patients with refractory bleeding and should be offered to these patients. The major problem with GAVE is continued blood loss requiring repeated blood transfusions. Ikeda and colleagues[217] presented a 10-year endoscopic follow-up study from discrete initial lesions to the full picture of GAVE. They reported that latent hemorrhage occurred at an early stage as the coalesced lesions formed and that the vascular lesions of GAVE should be eradicated at this stage. The underlying pathophysiology is unclear, and endoscopic ablative methods do not affect the origins of the problem, so there is a long-term potential for recurrent vascular lesions and bleeding.

Generally, Nd:YAG laser and APC are preferred over heater probe for the treatment of GAVE because of their ability to cover a greater surface area. However, the endoscopic therapeutic modality chosen also depends on the individual experience of the endoscopist and local availability.[189]

Other Endoscopic Techniques

Band Ligation

A retrospective study of thermal therapy (APC or multipolar electrocoagulation probe) compared with band ligation found that band ligation may offer a therapeutic option.[218] The use of band ligation requires meticulous efforts to band ligate all of the involved mucosa, which is technically challenging and expensive. At the present time, this form of therapy cannot be advocated as superior to existing therapies. Newer mucosal ablation techniques,[219] such as radiofrequency ablation and cryotherapy, have also been used to ablate GAVE in small pilot studies.

Cryotherapy

A study of 26 patients with various bleeding lesions (e.g., GAVE, arteriovenous malformations, radiation proctitis, radiation gastritis) were treated with cryotherapy with a mean of 3.6 sessions.[135] These patients had previously undergone treatment with multipolar electrocoagulation and heater probe but continued to have bleeding. Cryotherapy with nitrous oxide was efficacious in causing hemostasis in 77% overall, with follow-up of 6 months. Another report included 12 patients with a diagnosis of GAVE and documented iron deficiency anemia. Eight patients had a history of overt GI bleeding. Eight patients (67%) had previously been treated with APC (median 6 sessions, range 1 to 10 sessions) and failed to respond or had a recurrence. Six patients (50%) had a complete response, and six patients (50%) had a partial response.[220]

Preliminary data suggest that cryotherapy may be a reasonable option for diffuse GAVE lesions. Although the etiology of GAVE is poorly understood, histopathology results show distinct abnormalities limited to mucosa and lamina propria, including superficial fibromuscular hyperplasia with capillary ectasia and microvascular thrombosis. Cryotherapy seems to work in GAVE by causing a deeper injury compared with APC with necrosis of mucosa and superficial submucosa, followed

by reepithelialization. A major advantage of cryotherapy over APC is its ability to treat large areas of mucosa relatively quickly because ice formation occurs after 2 to 3 seconds of spraying the mucosa and is quickly followed by thawing.[135]

Effective and safe APC treatment requires an experienced endoscopist who is able to target the lesions accurately while maintaining a 1- to 3-mm distance from the mucosa for effective coagulation and avoidance of transmural injury especially because high-power settings are used. Cryotherapy treatment times for GAVE have not previously been reported. Cho and associates[220] were able to treat greater than 90% of affected mucosa in 89% of cases, with a mean of 5 minutes. Because of its ability to spray a large area quickly, there was no significant difference in the duration with respect to the extent of GAVE. A reduction in the duration of treatment was observed with subsequent cryotherapy sessions, which may reflect the endoscopists' learning curve with cryotherapy, the use of an overtube, and the reduction in the extent of the lesions to be treated. Limitations of cryotherapy include the need for specialized equipment and training. An overtube has been used to enable passive venting of carbon dioxide to reduce patient discomfort and the risk of perforation. The requirement for an overtube extends the duration of the procedure and adds technical difficulty and risk to the procedure.

The promising benefits of cryotherapy would suggest that a randomized controlled trial that compares endoscopic cryotherapy with APC is warranted. Documentation of different patterns of GAVE, patient characteristics, and histopathology of lesions before and after treatment for both responders and nonresponders to different treatment modalities may provide useful information regarding the optimal endoscopic management of this condition.

Radiofrequency Ablation

A pilot study of six patients with GAVE treated with the HALO90 device (Barrx Medical, Sunnyvale, CA) showed improved hemoglobin concentrations in all patients after one to three treatments. Five of six patients were no longer dependent on transfusions.[221] This device provided very superficial coagulation injury. Considerably more experience is needed to determine if this expensive form of therapy is justified.

SURGERY

In the study from Spahr and coworkers,[197] chronic bleeding was never controlled in one patient who underwent a surgical shunt despite a complete normalization of portal pressure. Similarly, it has been reported that portacaval shunt surgery proved ineffective in treating chronic GI blood loss related to GAVE in a patient with portal hypertension as a result of nodular regenerative hyperplasia.[222] Antrectomy provides the most definitive therapy for GAVE as illustrated by low rates of rebleeding and anemia recurrence.[223–225] Surgery carries a significant risk of mortality, however, in cirrhotic patients with portal hypertension. TIPS placement may make antrectomy easier and faster by avoiding operative blood losses related to the presence of collaterals secondary to portal hypertension. However, TIPS should be restricted to cirrhotic patients with good liver function, owing to the risk of TIPS-induced progressive liver failure.[197] Given the comorbid illnesses typically associated with GAVE and the advanced age of most patients, surgery is considered salvage therapy for patients who have not responded to a reasonable trial of endoscopic or pharmacologic therapies.[189]

Portal Colopathy

Clinical Manifestations

Over the past 2 decades, awareness of the association between portal hypertension and changes in the intestinal circulation has increased. The fundamental pathologic change is a vasculopathy. Portal hypertensive vasculopathy most often involves the stomach (PHG) and can be a source of bleeding. The significance of small bowel involvement (enteropathy) is unknown. Colonic involvement (colopathy) has been associated with bleeding. Several studies have described the colonic findings associated with cirrhosis and portal hypertension.[226–235] Colorectal lesions associated with portal hypertension and cirrhosis include hemorrhoids, varices (portosystemic collaterals that develop because of portal hypertension; **Fig. 16.7A**), focal and diffuse angiectases, and spiderlike vascular lesions. The term *portal colopathy* has been used to describe colonic lesions resembling the vascular lesions of portal gastropathy and the diffuse colitislike appearance seen in patients with portal hypertension (**Fig. 16.7B**).[226,227] There is confusion regarding the diagnostic criteria and clinical significance of this condition. This confusion might be attributable to imprecise terminology, lack of uniform endoscopic descriptions, interobserver variability, and the absence of distinctive histopathologic features.[236]

In previously published studies, the prevalence of colonic abnormalities in patients with cirrhosis varied widely (**Table 16.4**), and the true prevalence of portal colopathy is unknown. Because all patients in some studies were referred for colonoscopy based on clinical indications,[237] these reviews may have overestimated the true prevalence of portal colopathy. Conflicting data have been published regarding the relationship between the prevalence of portal colopathy and Child-Pugh classification in cirrhotic patients.[226–228,233,235,237,238]

In the study from Bini and associates,[237] portal gastropathy, 2+ or larger esophageal varices, Child-Pugh class C cirrhosis, and the use of β blockers were independent predictors of portal colopathy; the use of β blockers was protective. Portal hypertensive colopathy and gastropathy might not be distinct entities but rather regional manifestations of portal hypertension. These entities might share similar mechanisms with

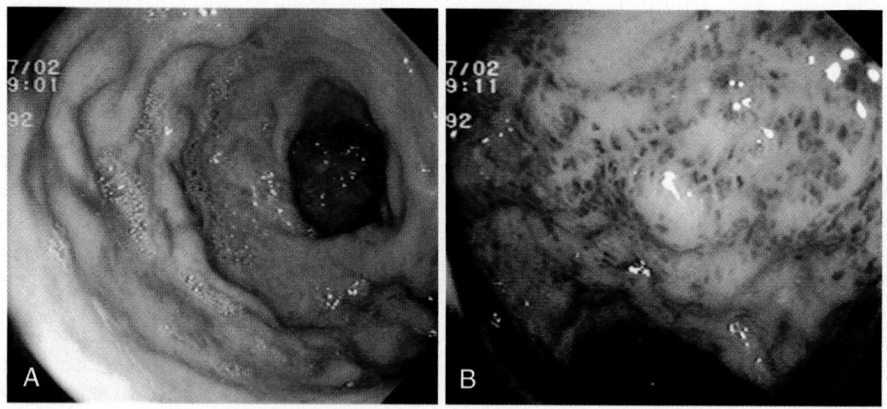

Fig. 16.7 Portal colopathy. **A,** Portal hypertension causing collateral circulation in the rectum. **B,** Colitis with granularity, erythema, friability, and cherry-red spots.

Table 16.4 Published Studies on the Prevalence of Colonic Abnormalities in Patients with Cirrhosis

Study	No. Patients	Colitislike Lesions (%)	Vascular Lesions (%)	Rectal Varices (%)	Hemorrhoids (%)
Kozarek et al[226]	20	20	70	25	NS
Naveau et al[227]	64	NS	25	20	NS
Chen at al[228]	35	NS	49	46	NS
Tam et al[229]	75	11	84	13	NS
Rabinovitz et al[230]	412	32	NS	4	25
Scandalis et al[231]	38	58	0	8	39
Goenka et al[232]	75	NS	12	89	41
Ganguly et al[233]	50	6	52	44	NS
Misra et al[234]	70	27	49	40	36
Bresci et al[235]	50	10	16	34	70
Bini et al[237]	437	38	13	9	46

NS, Not stated.

regard to pathogenesis. The histology of the colitislike mucosal abnormalities from most patients with portal hypertension is nonspecific, mild inflammation. Several studies have shown that the endoscopic appearance of colonic mucosal edema and erythema is not associated with significant inflammatory infiltrates but rather mucosal vessel changes.[227,237,239,240] Based on these findings, some authors suggest the use of the term *colopathy* when referring to the mucosal abnormalities of the colon in patients with cirrhosis.[237] This term avoids the suggestion of the involvement of inflammatory cells in the pathogenesis of a disease that lacks a definitive etiologic mechanism.

Several endoscopic classification systems exist to grade the severity of mucosal changes in patients with portal gastropathy.[161,163] To date, no classification systems exist for grading the severity of mucosal abnormalities in cirrhotic patients with portal colopathy, making comparisons between studies difficult. Based on their findings, Bini and associates[237] proposed that portal colopathy could be classified into three grades: *grade 1,* erythema of the colonic mucosa; *grade 2,* erythema along with a mosaiclike appearance of the mucosa; and *grade 3,* vascular lesions of the colon, including cherry-red spots, telangiectases, or angiodysplasialike lesions. The same authors[237] observed for the first time an increase in the prevalence of portal colopathy in cirrhotic patients who had undergone band ligation or sclerotherapy, or both, of esophageal varices. They suggested that, similar to PHG, it may be that portal colopathy is related to the levels of portal pressure and that obliteration of esophageal varices may cause a redistribution of blood flow in similar ways in the stomach and colon. Prospective studies are necessary to validate this observation.

Management

β-adrenergic blockers are usually the first-line therapy in patients with portal colopathy. The vascular lesions of portal colopathy are considered amenable to the same thermal therapies as GAVE and PHG, although no trials have been published at this time.[24,226] TIPS may be useful as a second-line treatment in patients with recurrent portal hypertensive bleeding from colonic angiodysplasialike lesions who do not tolerate or are unresponsive to treatment with β-adrenergic blockers.[241]

Hemangiomas

Clinical Manifestations

Hemangiomas are the second most common vascular lesion of the colon. Considered by some investigators to be true neoplasms, they are generally thought to be hamartomas because most are present at birth. They may be solitary or multiple lesions limited to one segment of the GI tract, or they may be part of diffuse GI or multisystem angiomatoses. Individual hemangiomas may be classified as cavernous, capillary, or mixed types. Most are small (**Fig. 16.8**), ranging from a few millimeters to 2 cm, but larger lesions do occur, especially in the rectum (see section on cavernous hemangioma of the rectum). In the presence of GI bleeding, hemangiomas of the skin should suggest the possibility of associated bowel lesions.[47] Hemangiomas causing upper GI hemorrhage are most commonly identified in the upper small intestine. These benign vascular tumors, almost all of which are cavernous hemangiomas, appear as single or multiple red, purple, or blue nodular lesions.

These lesions generally should not be treated endoscopically because they may be transmural, and treatment would result in perforation and induce bleeding from larger vascular elements. Angiographic therapy may stop bleeding; however, the most effective treatment is surgical. Bleeding from colonic hemangiomas usually is low in volume, producing occult blood loss with anemia or melena. Hematochezia is less common except in large, cavernous hemangiomas of the rectum, which may cause massive hemorrhage. Diagnosis is best established by endoscopy, including enteroscopy, because radiologic studies, including angiography, frequently are normal, although the presence of calcifications representing phleboliths within hemangiomas has been described.

Management

Hemangiomas that are small, solitary, or few in number can be treated by colonoscopic coagulation using laser or other thermal mode. Colonoscopic excision of small lesions has been described,[242] including removal of small lesions for the purpose of diagnosis in patients with multiple hemangiomas.[243] Amano and colleagues[244] reported electrosurgical snare polypectomy of a large, pedunculated, polypoid cavernous

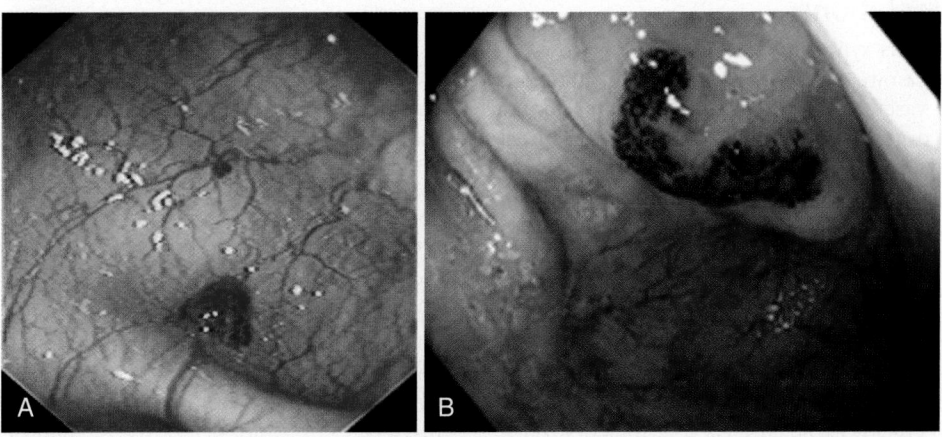

Fig. 16.8 **A,** Solitary hemangioma of the colon. **B,** Narrow band imaging of hemangioma of the colon.

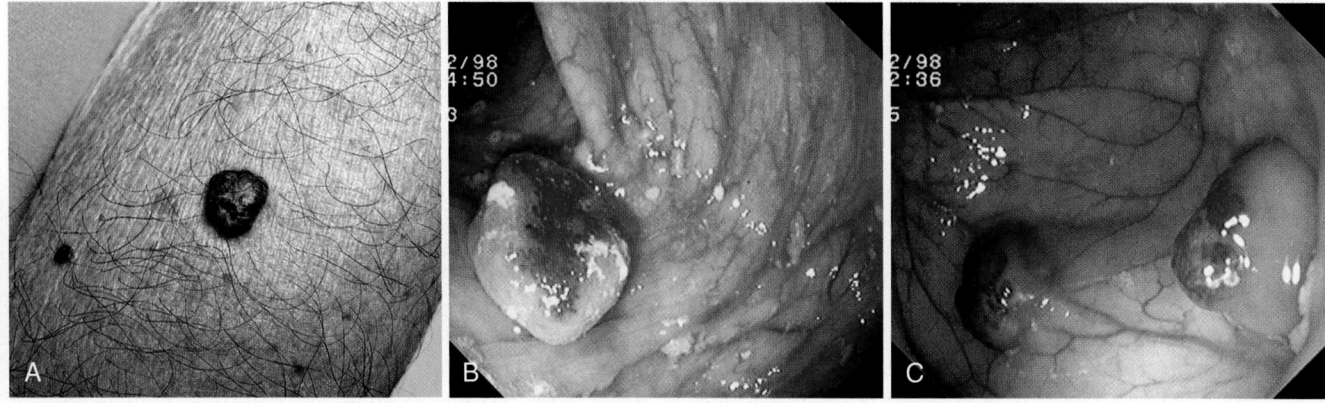

Fig. 16.9 Multiple hemangiomas of blue rubber bleb nevus syndrome. Typical dark blue nodular lesions of the skin **(A)** and involving the colon **(B** and **C)**.

hemangioma that arose in the sigmoid colon in a 28-year-old man who presented with prolapse of the lesion through the anus. Although complications of colonoscopic excision of hemangiomas seem to be rare, the number of reports is small, and it is difficult to determine the safety of colonoscopic treatment. Safety may depend on size and gross morphology of the lesion (e.g., sessile vs. pedunculated) and the technical feasibility of endoscopic treatment. Large or multiple lesions usually require surgical resection of either the hemangioma alone or the involved segment of colon.

Cavernous Hemangioma of the Rectum

A distinct form of colonic hemangioma is cavernous hemangioma of the rectum.[47] These lesions are usually not associated with other GI hemangiomas and are extensive, involving the entire rectum or portions of the rectosigmoid colon. The massive bleeding resulting from these rectal hemangiomas often necessitates excision of the rectum by either abdominal-perineal or low-anterior resection; ligation and embolization of major feeding vessels have been employed successfully. Attempts at local control have been valuable in some instances, but mostly these have been only temporarily effective.

Blue Rubber Bleb Nevus Syndrome

Clinical Manifestations

Blue rubber bleb nevus syndrome (BRBNS), also known as Bean's syndrome, is a rare entity, characterized by cutaneous hemangiomas and vascular tumors of the GI tract, that can also involve other organs such as the brain, kidneys, lungs, eyes, oronasopharynx, parotids, liver, spleen, heart, pleura, peritoneum, pericardium, skeletal muscles, bladder, penis, and vulva.[245–247] Although a familial history is infrequent, a few cases of autosomal dominant transmission have been reported,[24] and one analysis identified a responsible locus on chromosome 9. The lesions were thought to be hemangiomas, but they are now considered to be venous malformations,[24,248] which usually appear in early childhood and tend to increase in size and number with age. They are usually blue and raised, vary from 0.1 to 5 cm in diameter, have a wrinkled surface, and are easily compressible with light palpation. The con-

tained blood can be emptied by direct pressure, leaving a wrinkled blue sac that slowly refills over several seconds or minutes.[24] Skin lesions may be present throughout the body, particularly predominating on the upper limbs (**Fig. 16.9A**), trunk,[249] and face.

GI lesions are usually multiple and may involve any portion of the GI tract but are most common in the small bowel and in the distal part of the colon.[24] The characteristic GI lesion is a discrete mucosal nodule with an overlying central bluish red cap resembling a nipple, but a lesion may be a flat macular, dark bluish red spot or a frankly polypoid nodule with a central venous colored portion (**Fig. 16.9B** and **C**).[246,250] Most patients are asymptomatic. Loss of blood from the GI tract is the major problem and commonly causes chronic anemia.[250,251] The onset of GI bleeding may be at any time from early childhood to middle age.[145] The lesions can also cause intestinal intussusception[252] and numerous extraintestinal problems, such as orthopedic deformities associated with bone involvement,[245] neurologic defects secondary to central nervous system involvement[253] and spinal cord compression,[254] pulmonary hypertension owing to vascular obliteration, hemothorax and hemopericardium,[255] exophthalmos and loss of vision secondary to eye involvement,[247] and disseminated intravascular coagulation and thrombocytopenia.[256]

Diagnosis

When blue rubber bleb nevus syndrome is suspected and depending on the clinical manifestations, diagnostic studies should include gastroscopy, colonoscopy, capsule endoscopy,[257] enteroscopy,[246] intraoperative enteroscopy,[248] endoscopic ultrasound,[258] enteroclysis, ultrasound, CT,[251] magnetic resonance (MR) imaging,[249,253,259] radionuclide tagged red blood cell scan,[255] and angiography.[260]

Treatment

Most patients respond to supportive therapy, such as iron supplementation and blood transfusion when required.[250] For recurrent bleeding, medical, endoscopic, and surgical therapies have been used. Medical therapy includes the use of corticosteroids,[256,261] antifibrinolytic agents,[262] γ-globulin,[256] interferon,[248,261] and octeotride.[262] Endoscopic management seems to be safe and useful, although the lesions can be trans-

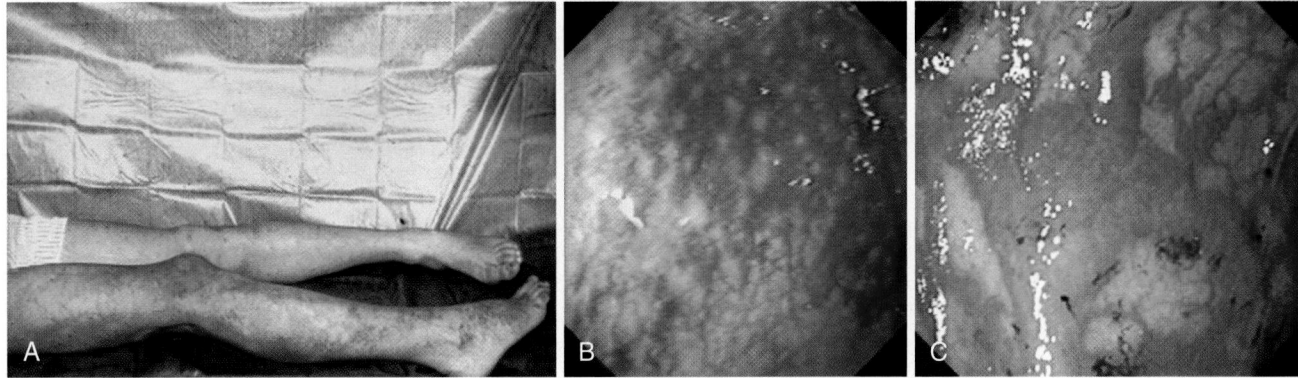

Fig. 16.10 Klippel-Trénaunay-Weber syndrome involving gastrointestinal tract. **A,** Hypertrophic leg caused by venous hypertension and stasis. **B,** Rectal hemangioma in the same patient. **C,** Rectal hemangiomas and venous varicosities in another patient with Klippel-Trénaunay-Weber syndrome.

mural, which implies a theoretical increase in risk for bowel perforation as a complication. There are several reports of endoscopic therapy, including sclerotherapy with absolute alcohol,[263] sodium morrhuate,[264] epinephrine and polidocanol,[265] band ligation,[251,265] polypectomy,[249,251,266] bipolar coagulation,[267] and laser therapy.[267,268]

Angiographic embolization can be useful for treating acute bleeding and preventing further bleeding.[269] Successful surgical excision of the bleeding lesions or segmental resection of the involved bowel segment has been performed[248,270] and can be aided by intraoperative endoscopy.[248,271] Patients with an overwhelming number of lesions may require staged operative procedures.[248]

Klippel-Trénaunay-Weber Syndrome

Clinical Manifestations

Klippel-Trénaunay-Weber syndrome, also known as nevus vasculosus hypertrophicus, is a rare congenital vascular malformation, secondary to a generalized mesodermal development abnormality.[272] Originally described by Klippel and Trénaunay in 1900, it is characterized by bony or soft tissue hypertrophy, usually affecting one extremity (**Fig. 16.10A**); hemangiomas or lymphangiomas or both; and varicosities or venous malformations, appearing at birth or in childhood.

Visceral hemangiomas have been described involving organs such as the GI tract (**Fig. 16.10B**), liver, spleen, bladder, kidney, lung, and heart.[273,274] Involvement of the GI tract may be more common than previously believed, occurring in 20% of patients.[274] GI hemorrhage is a potential serious complication secondary to diffuse vascular malformations involving the GI tract. GI bleeding usually begins in the 1st decade of life and may be recurrent and mild or severe.[273] The severity may be enhanced by a consumption coagulopathy owing to intravascular clotting within the venous sinusoids of the hemangiomas.[47] The most common reported cause of GI bleeding is attributed to diffuse cavernous hemangiomas of the distal colon and rectum,[275] found in 1% to 12.5% of cases.[273,276] Less frequent causes of GI bleeding are rectal or rectovaginal varices caused by obstruction of the internal iliac system, esophageal varices secondary to prehepatic portal hypertension owing to cavernous transformation or hypoplasia of the portal vein,[277] and jejunal hemangiomas.[278] Colonic obstruc-

tion and ascites secondary to massive hemangiomatous-lymphangiomatous retroperitoneal masses may occur.[279]

Diagnosis

Radiologic investigations play an important role in assessing colorectal involvement in Klippel-Trénaunay-Weber syndrome and occasionally finding the specific bleeding site. The presence of phleboliths on a plain abdominal radiograph in these very young patients suggests that they have angiomatosis.[273] Barium studies can show luminal distensible narrowing, with a scalloped mucosal outline caused by the presence of varicosities or submucosal hemangiomas.[47,280] CT and MR imaging of the abdomen and pelvis provide a simple, noninvasive means of assessing visceral hemangiomatous masses and identifying upward extension in the pelvis and abdomen.[274,280] Abdominal angiography is required preoperatively for defining the anatomy and extent of the intestinal involvement to guide surgical intervention.[278] At colonoscopy, the rectum and the lower part of the colon may show visible mucosal vessels or compressible nodules and extensive bluish angiomatous submucosal lesions. Biopsy of the lesions should be avoided because it may precipitate severe hemorrhage.[273] Lesions in deeper layers of the wall can be assessed by endoscopic ultrasound.[281]

Treatment

Treatment varies from conservative to surgical measures, depending on the clinical symptoms and risk of complications. Transfusion dependency, life-threatening bleeding episodes, and poor quality of life require definitive surgical therapy.[273,274] When the entire rectum is severely involved, surgery is sometimes necessary via an abdominoperineal resection of the involved rectum and colon, with a permanent colostomy[276] or with a colon pouch anal anastomosis.[282] Angiographic embolization may be useful if a specific active bleeding site is found[273] or preoperatively.[282] Endoscopic therapy has a limited role because of the commonly diffuse nature of the intestinal hemangiomas[283] and is reserved for management of localized lesions or ablation of postoperative residual disease. The use of argon[284] and Nd:YAG laser,[283] sclerosis with formaldehyde and absolute alcohol,[285] and placement of hemostatic clips in the rectum combined with arterial embolization[286] have been reported with success. APC and photodynamic therapy[273] may be very efficient, but their use in Klippel-Trénaunay-Weber syndrome has not yet been reported.

Radiation Injury of the Gastrointestinal Tract

Radiation Proctopathy

Clinical Manifestations

Radiotherapy is a common treatment modality used for several pelvic malignancies. Despite progress in radiation techniques, adjacent organs are still exposed to chronic radiation injury, which occurs in 2% to 25% of patients.[287]

The rectum, a fixed organ in the pelvis, has a glandular-type epithelium in which the cells undergo a rapid turnover. This organ is particularly vulnerable to ionizing radiation and to radiation-induced complications. The incidence of such complications is proportional to the dose and its degree of spreading and to the volume and method of irradiation (external or by brachytherapy).[287] Intracavitary radiation delivery has been shown to increase the risk of developing chronic radiation proctopathy.[288] Risk factors for radiation-induced damage include history of abdominal surgery, arteriosclerosis, obesity, diabetes, and concomitant chemotherapy.[287,289,290]

Radiation injury to the intestine has acute and chronic phases. Acute radiation injury occurs during or immediately after treatment and results from direct cellular damage. This injury inhibits division of the intestinal crypt stem cells, and the lamina propria becomes infiltrated with inflammatory cells resulting in loss of cellular function and mucosal inflammation. Clinical symptoms of acute radiation proctitis— diarrhea and tenesmus—are usually self-resolving, requiring only symptomatic treatment, and are not typically therapeutic challenges.[291] Chronic radiation proctopathy is histologically characterized by submucosal collagen proliferation, endarteritis of arterioles, and thrombi in vessel lumens, leading to submucosal fibrosis, chronic mucosal ischemia, and progressive epithelial atrophy.[292] Clinical symptoms of chronic radiation usually begin months to years after the initial radiation exposure, with a median of 8 to 16 months[292,293] but with latencies as long as 30 years.[294] Symptoms include rectal bleeding, diarrhea, rectal pain, fecal urgency, tenesmus, obstructed defecation (in patients who have developed stenosis), and less commonly fecal incontinence and fistulas. Many patients have multiple symptoms with a significantly negative impact on their daily activities.[291] Bleeding may be severe enough to require frequent hospitalizations and blood transfusions; 55% of patients may require support with blood transfusions before undergoing definitive therapy.[295]

Diagnosis

FLEXIBLE SIGMOIDOSCOPY AND COLONOSCOPY

Flexible sigmoidoscopy and colonoscopy aid in diagnosis and determine the extent and severity of radiation injury. The findings include distinctive angiectases accumulated in the distal rectum, extending to and often including the dentate line along with friability and spontaneous bleeding (**Fig. 16.11**). Less frequently, there may be ulceration, stenosis, and fistulas. There is often a distinct margin between normal and abnormal tissue that relates to the edge of the radiation field.[295]

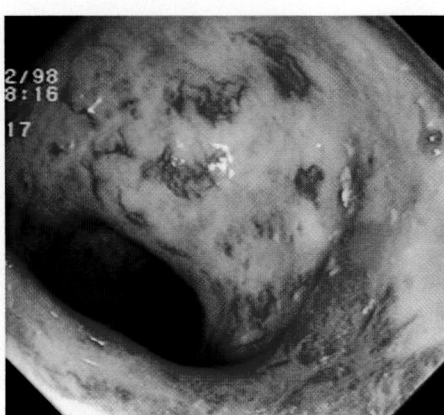

Fig. 16.11 Radiation proctopathy with pale mucosa, edema, and angiectasis.

In some patients, especially women who have undergone radiation therapy after surgery for a gynecologic malignancy, there may be an associated segment of sigmoid colon with identical findings.

BARIUM ENEMA

Barium enema may be helpful in investigating patients suspected to have fistulas or strictures. It may show distortion and narrowing of the colon and rectum, although it tends to underestimate the severity of radiation injury.[296]

MANOMETRY STUDIES

Anorectal physiology manometry studies reveal reduced rectal compliance, rectal volumes, and anal resting pressures and reduced internal anal sphincter length.[297,298]

Treatment

MEDICAL THERAPIES

The traditional approach to treatment of radiation proctopathy has been directed toward decreasing any inflammation with the use of antiinflammatory agents such as aminosalicylic acid derivatives and corticosteroids.[291] The response to such agents is disappointing. Other approaches such as promoting healing in damaged tissue with short-chain fatty acid enemas,[299] oral and rectal sucralfate,[293,300] antioxidants and vitamins,[291] or hormonal therapy with an estrogen-progesterone combination[301] have been tried without significant success. The use of hyperbaric oxygen has been shown more recently to be helpful in patients who are not controlled with endoscopic techniques such as formalin, laser therapy, and APC. The response rate was 68%.[302] The response rate for bleeding was 70% to 76%,[302,303] 48% showed complete resolution of bleeding, and 28% reported significantly fewer bleeding episodes.[303] Although this therapy is expensive and inconvenient, requiring 20 to 40 treatment sessions,[304,305] it should be offered to patients who fail conventional treatments.[306]

ENDOSCOPIC THERAPIES

Different endoscopic therapies have been described for rectal bleeding in this condition.

Topical Formalin

Topical formalin application for radiation injury was first reported in radiation-induced cystitis.[307] Its mechanism of action is likely to be due to a local chemical cauterization of the inflamed or fragile telangiectatic rectal mucosa.[295] The treatment is inexpensive and easy to perform. The technique involves the direct application of 4% formalin to the affected area in the rectum, either with formalin-soaked gauze[308] or by direct instillation and timed retention (typically approximately 10 minutes).[309] The application continues until mucosal blanching occurs, usually within 2 to 3 minutes.[310] The perianal area should be protected with careful draping and the application of petroleum jelly around the anus and perianal skin to avoid formalin injury.[296] The rectum is irrigated liberally after topical application to remove residual formalin. Formalin is contraindicated in the presence of fissures or ulceration. The short-term success of the technique with complete cessation of bleeding ranges from 59% to 100%.[295,311] Recurrent symptomatic relapses have been treated successfully with repeated applications.

In patients with severe radiation proctitis, the administration of topical formalin may be more effective than APC.[312] Complications have been described in 27% to 57% of patients[311,313] and include painful fissures of the anal margins, perianal ulcerations,[314] stool incontinence, and rectal ulcerations and strictures.[309] Some authors think that this technique should be reserved for severe hemorrhagic proctitis refractory to medical or endoscopic treatment and that it should be thoroughly discussed in cases of anorectal radiation–induced stricture, prior anal incontinence, or treated anal cancer.[311] Formalin offers an excellent option for patients who are on anticoagulation and have increased risk for bleeding from thermally induced ulceration after conventional coagulation therapies.

Bipolar Electrocoagulation and Heater Probe

Bipolar electrocoagulation and heater probe are more effective than medical therapy improving the quality of life.[315]

Laser

Argon,[316] Nd:YAG,[317] and KTP laser[318] have been reported to be effective with a marked decrease in bleeding in 87% of treated patients.[295] Repeated treatments were needed in the long-term because symptoms tended to recur.[316] Laser therapy has the advantage of being a precise technique that does not involve tissue contact, is well tolerated, and improves activities of daily life. Disadvantages include its high cost; the need for protective precautions; and the risk of rectal ulcer,[318] bowel perforation, and rectovaginal fistulas.[295]

Argon Plasma Coagulation

APC represents a safer, less expensive, and more widely available alternative to laser therapy.[313] Many authors consider APC to be first-line therapy for radiation proctopathy. When the lesions are circumferential and numerous, a staged treatment may be useful allowing a sufficient period of time for healing of the previously treated area of at least 4 weeks.[287] A median of 1.7 to 3.7 treatment sessions is necessary for control of bleeding.[295,319,320] APC is relatively ineffective in patients with excessive bleeding, owing to the absorption of current by blood on the surface. It is important to minimize contact-induced bleeding during endoscopy to maximize access to the vascular lesions.

Care must be taken not to overdistend the bowel with argon gas insufflations.[295] In the case of low rectal lesions, the use of a transparent cap at the tip of the colonoscope allows direct viewing of these lesions and of the upper part of the anal canal without the retroflexed position. Thanks to the cap, the endoscope remains close to the lesion but with sufficient distance to allow safe APC.[321] One of the most common reasons for failed endoscopic therapy is the failure to coagulate the lesions at and immediately above the dentate line. There was significant improvement in rectal bleeding in many patients, with complete cessation of bleeding in 81% to 98%,[319,322,323] providing long-lasting clinical remission.[324]

APC improves symptoms of diarrhea and tenesmus in 60% to 75% of cases[325] with no obvious reason apparent. Patients with diarrhea and tenesmus should be advised that these symptoms may seem worsened after bleeding is controlled owing to the greater awareness of the symptoms in the absence of bleeding. Because of its limited depth of penetration, morbidity is usually minor and consists of gas bloating, tenesmus, transient abdominal or anal pain, and diarrhea in about 20% of cases.[319] Major complications are exceptional but include rectovaginal fistula,[326] chronic rectal ulceration, anal or rectal stricture,[287] and perforation.[327] Deliberate care should be taken to use the lowest power setting that provides a coagulum and to avoid overtreating, especially with persistent oozing after initial coagulation.

Endoscopic Cryotherapy

Endoscopic cryotherapy using nitrous oxide has been described more recently in a small group of patients with radiation proctitis with complete control of bleeding in all patients.[135] It was also highly effective in patients with multiple angiectases (86%) and "watermelon stomach" (71%), but less effective in patients with radiation gastropathy and duodenopathy (40%). Cryotherapy was applied every 2 to 3 days until all lesions were ablated. The average number of therapeutic sessions needed to stop the bleeding was 3.6. Cryotherapy resulted in superficial tissue necrosis that was usually completely healed within 3 months after the final treatment sessions. Cryotherapy was remarkably safe with only benign self-limited adverse events.

SURGERY

Surgical treatment is now considered a last resort and should be reserved for patients who have intractable symptoms that have failed to respond to medical therapy and patients with rectal strictures and fistulas because it is associated with frequent morbidity (9% to 79%)[295,313] and mortality (3% to 13%).[313,328,329] Proctectomy and Hartmann's procedure, abdominoperianal resection, and coloanal anastomosis are the surgical options. Resection of the affected rectum necessitates dissection in an irradiated field with potential complications that range from bleeding to anastomotic leaks and sepsis.[293]

Radiation Gastropathy

Gastric complications secondary to radiotherapy are uncommon, but injury can occur when the stomach lies within the radiation field of an adjacent extragastric tumor.[330] A high total dose, usually greater than 5000 rad, and a high daily fraction seem to be the main risk factors.[331] There have been

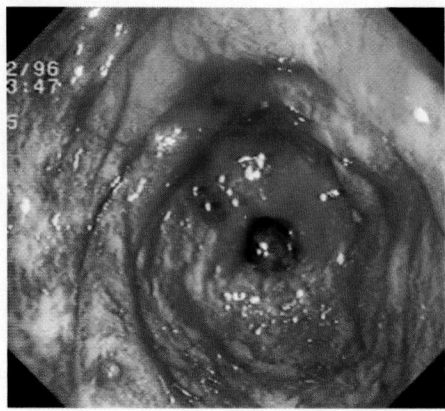

Fig. 16.12 Radiation-induced gastritis with erythema, friability, and ulcerated mucosa.

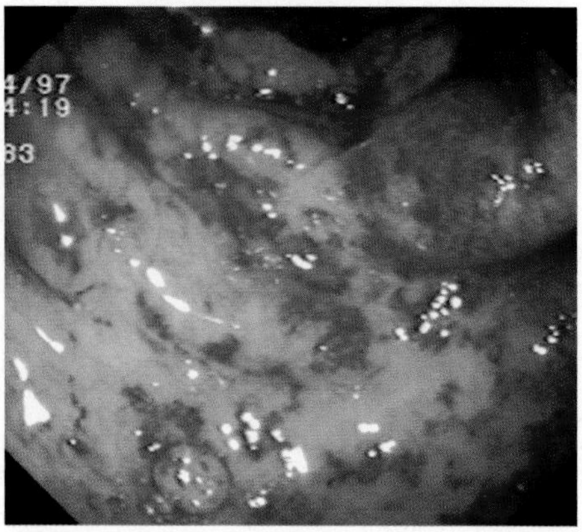

Fig. 16.13 Radiation-induced duodenopathy with edema, friability, and diffuse angiectases.

reports of chronic gastroduodenal ulcerations, gastritis, and duodenitis being diagnosed days to months after selective internal radiation therapy with resin-based microspheres loaded with yttrium-90. It is possible to find small spheres located inside the vessels in the biopsy specimens.[332,333] Acute vasculopathy may progress to a prolonged and progressive endarteritis obliterans, vasculitis, and endothelial proliferation, leading to mucosal ischemia, ulceration, mucosal angiectases and fibrosis.[334]

In contrast to radiation proctopathy, GI bleeding from chronic radiation gastropathy is rare with very few cases reported.[334–336] When it is present, there are multiple friable angiectases. These lead to melena and significant blood loss requiring multiple blood transfusions, prolonged hospitalizations, and repeated endoscopies. Endoscopically, the mucosa of the affected stomach (usually antrum) is friable and with multiple angiectases (**Fig. 16.12**). Other possible severe complications are perforation and gastric outlet obstruction.[292]

There is very little information in the literature on the management of radiation-induced complications in the stomach.[292] Prolonged blood loss needs to be treated with iron and folic acid supplements and with transfusions. Aminocaproic acid[334] and hyperbaric oxygen[335] have been reported to be effective in control of bleeding in a few patients. Bleeding can be controlled by any endoscopic coagulation technique, with APC preferred[336–338] and cryotherapy.[135] Surgery may be necessary if other treatment fails,[331,339] but is associated with high morbidity.[334]

Radiation Injury of the Small Bowel

The small intestine is particularly susceptible to radiation injury (**Fig. 16.13**).[330] Radiation injury to the small intestine most often occurs in the clinical setting of radiotherapy for rectal, urologic, gynecologic, or retroperitoneal malignancies. The degree of injury seems to be proportional to radiation dosage delivered to the segment of small bowel that lies within the radiation field. The relative fixed position of the duodenum and distal ileum within the abdominal cavity make these portions particularly vulnerable to radiation-induced injury. Predisposing factors in the progression of radiation injury include excessive radiation, previous abdominal surgery that fixes loops of bowel in place, underlying cardiovascular

disease, and an asthenic habitus.[340] The mechanism of injury is vascular damage with progressive localized ischemia. The ischemia leads to angiectases and ulceration of the mucosa, fibrosis with stricturing, and, less frequently, fistula formation or perforation.

The clinical manifestations of chronic radiation typically occur 1 to 2 years after exposure and range from malabsorption, hemorrhage, bowel obstruction, fistulas, and abscess formation secondary to perforation.[341] Bleeding can be managed with the same endoscopic techniques that are used in radiation proctitis. Balloon enteroscopy may be needed to access distal small bowel involvement and perform dilation of the diaphragmlike strictures, which resemble strictures seen with long-standing use of nonsteroidal antiinflammatory drugs. The treatment is difficult, and often surgery is necessary.[340] Resection of the involved small bowel segment is preferable to bypass.[137]

Cameron Ulcers and Erosions

Patients with large hernias may develop Cameron ulcers or erosions. These mucosal lesions are usually located on the crest of the mucosal folds that make up the distal hiatal hernia rosette, on the lesser curve of the stomach, or at the level of the diaphragmatic hiatus.[342] Cameron lesions can be found in 5% of all patients with hiatal hernias.[343] The cause of Cameron lesions is still unclear, but it is thought that mechanical trauma secondary to diaphragmatic contraction from respiratory excursions and, perhaps, ischemia and acid mucosal injury play a primary role in their pathogenesis.[344] Cameron lesions manifest clinically with chronic occult GI bleeding and associated iron deficiency anemia. These lesions can also manifest as acute upper GI bleeding in one-third of cases.[343] Treatment includes antisecretory therapy and supplemental iron. In about one-third of patients, Cameron lesions may persist or recur despite antisecretory medication, in which case surgical repair of the hiatal hernia is required.[343]

References

The complete reference list is available online at www.expertconsult.com.

Benign Strictures

Jason R. Taylor and Grace H. Elta

Introduction

Benign strictures occur throughout the gastrointestinal (GI) tract, although they are most common in the esophagus. This chapter focuses on endoscopic diagnosis and therapy of these strictures with a review of the long-term outcome data available.

Esophageal Strictures

The most common presenting symptom of an esophageal stricture is solid food dysphagia. Although there continues to be some debate about whether a barium esophagogram or upper endoscopy is the best initial test in patients with dysphagia,[1] many gastroenterologists favor endoscopy because the diagnoses that benefit from a barium x-ray, such as achalasia and Zenker's diverticulum, are uncommon, and endoscopy offers both diagnosis and treatment for most patients. Dysphagia can be a symptom of gastrointestinal reflux disease (GERD) without the presence of a stricture.[2] Dysphagia typically occurs when the esophagus narrows to a diameter of 13 mm or less (≤39-Fr). Mild degrees of stenosis can be missed endoscopically, and patients with persistent dysphagia after a normal endoscopy and a therapeutic trial of a proton pump inhibitor (PPI) should have a barium esophagogram subsequently performed. The most common etiology of benign esophageal stricture is GERD (**Fig. 17.1**).

Because of the widespread use of PPIs, peptic strictures are becoming less common[3] and are recurring less frequently.[4] They are usually at their worst at the initial presentation.[5] Another etiology of esophageal strictures is corrosive (or caustic) strictures, resulting from either alkali or strong acid ingestion. Compared with peptic strictures, corrosive strictures require more dilation sessions, and the chance of recurrence is higher.[6] Radiation-induced, infection-induced,[7] pill-induced,[8] sclerotherapy-induced,[9] and eosinophilic esophagitis–induced esophageal strictures are less common (**Table 17.1**).[10] Extrinsic compression of the esophagus can also cause symptomatic esophageal stenosis. The most common causes of extrinsic esophageal compression are mediastinal tumors, such as breast and lung cancer and lymphoma, although compression by lymph nodes in tuberculosis and histoplasmosis and by vascular structures such as an aberrant right subclavian artery (arteria lusoria)[11,12] also occurs.

Dilation of Esophageal Strictures

Most reported series on the treatment of benign esophageal strictures are composed predominantly or exclusively of patients with peptic strictures. Consequently, published guidelines on the management of strictures are based primarily on the results of studies of patients with peptic lesions.[1,13]

There are three primary types of dilator (**Table 17.2**). The first, and historically most widely used, type comprises the mercury-filled or tungsten-filled rubber bougies, either blunt-

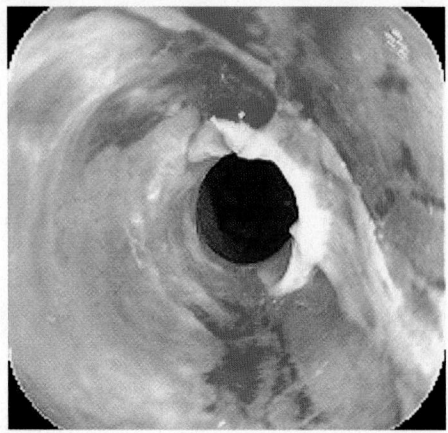

Fig. 17.1 Recurrent peptic esophageal stricture in a patient allergic to proton pump inhibitors who has had two failed fundoplications.

Table 17.1 Benign Diseases That Cause Dysphagia

Mucosal disease	Gastrointestinal reflux disease (peptic stricture)
	Caustic injury (corrosive ingestion, sclerotherapy)
	Radiation injury
	Pill-induced esophagitis
	Rings and webs
	Infectious esophagitis
	Eosinophilic esophagitis
	Anastomotic strictures
Motility disorders	Achalasia
	Scleroderma or CREST syndrome
	Hypothyroidism
	Other motility disorders
Mediastinal compression	Mediastinal infections (tuberculosis, histoplasmosis)
	Arteria lusoria

CREST, calcinosis, Raynaud's phenomenon, esophageal dysmotility, scleroderma, and telangiectases.

Table 17.2 Esophageal Dilators

Mercury- or tungsten-filled bougies	Maloney (tapered tip)
	Hurst (blunt tip)
Wire-guided polyvinyl bougies	Savary
	American Endoscopy
	Celestin (stepwise diameter increase)
Balloon dilators	Through the scope (TTS)
	Controlled radial expansion (CRE) through the scope
	Over-a-wire fluoroscopic control

tipped (Hurst) or with a tapered tip (Maloney). Except for home dilation performed by patients, weighted bougies have been replaced by wire-guided, tapered, polyvinyl bougies or by balloons in most endoscopy units. The major advantage to the wire-guided bougie is the security of knowing that the tip is directed through the stricture rather than into a side wall. This security is heightened by the use of fluoroscopy for wire-guided bougie dilation, although fluoroscopic guidance is unnecessary unless the stricture is extremely narrow or tortuous. There are several manufacturers of wire-guided bougies. The Celestin dilator has a series of short steps, which increase the diameter in a stepwise manner, rather than a smooth taper. In the United States, the Savary (Wilson-Cook) and American Endoscopy (Bard) bougies are the most popular. They differ in the length of the taper and the method for making them radiopaque. Available diameters range from 5 to 20 mm (15-Fr to 60-Fr).

There is insufficient evidence to support claims that fluoroscopic guidance improves the safety of esophageal dilation.[14] In a study of 145 patients treated with Maloney dilators, fluoroscopy was found to alter the dilation technique in 24%.[15] Fluoroscopy was found to be particularly useful for ensuring proper dilator passage in patients with large hiatal hernias. However, the wire-guided bougie alleviates the need for fluoroscopic control. Only in very tight, long, or tortuous strictures where the wire does not freely pass through the stricture is fluoroscopy needed. In a study of more than 300 patients using wire-guided bougienage, only 8% of the patients required fluoroscopically guided dilation.[16]

Balloon dilators can also be used over a wire under fluoroscopic control. At some institutions, this procedure is performed by interventional radiology. The most popular balloons are through the scope (TTS). TTS balloons are passed through the accessory channel of an endoscope and have a soft tip that is passed under direct vision through the stricture. The efficacy of the balloon is improved if water (or contrast medium), rather than air, is used for inflation because fluids are less compressible in tight strictures. TTS balloons range in length from 3 to 8 cm; longer ones (5 to 8 cm) are usually used for the esophagus. Available inflation diameters range from 6 to 20 mm (18-Fr to 60-Fr).

Controlled radial expansion (CRE) balloons are a more recent development in balloon dilation. Individual dilating balloon catheters have three different stepwise inflation diameters that achieve gradated dilation. An in vitro study showed that CRE balloons deliver a consistently reproducible and progressively greater dilating force.[17] The three dilation steps are 1 to 1.5 mm apart for all of the CRE balloon sizes. For example, the 6-mm or 18-Fr balloon achieves 12-Fr size at the first inflation step, 15-Fr size at the second step, and 18-Fr at the final dilation step. The 18-mm balloon has three steps at 16 mm, 17 mm, and 18 mm (48-Fr, 51-Fr, and 54-Fr).

Advantages for TTS balloons are that dilation can be performed immediately during the endoscopy and that the endoscope can be passed through the stricture after dilation. Complete endoscopic examination with biopsy and cytology is facilitated. The major disadvantage of balloons is that they are more expensive, and some are fragile. In bougienage, dilation is accomplished by the radial vector of an axially directed force. In contrast, balloon dilators deliver the entire dilating force radially and simultaneously over the entire length of the stenosis, rather than progressively from the proximal to the distal extent. There is less longitudinal shear stress

Table 17.3 Comparison of Balloon versus Wire-Guided Bougie Dilation

Study	No. Patients	Dilators Compared	Outcome
Scolapio et al (1999)[21]	251	Savary vs. 2 balloon types	No difference in immediate or 1-year relief of dysphagia
Cox et al (1988)[23]	65	Savary vs. balloon	Better relief of dysphagia with bougie
Shemesh and Czerniak (1990)[25]	60	Savary vs. balloon	Savary slightly more effective
Saeed et al (1995)[20]	34	Savary vs. balloon	Balloon slightly better for prevention of recurrence, less procedure discomfort, and required fewer treatment sessions
Tytgat (1989)[24]	60	Savary vs. balloon	Bougie modestly better than balloon for relief of dysphagia
Tulman (1981)[27]	93	Balloon vs. Celestin and Eder-Puestow	Bougie modestly better for relief of dysphagia and maintenance of patency

with balloons.[18] For balloons, the radial vector force is that exerted by the circumference of the balloon, and the magnitude of this force is related to the length and curvature of the balloon waist at the onset of dilation. The dilating force is greater if the stricture is tighter and longer.[19]

Relatively few patients have been studied in randomized trials comparing the efficacy and safety of the different dilator types.[20–27] Of six randomized controlled studies (**Table 17.3**) comparing wire-guided bougienage with balloon dilation, four concluded that a wire-guided bougie was modestly better than a balloon for reduction of dysphagia; one study found that balloon dilation was modestly better than bougienage for prevention of recurrence, required fewer sessions, and had less procedural discomfort; and one study found no difference with regard to relief of dysphagia or the need for repeat dilation. There seems to be no clear superiority in these various outcome measures for one technique over another. One study comparing the risk of perforation with Maloney dilators, wire-guided bougienage, and balloons concluded that Maloney dilation had a greater risk of perforation than the other two techniques.[22] Most endoscopy units have both balloon and wire-guided bougie devices available.

Esophageal Dilation Technique

Patient preparation for esophageal dilation should include holding warfarin or correcting coagulation defects before the procedure. Transient bacteremia is common with endoscopic procedures,[28] but routine antibiotic prophylaxis is not recommended as per the 2008 American Society for Gastrointestinal Endoscopy (ASGE) guidelines.[29]

There is no clear consensus on the optimal size to which a peptic stricture should be dilated. Dysphagia seems to occur when the esophagus is narrowed to less than 13 mm (<39-Fr). Most series report dilation to gauge diameters between 40-Fr and 60-Fr with good relief of symptoms and very low complication rates.[30,31] Although no study has documented a higher perforation risk with larger dilator sizes, it is generally assumed that little therapeutic benefit exists with dilation greater than 50-Fr to 54-Fr, and the possibility of increased risk exists.

When dilating a stricture with bougies, the initial dilator size chosen should approximately equal the estimated stricture diameter. It has been recommended that the stepwise increase in bougie size should be not more than three sizes above that at which significant resistance is felt—the "rule of threes." There are no studies to validate that adherence to this rule increases safety of the procedure. Reported series of patients treated by balloon dilation often use balloon diameters that are larger than the "rule of threes." Also, in a large series of more than 400 patients in which multiple dilators or a single large dilator (>45-Fr) was passed in a single session, only one perforation was observed.[32] Given the risks of perforation, however, it is prudent not to try to accomplish too much dilation in a single setting. Patients can be brought back in 1 to 2 weeks, or even shorter intervals of several days, for repeat sessions to achieve an adequate dilation.

Complications of Esophageal Dilation

The major complications of esophageal dilation are perforation and bleeding. Although there is considerable variation in the studies available, the overall serious complication rate seems to be 0.5%, with perforation and bleeding approximately equal in frequency.[33,34] It has been suggested that "blind" Maloney dilation has a higher perforation rate than wire-guided bougie.[22] However, if wire-guided techniques are reserved for tighter, longer, more difficult strictures, they may show more complications. Perforation usually is obvious with the patient exhibiting distress and in pain. Subcutaneous emphysema may not develop quickly. A chest x-ray and water-soluble x-ray contrast swallow examination should be performed if perforation is suspected. Surgical consultation is mandatory, although many confined perforations have been managed conservatively with no oral intake and intravenous antibiotics. Bleeding severe enough to require transfusions often leads to a repeat endoscopy to determine if endoscopic therapy is required, although most bleeding from esophageal tears stops spontaneously.

Antibiotic Prophylaxis

In 2008, the ASGE published a consensus guideline for antibiotic prophylaxis before endoscopy.[29] The recommendations state that routine antibiotic prophylaxis before endoscopic dilation is not indicated regardless of underlying cardiovascular pathology. Although three prospective trials showed the rate of transient bacteremia after esophageal dilation to be 12% to 22%,[35–37] activities of daily living are associated with higher rates of bacteremia. Chewing food is associated with a rate of bacteremia of 7% to 51%, and brushing and flossing the teeth are associated with rates of 20% to 40%.[38] The guidelines state that transient bacteremia is not a marker of persistent infection or infective endocarditis and that antibiotic prophylaxis before endoscopic dilation is not recommended.[29]

Stricture Recurrence

Before PPIs were available, approximately 60% of patients required repeat dilations for recurrent dysphagia.[39,40] With PPI therapy, 30% of patients with peptic strictures require repeat dilations within 1 year.[41] Factors that predict stricture recurrence depend on the type of stricture. One study evaluated 87 outpatients with either peptic or nonpeptic strictures undergoing initial dilation and followed them for 1 year. In multivariate analysis, narrower stricture diameter and nonpeptic strictures were predictors for early recurrence. The significant predictors for peptic stricture recurrence were the presence of a hiatal hernia and the persistence of heartburn after dilation.[42] The technique of self-bougienage can be taught to patients who require very frequent esophageal dilation despite intensive medical therapy and for whom surgery is either contraindicated or unacceptable. Published data on self-bougienage are very limited, but it seems to be both safe and effective.[43] Given the efficacy of PPIs, self-bougienage for peptic strictures may be primarily of historical interest.

Recalcitrant Esophageal Strictures

Refractory strictures are more commonly due to corrosive injury or surgical anastomoses than a peptic etiology.[44–46] Steroid injection has been recommended for refractory benign esophageal strictures.[47–53] Using a 22-gauge or 23-gauge sclerotherapy needle, four aliquots of 0.50 mL of triamcinolone acetonide are injected before dilation. The dilution of triamcinolone injectant can range from 10 to 40 mg/mL for a total dose of 40 to 100 mg of triamcinolone injected. Some studies report injecting proximal to the strictured segment in addition to within the strictured segment, whereas others report injecting into the strictured segment alone. Although most studies perform the injection before dilation, some experts believe that injection after dilation, once the stricture has been disrupted, is more effective. A study of 14 patients with corrosive strictures showed a marked decrease in the dilation requirement compared with their own historical control.[53]

Similar success was reported in a series of 31 patients with strictures resulting from various causes, including 12 patients with peptic etiology and 8 postsurgical anastomotic strictures, radiation therapy–induced strictures, pill-induced strictures, and sclerotherapy-induced strictures. Intralesional steroid injection led to a significant reduction in the number of dilation sessions in all subjects.[52] There has been one prospective, randomized, double-blind, placebo-controlled trial of endoscopic steroid injection for recalcitrant esophageal peptic strictures. In this study of 30 patients, 15 patients received sham therapy followed by TTS balloon dilation and were compared with another 15 patients who received endoscopic steroid injection with subsequent TTS balloon dilation. The groups were identical in pretreatment dysphagia frequency and severity, stricture length and location, use of PPIs, and presence of a hiatal hernia. Although the study was powered to only 60% given the lower than anticipated enrollment, only 2 of 15 patients in the steroid group compared with 9 of 15 patients in the sham group required repeat dilation at 1-year

follow-up.[47] This prospective randomized controlled trial further supports prior noncontrolled case series advocating the use of steroid injection for recalcitrant strictures.[48–53]

Removing staples and suture material from the anastomosis using a grasping forceps is thought to reduce stricture recurrence. Another endoscopic treatment that has been reported in the treatment of benign anastomotic esophageal stenosis is the use of electrocautery.[54,55] Approximately six radial incisions, each about 2 to 3 mm long, are made using a needle-knife sphincterotome. Hordijk and colleagues[55] enrolled 20 patients for treatment with electrocautery who had failed prior dilation therapy for anastomotic esophageal strictures. Of 12 patients with a stricture length of less than 1 cm, all remained symptom-free at 1 year. In eight patients with a stricture length of 1.5 to 5 cm, dysphagia recurred, and a mean of three treatments were necessary. Only two of these eight patients were treatment failures. The use of electrocautery has also been described in combination with balloon dilation[56] and argon plasma coagulation.[57] At this time, electrocautery should be considered an alternative treatment in short-segment (<1 cm) esophageal, anastomotic ringlike strictures. Whether this modality should be used as a solitary treatment or in conjunction with other modalities has not been determined.[58]

One novel approach to the treatment of benign, recalcitrant esophageal strictures was the use of endoscissors to cut the stenosed segment. Although this method was reported only as a case report and has not been studied in a randomized trial, endoscissors may be a device to use in refractory cases.[59]

Surgical treatment of refractory strictures is another alternative. There are two major approaches: (1) antireflux surgery with intraoperative stricture dilation and (2) esophageal reconstruction such as a gastric pull-through or colonic interposition. For peptic strictures that are associated with esophageal shortening, a lengthening procedure such as a Collis gastroplasty may be needed in addition to the antireflux surgery. Comparisons of surgical treatment for peptic strictures by antireflux surgery and intraoperative dilation versus nonsurgical therapy showed similar success rates.[60,61] The major advantage to surgery is the decreased need for long-term medical therapy. However, with long-term follow-up, most patients have reinstituted antireflux medications regularly.[62] One difficult subset of patients with esophageal peptic stricture comprises patients with esophageal motility disorders such as scleroderma. The abnormal esophageal motor function and mechanical obstruction caused by fundoplication can result in significant postoperative dysphagia, although there are reports of scleroderma patients with excellent surgical outcomes.[63] For severe strictures, often not resulting from peptic etiology, surgical resection and reconstruction is required with substantially higher morbidity and mortality.

The use of self-expanding metallic stents (SEMS) for the treatment of refractory benign esophageal strictures has been reported.[64] Early success rates are high, although late complications, primarily stricture above the stents, have been reported.[65,66] When stents are placed completely within the esophageal lumen, stricture formation also occurs at the distal end of the stent. SEMS generally are contraindicated for the treatment of benign strictures because of difficult long-term complications.

Self-expanding plastic stents (SEPS) have been studied for the treatment of benign esophageal strictures. The only current SEPS that is commercially available is the Polyflex stent, which is a silicone device with an encapsulated mono-filament braid made of polyester. An initial positive result with a Polyflex stent for benign esophageal strictures was reported by Repici and colleagues[67] in a study in which 12 of 15 patients had long-term relief of dysphagia at follow-up with only 1 patient experiencing stent migration. Several subsequent studies noted, however, that stent migration is common, the patient's dysphagia regularly returns, and there are serious complications associated with stent placement and removal. A review article by Siersema[68] summarized these nine studies (eight retrospective and one prospective) of 162 patients who underwent Polyflex stent placement for benign esophageal strictures. In this review, eight of nine studies showed migration in 60 of 129 patients (47%), and only 50 of 129 patients (39%) had long-term relief of dysphagia. Ten of 129 patients (6%) had major complications: two perforations, two fistulas, three bleeds, and three severe pain requiring stent removal. The last study in this review included a retrospective study by Holm and associates[69] at the Mayo Clinic from 2002 to 2006. In this study, 30 patients had 83 of 84 stents placed successfully. Migration occurred in 60% of all procedures, and only 17% of all patients had long-term resolution of symptoms.

Given their limited efficacy and high complication rate, we recommend considering SEPS as a last resort for patients with benign refractory strictures who have failed all other recommended therapeutic options and desire alternative treatment options. The availability of fully covered SEMS has reduced the need to use SEPS. SEPS may still have some role in treating tissue ingrowth and strictures within SEMS prior to SEMS extraction efforts.

Finally, biodegradable stents have been evaluated for the treatment of esophageal strictures. Two types of materials, natural and synthetic, have been tested with biodegradable stents. Natural materials such as catgut collagen and fibrin were shown to be of limited efficacy given the poor mechanical strength and poor conversion to the degradable form of fiber.[70] Three studies have been done with a polyactide-made biodegradable stent.[71–73] Although one study showed migration in 10 of 13 patients 10 to 21 days after placement, none of these 13 patients had dysphagia at follow-up 7 to 24 months later.[73] The results are promising with this synthetic material, but longer term studies with more technologically advanced stents are warranted before considering their use for benign esophageal strictures.

Esophageal Rings and Webs

Episodic and nonprogressive dysphagia without weight loss is characteristic of an esophageal web or a distal esophageal ring (Schatzki ring). The first episode often occurs during a hurried meal or with alcohol. The patient notes that the food is stuck in the distal esophagus and can often be passed by drinking large quantities of liquids. The offending food is frequently a piece of bread or steak and hence the description "steakhouse syndrome."[74]

Esophageal Rings

Two types of distal esophageal rings are described: the A and B (Schatzki) rings. The A or muscular ring is the proximal border of the lower esophageal sphincter. It is covered by squamous epithelium and can be shown only very rarely on esophagogram. If it is symptomatic, it can be treated by passage of a 50-Fr bougie or by injection of botulinum toxin.[75]

In contrast, the B ring, otherwise known as the mucosal or Schatzki ring, is very common and is found in 6% to 14% of subjects undergoing barium GI series.[76] It is a thin membrane that has squamous epithelium on its upper surface and columnar epithelium on its lower surface; it demarcates the squamocolumnar junction. The Schatzki ring is composed of mucosa and submucosa, and there is no muscularis propria. It is believed that most Schatzki rings are congenital in origin, although a relationship to GERD has been proposed.[77] It is unclear how many are truly scar tissue caused by acid reflux. Most rings shown at upper endoscopy or on barium esophagograms are asymptomatic. When the esophageal lumen is narrowed to less than or equal to 13 mm, rings can cause solid food dysphagia and food impactions.

Rings causing dysphagia are effectively treated by passage of a single large (50-Fr or 54-Fr) bougie or by a series of dilators of progressively larger diameter. Although passage of a single large dilator is the most popular means of therapy, there are no studies to confirm the superiority of this technique over the gradual dilation typically used for peptic strictures. Repeat dilations are required in most patients with Schatzki rings because 90% have recurrent dysphagia within 3 years. However, a prospective, randomized, placebo-controlled trial showed that acid suppressive therapy may prevent the relapse of lower esophageal (Schatzki) rings.[78] This trial enrolled 44 patients with symptomatic Schatzki rings. Patients who did not have GERD based on esophageal manometry and 24-hour ambulatory esophageal pH monitoring measurements were randomly assigned to receive 20 mg of daily omeprazole versus placebo. At 19-month follow-up, only 1 of 13 patients (7.7%) treated with 20 mg of omeprazole daily had recurrence of Schatzki ring compared with 7 of 12 (58.3%) patients receiving placebo. An alternative treatment for Schatzki rings is four-quadrant biopsy causing disruption of the ring. In a randomized study comparing this technique with passage of a single 52-Fr Maloney dilator, there was no difference in efficacy or in durability of response with 12-month follow-up.[79]

Electrocautery incision of Schatzki rings has also been reported.[80–82] In one case series study, 11 patients who had failed prior dilation were treated with dilation followed by endoscopic incision. The combination of treatments provided a longer dysphagia-free interval compared with repeated bougienage alone.[83] Further support for electrocautery was reported in a randomized, prospective trial, which found that electrosurgical incision provided longer dysphagia-free survival time than bougie dilation for patients with Schatzki rings.[84] Study limitations included that patients treated with bougie had higher pretreatment dysphagia scores than patients treated with incision, there were a limited number of patients in each group ($n = 25$), there was no diet score, and there was a high study dropout rate.[85] More randomized controlled trials comparing electrosurgical incision with dilation are needed before accepting incision therapy as superior to dilation alone for patients with Schatzki rings.

Esophageal Webs

Esophageal webs are one or more thin horizontal membranes of squamous epithelium within the upper and mid esophagus.

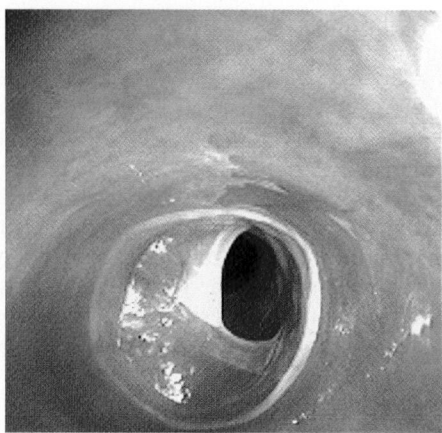

Fig. 17.2 Upper esophageal web in a patient with iron deficiency anemia.

In contrast to rings, they rarely encircle the lumen but protrude from the anterior wall extending laterally but not posteriorly. Webs may be asymptomatic but do cause solid food dysphagia and can manifest at any age. They are usually fragile membranes that respond well to dilation with bougienage after initial rupture by the endoscope (**Fig. 17.2**).[86] An association between cervical webs and iron deficiency anemia in adults (especially women) has been described as the Plummer-Vinson syndrome or Paterson-Kelly syndrome. This condition has also been associated with celiac sprue. The pathogenesis of this syndrome is unclear.

Eosinophilic Esophagitis

Eosinophilic esophagitis, also referred to as small-caliber esophagus, has been documented with increasing frequency over the last decade.[87–89] It is commonly seen in young patients who present with dysphagia or food impaction or both, but it can also mimic symptoms of reflux disease alone.[90,91] After treating the patient with a trial of a PPI, diagnosis requires endoscopic biopsies of the proximal and distal esophagus that show greater than 15 to 20 eosinophils per high-power field. Proximal esophageal biopsies are done to confirm the presence of eosinophils because distal esophageal eosinophils can also be seen with reflux alone.[92] Endoscopically, the esophagus may be normal in appearance or show ridges, furrows, or rings. The appearance of this ringed esophagus can be described as a "feline esophagus" because cats have similar-appearing esophageal rings. Other synonyms for a ringed esophagus include "corrugated esophagus" or "trachealization of the esophagus."[93] Although dilation may lessen dysphagia, there is an increased risk of mucosal tearing and perforation with dilation for patients with eosinophilic esophagitis, so dilation should be performed with caution.[93,94] Additional treatment of eosinophilic esophagitis includes swallowed fluticasone for a finite duration, consideration of referral to an allergist, avoidance of documented allergens, and a PPI.

Gastric, Pyloric, and Small Bowel Strictures

The major question for patients with nonesophageal strictures is the appropriateness of balloon dilation versus surgical therapy. This decision depends on the etiology of the stenosis and the long-term outcome for dilation therapy. When dilation therapy is chosen, most nonesophageal stenoses are best treated with balloon dilation. These can be placed over an endoscopically or radiographically placed wire or passed through the endoscope. Balloons passed through the endoscope (TTS or CRE) have the advantage of allowing completion of the endoscopic examination after dilation and are the most popular. Similar to esophageal balloons, CRE balloons allow three-step dilation with a single balloon, although the steps are only 1 mm apart, and the balloons are significantly more expensive than single-sized TTS balloons. Pyloric (and colonic) balloons are shorter in length than esophageal balloons with usual lengths of 3 to 4 cm. Some experts recommend the use of fluoroscopy and 10% to 25% contrast solution with endoscopic balloons to assess the bulb apex or C-loop wall better during inflation.[95] Technical variables such as the duration of balloon insufflation, the frequency and adequacy of dilation, and the size of balloons used have not been standardized. The successful use of Savary-Gilliard dilators for obstruction of the distal stomach and duodenal bulb has also been described in case reports.[96]

Causes of Nonesophageal Upper Gastrointestinal Tract Strictures

The most common site for nonesophageal, upper GI tract strictures is at the pylorus, although gastric, anastomotic, and duodenal strictures also occur. Peptic ulcer disease (PUD) is the most common cause of gastric outlet obstruction. PUD occurs most often due to a history of nonsteroidal anti-inflammatory drug (NSAID) use, whereas *Helicobacter pylori* infection infrequently causes PUD.[97] The initial technical failure rate of pyloric dilation, or an "intention-to-treat" analysis, is not reported in most case series. One report of 46 consecutive patients with benign gastric outlet obstruction had initial technical failure in 5 patients (11%).[98] A second series reported technical failure in 5 of 54 patients (9.3%).[95] In the patients in whom dilation therapy is technically possible, sustained relief was reported in only 16% to 50% of patients,[95,99] although most series[100,101] have long-term successful outcomes in 70% of patients. No prospective or controlled studies are available. Postoperative strictures may occur at any site, including efferent and afferent limb anastomoses in patients with prior Billroth II surgery and at gastric bypass sites for bariatric surgery. A report of fluoroscopic balloon dilation of gastric outlet obstruction after surgery for morbid obesity stated 50% of 28 patients experienced relief of symptoms.[102] The successful combined use of electrosurgical incision and balloon dilation was reported in five patients with refractory postoperative pyloric stenosis.[103]

Other causes of stomach or pyloric stenoses include a history of corrosive ingestion, prior radiation therapy, and Crohn's disease (**Box 17.1**). Three patients with gastric outlet obstruction resulting from prior corrosive ingestion were treated successfully with intralesional steroid injections combined with TTS balloon dilation.[104] There are several reports of balloon dilation for obstructive gastroduodenal Crohn's disease (Video 17.1).[105–107] Initial symptomatic relief is obtained, although a high rate of recurrence is reported. Repeat dilations may be required if there is a strong interest

---

Box 17.1 Benign Causes of Stomach or Pyloric Stenoses

Peptic ulcer disease (nonsteroidal antiinflammatory drugs, *Helicobacter pylori*)
Postoperative
Corrosive ingestion
Crohn's disease
Radiation therapy

Box 17.2 Benign Causes of Lower Gastrointestinal Stenoses

Surgical anastomoses
Crohn's disease (most often also at anastomoses)
Diverticular disease
Ischemia
Nonsteroidal antiinflammatory drug colopathy
Radiation-induced

---

in avoiding surgery. Long fibrous strictures resulting from Crohn's disease seem less likely to respond to endoscopic treatment.

Contraindications and Complications

Contraindications to balloon dilation include deep ulceration at the stenosis or uncorrectable coagulopathy. Although reported series are too small to assess the risk of active ulceration in the stricture, it is presumed that this does increase the risk of perforation. Perforation rates of 4% to 7.4% have been reported in small case series.[95,100] In one study of 54 patients, two of the four perforations occurred in patients with active ulceration, and all four occurred with large balloon diameters (16 mm and 20 mm).[95]

One frequently reported adverse outcome is ulcer and stricture recurrence. One retrospective review of 19 patients who had undergone balloon dilation for nonmalignant pyloric stenoses with a median follow-up of 45 months found that all patients had immediate symptomatic relief but that only 16% experienced sustained relief.[99] Symptoms of gastric outlet obstruction recurred in 84% of patients with the median time to recurrence being 9 months. NSAID intake was not studied in this group of patients with relapse; it was noted that recurrence was more likely in women.

In another series of 41 patients treated successfully with TTS dilation, only 14 patients (30%) remained disease-free at 3 years of follow-up.[98] Subsequent surgery was required in 21 patients; 18 patients underwent surgery for recurrent obstructions, 2 for interval perforations, and 1 for bleeding. These outcomes have led some experts to recommend initial surgical treatment for patients who are good operative candidates. In contrast, prolonged symptom relief is reported in up to two-thirds of treated patients, especially if they continue acid suppressive therapy.[100] It is reasonable to discuss these outcomes and potential complications with patients and to include them in the decision of trying endoscopic dilation treatment before surgery. Another possible adverse outcome of endoscopic dilation of gastric or duodenal stenoses is the potential for misdiagnosis of malignant obstruction resulting in delay in treatment.[95]

Benign Colonic and Ileocolonic Strictures

Similar to gastroduodenal strictures, the most important initial treatment decision for colonic and ileocolonic strictures is whether one should attempt balloon dilation or proceed directly to surgical treatment. This decision depends on the etiology of the stricture and the patient's wishes. An important caveat is that only symptomatic strictures require treatment. Many colonic strictures noted at colonoscopy are not causing obstructive symptoms and are best left untreated. TTS balloon dilators are available for use during colonoscopy. They are the same length (3 to 4 cm) as pyloric dilation balloons and are often marketed for both locations being sufficiently long for the colonoscope. CRE and TTS balloons are available in the standard 18-Fr to 54-Fr sizes, although larger "anastomotic" balloons at 20 mm (60-Fr) and 25 mm (75-Fr) are also available. Some data support a higher clinical success for colonic dilation when balloons of greater diameter than 51-Fr are used.[108] Successful radiologically guided balloon dilation has also been reported in lower GI tract strictures, as has dilation with polyvinyl over-the-guidewire dilators.[109,110] Case reports using SEMS in benign colonic strictures are available,[111] although use of SEMS is not routinely recommended because of the long-term patency problems associated with permanent metal stents in the GI tract.[112]

Causes of Benign Lower Gastrointestinal Tract Strictures

The most common site for lower GI tract strictures is at surgical anastomoses. Etiologies of benign lower GI stenoses include postoperative Crohn's disease (most of which occur at previous surgical anastomotic sites), diverticular, ischemic, NSAID-related colopathy, and radiation-induced (**Box 17.2**). More than 150 patients with lower GI strictures caused by Crohn's disease treated with endoscopic balloon dilation have been reported in case series.[113–117] No controlled studies are available. Most strictures occur at previous surgical anastomoses, although de novo Crohn's strictures have also been treated (**Fig. 17.3**). In the one prospective study of 55 patients submitted to 78 dilation procedures, the procedure was technically successful in 70 (90%).[114] The 13.6-mm diameter colonoscope was successfully passed through the stricture immediately after the dilation in 73% of the dilations. Another large retrospective case series reported that the median number of dilations per patient was one, although many patients underwent two or three sessions.[115] Long-term clinical benefit is reported in 41% to 62% of larger series[114,115] and 72% to 80% in some smaller ones.[116,117] There are three case series of combined local steroid injection and balloon dilation for a total of 44 patients.[118–120] The response rate from this combined therapy is similar to other series of balloon dilation alone. However, a more recent pilot study of intrastricture steroid versus placebo injection after balloon dilation showed that local steroid injection did not reduce the time to repeat dilation. In the steroid

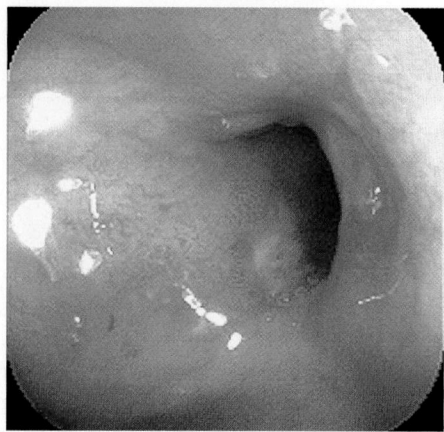

Fig. 17.3 Anastomotic ileocolonic stricture in a patient with clinically quiescent Crohn's disease. Two shallow ulcers are present at the stricture.

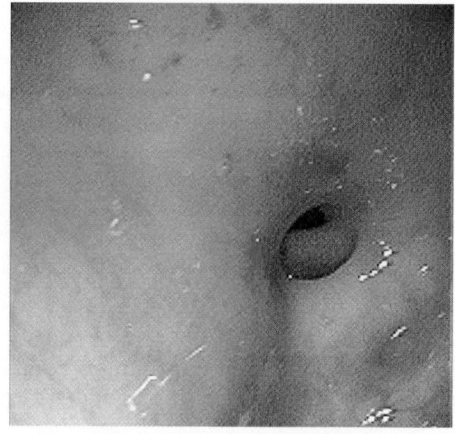

Fig. 17.4 Ascending colon stricture resulting from prior nonsteroidal antiinflammatory drug use.

arm, there was a trend toward earlier time to stricture relapse.[121] It is difficult to know if adding local steroid injection improves clinical outcome.

Sedation delivered by an anesthetist has been used for some procedures, but most patients have standard conscious sedation. Complications seem to occur infrequently with balloon dilation of strictures caused by Crohn's disease. Perforation has been the major concern and was reported in 1.6% to 8% of procedures. Colonic perforation usually requires surgical repair; however, this is not a dreaded outcome because surgery in a prepared bowel is the alternative treatment required for failure of treatment. However, the potential for perforation and surgical repair emphasizes the importance of not performing endoscopic dilation unless the lower GI stricture is symptomatic. Balloon dilation treatment of postoperative colorectal anastomotic strictures has been reported in more than 120 patients.[108,122–124] None of these are prospective or controlled trials; all are case series. Success rates seem to be slightly better than stricture dilation in Crohn's disease, although this may simply be reporting bias. Complications of perforation and bleeding occur in up to 7.8% of patients.[108] Refractory strictures have been treated with a combination of balloon dilation and endoscopic incision with an electrocautery needle-knife (6 patients) or with balloon dilation and endoscopic laser treatment (10 patients).[125,126] The success rate in both of these small series was 80% to 90%.

An alternative treatment was reported by Schubert and colleagues,[127] who used electrosurgical incisions and argon plasma coagulation to treat postoperative GI strictures with a 100% success rate at 23-month (mean) follow-up. Of the 49 patients treated, only 4 patients required more than one session of treatment to allow passage of a Fujinon videocolonoscope (diameter 12 mm, operative channel 3.2 mm; Fujinon). NSAID colopathy can also lead to colonic strictures, often with a "diaphragm-type" appearance.[128–130] These strictures are usually in the right colon and often are not narrow enough to cause obstructive symptoms. Multiple case reports exist, however, of successful balloon dilation as a viable option to surgical resection for tight NSAID strictures (**Fig. 17.4**). Discontinuation of NSAIDs is an important part of therapy.

Radiation-induced colorectal strictures are some of the most challenging stenoses to treat. Surgical management carries a high mortality, unless simple bypass with colostomy or ileostomy is performed. For this reason, endoscopic dilation has been attempted with Savary-Gilliard dilators,[131] balloon dilators,[132] and permanent metal stent placement.[133] The decision for the type of treatment for radiation strictures should be made after surgical consultation and careful consideration of patient wishes.

NSAID colopathy can also lead to colonic strictures, often with a "diaphragm-type" appearance.[128–130] These strictures are usually in the right colon and often are not narrow enough to cause obstructive symptoms. Multiple case reports exist, however, of successful balloon dilation as a viable option to surgical resection for tight NSAID strictures (see **Fig. 17-4**). Discontinuation of NSAIDs is an important part of therapy.

Radiation-induced colorectal strictures are some of the most challenging stenoses to treat. Surgical management carries a high mortality, unless simple bypass with colostomy or ileostomy is performed. For this reason, endoscopic dilation has been attempted with Savary-Gilliard dilators,[131] balloon dilators,[132] and permanent metal stent placement.[133] The decision for the type of treatment for radiation strictures should be made after surgical consultation and careful consideration of patient wishes.

Contraindications and Complications of Dilation of Benign Colonic Strictures

Contraindications to an attempt at lower GI dilation are coagulopathy, deeply ulcerated strictures, and long strictures. The major complications are bleeding and perforation. An additional adverse outcome is failure to respond to dilation therapy either initially or with frequent relapses.

References

The complete reference list is available online at www.expertconsult.com.

Achalasia

David A. Katzka and David C. Metz

Introduction

Achalasia is a relatively rare disease that affects both sexes and involves all races. It was described centuries ago; however, perhaps because of its relative rarity, little is known about it. There are still questions concerning the etiology, diagnosis, and management of achalasia. (1) What is the "gold standard" for the diagnosis of achalasia? (2) What is the best treatment algorithm for achalasia? (3) By what criteria should clinicians follow patients to determine whether treatment has been successful? This chapter provides an in-depth review of achalasia and a practical approach to answering these questions, or at least to determining why they may still be unanswerable at this time.

Etiology

The etiology of achalasia is unknown, but a reasonable theoretical construct that might explain the sequence of events is as follows: An external source of injury (infectious or otherwise) occurs in a genetically susceptible individual. This injury triggers an autoimmune response, which causes chronic damage to intramural esophageal and lower esophageal sphincter (LES) neurons possibly including central vagus nerve connections. The chronic neural damage results in depletion of all nerve elements, but there is a relatively greater loss of inhibitory nerve control of the LES, specifically, nitric oxide synthase, leaving a net increased stimulatory effect on LES function. This overall stimulatory effect causes incomplete LES relaxation and hypertonicity (i.e., spasm) of the sphincter. The neural dysfunction also causes a relative and often complete hypotonia of the esophageal body, but whether this is primarily from nerve injury or secondary to chronic

functional obstruction of the LES is unknown. With ongoing injury, secondary inflammation supervenes leading to neural destruction and fibrotic replacement with worsening LES dysfunction and esophageal hypotonia (i.e., loss of peristalsis). The result is progressive esophageal dilation, worsening dysmotility, and esophageal failure.

Fig. 18.1 illustrates the putative events in the development of achalasia. Extensive experimental data support this hypothesis. First, the neurotropic virus, varicella zoster, has been detected by in situ hybridization in cardiomyotomy specimens from patients with achalasia.[1] More recent data have also implicated herpes simplex virus type 1 as a cause of achalasia by showing a population of cells and cytokines in LES tissue typically found in herpes simplex virus infection.[2] In addition, Chagas' disease, a disease caused by *Trypanosoma cruzi*, a protozoan that is endemic in Central and South America, causes esophageal disease that may be indistinguishable from achalasia on manometric and radiographic grounds as a consequence of denervation of Auerbach's plexus.[3] Second, some investigators have shown an association between white patients with achalasia and the class II human leukocyte antigen (HLA) DQ1.[4] This genetic relationship has been characterized more specifically as an association with the DQB1*0602 and DRB1*15 HLA alleles.[5] Third, antimyenteric[6] and antimuscarinic cholinergic receptor autoantibodies[7] have been detected in patients with achalasia. Fourth, studies of surgical specimens from patients with achalasia have shown a chronic inflammatory infiltrate leading to ganglionic destruction and fibrosis.[8–12] Fifth, vagal dysfunction has been shown in natural and experimental animal models of achalasia.[13,14] Sixth, a selective deficiency of nitric oxide synthase, the predominant inhibitory neurotransmitter of the LES, has been shown in animal models and patients with achalasia.[15,16] Seventh, patients with less advanced forms of achalasia (from both a

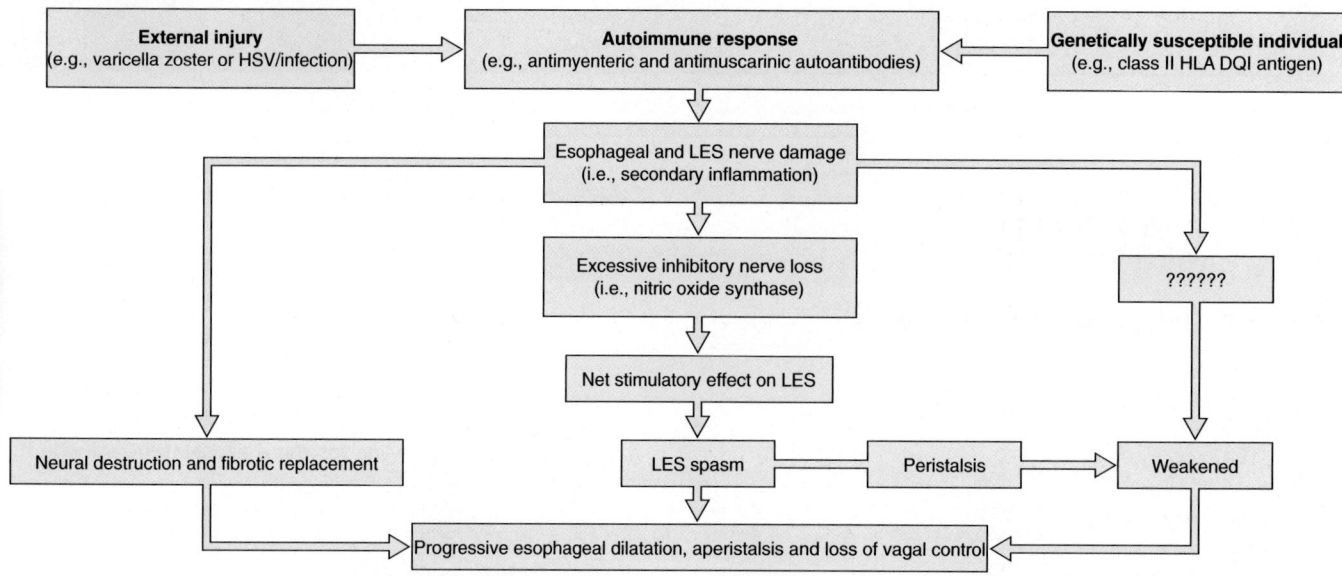

Fig. 18.1 Putative etiology of achalasia. LES, Lower esophageal sphincter.

clinical and a radiographic point of view) have more inflammation and less fibrosis in the ganglia of the LES than patients with more advanced forms of the disease,[11,17] suggesting that LES basal and residual tone may increase and esophageal body function deteriorates as the disease progresses.[18]

Much more data are needed to prove this hypothesis. The data referred to were generated from a relatively small number of patients, given the rarity of the disease. The abnormalities described are rarely identified in all patients with achalasia. Only 3 of 9 patients had detectable varicella zoster in the myenteric plexus,[1] and only 7 of 18 patients had antimyenteric neuronal antibodies.[5] These preliminary findings are encouraging, however, particularly because the general theory proposed here may apply to other gastrointestinal (GI) disease states in addition to achalasia (e.g., chronic idiopathic pseudoobstruction).

Diagnosis

The diagnosis of achalasia is based on clinical, radiologic, and manometric criteria because the pathologic equivalent is still being studied. In addition, pathologic specimens are not routinely accessible except after cardiomyotomy, in which case it is hoped that the diagnosis has already been made. Occasionally, the radiologic appearance (usually with barium swallow but occasionally with computed tomography [CT] scanning or routine chest x-ray film) or manometric tracing alone may be diagnostic of achalasia (in patients presenting with a compatible clinical syndrome). However, in most patients, the diagnosis is based on a constellation of findings using all three criteria.

Symptoms

The hallmark symptoms of achalasia are dysphagia, chest pain, and regurgitation (**Table 18.1**). Various series of patients with achalasia have reported dysphagia in 82% to 100% of cases, chest pain in 17% to 95%, and regurgitation in 59% to 81%.[19–24] Dysphagia occurs typically for both solids and

Table 18.1 Symptoms of Achalasia

Symptoms	Frequency (%)*
MAJOR	
Dysphagia	82–100
Chest pain	17–95
Regurgitation	59–81
Weight loss	32
MINOR	
Slow eating	
Stereotypic maneuvers during eating	
Halitosis	
Heartburn	
Accumulation of oral debris at night	
Staining of pillow during sleep	
Nocturnal coughing or choking	
Acute airway obstruction	
Inability to belch	
Postprandial syncope	
Dental caries	
Asthma	
Pneumonia	

*See text for references.

liquids, but solid food dysphagia often precedes liquid dysphagia. Some patients with early disease describe the need to "wash down their food with water," which possibly affords relief by raising a sufficient head of pressure above to overcome the LES spasm below. In others, there may be superimposed acute episodes of solid food dysphagia in which patients present with symptoms suggestive of food impaction that resolve spontaneously or are severe enough to warrant endoscopic removal.

Chest pain often occurs during ingestion and may signify food impaction. A spasmlike chest pain that may mimic gastroesophageal reflux disease (GERD) (i.e., heartburn) or cardiac pain (i.e., angina) may also occur spontaneously. The origin of the chest pain is generally unclear, and it may be independent of the mechanisms that cause dysphagia and regurgitation; this is suggested by data showing that chest pain commonly persists after achalasia treatment that is effective for the other two major symptoms.[24]

Regurgitation may occur minutes to hours after ingestion of a meal. Patients may even identify food that they ingested many days before in the regurgitant. Patients with severe symptoms may be unable to drink a glass of water without regurgitating. The nature of the regurgitant may be useful to differentiate achalasia from GERD. In achalasia, the regurgitant is typically described as nonsour or nonbitter, and patients may mention that it "tastes just like it did when it was initially swallowed." Because of the difficulty with eating, weight loss is also a common feature of achalasia; this was seen in 32% of patients in one more recent study.[25]

In our experience, a careful history emphasizing and dissecting the major symptoms of dysphagia, chest pain, regurgitation, and weight loss can be quite specific for the diagnosis of achalasia, although we are constantly surprised by the varied patterns of presentation of this unusual disease. As with many chronic disease states in which life-threatening consequences are rare and take months to years to develop, achalasia is a disease that lends itself to self-accommodation on the part of the patient. Behavioral adaptation may lead to the emergence of a whole host of subtle compensatory symptoms accompanied by the patient denying or downplaying the more classic symptoms described previously (see **Table 18.1**).

One more recent study[25] elicited numerous compensatory symptoms, including slow eating and other stereotypic maneuvers to aid swallowing such as walking, standing, sitting straight up, or arching of the neck during swallowing. Potential patients should also be interviewed about other subtle symptoms, including halitosis, heartburn, accumulation of oral debris or staining of the pillow during sleep, nocturnal coughing or choking, acute airway obstruction,[26,27] an inability to belch because of upper esophageal sphincter dysfunction,[28,29] and postprandial syncope.[30] Heartburn, the cardinal symptom of gastroesophageal reflux, is particularly important because its presence is often erroneously believed to be a strong negative indicator of achalasia. Although unproved, the sensation may be a consequence of bacterial fermentation of retained ingested foodstuff leading to lowering of the esophageal luminal pH mimicking GERD. Some studies have shown that heartburn and specialist referral of patients on proton pump inhibitors can be quite common in the early stages of achalasia.[25,31] Other important symptoms often erroneously ascribed to GERD include the presence of dental caries (from food bathing the teeth at night), asthma, and a history of pneumonia (presumably from microaspiration). Accurately differentiating between GERD and achalasia by history alone may be surprisingly difficult, given that the two diseases represent completely opposite ends of the pathophysiologic spectrum.

Radiography

Achalasia may be suspected on the basis of a routine chest x-ray film (particularly a lateral view) by the presence of an air-fluid level or a dilated esophagus or both. However, barium swallow is the most reliable radiographic method for making the diagnosis (**Fig. 18.2**). The pathognomonic findings include a smooth, tapered narrowing of the gastroesophageal junction (the so-called bird's beak appearance) with a proximally dilated esophagus that may be filled with fluid or food debris. Features of candidal infection, a consequence of long-standing esophageal stasis, may also be present. However, this basic template can include remarkable heterogeneity. The degree of esophageal dilation may vary from minimal to massive, and end-stage disease may reveal sigmoidization of the esophagus. Similarly, the diameter of the gastroesophageal junction may range from less than 1 mm to greater than 8 mm. Radiographs may also show single or multiple distal esophageal diverticula of varying sizes or a corkscrew or "spastic" appearance with several simultaneous lumen-obliterating contractions (this has been termed *vigorous achalasia*).

To assess and characterize these esophageal radiographic findings, various scoring systems have been devised.[19,25] Although these scoring systems help to standardize interpretation of radiographic appearance, which may be useful from a research point of view, there is generally very poor correlation between symptom severity and radiographic score.[25] This limitation is discussed further in the treatment section. Finally, there has been an old tenet in esophagology that a hiatal hernia is unusual in achalasia.[32] More recent data have questioned this dictum, showing the presence of a hiatal hernia in 10 of 71 radiographs reviewed from patients with achalasia (14.5%) compared with 9 of 35 patients (25.7%) 51 years old or older, a frequency that is similar to the normal population.[33] This finding makes intuitive sense because achalasia may develop at any age, sometimes in the presence of long-standing GERD with a hiatal hernia that preceded the development of the achalasia. Perhaps older studies had a bias of either underdiagnosis of hiatal hernia or overenrollment of younger patients.

Esophageal Manometry

In the absence of a true "gold standard," manometry is the best test for the diagnosis of achalasia (**Fig. 18.3**). However, manometric diagnosis of achalasia has undergone great revision in recent years. Classic teaching required the presence of a hypertensive LES with incomplete relaxation (i.e., an increased residual pressure) and esophageal body aperistalsis, whereas it is now clear that these classic criteria do not occur in all patients. Part of the reason for this reevaluation has been prolonged combined ambulatory pH and manometric recordings in which peristaltic contractions, complete LES relaxation, and acid reflux may be shown intermittently in patients who otherwise fulfill the classic criteria on stationary manometry.[34] As a result, it now seems conceivable that "normal" manometric findings might occur on stationary manometry as well in patients with achalasia, depending on the timing of the study.

Hirano and coworkers[35] in a study of 58 patients with achalasia proposed a manometric heterogeneity in patients with achalasia, including features such as a normal basal LES pressure, normal residual pressures, high-amplitude contractions, varying lengths of aperistalsis, and the presence of transient LES relaxations (the hallmark of GERD). In interpreting this important study, one might wonder what the "gold standard"

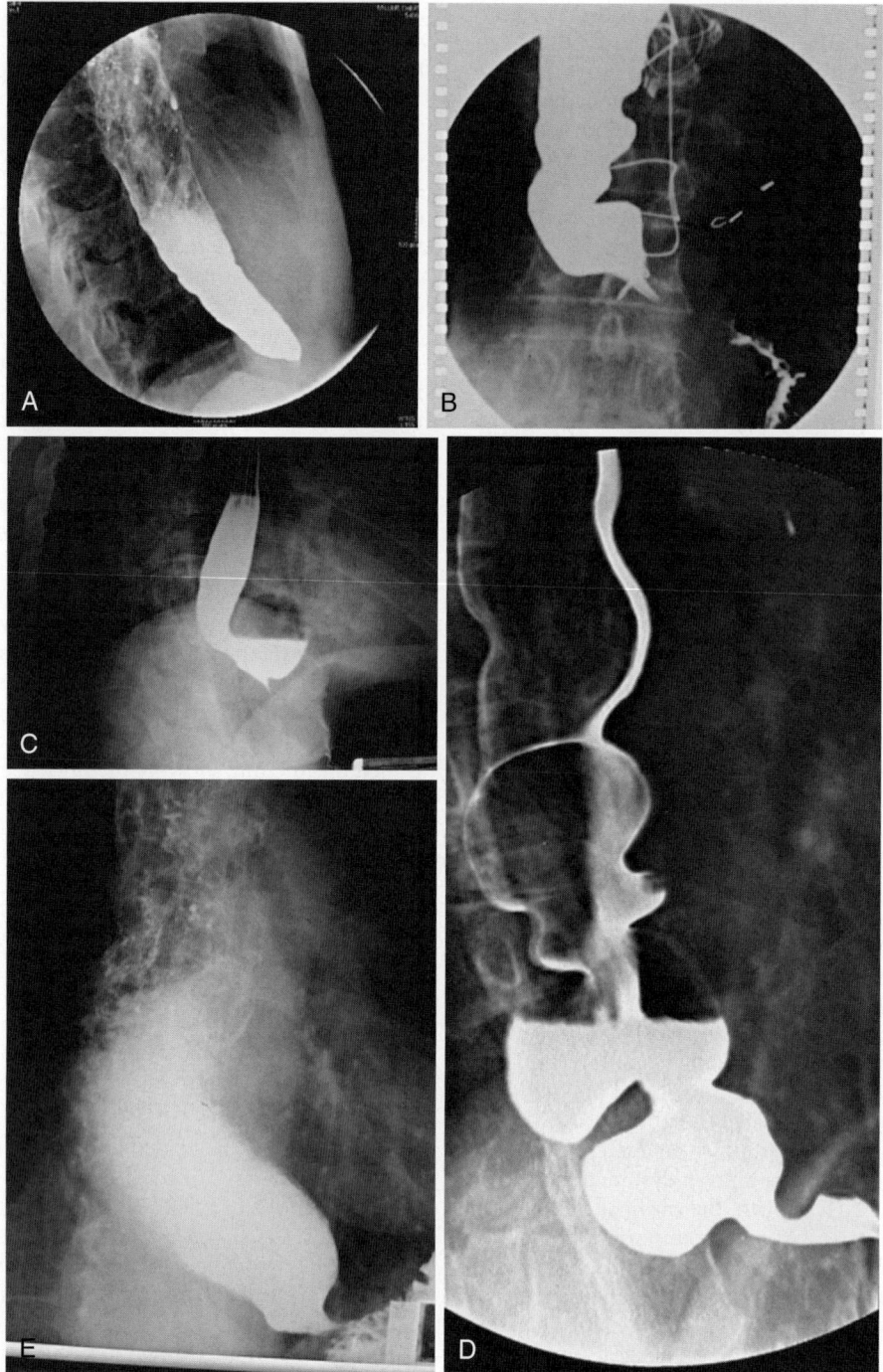

Fig. 18.2 Barium esophagograms in achalasia. **A,** Classic. **B,** Vigorous achalasia. **C,** Epiphrenic diverticulum. **D,** Multiple diverticula. **E,** Food retention and sigmoidization.

for the diagnosis of achalasia was in these "atypical" patients. This study shows the importance of making the diagnosis of achalasia based on a combination of compatible clinical, radiographic, and manometric findings in a specific patient rather than routinely relying on classic criteria. Similarly, Vantrappen and coworkers[36] in a landmark article proposed that diffuse esophageal spasm is in itself one end of the spectrum of achalasia. Several case reports have now shown spasm-type manometric (and perhaps radiographic) findings either as a component of established achalasia or as an early manifesta-

tion of dysmotility that may evolve into achalasia in due course.[37,38]

Currently, many esophagologists consider diffuse esophageal spasm a true variant of achalasia. Attention has also focused on the concept of vigorous achalasia, which is distinguished from classic achalasia by the presence of high-amplitude nonperistaltic esophageal body contractions. Vigorous achalasia may also represent an early manometric manifestation of the disease, before the development of complete aperistalsis. Although pathologic studies have shown progression of histologic injury within the myenteric plexus during the transition from vigorous to classic achalasia,[10] clinical studies comparing radiographic appearance and response to therapy in vigorous and classic achalasia have not borne out these differences.[39]

Significant advances have been made in motility testing of the esophagus in recent years with the advent of high-resolution manometry.[40–42] This technique expands on prior techniques by permitting simultaneous manometry measurements at centimeter intervals along the entire length of the esophagus. Three-dimensional color plots of change in pres-

sure measurements with time (pressure topography) allow more accurate recording of the upper esophageal sphincter and LES pressures and the proximal (striated) and distal (smooth) muscular contractions of the esophageal body. These sophisticated tracings have permitted a new manometric classification of achalasia as proposed by Kahrilas and colleagues.[40] This new classification divides achalasia into three manometric types: type I, achalasia with minimal esophageal pressurization, previously referred to as classic achalasia (with aperistalsis and an elevated LES pressure that fails to react; see **Fig. 18.3D**), occurring in roughly 21% of cases; type II,

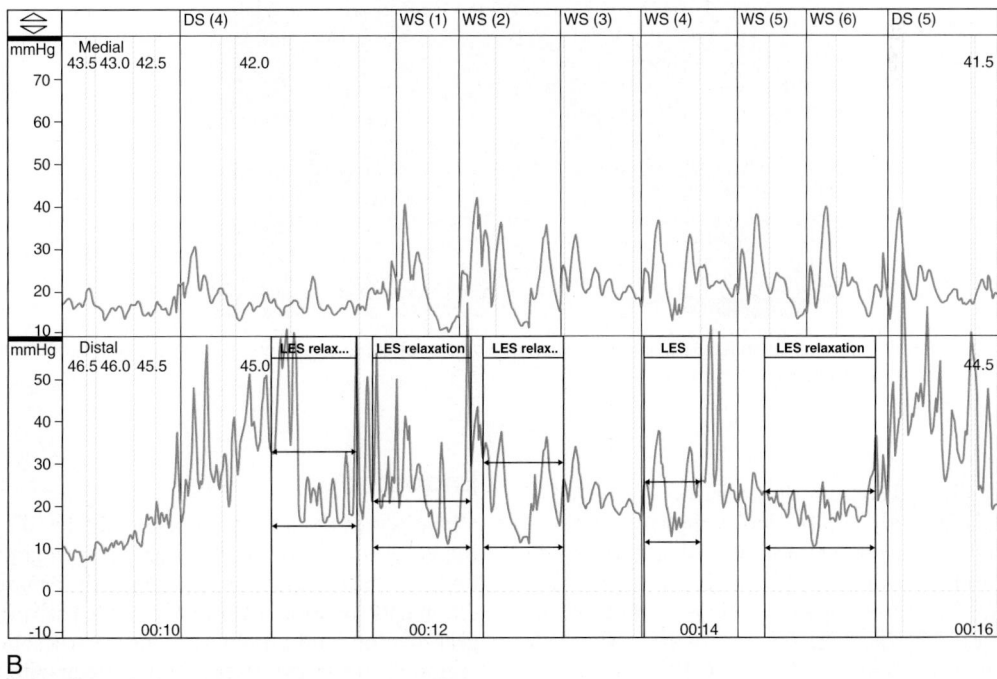

Fig. 18.3 Manometric tracings of achalasia. **A,** Hypertensive lower esophageal sphincter (LES). **B,** Incomplete LES relaxation.

Continued

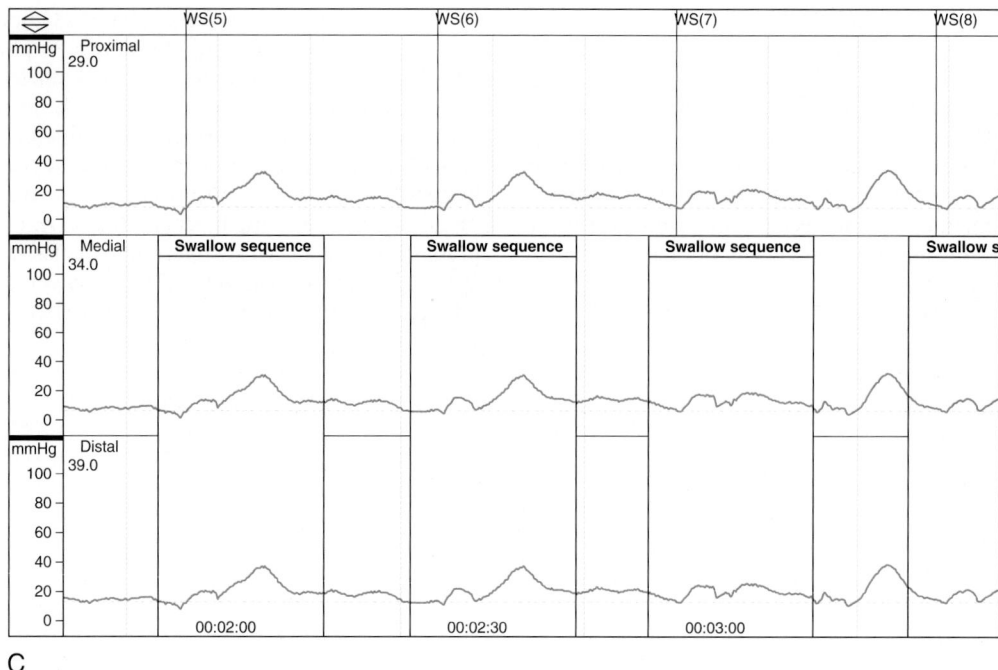

C

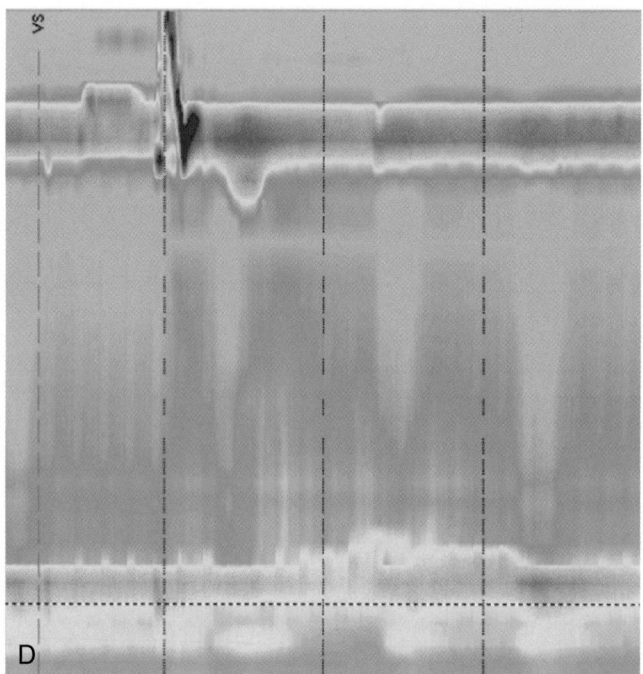

D

Fig. 18.3, cont'd C, Aperistalsis with mirror images. **D,** High-resolution manometry of entire esophagus in a patient with classic achalasia (aperistalsis with a high LES pressure that fails to relax).

achalasia with esophageal compression, previously referred to as vigorous achalasia (with swallow-induced pressurization), occurring in roughly 49% of cases; and type III, achalasia with spasm, a new variant characterized by high pressures in the distal esophageal body, occurring in roughly 29% of cases. The utility of this new classification has yet to be definitively shown, although proponents have suggested that it can be used prognostically (type II being more likely to respond to standard therapy than type I or III).

Endoscopy

Obvious achalasia may occasionally be diagnosed during upper GI endoscopy. As with barium radiography, endoscopic findings may include the presence of retained food in the esophagus (or, more commonly, pooled saliva), frank esophageal dilation, and a tight LES and gastroesophageal junction region that characteristically "pops" open with mild to moderate pressure. Endoscopy may appear completely normal in more subtle cases, however, discouraging its use for diagnosis.

Because endoscopy is now used more and more as a therapeutic modality for patients with achalasia, a firm diagnosis should preferably be made before endoscopic intervention (i.e., making a decision to perform botulinum toxin injection or pneumatic dilation requires advanced planning, which is best done before endoscopy). Upper GI endoscopy is of particular importance in the diagnosis of secondary achalasia, however, because of a gastroesophageal junction tumor, which may mimic primary achalasia in all of its manifestations. Secondary achalasia is discussed in more detail at the end of this chapter.

Several studies have also examined the role of endoscopic ultrasound in diagnosing achalasia.[43,44] Although some studies suggest that patients with achalasia may have increased LES and esophageal body wall thickness, these findings are not present in all patients. Currently, endoscopic ultrasound should be considered a research tool for patients with primary achalasia. Its role in secondary achalasia is discussed later.

Treatment

Many important therapeutic principles must be kept in mind before prescribing treatment options for patients with achalasia (**Box 18.1**). The first is the need to individualize the definition of a treatment threshold because no defined criteria exist. To date, investigators have been unable to define specific criteria for therapy or to evaluate treatment response. This controversy arises from data showing extremely poor correlation between symptoms and radiographic appearance before and after treatment. One more recent study[25] comparing the number and the severity of achalasia symptoms with radiographic scores (based on predefined radiographic parameters,

such as the degree of esophageal dilation, the LES diameter, and the presence or absence of sigmoidization or retained food debris) found no correlation at all between symptoms and x-ray appearance either before or after treatment. Other studies have had similar results.[45,46]

One has to decide whether treatment should be based on symptoms or x-ray appearance. For patients who are particularly symptomatic, treatment is usually indicated regardless of radiologic studies. However, does one treat a 30-year-old man with marked sigmoidization of the esophagus and retained debris who has stable weight and minimal symptoms? Similarly, does a patient without weight loss and minimal esophageal dilation on esophagogram who complains only of regurgitation thrice weekly merit surgical myotomy? These are some of the potential clinical decisions that need to be made purely based on best clinical judgment with little data for guidance.

In addition, one must keep in mind age when evaluating symptoms and treatment response. Studies have shown that older patients with achalasia (>45 to 60 years old depending on the study) tend to have better symptomatic responses to treatment. These improved responses have been shown with botulinum toxin injection[47] and with pneumatic dilation.[48] Whether the improvement is objective or subjective is unclear because older patients tend to have esophagi that are less sensitive to stimulation[49]; this population may be less reliable in conveying objective improvement. No outcome trials have been designed as yet to show whether or not early therapeutic intervention leads to an improved clinical outcome.

The second issue is whether one should standardize the criteria used for symptom assessment or radiographic evaluation. There is a wide variation in the way individual physicians take histories from patients with achalasia. Specific symptom scoring methods have been proposed to address this problem to allow standardized evaluation of treatment responses, but they have not been found to be very useful clinically.[25,50,51] Similarly, there is great variability in the way a barium swallow is performed in different radiology departments. Difference exists in terms of the amount and consistency of oral contrast medium given, the performance of video techniques versus static images, the use of double-contrast versus single-contrast imaging, and the number and rate of swallows administered.

Some investigators have studied the use of a standardized "timed" barium swallow.[45,52,53] The proposed technique requires ingestion of low-density barium sulfate suspension within 30 to 45 seconds (the maximum amount tolerated is measured) with spot films taken at 1 minute, 2 minutes, and 5 minutes. The height and width of the barium column is measured at each time point, and the rate of esophageal emptying from 1 to 5 minutes is recorded (**Fig. 18.4**).[51] In one of the studies using this technique,[52] 32 patients with near-complete symptom relief after therapy were followed. Initially, there was a significant association between patient symptoms and improvement in barium column height, although esophageal barium emptying was less predictive of the symptomatic response during longer term follow-up. Despite this limitation, patients whose symptom response correlated best with emptying were far less likely to have symptomatic relapse during follow-up.

Whether these standardized approaches, either symptomatic (i.e., subjective) or radiographic (i.e., objective), help

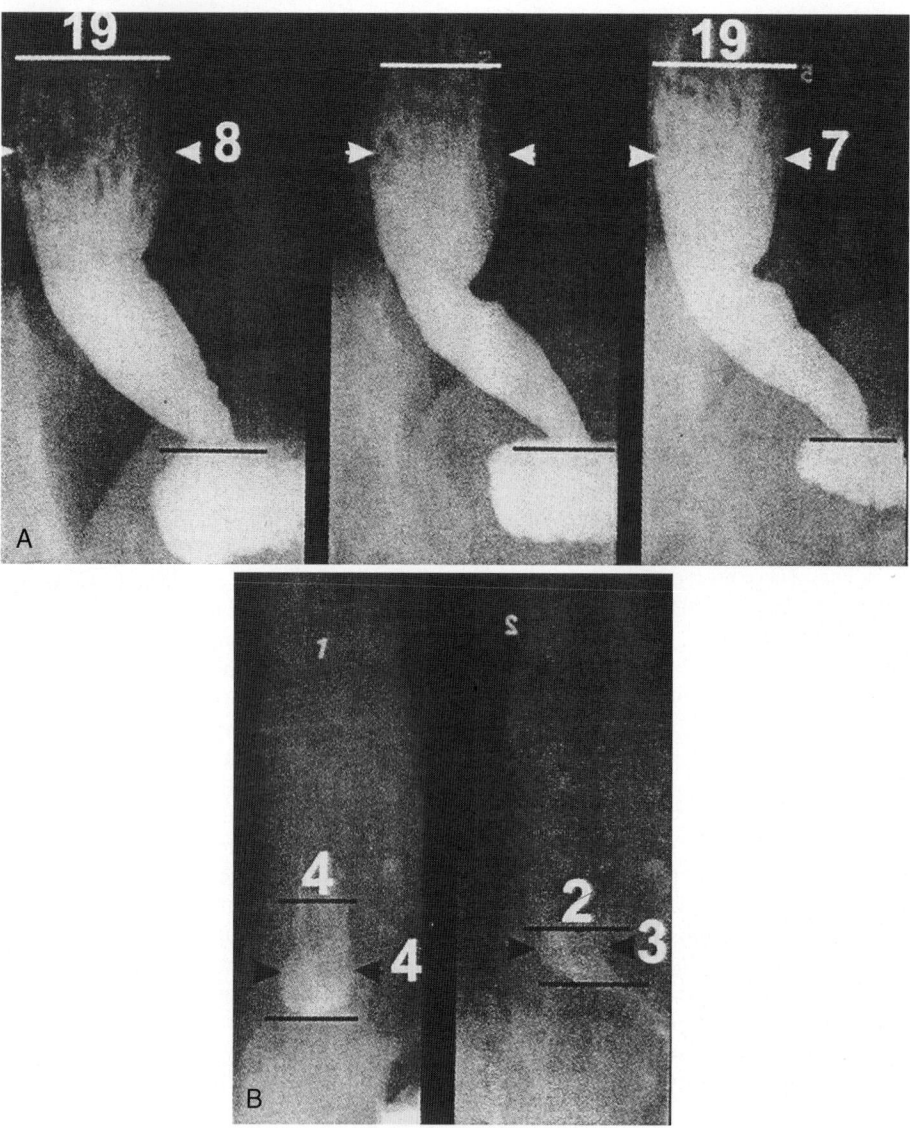

Fig. 18.4 Esophagogram after ingestion of 250 mL of barium. Height of barium column is indicated by transverse lines and numeric values. Width of barium column is indicated by arrows and numeric values. **A,** Barium columns at 1 minute, 2 minutes, and 5 minutes before myotomy. **B,** Post-myotomy barium columns at 1 minute and 2 minutes. *(From Kostic SV, Rice TW, Baker ME, et al: Timed barium esophagogram: A simple physiologic assessment for achalasia.* J Thorac Cardiovasc Surg *120:935–946, 2000.)*

improve patient outcome is unclear. In addition, in the face of an abnormal timed barium swallow but little symptomatic residual posttreatment, we may still be left with the question of whether to treat the x-ray film or the patient. We believe strongly, however, that standardization of symptoms and radiographic findings should be done for any type of achalasia research trial.

The third treatment principle is the need to weigh the risks of any planned procedure against the expected duration of treatment response for the individual patient. When choosing among the three standard treatment options (botulinum toxin injection, pneumatic dilation, and surgical myotomy), procedure risk seems to correlate with efficacy. In terms of initial treatment options, a healthy young patient may be viewed quite differently from an older patient or a patient considered to be a poor operative risk. The former would be a better candidate for pneumatic dilation or surgical myotomy with the expectation of a durable response, whereas the latter may

be a better candidate for repeated botulinum toxin injection at intervals.

Fourth, when evaluating the results of therapeutic studies, one must bear in mind that most studies deal with a heterogeneous population of patients with varying degrees of disease severity. Because of significant variability among patients in terms of specific symptoms,[25] extrapolating symptom response rates from clinical studies to individual patients may not always be valid. Because of the rarity of this disease, most achalasia studies group patients with all stages of severity together for analysis. These data include therapeutic responses ranging from patients with minimal esophageal dilation and some LES opening to patients with frank sigmoidization, complete aperistalsis, and severe LES spasm. Although the proportion of patients with end-stage disease may be similar among some studies, patients with end-stage disease are often excluded in other studies. In one study evaluating the efficacy of Heller myotomy for achalasia, symptomatic success was related to preoperative disease stage.[54] The relatively small numbers of achalasia patients in general also predisposes to type II errors in study design. Finally, the precise details of how therapeutic procedures (botulinum toxin injection, pneumatic dilation, and surgical myotomy) are performed often vary greatly among operators.

Fifth, many surgical series measure symptom response rates on a 4-point scale consisting of excellent, good, fair, and poor categories. However, when overall outcome is presented, these subgroups may be combined into two groups only to reflect satisfactory or successful outcomes (excellent plus good) as opposed to unsatisfactory or unsuccessful outcomes (fair plus poor). A study suggesting that two therapeutic modalities are equally effective for achalasia because a similar proportion of patients had successful outcomes may contain disparate numbers of patients with excellent versus good symptomatic responses because the two categories were combined to reflect equal success.

Botulinum Toxin Injection

From the innovative work of Pashricha and coworkers,[55] botulinum toxin injection into the LES has become a cornerstone of treatment for achalasia. Gastroenterologists have embraced this approach to treatment for three reasons: (1) It is easy to administer, (2) it is safe, and (3) it works. Because of its extremely favorable risk-to-benefit ratio, we commonly use botulinum toxin injection as a temporizing measure in patients presenting with severe disease who are concerned about undergoing more invasive procedures or in patients at poor risk for more invasive procedures.

The precise injection technique is unspecified. In Pashricha's original work, "the lower esophageal sphincter was visualized endoscopically by identification of the sphincteric rosette typically seen at the squamocolumnar junction. Botulinum toxin was injected through a 5-mm sclerotherapy needle into the region of the lower esophageal sphincter."[55] In a more recent report by Kolbasnik and colleagues,[56] botulinum toxin was administered "approximately 5 mm above the Z line." In a study by Annese and coworkers,[57] the toxin was injected into "the LES region identified at endoscopy." The fact that all these studies show similar efficacy for botulinum toxin injection suggests that the precise site of injection may not be critical to the success of the technique. The LES is generally longer in patients with achalasia (approximately 5 cm) compared with control subjects and patients with GERD. It is unknown whether clinical results vary with botulinum toxin injection into the proximal, mid, or distal LES region. In addition, there are no clear data to support an advantage to administering the injection using endoscopic ultrasound guidance or from a retroflexed position in the gastric cardia.

Our personal techniques for administering botulinum toxin for achalasia emphasize the following points. Good localization of the LES region is essential; this is best achieved by straddling back and forth between the stomach and distal esophagus to check position before injection because the increased LES tone may "grab" the endoscope making the proximal border of the LES appear higher at times. The endoscope is kept approximately 5 mm above the squamocolumnar junction and then is swung in the direction of the anticipated injection site to permit an en face angle of injection. The sclerotherapy injection catheter is used to push the

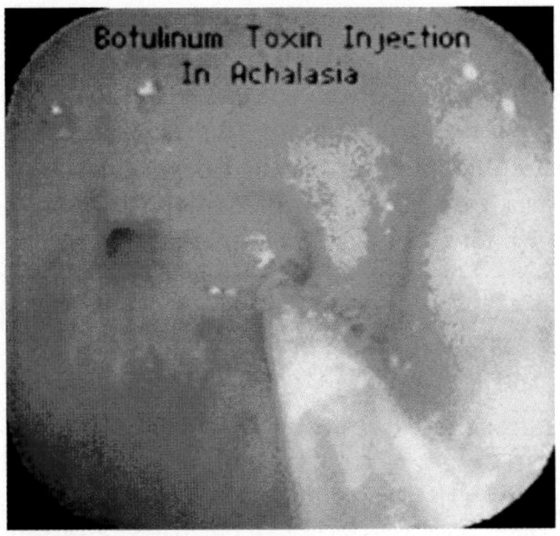

Fig. 18.5 Photograph of botulinum toxin injection.

wall of the LES region away from the endoscope, maintaining a perpendicular relationship to the esophageal wall (to avoid a tangential injection). With the tip of the catheter firmly opposed to the mucosa, the needle is deployed, and a submucosal injection is administered. We generally use 20 U of toxin injected sequentially into each quadrant with the final injection being administered from a retroflexed position below (i.e., 100 U in total).

Additional important aspects of botulinum toxin administration include not preparing the solution until just before its use (because it is extremely expensive), using nonbacteriostatic saline without preservatives (preservatives may destroy the toxin), admixing the toxin with the saline solution by slowly injecting the saline into the vial followed by gently rolling the vial back and forth (to prevent denaturing of the toxin), and ensuring that the sclerotherapy catheter is fully flushed before injection (to prevent submucosal injection of air). **Fig. 18.5** illustrates performance of an injection using this technique.

That botulinum toxin works well for patients with achalasia has been clear from the first published trial.[58] Numerous subsequent trials[59–61] have confirmed this fact. The symptom response after one injection ranges from 64% to 100%,[57–61] and a more recent meta-analysis showed a 78.7% efficacy of botulinum toxin injection in 315 patients described in nine articles.[62] Manometric and radiologic parameters in these studies also improve significantly. There is a 33% to 49% reduction in basal LES pressure and a 35% to 47% reduction in esophageal retention. The duration of response ranged from 7.1 to 11 months with overall efficacy of 68.3% at 12 months in the aforementioned meta-analysis.[62] Prolonged responses (>2 years) have been documented in several patients. In addition, patients who respond well to their initial injection also seem to respond well to a second injection. Studies vary, however, on the symptomatic response to a second injection in initial nonresponders (from 0% to 33%).

We believe a second injection is worthwhile in patients who initially fail to respond, particularly if the patient is elderly or a poor operative risk. Data on the efficacy of a third or fourth injection are scant, but anecdotal and published data suggest it may still work. As discussed, age may be an important predictor of response to botulinum toxin injection. In the initial study by Pashricha and coworkers,[55] 53 patients older and younger than 50 years had an 82% (>50 years old) and 43%

(<50 years old) chance of responding symptomatically. Other, but not all, studies show similar trends.[59] Another predictor of success is the presence of vigorous achalasia, although the number of patients available for analysis is very small.[58] This smaller patient population is not unexpected because vigorous achalasia may represent an earlier form of the disease process in which esophageal peristalsis is less impaired.

The most important predictor of initial and long-term symptomatic response is a documented reduction in LES pressure (this holds true in general for all achalasia treatment modalities). One study[59] showed that a decrease in basal LES pressure to less than 20 mm Hg predicted a 100% symptomatic response. One study[60] suggested only that a low basal LES pressure before treatment was also predictive of a better outcome (see figures presented by Pashricha and coworkers[55]). Side effects of botulinum toxin injection are infrequent. Studies have reported transient chest pain, heartburn-type symptoms, and rash. In one case report,[63] a 10-year-old girl with achalasia developed a sinus tract between the esophagus and fundus, but this occurred after six botulinum toxin injections. One other potential side effect of this type of therapy is its potential impact on future surgical therapy. Specifically, several surgical studies have shown more difficult surgical dissection and perhaps poorer surgical outcome.[64] Whether a poorer surgical outcome is uniformly accepted is unclear, but one should not use botulinum toxin without considering the possibilities of its effect on subsequent myotomy.

Pneumatic Dilation

In evaluating studies of pneumatic dilation for achalasia, evaluation of the precise method used and the age of the study are paramount for two reasons. First, as discussed previously, there is marked variation in the precise details of the technique used. Methods vary from brief 3- to 5-second dilations at 12 to 15 pounds per square inch (PSI),[65] to maintaining an average dilation pressure of 7 PSI for less than 30 seconds, to maintaining a pressure of 6 to 12 PSI for up to 2 minutes. Whether such variations in technique influence outcome has not been well studied. Studies specifically examining the effect of the dilator size or the duration or number of inflations have not shown any clear differences,[66,67] although one early study showed an increased benefit if a larger balloon size was used (35 mm vs. 30 mm),[67] and another showed a benefit to inflating the balloon to a pressure of greater than 7 PSI.[65]

Second, there has been a progressive change in the types of dilators used over time. Earlier studies described the use of the bulky, cumbersome Brown-McCarty or Mosher bags. However, these have been replaced over the past decade by Rigiflex dilators. Although the Rigiflex dilator is considered easier to use, few data suggest that it actually yields superior results.[68] There is no agreed-on method for balloon dilation, and many methodologic variations exist based mainly on anecdotal, personal experience. The following points regarding performance of balloon dilation for achalasia should be emphasized. We always start with a 30-mm balloon Rigiflex dilator. Although data suggest that there may be an incremental benefit to using a larger diameter balloon,[66] we prefer to start off with the smaller 30-mm balloon in the hopes of limiting the likelihood of perforation. We are willing to repeat the procedure with a 35-mm balloon at a later setting if the initial dilation is unsuccessful, but we are very averse to using the 40-mm balloon given its

high rate of perforation and the fact that alternative therapies (especially laparoscopic myotomy) are so successful.

Balloon dilations are always performed under fluoroscopic guidance. Before the actual procedure, it is essential to test the balloon for leaks by inflating it fully with saline or water. It is also important to check the location of the radiopaque markers on the balloon surface for later reference during the procedure because they are commonly not located in the center of the balloon. The actual dilation is always preceded by an upper GI endoscopy to ensure that the esophagus is clear of luminal contents, to exclude an obvious carcinoma, to gauge the extent of esophageal tortuosity, and to identify the presence or absence of a hiatal hernia to permit appropriate LES location fluoroscopically. The balloon is passed under fluoroscopic guidance over a rigid guidewire with a soft flexible tip. It is important to confirm that the guidewire traverses the diaphragm before deployment of the balloon dilator. The balloon is maneuvered until it traverses the LES region, and the position is verified fluoroscopically.

We first inflate the balloon to about 2 to 3 PSI to confirm appropriate positioning of the balloon looking for a "waist" in its center. This commonly is just below, not at, the diaphragm. The catheter is fixed in place by grasping it firmly against the bite-block. If there is too much give on the catheter, it is squeezed inferiorly by the hypertensive LES during inflation. The balloon is inflated slowly up to a limit of 10 PSI. During the process, we attempt first to identify the waist and then notice its obliteration to confirm that the balloon has reached its full diameter. We prefer to deflate the balloon as soon as the waist is obliterated rather than maintaining full inflation for any set amount of time. We do not exceed a balloon pressure of 10 PSI based on data suggesting an increased chance of perforation above this limit.[69] The dilator and guidewire are removed and examined for blood to confirm that the LES region has been torn. We generally do not reintubate the esophagus endoscopically, but we always follow therapeutic dilation with a Gastrografin oral solution swallow immediately after the patient has awakened from the intervention. Gastrografin oral solution is primarily administered to exclude a procedural perforation rather than as an attempt to document efficacy; postdilation spasm may hide a perforation that manifests later as the spasm resolves.

There is general consensus among most authorities that a single, successful balloon dilation has a duration of efficacy of a few years. Specifically, 5-year follow-up data show that the effect of a single dilation remains effective in 30% to 50% of patients.[67,69–71] Typically, patients require two to three dilations over a 5-year period to stay in remission. In the classic study by Parkman and associates,[72] three dilations maintained remission in 90% of patients after 5 years of follow-up (**Fig. 18.6**). Only 15% of patients required myotomy during this period (although two of these were a consequence of procedurally induced perforation). Longer term follow-up studies have also been reported. In one of these,[73] pneumatic dilation was effective in 61 of 72 patients followed for a mean length of 6.5 years, and a second dilation was required in only 4 patients. One patient responded for 25 years with a single procedure. Another series[67] followed patients for more than 15 years, at which time the therapeutic response to balloon dilation was classified as excellent in 12%, good in 28%, moderate in 20%, and poor in 40% with a requirement of a median four dilations.

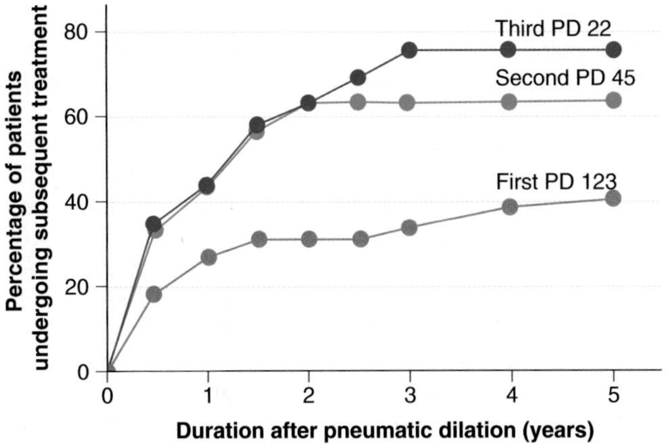

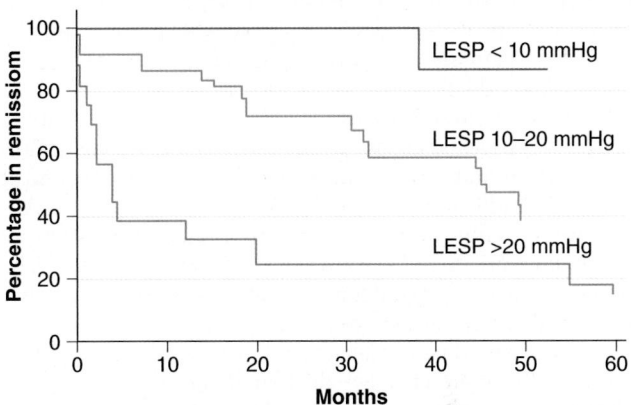

Fig. 18.6 Efficacy of repeated balloon dilations in patients with achalasia. PD, Pneumatic dilation. *(From Parkman HP, Reynolds JC, Ouyang A, et al: Pneumatic dilatation or esophagomyotomy treatment for idiopathic achalasia: Clinical outcomes and cost analysis.* Dig Dis Sci *38:75–85, 1993.)*

Box 18.2 **Predictors of Response to Balloon Dilation**

Durable first response
Absence of early relapse (within 2 months)
Older age (older patients do better)
Absence of advanced disease
LES pressure
? Complete balloon distention

LES, Lower esophageal sphincter.

Fig. 18.7 Correlation between postdilation lower esophageal sphincter pressure (LESP) and clinical outcome. *(From Eckardt VF, Aignherr C, Bernhard G: Predictors of outcome in patients with achalasia treated by pneumatic dilation.* Gastroenterology *103:1732–1738, 1992.)*

Two caveats must be kept in mind when evaluating these long-term follow-up studies. First, a significant number of patients were lost to follow-up, which hampers the quality of the report.[74] Second, one of the reports[75] describes the personal experience of one of the most experienced esophagologists in the world, and it is unclear whether or not physicians with less experience can expect similar outcomes. Finally, some authors have advocated the use of endoscopically guided pneumatic dilation without fluoroscopy.[76] In this technique, a colored mark is placed on the center of the balloon for visualization; whether or not this is an advantageous approach is unclear.

As with botulinum toxin injection, pneumatic dilation works well for patients with achalasia. An effective symptom response occurs in most patients, and, in contrast to botulinum toxin injection, the effect may be quite durable. Also, objective data show that the technique is effective in terms of producing a reduction in LES pressure and esophageal diameter and improved esophageal emptying by scintigraphy.[66,67] Patients commonly require repeated procedures, and some patients have little, if any, response. One study[67] showed little or no improvement in 12 of 54 patients (23%) 4 weeks after dilation. There is a wide range of potential outcomes from no response at all to long-term resolution of symptoms.

Several factors have been proposed as useful predictors of a response to balloon dilation (**Box 18.2**). First (and intuitively), the more frequent the dilations are needed to induce remission, the less likely they are to provide long-term responses. This has been shown in 5-year studies when multiple dilations were required for symptom control.[67] Second, early relapse (i.e., within 2 months) predicts a poor long-term outcome.[65,67] Third, age is an important predictor of success. In various studies, older age may be defined as older than 40 years,[65,67] older than 45 years,[69] or older than 60 years.[71] In one of these studies,[65,67] four of five patients younger than 18 years had symptomatic relapse within 2 months. In another study of 132 patients,[71] patients younger than 60 years were much more likely to need myotomy (14 patients) than patients older than 60 years (1 patient). Fourth, advanced stage achalasia is also less likely to respond to dilation. Many studies evaluating balloon dilation specifically exclude patients with sigmoidization of the esophagus because such patients are believed to have end-stage disease that is unlikely to respond to any therapeutic modality other than esophagectomy.

From an objective point of view, neither radiographic findings nor the degree of esophageal emptying after dilation can predict long-term clinical course.[70] However, absolute LES pressure does seem to correlate with long-term clinical benefit (**Fig. 18.7**), and a reassessment of LES pressure after the procedure may be helpful in some cases.[70] As discussed previously, newer balloons and balloons with a greater diameter have not been shown to influence outcome, although one study suggested that higher balloon inflation pressures and radiographic visualization of a fully expanded balloon diameter predicted greater success.[70]

Pneumatic balloon dilation of the LES for achalasia is by no means a risk-free procedure. The most concerning complication is esophageal perforation. Most studies quote a perforation rate of 0% to 6%.[66,71,77–80] This complication is particularly important because esophageal perforation may have a poor outcome even with rapid careful management. The quoted mortality rate from traumatic esophageal perforation is 10%.[81,82] Factors associated with an increased likelihood of esophageal perforation after balloon dilation include (1) a first dilation, (2) high-amplitude esophageal contractions, and (3) malnutrition.[65,83,84]

Perforation rates may be lower in the Rigiflex era,[83] possibly as a result of the use of lower inflation pressures and shorter inflation times compared with prior reports. A more recent meta-analysis of 15 articles including 1065 patients who underwent pneumatic dilation quoted only a 1.6% perforation rate.[85] Patients still must be cautioned very carefully before dilation. They especially need to be made aware that the operative management of a traumatic esophageal perforation generally requires an open approach through either the chest or the abdomen, whereas a primary Heller myotomy is easily accomplished laparoscopically in most cases. For this reason, many esophagologists are moving away from recommending pneumatic dilation as the primary modality for therapy, unless patients have a particular aversion or contraindication to surgery. Other worrisome complications of balloon dilation include hematomas (which rarely may cause esophageal obstruction[68]) and chest pain. As expected, chest pain is quite common, and sometimes it may be severe enough to warrant hospitalization even if contrast studies fail to show a perforation. Patients with achalasia who present initially with chest pain are more likely to develop severe chest pain after balloon dilation.[65]

Long-term complications may also develop after dilation. Gastroesophageal reflux is common when measured by ambulatory pH monitoring,[86] but it usually is not severe, and it responds readily to proton pump inhibitor therapy. Nevertheless, severe reflux complications such as esophageal stricture formation and Barrett's esophagus have been reported.[65] The development of a diverticulum in the distal esophagus after balloon dilation has also been described,[65] but whether this represents true diverticular formation or an esophageal ballooning from an effective dilation-induced myotomy[87] is unclear.

Surgical Myotomy

Surgical cardiomyotomy (the Heller procedure) is an important and effective therapy for achalasia. It has stood the test of time (many long-term series have been published), it is relatively safe, and it has been successfully adapted to a minimally invasive laparoscopic approach.[88–113] Patient satisfaction remains high 5 to 10 years after surgery with good to excellent results persisting in 85% to 90% of patients. Laparoscopic myotomy, a newer technique for which the available duration of follow-up is shorter by necessity, seems to be associated with similar outcomes to traditional open myotomy. Compared with pneumatic dilation, myotomy (whether performed in an open or laparoscopic fashion) outperforms dilation.[77,88–91] However, there are two important limiting factors that keep pneumatic dilation a viable option. First is the ever-present, albeit small, risk of perioperative complications. Second is the steep learning curve involved in learning to perform laparoscopic myotomy reliably (at least 20, but probably more, cases). Several series note that most, if not all, serious complications occur within the first 20 to 30 patients.[102,114] Similar to many other foregut surgical procedures, the results of laparoscopic myotomy are best if the procedure is performed by an expert, experienced surgeon.

We currently believe that laparoscopic myotomy (usually with a fundoplication) is probably the primary therapeutic modality of choice for achalasia when performed by an expert, experienced esophageal surgeon. The mortality from Heller myotomy is low, rarely exceeding 1% in expert hands. Common major early complications include inadvertent mucosal perforation (up to 25%), pneumothorax, inadvertent splenectomy (<4%), and vagotomy. Most of these complications are managed easily without significant long-term sequelae. Longer term technical complications include an incomplete myotomy, which fails to cure the problem (in approximately 5% to 10% of cases) or, conversely, GERD (which in a small percentage of cases may lead to Barrett's esophagus or stricture formation or both).

Prior surgical controversies regarding the performance of a Heller myotomy have largely been resolved in recent years. Most esophagologists currently believe that a laparoscopic approach is superior to a thoracoscopic approach, and most believe a loose antireflux procedure should be performed at the same time, although debate still rages regarding what type of antireflux surgery is best. Esophagologists who argue against the need for an antireflux procedure point out that a carefully performed thoracoscopic or laparoscopic myotomy permits excellent visualization of the gastroesophageal junction allowing preservation of the vagus nerve and oblique sling fibers of the cardia, resulting in only minor traumatic mobilization of the lower esophagus through the diaphragmatic crural sphincter. As a consequence, reflux is unlikely to occur,[114] as is borne out by some studies that show no differences in the development of reflux symptoms whether or not an antireflux operation is performed.[96]

Numerous other series have identified a high incidence postoperatively of reflux symptoms, abnormal ambulatory pHmetry scores, and subsequent development of peptic strictures and Barrett's esophagus.[109] In particular, over long-term follow-up, patients studied for greater than 6 years even with fundoplication have a greater than 40% chance of developing reflux manifest by esophagitis or abnormal pH monitoring or both.[115,116] Surgeons continue to debate whether to perform a loose, but complete, fundoplication (i.e., a Nissen operation) or a partial fundoplication (e.g., a Dorr or Toupet procedure), and no clear recommendations have emerged to date. There is a fine line between not extending the myotomy too far down the cardia (leading to reflux) and paying the price with an incomplete myotomy (leading to failure and requiring a repeat operation). Consequently, we believe that most patients, if not all, should undergo an antireflux procedure with an extended (at least 8 cm above the LES and 2 cm below it) laparoscopic myotomy specifically. We do not favor a thoracoscopic approach, given the ease, lower complication rate, shorter hospital stay, and less postoperative pain associated with the laparoscopic approach.

Occasionally, patients with end-stage achalasia require esophagectomy. Numerous studies have shown that a favorable surgical outcome is closely related to the preoperative stage of disease.[54] Patients with marked sigmoidization and dilation of the esophagus may not respond well to sphincter-directed therapy alone, although some investigators still advocate an attempt at surgical myotomy first.[117] The few data available regarding these end-stage patients suggest that esophagectomy (preferably with a gastric pull-up rather than a colonic or jejunal interposition) enables most of these patients to regain their weight and eat within the expected limitations of any patient undergoing a total esophagectomy.[118,119] Finally, successful robot-assisted laparoscopic Heller myotomy has been described.[120] This technique provides further potential advances over a standard laparoscopic approach by providing a three-dimensional view of the gastroesophageal junction, restoring depth perception to the operator, and by improving precision by scaling down the surgeon's movements so that large movements of the robotic console are translated into smaller movements in the patient.

Table 18.2 Advantages and Disadvantages of Initial Approaches for Treatment of Achalasia

Therapy	Advantages	Disadvantages	Comments
Botulinum toxin injection	Easy to perform	Short effect duration	Useful for poor surgical risks, elderly patients, or acute management of malnourished patients
	Generally effective		
	Safe		
	Repeatable		
	? Diagnostic utility		
Balloon dilation	Avoids anesthesia	? Surgery better	Requires expert operator and surgical backup
	Generally effective	Perforation risk	Reserve for poor operative risks or patients reluctant for surgery
	Outpatient procedure	Perforation requires open repair	
	More effective in elderly patients		
Surgical myotomy	Effective	Inpatient stay	Ideal approach in healthy young patients
	Safe	Not 100% effective	
	Can be combined with antireflux surgery	Anesthesia risk	

Robotic surgery also eliminates hand tremor. Whether or not these theoretical advantages result in better long-term outcomes remains to be shown.

Miscellaneous and Emerging Treatments

Pharmacologic therapy for achalasia has been used in the past and is presently undergoing further investigation. Sublingual nifedipine has been reported to improve symptoms, esophageal retention, and LES pressures.[121,122] This approach may be useful in isolated, rare instances, but potential side effects and lack of published long-term efficacy limit its use. Similarly, sildenafil, by augmenting nitric oxide effects, lowers the LES pressure and improves some manometric measurements in patients with achalasia.[123] Symptoms are not improved significantly, however, so there are no indications for its use at this time. Finally, expandable metal stents have been attempted in six poor surgical candidates with achalasia.[124] There was no sustained symptom relief, and the 1-month mortality was extremely high, suggesting no role for this approach at the present time.

One of the newest and potentially useful methods of therapy for achalasia may be the use of peroral endoscopic myotomy (POEM). This method of myotomy is performed completely endoscopically without the need for breaching the abdomen. The seeds of success for this operation were first developed with the ability to perform submucosal endoscopy with mucosal flap safety valve (SEMF), at first used for access to the abdominal cavity.[125] Following this breakthrough technique, the first successful POEM was performed in pigs.[126] Most recently, this technique was adapted successfully to a series of 17 patients with achalasia.[127] In this study, a submucosal myotomy, on average 8.0 cm in length including a 2-cm extension onto the cardia, leg to significant improvement of dysphagia score and reduction in LES pressure without serious complications. The follow-up for this group of patients was

only 5 months, however. Whether this will become an effective long-term treatment comparable to laparoscopic myotomy has yet to be determined. It is also important to keep in mind that a fundoplication is not performed with this technique.

Treatment Summary

Trying to reach consensus on the appropriate initial treatment strategy for achalasia is one of the great debates in esophagology. Even decision models cannot agree, with one recent study recommending pneumatic dilation[128] and another recommending laparoscopic cardiomyotomy.[129] The latter publication indicated a preference for botulinum toxin injection over balloon dilation.[130] Each of the three major approaches has its own advantages and disadvantages (**Table 18.2**). Botulinum toxin injection is easy to perform, generally works well, has only a small chance of significant complications, and can be given multiple times. One placebo-controlled trial showed similar outcomes for symptom control and objective measurements of changes in LES pressure and esophageal retention in patients randomly assigned to pneumatic dilation or botulinum toxin injection,[57] although the number of patients studied was small (16), and the trend was in favor of dilation. The duration of effect with botulinum toxin is much shorter than with either balloon dilation or surgical myotomy requiring either repeated injections or ultimately a more definitive intervention such as balloon dilation or surgical myotomy.

In comparing balloon dilation with surgical myotomy, the available data favor a surgical approach, especially when one factors in the advantages afforded by using the laparoscopic approach. Although anecdotal evidence[130] has suggested that dilation-induced esophageal perforation may be repaired laparoscopically with little lost compared with an elective procedure, this is by no means generally accepted. The disadvantages of balloon dilation over surgical myotomy include a poorer efficacy and a potentially missed opportunity to undergo a minimally invasive procedure. Some medical centers have all but abandoned pneumatic dilation in favor of laparoscopic myotomy. We have not yet embraced this approach completely, but the number of dilations we are performing currently has decreased markedly.

Our general approach for the management of patients with achalasia is as follows. Botulinum toxin injection is our preferred initial management strategy for patients who are elderly, who are poor operative risks, or who have an unclear or atypical form of achalasia (i.e., as a diagnostic approach[131]). We also favor this approach initially for patients who present in extremis to permit stabilization of their condition before definitive therapy is undertaken later or for patients who are reluctant to undergo definitive therapy until we can show the likely benefit of lowering LES pressure by another means later on. For young, healthy patients (arbitrarily, one might say, <25 years old), laparoscopic myotomy is indicated initially. We favor combining cardiomyotomy with a loose fundoplication at the same time. For older patients (arbitrarily >60 years old) who are otherwise in good health, pneumatic dilation may be indicated initially.

The initial management of choice in healthy patients 25 to 60 years old (actually most patients seen in clinical practice) is not clearly defined. It is important to offer all the available options in as unbiased a manner as possible, which requires consultation with both a gastroenterologist and a laparoscopic surgeon; it is also important to stress the lack of durability with botulinum toxin injection, which otherwise seems a quick, easy fix. We are leaning more and more toward recommending cardiomyotomy as primary therapy in this group, too. For patients who respond poorly initially or in whom there is a rapid return of symptoms after a less risky procedure, the next step up should be offered early in the treatment process rather than performing the previously ineffective approach repeatedly. Finally, we also believe it worthwhile to offer patients presenting with apparently end-stage disease an initial attempt at sphincter-directed therapy before resorting to an esophagectomy because of the poor relationship between radiologic findings and outcome. Under these conditions, we favor botulinum toxin injection as a safe, initial diagnostic approach in determining the likely efficacy of future sphincter-directed therapy.

Achalasia and Cancer

The relationship of achalasia with cancer warrants special mention (**Box 18.3**). The disease has two important associations with malignancy. First is the development of an achalasialike syndrome as a consequence of malignancy (i.e., secondary achalasia), and second is the development of malignancy in patients with long-standing achalasia (i.e., secondary malignancy).

Box 18.3 Achalasia and Malignancy

Secondary achalasia
    Gastroesophageal junction tumor
    Paraneoplastic achalasia
Secondary malignancy

Secondary Achalasia

Secondary achalasia accounts for approximately 2.4% to 4% of all cases of achalasia.[131,132] Malignancy may cause an achalasialike syndrome through two unrelated mechanisms. The first is through direct anatomic compression or infiltration of the LES[133] mandating the performance of a careful upper GI endoscopy with careful retroflexion in all patients. The second is through an antibody-mediated paraneoplastic effect on esophageal function. In a study of 13 patients with tumor-induced achalasia,[134] 11 cases had direct involvement of the LES with penetration into the muscularis propria. Three of these cases showed extensive neoplastic involvement of the myenteric plexus of the LES. Ganglion cells appeared normal suggesting that the effect is purely due to an obstruction to esophageal outflow. That some of these malignancies induced achalasia through extrinsic compression alone is supported by case reports of benign processes, such as mediastinal fibrosis, surgical procedures, or large pancreatic pseudocysts, also causing achalasialike syndromes.[135,136] In one of the patients in the aforementioned series, anti-Hu antibodies (antineuronal nuclear antibody type 1) were detected. Histologic analysis of the LES in this patient revealed marked lymphocytic myenteric plexus inflammation and marked depletion of ganglion cells identical to that seen in primary achalasia.

Several types of malignancy cause secondary achalasia. Their distribution depends partly on the mechanism involved. For malignancies that cause achalasia by direct involvement of the distal esophagus, adenocarcinoma of the cardia or gastroesophageal junction (with or without Barrett's esophagus) predominates,[129] but many other types of cancer have also been described, including cancer of the breast, liver, prostate, lung, pleura, pancreas, cervix, and uterus.[134,137–141] For paraneoplastic achalasia, small cell carcinoma of the lung predominates, but other cancer types including lymphoma have also been described.[134,142]

The diagnosis of secondary achalasia requires a high index of suspicion. Although these patients tend to be older, have a shorter duration of symptoms, and commonly exhibit weight loss, studies have shown that even with these "red flags" primary achalasia is still statistically much more common.[143] The onset of achalasia symptoms may precede signs of cancer by months or years[144] in patients with paraneoplastic achalasia. One clue may be the presence of other neurologic symptoms or the presence of a more global GI motility syndrome (e.g., colonic pseudoobstruction) together with the presence of achalasia symptoms. In addition, although patients with paraneoplastic achalasia may appear radiologically and endoscopically identical to patients with primary disease, patients with secondary achalasia from direct tumor involvement tend to have longer areas of distal esophageal narrowing and less esophageal dilation than patients with primary achalasia.[145] Endoscopically, as opposed to the characteristic "pop" that one feels on traversing the LES with primary achalasia, there is moderate to severe resistance during passage of the endoscope.

Despite the absence of firm data, we favor careful anatomic evaluation of the LES region with endoscopic ultrasound or CT scanning or both in elderly patients with significant weight loss who present with the new onset of rapidly progressive symptoms. We favor performing endoscopic ultrasound at the time of initial optical endoscopy in such patients unless there is a clear infiltrative lesion on optical endoscopy. CT scanning should also be considered in patients with a long history of cigarette smoking or associated pulmonary symptoms because paraneoplastic achalasia associated with the anti-Hu antibody syndrome is most commonly seen in patients with lung malignancies.

Treatment for secondary achalasia is usually directed at the tumor. The one exception might be patients with paraneoplastic disease, especially patients with antibody-confirmed disease but no obvious primary tumor in whom a botulinum toxin injection may be effective[144] (anecdotal personal observation).

Secondary Malignancy

The second association of achalasia with malignancy is the increased risk of squamous cell carcinoma and perhaps adenocarcinoma of the esophagus in patients with long-standing primary disease. The estimated relative risk of developing squamous cell carcinoma of the esophagus in achalasia is 8-fold to 140-fold higher than in the normal population.[146–149] In a long-term follow-up study of 249 patients with achalasia (a mean of 12 years), 6 (2.4%) developed esophageal cancer.[149] A more recent study similarly showed the occurrence of squamous cell carcinoma in 5 of 228 consecutive patients with achalasia studied over a median of 18.3 years.[150]

Esophageal cancer generally develops at a younger age in patients with achalasia. Symptoms of achalasia generally precede the development of squamous cell carcinoma of the esophagus by 17 to 20 years.[146–149] Consequently, there has been a long debate regarding the role, if any, of endoscopic surveillance in patients with achalasia, which remains unresolved. One more recent report described the potential role of flow cytometric analysis of esophageal biopsy specimens as a means of surveying these patients, but this recommendation was based on a single case report.[151] No data are available to show whether effective treatment of achalasia reduces the development of esophageal cancer.[150]

References

The complete reference list is available online at www.expertconsult.com.

Chapter **19**

Ingested Foreign Objects and Food Bolus Impactions

Ian Grimes and Patrick R. Pfau

Video related to this chapter's topics can be found online at expertconsult.com.

Introduction

Ingested gastrointestinal (GI) foreign bodies and food bolus impactions occur frequently and are the second most common endoscopic emergency after GI bleeding. The actual incidence of foreign bodies and food impaction is unknown, and few controlled data exist on the management of foreign body ingestions. Although most GI foreign bodies do not result in serious clinical sequelae or mortality,[1] it has been estimated that 1500 to 2750 patients die annually in the United States because of the ingestion of foreign bodies.[2-4] More recent studies have suggested the mortality from GI foreign bodies to be significantly lower, with no deaths reported in more than 850 adults and one death in approximately 2200 children with a GI foreign body.[5-11] As a result of the frequency of this problem and the rare but possible negative consequences, it is important for the gastroenterologist and endoscopist to understand the patients at risk for ingestion of foreign bodies, the best method for a prompt diagnosis, and the correct management with avoidance of unwanted complications.

Epidemiology

True foreign bodies may be the result of either unintentional or intentional ingestion. The most common patient group that unintentionally ingests foreign bodies is children. Of foreign body ingestions, 80% occur in children, with most occurring between the ages of 6 months and 3 years.[12,13] Pediatric ingestions are almost always accidental, resulting from the child's natural oral curiosity.[14] The most common items ingested by children are coins followed by small

toys, crayons, buttons, pins, jewels, nails, and disc batteries.[6,9,10,15,16]

Accidental ingestion in adults occurs in various groups of patients. Dentures and the presence of dental appliances are a common risk factor for accidental foreign body ingestion secondary to impaired tactile sensation during swallowing.[17,18] A common occurrence is a patient mistakenly ingesting his or her own dentures.[19] The other large patient group in which accidental ingestion of foreign bodies occurs includes individuals with compromised judgment or senses, such as very elderly, demented, or intoxicated individuals. Accidental coin ingestion has been encountered in young college students secondary to an increasingly popular beer drinking game, "Quarters," where a quarter may inadvertently be swallowed and become lodged in the esophagus.[20] Roofers, tailors, carpenters, and seamstresses have increased rates of foreign body ingestion because of accidental swallowing of nails or needles placed in the mouth during work. Intentional ingestion of foreign bodies is frequent in psychiatric patients or prisoners (**Fig. 19.1**).[21,22] These patients ingest foreign bodies for a secondary gain and often have a history of previous foreign body ingestion, ingest multiple objects, and often ingest very complex objects.

Iatrogenic foreign bodies related to GI endoscopy procedures are becoming an increasing problem. Symptoms and complications have been reported as a result of capsule endoscopy; migrated esophageal, luminal, or biliary stents; and migrated gastrostomy buttons and catheters.[23,24]

Esophageal food impaction is a much more common problem than true foreign body ingestion with an estimated annual incidence of 13 to 16 episodes per 100,000 people.[25] Most (75% to 100%) patients who present with a food

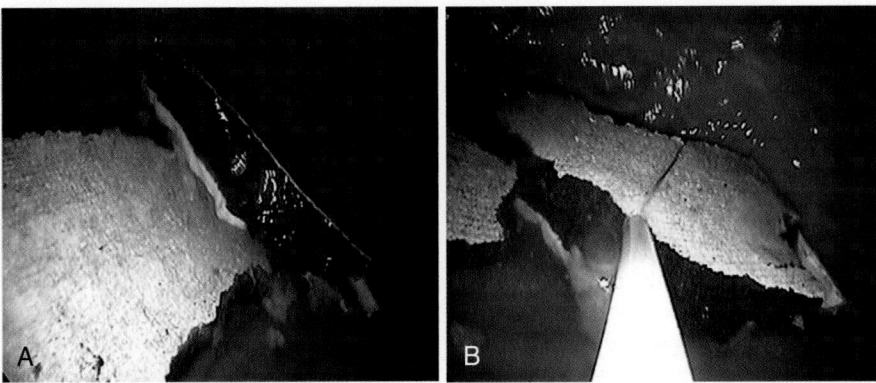

Fig. 19.1 Endoscopic image of tennis shoes that a prisoner with a psychiatric history ingested. These were successfully removed with a snare.

impaction have some type of predisposing esophageal pathology.[5,25–28] The most commonly observed abnormalities associated with food impaction are Schatzki rings or peptic strictures and, increasingly, eosinophilic esophagitis.[29] Less commonly found as a predisposing cause are webs, extrinsic compression, surgical anastomoses, fundoplication wraps, and bariatric gastroplasties.[30] Esophageal cancer very rarely manifests with acute food bolus impaction.[31] Motility disorders such as achalasia, diffuse esophageal spasm, and nutcracker esophagus are infrequent causes of food impactions.[32]

Food impaction most commonly occurs in adults in their 4th or 5th decade but is becoming more prevalent in young adults because of the increasing incidence of eosinophilic esophagitis. The type of food impacted correlates with cultural and regional dietary habits. In the United States, hot dogs, pork, beef, and chicken are the most common foods resulting in impaction, whereas fish and fish bones are the most common food to result in impaction in Asian countries and coastal areas.[33–35]

Pathophysiology and Pathogenesis

Most (80% to 90%) ingested foreign bodies and food bolus impactions pass spontaneously without clinical sequelae.[1] However, 10% to 20% of GI foreign bodies require endoscopic intervention, and 1% may require surgical intervention.[5,31,36] It is important to understand how ingested foreign bodies can result in significant disease, which patients are more likely to ingest complex foreign bodies, and in which parts of the GI tract foreign bodies are most likely to cause damage (**Fig. 19.2**). This understanding ensures appropriate use of endoscopic and surgical interventions.

The most common complications related to foreign bodies are obstruction and perforation, which can occur in any area of the GI tract where there is narrowing, angulation, anatomic sphincters, or previous surgery.[37] The posterior hypopharynx is the first area of the GI tract in which a foreign body may become lodged, particularly small sharp objects such as chicken or fish bones.[38,39] In the esophagus, there are four areas of physical narrowing where a food bolus or foreign body is likely to impact: the upper esophageal sphincter, the level of the aortic arch, the crossing of the main stem bronchus, and the lower esophageal sphincter (LES) and gastroesophageal junction. All of these areas have been shown to be areas of true

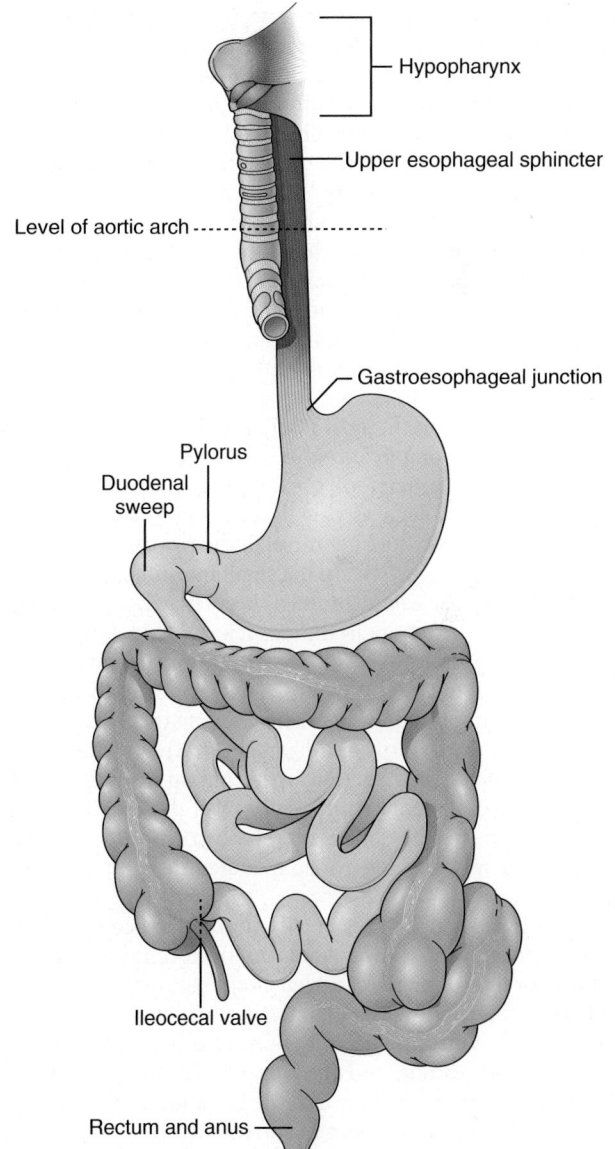

Fig. 19.2 Gastrointestinal areas of luminal narrowing and angulation that predispose to foreign body impaction and obstruction. (*From Feldman M, Friedman LS, Sleisenger MH, editors: Sleisenger & Fordtran's Gastrointestinal and Liver Disease: Pathophysiology, Diagnosis, Management, vol 1, ed 7, Philadelphia, 2002, Saunders, p 387.*)

luminal narrowing with diameters of 23 mm or less in adult patients.[40]

Independent of the physiologic areas of narrowing, most food boluses are associated with esophageal pathology, including rings, webs, diverticula, and peptic strictures.[2] Multiple esophageal rings associated with eosinophilic esophagitis have led to esophageal food impaction at much greater incandescence in young adults.[41,42] Uncommonly, esophageal motor disturbances, such as achalasia, diffuse esophageal spasm, or segmental variations in peristalsis, may contribute to food and foreign body impactions.[43–46]

Foreign bodies and food impactions in the esophagus generally have the highest incidence of complications with the rate of complication being directly proportional to the time the object spends in the esophagus. Esophageal foreign bodies may lead to perforation, abscess, mediastinitis, pneumothorax, fistula formation, and cardiac tamponade.[47,48] Once through the esophagus, most objects, including sharp objects, pass through the intestinal tract without consequence.[1,37] However, among patients presenting with symptoms related to a foreign body, the perforation rate has been estimated to be 5% overall and up to 35% for sharp and pointed objects.[31,49] Esophageal perforation is the most frequent cause of significant morbidity and mortality.[47] The risk of perforation of the esophagus increases dramatically when foreign bodies or food boluses are left impacted in the esophagus for more than 24 hours. Other reported complications, including complications that have been reported to lead to fatalities, include GI bleeding, aortoenteric fistulas, aspiration, abscess formation, and true rarities such as perforation of the heart and lead and zinc toxicity.[50–56]

Once in the stomach, most foreign bodies pass through the GI tract without complications in 1 to 2 weeks. Exceptions are objects with a diameter of greater than 2 cm and objects longer than 5 cm, such as pencils, pens, and eating utensils, which have difficulty passing through the pylorus or the duodenal bulb and sweep.[37,38,57] In the small intestine, three points of impedance exist where a foreign body may become lodged and result in obstruction: In the duodenal C-loop, long objects may get "hung up" and result in perforation. The narrowing and angulation of the ligament of Treitz can result in foreign body obstruction, and even smaller objects that were able to pass through the pylorus and ligament of Treitz may cause a distal small bowel obstruction by becoming impacted at the ileocecal valve. Patients with small bowel disease, history of adhesions, or partial small bowel obstructions may have greater difficulty passing foreign bodies through the small intestine.

Most objects, once in the small intestine and colon, do not cause damage. The bowel tends to protect itself naturally against foreign bodies. A foreign body stimulates peristalsis and axial flow in the small intestine, which results in the foreign body concentrated in the center of fecal residue with the blunt end leading and the sharp end trailing.[58,59] As the foreign body travels further into the large intestine, it usually becomes centered in the lumen surrounded by stool, making a complication even less likely.[2] Rectal foreign bodies rarely result from ingestion and more frequently are inserted into the rectum through the anus. However, occasionally an ingested foreign body may traverse the entire GI tract to the rectum before further passage is impaired by the rectal valves of Houston or the internal and external sphincters.

Clinical Features: History and Physical Examination

For adults who are able to communicate, a history of ingestion including timing, type of foreign body ingested, and onset of symptoms is usually reliable. History is particularly reliable for food impactions because patients are almost always symptomatic and can detail the exact onset of symptoms. Small sharp objects or fish bones often manifest with a foreign body sensation or odynophagia in the posterior pharynx or cervical esophagus; this occurs even if the foreign body has passed to the stomach because of a small mucosal laceration. Partial or complete esophageal obstruction almost always results in symptoms. Esophageal obstruction may cause substernal chest pain, dysphagia, gagging, vomiting, or a sensation of choking.[60] More complete obstruction can lead to drooling and the inability to handle oral secretions.

The type of symptoms may aid in determining whether an esophageal foreign body is still present and where in the esophagus it may be located. If the patient presents with dysphagia, dysphonia, or odynophagia, there is almost an 80% chance that a foreign body or food impaction is present. If the symptom is retrosternal pain or a pharyngeal discomfort only, less than 50% of patients have an identifiable foreign object.[61] The patient may be able to localize the object successfully in the posterior pharynx or at the level of the cricopharyngeal muscle. However, for objects located more distally in the esophagus and in the stomach, patient localization becomes poor with an accuracy of 30% to 40% in the esophagus and almost 0% in the stomach.[62,63] Once in the stomach, small intestine, or colon, the only symptoms described would be secondary to a complication resulting from the foreign body, such as obstruction, perforation, or bleeding.

The history and symptoms for true foreign bodies are often less reliable than food impaction because true foreign bodies are often ingested by children, mentally impaired adults, or adults who have ingested the foreign body for secondary gain. Even with esophageal foreign bodies, 20% to 38% of children are asymptomatic.[62,64] In children and adults unable to communicate, there may be no history of a foreign body ingestion from the patient or the caregiver in up to 40% of cases,[65] necessitating a high degree of suspicion. Symptoms are more subtle and include drooling, poor feeding, blood-stained saliva, or a failure to thrive.[65,66] Respiratory compromise may occur with aspiration or a proximally located esophageal foreign body that compresses the trachea causing wheezing and stridor.[65,67]

Past medical history is important in regard to previous episodes of either food impaction or foreign body ingestion. Previous food impaction or a previous need for esophageal dilation makes recurrent episodes more likely. Patients with previous true foreign body ingestion are often multiple ingestors who are more likely to ingest multiple objects and complex objects.

Physical examination aids little in determining the presence or location of a foreign body but is important to detect potential ingestion-related complications. Determination of airway and level of consciousness is crucial before any endoscopic or nonendoscopic intervention. Lung examination should be performed to detect the presence of wheezing or aspiration. Esophageal or oropharyngeal perforation may result in swell-

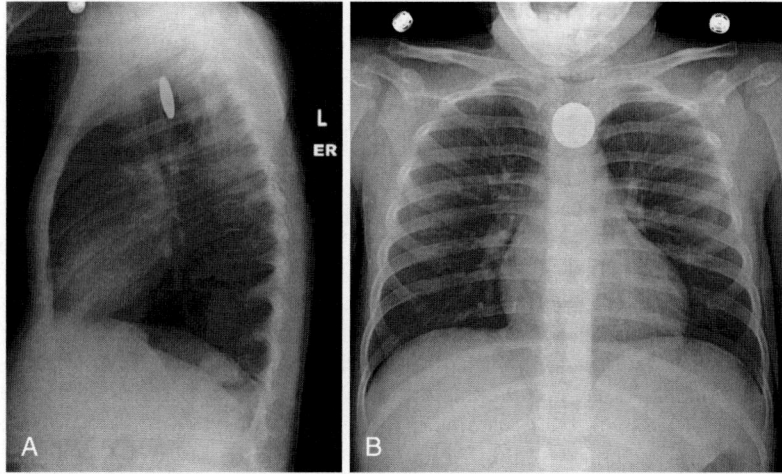

Fig. 19.3 Anteroposterior and lateral chest x-rays of a child with suspected coin ingestion show the coin clearly in the proximal esophagus. *(Image courtesy of Dr. Ken L. Schreibman, Department of Radiology, University of Wisconsin Medical School.)*

ing, erythema, or crepitus of the neck or chest region. Abdominal examination aids in determining the signs of an obstruction or perforation.

Diagnosis

Diagnostic evaluation should begin with plain film radiographs. Patients with suspected foreign body ingestion should undergo anteroposterior and lateral radiographs of the chest and abdomen to help determine the presence, type, and location of a foreign body.[49] Anteroposterior and lateral neck and chest films are suggested if there is a suspicion of a foreign body in the esophagus versus the trachea or if there is a foreign object that may be obscured by overlying spine (**Fig. 19.3**).[65,68] Plain films also aid in detecting complications such as aspiration, abdominal free air, or subcutaneous emphysema.[60,69] Radiographic studies are more controversial in children. Because history from children is often poor, mouth-to-anus screening films have been advocated in suspected foreign body ingestions.[49]

Other authors have suggested a more directed approach or nonradiographic methods to determine the presence and location of foreign bodies in children.[70] To limit radiation, hand-held metal detectors have been used with a sensitivity of greater than 95% for the detection and localization of metallic foreign bodies.[71] Plain films are satisfactory in some cases of true foreign bodies and occasionally in cases of food ingestions with larger bones. Smaller bones or thin metal objects are not readily seen, however, and many objects, including plastic, wood, and glass, are not radiopaque.[6] False-negative rates with plain films can be 47% and false-positive rates are close to 20% in the investigation of foreign bodies.[61,72] Of films read by a nonradiologist for the presence of foreign bodies, 35% have been found to be misread.[73] Generally, it is accepted that barium studies should not be performed in the evaluation of GI foreign bodies. If aspiration occurs, the hypertonic contrast agents used can cause acute pulmonary edema.[74] Barium evaluation can delay a necessary therapeutic endoscopic procedure by interfering with endoscopic visualization and complicating removal of a foreign body.[75]

Advanced imaging such as computed tomography (CT) or magnetic resonance (MR) imaging may be used in unusual or difficult-to-diagnose cases and may aid in detecting soft tissue inflammation or the presence of an abscess. Three-dimensional CT has been used to diagnose foreign bodies not seen with other imaging and may aid in detecting complications of foreign body ingestion such as perforation or abscess before the use of endoscopy, and MR imaging may have a role in showing soft tissue periesophageal pathology.[65,76,77]

Diagnostic endoscopy provides the most accurate diagnostic modality in suspected ingested foreign bodies and food impactions. Any patient with persistent symptoms and a continued clinical suspicion of a GI foreign body should undergo upper endoscopy even after negative or unrevealing radiographic evaluation.[78] This approach ensures the correct diagnosis of food impactions, nonradiopaque objects, and radiopaque objects that are obscured by overlying bony structures.[37] Endoscopy is the best method to detect underlying pathologic conditions, such as esophageal strictures, that contribute to a food impaction or foreign body that does not pass readily through the GI tract. Endoscopy also can closely examine the GI mucosa to assess for laceration or damage that may contribute to continuing symptoms after a foreign body has spontaneously passed. Most importantly, diagnostic endoscopy is directly linked to when endoscopy is used for therapy—treatment or extraction of a known or suspected foreign body. Diagnostic endoscopy is not indicated when small, blunt objects are known to have passed into the stomach and the patient is asymptomatic. These objects traverse the pylorus and the rest of the GI tract without complications. If a foreign body is known to have passed the ligament of Treitz, diagnostic and therapeutic endoscopy would be of little added benefit. Rare exceptions are sharp objects that can be safely extracted with an enteroscope. More recently, double-balloon enteroscopes have been used for the retrieval of ingested foreign bodies and retained endoscopy capsules in the small bowel.[79,80] Finally, diagnostic endoscopy is contraindicated when there is physical examination or radiographic evidence of a bowel perforation anywhere in the GI tract or a small bowel obstruction beyond the ligament of Treitz secondary to the foreign body.

Treatment

Of GI foreign bodies, 75% to 90% pass through the GI tract spontaneously without complication.[5,81] Two more recent studies have emphasized conservative management with 86% to 97% of foreign bodies passing spontaneously with minimal complications.[82,83] Esophageal foreign bodies were excluded from the above-mentioned studies. Although conservative management is successful in most nonesophageal foreign bodies, a more appropriate treatment plan if immediate endoscopy is not performed is to have a policy of expectant management and then selective endoscopy based on type, size, and location of the ingested object.[84,85]

Numerous medical therapies for esophageal foreign bodies or food impactions have been studied as primary treatment or in conjunction with endoscopic therapy. The most frequently used medication is glucagon, a smooth muscle relaxant that significantly reduces LES pressure with doses of 0.25 mg.[86] Glucagon has treated esophageal food impactions successfully in 12% to 58% of cases.[87-89] However, a randomized trial found glucagon no better than placebo in treating children with coins lodged in the esophagus.[90] Glucagon is generally safe but may result in nausea, abdominal distention, and, rarely, vomiting. Glucagon would not work with a fixed obstruction present, which is often found with esophageal foreign bodies and food impactions. Glucagon does not provide definitive examination and treatment of coexisting esophageal pathology as does flexible endoscopy. Finally, glucagon may help when used with endoscopy by lowering LES pressure and facilitating the endoscope pushing a food impaction into the stomach.[91] Nitroglycerin and nifedipine are other smooth muscle relaxants that have been anecdotally described as promoting passage of esophageal impactions into the stomach.[49]

Medical methods that have been described but should be avoided are gas-forming agents, emetics, and papain meat tenderizer. Gas-forming agents combined with a smooth muscle relaxant have been reported to have success rates of almost 70% in clearing esophageal foreign bodies into the stomach.[92] However, esophageal rupture and perforation have occurred with these agents, particularly if there is a fixed obstruction or the foreign body has been present more than 6 hours.[93,94] Papain, a meat tenderizer, and emetics for the treatment of food impaction are two methods that should never be used because of the risk of esophageal necrosis, perforation, and aspiration.[2,95,96]

The radiologic literature has multiple descriptions of methods to remove esophageal foreign bodies under fluoroscopic guidance. Reported methods include extraction with Foley balloon catheters, suction catheters, wire baskets, or a magnetic catheter to extract ferromagnetic metal objects.[69,97] The largest experience has been with Foley catheters where the catheter is passed either nasally or orally into the esophagus and past the foreign body. The balloon is inflated and withdrawn to deliver the foreign body to the oropharynx where it can be retrieved. Although high success rates have been reported, the major drawback is loss of control of the foreign body, particularly at the level of the upper esophageal sphincter and laryngopharynx. Complications reported include nosebleeds, dislodgment of the foreign body in the nose, laryngospasm, vomiting, and, of largest concern, aspiration with resultant airway obstruction and death.[98,99] Because

radiologic methods do not match the efficacy or safety of endoscopy, few indications exist for their use. Radiologic methods to remove foreign bodies or food impactions should be limited to when endoscopy is unavailable or cannot be available within 12 to 24 hours.

Flexible endoscopy has become the diagnostic and therapeutic method of choice in both true GI foreign bodies and food boluses in pediatric and adult patients. This recommendation is based on multiple large series using endoscopy for the treatment of GI foreign bodies with success rates greater than 95% and associated morbidity and mortality reported at 0% in most studies but always less than 5%.[5,9,25-27,75,100-103] Although treatment failures are rare, predictors of endoscopic failure and complications include intentional ingestion, ingestion of multiple complex foreign bodies, and lack of patient cooperation.[49]

Because most GI foreign bodies pass through the GI tract uneventfully, the indication and timing for intervention with endoscopy is important. Generally, if a patient is symptomatic, intervention is required. For esophageal foreign bodies, this includes patients with odynophagia, dysphagia, vomiting, inability to handle secretions, drooling, chest pain, or the sensation of a present foreign body. Once past the esophagus, symptoms of obstruction or perforation may necessitate surgical rather than endoscopic intervention. If the patient is not overtly symptomatic or cannot accurately give a history concerning symptoms, the location and characteristics of the foreign body define the need for intervention. Generally, all esophageal foreign bodies and food impactions require intervention in an urgent or emergent fashion. No foreign body should be allowed to remain lodged in the esophagus longer than 24 hours. The time a foreign body is present in the esophagus is directly related to an increase in complications (**Fig. 19.4**).[104,105]

For most objects that reach the stomach, observation is acceptable because the risk of complications once the object is out of the esophagus is greatly diminished. Sharp objects are the primary exception and should be removed from the stomach and duodenum if they are within reach of the endoscope because the risk of perforation can be 15% to 35%.[106] Objects longer than 5 cm and objects larger than 2 cm in diameter are unlikely to pass the duodenal sweep or pylorus, and attempts to remove them should be made. Observation is recommended for small blunt objects in the stomach, which almost always pass without complication. Even sharp or complex foreign bodies that fail endoscopic retrieval can initially be observed because only a few of these objects result in significant complications.[82,83]

In cases of more complex foreign bodies that are not extracted with the endoscope, periodical radiographs should be obtained to document progression through the GI tract. Close attention should be paid to symptoms such as fever, distention, vomiting, or abdominal pain that could suggest obstruction or perforation. For objects that are not extracted, the amount and timing of observation and radiographs should be individualized because transit time varies greatly based on patient and type of object ingested.[107]

Ensuring proper procedure, equipment, and patient preparation before initiating endoscopic therapy for foreign bodies and food boluses increases the success rate while maintaining a low complication rate. The endoscopist should be aware of the type of foreign bodies that may be encountered in that

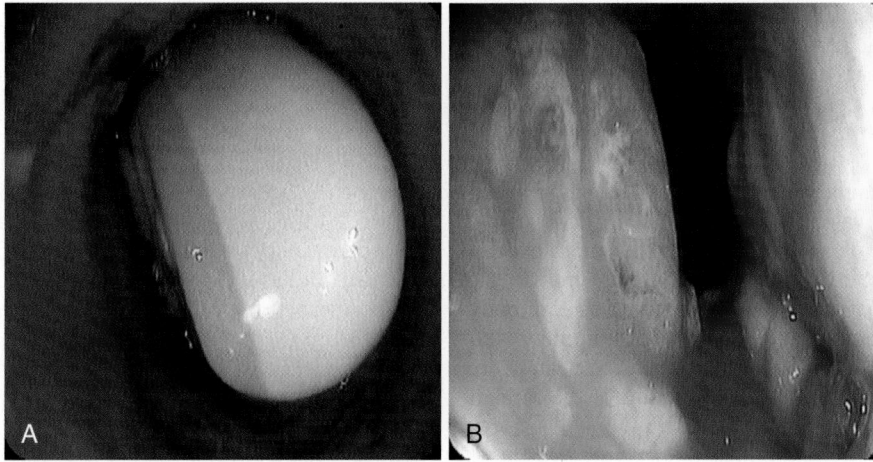

Fig. 19.4 A, Endoscopic image of ingested hearing aid that remained in the esophagus for more than 24 hours. **B,** Significant edema, erythema, and ulceration were seen in the esophageal mucosa after removal of the foreign body.

Table 19.1 Equipment for Treatment and Removal of Gastrointestinal Foreign Bodies and Food Impactions

Endoscopes	Overtubes	Accessory Equipment
Flexible endoscope	Standard esophageal overtube	Retrieval net
Rigid endoscope	45–60 cm foreign body overtube	Alligator or rat-tooth forceps
Laryngoscope		Dormia basket
Kelly or McGill forceps		Polypectomy snare
		Three-pronged grabber
		Magnetic extractor
		Steigmann-Goff variceal ligator cap
		Latex protector hood

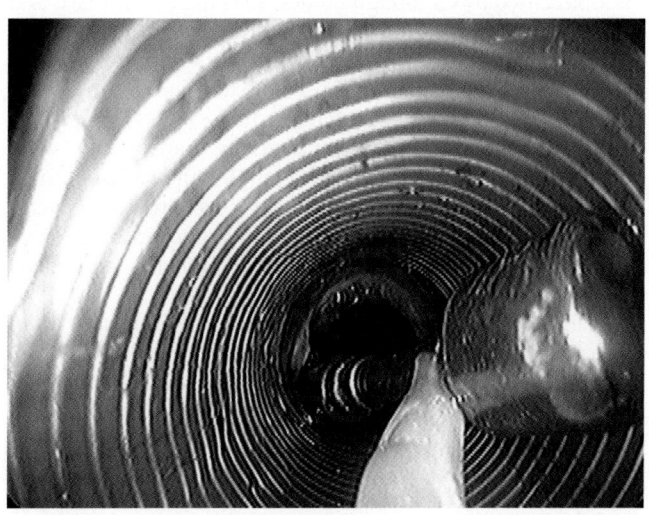

Fig. 19.5 A broken sharp antenna being safely removed through an esophageal overtube. The overtube prevented the antenna from causing tears or lacerations in the esophagus.

particular patient and the safest method to remove these objects. Before endoscopy, it is beneficial to perform a "dry run" on a similar object ex vivo[5]; this allows selection of a proper retrieval device and makes the extraction safer and easier. **Table 19.1** lists endoscopes, endoscopic retrieval devices, and accessory equipment available to assist in removal of foreign bodies and food impactions. Before an attempt at removal of a complex foreign body, an endoscopy suite should be equipped with a minimum of a rat-tooth forceps, polypectomy snares, Dormier baskets, and retrieval nets.[1,108] Standard size overtubes that extend past the upper esophageal sphincter and overtubes 45 to 60 cm in length that extend past the LES should be available. An overtube provides airway protection, allows frequent passes of the endoscope, and protects the mucosa from superficial and deep lacerations (**Fig. 19.5**).[109] The longer overtube can aid in removing sharp objects and objects that cannot be pulled backward through the LES. A latex protector hood that can be simply attached to the end of

the endoscope also helps prevent mucosal trauma in retrieval of sharp objects when overtubes are unavailable or when objects cannot easily be pulled through an overtube.[110,111]

The flexible endoscope is the preferred endoscopic method for treating GI foreign bodies and food impactions because of the high success rate, low complication rate, availability, patient comfort, affordability, and lack of need for general anesthesia.[37,112] Rigid esophagoscopy has equal efficacy to flexible endoscopy in the treatment of esophageal foreign bodies but always requires general anesthesia, and few endoscopists have experience with the rigid endoscope.[113] Flexible nasoendoscopes have been suggested as an alternative to standard flexible endoscopes but have been shown to have no additional benefit and may fail more frequently for foreign bodies below the cricopharyngeus.[114] Laryngoscopes with the aid of a Kelly or McGill forceps should be available and may help in the removal of small sharp objects at the hypopharynx.

Intravenous conscious sedation provides sufficient sedation in most adult patients with foreign bodies or food impactions. General anesthesia with endotracheal intubation in certain patients is preferred because it provides complete control over the airway and the patient. General anesthesia should be used in most pediatric patients and should be considered in uncooperative patients and patients with multiple or complex foreign bodies in whom removal would take an extended period of time.

Finally, an ex vivo study has shown that success and speed of foreign body retrieval is directly related to endoscopist experience.[109] For complex foreign bodies, the most experienced endoscopist at an institution should attempt endoscopic retrieval. If concern exists about experience with foreign body retrieval or a lack of necessary endoscopic equipment and accessories, the patient should be transferred to a tertiary care center for successful treatment and extraction of the foreign body.

Sharp Objects

Sharp and pointed objects account for one-third of all perforations caused by GI foreign bodies; 15% to 35% of sharp and pointed foreign bodies left untreated may lead to a GI complication. Sharp objects, particularly toothpicks and animal bones, are the most likely to cause a perforation leading to the need for surgical management.[115] Bones, toothpicks, and dental bridgework are the most common inadvertently swallowed sharp foreign bodies. More complex and varied pointed objects are seen in patients with psychiatric illnesses or incarcerated patients; common objects ingested include razor blades, pins, needles, nails, writing instruments, and metal wires (**Fig. 19.6**).

Sharp objects in the esophagus should be addressed in an emergent fashion with an attempt to remove the object within at least 24 hours. Because of the risk of perforation, attempts should be made to retrieve any sharp object within the reach of the endoscope. When removing sharp ingested foreign bodies Jackson's axiom should be remembered: "advancing points puncture, trailing points do not."[116] When removing sharp objects, the foreign body should be grasped in a position so that the sharp or pointed end trails distally to the endoscope, reducing the chance of a significant procedure-related perforation or mucosal trauma during extraction.

Polypectomy snares and foreign body retrieval forceps such as a rat-tooth or alligator forceps are the most commonly used devices for removing sharp foreign bodies with the most endoscopic control. If the size and shape of the foreign body prohibit easy withdrawal of the object, a standard-size overtube or a foreign body overtube (45 to 60 cm) should be used to protect the esophagus, airway, and oropharynx.[111] An alternative is a soft latex protector hood that provides mucosal protection. The hood is simply placed and sometimes tied to the end of the endoscope with suture and folded back on itself to obtain endoscopic visualization. The foreign body is grasped, and as it is pulled through the LES or upper esophageal sphincter, the hood flips over the end of the endoscope and the tightly grasped foreign body, which is protected within the hood (**Fig. 19.7**). Hoods are commercially available, or alternatively a modified latex glove has been described to be used with similar methodology for the removal of sharp gastric foreign bodies.[117]

Sharp objects that are beyond the reach of the endoscope or cannot be safely removed with the endoscope still can be observed with a relatively low risk of complication. Sharp objects should be followed more closely, and surgery should

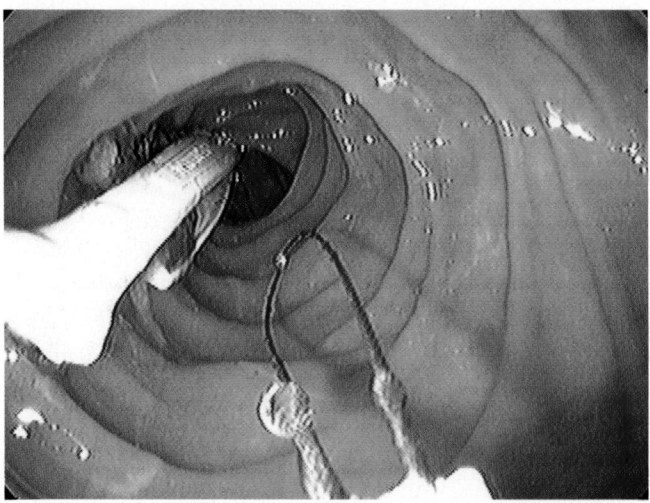

Fig. 19.6 Endoscopic photograph of a prisoner who swallowed multiple sharp objects including a nail and plastic forks that passed to the duodenum. All the objects were removed with a snare in conjunction with an esophageal overtube.

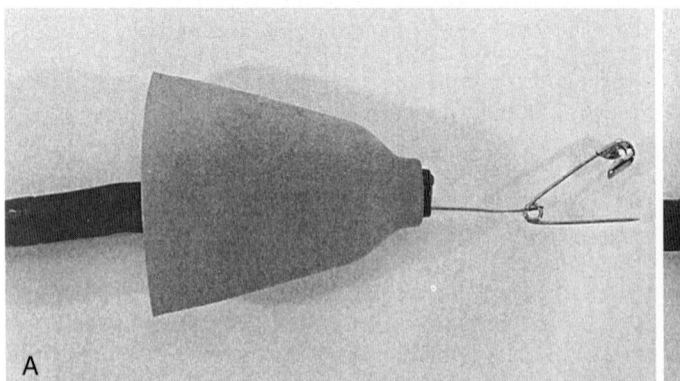 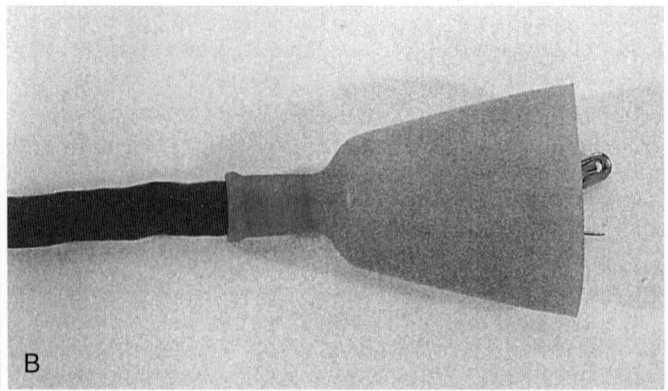

Fig. 19.7 A, Latex protector hood with the hood pulled back providing full visualization and allowing the endoscopist to grasp a sharp object easily. **B,** As the protector hood is pulled back through the lower esophageal sphincter, the hood flips forward protecting the gastrointestinal mucosa from the sharp object. *(From Feldman M, Friedman LS, Sleisenger MH, editors: Sleisenger & Fordtran's Gastrointestinal and Liver Disease: Pathophysiology, Diagnosis, Management, vol 1, ed 7, Philadelphia, 2002, Saunders, p 393.)*

be considered if the object does not progress on serial radiographs or if there is any evidence of abdominal pain; fever; or overt signs of obstruction, perforation, or bleeding.

Coins, Button Batteries, and Magnets

Coins and button batteries are the most common and among the most dangerous foreign bodies ingested by children. Coins in the esophagus that are not promptly removed can result in pressure necrosis of the esophageal wall with possible perforation or fistulization. Airway protection should be provided via endotracheal intubation before attempted endoscopic removal of lodged esophageal foreign objects in children. In adults, dimes and pennies, measuring 17 mm and 18 mm, pass through the esophagus, but larger coins may become lodged. An overtube can be used for airway protection in adults if the coin can be retrieved through it. Pinch biopsy forceps should be avoided because greater control is provided with a rat-tooth forceps or a basket.

The preferred retrieval device for coins is a retrieval net, which allows easy snaring of the coin and additionally protects the airway as the coin is pulled past the larynx.[109] Retrieval with a net can be performed by directly snaring the coin in the esophagus and then pulling out the endoscope, net, and coin in toto. Alternatively, if there is no resistance, the coin can be gently pushed into the stomach and then more easily secured and retrieved by the net and subsequently removed via the mouth. Objects 2.5 cm or less can pass through the pylorus; this includes all coins except half dollars (30 mm) or silver dollars (38 mm). Once a coin enters the stomach, observation with conservative management is sufficient in most patients.[118] Patients may maintain a regular diet, but if the coin does not pass in approximately 4 weeks or if more than one coin has been ingested, endoscopic removal is indicated.[118,119]

Button batteries are of special concern because they may contain an alkaline solution that can rapidly cause a liquefaction necrosis of esophageal tissue resulting in perforation or fistula formation. Ingested button batteries become symptomatic in 10% of cases, with children younger than 5 years being the most common patients.[120] The mechanisms of injury include direct corrosive action, low-voltage burns, and pressure necrosis.[5] Any clinical suspicion or radiographic evidence of a disc battery localized in the esophagus should lead to emergent endoscopy. In the retrieval of button disc batteries, it is crucial to protect the airway with endotracheal tube intubation in young children or an overtube in adults or older children.

Traditionally, a high endoscopic failure rate of up to 60% was associated with cases of button battery ingestion because the shape and contour made it difficult to grasp.[121] The use of the Roth retrieval net has solved this problem making retrieval of button batteries successful in almost all cases. The battery can be retrieved from the esophagus or pushed into the stomach and retrieved. A stone retrieval basket also works with a high success rate but slightly less control than a retrieval net. Once in the stomach and beyond, button batteries rarely cause problems and are generally treated with observation.[122] Of batteries that reach the duodenal sweep, 85% pass through the GI tract within 72 hours.[123] Batteries located beyond the esophagus require endoscopy if the patient develops symptoms or the battery remains in the stomach for 48 hours on repeat radiograph.[96]

Ingested magnets within the reach of the endoscope should also be removed on an urgent basis. Single magnets rarely cause symptoms. However, concern should exist if multiple magnets were ingested or if magnets were ingested with other metal objects. These scenarios can lead to transmural magnetic attraction with subsequent pressure necrosis, fistula formation, and bowel perforation.[124,125] Magnets can be removed with rat-tooth forceps, retrieval nets, or wire baskets. Using metal retrieval devices that attract the magnet may also make it easier to remove the magnets.

Long Objects

Objects longer than approximately 5 to 10 cm may have difficulty passing the duodenal sweep resulting in perforation or obstruction. Objects of concern are toothbrushes, spoons and forks, and pens and pencils. Long objects can easily be grasped with a snare or basket. The object must be grabbed at the end to allow retrograde removal through the LES, esophagus, and upper esophageal sphincter. Grasping the object near the center orients the object in a horizontal plane prohibiting pulling the long object through the LES or the esophagus. A long overtube that passes the gastroesophageal junction is beneficial because the object can be pulled into the overtube, and the foreign body, overtube, and endoscope all can be removed as a single entity.

Narcotic Packets

Ingested narcotic packets are found in two types of patients—the "body stuffer" and the "body packer." The body stuffer is a user or dealer who "stuffs" varying amounts of drugs into often poorly made packets before ingesting them to avoid arrest. The "body packer," in the process of smuggling drugs, "packs" much larger amounts of drugs into carefully prepared, usually latex or plastic, packages that are designed to withstand GI tract transit.[126,127] Diagnosis is usually made because of an arrest and confession by the patient.

Patients may present with intestinal obstruction or experience toxic effects of the drugs they have ingested. Up to 26% of patients who have ingested narcotic packets may have symptoms related to the narcotic ingested with serious symptoms including death in almost 5%.[128] Toxicology screens may identify the drug, detect leakage, and allow the correct reversal agent to be administered. Abdominal radiographs and CT scans of patients with ingested narcotic packets show multiple round or sausage-shaped radiopacities, but false-negative imaging is well described.[127–129] Endoscopy for removal of narcotic packets is contraindicated because of the danger of rupture of the package resulting in a toxicologic emergency.[1] Observation with a clear liquid diet is recommended; lavage and purgatives are best avoided because of the risk of the rupture. Surgery is indicated for failure of the packets to progress, intestinal obstruction, and occasionally acute rupture.[37]

Food Bolus Impaction

Esophageal food bolus impaction is the most common "foreign body" in adults that can cause symptoms and require endoscopic intervention. In the United States, the most common impacted foods are meat products such as beef, chicken, pork, and hot dogs (**Fig. 19.8**).[30,31] Food impaction may occur in

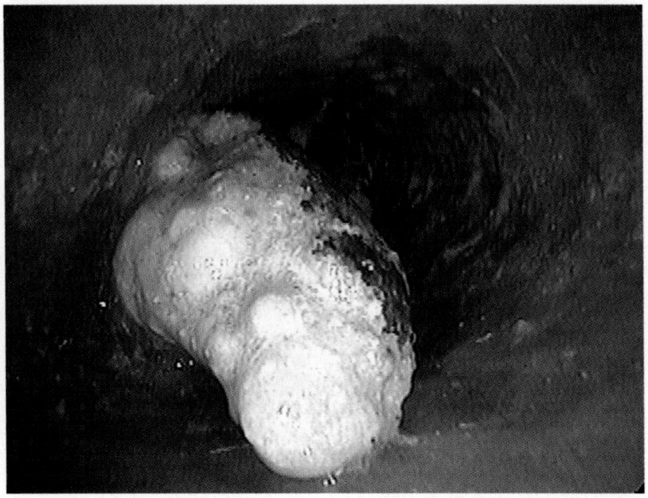

Fig. 19.8 Endoscopic image of a large bratwurst that had caused acute impaction in the distal esophagus. This was treated with the push technique.

association with alcohol ingestion, during which the patient may not chew food as carefully, leading to the terms "steakhouse syndrome" and "backyard barbecue syndrome." In Asia and coastal areas, the most common food foreign bodies are fish bones. Fish bones rarely cause food impaction but cause symptoms because of the sharp and pointed ends of bones.

Food boluses may pass spontaneously; endoscopic intervention needs to be based on symptoms. If there is evidence of near or complete obstruction with the patient unable to handle secretions, salivating, or drooling, endoscopy should be performed on an urgent basis. If the patient has the sensation of the food bolus passing either spontaneously or after preendoscopy glucagon, a gentle trial of fluids then solids may be sufficient, and endoscopy can be avoided. However, if there is any concern that the food bolus remains, endoscopy should be performed because all esophageal food impactions should be removed in 24 hours owing to increased complications, with ideal removal in the first 6 to 12 hours after the onset of symptoms.[1,130,131]

Endoscopy is indicated because of the high esophageal-related pathology associated with food impactions. The accepted first endoscopic method used for the treatment of esophageal food impactions is the "push technique" with success rates greater than 90% and minimal complications.[27] This technique entails gently pushing the esophageal food bolus into the stomach with the endoscope. Before pushing the food bolus into the stomach, an attempt should be made to steer the endoscope around the impaction and into the stomach; this allows assessment of the nature and degree of any obstructive esophageal pathology beyond the food bolus. Generally, if an endoscope can be advanced around a food bolus and past any obstruction, the push technique should be successful. After steering around the food bolus, the endoscope is pulled back proximal to the food impaction, and the impaction is gently pushed forward. This movement is aided by esophageal muscle relaxation induced by sedation, expansion of the esophageal lumen with endoscopic air-insufflation, and intravenous glucagon if it has been given.[49]

Even if the endoscope cannot be initially maneuvered around the impaction, a trial of gently pushing the food bolus

can be safely attempted. Forcefully pushing the endoscope or blindly advancing dilators or retrieval devices past the food bolus is not recommended, however, because of the high percentage of patients with esophageal pathology.[1,49] For larger food impactions, particularly meats such as chicken or beef that can be broken apart, the push technique can be performed after breaking the bolus into smaller pieces with a forceps or snare. With the increasing prevalence of eosinophilic esophagitis, extra care should be taken pushing food through the esophagus because of the potential increased chance of perforation and mucosal tears.[132] However, more recent studies have suggested that food impaction in patients with eosinophilic esophagitis can be treated effectively and safely with the push method.[29]

Certain food impactions cannot be safely pushed into the stomach and must be retrieved with the endoscope via the mouth. An overtube is useful to protect the airway and allow multiple passes of the endoscope. This approach is particularly useful in meat impactions in which the bolus shreds and breaks into multiple pieces before it can be completely removed. Standard endoscopic grasping forceps, snares, and baskets used under direct visualization can be employed alone or together. The Roth retrieval net can be particularly useful in managing food impactions because the food bolus can be contained completely within the net avoiding the use of an overtube and minimizing the risk of aspiration.[133] For well-impacted food boluses, a Steigmann-Goff endoscopic ligator can be used to suction up large pieces of food that can be removed via the mouth.[134,135]

Greater than 75% of patients with food impactions are found to have esophageal pathology at the time of the index or follow-up endoscopy.[5,25,27] More than half of patients with food bolus impactions have abnormal 24-hour pH studies, and almost half have abnormal esophageal manometry tests.[28] In most patients, if a benign stricture or Schatzki ring is visualized after clearance of the food bolus, the narrowing can be effectively and safely dilated during the same endoscopy. If multiple esophageal rings are present, biopsy specimens should be obtained to evaluate for eosinophilic esophagitis, but dilation should generally be avoided.

Occasionally, esophageal mucosal erythema, edema, and abrasions from the food bolus or the endoscope may interfere with accurate endoscopic diagnosis and safe dilation treatment. These patients can be placed on acid suppression therapy and have an elective endoscopy with possible dilation in approximately 4 to 6 weeks.

Colorectal Foreign Bodies

Although most rectal foreign bodies occur secondary to retrograde insertion through the anus, some objects that are ingested may traverse the entire GI tract and become lodged in the colon, particularly the rectum. Radiographs should be obtained before removal of colorectal foreign bodies. Radiographs allow determination of the location of the object, orientation of the object, and type of object. Manual removal or digital rectal examination is not recommended until a film has been obtained because of concern about performing a digital rectal examination with the presence of a sharp or pointed rectal foreign body.

If the object is in the distal rectum and is blunt and small, manual removal should be attempted. The ability to palpate the foreign body on rectal examination increases the chance that it can be removed successfully with manual extraction. Conscious sedation is usually adequate for manual removal, but in some cases general anesthesia may be needed to allow greater anal sphincter relaxation and ensure removal. Objects that are more proximally located and sharp or pointed objects should be removed under direct visualization with the use of a rigid proctoscope or flexible sigmoidoscope.[110] Standard retrieval devices can be used to remove the object from the rectum. A latex hood or overtube can be particularly useful in removing longer and sharp objects to protect the rectal mucosa from laceration and to overcome the tendency of the anal sphincter to contract on removal of objects. Although conscious sedation often facilitates removal, general anesthesia can allow maximum dilation of the anal sphincter and allow removal of longer, more complex objects.[111] Surgery is indicated for any complications secondary to a rectal or colon foreign body, including perforation, abscess, and obstruction, and may be more likely required when the object is proximal to the rectum.[112]

Postoperative Care

For uncomplicated removal of true foreign bodies or food bolus impactions, postoperative care should be no different than care after standard endoscopy. Each institution should follow its routine postprocedure recovery guidelines according to whether the procedure was performed under conscious sedation or general anesthesia. Most patients with foreign bodies and food impactions can be treated as outpatients. If the patient recovers without sequelae, the patient, family, or parents should observe the patient for any sign of complications in the next 24 hours. Patients with a food bolus impaction should be educated in methods of reducing further impactions, including eating more slowly, chewing foods thoroughly, and avoiding troublesome foods.[49] Admitting certain patients for 24-hour observation postprocedure should be considered. These include young children, patients with multiple or complex foreign bodies, and patients in whom extraction and treatment of the foreign body was technically difficult.

A patient requires observation and further investigation if the extraction was difficult, if there was any evidence on endoscopy of a complication secondary to the foreign body or the endoscope, or if the patient shows signs of a complication postprocedure. The greatest concern is esophageal perforation, and the best outcomes and survival occur when this is recognized early.[5] Any evidence of postprocedure fever, tachy-cardia, shortness of breath, chest or abdominal pain, or crepitus should lead to prompt plain films followed by contrast radiographic studies and surgical consultation.

Complications

The complication rate of endoscopic treatment of GI foreign bodies or food impactions ranges from no complications found in most studies to 1.8%.[5,9,25,27,31,75,136] The most common complication associated with endoscopic removal of foreign bodies is esophageal perforation. Although no prospective data exist, patients with risk factors thought to increase the complication rate include uncooperative patients, patients with multiple ingestions, patients with deliberate ingestion such as prisoners or psychiatric patients, and patients with removal of sharp and pointed objects. Other complications reported with endoscopic removal of foreign bodies are GI bleeding, aspiration, and cardiopulmonary complications secondary to sedation. These complications do not occur at a rate significantly different than the complication rate found in standard upper GI endoscopy.

Future Trends

Paralleling the development and availability of flexible endoscopes, endoscopy has become the diagnostic modality of choice and the standard of care for the treatment of ingested foreign bodies and impacted food boluses. No rival technology or method used in the treatment of foreign bodies exists, and no such technology is likely to match the efficacy or safety of endoscopic methods in the future. However, despite the frequency of foreign bodies treated with upper GI endoscopy, data are lacking on the actual incidence of foreign bodies, and treatment recommendations are still based primarily on retrospective collections of data. The main challenge for the future is the thorough collection of prospective data concerning patients with foreign bodies and food boluses and how these patients may best be treated with GI endoscopy both in the community and at tertiary endoscopy centers. With these data, endoscopists will be able to offer optimal treatment to the frequently encountered patients with ingested foreign bodies or food impactions.

References

The complete reference list is available online at www.expertconsult.com.

Chapter 20

Zenker's Diverticula

Kiyoshi Hashiba

Video related to this chapter's topics can be found online at expertconsult.com.

Introduction

Zenker's type is the most important diverticulum of the esophagus and usually causes symptoms that require surgical treatment. Zenker's diverticulum (ZD) is an indication for minimally invasive endoscopic treatment, which is important as an alternative to operative therapy because most patients with ZD are elderly.

Epidemiology

ZD is a false diverticulum first described by Ludlow in 1769.[1] X-ray studies have shown its incidence to be around 0.1% of upper gastrointestinal (GI) barium studies.[2] Of patients, 80% are older than 60 years.[3] ZD is more frequent in men than in women.[3] The occurrence in children is rare,[4] and no differences have been mentioned concerning race or geographic areas.

Pathogenesis

ZD develops as a result of the cooccurrence of weak points in the posterior wall of the hypopharynx and a lack of coordination between the pharyngeal constrictor and the cricopharyngeal muscles.[5] Fibrosis of the cricopharyngeal muscle and the striated muscle of the upper esophagus has been shown more recently as the cause of such incoordination.[6,7] Contraction of the pharyngeal constrictor muscle combined with the absence of relaxation of the cricopharyngeal muscle results in difficult passage of a food bolus and an increase in local pressure, which makes the mucosa and submucosa bulge through the weak sites between the descending fibers of inferior constrictor and transverse cricopharyngeal muscles, which constitute

the distalmost part of the inferior constrictor (**Fig. 20.1**). Some authors believe that the incomplete sphincter opening is more likely than the incoordination to cause dysphagia.[6] The mucous membrane sac can also pass through or immediately beneath the cricopharyngeal muscle.

Clinical Features

There is a well-established relationship between the anatomic changes and clinical symptoms.[8] When a ZD is small, the patient has the sensation of having a foreign body in his or her throat. Throat irritation with excessive mucus is also common. As the ZD increases in size, regurgitation of food and mucus begins to occur after meals and when the patient lies down. If the sac is very large and the opening is transverse, the preferential route of food would be into the ZD. Symptoms of obstruction appear in this case, and many patients lose a significant amount of weight. In the second and third phases of the disease, pulmonary complications are common and sometimes repetitive, usually obliging the patient to seek treatment. Difficulty swallowing large food boluses, medication, or devices such as endoscopic capsules can be the earliest indicators for the detection of ZD.[9]

Pathology

The diverticulum arises as a protruding area at the weak points of the muscular structures of the hypopharynx and then increases progressively. The wall of the sac is formed only by the mucosa and submucosa. In contrast to esophageal diverticula, ZD is not a true diverticulum. As a diverticulum, ZD forms a pouch and descends along the left side of the neck; however, it may be present on either side. In advanced phases

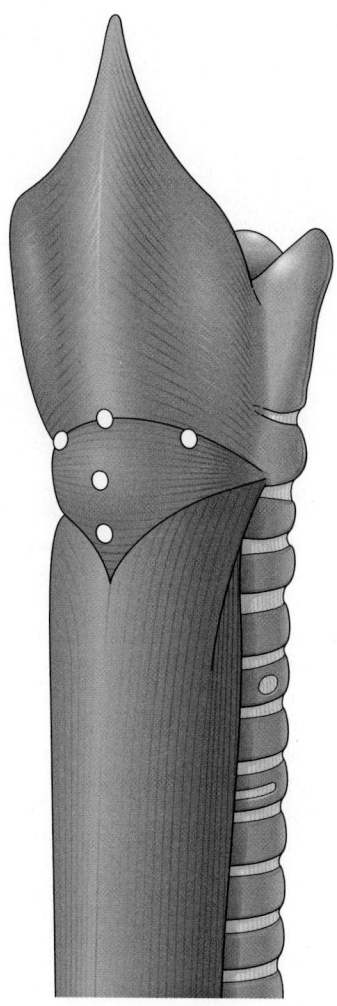

Fig. 20.1 Schematic view of hypopharynx. *Dots* show sites of weakness from which a Zenker's diverticulum can develop.

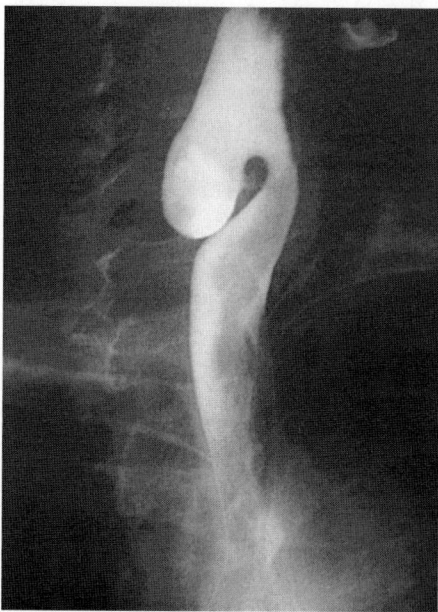

Fig. 20.2 Lateral x-ray study of esophagus showing a Zenker's diverticulum.

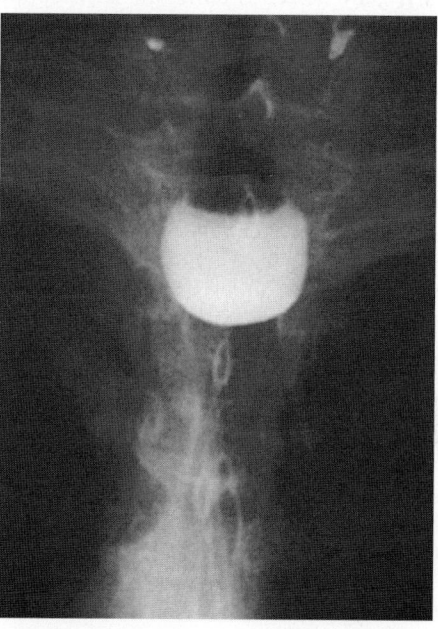

Fig. 20.3 Frontal upper gastrointestinal barium study of esophagus showing a Zenker's diverticulum (ZD). The contrast material remained in the ZD.

of the disease, the mucosa may show esophagitis. The incidence of cancer seems to be higher in patients with ZD than in patients without this disease.[10,11] ZD is usually found in association with some other esophageal disease, such as hiatal hernia, gastroesophageal reflux, esophageal membranes in 50% of cases, achalasia, and polyps.[12,13]

Differential Diagnosis

Radiography is very useful when the patient experiences some difficulty in swallowing solid medication, such as a pill, and it is important in advanced phases of ZD. If the sac is not small, the diagnosis is easily established in the anteroposterior projection (**Fig. 20.2**).[14] The sac lies in the midline and extends to the left. However, in the case of a small and nonretentive ZD, the lateral projection is important (**Fig. 20.3**). When aspiration of a bolus is suspected, an x-ray study without barium is needed. In such a case, iodine contrast material should be used to avoid complications secondary to aspiration of barium into the lung. Sometimes it is necessary to clear the ZD lumen from retained foods to avoid filling defects that may look like mucosal lesions on imaging.

Endoscopy is the alternative diagnostic test. For many years, endoscopy was not recommended; however, it is a very important means of diagnosis and treatment. Even when the diagnosis of ZD has been established, endoscopy should be performed because alterations in the mucosa can occur, and a biopsy is essential (**Fig. 20.4**). The incidence of cancer is higher in ZD mucosa than in normal esophageal mucosa. In early phases of the disease, when ZD cannot yet be detected, the difficulty found in inserting the endoscope into the esophagus is the most common basis for the suspicion of ZD. Because endoscopy is the first option of most physicians, when a patient presents with upper GI tract symptoms, the possibility of a ZD must be considered in case of such difficulty.

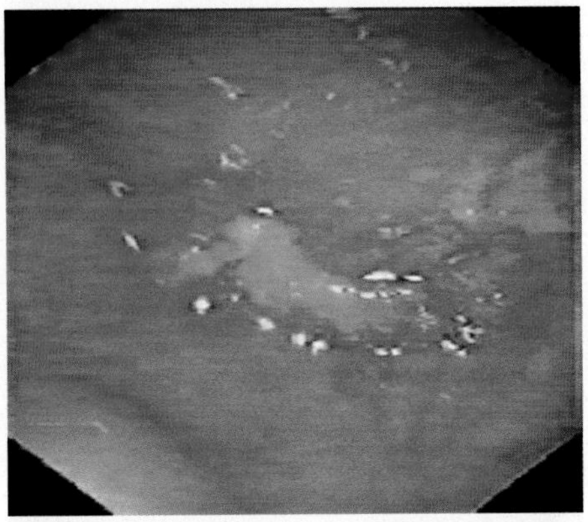

Fig. 20.4 Ulcerated lesion in a Zenker's diverticulum.

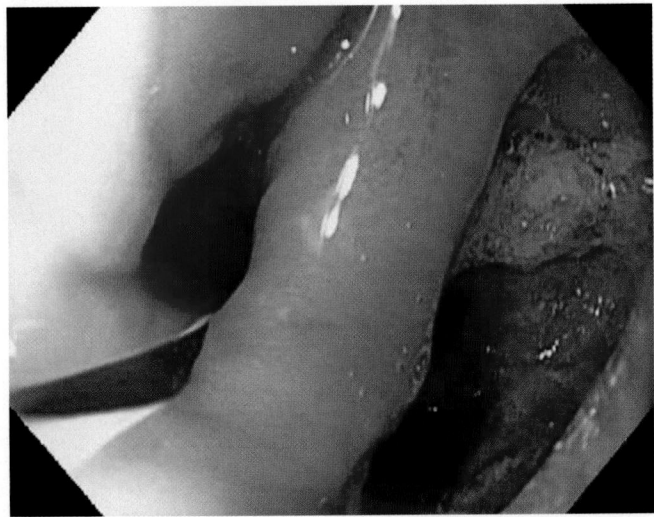

Fig. 20.5 Endoscopic view of hypopharynx in a patient with a Zenker's diverticulum. A guidewire is inserted in the esophageal lumen.

The endoscopy procedure is not dangerous in experienced hands, and insertion of the endoscope into the esophageal lumen is usually achieved often with the help of a flexible accessory used as a guide (**Fig. 20.5**). This method allows examination of the ZD mucosa and even the biopsy specimen. As the ZD increases progressively from a small protruding area to a sac, it usually descends down the left side of the neck. However, it may manifest on either side of the neck where an alteration is detected. A long fast period should be always recommended before the endoscopy procedure. During the diagnostic procedure, in cases of superficial trauma or biopsy, antibiotics should be prescribed. If a perforation is suspected in the case of failure in attempting to perform an endoscopy in a patient with a ZD, an upper GI barium study is not advised because the preferential way for the contrast material to flow would be the perforation opening secondary to the alteration and dysfunction of the cricopharyngeal muscle. Although endoscopic examination is helpful, it can increase pneumomediastinum.

Treatment

When the initial complaint of the patient is difficulty swallowing and ZD can be suspected from the x-ray study, improvement may result from dilation. In advanced cases, the classic treatment has been surgery. Resection of ZD and cricopharyngeal myotomy is the "gold standard," although inversion of the sac has been performed by some surgeons. Cricopharyngeal myotomy is a fundamental part of the procedure, and this is probably the reason for the failure of treatment with resection of the diverticulum only.[15]

For many years, surgery was performed in two stages to avoid mediastinitis and pulmonary complications. However, most surgeons prefer a one-stage operation using a tube inside the esophagus or an endoscope inside the diverticulum to determine the ZD position, preventing excessive resection of tissue with subsequent stricture. For a small ZD, some authors recommend cricopharyngeal myotomy only. Although this procedure is associated with diverticulopexy or diverticulotomy, it is an important step for the treatment of large ZD. The most frequent complication of surgery is the development of a pharyngocutaneous fistula in the early postoperative course. When spontaneous healing does not occur, endoscopic dilation of the esophagus and fibrin injection around the internal

orifice with or without placement of clips at the same site have been successful. A randomized study by Bowdler and Stell[16] compared inversion with resection in association with cricopharyngeal myotomy. Better results and lower incidence of fistulas were obtained with inversion. Other complications of the conventional approach are mediastinitis, laryngeal paralysis, stricture, and recurrence.

Endoscopic treatment is not new. In 1917, Mosher[10] had described an endoscopic transoral diverticulotomy, but this method was soon abandoned because of complications. In 1960, Dohlman and Mattson[17] presented their endoscopic technique using electrocoagulation to divide the wall between the esophagus and the diverticulum. Another transoral technique was proposed by Collard and associates[18] in 1993 using an Endo GIA 30 2.5-cm stapler to cut the muscle bar. In this case, the cut edges were stapled with metallic clips, which avoids contamination of the mediastinum and ensures hemostasis of the wound edges. However, this procedure requires general anesthesia, and the postoperative course can be uncomfortable. In addition, it is uncertain if a sufficient myotomy can be performed. Because of the design of this device, usually a small pouch remains at the bottom of the ZD. More recently, a simple, low-cost endoscopic technique was described that is performed without general anesthesia and can be used in most cases with good results and a low morbidity rate.

Endoscopic Treatment of Zenker's Diverticulum
Technique
PREPARATION

Endoscopic treatment of ZD[19] should be performed in fasted patients. Patients with a deep ZD must have only liquid foods on the day preceding the endoscopic treatment, and just before the operation, all patients must use a liquid antiseptic mouthwash and gargle repeatedly. Antibiotic (2 g cephalosporin) is given intravenously before the procedure. Diverticulotomy can be performed under monitored anesthesia care and topical anesthesia with lidocaine.

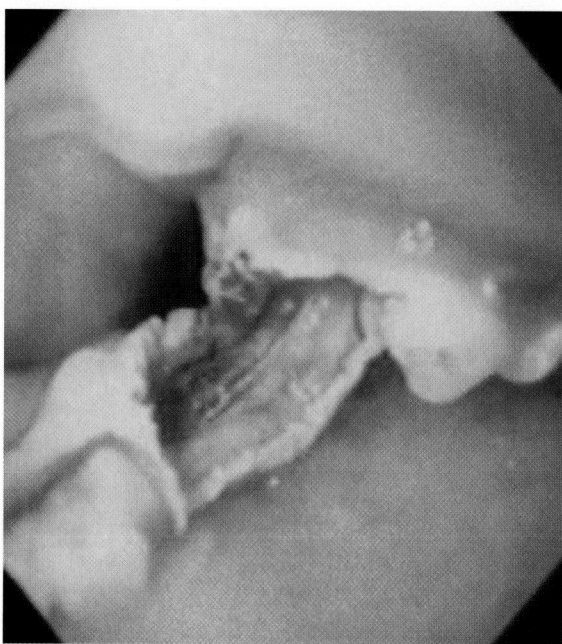

Fig. 20.6 Near the end of the cutting, cricopharyngeal muscle fibers are clearly seen.

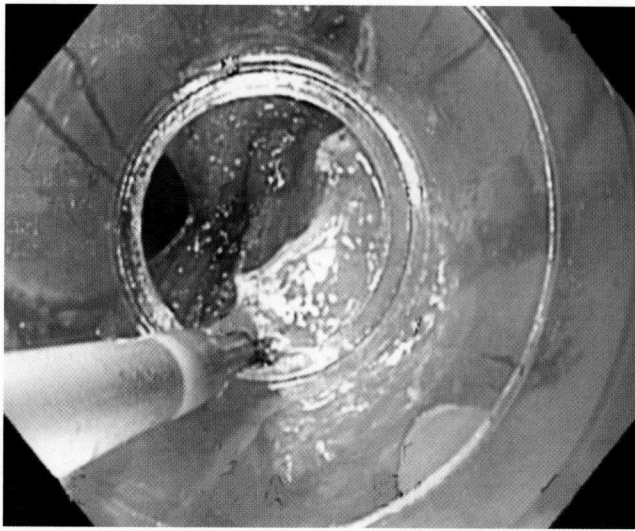

Fig. 20.7 A transparent cap sometimes improves the visual control.

DIVERTICULOTOMY

Diverticulotomy is performed with a forward-viewing endoscope. If the patient has not had an upper GI endoscopy recently, an endoscopic examination of the diverticulum is needed. This examination is important not only to develop the treatment plan but also to detect any mucosal alterations, including neoplasia. Alterations in the esophagus and stomach for which diverticulotomy of ZD is not recommended, such as malignant disease, must be excluded. Mucosal lesions caused by gastroesophageal reflux are very common, however.

A 0.035-inch wire is inserted into the esophagus as a guide to introduce a 12-Fr semiflexible tube. The purpose of the tube is to optimize exposure of the wall between the ZD and the esophageal lumen and to protect the anterior wall from thermal injury. The diverticulotomy (septotomy) is performed with a needle-knife papillotome (Olympus KD-630 L; Olympus, Tokyo, Japan) and electrical monopolar cautery set to cut and coagulate. The operative field is not wide, so it is important to avoid hemorrhage because even a small amount of blood makes it difficult to visualize the site of cutting. It is convenient to make an electrocoagulation mark in the distalmost point of the intended incision because edema and coagulation tissue changes make it hard to identify the bottom of the ZD septum accurately. It is easiest to initiate the incision at the top of the septum and divide it distally to the coagulation mark. Experienced endoscopists may make the first cut near the electrocoagulating mark placed previously.

The transverse fibers of the cricopharyngeal muscle are important to target as the endpoint of the septotomy and are usually clearly seen across the bottom of the diverticulum (**Fig. 20.6**). Analgesics are needed after the procedure. Patients are allowed to resume oral intake of liquid about 18 hours after the procedure and proceed to a regular diet as tolerated. Some authors suggest that a dilation procedure before diverticulotomy makes the procedure easier.

Interest in the endoscopic treatment of ZD has been increasing. Technique variations are available that may make the septotomy easier and safer. However, some of these alternative options increase the cost of the procedure. If the endoscopist detects a good exposure and has a reasonable experience, he or she should perform the endoscopic treatment of ZD without using other devices. Noncontact cutting has been reported using the argon plasma coagulator.[20] The simplest accessory is described by Sakai and colleagues.[21] The device is a transparent cap (MH589; Olympus, Tokyo, Japan) that can be attached to the distal end of the forward-viewing endoscope similar to caps used for mucosectomy during the cut.[21] The cap concept has been developed further with the addition of cutting wires that allow the septum to be straddled with a gap in the cap cylindric wall at the upper end of which is an electrosurgical cutting wire.[22] It improves the septum exposure almost without trauma (**Fig. 20.7**). Another device is a diverticuloscope[23,24]; it consists of a soft rubber or plastic overtube with a distal end designed to provide good septum exposure and protect the walls.

The pig pharyngeal pouch anatomy accurately mimics ZD. This pouch has been shown to serve as an effective training model to learn the septotomy technique.[25]

Results

Endoscopic diverticulotomy has been performed in one session with complete section of the cricopharyngeal septal bar. Dysphagia disappeared after the procedure, even when complete incision of the septum had not been performed. Other symptoms, including regurgitation, halitosis, coughing at night, and respiratory distress, also disappeared after the procedure. In our first series, 17 of 47 (36%) patients underwent endoscopic diverticulotomy in one session; 30 (64%) patients needed more than one session (mean value 2.2). A noticeable improvement in symptoms after the first session occurred in 45 (96%) patients; all experienced minimal to no dysphagia. Cough and halitosis also disappeared after the treatment. Sectioning of the septum was incomplete in 17 patients after the first session, but the improvement of

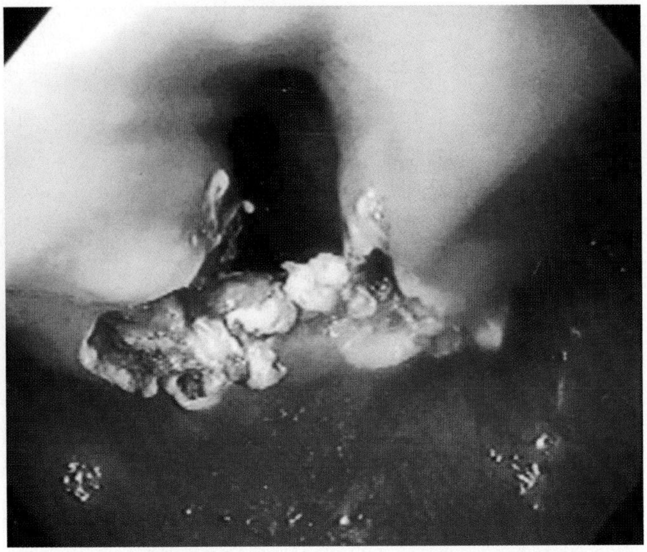

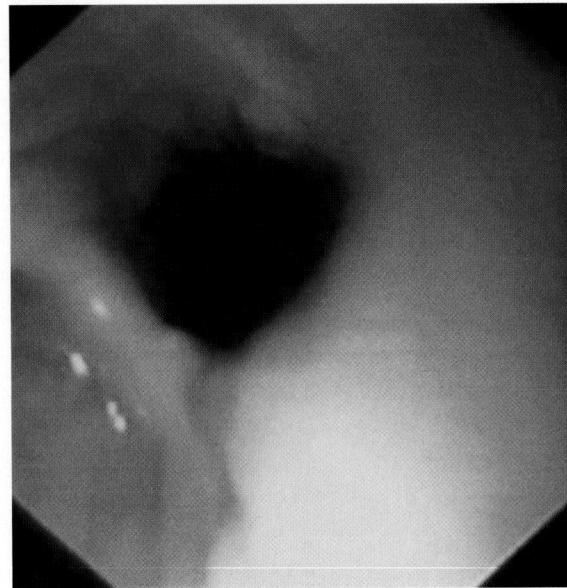

Fig. 20.8 Two sections, lateral to the middle line, performed in a symptomatic patient after endoscopic complementary diverticulotomy.

Fig. 20.9 Endoscopic postoperative control in an asymptomatic patient.

dysphagia was marked. Bleeding usually occurred during the procedure, but was always self-limited.

In the postoperative course, bleeding is rare and has been controlled endoscopically. Cervical emphysema is not rare and can be encountered when there has been complete section of the septum. It may increase if the patient coughs just after the incision has been made. In our first series, 83% of the patients began oral intake of liquids and ice cream on the first day after the endoscopic diverticulotomy and of solid food in the subsequent days. In two patients, endoscopic control 1 month later revealed stenosis of the esophageal entrance, and a new section had to be performed for resolution of the dysphagia recurrence. In case of recurrence, the preference now is to perform two lateral incisions, not only one in the middle (**Fig. 20.8**). However, it is important that the incisions be performed not far from the middle line to avoid laryngeal alterations. Serious complications such as mediastinitis and fistula can occur, but they are rare with endoscopic treatment.

Follow-up for our first series ranged from 1 day to 1 year. In many cases, endoscopic therapy results in a shallow remaining pouch at the bottom of the ZD, despite an apparent complete section (**Fig. 20.9**). Rarely, a residual septum is not seen. Even in patients without symptoms, contrast study has shown that the ZD has not disappeared completely and is not a useful long-term follow-up assessment tool; because of this, some authors distinguish between clinical and radiologic recur-

rence.[26] In successful cases, manometry has revealed a reduction of the upper esophageal sphincter pressure.[15] Despite various technique modifications, it is impossible to determine the best treatment for symptomatic patients with ZD because comparative studies are difficult to accomplish given the rare prevalence of the disorder.

Future Trends

Endoscopic treatment should be a strong consideration with available expertise in interventional endoscopy. The porcine pharyngeal pouch should be included in training and competency for septotomy. Conventional surgery can be reserved for failure of septotomy. Stapling or suturing of the septotomy edges is desirable, as in the endoscopic staple-assisted esophagodiverticulostomy proposed by Collard and colleagues[18] and Scher and Richtsmeier.[27] The development of freehand suturing may allow the closing of the edges of the septum once the endoscopic device becomes clinically available.[28] This closure would ensure hemostasis and avoid perforation, which is the main complication of the endoscopic treatment of ZD.

References

The complete reference list is available online at www.expertconsult.com.

Inflammatory Bowel Disease

Jesse K. Liu and Gary R. Lichtenstein

Introduction

Inflammatory bowel disease (IBD) is an idiopathic, chronic intestinal disorder characterized by episodes of relapse and remission. The diagnosis of Crohn's disease or ulcerative colitis depends on the clinical presentation and the findings on imaging studies.

Endoscopy is the most sensitive method to evaluate mucosal changes and is the only method available for providing histologic information. It is indicated to evaluate unexplained diarrhea and to aid in the differential diagnosis of IBD. Endoscopy is used to investigate radiographic abnormalities, such as mass lesions and strictures. In patients with IBD, it is crucial to determine the extent of disease and the disease activity and to have a good working knowledge of the efficacy of various medical therapies used to treat patients with IBD so that the appropriate medication can be applied in the correct clinical scenario. Endoscopy also is indicated in the screening and

surveillance for dysplasia and cancer. Colonoscopy, flexible sigmoidoscopy, and esophagogastroduodenoscopy (EGD) offer therapeutic benefits as well, including stricture dilation, stent placement, and bleeding control. Endoscopic retrograde cholangiopancreatography (ERCP) is often used to evaluate for the potential of primary sclerosing cholangitis. More recently, the role of video capsule endoscopy in patients with known or suspected IBD has begun to evolve.

Normal Appearance of the Bowel

Endoscopically, the normal colon appears to glisten and is salmon-pink in color. There is a visible network of branching vessels identified throughout the colon. The smoothness of the mucosal surface and the absence of nodules or irregular polyps are the hallmarks of a healthy colon. There is a classic triangulated or semicircular configuration of the interhaustral markings. Contact bleeding or friability is not seen in a normal, healthy colon.

The rectum has a more vascular appearance. Its vessels increase in caliber the further distal they are, producing more prominent vasculature.

Early Lesions of Inflammatory Bowel Disease

Crohn's Disease

The earliest endoscopic lesions in Crohn's disease are considered to be tiny punched-out ulcers in an otherwise normal-appearing mucosa. These tiny ulcers enlarge and aggregate to form larger surface ulcerations. Normal mucosa surrounds the ulcerations until late in the disease. Scanning electron microscopy has identified surface erosions of 100 to 200 μm surrounded by M cells, which may be the entry point for whatever the etiologic agent is found to be in Crohn's disease.[1]

Ulcerative Colitis

Ulcerative colitis triggers an increase in the surface blood flow, which causes the earliest lesions endoscopically to be diffuse erythema and vascular congestion. The mucosa looks like "wet sandpaper"; the edema produces a fine granular appearance and dulls the mucosal vascular architecture. The engorged mucosa bleeds readily when touched by the endoscope (termed *mucosal friability*), and as inflammation progresses, spontaneous bleeding occurs secondary to minute surface ulcerations that have been formed.

Importance of Assessing Extent of Disease

Establishing the extent of intestinal inflammation is essential in attempting to differentiate Crohn's disease from ulcerative colitis. This effort may be helpful to help guide medical therapy, to establish the risk of colorectal carcinoma, and to decide when to consider surgery. Colonoscopy with multiple biopsies is the standard for defining the extent of disease and excluding other forms of inflammation. Biopsies are more sensitive than macroscopic evaluation in determining the degree of inflammation and increase the diagnostic yield of an endoscopy considerably; biopsy specimens from macroscopically normal mucosa can reveal microscopic areas of inflammation. Skip lesions are suggestive of Crohn's disease, whereas ulcerative colitis tends to be a more circumferential and contiguous disease. Biopsies of the terminal ileum are often crucial in the differentiation of Crohn's disease from ulcerative colitis. Involvement of the ileum is highly suggestive of Crohn's disease. Proximal biopsy specimens often are revealing in a patient with resistant proctitis and a normal-appearing barium study. Proximal inflammation can be present in biopsy specimens in 50% of these patients. In addition, proximal biopsy specimens that are negative for inflammation identify patients with primarily rectal or left-sided colonic involvement; these patients usually respond to medicated suppositories or enemas, and evidence shows that the

addition of topical therapy offers significant benefit for these patients.[2]

Assessing Disease Severity

Many disease activity indices have been formulated over the past 30 years. None of these indices have been formally validated. These indices are useful mostly in clinical trials, in which the necessity to characterize severity and response to treatment in a reproducible fashion from institution to institution and from study to study is imperative. They also allow for enrollment of homogeneous groups of patients. An ideal index of disease activity would be simple to use, encompass the variability of disease manifestations, and be easily reproducible. No index so far has been widely adopted by gastroenterologists in their clinical practice, and no index can replace a good clinical history and clinical judgment.

Crohn's Disease

The Crohn's Disease Activity Index (CDAI) was developed in 1976 by Best and coworkers[3] as part of the National Cooperative Crohn's Disease Study. It is the "gold standard" index for any Crohn's disease clinical trial. A multivariant regression analysis was performed, and eight variables were identified as predictors of disease activity: number of stools, abdominal pain, general well-being, extraintestinal complications, antidiarrheal agents used in the previous 7 days, abdominal mass felt on palpation, hematocrit, and body weight (**Table 21.1**). CDAI scores range from 0 to 600. A score of less than 150 corresponds to relative disease quiescence (remission); 150 to 219, mildly active disease; 220 to 450, moderately active disease; and greater than 450, severe disease. A decrease in greater than 100 points indicates a clinically significant improvement in disease activity (termed *clinical response*). Older literature suggests that a clinical response is defined by a decrease in CDAI by greater than 70 points. The limitations of the CDAI include the complexity of the calculation needed by the physician, the weight placed on subjective complaints such as general well-being and abdominal pain, and the requirement of the patient to keep a diary for 7 days.

The Harvey-Bradshaw Index,[4] or the Simple Index, is less complicated than the CDAI and uses five variables recorded on one occasion (**Table 21.2**). No diary and no laboratory values are required. The five variables are general well-being, abdominal pain, abdominal mass, number of liquid stools, and systemic complications. Each variable is weighted the same. Studies have found that the Harvey-Bradshaw Index correlates well with the CDAI.[5]

The Crohn's Disease Endoscopic Index of Severity (CDEIS)[6] is a third index and the first to use endoscopic data in assessing disease severity. This prospectively developed index was established in 1989 by the French group Groupe d'Etudes Therapeutique des Affections Inflammatoires du Tube Digestif (GETAID). The CDEIS was validated in a large multicenter trial[6] and is the "gold standard" for evaluation of endoscopic, rather than clinical, activity. The bowel is divided into five segments (rectum, sigmoid and left colon, transverse colon, right colon, and ileum), and a numerical score is assigned based on objective endoscopic criteria: the presence or absence of deep or superficial ulcerations and the extent of the surface

Table 21.1 Crohn's Disease Activity Index

Variable	Description	Scoring	Multiplier
No. liquid stools	Sum of 7 days		×2
Abdominal pain	Sum of 7 days ratings	0 = none 1 = mild 2 = moderate 3 = severe	×5
General well-being	Sum of 7 days ratings	0 = generally well 1 = slightly under par 2 = poor 3 = very poor 4 = terrible	×7
Extraintestinal complications	No. listed complications	Arthritis or arthralgia; iritis or uveitis; erythema nodosum; pyoderma gangrenosum; aphthous stomatitis; anal fissure, fistula, or abscess; fever >37.8° C	×20
Antidiarrheal drugs	Use in previous 7 days	0 = no 1 = yes	×30
Abdominal mass		0 = no 2 = questionable 5 = definite	×10
Hematocrit (Hct)	Expected − observed Hct	Males: 47 − observed Females: 42 − observed	×6
Body weight	Ideal/observed ratio	[1 − (ideal/observed)] × 100	×1 (not <−10)

From Best WR, Becktel JM, Singleton JW, et al: Development of a Crohn's disease activity index. National Cooperative Crohn's Disease Study. Gastroenterology 70:439–444, 1976.

Table 21.2 Harvey-Bradshaw Index (Simple Index)

Variable	Scoring	Total
General well-being	0 = very well 1 = slightly below par 2 = poor 3 = very poor 4 = terrible	
Abdominal pain	0 = none 1 = mild 2 = moderate 3 = severe	
No. liquid stools daily	—	
Abdominal mass	0 = no 1 = dubious 2 = definite 3 = definite and tender	
Extraintestinal complications	Arthritis or arthralgia; iritis or uveitis; erythema nodosum; pyoderma gangrenosum; aphthous stomatitis; anal fissure, fistula, or abscess	

From Harvey RF, Bradshaw JM: A simple index of Crohn's disease activity. Lancet 1:514, 1980.

involved by the disease (**Table 21.3**). Scores range from 0 to 44, with higher scores indicating more severe disease. The CDEIS is reproducible, but it is time-consuming for the physician to calculate a score, which hinders its use outside of clinical trials. It also has failed to correlate with patient symptoms or other indicators of clinical activity.[7]

The main goal of therapy in Crohn's disease has been to achieve remission from disease symptoms rather than to achieve endoscopic remission. Endoscopic severity previously had not been shown to correlate reliably with prognosis or to predict a clinical response to therapy.[8] However, more recent studies with infliximab treatment imply that there is a longer remission and fewer disease events in patients achieving endoscopic remission.[9,10] This finding may alter the role that endoscopy plays in the evaluation of the clinical course of Crohn's disease.

In 2002, a second severity index based on endoscopic findings was proposed: the Simple Endoscopic Score for Crohn's Disease (SES-CD).[11] Because endoscopic remission has become one of the goals for monitoring treatment in clinical trials, a simpler endoscopic activity assessment than the CDEIS is needed. The bowel is divided into the same five segments as in the CDEIS, and a score of 0 to 3 is assigned based on endoscopic criteria—presence of ulcers, degree of ulcerated surface, degree of affected surface, presence of narrowings, and number of affected segments (**Table 21.4**). This index is easier and faster to calculate than the CDEIS. The reproducibility of the SES-CD was as good as the CDEIS, and it reliably correlated with the CDEIS, the present "gold

Table 21.3 Scoring System for Crohn's Disease Endoscopic Index of Severity

Scoring	Rectum	Sigmoid and Left Colon	Transverse Colon	Right Colon	Ileum	Total
Deep ulcerations (12 if present)						Total 1
Superficial ulcerations (12 if present)						Total 2
Surface involved by disease (cm)						Total 3
Surface involved by ulcerations (cm)						Total 4
Total 1 + Total 2 + Total 3 + Total 4 =						Total A
No. segments totally or partially explored =						n
Total A/n =						Total B
If ulcerated stenosis is present anywhere, add 3 =						C
If nonulcerated stenosis is present anywhere, add 3 =						D
Total B + C + D =						CDEIS

From Mary JY, Modigliani R: Development and validation of an endoscopic index of the severity for Crohn's disease: A prospective multicentre study. Groupe d'Studes Therapeutiques des Affections Inflammatoires du Tube Digestif (GETAID). Gut 30:983–989, 1989.

Table 21.4 Definitions of the Simple Endoscopic Score for Crohn's Disease Variables

Variable	0	1	2	3
Presence of ulcers	None	Aphthous ulcers (0.1–0.5 cm)	Large ulcers (0.5–2.0 cm)	Very large ulcers (>2.0 cm)
Ulcerated surface	None	<10%	10%–30%	>30%
Affected surface	Unaffected segment	<50%	50%–75%	>75%
Presence of narrowings	None	Single, can be passed	Multiple, can be passed	Cannot be passed
No. affected segments	All variables = 0	At least one variable ≥1	—	—

To determine the simple endoscopic score for Crohn's disease (SES-CD), the equation is SES-CD = sum of all variables − 1.4 × (no. affected segments).
From Daperno M, Van Assche G, Bulois P, et al: Development of Crohn's disease endoscopic score (CDES): A simple index to assess endoscopic severity of Crohn's disease [abstract]. Gastroenterology 122:A216, 2002.

standard." However, similar to the CDEIS, the correlation of SES-CD results with clinically active disease was weak.

The role of endoscopic assessment of severity of disease in clinical practice is still being developed. It is currently well accepted that if a patient with Crohn's disease has symptoms of active disease it is appropriate to assess if there is mucosal inflammation because numerous other factors may cause patients to have similar symptoms, including bacterial overgrowth; intestinal fistulas; infectious diseases including *Clostridium difficile*, cytomegalovirus (CMV), and enteric infections; and other conditions, such as intestinal fibrotic strictures. It has not yet become the standard of practice to reassess the intestinal mucosa if a patient enters remission from a specific medical therapy.

Ulcerative Colitis

The first qualitative grading system for ulcerative colitis was developed by Truelove and Witts[12] in 1955. This classification system divides patients into mild, moderate, or severe disease categories based on five criteria: temperature, heart rate, hemoglobin, erythrocyte sedimentation rate, and diarrheal symptoms (**Table 21.5**). When this index was initially described, only definitions for patients with mild and severe disease were provided. This index is simple, quick, and easily applied and can identify rapidly the sickest patients with ulcerative colitis. Powell-Tuck and coworkers[13] developed a scoring system to be used in their clinical trial that incorporated clinical data and endoscopic criteria. This scoring system includes a wider range of symptoms than the Truelove and Witts scoring system and includes examination for abdominal tenderness and a sigmoidoscopic scoring system. Assessment of the macroscopic sigmoidoscopic appearance is subjective, and studies have found poor correlation between the colonoscopic findings and the Powell-Tuck Activity Score.[14] This finding suggests that sigmoidoscopy is not the most accurate method of assessing disease activity once the diagnosis of ulcerative colitis has been established.

The Simple Colitis Activity Index[15] was developed to aid in the initial evaluation of exacerbations of ulcerative colitis by outpatient physicians. It was compared with the established Powell-Tuck Activity Score, and the authors found good correlation between the two indices ($P < .0001$). This simpler index includes six clinical criteria: bowel frequency during the day, bowel frequency during the night, urgency of defecation, blood in stool, general well-being, and extracolonic manifestations (**Table 21.6**). Because this index does not employ endoscopic or laboratory data, it may be used as an initial assessment in the outpatient setting and possibly by patients themselves

Table 21.5 Truelove and Witts' Classification of Severity in Ulcerative Colitis

Mild	Diarrhea: <4 bowel movements daily, with only small amounts of blood
	No fever
	No tachycardia
	ESR <30 mm/hr
Moderate	Activity between mild and severe
Severe	Diarrhea: ≥6 bowel movements daily, with blood
	Fever: Mean evening temperature >37.5° C or temperature >37.5° C on at least 2 of 4 days at any time of day
	Tachycardia: Mean pulse >90 beats/min
	Anemia: Hemoglobin <7.5 g/dL compared with normal, allowing for recent transfusions; ESR >30 mm/hr

ESR, erythrocyte sedimentation rate.
From Truelove SC, Witts LJ: Cortisone in ulcerative colitis: Final report on a therapeutic trial. BMJ 2:1041–1048, 1955.

Table 21.6 Simple Colitis Activity Index

Symptoms	Score
Bowel frequency (day)	
1–3	0
4–6	1
7–9	2
>9	3
Bowel frequency (night)	
1–3	1
4–6	2
Urgency of defecation	
Hurry	1
Immediately	2
Incontinence	3
Blood in stool	
Trace	1
Occasionally frank	2
Usually frank	3
General well-being	
Very well	0
Slightly below par	1
Poor	2
Very poor	3
Terrible	4
Extracolonic features	1 per manifestation

From Walmsley RS, Ayres RC, Pounder RE, et al: A simple clinical colitis activity index. Gut 43:29–32, 1998.

as a guide to modifying treatment and the need to seek further medical advice.

The Ulcerative Colitis Disease Activity Index (UCDAI) was designed in 1987 by Sutherland and coworkers[16] to provide an objective basis for assessing drug efficacy. Four variables are measured, with each receiving a numerical value of 0 (normal) to 3 (most severe); a total value of 12 indicates the most severe disease. The four variables are stool frequency, amount of blood in stool, endoscopic appearance of colonic mucosa, and physician's assessment of disease severity. A potential strength of this index is its incorporation of endoscopic appearance. A clinical response to therapy is defined as a reduction in the UCDAI score by 2 or more points. This index is very similar to another well-accepted index, often called the "Mayo score," developed by investigators at the Mayo Clinic.[17] None of the aforementioned indices that have been described for patients with ulcerative colitis has been validated. They have been accepted as being appropriate without proper formal validation.

Preparation of Patients for Gastrointestinal Endoscopy

Lower Flexible Gastrointestinal Endoscopy (Colonoscopy and Flexible Sigmoidoscopy)

The quality of colonoscopy or flexible sigmoidoscopy depends on the effectiveness of the bowel preparation. Bowel cleansing should leave no residual fecal material and only very little fluid. An inadequate bowel preparation has many repercussions: It impairs visualization and colonoscopic diagnosis; it may require the procedure to be rescheduled; and it prolongs insertion time, which not only adds to patient discomfort[18] but also increases the cost of the procedure.[19]

In a study comparing GoLYTELY, NuLytely, and Fleet Phospho-soda, Ell and colleagues[20] showed a statistically sig-

nificant benefit to using GoLYTELY over the other two preparations in achieving effective cleansing of the entire colon before colonoscopy. There was no difference in patient satisfaction between the three preparations. In this study, the patients ate a regular breakfast on the day before the examination and thereafter had only clear fluids; they were not to eat anything on the day of the colonoscopy. The bowel cleansing regimen occurred in two stages, with divided doses the day before and on the morning of the procedure. A short interval between bowel preparation and colonoscopy has yielded better cleansing results.[21] The GoLYTELY preparation in the past had been considered to be the "gold standard" for bowel cleansing before colonoscopy. None of these studies were performed in patients with IBD, and Fleet Phospho-soda enemas have been implicated in the development of an acute colitis.

For flexible sigmoidoscopy, patient studies have not shown a clearly superior method for bowel preparation. The addition of magnesium citrate to the regimen seems to improve the quality of the study over enemas alone.[22,23] Patients may consider a completely oral regimen more easily tolerated than one that includes enemas,[24] but the best preparation probably would be one that includes both oral magnesium citrate and one to two Fleet enemas.[25] These have yet to be adequately assessed in blinded controlled trials for patients with IBD.

Upper Endoscopy

No preparation is required for a patient to undergo an upper gastrointestinal (GI) endoscopy. Patients should ingest no solids for at least 6 hours before the procedure and no liquids for at least 4 hours. If a patient has a gastric emptying disorder, a longer period of fasting may be required.

Indications for Gastrointestinal Endoscopy in Inflammatory Bowel Disease

Lower Flexible Gastrointestinal Endoscopy

Endoscopy plays a key role not only in the diagnosis of Crohn's disease but also in its management. Although other radiologic modalities often are complementary to the diagnosis and treatment of Crohn's disease, endoscopy is the only method that allows for biopsy specimens to be taken. **Box 21.1** lists indications for colonoscopy in IBD. Colonoscopy is usually performed during the initial evaluation of ulcerative colitis and Crohn's disease to confirm the diagnosis, assess disease severity, and determine the extent of the disease. It also plays an important role in assessing the disease response to therapy and is important in performing endoscopic surveillance for dysplasia or cancer. Colonoscopy and flexible sigmoidoscopy are contraindicated in patients with known or suspected peritonitis, bowel perforation, or colonic necrosis.[26] Severe coagulopathy, thrombocytopenia, and neutropenia also are contraindications for the procedure. In addition, toxic megacolon and fulminant colitis generally are relative contraindications for the procedure secondary to their increased risk of colonic perforation.

Upper Gastrointestinal Endoscopy

Upper GI endoscopy is used to evaluate upper GI symptoms in patients with IBD. Biopsy specimens of normal gastric mucosa in patients with indeterminate colitis may aid in the diagnosis of Crohn's colitis. In patients with known Crohn's disease, upper GI endoscopy allows for the diagnosis of Crohn's disease of the esophagus, stomach, and duodenum. It also can treat strictures or upper GI bleeding.

Crohn's Disease

Lower Gastrointestinal Endoscopy

Colonoscopy is performed in the initial diagnosis of Crohn's disease to confirm the diagnosis and assess the extent of the disease. Intubation of the terminal ileum should be attempted in all patients; there is an 80% to 97% success rate of insertion of the colonoscope into the distal ileum.[27,28] Biopsy specimens of the terminal ileum should be taken because Crohn's ileitis can appear macroscopically normal. Endoscopic involvement of the ileum is usually associated with Crohn's disease, but patients with pancolonic involvement who have ulcerative colitis can have backwash ileitis, a patchy inflammation without ulceration that extends a few centimeters into the terminal ileum. Biopsy specimens are required to differentiate the two diagnoses.

Flexible sigmoidoscopy may be appropriate to perform when a colonoscopy was recently performed or when the inflammation is known to be limited to the left side of the colon.[29] In patients with severe disease activity, colonoscopy may be contraindicated secondary to the severe degree of inflammation, whereas flexible sigmoidoscopy can be useful to confirm that a patient's symptoms are related to Crohn's disease and not to an infectious or other form of colitis. Flexible sigmoidoscopy can also be used to confirm a diagnosis of irritable bowel syndrome (IBS) by excluding other inflammatory or neoplastic disorders. In IBS, there is normal colonic anatomy, but there may be nonspecific findings of increased colonic mucus, mural spasm, and increased sensitivity to painful stimuli during flexible sigmoidoscopy.[30]

Colonic perforation is the most common major complication of diagnostic colonoscopy, with a risk of approximately 0.25%.[31,32] In patients with severe colitis, a suspected abscess, toxic megacolon, or signs or symptoms of a bowel obstruction, colonoscopy is generally not recommended because the risk of perforation is greatly increased. A very small scope (6-mm outer diameter) can be used to assess the rectum and sigmoid; this technique practically eliminates the risk of colonic perforation. The proximal extent of disease can be evaluated by computed tomography (CT) scan. The most common reason to abort a colonoscopy in patients with Crohn's disease is related to the presence of severe inflammation with large, deep ulcerations, which carry an increased risk of perforation.

The endoscopic appearance of IBD usually is not specific enough to make the definitive diagnosis of ulcerative colitis versus Crohn's disease; the accuracy of colonoscopy in differentiating between the two forms of inflammatory colitis is 85% to 90%.[33] Some features favor one diagnosis over the other (**Table 21.7**). Endoscopically, Crohn's disease tends to vary with disease duration and severity. The rectum is typically spared, with the most severe involvement occurring in the cecum and right colon; the most common patterns of disease distribution are ileocolitis in 40% to 50%, ileitis in 30% to 40%, and colitis in 15% to 25%. Classically, the disease is discontinuous, forming skip areas—areas of disease that are separated by normal mucosa. In early Crohn's disease, small punched-out aphthous ulcers are typically seen on the background of normal mucosa (**Fig. 21.1**). Aphthous ulcers are a result of submucosal lymphoid follicle expansion and penetration through the mucosa. As the disease progresses,

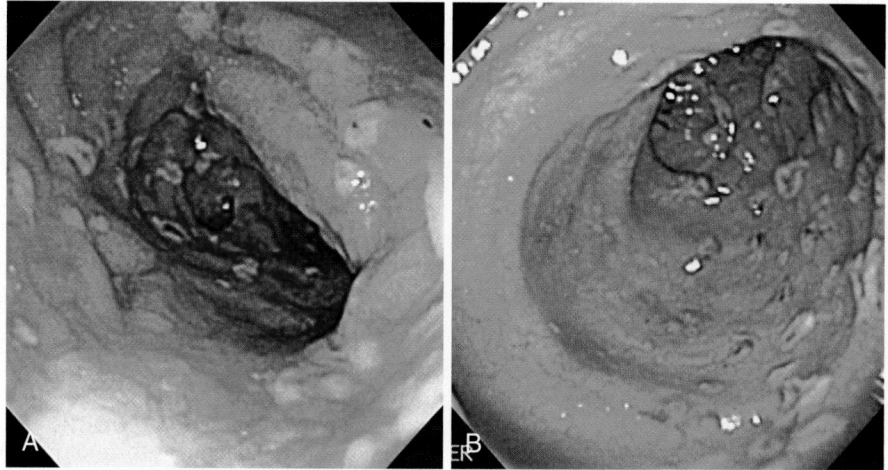

Fig. 21.1 A and **B,** Multiple aphthous ulcers seen in recurrent Crohn's disease in the neoterminal ileum of ileocolic anastomosis 3 months after resection.

Table 21.7 Endoscopic Appearance of Crohn's Disease and Ulcerative Colitis

Endoscopic Appearance	Crohn's Disease	Ulcerative Colitis
Rectum	Spared	Involved
Vascular pattern	Normal	Early loss of vascular markings
Mucosal involvement	Skip lesions	Continuous
Ulcers	Within inflamed mucosa	Within normal mucosa
Mucosal granularity	Present	Present ("wet sandpaper")
Mucosal friability	Present	Present
Cobblestoning	Present	Absent
Thick interhaustral septum	Present	Present
Pseudopolyps	Present	Present
Narrowing of lumen	Present	Present
Strictures	Present	Present
Fistula	Present	Absent
Ulcerations in terminal ileum	Present	Absent
Mucosal bridge	Present	Present

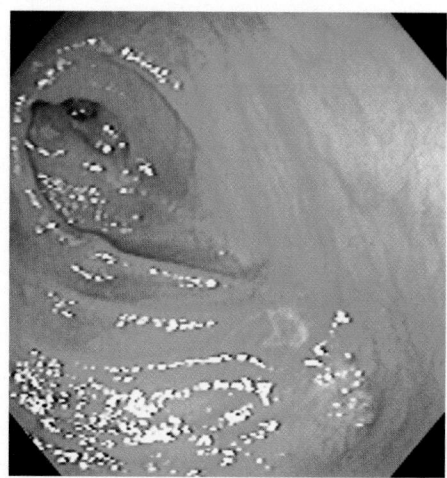

Fig. 21.2 Stellate colonic ulcers in a patient with Crohn's disease.

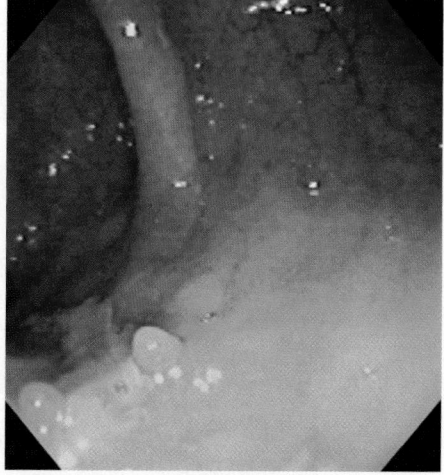

Fig. 21.3 Irregularly shaped ulcerations in a patient with Crohn's disease.

these superficial ulcerations enlarge and coalesce to become long and linear and may take on the appearance of a star ("stellate ulcers") (**Fig. 21.2**). These ulcerations can deepen throughout the bowel wall to lead to abscess and fistula formation. With increasing chronicity, submucosal edema and injury results in a cobblestoning appearance, which practically is pathognomonic for Crohn's disease; cobblestoning consists of uniform nodulations that are low in height with a broad base.

Patients with severe disease can have large linear ulcers ("bear claw" ulcers) and deep serpiginous ulcers (**Figs. 21.3 and 21.4**). Strictures can form in areas with transmural circumferential inflammation. Patients with moderate to severe

disease activity may be endoscopically indistinguishable from patients with ulcerative colitis and many other similar diseases (**Fig. 21.5**). Histologically, there is transmural inflammation with predominantly lymphocytic infiltration. Granulomas are the hallmark of Crohn's disease, although

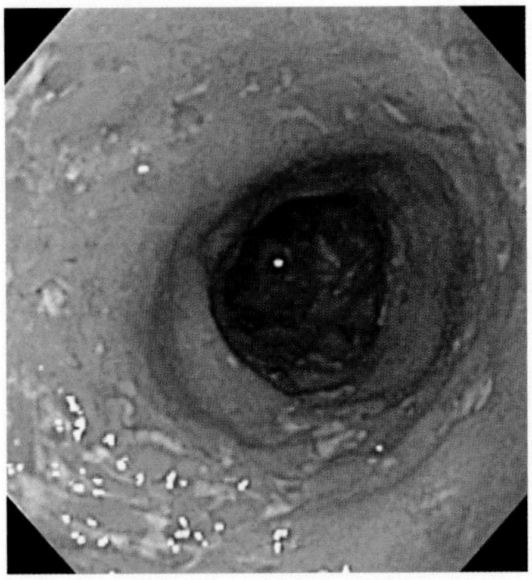

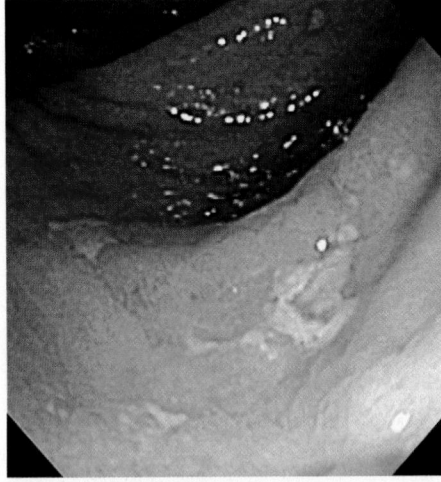

Fig. 21.4 Multiple serpiginous ulcerations of the rectum in a patient with Crohn's disease.

Fig. 21.5 Ulcers in the colon in patients with Behçet's disease cannot be differentiated endoscopically from patients with Crohn's disease.

they are present in only 10% to 25% of biopsy specimens. They are more common in the early stages of the disease.[34] Granulomas can be found throughout the GI tract and in macroscopically normal areas. For this reason, it is recommended that upper GI endoscopy with mucosal biopsy be performed when the differentiation between ulcerative colitis and Crohn's disease is unclear.

Upper Gastrointestinal Endoscopy

A hallmark of Crohn's disease is that it can affect the entire GI tract, from the mouth to the anus. The upper GI tract was previously thought to be an uncommon site of disease, with a prevalence of less than 4%.[35,36] Routine use of endoscopy has found a prevalence closer to 50% to 60%.[37] Dysphagia, odynophagia, epigastric pain, and stomatitis are the most common symptoms, although most patients are asymptomatic.[38–40]

Endoscopic features of Crohn's disease in the esophagus tend to be nonspecific and may include aphthous ulcers, cobblestoning, stricture formation, friability, and granularity. Huchzermeyer and coworkers[41] described two different stages of esophageal involvement. The first stage is a milder and earlier form of the disease. Erythema and edema progress to aphthous ulcerations with intervening normal mucosa, resembling a cobblestoning appearance. In the second stage, esophageal strictures and stenosis occur. Histologically, it is rare to see a granuloma on a biopsy specimen of the esophagus; 75% of biopsy specimens show active chronic inflammation, and 30% show ulcerations.[38]

The antrum and duodenum are the most common sites of involvement of the upper GI tract (**Fig. 21.6**). Gastroduodenal disease is contiguous in approximately 60% of patients, with only 40% having duodenal disease solely.[42] In contrast to the round and oval ulcers seen in peptic ulcer disease, the ulcerations in gastroduodenal Crohn's disease tend to be more serpiginous and longitudinal.[35] Mucosal erythema and nodularity, cobblestoning, and strictures have also been described.[36,42] The descending duodenum is often the most severely affected. The pathognomonic granulomas are found in approximately 40% of biopsy specimens taken from the duodenum.[42]

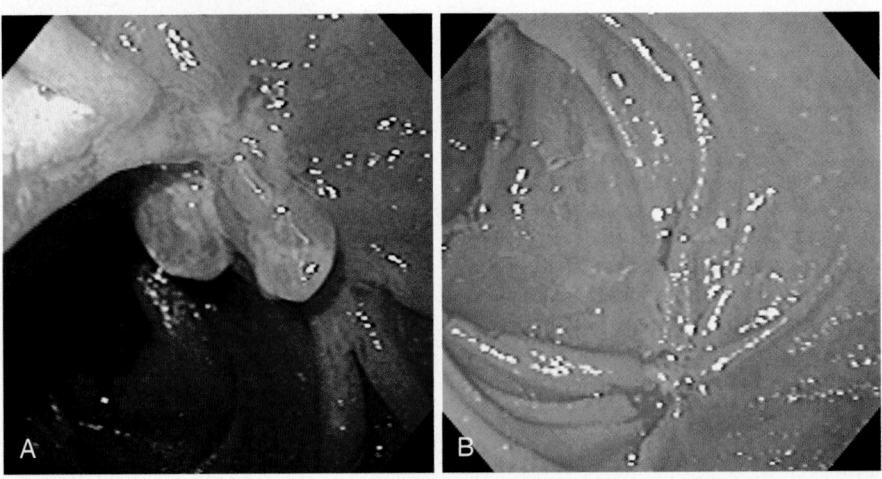

Fig. 21.6 A, Duodenal active ulceration in a patient with Crohn's disease. **B,** Duodenal bleeding in an active ulcer in the same patient with Crohn's disease.

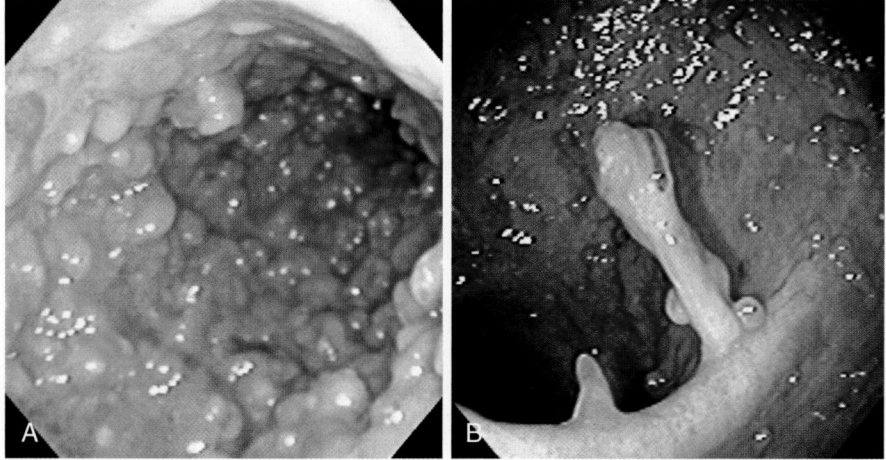

Fig. 21.7 **A** and **B,** Pseudopolyps in a patient with ulcerative colitis.

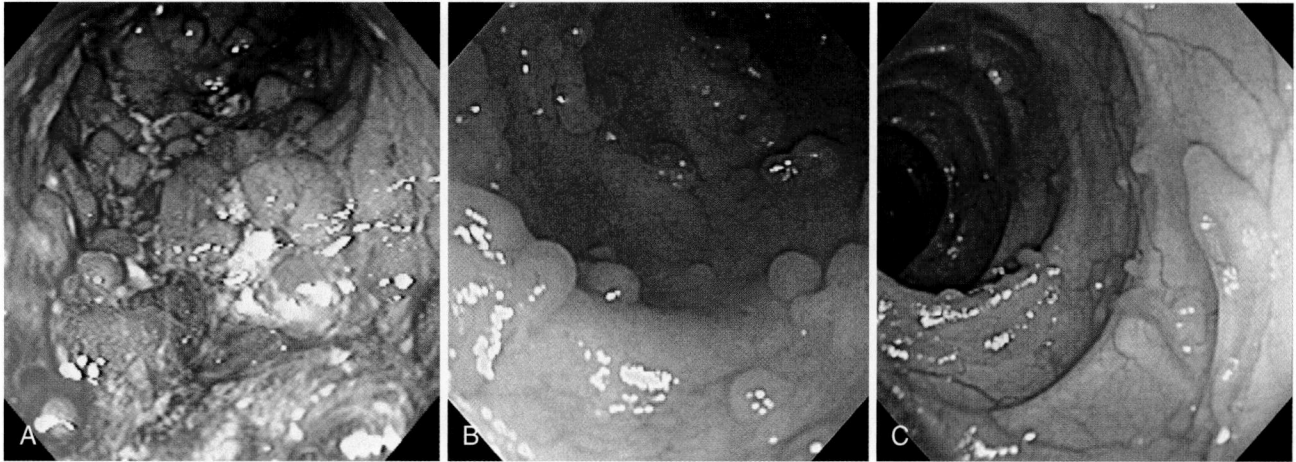

Fig. 21.8 **A,** Pseudopolyps in a patient with severe ulcerative colitis. **B** and **C,** Pseudopolyps in the same patient after treatment.

Ulcerative Colitis

Lower Gastrointestinal Endoscopy

In ulcerative colitis, the inflammatory response is directed solely at the colon and is limited to the mucosa and submucosa. The disease starts in the rectum in 95% of cases, which should cause one to reconsider the diagnosis of ulcerative colitis in any patient with rectal sparing. The inflammation usually occurs in a circumferential, contiguous pattern.

Early in the disease, there is loss of the vascular pattern and congestion. The smooth and glistening appearance of normal colonic mucosa is replaced by a more granular-appearing mucosa caused by disruption of the normal light reflection. There is blunting of the normal, finely branched mucosal vascular pattern, blunting of the intrahaustral folds caused by mucosal edema, and diffuse mucosal erythema. At later stages, the edematous mucosa acquires a sandpaperlike appearance and becomes very friable; this leads to easy mucosal bleeding, even in response to being brushed lightly by the endoscope or a cotton swab. With severe disease, mucopus, a yellow-white exudate, may be present. The colonic mucosa is disrupted, and small shallow ulcers can develop and progress to large deep ulcerations. These large ulcerations can coalesce to form areas

of completely destroyed mucosa; pseudopolyps or mucosal bridges can form from the congested mucosal remnants present in the denuded areas (**Figs. 21.7 and 21.8**).[43] Usually pseudopolyps are not clinically significant, but in patients with long-standing ulcerative colitis, biopsy of pseudopolyps is needed because they resemble adenomatous and malignant polyps (**Fig. 21.9**).

Toxic megacolon is a dreaded complication of colitis; although seen more often in patients with ulcerative colitis, it is found in Crohn's disease as well. In severe colitis, damage to the neural plexus and muscularis propria can lead to neuromuscular dysfunction. Progressive colonic dilation can result leading to a toxic megacolon. In chronic ulcerative colitis, the colon appears smooth, shortened, and noncompliant (rigid) on colonoscopy. There is loss of the haustral folds caused by thickening of the muscularis mucosae and submucosal fibrosis. The colon has a characteristic pipelike appearance. The terminal ileum can also be involved in 10% to 20% of patients with ulcerative pancolitis. There is erythema, an abnormal vascular pattern, and superficial erosions in the distal 5 cm of the terminal ileum secondary to backwash ileitis. This backwash ileitis is almost always found in the setting of a dilated and incompetent ileocecal valve. Although this ileitis does not cause any clinical symptoms, retrospective

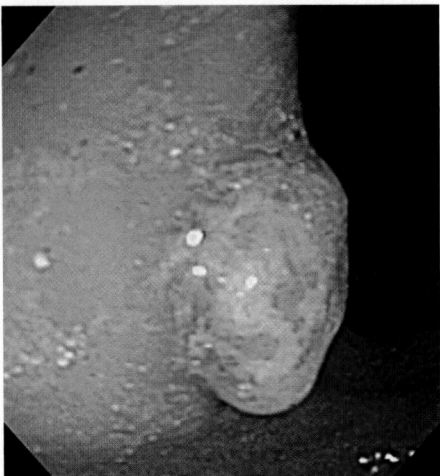

Fig. 21.9 Large pseudopolyp in the rectum of a patient with long-standing ulcerative colitis.

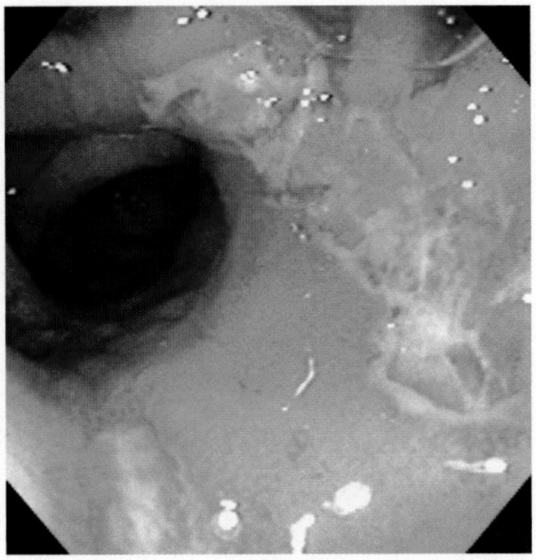

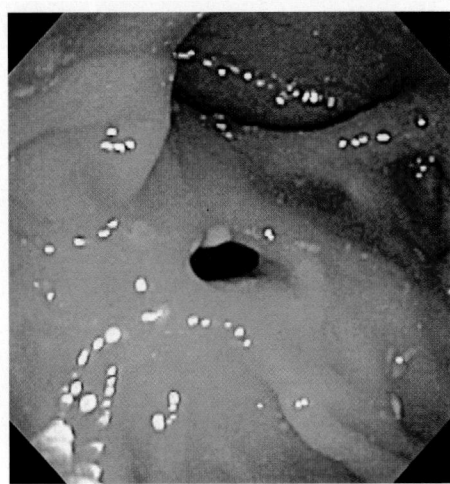

Fig. 21.10 Multiple active ulcers in a patient with fibrostenotic Crohn's disease.

data suggest that backwash ileitis is associated with an increased risk of colorectal cancer (CRC).[44]

Upper Gastrointestinal Endoscopy

Because ulcerative colitis, by definition, does not affect the upper GI tract, upper endoscopy would not be performed routinely. One of the few reasons to perform upper GI endoscopy is if the diagnosis of ulcerative colitis is in question; this test can look for evidence of inflammatory disease elsewhere in the GI tract to establish the diagnosis of Crohn's disease.

Strictures and Mass Lesions

Differentiating Malignant from Benign Strictures

The healing response to the chronic inflammation found in IBD is thought to result in intestinal strictures. It is believed that there is recruitment of fibroblasts and other structural components in healing, which promote fibrosis and luminal narrowing leading to strictures (**Fig. 21.10**).[45] The sheer number and diversity of cell types in the intestine make it difficult to identify a solitary cell responsible for the fibrosis seen in IBD. Stricture formation is found more often in patients with Crohn's disease than in patients with ulcerative colitis because of the transmural nature of inflammation seen in Crohn's disease (**Figs. 21.11 and 21.12**). The prevalence of colonic strictures in Crohn's disease ranges from 4% to 5% in surgical series[46] to 8% to 9% in endoscopic series.[47] With all strictures, it is imperative to assess for any evidence of malignancy. Although strictures are found more often in patients with Crohn's disease, the strictures that are associated with ulcerative colitis have a higher frequency of malignancy. The rate of malignancy in patients who have strictures is 7% to 11% in Crohn's disease[48] compared with approximately 25% in ulcerative colitis.[49]

Efforts should be made to exclude malignancy when performing a colonoscopy (**Fig. 21.13**). Such efforts include visualizing the entire length of the stricture and beyond and using a narrower pediatric colonoscope, push enteroscope, or gas-

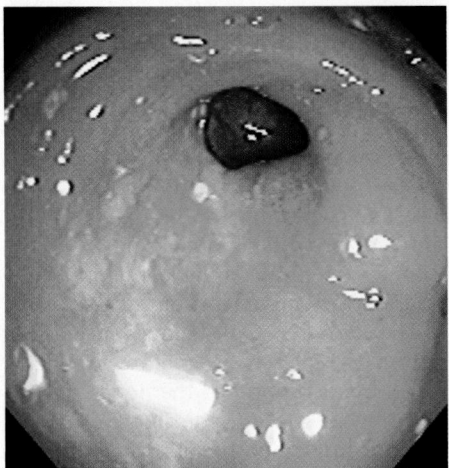

Fig. 21.11 Crohn's stricture at the anastomosis.

Fig. 21.12 Stricture at the ileocolic anastomosis.

troscope if necessary. Biopsy specimens should be obtained from the edge and the core of the stricture. Endoscopic features suggesting malignancy within a stricture are rigidity of the edge, an eccentric lumen, nodularity within the stricture, and an abrupt shelflike margin. Even if the biopsy specimen

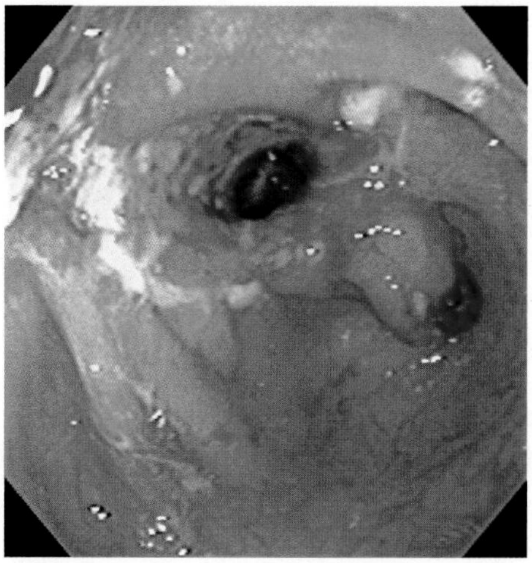

Fig. 21.13 Ulceration and nonmalignant stricture in a patient with active Crohn's disease in the descending colon.

is negative for malignancy, these highly suspicious lesions should be treated as if they were malignant because carcinoma complicating IBD can extend submucosally. Surgery should be considered in all patients with biopsy-proven malignant strictures, patients with highly suspicious lesions based on gross endoscopic assessment, and patients in whom a colonoscope is unable to pass to survey the remainder of the colon.

Role of Balloon Dilation of Strictures

Strictures that are deemed to be benign may be treated without surgical resection by using through-the-scope (TTS) balloon dilation. Strictures most amenable for endoscopic therapy are short (typically <8 cm), isolated, and located in areas of only mild inflammation. The overall success rate of TTS balloon dilation ranges from 50% to 85%.[50–56] Dilation can be repeated in cases of symptomatic recurrence; both Couckuyt and colleagues[50] and Sabate and coworkers[57] found a 40% success rate of TTS dilation, but they also found a 40% probability of patients requiring surgery at 5-year follow-up. The complication rate of TTS balloon dilation ranges from 2.9% to 8%, with colonic perforation being the most common complication.[50,54,57] No prospective randomized controlled studies have been performed to compare endoscopic treatment of strictures directly with surgical strictureplasty.

Endoscopic dilation for Crohn's disease has been evaluated only in some small, heterogeneous studies. A more recent systematic review of the literature evaluated the efficacy of pneumatic dilation in Crohn's disease.[58] The authors reviewed 13 studies enrolling 347 patients with Crohn's disease. Endoscopic dilation was mainly applied to postsurgical strictures and was technically successful in 86% of the cases. Long-term clinical efficacy was achieved in 58% of the patients. Mean follow-up was 33 months, corresponding to 800 patient-years of follow-up. The major complication rate was 2%; it was greater than 10% in two series. Multivariate analysis showed that a stricture length less than or equal to 4 cm was associated with a surgery-free outcome (odds ratio 4.01, 95% confidence interval 1.16 to 13.8, $P < .028$). The overall conclusion was that endoscopic balloon dilation is effective and safe for treatment of short strictures caused by Crohn's disease.

Steroid injections at the time of dilation have been proposed to improve the results of balloon dilation. Ramboer and coworkers[52] treated 13 patients with symptomatic strictures that precluded the passage of a standard 13-mm colonoscope. Although there was no control group, this study offered promising results because all 13 patients experienced immediate relief, and none required surgery at 47 months of follow-up. The success of the combined therapy may be secondary to a local antiinflammatory effect of the corticosteroids or a decrease in the tendency toward fibrosis after dilation or both. Intrastricture steroid injection after balloon dilation has been reported to reduce the need for repeat stricture dilation in patients with Crohn's disease in retrospective series.

There is only one randomized pilot series performed to date. The pilot study was performed comparing local injection of triamcinolone (40 mg total dose) after endoscopic balloon dilation of Crohn's ileocolonic anastomotic strictures versus saline placebo. The primary endpoint was time to repeat dilation or surgery. Patients were followed up for 52 weeks. In this pilot study, 13 patients were randomly assigned—7 to steroid and 6 to placebo. These groups were well matched for baseline and dilation characteristics. When evaluated by intention-to-treat analysis, one of six patients in the placebo group and five of seven patients in the steroid group needed repeat dilation (log-rank test $P = .06$, Cox regression $P = .10$, hazard ratio 6.1; 95% confidence interval 0.7 to 53.0). When analyzed by per-protocol analysis, the differences were more significant (log-rank test $P = .03$, Cox regression $P = .07$, hazard ratio 7.7; 95% confidence interval 0.9 to 67.9). The overall conclusion was that a single treatment of intrastricture triamcinolone injection did not reduce the time to repeat dilation after balloon dilation of Crohn's ileocolonic anastomotic strictures, and there was a trend toward a worse outcome. The investigators cautioned that the use of intrastricture steroid injection after balloon dilation in clinical practice should be considered carefully until more data are available.[59]

Differential Diagnosis

Differentiating Crohn's Disease from Ulcerative Colitis

The accuracy of colonoscopy in differentiating Crohn's disease from ulcerative colitis is approximately 85% to 90%.[33] Establishing an accurate diagnosis is important because the treatment, surgical options, and prognosis often differ significantly between the two forms of colitis. It is also important to reevaluate the original diagnosis and to continue to evaluate patients with an "indeterminate colitis" because these diseases often evolve over time. Two studies looked at this phenomenon. Moum and coworkers[60] studied 527 patients with ulcerative colitis, and 88% had their diagnosis confirmed at 2 years' follow-up; 91% of the 228 patients with Crohn's disease had their diagnosis confirmed. In 36 patients who were originally listed as "indeterminate colitis," 33% and 17% were reclassified at 2 years as having ulcerative colitis and Crohn's disease. Langevin and colleagues[61] studied 96 patients with ulcerative proctitis; over a 29-month period, 14% developed features more consistent with Crohn's disease.

The expression of perinuclear antineutrophil cytoplasmic antibodies (pANCA) is present in most patients with ulcerative colitis, but 10% to 30% of patients with Crohn's disease also have this antibody; these appear to be a subset of patients with Crohn's disease who have a more ulcerative colitis–like pattern of disease: left-sided colitis, rectal bleeding, and mucus discharge.[62] The anti–*Saccharomyces cerevisiae* antibody (ASCA) also is helpful in IBD. ASCA is present in 50% to 70% of patients with Crohn's disease and in only 7% to 14% of patients with ulcerative colitis.[63] These serologic tests have not been proven to play a significant role in establishing a diagnosis for an indeterminate colitis. In the rare case in which an individual has IgG and IgA ASCA positivity (the so-called double ASCA positive), there has been an excellent correlation with the presence of Crohn's disease. Other serologic tests have been evaluated more recently. Serum markers that are available for assessing IBD include ASCA, anti-OmpC (a human antibody specific for the outer membrane porin C of *Escherichia coli*), ANCA, pANCA, and DNAse-sensitive pANCA (when the pANCA stain is sensitive to treatment with DNAse, it is associated with ulcerative colitis).[64]

Another serologic marker also has been described, anti-CBir1. The anti-CBir1 assay was developed at Cedars-Sinai Medical Center. Results of studies showed that 50% of patients with Crohn's disease had concentrations of anti-CBir1 that were greater than the reference range, suggesting that anti-CBir1 had good sensitivity as a single marker for Crohn's disease. Targan and colleagues[65] showed that in a cohort of patients with Crohn's disease who had defined serologic profiles, 46% of the patients who were nonreactive to ASCA expressed antibody to CBir1. Anti-CBir1 adds benefit to IBD serology testing. Additionally I2 antibodies have been investigated. I2 is associated with the organism *Pseudomonas fluorescens*. The use of serologies in the diagnosis of IBD is an area that is evolving.

Lesions such as inflammatory polyps (pseudopolyps) and mucosal bridges can occur in both forms of IBD. Mucosal bridges develop when two adjacent ulcers meet by burrowing beneath an area of inflamed mucosa, and as the area heals, reepithelialization of the ulcers and the undersurface of the mucosal strip produces a mucosal covered tube connected at both ends. There is a loss of haustral folds and linear scar formation in the healing process of both forms of colitis. The endoscopic recognition of inflammatory polyps, mucosal bridges, loss of haustral folds, or linear scarring does not offer any mechanism to differentiate ulcerative colitis from Crohn's disease. It is most difficult to distinguish between ulcerative colitis and Crohn's disease when there is severe and active disease present. In the later stages of both diseases, the two forms of colitis can resemble each other so closely endoscopically that the diagnosis may be impossible until more time has passed and the patient is reexamined. The most helpful distinguishing features in Crohn's disease are the presence of aphthous ulcers, the cobblestoning appearance, and the focal and asymmetric distribution of the colitis. In ulcerative colitis, more important differentiating endoscopic features are the small ulcers in a diffusely inflamed mucosa and the granularity and friability of the mucosa.[33]

Multiple biopsy specimens are needed to make an accurate diagnosis. Each biopsy specimen is labeled according to its location in the colon because the pattern of inflammation is often very important in establishing a diagnosis. Focal inflammation is more consistent with Crohn's disease, whereas progressively increasing inflammation of the distal colon is more

suggestive of ulcerative colitis. Intubation of the terminal ileum and a biopsy of the small bowel are imperative in establishing a diagnosis. Although there may be backwash ileitis in patients with pancolonic involvement who have ulcerative colitis, no actual ulcerations are seen, and most often the ileum is free of disease in patients with ulcerative colitis; up to two-thirds of patients with Crohn's disease have ileal involvement. The ileocecal valve is often patent in ulcerative colitis, whereas in Crohn's disease it is contracted and difficult to intubate.

Differentiating Crohn's Disease and Ulcerative Colitis from Infectious Colitis

The initial diagnosis of IBD can be challenging because many conditions share the same clinical presentation (**Box 21.2**). In a patient with a diarrheal illness that lasts for more than 2 weeks, IBD and infectious colitis are important considerations. A careful history including travel information, diet, and antibiotic usage and stool studies and an endoscopy with biopsy specimens often are required to make the diagnosis. It may be difficult initially to distinguish idiopathic IBD from infectious colitis because many of the clinical symptoms are similar. The endoscopic appearance of the colonic mucosa and the histologic changes in inflammatory bowel disease and infectious colitis may also be practically identical. Determining the accurate diagnosis depends on an experienced endoscopist, a reliable pathologist, and subsequent visits with the patient to observe the disease progression.

Flexible sigmoidoscopy and rectal biopsy are often adequate to distinguish between inflammatory and infectious colitis; a complete colonoscopy usually is not required.[66] However, if a diagnosis cannot be made based on flexible sigmoidoscopy alone, both proximal and distal biopsy specimens of the right colon can be useful. In a patient with unexplained diarrhea of at least 4 to 6 weeks' duration who has severe symptoms, nocturnal or frequent watery stools, weight loss, an elevated erythrocyte sedimentation rate or who is immunocompromised, it is reasonable to perform a colonoscopy with multiple biopsies.[67]

Approximately 30% of patients with mucoid bloody diarrhea and suspected IBD have an infectious etiology for the diarrhea.[68] Many patients who present with IBD also are superinfected.[69] In one study, 36% of patients with refractory ulcerative colitis had CMV found on a rectal biopsy specimen.[70] Endoscopic features seen more commonly in infectious

---

Box 21.2 Differential Diagnosis of Inflammatory Bowel Disease

Behçet's syndrome
Diversion colitis
Diverticulitis
Graft-versus-host disease
Infectious colitis
Ischemic colitis
Malignancy
Microscopic colitis
Pseudomembranous and drug-induced colitis
Radiation colopathy

colitis include free pus, intense reddening of the surface mucosa, and yellowish exudates that partially or completely cover the mucosal surface. Patchy inflammation within the same colonic segment that consists of multiple small areas of inflammation with intervening normal-appearing mucosa is a characteristic endoscopic feature of infectious colitis.[68] A brief description follows of some of the most common causes of infectious colitis and their distinctive endoscopic findings.

Actinomycosis

Actinomyces israelii is an anaerobic gram-positive bacterium that is found in the mouth, lungs, and GI tract. The most common site of GI tract involvement is the ileocecal region, and it can produce a suppurative, granulomatous infection with a propensity for fistula formation and a release of "sulfur granules."[71] Symptoms include weight loss, night sweats, draining fistulas, and abdominal masses.[72] The diagnosis is confirmed by culture and histopathologic evaluation.

Amebiasis

Amebic colitis (*Entamoeba histolytica*) is a protozoan infection that primarily affects the large bowel.[73] It is most often seen in patients who recently emigrated from developing countries and who recently traveled to developing countries. Symptoms vary from none to explosive diarrhea, tenesmus, fever, and abdominal cramps. The colonoscopic appearance during the acute phase resembles ulcerative colitis, but in the chronic phase it resembles Crohn's disease. The most common segments involved are the cecum and right colon, with the rectum and sigmoid involved less often.[74] Toxic megacolon may develop in severe cases of amebiasis. Colonoscopy reveals granular, friable, and erythematous mucosa with discrete large ulcers covered by yellowish, mucopurulent exudates.[75] Biopsy specimens of the margins of the ulcers provide a 60% to 90% yield of trophozoites to make the diagnosis.[76]

Balantidium coli

Balantidium coli is a protozoan transmitted by pigs that only rarely affects the colon. This infection causes varying degrees of inflammation in the rectosigmoid that initially may resemble Crohn's disease or amebiasis. Ulcers vary from scattered and superficial to multiple and deep. To make the diagnosis, the characteristic trophozoites can be found in scrapings from the rectal ulcers or in tissue samples.

Campylobacter jejuni

Campylobacter jejuni is a bacterial pathogen that typically causes a self-limited infectious diarrhea. It is the most commonly identified bacterial pathogen in cases of diarrhea in the United States.[77] It can resemble both ulcerative colitis and Crohn's disease.[78,79] Typically, *C. jejuni* produces mucosal erythema and friability in the early stages and diffuse exudates over the mucosa that makes the infection indistinguishable from ulcerative colitis. The rectum is usually involved, and the right colon is rarely affected; 50% of patients may present with rectal bleeding and tenesmus similar to ulcerative colitis. Less commonly, the colonoscopic appearance resembles Crohn's disease with hyperemia, friability, edema, and scattered small

ulcers. Extraintestinal manifestations, such as erythema nodosum and peripheral arthritis, may be present.[80] Hepatosplenomegaly may occur from *Campylobacter* infections.[81] Of patients, 20% may relapse or have a prolonged illness that may mimic IBD. Dark-field or phase-contrast examination of fresh stool may be diagnostic.[78]

Chlamydia trachomatis

Chlamydia trachomatis is the etiologic agent for lymphogranuloma venereum (LGV), a sexually transmitted infection that may cause proctitis and rectal strictures. Discrete ulcers and friable mucosa often are seen in the rectum and may extend to the descending colon. The presence of stenosis and fistula formation may make *C. trachomatis* infection difficult to distinguish from Crohn's disease. Cultures, serologic tests, or both are needed to establish the diagnosis.

Clostridium difficile *or Pseudomembranous Colitis*

C. difficile is a bacterial infection that typically manifests with watery diarrhea and crampy abdominal pain after a course of antibiotic therapy.[82] The characteristic colonoscopic finding is a pseudomembrane consisting of raised, yellow-white adherent plaques that range from 2 to 8 mm in diameter[83]; these pseudomembranes stud the surface of a moderately inflamed mucosa. The plaques typically occur in the rectum but occasionally occur exclusively in the proximal colon.[84] The diagnosis is confirmed by fecal assay for *C. difficile* toxin A or B.[85] When assessing for the presence of *C. difficile*, it is important to assess for the presence of both toxin A and toxin B.

Cytomegalovirus

CMV is an opportunistic viral infection that affects immunocompromised patients, most commonly patients with acquired immunodeficiency syndrome (AIDS) whose CD4 count is less than 100. Patients can be asymptomatic or may complain of abdominal pain and bloody diarrhea. The presence of discrete, punched-out, shallow ulcerations is a hallmark for this disease (**Fig. 21.14**). This appearance can be difficult to distinguish from Crohn's disease because there may be normal-appearing mucosa adjacent to these ulcerations; in contrast to Crohn's disease, CMV ulcers are usually single and vary in size from 2 to 6 mm. Isolated right-sided disease is common. The diagnosis is made with a biopsy of the ulcer edges and finding CMV inclusion bodies on hematoxylin and eosin staining.[86] Multiple biopsy specimens may be required because of the low density of infected cells.[87]

Escherichia coli O157:H7

E. coli O157:H7 is a bacterial infection that produces a hemorrhagic colitis and can lead to hemolytic uremic syndrome and thrombotic thrombocytopenic purpura. It is associated with contaminated undercooked beef products. Endoscopically, the mucosa appears edematous, hyperemic, and friable, mimicking Crohn's disease.[88] When assessing for the presence of *E. coli* O157:H7, histology is not specific and is unable to establish the presence of this versus other infectious etiologies.

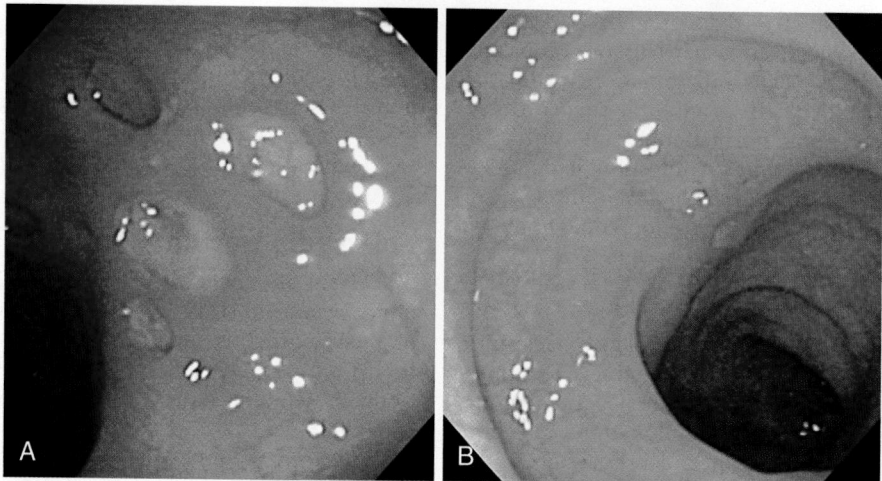

Fig. 21.14 A and **B,** Cytomegalovirus ulceration in immunocompromised host after a renal transplant.

Definitive diagnosis is established by the finding of a positive stool culture (although stool culture has a very low yield) or detection of the molecular probes Shiga toxin A or B.

Herpes Simplex

Herpes simplex proctitis, another sexually transmitted viral infection, produces anal pain, tenesmus, rectal discharge, and constipation. It rarely affects any part of the colon more proximal than the rectum. The combination of external perianal vesicles and rectal lesions with mucosa that is erythematous, friable, and ulcerated in the distal 10 cm of the rectum is highly suggestive of herpes simplex infection. These perianal vesicles can progress to deep ulcerations. Lymphadenopathy, impotence, urinary retention, and lumbosacral dysesthesia can develop.[89] To diagnose this infection, viral cultures of rectal swabs or biopsy specimens are performed.[90]

Histoplasma capsulatum

Histoplasmosis is a mycotic infection that rarely infects the colon. When it is present, there is usually mucosal hyperemia, friability, ulcerations, lymph node hypertrophy, and pseudopolyps in the ileocecal region.[91] Histoplasmosis mimics Crohn's disease in its predominantly right-sided distribution and its noncontiguous nature.[92] The diagnosis should be considered in immunocompromised hosts and travelers from endemic areas. The organism is identified by serology, culture, or DNA probe.

Mycobacterium tuberculosis

Mycobacterium tuberculosis can affect any part of the large bowel and terminal ileum.[93] The rectum is often spared. A deformity of the ileocecal valve and luminal narrowing in the ileocecal area are usually present. It often can be difficult to distinguish colonic tuberculosis from Crohn's disease on colonoscopy. Both conditions produce ulcerations bordered by edema and erythema, and the ulcers are often located in areas of otherwise normal-appearing mucosa. There may be cobblestoning as a result of submucosal involvement, thickening of the bowel wall, and inflammatory pseudopolyps. Two distinc-

tions between Crohn's disease and *M. tuberculosis* endoscopically are that in the later stages the ulcers often have a rolled edge and lack the sharp definition that is seen in Crohn's disease, and the areas of normal mucosa are shorter in colon affected by *M. tuberculosis*. Mass lesions or tuberculomas can develop, and fistulization may be present between loops of bowel. Caseating granulomas can be found on biopsy specimens to diagnose *M. tuberculosis*.[94]

Neisseria gonorrhoeae

Neisseria gonorrhoeae, similar to other sexually transmitted diseases such as herpes simplex virus and lymphogranuloma venereum, produces a proctitis. A creamy rectal discharge or rectal bleeding, rectal friability, and erythema are usually present.[95] Anal intercourse is the largest risk factor for developing this proctitis. Cultures are required to distinguish *N. gonorrhoeae* infection from ulcerative colitis.[96]

Salmonella

Salmonellosis is a bacterial diarrheal illness that usually lasts less than 2 months. It primarily involves the small bowel, spares the rectum, and affects the colon only sporadically. Early in the disease, there is edema, hyperemia, and granularity of the mucosa, which progresses to petechial hemorrhages and mucosal friability. Typhoid fever, a distinctive acute systemic febrile infection caused by *Salmonella*, is a result of a heat-labile enterotoxin that on invasion of the mucosa causes an influx of water and electrolytes into the lumen of the bowel.[97,98] As invasion occurs, localized infections develop, and the bacteremia may produce fever, headache, delirium, maculopapular rash ("rose spots"), leukopenia, and splenomegaly.[99] On endoscopy, volcanolike ulcerations with a surrounding border of erythema can be seen.[100]

Schistosoma mansoni

Schistosoma mansoni is a parasite that is found mostly in tropical climates and may be difficult to diagnose because it is not found on routine ova and parasite examination; the encysted schistosomes are found in resected polyps or biopsy specimens.[101] Schistosomiasis produces a severely inflamed colon with multiple proximal polyps that have a whitish surface exudate. The polyps are produced by the inflammatory response to the degenerating ova. Often the rectum and sigmoid colon are completely normal, but when they are involved, this disease mimics ulcerative colitis; in these cases, there are shallow ulcerations with hyperemia, friability, and edema of the mucosa.

Shigella dysenteriae

Shigella dysenteriae is a gram-negative bacterium that causes bacillary dysentery or shigellosis. The disease can be divided into two phases.[102] The first phase, occurring in the first 1 to 2 days, consists of watery diarrhea and cramping; this phase is mediated by an enterotoxin. The second phase is caused by invasion of the organism into the large intestine and produces fever, cramps, bloody diarrhea, and tenesmus. Although patchy in appearance, the endoscopic appearance often resembles ulcerative colitis because there are multiple ulcers with considerable exudate. The mucosa often appears magenta-colored because of the intense erythema. *S. dysenteriae* infection is diagnosed with stool culture, which is positive in only 50% of cases.

Strongyloides stercoralis

Strongyloides stercoralis is a helminth infection that has ongoing cycles of autoinfection resulting from the internal production of infective larvae. It is found mostly in tropical climates. It produces nausea, diarrhea, GI bleeding, and weight loss. Endoscopically, it may produce a brown pigmentation in a speckled distribution. The diagnosis is made by detecting the rhabditiform larvae in the stool or by detecting the organism in biopsy specimens.

Treponema pallidum

Treponema pallidum causes syphilis and is another sexually transmitted infection that leads to proctitis. Lesions in the anal or anorectal region can resemble both Crohn's disease and ulcerative colitis.

Yersinia enterocolitica

Yersinia enterocolitica is an enteroinvasive bacterium that produces abdominal pain, fever, and diarrhea; symptoms can last for months. Diffuse erythema, friability, and edema throughout the entire colon produce a similar appearance to ulcerative colitis.[103] Less often, there is involvement of the ileum with aphthous ulcers adjacent to normal mucosa, which resembles Crohn's disease.[103] Extraintestinal symptoms, such as arthritis, erythema nodosum, and aphthous stomatitis, can also occur. The diagnosis can be challenging because the laboratory must inoculate the proper medium for this bacteria to grow, and it can often take several weeks to show growth of the organism.

Other Inflammatory Disorders of the Colon
Disinfectant Colitis

Colonic mucosal damage can occur from the inadequate rinsing of the cleaning solutions that are used to disinfect colonoscopes.[104] Colonoscopic instillation of fluid containing residual hydrogen peroxide instantaneously causes compromise to the mucosal stroma, resulting in mucosal blanching and effervescence; these white, plaquelike lesions form a pseudolipomatosis colitis and produce the "snow white" sign.[105] Glutaraldehyde solution is also used in disinfecting the colonoscope; this causes direct injury to the crypt epithelium. Disinfectant colitis is a rare complication of colonoscopy.

Diverticular Disease–Associated Colitis

Colonoscopy is not usually warranted in acute diverticulitis and often is contraindicated because there can be resistance to the passage of the colonoscope secondary to the pronounced tortuosity, fixation, and redundancy of the colon. When colonoscopy is performed, exuding pus and inflammation around the orifice of a single diverticulum may be present. There is often severe spasm of the diseased segment without the typical redness, granularity, or friability found in most forms of inflammatory colitis. In diverticular disease, the mucosa found on the tips of several adjacent hypertrophied folds may be patchy, mottled, and reddened. The redness is actually many tiny petechial dots; pressure generated by the muscular activity of the narrowed and hypertrophied colon leads to capillary rupture. In contrast to IBD, this mucosa is not friable and does not bleed easily when touched by the tip of the colonoscope. When a large enough segment is involved, the mucosa may become friable, and spontaneous bleeding can occur.

Inflammatory cell response is lacking in a biopsy specimen. Instead, there is a characteristic hemorrhagic infiltration that is diagnostic of diverticular colitis.

Ischemic Colitis

Acute ischemic colitis manifests with symptoms of severe abdominal pain, rectal bleeding, and abdominal distention. Atherosclerosis is the most common risk factor, but atrial fibrillation, congestive cardiomyopathy, recent aortic surgery, and hypercoagulability have also been associated with it.[106] The most common sites of ischemia are the descending colon distal to the splenic flexure, the sigmoid colon, and the rectum.[107] There are varying degrees of ischemic injury; there can be complete full-thickness necrosis, transient mucosal necrosis with partial resolution and residual scarring and stricture formation, or simply transient mucosal necrosis with complete resolution of the ischemia. On endoscopy, mild ischemia produces only slightly edematous mucosa. Severe ischemia causes hemorrhagic, friable, and ulcerated mucosa and often has a characteristic plum-red to blue-black coloration. These ulcerations resemble aphthous ulcers, but the clinical history and acuity usually exclude Crohn's disease from the differential diagnosis. A biopsy can also differentiate ischemic from inflammatory colitis; ghost cells are pathognomonic for ischemia but are rarely seen.[108] Usually, there are nonspecific findings of submucosal hemorrhage, vascular congestion, and interstitial edema.

Nonsteroidal Antiinflammatory Drug Colopathy

Nonsteroidal antiinflammatory drugs (NSAIDs) have been associated with reactivation of quiescent ulcerative colitis and

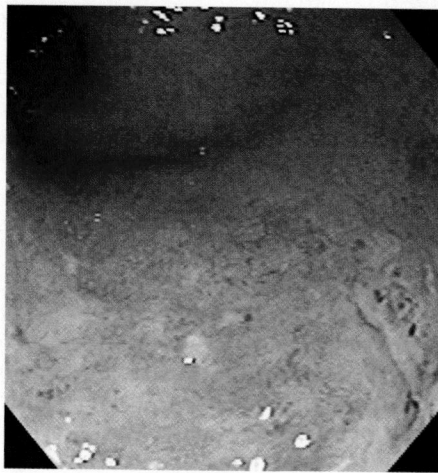

Fig. 21.15 Moderately severe radiation proctitis.

Crohn's disease.[109] In addition to this form of colitis, NSAIDs are also associated with their own de novo nonspecific colitis. The mechanism for this colitis is unclear, but it is thought to relate to prostaglandin inhibition and increased intestinal permeability. Symptoms include hematochezia, diarrhea, ulcerations, perforations, abdominal pain, and iron deficiency anemia.[110] The diagnosis is based on history in conjunction with endoscopic evidence of submucosal fibrosis and focal inflammatory lesions.

Preparation-Related Colitis

Toxic or caustic materials introduced into the rectum by enema or suppository can cause colitis. Fleet Phospho-soda enemas cause a loss of normal vascular pattern, granularity, and friability in the distal colon.[111] Oral sodium phosphate has also been shown to cause mucosal abnormalities.[112] Small aphthouslike ulcerations are formed, which macroscopically can resemble Crohn's disease but pathologically are easily differentiated.

Radiation Colitis

Colonic mucosa can be damaged by radiation to the pelvis and abdomen. Radiation colitis most commonly occurs in the treatment of cervical and prostate cancers. Most commonly, the distal sigmoid and proximal rectum are involved. Acutely, a patient often experiences a self-limited illness that consists of diarrhea, tenesmus, and occasional rectal bleeding. Chronic radiation colitis produces rectal bleeding that can present 20 years after the initial radiation. The mucosa is granular and friable on colonoscopy with evidence of spontaneous bleeding and telangiectasias in the rectum and sigmoid (**Fig. 21.15**). Radiation colitis can resemble ulcerative colitis and idiopathic proctitis.

Solitary Rectal Ulcer Syndrome

Solitary rectal ulcer syndrome (SRUS) is a rare disorder of unknown etiology whose cardinal feature is isolated erythema or ulceration of a part of the rectal wall. Rectal bleeding, mucus production, constipation, rectal discomfort, and urgency also are usually present. SRUS may be initially misdi-

agnosed in 26% of patients.[113] Ulcerated SRUS may be mistaken for IBD, and some patients have been treated with high-dose steroids. Polypoid lesions (colitis cystica profunda, seen in association with SRUS), usually found on the anterior rectal wall, have been mistaken for neoplasms. Histologically, SRUS is unique; there is evidence of fibromuscular obliteration of the lamina propria with disorientation of the muscularis mucosae and extension of smooth muscle fibers into the lamina propria.

SRUS affects men and women equally, and the mean age of onset is 49 years.[114] The mean reported duration of symptoms before diagnosis ranges from 3 to 5 years.[114–116] The diagnosis can often be made on sigmoidoscopy. Ulceration is not universally present, with polypoid, nonulcerated lesions, and erythematous areas also seen; in one series, the prevalence of ulceration was 57%, the prevalence of polypoid lesions was 25%, and the prevalence of patches of hyperemic mucosa was 18%.[115]

There is no specific cure for SRUS. Topical steroids and sulfasalazine enemas are ineffective.[115,117] Sucralfate enemas have been used, which lead to symptomatic and macroscopic improvement, but the histologic changes persisted.[118] Biofeedback techniques such as correction of pelvic floor defecatory behavior; regulation of toilet habits; and encouragement to stop laxatives, suppositories, and enemas have been shown to be useful[119,120] and should be the first-line therapy for patients with SRUS. Surgery plays only a minor role in the treatment of SRUS and should be reserved for patients with intractable symptoms and patients with evidence of rectal prolapse; there is symptomatic improvement in approximately 56% of patients, but 33% are often unchanged or worse.[121]

Cancer in Inflammatory Bowel Disease

Both ulcerative colitis and Crohn's disease are associated with an increased risk for developing precancerous dysplastic epithelial changes and CRC. In the general population, CRC is the third leading cause of death in the United States in both men and women and the second leading cause of cancer death overall. CRC may be one of the most preventable forms of cancer because routine colonoscopies allow detection and removal of precancerous polyps. Knowledge of CRC risk in patients with IBD is inadequate, despite the obvious conclusion that this is one of the most frightening aspects of the diagnosis of IBD. Physicians need to educate their patients and stress the importance of screening. There is no debate that ulcerative colitis bears a high risk for the development of CRC. A meta-analysis of 116 studies by Eaden and coworkers[122] showed that the prevalence of CRC in patients with ulcerative colitis is approximately 3.7%. The risk for CRC increased with duration of disease: There was a 2% incidence of cancer after 10 years, a 9% incidence after 20 years, and a 19% incidence after 30 years of disease. The development of cancer accounts for one-third of deaths related to ulcerative colitis.

In contrast, data exist that both support and refute the hypothesis that Crohn's disease is associated with an increased risk of CRC. However, increasing data show a similar risk for CRC in Crohn's disease as in ulcerative colitis. Gillen and coworkers[123] studied patients with extensive Crohn's disease of the colon and equally extensive ulcerative colitis and found that the relative and the absolute 20-year cumulative incidence of CRC were virtually identical in both groups. Earlier studies did not adjust for the absence of colonic disease, a history of colonic resection, or the duration or extent of disease,[124–126] and this probably resulted in the apparently lower risk of CRC in Crohn's disease. Ekbom and colleagues[127] found that the relative risk of CRC in patients with Crohn's disease regardless of disease localization was approximately 2.5, but in Crohn's colitis the relative risk was 5.6, which is similar to the relative risk seen in ulcerative colitis.

Several factors have been suggested to be associated with a higher risk for CRC in patients with IBD (**Box 21.3**). Most studies have examined risk factors for patients with ulcerative colitis, but it is generally extrapolated that these are probably risk factors in patients with Crohn's disease also. Young age at diagnosis and increasing duration of disease are risk factors, with CRC rarely being diagnosed when ulcerative colitis has been present for less than 8 years; typically, surveillance with colonoscopy does not begin until after 8 years of pancolonic disease. The age of onset has been suggested to be related to the risk of developing CRC.[128,129] A family history of CRC is also a risk factor. Patients with IBD have a relative risk of 2.5 for developing CRC, and patients with IBD who have a first-degree relative with CRC have a relative risk of 3.7; the relative risk is 9.2 if the first-degree relative was diagnosed before age 50 with CRC.[130] The severity of inflammation and extent of the disease are also risk factors for developing CRC in most studies. It has been reported that the incidence ratio for the risk of CRC in patients with proctitis is 1.7; for patients with disease extending beyond the rectum but no further than the hepatic flexure, the incidence ratio is 2.8; and for patients with disease beyond the hepatic flexure, the incidence ratio is 14.8.[129]

Patients with ulcerative colitis and primary sclerosing cholangitis (PSC), a progressive, fibrotic, cholestatic hepatobiliary inflammatory disease, seem to be at increased risk for CRC. Soetikno and coworkers[131] performed a meta-analysis of 11 studies to study this association further. They found an approximate fourfold increased risk for CRC in patients with ulcerative colitis and PSC compared with patients with ulcerative colitis alone. The explanation for this association is unknown. The detection of colitis-associated CRC during colonoscopy is difficult because the dysplasia may be present in macroscopically normal mucosa; it has been suggested that only 20% to 50% of intraepithelial neoplasias can be detected by routine colonoscopy.[132] Cancers in ulcerative colitis grow in a diffusely infiltrating pattern, also hindering the macroscopic diagnosis of dysplasia.[133]

Dysplasia is broadly classified as flat or raised based on its appearance endoscopically. Flat dysplasias occur most often in macroscopically normal mucosa and represent 95% of the dysplasia found.[134] When macroscopically detectable, there is thickened mucosa with mild discoloration and a velvety appearance with evidence of nodularity. If flat dysplasia is found in a biopsy specimen, the patient should undergo a colectomy. Raised dysplasia, or a dysplasia-associated lesion or mass (DALM), is found in less than 5% of patients with dysplasia. DALMs can be subdivided further into adenomalike and non-adenomalike dysplasia. The latter are composed of plaques, masses, or strictured lesions and are prone to progress to colon cancer[135]; these patients, similar to patients with flat dysplasia, should undergo total colectomy. Adenomalike DALMs appear as discrete, sessile or pedunculated polyps. If these lesions are noted on colonoscopy, the patient should undergo polypectomy and biopsy; if the biopsy is negative for adenocarcinoma, the patient does not require a colectomy but rather only increased surveillance. Further studies with long-term follow-up are required to determine the natural history of these lesions. Surveillance programs that focus on colonoscopy with biopsies have been the main method used to detect dysplasia and early cancers in patients with IBD.

In contrast to sporadic CRC, carcinogenesis in IBD does not always follow the typical dysplasia-adenoma-cancer progression. This unpredictable and highly variable sequence of events underlies the importance of increased vigilance and surveillance for CRC in a particularly high-risk population.[136] Although there are no randomized controlled trials, prospective cohort studies, or case-control studies that definitively prove a benefit for surveillance colonoscopy, anecdotal and circumstantial evidence seems to suggest one. Randomized controlled trials are not likely ever to be done because most physicians would consider it unethical to withhold surveillance colonoscopy from a patient with IBD.

Endoscopic Imaging Modalities

Although more recent studies have suggested that dysplasia in IBD may be endoscopically visible,[137,138] it nevertheless can be challenging to determine macroscopically if dysplasia is present. The current standard of care is to obtain four-quadrant jumbo biopsy specimens every 10 cm between the rectum and the cecum, for a total of 40 to 50 random biopsy specimens per colonoscopy in patients with ulcerative colitis. It has been estimated that 33 biopsy specimens are required to give 90% confidence in the detection of dysplasia if it is present.[139] Besides the time-consuming nature and potential increased risk of procedure-related complications with increased numbers of biopsy specimens, this random biopsy approach is most limited by its nondirected technique. As a result, more recent investigative efforts are looking into newer, adjunctive endoscopic imaging modalities to direct biopsies with the goal to enhance detection and discrimination of dysplastic and neoplastic lesions.

Chromoendoscopy may prove to be a more efficient way to obtain biopsy specimens of the colon (**Table 21.8**). In chromoendoscopy, various dyes, such as indigo carmine or methylene blue, are sprayed onto the colonic mucosa to allow for more detailed evaluation of the mucosal surface (**Fig. 21.16**). The rationale is to enhance the sensitivity of detection of otherwise subtle lesions, particularly in the setting of colitis. A secondary aim is to enhance the specificity via enhanced characterization of lesions (**Figs. 21.17 and 21.18**). Studies have shown that not only does chromoendoscopy allow for better differentiation between the neoplastic and nonneoplastic changes in the colon based on the staining pattern,[140] but it also improves early diagnosis of adenomas and CRCs.[141] In a randomized, controlled trial, Kiesslich and colleagues[142] showed that methylene blue–aided chromoendoscopy permitted more accurate diagnosis of the extent and severity of the inflammatory activity in ulcerative colitis compared with conventional colonoscopy. More targeted biopsies were possible, and a statistically significant higher number of intraepithelial neoplasias were detected in the chromoendoscopy group—32 versus 10 in the conventional colonoscopy group (**Fig. 21.19**).

Marion and colleagues[143] provided further evidence in a prospective study of patients with chronic ulcerative colitis or Crohn's colitis comparing methylene blue dye–spray technique with standard colonoscopic surveillance in detecting dysplasia.

Their results showed that specimens obtained with targeted biopsies with dye spray revealed significantly more dysplasia (16 patients with low-grade dysplasia, 1 patient with high-grade dysplasia) than a targeted biopsy protocol (3 patients with low-grade dysplasia). Both techniques were better than conventional random biopsy specimens (four-quadrant every 10 cm), with statistical significance (**Fig. 21.20**).

Chromoendoscopy may prove to be extremely beneficial in the diagnosis of early CRCs in patients with IBD. Although the colonoscopies take longer to perform, with more experience and increasing sensitivity of the biopsy specimens, it still would seem to be a superior surveillance method to standard colonoscopy. The accurate prediction of histology through endoscopic visualization would be of immense value. The Crohn's and Colitis Foundation of America Colon Cancer in IBD Study

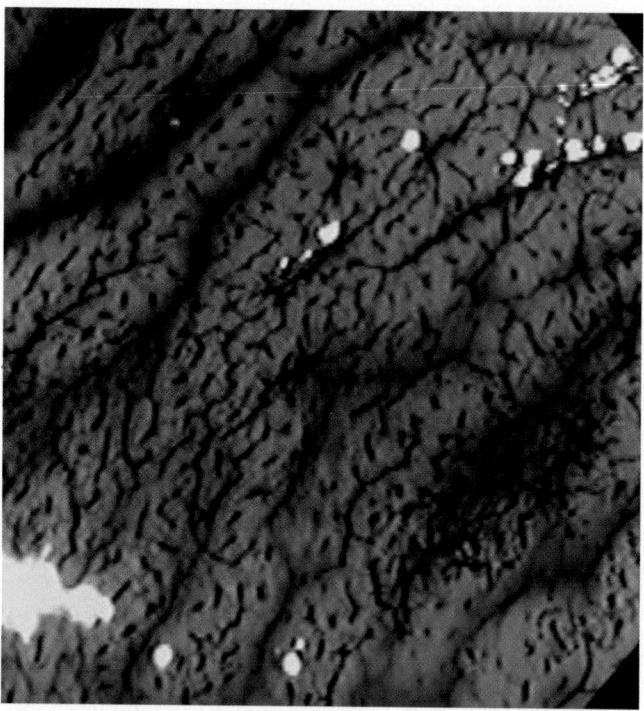

Fig. 21.16 Normal-appearing mucosa with magnification and chromoendoscopy.

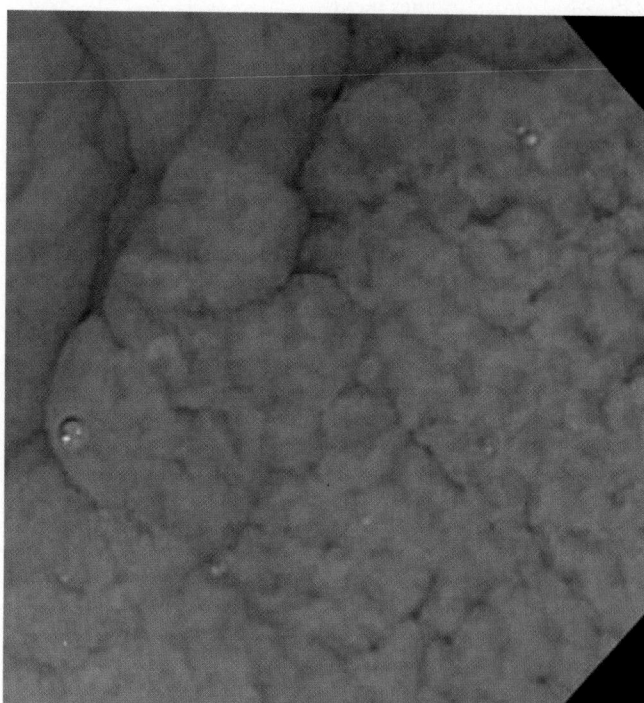

Fig. 21.18 Hyperplastic polyp with magnification and chromoendoscopy.

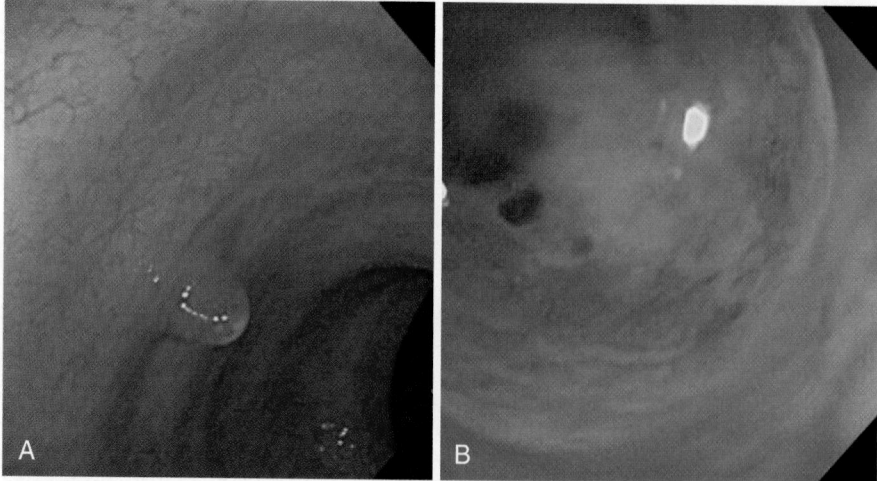

Fig. 21.17 A, Pseudopolyp without magnification and chromoendoscopy. **B,** Pseudopolyp with magnification and chromoendoscopy.

Group endorses the use of chromoendoscopy in surveillance colonoscopy for appropriately trained endoscopists.[144] Consensus incorporation into general guidelines for CRC screening in IBD remains to be established, however, particularly considering the additional endoscopic training required.

Newer techniques are under investigation. Narrow band imaging (NBI) is an optical technology using filters to visualize the microvascular structure of the mucosal layer.[145] NBI and chromoendoscopy showed the same sensitivity (100%) and specificity (75%) to differentiate neoplastic from nonneoplastic lesions (see **Table 21.8**). Comparatively, NBI achieved better visualization of the vascular network, whereas chromoendoscopy achieved more precise characterization of mucosal surface pit pattern. The value of NBI in ulcerative colitis has not yet been established, particularly in mucosa with inflammation affecting vascular structures. Less proven but promising techniques include optical coherence tomography, an optical analogue of ultrasound; fluorescence endoscopy, a technique to reveal neoplastic lesions using autofluorescence or self-induced fluorescence; and confocal laser endomicroscopy, a novel technology allowing subsurface analysis of intestinal mucosa and in vivo histologic examination. Future studies into these newer techniques and refinement of existing ones will continue to aid in further establishing appropriate guidelines and surveillance recommendations. Standardized procedure recommendations are lacking for all of the above-mentioned imaging technologies.

Pouchitis

Pouchitis is an acute inflammatory condition of a pouch or reservoir occurring after a restorative proctocolectomy or continent ileostomy. Pouchitis occurs in 30% to 46% of patients 10 years after surgery.[146,147] Symptoms of pouchitis include diarrhea, urgency, abdominal pain, tenesmus, bleeding, and incontinence. If a patient previously had experienced extraintestinal symptoms of ulcerative colitis, these may often recur during an episode of pouchitis.

The cause of pouchitis is unknown. It has been related to stasis of intestinal contents and bacterial proliferation within the ileal reservoir. This hypothesis is strengthened by data that treatment with metronidazole or ciprofloxacin decreases patients' symptoms; recurrence may arise after cessation of the antibiotics.[148] Impaired use of short-chain fatty acids[149] and recurrent colitis in an ileal mucosa that has undergone colonic metaplasia[150] have also been suggested in the etiology of pouchitis. Women may experience pouchitis more often than men—74% versus 47%.[151] For unclear reasons, smoking may be protective against pouchitis.[152]

Pouchitis is diagnosed by endoscopy and biopsy (**Fig. 21.21**). Endoscopically, the mucosa appears erythematous, friable, and nodular. There is a loss of the normal vascular pattern and contact bleeding. Aphthous ulcers may also be found within the pouch; for this reason, Crohn's disease may resemble pouchitis on endoscopy and should be considered in the differential diagnosis of pouchitis. The differential diagnosis in a patient with pouchitis is either pouchitis with Crohn's disease–like features or Crohn's disease in a patient with a misdiagnosis of ulcerative colitis before surgery; the latter occurs in up to 10% of patients.[153] The endoscopist should always advance the scope proximal to the pouch to the ileum above the pouch, and biopsy specimens should be taken from there. Pouchitis should never spill over into the ileum above the pouch, and if inflammation is found in the ileum above the pouch, the diagnosis of Crohn's disease should be seriously considered.

Dysplasia can occur in the rectal mucosa adjacent to the ileorectal anastomosis because a small amount (usually

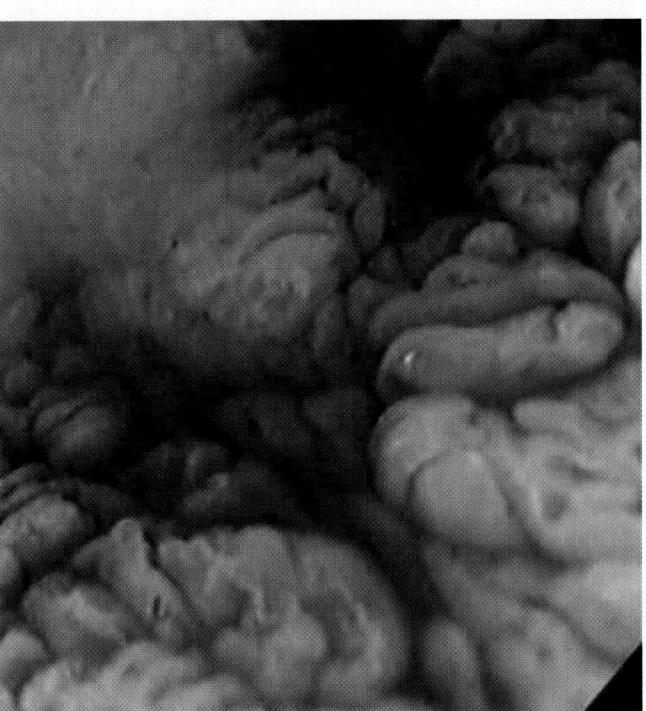

Fig. 21.19 Dysplasia-associated lesion or mass with magnification and chromoendoscopy.

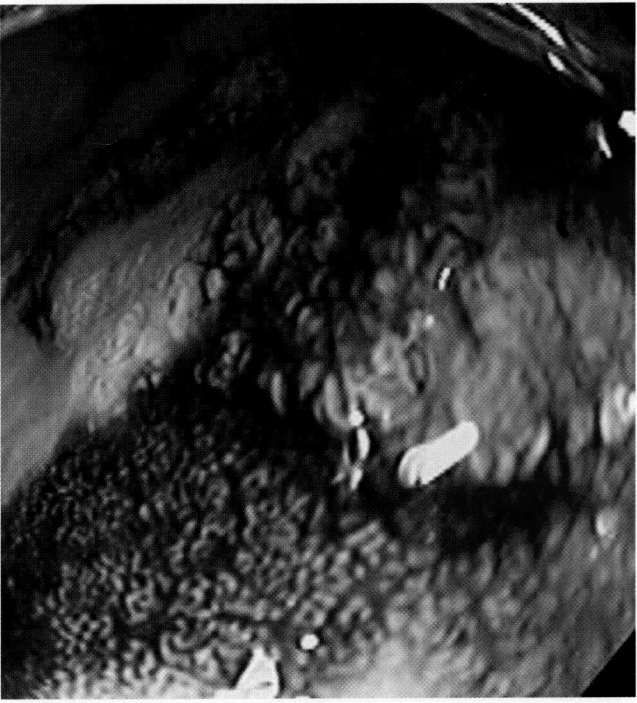

Fig. 21.20 Dysplasia-associated lesion or mass and adjacent normal mucosa.

Table 21-8 **Advantages and Disadvantages of Endoscopic Imaging Techniques**

Imaging Technology	Advantages	Disadvantages
Chromoendoscopy	High sensitivity and specificity for detection of dysplasia	Requires specific endoscopic training for competency
		Increase in DNA lesions with methylene blue-light treatment but unlikely to have biologic significance in vivo
		No standardized procedure recommendations
Magnification endoscopy	May further improve detection of intraepithelial neoplasia, particularly in combination with chromoendoscopic techniques	Inflammation can cause significant image disturbance
		False positivity
		Not useful or practical to use zoom mode permanently when screening lower GI tract
		Difficult to use at high magnification levels, particularly with peristaltic and respiratory movements
		No standardized procedure recommendations
Narrow band imaging	Uniquely visualizes microvascular structure of mucosal layer	Possible difficulty in visualizing microvasculature in the setting of background mucosal inflammation
	Similar sensitivity and specificity to chromoendoscopy for neoplastic lesions	May not be as precise as chromoendoscopy in characterization of surface pit pattern
Optical coherence tomography (OCT)	Provides imaging depth beyond mucosal surface based on similar principles of ultrasound	Resolution of current OCT probes is unsatisfactory
	May be able to predict malignant infiltration into submucosa, helping to guide decision making for mucosal resection	
Fluorescence endoscopy	May allow unmasking of neoplastic lesions by fluorescent technology	Very early technology, limited studies
Confocal laser endomicroscopy	Allows detailed submucosal analysis and in vivo histologic examination during endoscopy	Very early technology, limited studies
	Early studies suggest very high sensitivity, specificity, and accuracy for detection of presence of neoplastic lesions	

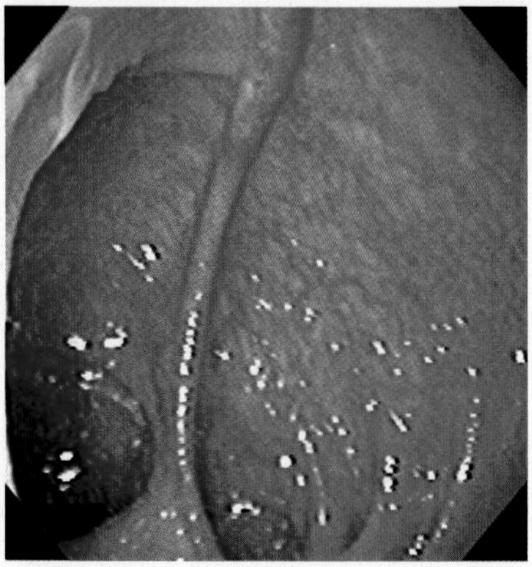

Fig. 21.21 Mild pouchitis in a patient with ulcerative colitis.

approximately 1 to 2 cm of rectal mucosa) of rectum remains in patients who have had ileal pouches. For this reason, patients should undergo periodic surveillance sigmoidoscopy with rectal mucosal biopsy for the evaluation of dysplasia. Risk factors that have been suggested for the development of dys-plasia include a history of primary sclerosing cholangitis, prior colorectal carcinoma, or pouchitis.[154]

Intraoperative Endoscopy

Intraoperative endoscopy has been performed to locate areas of inflammation in the small bowel that are not well defined by radiography before surgery. The endoscope is inserted in a retrograde fashion from the distal opening of the small intestine up to the ligament of Treitz. The benefit of this procedure is questionable because, although more lesions are found intraoperatively than in radiography preoperatively, the findings do not relate to postoperative recurrence of Crohn's disease.[155] In one study, more than half of the lesions found on intraoperative endoscopy were not found radiographically before surgery; however, this endoscopic data modified surgery in only 2 of 20 patients.[156]

The endoscopic findings usually do not alter the decision of the surgeon.[157] The anastomosis can be made in an area of relatively inflamed bowel or at areas of microscopic involvement because this does not seem to be a factor in the postoperative recurrence rate of Crohn's disease.[158–160] Patients treated with radical resections and patients treated with nonradical

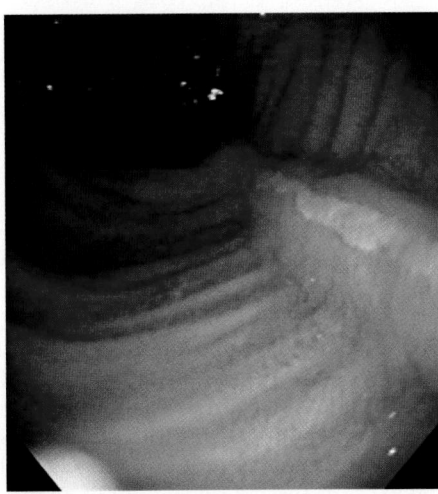

Fig. 21.22 Granulation and ulceration along the suture line in a patient with ileoanal pouch.

resections have the same recurrence rate; a nonradical resection is the preferred surgery for patients with Crohn's disease.[161]

Endoscopy and Ileostomy

When the entire colon is removed in a patient with IBD, the patient can be left with a standard Brooke ileostomy, an ileoanal anastomosis with a pouch, or a continent ileostomy. An upper endoscope is often used for examination of the stoma because of its thin diameter and small radius of tip deflection. The endoscope usually can visualize the distal 10 to 20 cm of the ileostomy stoma (**Fig. 21.22**). Ileoscopy can be beneficial in evaluating a patient with indeterminate colitis who has undergone colectomy and is scheduled for an ileoanal anastomosis. If there is evidence of Crohn's disease, this would argue against proceeding with the ileoanal procedure. This examination is best performed when the patient is in the supine position and can often be done without sedation.

Capsule Endoscopy

Imaging the small bowel is always a challenge for the gastroenterologist, and the methods used to visualize the small intestine were unsatisfactory until more recently. CT scan of the abdomen can show transmural thickening and extramural complications, including periintestinal fat stranding and mesenteric lymphadenopathy, but it is not sensitive enough to detect mucosal inflammation. Push endoscopy has been used more often, but it is extremely uncomfortable, can take 15 to 45 minutes, and requires sedation and analgesia, and there is a danger of perforation.[162] Conventional endoscopic techniques are limited by the length of the small bowel; the endoscope can examine only 10 to 20 cm beyond the ligament of Treitz. Another approach is examination of the entire small intestine by intraoperative endoscopy; this is a more invasive method that carries the standard complication risks of general anesthesia and surgery.[163]

The development of wireless capsule endoscopy (video capsule endoscopy) has offered a new modality for visualizing the small bowel and more recently the upper GI tract (esophagus and stomach) and the colon. It was initially marketed in 2001. The capsule enteroscope contains a miniature video camera, a light source, batteries, and a radio transmitter. Video images are transmitted by radio waves to the sensor array that is attached to the patient. Images of the entire GI tract (for a period of up to 8 hours) can be captured and stored in a portable recorder. Capsule endoscopy has been shown to be superior to standard small bowel examination with barium for suspected small bowel disease.[164] For obscure GI bleeding, evaluation with a small bowel follow-through (using barium) was less effective compared with capsule endoscopy in making a diagnosis—5% versus 31%.[164] In 20 patients with suspected small bowel disease, small bowel follow-through was diagnostic in 20% of patients, whereas capsule endoscopy was diagnostic in 45% of patients, suspicious in 40%, and nondiagnostic in 15% of patients.[164]

In Crohn's disease, capsule endoscopy has been shown to be a superior diagnostic tool compared with small bowel follow-through and CT. Perhaps its greatest utility lies in detection of early small bowel lesions and in diagnostic situations with negative upper and lower endoscopies, along with negative findings on traditional radiographic studies. Eliakim and coworkers[165] found that capsule endoscopy established new diagnoses, confirmed existing diagnoses, established the presence of more extensive disease, and excluded the suspicion of having Crohn's disease in 70% of patients. Small bowel follow-through accomplished this in only 37% of patients. In addition, capsule endoscopy detected all of the lesions detected by small bowel follow-through and CT and found additional lesions in 47% of cases. Capsule endoscopy was also able to rule out lesions found in other modalities in 16% of cases, making capsule endoscopy both more sensitive and more specific than barium follow-through and CT. Fireman and colleagues[166] evaluated the effectiveness of wireless capsule endoscopy in patients with suspected Crohn's disease of the small bowel that had previously been undetected by small bowel follow-though and CT radiography and established a diagnostic yield of 71%. The capsule was able to detect mucosal erosions, ulcers, and strictures, and the degree of severity ranged from mild to severe.

Overall, capsule endoscopy is proving to be a useful modality in a select group of patients with suspected or known inflammatory bowel disease and can aid in defining the diagnosis, extent of disease, and disease activity over time, affecting therapeutic and management decisions. Capsule endoscopy is generally well tolerated by patients. A limitation of the procedure is possible retention of the capsule in patients with Crohn's disease with small bowel strictures or fistulas. In these scenarios, capsule endoscopy is contraindicated. Another disadvantage of the procedure is the time that is required for the physician to review all of the images; the images should be reviewed by individuals who are experienced in viewing and interpreting endoscopic images. Finally, at the present time, there is no validated endoscopic scoring system when describing small bowel inflammatory lesions in patients with Crohn's disease. Proposed variable definitions are based on mucosal villous appearance, ulceration, and stenosis, with each variable additionally characterized by size and extent of change. This endeavor is now ongoing. In the future, capsule endoscopy could potentially play roles in assessing mucosal healing after medical therapy, assessing early postoperative recurrence, and contributing to a better understanding of the natural history of inflammatory bowel disease. Further research is needed to address these nascent avenues.

Endoscopic Retrograde Cholangiopancreatography

PSC is one of the most devastating complications of IBD, occurring in up to 5% of patients with ulcerative colitis and less commonly in Crohn's disease. PSC is a cholestatic disease in which a nonsuppurative, chronic inflammation involves the biliary tree leading to progressive strictures. ERCP is the "gold standard" for diagnosis of PSC. Findings on ERCP include diffuse multifocal annular strictures of the intrahepatic and extrahepatic bile ducts and a characteristic "beads on a string" appearance on cholangiography. ERCP offers the ability to obtain biopsy and brush specimens of these strictures to exclude the diagnosis of cholangiocarcinoma.[167] It also plays a key role in the nonoperative management of cholangitis associated with stricture formation, by allowing for dilation and stenting of dominant strictures.[168,169] PSC can develop before any evidence of colitis is found. Up to 80% of cases of PSC are associated with IBD, most with ulcerative colitis. It is recommended that patients undergo colonoscopy with surveillance biopsy specimens to assess for the presence of subclinical colitis. If either ulcerative colitis or Crohn's colitis is present, it is recommended that annual surveillance colonoscopic evaluation be performed in search of dysplasia.

Conclusions

Although other radiographic imaging modalities are complementary in the diagnosis of IBD, endoscopy plays a key role in diagnosing and managing IBD. Colonoscopy with biopsy is the most sensitive method to detect, diagnose, and differentiate Crohn's disease and ulcerative colitis from all other forms of colitis. Endoscopy is integral in treating many complications of IBD, including stricture formation and bleeding. As the diseases progress, both patients with ulcerative colitis and patients with Crohn's colitis must be routinely evaluated by colonoscopy to assess for any evidence of dysplasia. The gastroenterologist must be well trained to recognize the multitude of endoscopic appearances of IBD. These images and a solid clinical history are crucial in the diagnosis and management of patients with IBD.

References

The complete reference list is available online at www.expertconsult.com.

Infections of the Luminal Digestive Tract

C. Mel Wilcox

Introduction

The management of luminal gastrointestinal (GI) tract infections has been an essential component of the practice of gastroenterology since the birth of the subspecialty. The emergence of endoscopy with mucosal biopsy as a safe and accurate diagnostic tool for patients with suspected infection has elevated the GI endoscopist to a key partner in the management team. The importance of the endoscopist is best appreciated for patients who develop GI complications after organ transplantation and for patients with acquired immunodeficiency syndrome (AIDS). In these settings, infections are the most frequent complications, and the differential diagnosis and diagnostic approach to GI symptoms often differ from the normal host. This chapter provides an overview of GI infections from the endoscopist's perspective based on organ system because the clinical presentation generally points to the site of gut involvement and dictates the diagnostic strategy. The following common themes that are applicable to all GI infections emerge:

1. The clinical presentation is dictated by the infecting pathogen.
2. The severity and chronicity of infection for an immunosuppressed patient are dictated by the cause, duration, and type of immunodeficiency.
3. The endoscopic features of any GI infection are variable and overlapping making definitive diagnosis by biopsy essential.

Epidemiology

The prevalence, incidence, and etiology of luminal GI tract infections are influenced by many factors (**Box 22.1**). In the normal host, luminal GI infections generally occur randomly after exposure to a pathogen and are self-limited. Exposure may take many forms, such as occupational (day care centers), dietary, and environmental (contaminated water). Coexisting host factors may promote the clinical expression of infection and either attenuate or exacerbate the disease. For immunosuppressed patients, the incidence and severity of infection are linked to the cause and degree of the immunodeficiency state. Patients undergoing solid organ transplantation are at the highest risk of infection early on after transplantation because of profound medication-induced immunodeficiency. Latent infections become manifest during this period, and susceptibility to infections is greatest. Over time, however, as drug-induced immunosuppression is tapered, the incidence of infections decreases. For patients infected with human immunodeficiency virus (HIV), the incidence of GI infections increases markedly as immune function deteriorates, and the infection risk can be accurately stratified by the absolute CD4 lymphocyte count and HIV-1 RNA levels.[1,2]

Two additional factors that commonly play a role in the genesis of infection in both immunosuppressed and normal hosts are medication exposure, such as to antibiotics or corticosteroids, and hospitalization; both of these factors may predispose to the development of infection. The array of luminal GI infections is broad and parallels the unique epidemiologic factors of each patient. Numerous infectious pathogens are termed *opportunistic* because they generally complicate only immunodeficiency states. The specific immunodeficiency state, its pathophysiology, and severity dictate the spectrum of complicating pathogens. Within a specific risk group (e.g., solid organ transplantation), the causes and frequency of infections differ because of the variable levels of immunosuppression. Infections are more commonly observed after heart transplantation than liver transplantation because more potent and prolonged drug-induced immunosuppression is required to prevent cardiac rejection.

Rarely, opportunistic infections have been observed in the apparently normal host, but in contrast to an immunodeficient patient, these infections are typically self-limited.[3,4] Generally, the more severe the immunodeficiency state required for development of an opportunistic infection, the less likely the pathogen will be observed in the normal host. Although herpes simplex virus (HSV) is a well-recognized pathogen in otherwise healthy people,[3] HSV esophagitis occurs most often in patients with some predisposing factor. In contrast, until the advent of transplantation, cytomegalovirus (CMV) was a rare pathogen, and its identification in any patient suggests some type of immune dysfunction.[4,5] CMV is regarded as one of the most common opportunistic infections. This frequency of infection relates to the high prevalence of prior exposure to CMV, as reflected by seropositivity rates of more than 90% in developed countries,[6] and to the fact that CMV disease generally occurs from recrudescence of latent infection during periods of profound immunosuppression.

Overall, the frequency of GI infections has been decreasing in immunosuppressed patients. Extensive research has defined the time course and spectrum of infections that complicate immunodeficiency states.[7] Based on these observations, targeted preemptive antimicrobial prophylaxis has become the standard of care against many of these infections during periods of greatest vulnerability. Different classes of agents are used at varying time points depending on the infection risk and pathogens associated with the level of immune impairment. However, antimicrobial prophylaxis is associated with an increased risk for other infections and the development of drug resistance. The use of prophylaxis for *Pneumocystis carinii* infection in AIDS is associated with an increase in the prevalence of other opportunistic infections, such as viral disease, because patients are now living longer.[8] The implementation of *Candida* prophylaxis in selected patients undergoing transplantation and the widespread use of oral antifungal therapies in AIDS has reduced the incidence of fungal infec-

tions in these settings but has been linked with drug resistance to *Candida* species.[9]

The use of highly active antiretroviral therapy for HIV-infected patients has drastically reduced the frequency of GI complications, including infections and neoplasms.[10-12] More selective immunosuppressive therapy, such as with cyclosporine, has been beneficial in reducing the incidence of infections after transplantation.[13] Methods for prophylaxis other than use of antimicrobials have also played a beneficial role in the reduction of opportunistic infections. In high-risk transplant patients, the use of CMV-seronegative organs and blood products for seronegative recipients, the use of leukocyte-depleted platelets for patients after bone marrow transplantation, and the administration of preemptive antiviral therapy all have reduced the incidence of CMV disease.[14,15]

With the increase in international travel for both business and pleasure, geography plays an increasingly important role in the prevalence of some GI infections. Pathogens are endemic in certain portions of the world and in specific regions within countries. In the United States, histoplasmosis is endemic in the Midwest and Mississippi Valley, and coccidioidomycosis is endemic in the Southwest. *Mycobacterium tuberculosis* (TB) is endemic in Third World countries and involvement of the GI tract is well recognized. *Penicillium marneffei* has been described as a pathogen more recently and appears to be limited geographically to Southeast Asia.[16] Traveler's diarrhea, usually caused by enteropathogenic *Escherichia coli*, is characteristically seen with travel to Mexico and other developing countries.[17]

The frequency of luminal GI infections, spectrum of pathogens, severity of infection, and organ involvement are dictated by the combination of exposure, predilection (host factors), and organ-specific tropism of the infecting pathogen. A careful history regarding potential exposures; cause and stage of immunodeficiency, if present; and specific epidemiologic factors germane to the clinical presentation determine the potential causes of infection.

Pathogenesis

The pathogenic mechanisms of luminal GI infections are (1) exposure to a pathogen, (2) reactivation of prior infection (recrudescence), (3) overgrowth of a commensal organism, and (4) local spread or dissemination. The specific organ involved with any infectious process, other than local spread, is dictated by the organ-specific tropism of the infecting pathogen. *Candida* and HSV almost exclusively infect squamous epithelium, whereas *Campylobacter jejuni* and *Shigella* species are colonic pathogens. Inherent to any discussion of pathogenesis is the issue of host-related factors. Numerous nonspecific and immune-based defense mechanisms both prevent and attenuate GI infections.[18] These defenses may be altered by disease, by medications, or as a part of the aging process. Saliva provides an effective physical barrier because of its physical properties, and immunoglobulins that are present in saliva and in intestinal secretions provide an important early line of defense. Gastric acid is a barrier to enteropathogens, and hypochlorhydria has been shown to be a risk factor for the development of cholera and other GI infections.[19] GI motility moves ingested pathogens through the gut and prevents stasis, which can lead to bacterial overgrowth.

Inherent antibacterial proteins secreted by Paneth cells, termed *defensins*, seem to play a key role in the host response to bacterial infections of the gut.[20]

The mucosal immune system is composed of inflammatory cells, most notably T cells.[18] After exposure to a foreign antigen, these cells differentiate into helper or cytotoxic cells depending on whether the cells express the CD4 or CD8 receptor. The release of cytokines by these cells plays a key role in limiting infection but can also result in tissue damage. The critical role of the mucosal immune system in preventing and controlling infections is best shown by the array and severity of luminal GI infections that occur in AIDS, in which a progressive loss of CD4 lymphocytes from both the systemic circulation and the mucosal-based immune system occurs.[21] Loss of these cells predisposes to small intestinal infections by opportunistic infections such as cryptosporidiosis and microsporidiosis. Likewise, lymphocyte dysfunction, either medication-induced or as part of an immunodeficiency state, predisposes to symptomatic primary infection or recrudescence (e.g., CMV).

Most viral GI infections considered here result from recrudescence of infection rather than recent exposure (primary infection). Normally, exposure to these infections occurs during childhood, and the systemic and mucosal-based immune systems keep these infections controlled. However, with immunodeficiency, disease may become overt. *Candida* is a commensal organism of the oropharynx and esophagus. Although *Candida* is usually present in small numbers, overt disease can be observed even in the normal host under certain conditions, such as antibiotic use; use of inhaled or ingested corticosteroids; antacid therapy or hypochlorhydria states; diabetes mellitus; alcoholism; malnutrition; old age; radiation therapy to the head, neck, and chest; and esophageal motility disturbances. Alterations in cellular immunity lead to candidal colonization and superficial infection, and humoral immunity (granulocytes) prevents invasive disease and dissemination.

Bacterial esophagitis is a polymicrobial infection consisting of oral flora, particularly gram-positive organisms, including *Streptococcus viridans,* staphylococci, and other bacilli. This rare cause of esophagitis occurs under conditions of absolute granulocytopenia or severely impaired granulocyte function in which these commensal bacteria invade mucosa that has been damaged from reflux disease, from radiation therapy, or from chemotherapy, leading to an active local infection and potential dissemination.[22] GI infections may result secondarily from active disease in adjacent organs. Esophageal disease may be caused by contiguously infected mediastinal lymph nodes or pulmonary parenchymal infection[23] and by spread of infection via a draining fistula or obstructed lymphatics, resulting in tracheoesophageal fistula.[24] Widespread lymphohematogenous dissemination of opportunistic infections causes either diffuse or focal disease anywhere in the gut; this process is generally limited to only the most severely immunocompromised patients.[25,26]

Most intestinal infections result in tissue inflammation of varying degrees. Local upregulation of cytokines plays a central role in the local immune response to the pathogen but may also cause tissue injury. CMV esophagitis is associated with high mucosal concentrations of the proinflammatory cytokine tumor necrosis factor.[27] Toxin production and virulence factors play a key role in the clinical expression and tissue damage caused by many GI infections, especially bacterial infections.[28]

Luminal digestive tract infections occur under specific epidemiologic conditions and in the appropriate host. The tissue-based immune system is crucial for preventing opportunistic infections; when this system is absent, infection with such pathogens may be chronic and potentially life-threatening. Exposure to the pathogen is important; however, concurrent predisposing factors that were elucidated previously, such as antibiotic or chemotherapy exposure, can play a pathogenic role in both the normal and the immunosuppressed host.

Clinical and Endoscopic Features

Numerous factors guide the approach to a patient with suspected GI infection. Given the breadth of potential etiologic pathogens, the diagnostic strategy should be based on the character and chronicity of the symptoms, the organ systems involved, and the findings on physical examination. As noted previously, for an immunosuppressed patient, the cause and severity of the immunodeficiency syndrome play an important role in the diagnostic approach.

Esophagus
Clinical Features

The most prevalent cause of esophageal infection in both the normal host and the immunosuppressed patient is *Candida* followed by the herpesviruses.[5,29,30] CMV occurs more commonly in patients with AIDS, whereas HSV is more often observed in the normal host and non–HIV-infected immunosuppressed patients. Odynophagia is the characteristic symptom of esophageal infection, and infections resulting in esophageal ulceration almost uniformly cause odynophagia.[5,31] Although less common, dysphagia may be observed with esophageal infections, especially *Candida* esophagitis, or may represent esophageal obstruction or dysmotility from the infection or its sequelae. Bleeding is generally observed only when there is ulceration, and although generally mild, it can be severe if there is an associated coagulopathy. Pulmonary symptoms may predominate when there is fistula formation to the tracheobronchial tree or coexistent pulmonary involvement. Patients with AIDS often have multiple coexisting esophageal disorders, which complicate management further.[5,32]

Physical examination, particularly of the oropharynx, may be helpful in suggesting the diagnosis of esophageal infection. Approximately two-thirds of patients with AIDS and esophageal candidiasis have oral candidiasis (thrush).[33] In other immunocompromised patients, oropharyngeal candidiasis is also commonly associated with esophageal candidiasis.[5] Thrush may be absent, however, if antifungal therapy, such as nystatin, is currently administered. The presence of oropharyngeal candidiasis does not prove that *Candida* is the only cause of symptoms, and the absence of oropharyngeal candidiasis does not exclude *Candida* esophagitis. Patients with chronic mucocutaneous candidiasis may have fungal involvement of various mucous membranes, hair, nails, and skin and have a history of adrenal or parathyroid dysfunction. Coexistent oropharyngeal ulceration is common in patients with HSV esophagitis but is infrequent in patients with CMV esophagitis or other systemic infections.[34,35]

After *Candida* species, herpesviruses are the most frequent infectious agents that cause esophagitis. After transplantation, HSV and CMV occur with equal frequency as causes of esophagitis,[5] whereas in patients with AIDS, HSV esophagitis is uncommon and far less frequent than CMV. In a study of 100 HIV-infected patients with esophageal ulcer, HSV was found in only 9 (in 4, it was a copathogen with CMV).[30] HSV esophageal infection commonly manifests with the sudden onset of severe odynophagia, heartburn, or chest pain.[3,34] Autopsy studies suggest that esophageal symptoms may be absent. Herpes labialis (i.e., cold sores) and oropharyngeal ulcers may coexist, antedate, or develop during the esophageal infection, whereas skin infection is rare.[5] Numerous systemic manifestations, including low-grade fever or upper respiratory symptoms, may precede the onset of esophageal symptoms. In untreated immunocompetent persons, spontaneous resolution of HSV esophageal infection occurs within 2 weeks of the onset of symptoms. Rarely, bleeding is the initial presentation and may be observed in the absence of esophageal complaints.

Odynophagia is almost uniformly present and is characteristically severe with CMV esophagitis. Chest pain, weight loss, and fever may be reported. The onset of symptoms is often more subacute than the acute presentation of HSV. A prior or coexistent diagnosis of CMV infection in other organs (e.g., retinitis or colitis) is frequent. Although rare in transplant patients, retinitis may be observed in approximately 15% of AIDS patients at the time of diagnosis of GI disease.[35] The frequency of esophageal involvement with other pathogens is rare. Bacterial esophagitis has been observed in patients with severe neutropenia, usually patients with hematologic malignancies, but occasionally it is observed after bone marrow transplantation,[36] diabetic ketoacidosis,[37] or steroid therapy. The presentation is similar to the presentation with other infection agents.

Bacteria reported to involve the esophagus include *Brucella,*[38] *Actinomyces,*[39] *Nocardia,*[40] and *Bartonella henselae.*[41] The symptoms of esophageal TB depend on the degree and type of involvement.[24,42,43] Systemic symptoms of fever and weight loss are common. Pulmonary complaints often predominate because of a fistula to the trachea, bronchus, or pleural space. Dysphagia may be prominent with the formation of long strictures or traction diverticula resulting from the fibrotic response. Upper GI hemorrhage caused by esophageal ulcers or tuberculous arterioesophageal fistulas may be the primary manifestation. Bleeding caused by extensive mucosal disease has been described in an AIDS patient with esophageal *Mycobacterium avium* complex (MAC).[44,45] Fungi other than *Candida* species and parasitic diseases have rarely been reported to involve the esophagus.[46-51]

Barium radiography plays a minor role in the diagnosis of esophageal infection. In any patient, the presence of severe odynophagia limits the ability to drink barium, hampering the adequacy of the examination. Although specific barium esophagogram findings may be more typical for certain disorders,[52] given the potential overlap, many of the findings are nonspecific, and endoscopy with biopsy is generally indicated. The wide spectrum of causes coupled with the specific antimicrobial regimens that are required necessitates a definitive diagnosis rather than empiric antimicrobial therapy. Nevertheless, a sinus tract or fistulous connection to the bronchial tree or mediastinum at the level of the hilum is highly sugges-

tive of TB, although it also may be the result of malignancy. An esophageal neoplasm may be mimicked by an ulcerated tuberculous granulomatous mass or CMV ulcer.[42,53] Chest radiography or computed tomography (CT) scan of the chest may support the diagnosis of TB.

Endoscopic Features

The characteristics of the esophageal lesions provide very important diagnostic clues. The location, size, and appearance of all endoscopic abnormalities should be documented because these features form the basis of the differential diagnosis and are useful for comparison on follow-up endoscopic examinations. The differential diagnosis of the lesion dictates how lesions should be sampled and what recommendations for diagnostic testing should be made on the biopsy or cytologic specimens (discussed later). Serologic testing plays no significant role in the diagnosis of acute infectious esophagitis. Endoscopic examination of the esophagus is the most sensitive and specific method for diagnosing esophageal candidiasis (**Table 22.1**).

The gross endoscopic appearance of *Candida* esophagitis is pathognomonic (**Fig. 22.1**) and may be graded according to published criteria.[54] A large, well-circumscribed ulceration should not be attributed to *Candida*. The endoscopic characteristics of HSV esophagitis reflect the pathologic changes. HSV esophagitis appears as discrete, usually small (<1 cm), well-circumscribed shallow ulcers; a diffuse erosive esophagitis; or rarely vesicles (**Fig. 22.2**).[5,55] Small, scattered lesions covered with exudate mimic esophageal candidiasis. Deep ulcers, as seen with CMV, are very rare. CMV esophagitis is characteristically associated with one or more ulcerations that can be quite striking in patients with AIDS. Nevertheless, as with other infections, variability has been reported with appearances ranging from multiple shallow ulcers, to solitary giant ulcers, to a diffuse superficial esophagitis (**Fig. 22.3**).[56] Although serologic testing is not helpful because of the high rate of prior exposure to CMV, the absence of CMV DNA or antigenemia in the blood would suggest an alternative diagnosis. Esophageal TB can manifest with a fistula to the

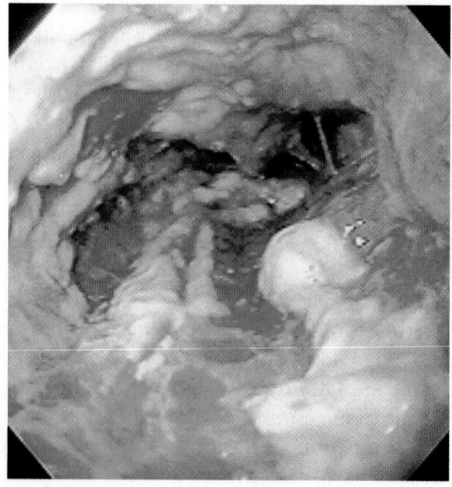

Fig. 22.1 *Candida* esophagitis. Multiple yellow plaques coat the esophageal lumen. In several areas, the plaque has been removed, showing a normal-appearing underlying mucosa.

Table 22.1 Differential Diagnosis of Endoscopic Findings Based on Organ System and Pathogen

Finding	Esophagus	Stomach	Small Bowel	Colon
Plaque	*Candida*	*Cryptococcus*	MAC	*Clostridium difficile*
	HSV	MAC	*Cryptococcus*	CMV
Inflammation*	HSV	CMV	*Cryptosporidium*	Bacteria
	CMV	*Cryptococcus*		CMV
		Cryptosporidium		
Erosion or ulcer	Any infection	CMV	CMV	Bacteria
		TB	*Cryptosporidium* and *Cryptococcus*	CMV
		Syphilis		*Histoplasma*
				Amebae
				Strongyloides
Stricture	CMV	*Cryptosporidium*	CMV	CMV
	TB	TB	TB	TB
	Histoplasma			
	Blastomyces			
Mass	CMV	CMV	CMV	CMV
	TB			*Histoplasma*

*Edema, subepithelial hemorrhage.
CMV, cytomegalovirus; HSV, herpes simplex virus; MAC, *Mycobacterium avium* complex; TB, *Mycobacterium tuberculosis*.

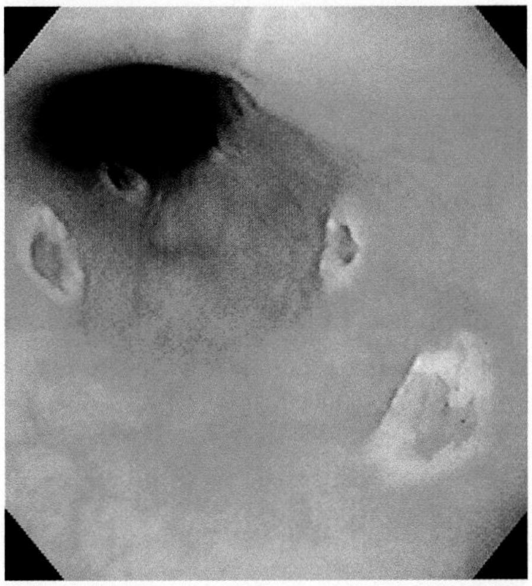

Fig. 22.2 Herpes simplex virus esophagitis. There are multiple small ulcers, some of which have a "volcano" appearance typical for herpes simplex virus. The intervening mucosa is normal.

tracheobronchial tree easily visualized endoscopically and rarely as an ulcer or mass lesion resembling a neoplasm. In normal hosts from endemic areas in South America, *Trypanosoma cruzi* may involve the myenteric plexus of the esophagus resulting in Chagas' disease and an appearance that is indistinguishable clinically, radiographically, manometrically, and endoscopically from idiopathic achalasia.[57] This diagnosis may be established by antibody testing. The endoscopic appearances of other rare infections have been described in case reports and resemble other infections.

Stomach
Clinical Features

Symptomatic gastric infections are much less prevalent than infections of the esophagus. The primary gastric pathogens are *Helicobacter pylori* and CMV; parasites and mycobacteria are also reported but are uncommon.[58] Because of the relative infrequency of gastric infections, understanding of the presentation and endoscopic findings of most of these infections is based on case reports or small series. With the exception of *H. pylori*, most infections of the stomach occur in the setting of an immunodeficiency state. Gastric infections are typically manifested by upper abdominal pain that is generally steady and may radiate to the back. Associated symptoms may include nausea with or without vomiting; vomiting may be prominent when mucosal infection is severe. Infrequently, nausea alone in the absence of abdominal pain may be observed. Fever and weight loss are variable. Diarrhea may be the prominent symptom if the infecting pathogen also involves the small bowel (e.g., *Cryptosporidium*). Bleeding, both occult and overt, is usually a marker of mucosal ulceration. However, because most gastric infections are superficial, severe bleeding is unusual unless there is an associated coagulopathy.

As in the esophagus, the primary symptom is dictated by the infecting pathogen. CMV gastric infection typically produces ulceration; abdominal pain with or without bleeding is the most frequent presentation. Mucosal infections that result in gastritis without ulceration such as cryptosporidiosis more commonly manifest with nausea without pain or may be asymptomatic. *H. pylori* infection of the stomach is generally considered an asymptomatic infection in most people regardless of immune status. Physical examination is generally unrevealing. Mild abdominal pain may be elicited on palpation of the epigastrium. A Hemoccult-positive stool is nonspecific.

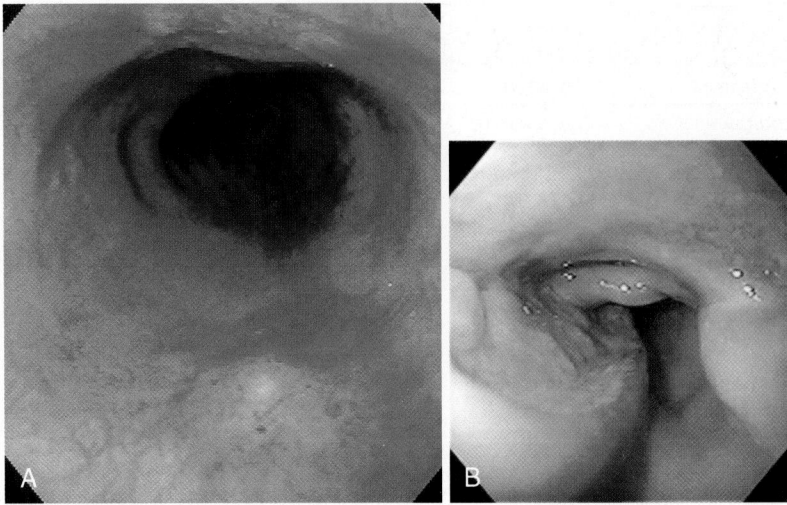

Fig. 22.3 Cytomegalovirus esophagitis. **A,** Two ulcers in the midesophagus with normal surrounding mucosa. **B,** Large hemicircumferential ulcer in the midesophagus with heaped-up margins.

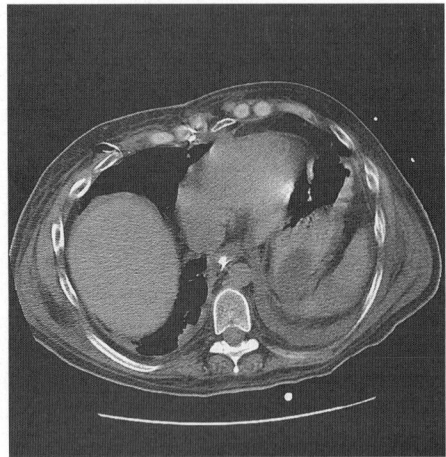

Fig. 22.4 Gastric mucormycosis. Computed tomography (CT) scan shows a large hypodense area in the gastric wall.

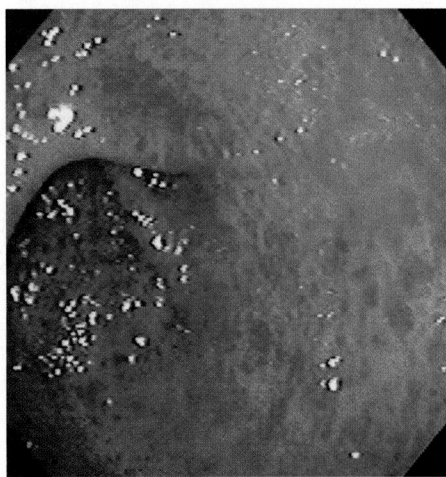

Fig. 22.5 Cytomegalovirus gastritis. There is diffuse subepithelial hemorrhage, some of which is confluent in the gastric antrum. Several small erosions were also present in this patient.

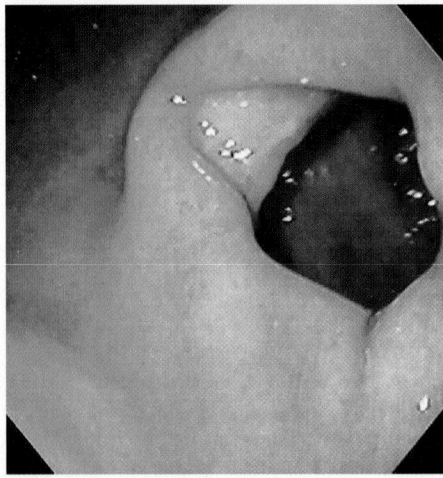

Fig. 22.6 Pyloric channel ulcer resulting from cytomegalovirus. Hemicircumferential ulceration with a clean base in the pyloric channel. This lesion resembles a peptic ulcer.

Radiologic studies may suggest the presence of gastric infection. Although abnormalities can often be identified, the findings are typically nonspecific, and further investigation with endoscopy is often required. Barium findings of gastric infection may include fold thickening or ulceration, whereas the most common CT finding is wall thickening, usually diffuse, and focal lesions mimicking a mass lesion (**Fig. 22.4**).

Endoscopic Features

Similar to all GI infections, the primary endoscopic abnormality is dictated by the infecting pathogen, and the severity of disease clinically and endoscopically depends on the presence and degree of immunodeficiency. CMV, the most common opportunistic gastric pathogen, generally manifests with a diffuse gastritis characteristically with a hemorrhagic component (**Fig. 22.5**). Mucosal breaks are typical with focal or diffuse erosions or frank ulcerations (**Fig. 22.6**) that may be large, are usually well circumscribed, and may mimic a malignancy.[53,59] Ulcerations have also been described with fungi, secondary to syphilis.[60–63] The endoscopic features of gastric cryptosporidiosis and mycobacterial infection may appear as inflammation, polyps, or antral narrowing.[64–66] In the normal host, gastric anisakiasis has been associated with ingestion of raw fish, and the *Anisakis* larvae may be visualized and removed at the time of endoscopy (**Fig. 22.7**).[67]

Small Intestine
Clinical Features
Parasitic disorders are the predominant cause of small bowel infection. In the normal host, *Giardia* infection predominates.

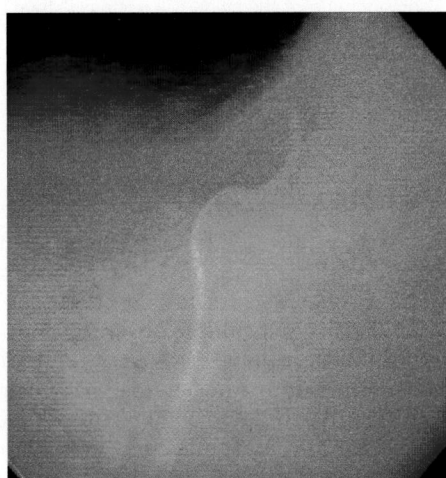

Fig. 22.7 Anisakiasis. A well-circumscribed area of subepithelial hemorrhage is seen with a small worm emanating from the center of the hemorrhage. The worm was removed with biopsy forceps.

With the exception of CMV, opportunistic small bowel infections are uncommon in transplant patients, but they are a hallmark of AIDS, where *Cryptosporidium* and microsporidia are frequent pathogens. Although typically a pathogen complicating immunodeficiency syndromes, self-limited cryptosporidiosis has been observed in the normal host usually during single-source outbreaks and may be a more common cause of acute diarrhea than previously thought.[68] MAC, a pathogen principally restricted to patients with AIDS, is a common small bowel pathogen that is widely disseminated at the time of diagnosis (**Fig. 22.8**). A localized proximal small bowel infection can occur with CMV, and distal ileitis has been reported with CMV, bacteria, mycobacteria, fungi, and parasites.[26,69–75]

Diarrhea is the hallmark of small bowel infections; the severity and chronicity depend on the etiology and the host. Severe watery diarrhea causing dehydration is characteristic of intestinal cryptosporidiosis, whereas less severe diarrhea is observed with most other pathogens. Although crampy abdominal pain may be seen with any diarrheal disorder, more constant discomfort would be most typical for CMV enteritis and MAC.[44] Symptoms of malabsorption may be prominent when the infection is diffuse and severe, although overt steatorrhea suggests pancreatic rather than small intestinal disease. Significant borborygmi may occur when the diarrhea is more voluminous. Because CMV generally causes focal mucosal ulceration sparing the intervening mucosa, abdominal pain and overt bleeding can be observed in the absence of diarrhea.

Weight loss may be profound with some infections. As noted, a distal ileitis, as reported from CMV, bacteria, TB, MAC, and parasites including *Isospora,* may result in a right lower quadrant pain syndrome. An acute abdomen can result

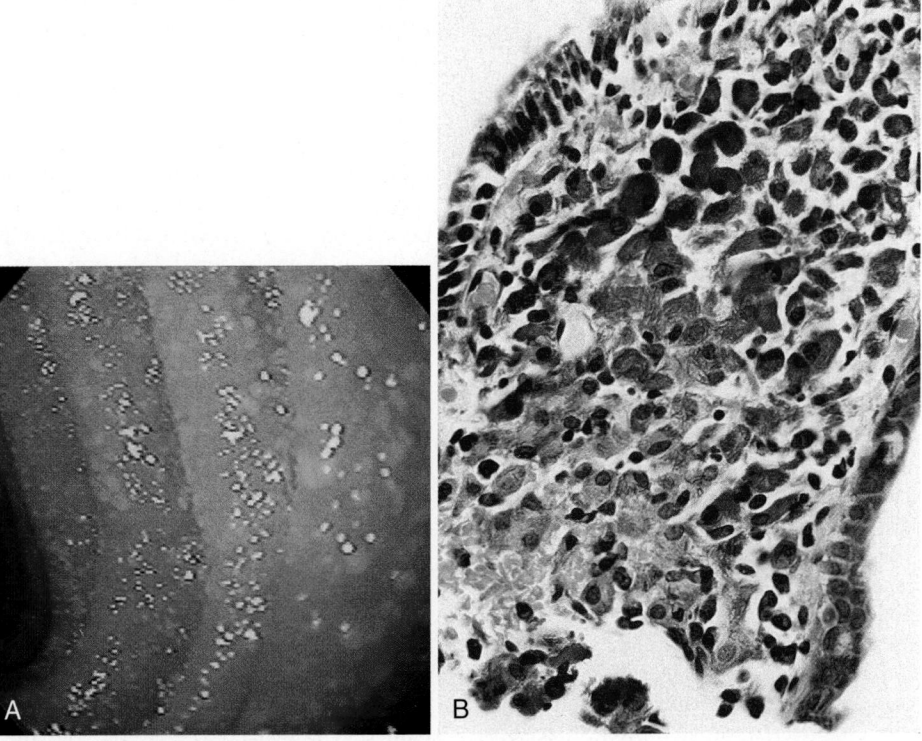

Fig. 22.8 Duodenal *Mycobacterium avium* complex (MAC). **A,** Multiple well-circumscribed papular lesions typical for intestinal MAC. **B,** Acid-fast staining of mucosal biopsy specimens shows numerous mycobacteria filling the lamina propria.

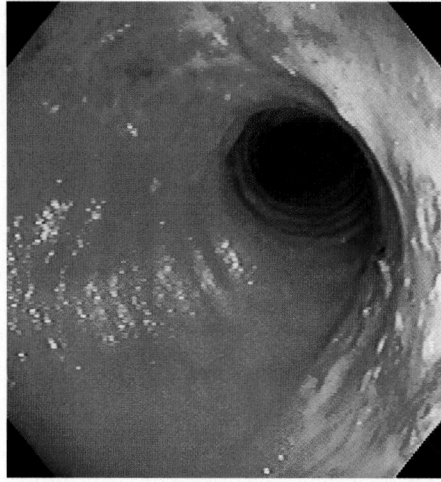

Fig. 22.9 Cytomegalovirus ileitis. There is well-circumscribed hemicircumferential ulceration at the ileocolonic anastomosis after heart transplant and right hemicolectomy.

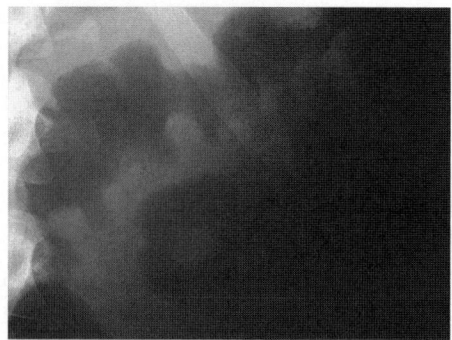

Fig. 22.10 Thumbprinting of the colon. Characteristic thumbprinting is seen on this plain abdominal radiograph of a patient with bacterial colitis.

from intestinal perforation and is most commonly due to CMV.[76] The physical examination is variable from normal to cachexia and dehydration. Dehydration and electrolyte abnormalities would suggest a more severe process, such as cryptosporidiosis. Abdominal tenderness may be elicited and would suggest CMV or perhaps MAC. Occult blood in the stool is nonspecific. Extraintestinal signs and symptoms may be associated with infection by *Yersinia* species.[75] Radiologic studies are of limited use in the setting of suspected small bowel infection. Small bowel barium studies may obscure stool studies and should be avoided. CT can be helpful if thickened small bowel segments are visualized, although the differential diagnosis is broad.[73,76,77]

Endoscopic Features

The endoscopic findings of small bowel infections vary from normal to widespread hemorrhage and ulceration. Focal erosions and ulcerations are typical for a viral infection with CMV, whereas minimal mucosal changes, if any, are common with parasitic diseases. Ulcers have also been reported with *Toxoplasma*.[72] Small bowel atrophy is associated with some of these infections and endoscopically mimics celiac sprue.[78] MAC infection has a characteristic appearance of small to confluent nodular lesions often with a yellow color resembling Whipple's disease (see **Fig. 22.8**). Disseminated fungal infections can also manifest with small nodular lesions.[79] Rarely, obstructive symptoms may predominate if there is an obstructive process. Stricture and ulceration of the ileum is typical for TB and rare for CMV (**Fig. 22.9**); these are best characterized by radiographic rather than endoscopic examination.[80,81] Ileitis can also be observed with some bacterial infections, including *Yersinia* species and *Salmonella* species.[74,82] The endoscopic and radiographic features of any severe ileitis may mimic Crohn's disease. The diffuse nature of most small bowel infections highlights the importance of ileal examination with mucosal biopsy if colonoscopy is performed. Capsule endoscopy may also help characterize small bowel infections, although mucosal biopsy would require double-balloon enteroscopy.

Colon
Clinical Features

In contrast to the upper GI tract, bacteria are the most common colonic pathogens. *Campylobacter* is the most prevalent isolate in most series of acute infectious diarrhea and colitis.[28] Depending on the clinical setting, CMV is the most frequent opportunistic pathogen, whereas *Clostridium difficile* remains an important pathogen in all patients regardless of immune status. Diarrhea and abdominal pain are the cardinal manifestations of colonic infection. Acute diarrhea with urgency, tenesmus, and small-volume bleeding is typical for bacterial colitis in any patient regardless of immune status. Although colonic infection is typically acute, especially in the normal host, chronic or recurrent diarrhea may be observed in immunodeficient patients. If the proximal colon is preferentially involved, right-sided abdominal pain may predominate. Bleeding is uniformly present with *E. coli* O157H7 enteritis, and this infection should not be considered in its absence.[83] Parasitic diseases can involve the colon and manifest either acutely (amebic disease) or with a chronic watery diarrhea (cryptosporidiosis); concomitant small bowel disease is seen with cryptosporidiosis. Microsporidia do not infect the colon.[84] Colonic CMV infection characteristically manifests as a chronic watery diarrhea; pain is often a prominent feature, and occult and overt bleeding may occur. Fever is common in bacterial infection, less so with CMV, and absent in most parasitic disorders. MAC can involve the colon; although rare in developed countries, TB involvement of the colon is well recognized.[80] Toxic megacolon and perforation may complicate severe infection with either bacteria or viruses.[85]

The physical examination is generally dictated by the infecting pathogen. With acute bacterial colitis, the patient may appear toxic and have significant abdominal tenderness suggesting an acute abdomen, and the pain may predominate over the diarrhea. Fever and abdominal pain may also be the main features of severe *C. difficile* colitis. Laboratory studies may show a leukocytosis with left shift, which may approach a leukemoid reaction, but are otherwise nonspecific. The most common radiographic study used in colonic infection is CT scanning. CT scans are often performed because of the marked pain that is observed. Colonic wall thickening, which may be dramatic, is the typical finding for any colitis and may be found on routine abdominal radiographs (**Fig. 22.10**).

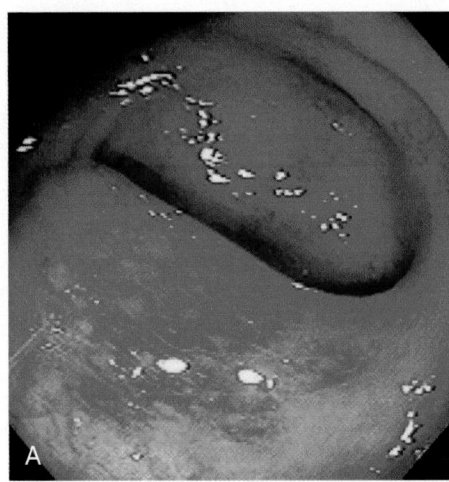

Fig. 22.11 *Campylobacter* colitis. **A,** Focal area of subepithelial hemorrhage and erosion in the cecum. **B,** Hematoxylin and eosin staining of cecal biopsy specimens shows preserved architecture, mucosal edema, subepithelial hemorrhage, and acute inflammatory cells. These findings are typical for acute self-limited colitis resulting from a bacterial infection.

Additional findings on CT may include small bowel thickening or lymphadenopathy.[85,86] Depending on the infectious cause, radiographic abnormalities may be either focal or diffuse. Barium enema examination, if indicated, should not be performed in patients with suspected colonic infection until all stool studies are collected.

Endoscopic Features

The endoscopic findings in colonic infection range from normal to severe pancolonic edema and ulceration typical for a fulminant ulcerative colitis. *Campylobacter, Shigella,* and *Salmonella* infections may appear similar endoscopically with mucosal edema, subepithelial hemorrhage, erosions, and ulcers of varying size (**Fig. 22.11**). Distal disease is typical for *Campylobacter* and *Shigella* infections, whereas infections with *Salmonella* and *Yersinia* preferentially involve the right colon and ileum.[87–89] *Salmonella typhi* infection results in lymphoid hyperplasia leading to ulceration at the site of Peyer's patches; this may explain the geographic location in the bowel.[90]

With any bacterial colitis, the colitis may be patchy, segmental, or diffuse. *C. difficile* colitis has a well-recognized appearance of plaquelike lesions that are typically confluent and are generally present in the distal colorectum (**Fig. 22.12**). When the disease is severe, mucosal edema is prominent. Subepithelial hemorrhage is characteristic of CMV infection, as is ulceration of variable distribution (**Fig. 22.13**). An appearance of inflammatory bowel disease, either ulcerative colitis or Crohn's disease, has been described with bacteria and CMV.[91] HSV can rarely involve the colon, but generally only the distal rectum and anus are involved given the tropism of HSV for squamous mucosa. Amebic colitis may resemble a fulminant colitis or more commonly cause multiple ulcers that can be mistaken for idiopathic inflammatory bowel disease (**Fig. 22.14**).[92] The colonoscopic findings of cryptosporidiosis may be minimal edema or normal-appearing colon. TB may manifest with a mass lesion or serpiginous ulceration and nodularity.[80] Fungi have rarely been reported to involve the colon with histoplasmosis noted to cause ulceration or mass lesions resembling carcinoma.[26,93] Helminthic and other pathogens of the colon

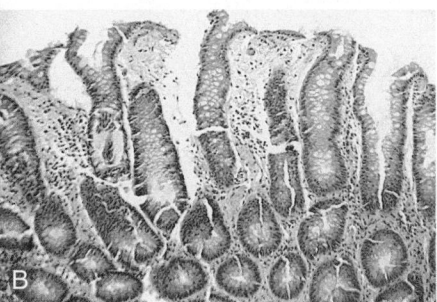

Fig. 22.12 *Clostridium difficile* colitis. Typical yellow plaques are in the distal colon.

have also been described.[94,95] Abdominal CT may be helpful when evaluating for complications such as toxic megacolon.

Pathology

The pathologic features of GI infections depend on the infecting pathogen, and tissue tropism dictates the organs of involvement. The gross pathologic appearance of esophageal candidiasis ranges from a few white or yellow plaques on the mucosal surface to a dense, thick plaque coating the mucosa and encroaching on the esophageal lumen. Although potentially misinterpreted as "ulcer," this plaque material is composed of desquamated squamous epithelial cells, admixed with fungal organisms, inflammatory cells, and bacteria.[54] True ulceration (granulation tissue) is rarely caused by *Candida* alone and has been documented most commonly in patients with profound granulocytopenia or when *Candida* is a coinfection with another cause of ulceration.[32] More deep-seated submucosal infections can occur with some fungi, and disseminated fungal infections can lead to ulceration.

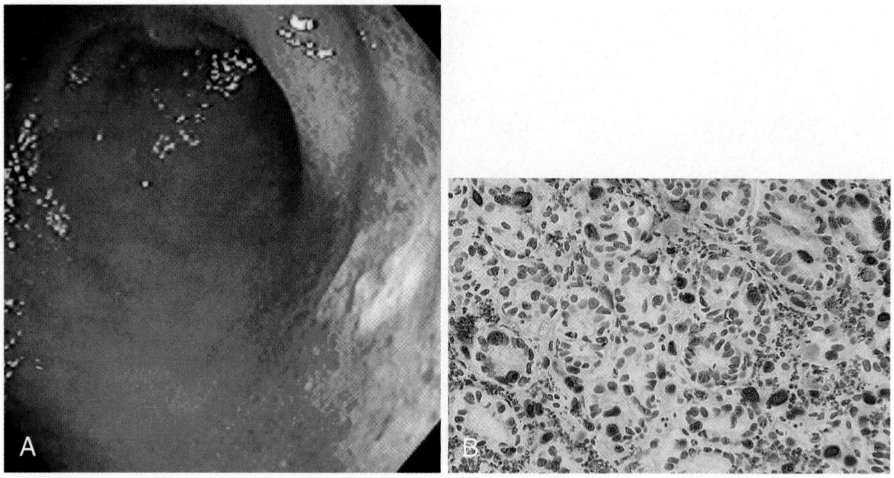

Fig. 22.13 Cytomegalovirus (CMV) colitis. **A,** Diffuse subepithelial hemorrhage typical for CMV infection. **B,** Immunohistochemical stain for CMV antigens highlights the numerous infected cells.

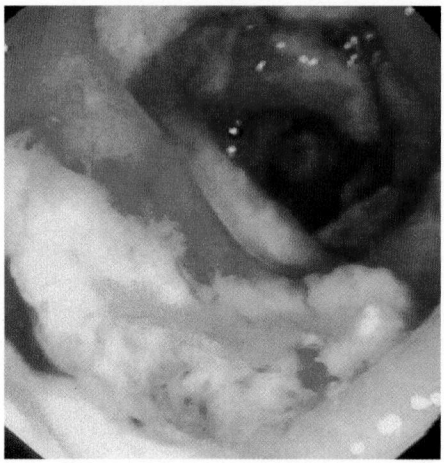

Fig. 22.14 Amebic colitis. Patchy erosions and ulcer are suggestive of inflammatory bowel disease. *(Courtesy of John L. Meisel, MD.)*

Viral infection characteristically results in mucosal erosion and ulceration regardless of the site of infection. HSV infection is generally limited to squamous mucosa, where the earliest manifestation is a vesicle. As these vesicles enlarge and ulcerate, they coalesce to form larger superficial lesions, which are typically focal leaving the intervening mucosa normal. Microscopic examination of the squamous epithelial cells at the ulcer edge reveals multinucleation, ground-glass nuclei, and eosinophilic Cowdry's type A inclusion bodies that may take up half of the nuclear volume. With progression, these inclusion bodies may be surrounded by halos and may become more basophilic, filling, enlarging, and deforming the nucleus.

The histologic hallmark of CMV esophagitis is mucosal ulceration. Although variable, deep ulcers are very characteristic for disease in patients with AIDS, whereas in other immunocompromised patients, lesions tend to remain more superficial. Despite the depth of the lesions, perforation is rare. In contrast to HSV, the viral cytopathic effect of CMV is located in endothelial and mesenchymal cells in the granulation tissue of the ulcer base rather than in squamous cells. Inclusions are large (cytomegalic) and often have an eosino-philic appearance that may be located either in the nucleus or in the cytoplasm.[96] The inclusions can assume an atypical appearance especially in patients with AIDS[97]; immunohistochemical stains play a valuable role in selected patients to confirm the presence of CMV, and they often highlight more infected cells than are appreciated by routine hematoxylin and eosin staining (see **Fig. 22.13B**).[98] CMV may coexist with HSV or *Candida* or other pathogens in patients with AIDS. The gross pathologic appearance of bacterial esophagitis depends on the etiologic pathogen and ranges from diffuse, shallow ulcerations to ulcers associated with erythema, plaques, pseudomembranes, nodules, or hemorrhage.

Microscopic examination reveals pseudomembranes and bacterial invasion that may be superficial and limited to squamous epithelium or may be invasive and transmural with infiltration of blood vessels (i.e., phlegmonous esophagitis). Esophageal actinomycosis is characterized by ulceration and sinuses leading from abscess cavities with sulfur granules and filamentous gram-positive branching bacteria seen on tissue biopsy specimens.[39] In the one reported case, *B. henselae* esophagitis resulted in multiple nodules resulting from a lobulated proliferation of capillary vessels lined by plump endothelial cells.[41] Bacterial infection of the stomach is generally limited to *H. pylori* infection, which has the characteristic active chronic gastritis often with lymphoid aggregates.[99] Phlegmonous gastritis, whose pathogenesis is not well understood, may involve gram-positive and gram-negative bacilli.[100] Acute bacterial colitis is pathologically shown by crypt abscess with a preponderance of polymorphonuclear leukocytes and preservation of the mucosal architecture. These features help distinguish these processes from idiopathic inflammatory bowel disease.[101]

TB generally results in disease secondarily from paraesophageal infected nodes in the midesophagus at the level of the carina or tracheoesophageal fistula. In other parts of the gut, primary mucosal infection can occur. Histologically, granulomas are often present in ulcer tissue, with mycobacteria identifiable by mycobacterial staining. MAC, in contrast to TB, may not result in well-formed granulomas. Staining for MAC often yields an abundance of organisms (see **Fig. 22.8B**), whereas tuberculous bacilli may be few in number even in patients with AIDS.

Table 22.2 Suggested Regimens for Treatment of Luminal Gastrointestinal Infections

Pathogen	Drug	Dosage	Route	Duration	Efficacy (%)
Candida	Ketoconazole	200–400 mg/day	PO	7–14 days	<80
	Fluconazole	100 mg/day	PO/IV	7–14 days	~80
	Itraconazole	200 mg/day	PO	7–14 days	~80
	Voriconazole	400 mg for 2 doses then 200 mg bid	—	—	—
	Caspofungin	70 mg loading dose then 50 mg/day	—	—	—
	Amphotericin B	0.5 mg/kg/day	PO/IV	7 days	>95
Histoplasma	Amphotericin B	—	IV	—	>90
	Ketoconazole	—	—	—	—
Other fungi	Amphotericin B	—	—	—	—
CMV	Ganciclovir	5 mg/kg bid	IV	2–4 wk	~75
	Foscarnet	90 mg/kg bid	IV	2–4 wk	~75
	Valganciclovir	900 mg bid	PO	14 days	>90
HSV	Acyclovir	400 mg five times/day	PO/IV	14 days	>90
	Valacyclovir	1 g tid	PO	14 days	>90
	Famciclovir	500 mg tid	PO	14 days	>90
	Foscarnet	90 mg/kg bid	IV	14 days	>95
	Ganciclovir	5 mg/kg bid	IV	14 days	>95
Mycobacteria	Same as for pulmonary disease				
Bacteria	Based on infecting species				
Idiopathic ulcer	Prednisone	40 mg/day, taper	PO	4 wks	>90
	Thalidomide	200–300 mg/day	PO	4 wks	>90

CMV, cytomegalovirus; IV, intravenous; HSV, herpes simplex virus; PO, oral (per os).

Although generally an excellent stain, hematoxylin and eosin staining may not identify all pathogens. Various pathogen-specific stains are available to aid in the identification of nearly all common GI infections (with the exception of non-herpesviruses). These stains highlight infecting pathogens and make identification easier. Immunohistochemical stains for viral antigens are very helpful when examining for herpesviruses.[102] Because a battery of stains is not routinely performed on all biopsy specimens, communication with the pathologist is essential to ensure appropriate pathologic evaluation.

Differential Diagnosis

Diagnostic considerations are determined by the clinical presentation, risk group and severity of immunodeficiency, and specific endoscopic findings. Although overlap is broad, some endoscopic abnormalities are typical for a specific pathogen and may be organ-specific (see **Table 22.1**). In the esophagus, CMV esophagitis and the idiopathic esophageal ulcer of AIDS are difficult to differentiate.[35,103] These two processes generally result in one or more large ulcers. Pill-induced esophagitis must be excluded by history because the pathologic findings of esophageal biopsy specimens are similar. Likewise, distal esophageal ulcer may suggest gastroesophageal reflux disease, and the histopathologic features cannot distinguish idiopathic esophageal ulcer from gastroesophageal reflux disease. The

clinical history is different, however, and the endoscopic appearance helps suggest gastroesophageal reflux. Small esophageal ulcers can be observed in the acute phase of HIV infection, which can mimic viral or pill-induced esophagitis.[104] Esophageal strictures can result from opportunistic infections.[105] The history coupled with mucosal biopsy helps differentiate infection from gastroesophageal reflux disease.

The appearance of the small bowel is similar in many infections and can be normal. The cause of bacterial colitis, with the exception of *C. difficile*, can rarely be differentiated by presentation or endoscopic appearance alone, although some infections may favor a proximal or distal location. In this setting, stool culture and blood culture may be diagnostic. In an immunosuppressed patient with chronic diarrhea, one or more colonic ulcers associated with subepithelial hemorrhage are highly suggestive for CMV, but this appearance can result from other disorders as well.

Treatment

Effective antimicrobial therapies are available for most GI infections (**Table 22.2**). The pathogen rather than the organ of involvement dictates the treatment regimen. Systemic therapy should be provided for patients with severe disease and associated immunodeficiency. In the normal host, many infections are acute and self-limited and require no specific therapy. Antimicrobial therapy may be contraindicated and potentially harmful with some infections, such as *E. coli* O157H7, in which antibiotic therapy may be associated with hemolytic uremic syndrome in children.[106] For HIV-infected patients, treatment of the underlying immunodeficiency with highly active antiretroviral drugs is quite effective and is fundamental to the treatment of any opportunistic infection in this setting. Antiretroviral therapy alone can result in remission of some opportunistic infections and AIDS-associated neoplasms, which underscores the importance of immune reconstitution in any setting.[107,108] Likewise, in a transplant patient, reducing the dosage of immunosuppressive drugs, when possible, plays an important adjunctive role in the management of any opportunistic infection.

Indications and Contraindications

Luminal GI infections are generally suspected clinically, and the diagnosis can often be established by noninvasive studies. Small bowel and colonic infections, which are manifested by diarrhea, can be diagnosed by routine stool studies. Blood cultures in a febrile patient may be diagnostic, and bone marrow examination may be helpful in certain situations in which a disseminated infection is suspected. In the appropriate setting, endoscopic evaluation may not be indicated initially; instead, empiric therapy directed at suspected pathogens may be the best initial strategy. For HIV-infected patients at risk for esophageal candidiasis, in whom oropharyngeal candidiasis is found, an empiric trial of fluconazole therapy should be performed first, and endoscopic evaluation should be reserved for nonresponders (discussed later). Although stool studies may identify a pathogen in a patient who is not severely ill and in whom diarrhea is chronic, when the infection is acute and severe, early endoscopy may be helpful in suggesting the etiology and directing therapy until the biopsy results return.

The contraindications for endoscopic evaluation are generally similar to contraindications for any other patient. Severe coagulopathy must be recognized and treated appropriately if mucosal biopsies are anticipated. However, the endoscopic appearance alone, as noted previously, may be diagnostic in some cases, obviating a need for routine biopsy in this setting.

Preoperative History and Considerations

The clinical history and epidemiologic features dictate the potential cause of intestinal infection. Patients at risk for pulmonary TB must be recognized before upper endoscopy is performed so that the appropriate respiratory precautions are taken. Specialized media for endoscopic biopsies may be required in some settings. Culture media for mycobacteria should be available when TB is considered. Coagulopathy must be recognized before endoscopy.

In patients with AIDS and thrush, the presence of dysphagia or odynophagia usually indicates *Candida* esophagitis. In a symptomatic patient with associated thrush, an empiric trial of antifungal therapy should be instituted, reserving endoscopy for patients who fail to respond. Further evaluation should be delayed no longer than 1 week for patients with severe persistent symptoms because the response to antifungal therapy is rapid, with clinical improvement occurring in most patients within days.[109,110] If patients fail to improve with empiric antifungal therapy, endoscopy should be performed because disorders other than *Candida* are identified in most

patients.[111] This empiric strategy has not been critically studied in the transplant setting; however, clinical experience suggests it is effective. Empiric therapy for acute diarrhea in other immunosuppressed patients is commonly practiced, but few studies exist.

Description of Techniques

No specific techniques are generally required for the endoscopic evaluation of GI infection. Based on the suspected cause clinically, endoscopically, and pathologically, additional stains may be required, necessitating close collaboration with the pathologist to diagnose these infections accurately. Because most infections can be diagnosed on tissue biopsy alone, multiple biopsy specimens of endoscopic abnormalities should be obtained to increase diagnostic yield. Even when the mucosa appears normal, multiple biopsy specimens should be taken when infection is suspected. During endoscopy, mucosal lesions can be brushed and submitted for cytologic evaluation, or biopsy specimens can be obtained for histologic diagnosis. Esophageal brushings with cytologic evaluation may be diagnostically helpful in certain diseases, such as those resulting from *Candida* and HSV, but are not helpful for diagnosis of CMV disease.

Viral culture of biopsy specimens may increase the diagnostic yield, although false-positive and false-negative results occur, and viral cultures are less sensitive than multiple biopsy specimens. Use of shell vial techniques improves the turnaround time for CMV culture to 48 hours. Bacterial culture of colonic biopsy specimens has been found in some series to enhance the diagnostic yield. Cytologic brushings and endoscopic mucosal biopsy specimens should be taken from the ulcer edge when HSV disease is suspected because the viral cytopathic effect is best identified in epithelial cells rather than in granulation tissue in the ulcer bed.[112] In contrast, a biopsy specimen of the ulcer base must be obtained when viral infection is suspected with CMV (**Fig. 22.15**). Multiple biopsy specimens (up to 10) may be required to establish the diagnosis in patients with AIDS and should be taken from the base of the ulcer.[113] Overall, mucosal biopsy for histologic diagnosis is the preferred method to distinguish the cause of ulcer.[114] Culture of an aliquot of stool obtained at colonoscopy and bacterial culture of mucosal biopsy specimens may increase the diagnostic yield.[115]

As mentioned previously, many histologic stains are available to identify pathogens. Immunohistochemical staining on biopsy samples using specific monoclonal antibodies to viruses such as HSV and CMV helps confirm the diagnosis when the viral cytopathic effect is difficult to appreciate. We generally rely on histology for the diagnosis of viral GI infections and use brushings and viral culture selectively. A technique first described for gastric biopsies, whereby the forceps are tilted into the lesion and the tissue is avulsed, is especially useful for taking samples from esophageal lesions (**Fig. 22.16**). Lastly, as noted previously, communication with the pathologist is essential so that appropriate attention can be drawn to specific pathogens and so that special stains can be performed.

Variations and Unusual Situations

Although the endoscopic findings are well recognized for some pathogens, numerous peculiar endoscopic

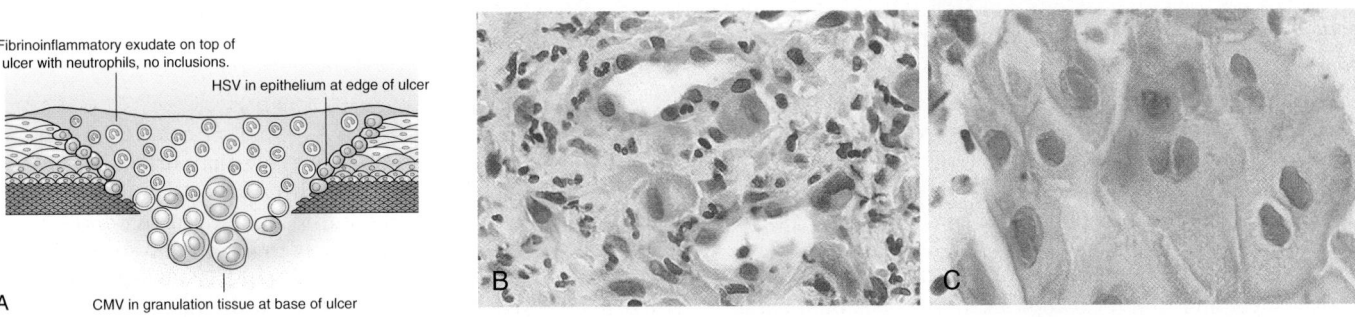

Fig. 22.15 A, Location of viral cytopathic effect in mucosal ulceration. Herpes simplex virus (HSV) can be found at the ulcer edge, whereas cytomegalovirus (CMV) is located in granulation tissue deep in the ulcer bed. **B,** Large cells with intranuclear inclusions typical for CMV. **C,** Multinucleated cells in squamous tissue typical for HSV. *(From Lazenby AJ: Gastroenterologist/pathologist partnership. Tech Gastrointest Endosc 4:95–100, 2002.)*

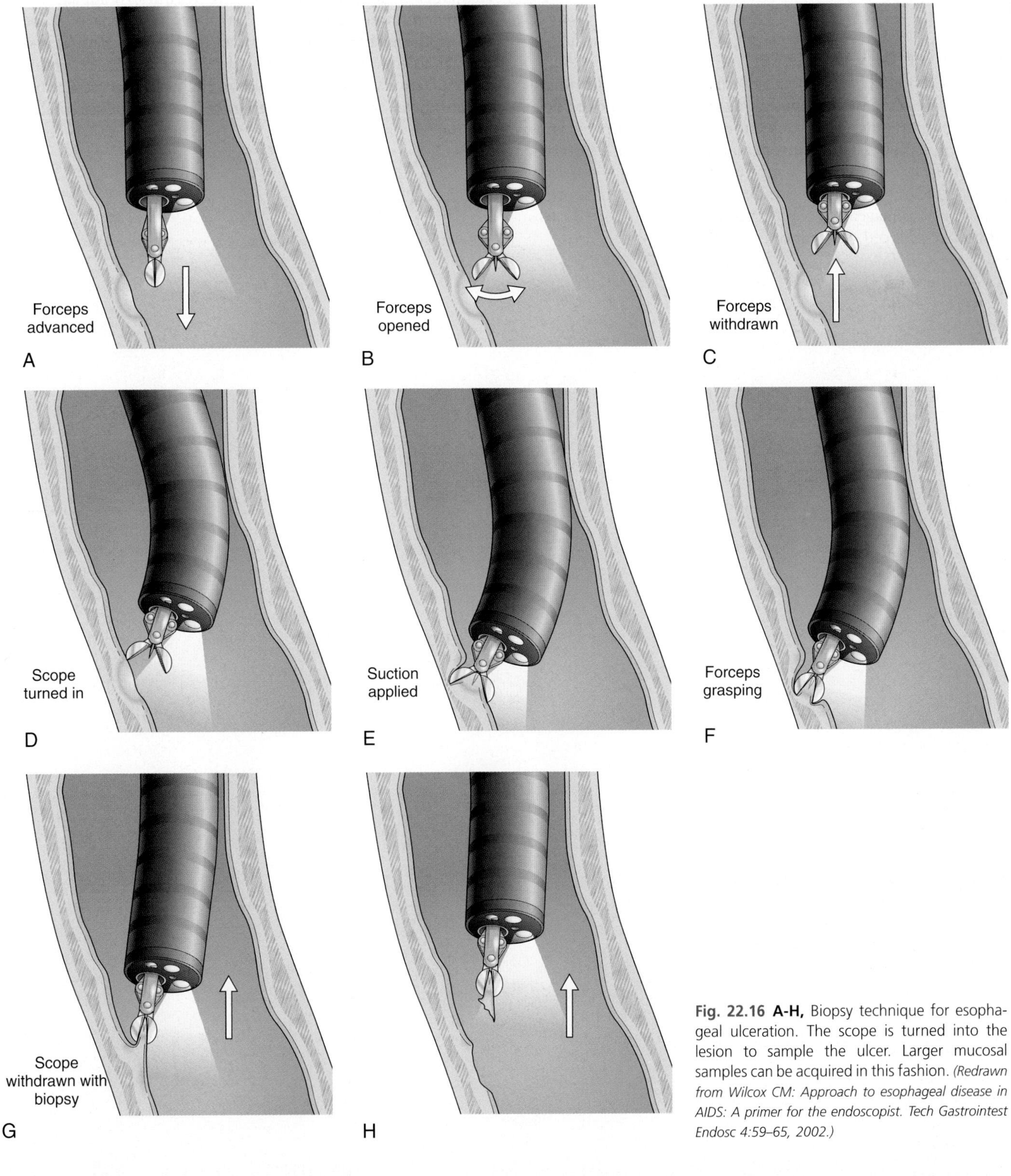

Forceps
advanced

A

Forceps
opened

B

Forceps
withdrawn

C

Scope
turned in

D

Suction
applied

E

Forceps
grasping

F

Scope
withdrawn with
biopsy

G

H

Fig. 22.16 A-H, Biopsy technique for esophageal ulceration. The scope is turned into the lesion to sample the ulcer. Larger mucosal samples can be acquired in this fashion. *(Redrawn from Wilcox CM: Approach to esophageal disease in AIDS: A primer for the endoscopist. Tech Gastrointest Endosc 4:59–65, 2002.)*

abnormalities have been previously reported. Generally, if an infection is suspected, a systematic endoscopic approach as noted previously should be taken.

Postoperative Care

Management after the endoscopic examination should parallel postoperative care of any other patient. Close follow-up with the pathologist may yield a preliminary diagnosis within 24 hours.

Complications

Complications from endoscopy in immunocompromised patients are similar to complications in the normal host. There have been rare reports of bacteremia after endoscopic examination in patients with neutropenia. In this setting, antibiotic therapy before endoscopy is appropriate. Bleeding is generally self-limited but may occur in anticoagulated patients. Vigorous biopsy of esophageal ulceration is safe with no reported cases of biopsy-induced perforation.[113]

Future Trends

The GI endoscopist will continue to play an important role in the management of GI infections because of the ability to visualize the GI tract directly and to obtain mucosal biopsy specimens. Future advances are likely to involve most notably molecular techniques to identify infections. These techniques could involve specific use of markers in the blood or, more likely, use assays on mucosal tissue to search for microbial DNA fingerprints. These technologies should expedite the diagnosis and improve both sensitivity and specificity. Further refinements in immunosuppressive regimens coupled with tailored antimicrobial prophylaxis are expected to reduce further the incidence of infections in the transplant setting. Similar to the advent of HIV-1 decades ago, further unforeseen infections are likely to arise in the future, necessitating a collaborative approach involving various disciplines, including the GI endoscopist.

References

The complete reference list is available online at www.expertconsult.com.

Techniques in Enteral Access

Stephen A. McClave and Wei-Kuo Chang

Video related to this chapter's topics can be found online at expertconsult.com.

Introduction

Using the gut and providing nutritional therapy by the enteral route play a pivotal role in patient outcome in the critical care setting. When there is failure to obtain enteral access and gut disuse ensues, the gut becomes a proinflammatory organ, increasing oxidative stress and the risk of complications.[1] Early enteral access and use of the gut promote or support the mass of gut-associated lymphoid tissue and mucosal-associated lymphoid tissue at distant sites such as the liver, lungs, and kidney.[2] This process contributes to an appropriate immune response, downregulation of inflammation, and a reduction in the rate of long-term complications. The sicker the patient, the greater the need to maintain gut integrity, and enteral nutrition support becomes a therapeutic tool or pharmacologic agent capable of changing outcome by reducing nosocomial infection, multiple organ failure, and hospital length of stay.[3,4]

The literature confirms that aggressive enteral tube feeding decreases the rate of complications compared with "standard therapy" (patients advance to oral diet on their own as tolerated) or total parenteral nutrition.[5,6] However, obtaining enteral access early in the course of a critically ill patient may be difficult. Patients in this setting are at the height of the hypermetabolic response, often requiring high doses of narcotic analgesia and sedation; they are prone to ileus, gastroparesis, and high gastric residual volumes. Transporting these patients to the radiology suite for placement of feeding tubes is difficult because they are unstable. Transport leads to delays in getting tubes placed and has been shown to increase the risk of complications (e.g., aspiration, hemodynamic instability, and new cardiac dysrhythmias).[7,8] Bedside techniques to place feeding tubes are essentially blinded, which carries some additive risk. Although bedside techniques may be sufficient in many patients in the critical care setting, the success rate for bedside placement decreases as disease severity increases, and there is greater need to place the tube lower in the gastrointestinal (GI) tract.

In long-term acute care and in the long-term management of patients recovering from stroke and neurologic injury, percutaneous endoscopic techniques provide a more reliable semipermanent enteral access, affording numerous options in a variety of patients. Getting a tube down below the stomach into the small bowel has been shown to reduce the incidence of regurgitation and aspiration.[9,10] In a meta-analysis, small bowel feeding was shown to reduce significantly the incidence of aspiration pneumonia compared with gastric feeding.[11] In patients with severe gastroparesis, percutaneous endoscopic techniques may provide a gastrostomy tube for decompression and a direct jejunostomy tube for continued enteral feeding. In patients with recurrent flares of chronic pancreatitis, placement of an endoscopic jejunostomy tube may provide therapeutic options that preserve nutritional status, decrease dependence on narcotic analgesia, and reduce the number of hospitalizations per year. In patients with dysphagia resulting from neurologic injury, percutaneous endoscopic feeding tubes are easily removable should the patient recover function and resume adequate volitional oral intake.

The role of the endoscopist with the skills to place the tube at the appropriate level in the GI tract is critical in these settings. Most techniques can be performed at the bedside in the intensive care unit (ICU) without transport to the radiology suite. The endoscopist has expertise in gut physiology, enabling monitoring of enteral nutrition therapy and the detection of tolerance versus intolerance of feedings. Endoscopists can provide simple techniques by which to manage complications. In the absence of such expertise for enteral access, the use of total parenteral nutrition increases significantly, a change in management strategy that may negatively affect patient outcome.

How to Establish an Endoscopy Service for Enteral Access

Several important steps should be taken to set up an effective endoscopic enteral "tube service." The nutrition literature is so strong regarding the beneficial effects of enteral feeding in the critical care setting that multidisciplinary nutrition teams are under significant pressure to get tubes in early and get feeds started quickly. The endoscopist should establish rapport with the multidisciplinary nutrition team and provide a timely response to consultations for enteral access. This timely response can be facilitated by flexibility with potential time slots in the endoscopy schedule to make room for add-on cases for enteral access. It is important to provide same-day service when a request for access is placed to deliver the best patient care. Generally, it helps to treat a request for enteral access for a patient in the ICU as one would respond to a request to evaluate a patient with a GI hemorrhage.

The two most important endoscopes needed to outfit an endoscopy enteral "tube service" are a pediatric colonoscope and a small-caliber gastroscope with an insertion tube outer diameter less than 6 mm. A pediatric colonoscope is usually the best choice for endoscopic nasoenteric tube (ENET), percutaneous endoscopic gastrojejunostomy (PEGJ), and direct percutaneous endoscopic jejunostomy (DPEJ) because of its length and relative stiffness. Although a push enteroscope is an adequate substitute for a pediatric colonoscope, the greater flexibility of the small bowel enteroscope promotes looping or curling in the stomach. The small-caliber gastroscope has the advantage that it can be passed via the transnasal route at the bedside with no sedation, making it an ideal choice in cases requiring ENET placement. When a 28-Fr percutaneous endoscopic gastrostomy (PEG) is in place, the same endoscope may be passed through the PEG for purposes of conversion to a PEGJ. The endoscopist is encouraged to learn one technique

well for each of the four procedures (ENET, PEG, PEGJ, and DPEJ) and then experiment with many other techniques to find his or her personal favorite.

Fluoroscopy is valuable early in the learning curve, but all of these techniques may be performed easily at the bedside or in the endoscopy suite without fluoroscopy. The ability to come to the ICU and place these tubes endoscopically without fluoroscopy avoids the need to transport the patient out of the ICU, increases flexibility in scheduling, and avoids the cost and exposure to radiation involved with fluoroscopy. Having appropriate ancillary devices such as wires, biopsy forceps, and snares that are long enough (such that they can be passed out through the colonoscope and still have a workable length beyond the tip of the scope) and having key accessories such as a hemoclip (to secure the distal tube tip to the intestinal mucosa) or bandage clips (to secure the proximal end of the tube to the skin) improve the efficiency and success rate for these procedures. It is important to maximize lubrication when working with feeding tubes by activating the hydrophilic lubricant on the inner surface of the tube by water infusion and by applying a vegetable spray or surgical lubricant to the outer surface.

Endoscopic Nasoenteric Tubes

ENET placement is most commonly required in the critical care setting. Severity of critical illness, complications of sepsis and multiple organ failure, and therapeutic strategies such as placement on mechanical ventilation all are factors indicating the need for early enteral access. Establishing enteral access and initiating enteral feeds is considered part of the basic resuscitation of these patients. ENET placement deep into the jejunum is specifically reserved for critically ill patients unable to tolerate initial nasogastric feeding (owing to poor gastric emptying, ileus, regurgitation, or aspiration) and patients who require jejunal feeding because of acute pancreatitis. Several techniques have been described for ENET placement.

Over-the-Guidewire Technique

The over-the-guidewire technique may be more difficult technically than other ENET procedures because of the oronasal transfer and wire exchanges (removing the endoscope from the wire and placing the feeding tube over the wire). However, this technique is the one ENET procedure that most reliably places the feeding tube at or below the ligament of Treitz. Before performing endoscopy, the oronasal transfer tube is placed through one nostril, brought out the mouth, and clamped to the side using a hemostat. The pediatric colonoscope is passed through the mouth down the esophagus and stomach into the small bowel. As the endoscopist traverses the duodenum, it is important to pay attention to landmarks of the duodenal bulb and the C-loop. The long straight segment immediately after the duodenal C-loop is the distal duodenum leading up to the ligament of Treitz. The ligament of Treitz is the first turn after this long segment. Paying attention to these landmarks helps assure the endoscopist of the location of the tip of the endoscope within the GI tract. Passing the endoscope one to two loops below the ligament of Treitz helps to anchor the tip of the wire ultimately during subsequent wire exchanges (**Fig. 23.1A**). Once the endoscope has been passed as deep as possible, the wire is extended out from the end of the endoscope until it meets gentle resistance.

The first wire exchange involves removing the endoscope off of the wire without displacing the tip. The key point to this aspect of the procedure is that the endoscopist places one hand on the endoscope as he or she removes it from the mouth and the other hand on the wire as it is passing into the operating channel of the endoscope at the other end (**Fig. 23.1B**). An assistant may support the weight of the scope, keeping it from bowing in the middle during the wire exchange. The point at which the colonoscope has been withdrawn off the wire, the tip of the wire is protruding from the patient's mouth. If done incorrectly, the oronasal transfer of the wire causes a loop to form in the mouth or displacement of the tip of the wire from the small bowel back into the stomach or both. The tip of the wire is placed through the oronasal transfer tube, passing the excess wire out of the end of the transfer tube protruding from the nose (**Fig. 23.1C**).

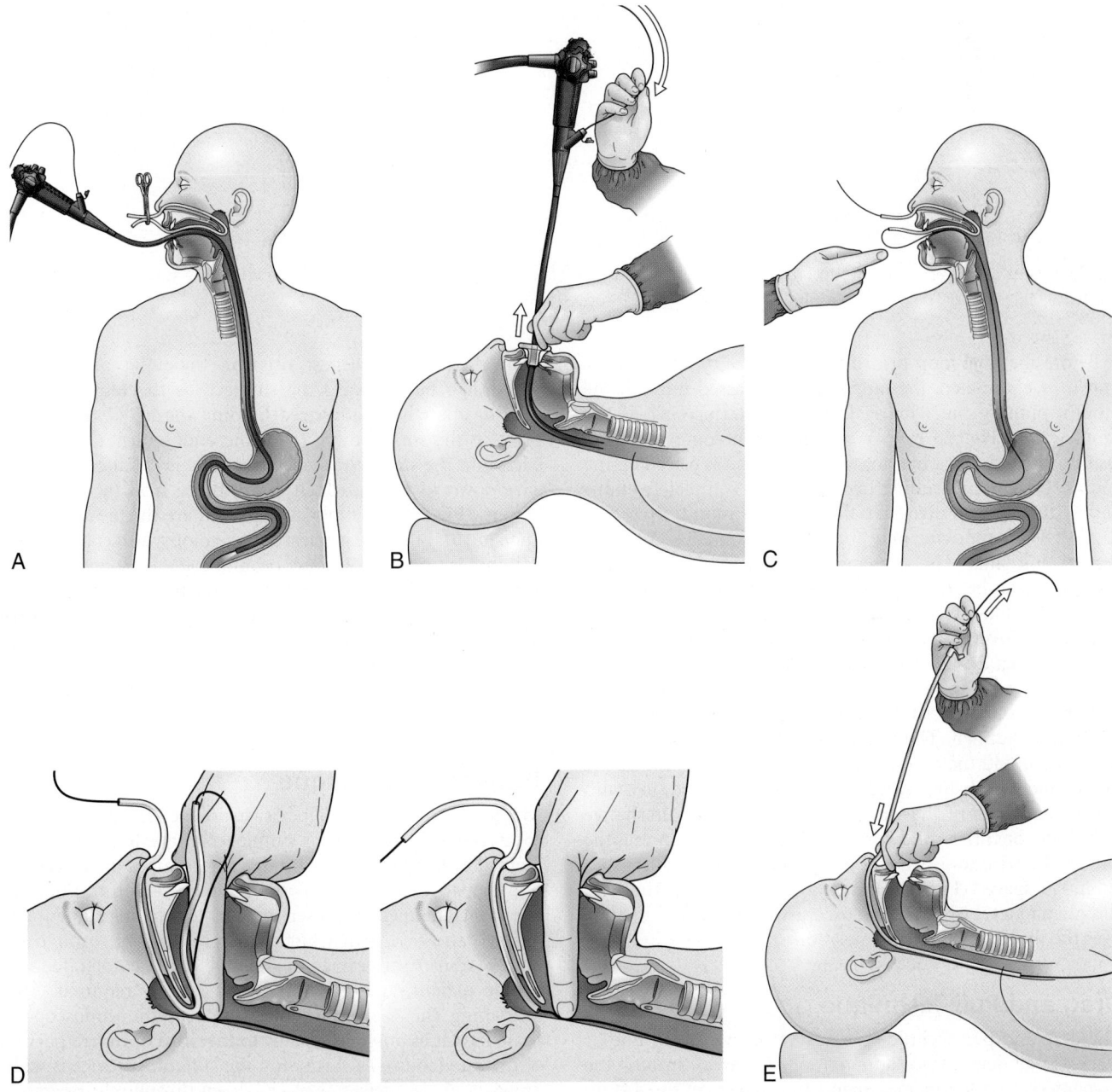

Fig. 23.1 Over-the-guidewire endoscopic nasoenteric tube (ENET) technique. **A,** The pediatric colonoscope is passed down below the ligament of Treitz, and the wire is extended out beyond the end of the scope. **B,** In the initial wire transfer, the scope is withdrawn from the mouth at the same rate the guidewire is passed down through the operating channel, to prevent displacement of the wire tip from its position in the small bowel. **C,** With the wire protruding out through the mouth, the tip of the wire is passed through the oronasal transfer tube. **D,** The index finger is used to pin the wire against the posterior pharyngeal wall, while traction is placed on the wire protruding out through the nose, pulling on the wire until the wire is straight and tension is felt against the finger in the posterior pharynx. **E,** In one technique for the final wire transfer, the feeding tube is passed over the wire down through the nares at the exact same rate that the wire is withdrawn out from the distal end of the feeding tube, again to avoid displacing the wire tip.

Continued

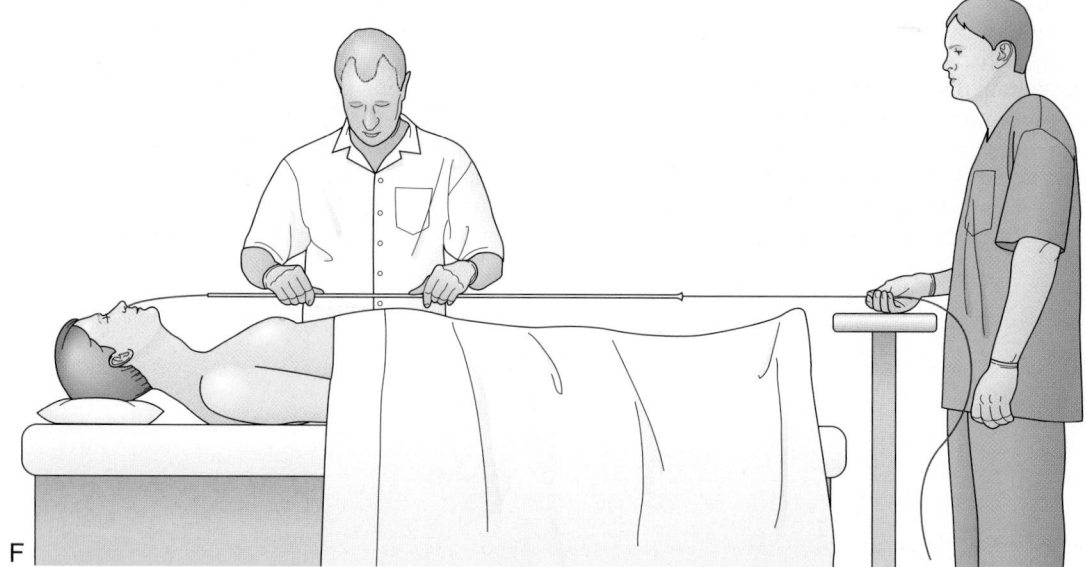

Fig. 23.1, cont'd **F,** In an alternative technique for the final wire transfer, an assistant pins the wire to a "point in space" (using a bedside table), and the tube is slid over the fixed wire into final position.

Before the final loop protruding from the mouth is withdrawn or eliminated, the index finger is passed through the mouth, pinning the wire against the posterior wall of the oropharynx (**Fig. 23.1D**). While firmly holding the wire against the posterior pharyngeal wall, traction is placed on the end of the wire protruding from the nose, completely eliminating the loop protruding through the mouth (see **Fig. 23.1D**). With the wire now protruding from the nose, the second and final wire exchange is made. This latter wire exchange may be accomplished using one of two different techniques. One technique involves carefully passing the feeding tube over the wire in a manner similar to the first wire exchange (**Fig. 23.1E**). The endoscopist is careful to place one hand at the nose as he or she inserts the tube, with the other hand at the opposite end of the feeding tube where the wire is being withdrawn. The rate of the tube passing down into the nose should match exactly centimeter for centimeter the rate of the wire being withdrawn at the other end, to avoid deflecting the tip of the wire (see **Fig. 23.1E**). An alternative technique for this second wire exchange involves pinning the end of the wire to a bed rail or bedside table to establish a "point in space" (**Fig. 23.1F**). Assistants help keep the wire straight and level while the endoscopist slides the feeding tube over the fixed wire into final position.

Drag and Pull Technique

The drag and pull technique is facilitated by placing one or two extra guidewires (for a total of two or three) through the nasoenteric tube before placement. Two to 3 cm of the soft tip of one wire should protrude out through the distal end of the tube. This assembly is passed down through the nose into the stomach, followed by passage of the endoscope alongside the tube down through the mouth into the stomach. Once in the stomach, a long biopsy forceps is used to grab the soft tip of the wire protruding from the feeding tube. The endoscope holding the wire is passed into the small bowel, it is hoped down to or beyond the ligament of Treitz (**Fig. 23.2A**).

From the point of deepest insertion, the endoscope is slowly withdrawn back toward the stomach as the biopsy forceps holding the wire is advanced holding the tip of the wire in place in the small bowel. Once the endoscope is positioned back into the stomach, the feeding tube is advanced over the wire down to its tip, which is still being held by the biopsy forceps (**Fig. 23.2B**). Only at this point are the biopsy forceps opened, and the wire is released. The biopsy forceps are withdrawn back into the endoscope, and the endoscope is slowly withdrawn back out through the esophagus and mouth. The keys to success for this procedure are a pair of biopsy forceps that are long enough (≥240 cm) and the stiffening of the feeding tube with extra guidewires (which facilitates removal of the endoscope without displacing the tube back into the stomach) (see **Fig. 23.2B**).

Transnasal Technique

Availability of a small-caliber gastroscope affords the endoscopist the opportunity for a simple technique for ENET placement. The key to success with this technique is the placement of a biopsy forceps or a Savory guidewire down through the operating channel, which serves to stiffen the instrument and increase the ease with which it may be passed through the bowel. Transnasal passage of the endoscope is tolerated well by the patient, and sedation is not usually required. After intubating the esophagus and stomach, the endoscope is passed as far as possible, usually to the third or fourth portion of the duodenum. At this point, the stiffening device is withdrawn, and a guidewire is placed down through the operating channel out as far as possible until meeting gentle resistance (**Fig. 23.3**). Using the wire exchange system described in the section on the over-the-guidewire technique, the small-caliber gastroscope is withdrawn off the wire. No oropharyngeal transfer of the wire is required, and the feeding tube may be passed immediately directly over the wire. Wire exchanges are more tenuous and difficult with this procedure because the wire is usually not passed as deep into the small bowel as in

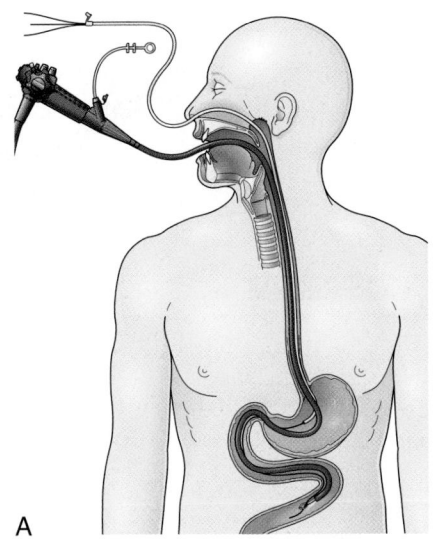 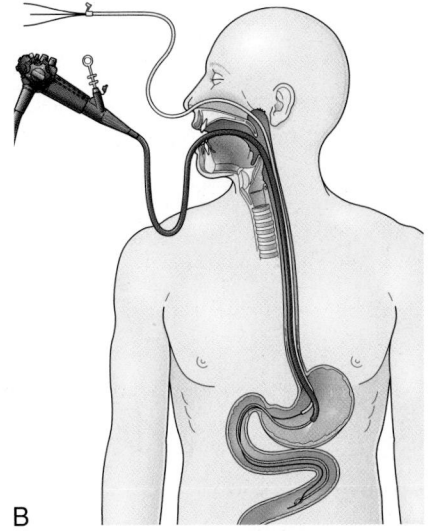

A B

Fig. 23.2 Drag and pull endoscopic nasoenteric tube (ENET) technique. **A,** The feeding tube is stiffened with three guidewires and passed into the stomach, where one of the three guidewires is passed out beyond the end of the feeding tube. This one wire is grabbed with biopsy forceps, and the pediatric colonoscope drags the wire down below the ligament of Treitz. **B,** As the endoscope is withdrawn back into the stomach, the biopsy forceps are pushed out to hold the wire in position below the ligament of Treitz. With the endoscope still positioned in the stomach, the feeding tube is advanced over the wire until it meets the biopsy forceps at the distal end. The endoscope is withdrawn through the mouth before all of the guidewires are removed.

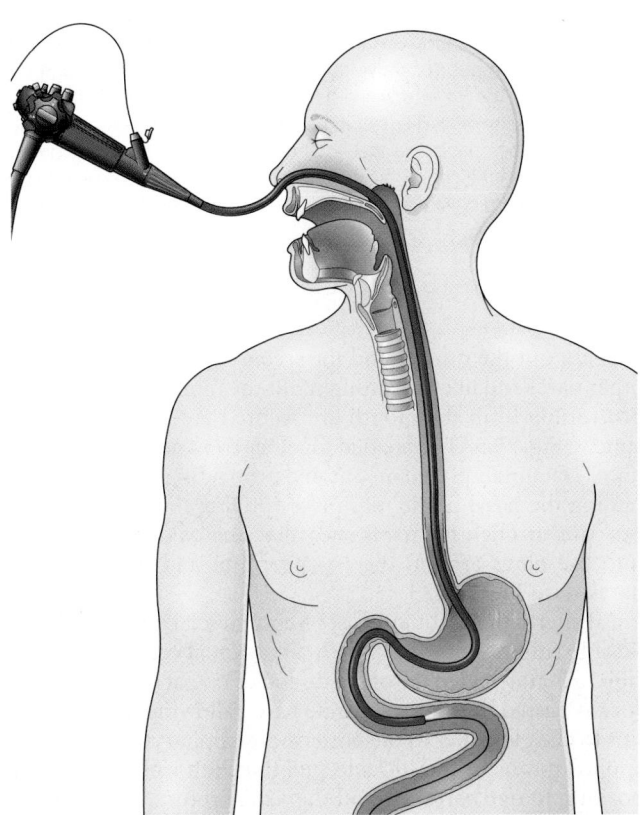

Fig. 23.3 Transnasal endoscopic nasoenteric tube (ENET) technique. After first placing biopsy forceps down through the operating channel to stiffen the endoscope, a small-caliber (<6 mm diameter) gastroscope is passed through the nares down into the stomach and beyond the pylorus. A guidewire is passed through the operating channel out beyond the end of the endoscope, and the endoscope is subsequently withdrawn. The final feeding tube is passed over the wire.

the over-the-guidewire technique, and the tip may be displaced more easily back into the stomach.

Alternative Options

In a simpler version of the previously mentioned drag and pull technique, knotted suture line is attached to the distal end of the feeding tube, and the tube is passed through the nares down into the stomach. The endoscopist passes the endoscope alongside the tube through the mouth down into the stomach, grabbing the knotted suture with biopsy forceps (**Fig. 23.4A**). It can be difficult and frustrating to drag the tip of the feeding tube through the pylorus and down into the duodenum. The success of this sometimes awkward procedure is improved by using knotted suture line instead of a loop or single strand on the tip of the tube (**Fig. 23.4B**), by adding a second guidewire to stiffen the tube to prevent displacement on withdrawal of the endoscope, and by keeping the biopsy forceps 1 to 2 cm out away from the tip of the endoscope to enhance visualization (see **Fig. 23.4A**).

In another alternative technique, one or two extra guidewires (for a total of two or three) are added to the feeding tube to increase stiffness, and the tube is passed through the nares down into the esophagus and stomach. The endoscope is passed through the mouth alongside the tube down into the stomach, and the tip of the stiffened tube is simply pushed or nudged using open biopsy forceps through the pylorus into the duodenal bulb (**Fig. 23.4C**). Continuing to watch endoscopically from the stomach, the endoscopist pushes the stiffened feeding tube from the outside proximal end in an effort to pass the distal tip around the C-loop and into the third and fourth portion of the duodenum (see **Fig. 23.4C**). The most reliable of the three alternative methods uses an 8-Fr nasoenteric tube, which is passed through the operating channel of the endoscope after it has been passed through the esophagus and stomach into the small bowel. The success of this

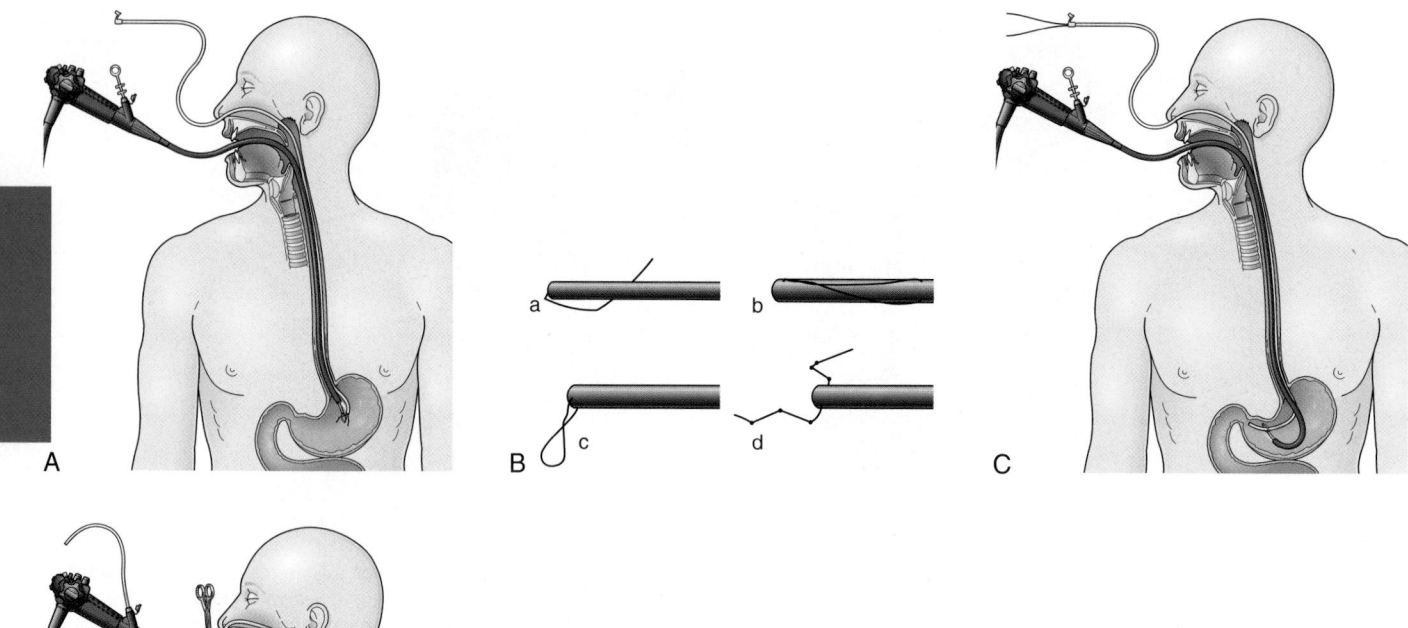

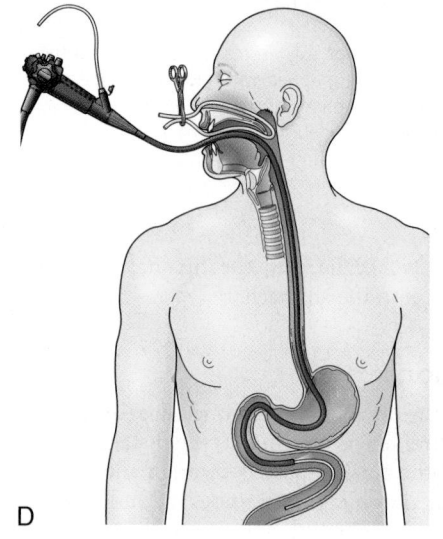

Fig. 23.4 Additional endoscopic nasoenteric tube (ENET) options. **A,** One option involves two knotted sutures, attached to the distal end of the feeding tube, which is passed through the nares down into the stomach. Biopsy forceps passed through the gastroscope grab the knotted suture and drag the tube down below the pylorus into the distal duodenum. **B,** This figure shows how the knotted suture is superior to a single or double suture line (which may adhere with gastric juices and mucus to the feeding tube) and a loop of suture (which may become tangled and twisted). **C,** A second option involves two or three guidewires passed through the feeding tube, which is subsequently passed through the nares down into the stomach. The endoscope is passed through the mouth down into the stomach where biopsy forceps are used to push or shove the stiffened feeding tube through the pylorus. The tube can be advanced further down into the distal duodenum by pushing from the outside. **D,** Another option involves the passage of an 8-Fr feeding tube through the operating channel of a therapeutic gastroscope, which has been passed to the distal duodenum or proximal jejunum. After advancing the feeding tube out beyond the end of the endoscope, the endoscope is withdrawn out from the mouth, and the tube is transferred via a larger oronasal transfer tube out through the nose.

procedure is enhanced by using a large-channel therapeutic endoscope and a small-bore (8-Fr) nasoenteric tube whose proximal feeding cap can be removed. Because the endoscope is passed through the mouth, it requires placement of an oronasal transfer tube and the subsequent transfer of the tube from the mouth out through the nose (**Fig. 23.4D**) using the method described in the over-the-guidewire technique.

Securing Tube with Nasal Bridle

For any case in which the time and expense of endoscopic placement of a nasoenteric tube is required, consideration should be given to securing the tube with a nasal bridle. Although this technique may seem barbaric and overly punitive to the patient, selection of the proper tube for the nasal bridle results in a degree of discomfort that is no different than the presence of the nasoenteric tube alone. The timing of the nasal bridle placement is important; placement should be done initially before endoscopy is performed (before the patient is agitated from the passage of the endoscope). Two separate but similar techniques may be used to establish a nasal bridle. In one technique, two 5-Fr neonatal feeding tubes are used. The first tube is passed through one nares and

brought out the mouth, and the second is passed through the other nares and likewise brought out the mouth. The two ends protruding from the mouth are secured together by a single suture (**Fig. 23.5A**) or are tied together by hand using a square knot. Traction is placed on one end protruding from the nares, pulling the nasal bridle into place (pulling the knotted juncture out through the nares such that one of the tubes passes into the nares around the nasal septum and out the other nares) (see **Fig. 23.5A**).

An alternative technique uses a commercial device with two flexible rubber sticks, each with a magnet at one end. A cloth ribbon is attached to the opposite end of one of the sticks. Each stick is passed through a separate nares, allowing the magnetic tips to click together in the posterior hypopharynx. Traction is applied to one of the sticks to pull the cloth ribbon into final position in one nares, around the nasal septum, and then out the other nares (**Fig. 23.5B**). The oronasal transfer tube is placed, and the rest of the ENET procedure commences thereafter. At the completion of the ENET placement, the feeding tube is taped to the 5-Fr nasal bridle tube (beginning 1 cm below the nose and wrapping the tape downward over the feeding tube and bridle until the bridle is completely covered; see **Fig. 23.5A**) or clipped to the cloth ribbon (see **Fig. 23.5B**).

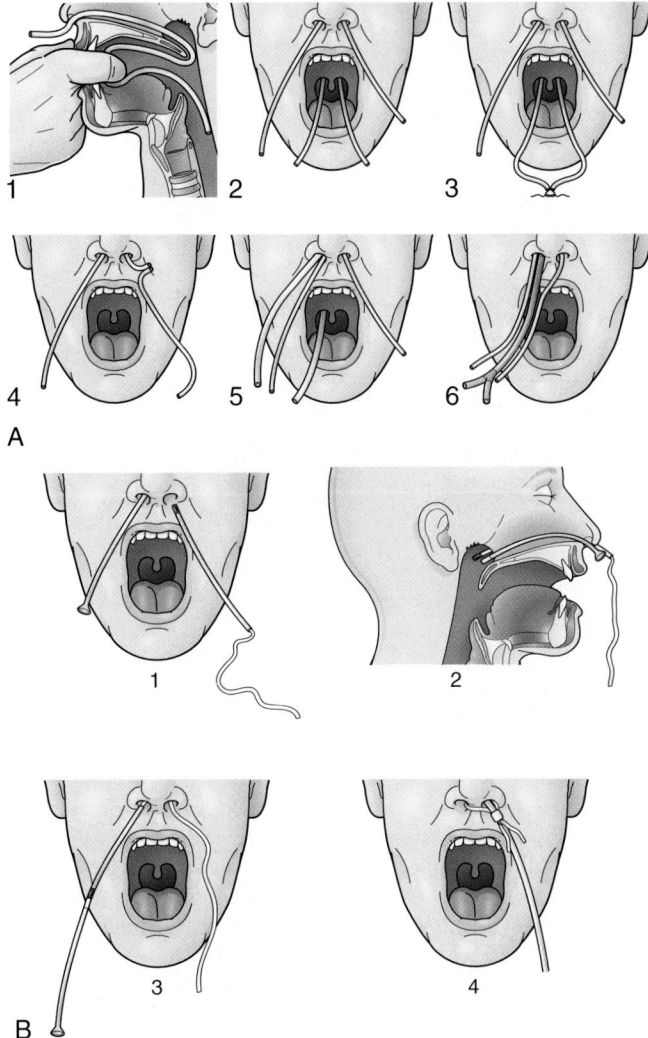

Fig. 23.5 Bridle technique for securing endoscopic nasoenteric tube (ENET), using two 5-Fr neonatal feeding tubes (**A**) or a commercial device using two flexible sticks with magnetic ends (**B**).

Percutaneous Endoscopic Gastrostomy

Placement of a PEG tube provides a more reliable and semi-permanent enteral access compared with the ENET and should be considered in any patient requiring specialized nutrition therapy for greater than 4 weeks' duration. Because an incision is made, patients who are not already receiving antibiotics need a single dose for antibiotic prophylaxis (a third-generation cephalosporin is appropriate) at the time of the initial procedure. Identifying landmarks such as the midline and the left costal margin with an indelible marker provides good orientation during the procedure and avoids the possibility of lacerating the left lobe of the liver with placement too close to the left costal margin. Antiplatelet or anticoagulant therapy is not a contraindication to these percutaneous techniques. Aspirin does not have to be stopped before the procedure. Patients receiving warfarin (Coumadin) may be switched to low-molecular-weight heparin (Lovenox) 1 week before the procedure (holding the dose on the morning of the procedure). If patients receiving clopidogrel (Plavix) cannot be switched to aspirin alone 5 days before the procedure, the procedure may still be performed with caution (adding epinephrine to the anesthetic used for the initial skin incision).

In the past, the traditional location for PEG placement was in the left upper quadrant in the vortex formed by the midline and left costal margin (**Fig. 23.6A**). Relocating the site of routine PEG placement down lower close to the umbilicus and to the right of the midline should be considered for two good reasons. First, as shown on computed tomography (CT) scan (**Fig. 23.6B**), the area of greatest interface between the stomach and anterior wall that provides the shortest, most direct passage into the stomach is located at this site. The traditional site in the left upper quadrant creates a tract that is longer and more tangential as it enters the stomach. Even more importantly, this lower position on the abdomen places the PEG in the antrum, which facilitates conversion of the PEG to a PEGJ should the patient develop intolerance to gastric feeding later on.

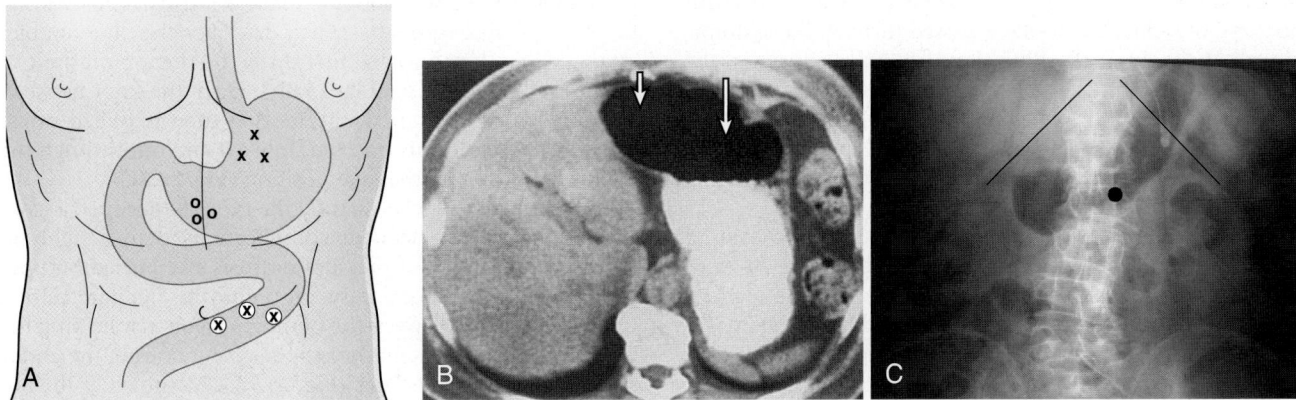

Fig. 23.6 Steps to localize percutaneous endoscopic gastrostomy (PEG), percutaneous endoscopic gastrojejunostomy (PEGJ), and direct percutaneous endoscopic jejunostomy (DPEJ) sites. **A,** The traditional PEG site is marked by the x's in the left upper quadrant. Better placement is above the umbilicus, close to the midline, or slightly to the patient's right of midline position. The PEG is in the gastric antrum, which is ideal should the patient require conversion later to a PEGJ. *Circled x's* show the tremendous variability in the site for DPEJ placement, which can occur anywhere from the left costal margin down to the left iliac crest. **B,** Computed tomography (CT) scan shows that the PEG site slightly above or to the patient's right of the umbilicus coincides with the area with the most direct, perpendicular, and shortest tract into the gastric antrum. Traditional sites in the left upper quadrant have a longer, more tangential tract into the midbody or lower fundus. **C,** Placing a coin in the umbilicus and injecting 500 mL of air through a nasogastric tube before PEG placement helps identify the gastric antrum, simplifying selection of the PEG site.

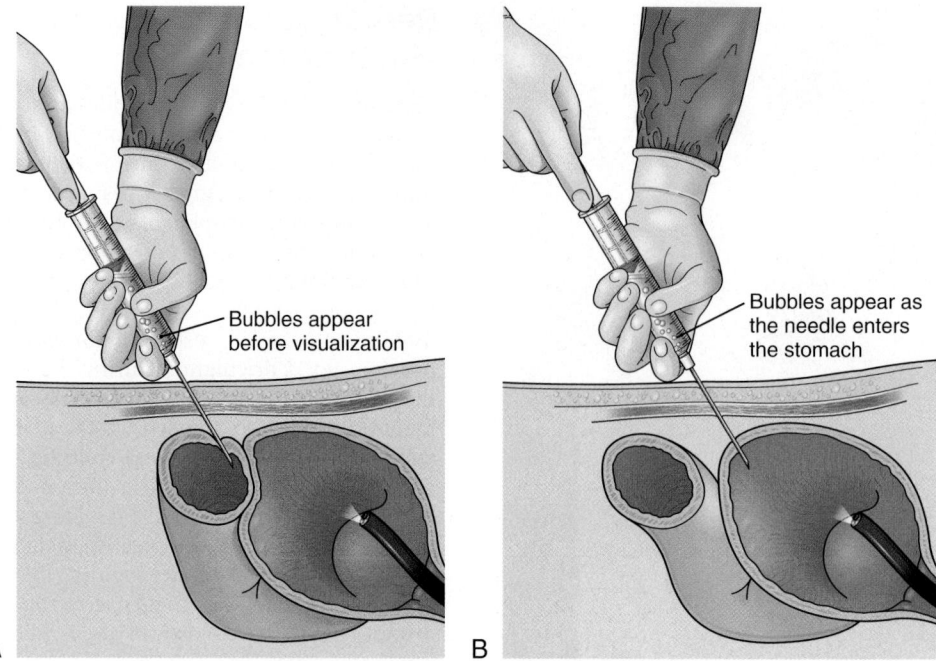

Fig. 23.7 Safe tract technique for percutaneous endoscopic gastrostomy (PEG) placement helps avoid inadvertent tracking through an adjacent loop of bowel before passage into the stomach.

Site selection is enhanced further by instilling 500 mL of air through the nasogastric tube into the stomach and obtaining an abdominal film 1 hour before PEG placement. Putting a coin in the umbilicus serves as an obvious landmark on the abdominal film, the position of which can be compared with the costal margin. The position of the air bubble with respect to the coin and the costal margins helps select the specific PEG site (**Fig. 23.6C**). Palpating the stomach and obtaining translumination through the abdominal wall is a valuable reassurance for proper PEG site selection. If there is any question (especially in cases of obesity), a safe tract technique may be used to ensure that no intervening loop of bowel exists between the stomach and the anterior abdominal wall (**Fig. 23.7**). Using a 21-gauge to 23-gauge spinal needle and a syringe with 1 to 2 mL of saline, the needle is passed through the abdominal wall at the proposed PEG site. If bubbles appear in the saline while aspirating just as the needle passes into the lumen of the stomach (as seen by endoscopy), there is some reassurance that the tract is appropriate. If bubbles appear before the needle passes into the stomach, there may be an intervening loop of bowel present (see **Fig. 23.7**).

PEG tubes should be selected that can be easily converted to a PEGJ should intolerance develop, and at least 20-Fr to 24-Fr diameter may be selected to minimize chance of clogging. The length of the skin incision should be adequate just to accommodate the diameter of the feeding tube.

Ponsky Pull and Sachs-Vine Push Technique

The Ponsky pull and Sachs-Vine push techniques are virtually indistinguishable, with one providing no real advantage over the other, and may be selected based on personal preference of the operator. After the PEG site is selected, the skin is anesthetized, a small incision is made, and the initial trocar is passed into the stomach. In the Sachs-Vine push technique, a single-stranded wire is passed through the trocar in the stomach and secured by a snare passed through the endoscope. With the Ponsky pull technique, a blue double-stranded wire loop is passed through the trocar and grabbed by the snare (**Fig. 23.8A**). The wire passed by either technique is brought out the mouth. In the Sachs-Vine push technique, a long 2- to 3-foot plastic pointed leader is fused to the proximal end of the feeding tube, facilitating passage over the single-stranded guidewire. This assembly is pushed down the wire through the esophagus and out through the gastric and abdominal wall (**Fig. 23.8B**). The Ponsky pull technique involves a loop on the end of the feeding tube that is affixed to the double-stranded blue loop of wire protruding from the patient's mouth. Attaching the two wire loops is made easier by remembering the phrase "blue through," which describes the blue double-stranded wire being passed first through the loop on the end of the feeding tube (see **Fig. 23.8B**). Once the knot between the wire loops is secured, the feeding tube is pulled down through the esophagus into the stomach and out through the abdominal wall into the final position (**Fig. 23.8C**).

As a general rule when setting the external bumper, a close fit causes fewer subsequent complications than a tight fit, which can later lead to pressure necrosis and buried bumper syndrome. A quick and easy procedure to facilitate setting adequate tension between the bumpers involves following the PEG tube down through the esophagus by snaring the endoscope to the enteral bolster (**Fig. 23.9A**). As shown at the top of **Fig. 23.9A**, snaring one-third of the enteral bolster makes it easy to release the bolster when the endoscope is led down into the stomach. As the tube is pushed or pulled down through the esophagus and stomach, the endoscope is brought down easily with it into position into the stomach. Once the snare is released, the external bolster may be set with the enteral bolster under direct endoscopic visualization (**Fig. 23.9B**). Drawing a figure and marking the exact number on

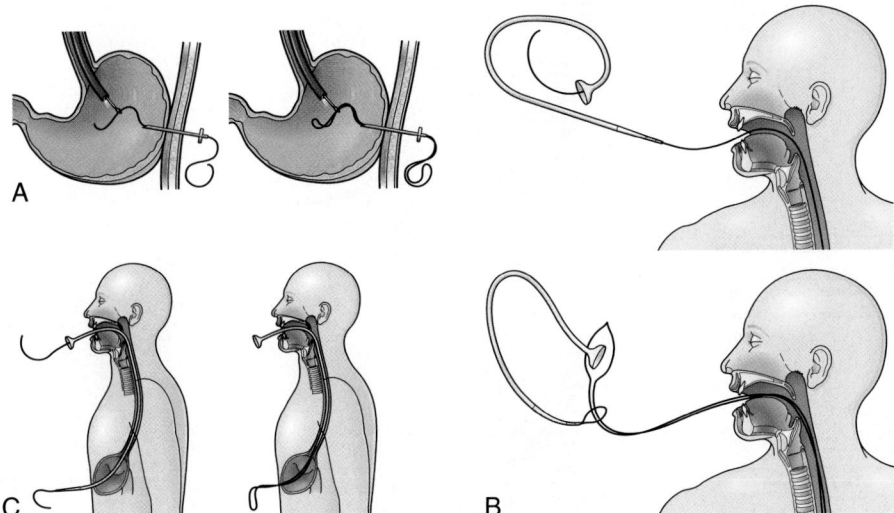

Fig. 23.8 Comparison of the Sachs-Vine push versus the Ponsky pull technique for percutaneous endoscopic gastrostomy (PEG) placement. **A,** In the Sachs-Vine technique, a single wire is passed through the trocar and grabbed with the snare, whereas a wire loop is passed through the trocar in the Ponsky pull technique. **B,** A long, 2-foot plastic leader attached directly to the feeding tube allows the entire ensemble to be passed or pushed over the wire in the Sachs-Vine push technique, whereas the blue wire loop can be attached to a wire loop on the end of the feeding tube in the Ponsky pull technique allowing the tube to be pulled into position. **C,** In the Sachs-Vine technique, the tube attached to the plastic leader is pushed through the esophagus and out through the gastric wall, whereas in the Ponsky pull technique, the wire loop pulls the feeding tube down through the esophagus and out through the gastric wall.

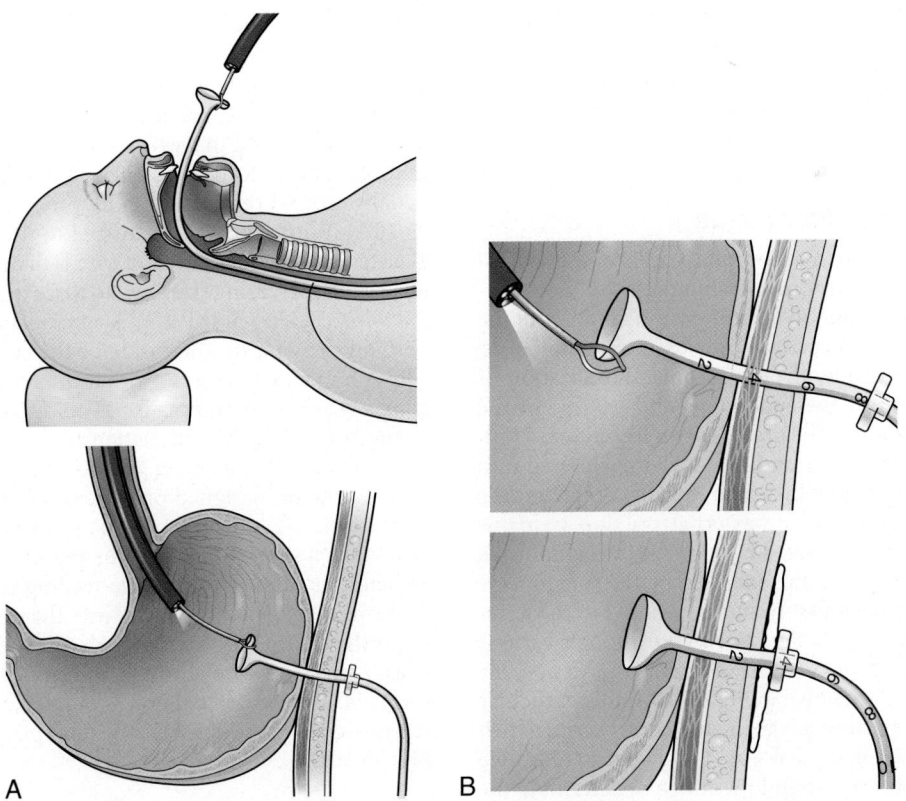

Fig. 23.9 Following the percutaneous endoscopic gastrostomy (PEG) tube down into place and positioning the external bolster for appropriate tension. **A,** Just before the feeding tube is pushed or pulled down through the oropharynx and esophagus, a snare passed through the endoscope is attached to the enteral bolster of the feeding tube securing the endoscope to the tube. The endoscope is pulled down through the oropharynx and esophagus as the PEG is brought down into position. **B,** Once in the stomach, the snare is released, and the bumper is positioned gently up against the gastric wall. The external bumper is positioned with a single layer of gauze underneath. A final figure indicating the appropriate number on the feeding tube for position of the external bolster may be drawn and recorded on the patient's chart.

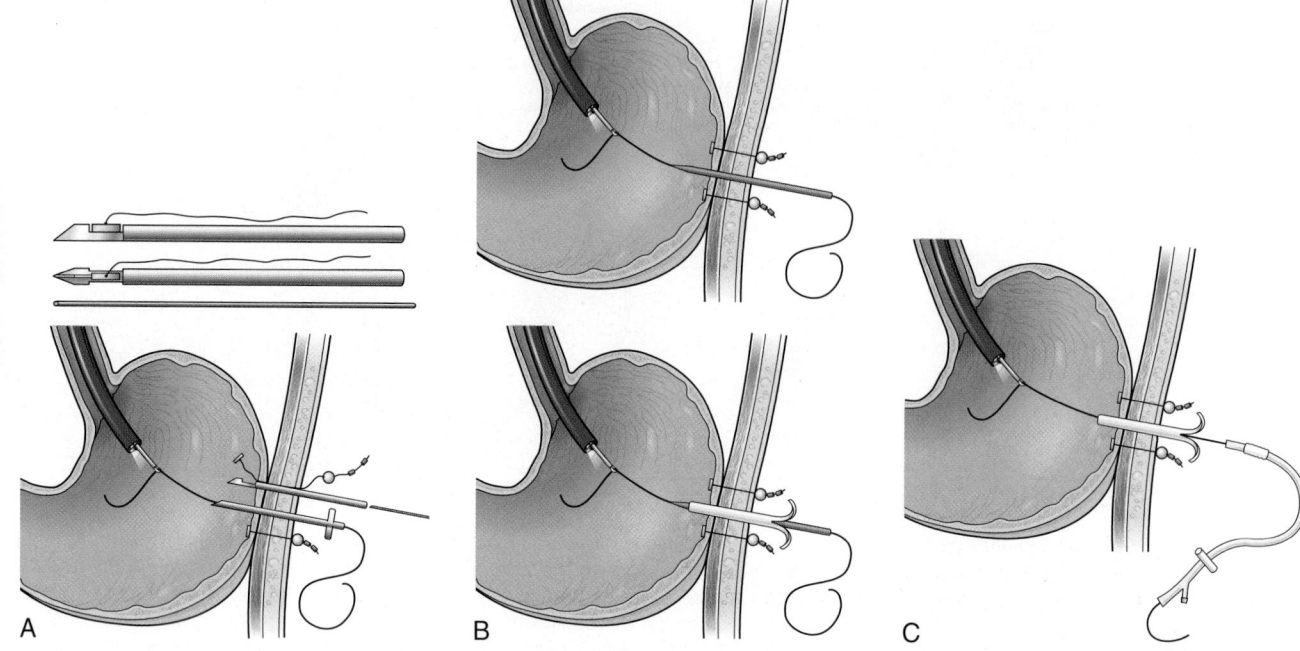

Fig. 23.10 Russell introducer percutaneous endoscopic gastrostomy (PEG) technique. **A,** After initial placement of the trocar and passage of a single-stranded wire, the wire is held with some tension against external traction by a snare passed through the endoscope within the stomach. T-fasteners are passed to secure the stomach up against the anterior abdominal wall. The top of this figure shows how the T-fasteners with attached suture are released by the cannula device. **B,** Once the stomach is secured to the anterior abdominal wall, the tract is dilated over the guidewire by three Seldinger dilators of increasing size. After the last dilation, a peel-away sheath over the final dilator is passed into position, and the dilator is removed. **C,** After first preloading an external bumper on the feeding tube, the feeding tube is passed over the wire through the peel-away sheath into the stomach where the enteral bolster is inflated, the peel-away sheath is removed, and the external bolster is positioned down against the skin.

the tube for the position of the external bolster is a valuable aid for nursing care and may be placed on the chart for reference at any time (see **Fig. 23.9B**).

Russell Introducer Technique

In patients with a large exophytic oropharyngeal or esophageal carcinoma, the Russell introducer technique should be considered to reduce the likelihood for tumor implantation of the PEG site. This is a technique commonly used by radiologists, but it is easily performed by the endoscopist. Localization of the PEG site, position of the endoscope, and passage of the initial trocar are identical to the previous two techniques. With the trocar in place, a single-stranded guidewire is passed into the stomach and held firmly by a snare protruding from the endoscope (**Fig. 23.10A**). Gentle external traction is maintained on the wire from outside the abdomen throughout the procedure by pulling against the end held by the snare inside the stomach. The stomach first has to be secured to the anterior wall by T-fasteners (see **Fig. 23.10A**). Although various commercial models of these fasteners exist, the design for deployment is similar. As shown in **Fig. 23.10A**, this particular technique involves a narrow-gauge introducer trocar in which the T-fastener is placed in a distal slot. A 21-gauge to 23-gauge spinal needle is helpful as a sounding device to determine the appropriate tract for each T-fastener. After making a nick in the skin with a scalpel blade, the device is passed through the abdominal wall.

The T-fastener is deployed in the stomach by a central cannula. After removing the small trocar and cannula for the T-fastener, a cotton roller ball and two metal fastening devices

are cinched down until there is mild tension on the outer abdominal wall against the T-fastener on the inside of the stomach. Crimping the two metal fasteners holds the T-fastener in place. Two to four T-fasteners should be placed circumferentially around the trocar before proceeding further (see **Fig. 23.10A**). With the stomach affixed to the anterior wall by the T-fasteners, the tract over the wire is dilated by Seldinger-type dilators of increasing size. Two to three dilators are passed over the wire as external traction is again placed against the snare holding the wire on the inside of the stomach (**Fig. 23.10B**). After the tract has been fully dilated, a peel-away sheath overlying a larger bore cannula is passed over the wire and into the stomach (see **Fig. 23.10B**, *bottom*).

Most Russell introducer kits do not come with an external bolster and are designed or anticipated instead to be sutured to the skin. A simple homemade external bolster may be created by a short segment from any small Salem sump, Foley catheter, or other larger gauge feeding tube and placed over the feeding tube before passage into the stomach (**Fig. 23.10C**). Once the external bolster is in place, the feeding tube may be placed over the wire through the peel-away sheath into the stomach. The enteral balloon is inflated, the peel-away sheath is removed, and the external bolster is placed into position (see **Fig. 23.10C**).

Percutaneous Endoscopic Gastrojejunostomy

For patients with documented intolerance to gastric feeding with nausea, vomiting, high gastric residual volumes, or

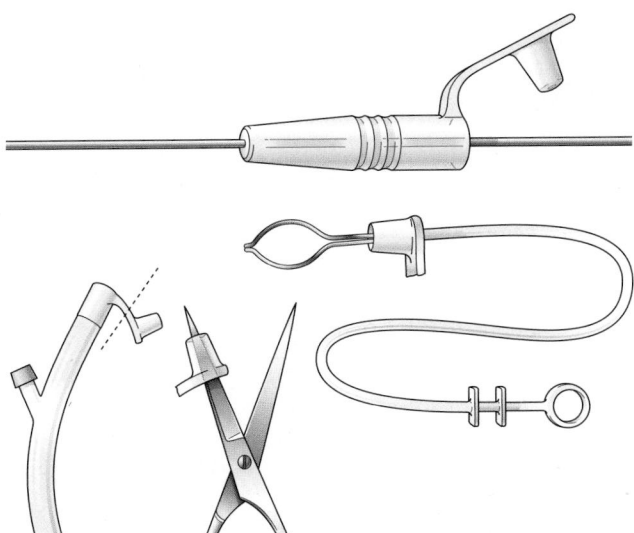

Fig. 23.11 Commercial and homemade air valves. At the top is a commercial air valve passed over the guidewire, which is used most often during percutaneous endoscopic gastrojejunostomy (PEGJ) conversions. A homemade air valve may be created by cutting off the valve plug on a feeding tube, coring the valve out with a pair of scissors, and passing a snare or wire through the valve.

evidence of gastroparesis, the PEGJ provides an easy, although less reliable access to the small bowel. The success of this procedure is related to many factors. Localization of the PEG in the antrum is most important. The PEG should be cut down to approximately 10 cm in length to afford a maximum length of the jejunal tube for passage into the small bowel. If the PEGJ is performed at the time of initial PEG placement, antibiotic prophylaxis should be used. A site just to the right and above the umbilicus is the best site for placement into the antrum. Use of a pediatric colonoscope is important to try to get one to two loops below the ligament of Treitz. Use of long biopsy forceps of at least 240 cm in length is important to have a sufficient working length beyond the tip of the colonoscope. The endoscopist should not use a snare to place wires in this procedure because it can be difficult to extract the snare from the tip of the wire after it is positioned in the small bowel.

One of the most important elements in the success of this procedure is the function of an air retention valve (**Fig. 23.11**). Although numerous commercial models are available (see top of **Fig. 23.11**), a homemade air valve can be made from the cap of the feeding tube (creating a hole with a pair of scissors) (see bottom of **Fig. 23.11**). The air valve allows passage of a wire or a snare through the PEG into the stomach without losing air insufflation. Failure to use or create an air valve significantly prolongs the procedure and can make visualization very difficult when passing the endoscope from the stomach into the small bowel.

Through-the-Snare Technique

The through-the-snare technique is the most reliable way to place a PEGJ tube successfully in the proximal jejunum at or below the ligament of Treitz. After cutting the PEG down to 10 cm, an air retention valve is fashioned, and the snare is passed through the hole in the air valve positioned in the PEG

and on into the stomach. The snare is opened allowing the pediatric colonoscope to be passed down through the esophagus and stomach, through the snare, and on into the small bowel. After the endoscope has been passed into the small bowel, the snare is closed once to ensure the endoscope has passed through the snare, and then reopened to allow further passage. The air valve may be backed out of the PEG at this point to decompress the stomach and prevent looping or curling of the endoscope. The endoscope is passed, it is hoped, one to two loops beyond the ligament of Treitz. At its deepest penetration, a guidewire is passed out further into the jejunum until gentle resistance is met.

The key to success of this technique is the selection of a very long 480-cm standard guidewire. The usual wire that comes with PEG and PEGJ kits is usually substantially shorter than this (**Fig. 23.12A**). Using proper wire exchange techniques, the endoscope is withdrawn back to the proximal stomach above the level of the snare, keeping the tip of the wire in position in the small bowel (**Fig. 23.12B**). Once the endoscope has been brought back to approximately 45 cm (from the incisors), the air valve is placed back into the PEG to insufflate the stomach and confirm the position of the endoscope above the snare (see **Fig. 23.12B**). The snare is closed on the wire, and a loop of the wire is pulled out through the PEG to the outside (**Fig. 23.12C**). The endoscopist manually separates the loop and has an assistant pull on the proximal wire extending out from the proximal operating channel of the endoscope. The movement of one side of the loop helps identify that end of the wire coming from the endoscope (see **Fig. 23.12C**). This end of the wire is pulled out through the PEG, resulting in a straightened single-strand guidewire passing through the PEG and down into the small bowel (**Fig. 23.12D**). The jejunal tube is passed over the wire (using good wire exchange technique) into position in the small bowel. Having an assistant provide a "point in space" above the abdomen secures or fixes the guidewire, facilitating passage of the jejunal tube into final position.

Over-the-Guidewire Technique

Although the over-the-guidewire technique appears to be more simplified than the through-the-snare technique, it may be slightly more frustrating for getting proper placement of the jejunal tube well down into the small bowel. For this technique, an air retention valve is placed over a wire, and the wire is passed through the PEG into the stomach. After passing the endoscope through the esophagus into the stomach, biopsy forceps are used to grasp the wire and walk it on down into the small bowel. The key to the success of this procedure is using biopsy forceps that are at least 240 to 320 cm in length to afford a sufficient working length out beyond the end of the colonoscope. The colonoscope is passed, it is hoped, down to a level at or below the ligament of Treitz (**Fig. 23.13A**). While still holding the wire in place at its distal tip, the biopsy forceps are slowly advanced as the endoscope is withdrawn back into the proximal stomach. The jejunal tube is passed over the wire all the way down until it strikes the biopsy forceps still holding the tip of the wire in the small bowel (**Fig. 23.13B**). Only at this point are the biopsy forceps opened, releasing the wire. The biopsy forceps are withdrawn back into the endoscope. If shorter biopsy forceps are used, the jejunal tube may strike the forceps holding the end of the wire while

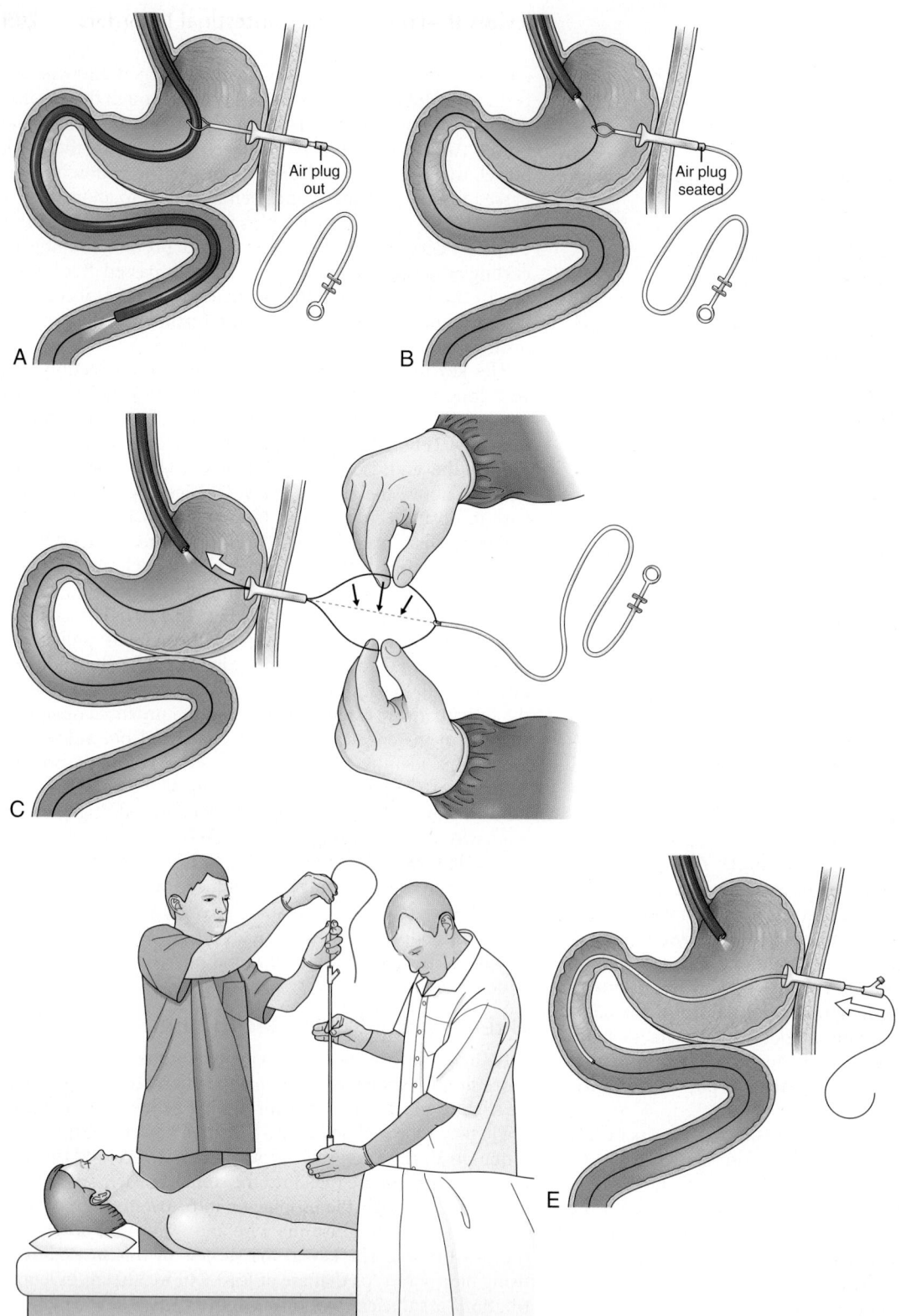

Fig. 23.12 Through-the-snare percutaneous endoscopic gastrojejunostomy (PEGJ) technique. **A,** After initial placement of the percutaneous endoscopic gastrostomy (PEG), the PEG tube is cut down short to approximately 10 cm, and a snare placed through a homemade or commercial air valve is passed into the stomach. A pediatric colonoscope is passed into the stomach, through the snare, and down into the small bowel below the ligament of Treitz (after which the wire is extended beyond the end of the scope). **B,** Using careful wire transfer technique, the endoscope is withdrawn back to the proximal stomach, keeping the tip of the wire in place below the ligament of Treitz. The air plug may be seated to allow visualization of the snare within the stomach. The snare is closed on the wire, which is pulled out through the PEG. **C,** While the assistant holds the wire loop coming out from the PEG, the operator pulls on the wire extruding from the operating channel of the scope, to indicate which side of the wire loop represents the proximal end of the wire. That loop is pulled out through the PEG. **D,** An assistant provides a "point in space" to secure or fix the guidewire as the operator passes the jejunal tube down through the PEG. **E,** The jejunal extension tube is passed down into final position, with the tip located well below the ligament of Treitz.

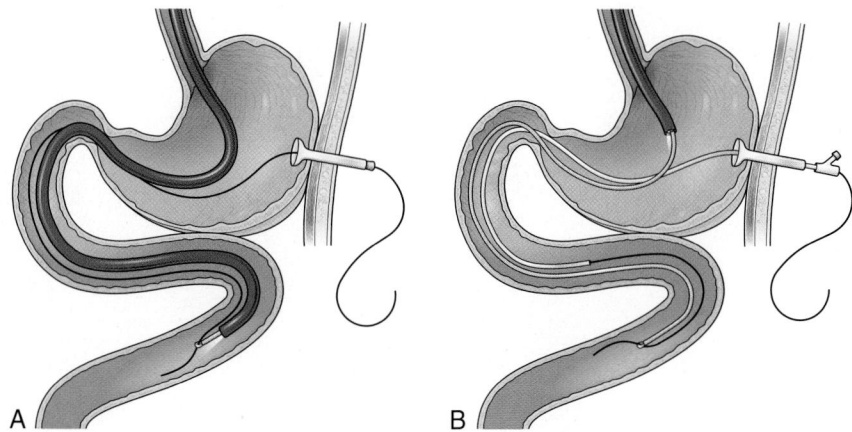

Fig. 23.13 Over-the-guidewire percutaneous endoscopic gastrojejunostomy (PEGJ) technique. **A,** A single-stranded guidewire passed through a valve (which is seated in the percutaneous endoscopic gastrostomy [PEG]) is grasped by biopsy forceps (passed down through a pediatric colonoscope). The endoscope holding the wire (via biopsy forceps) is passed down into the small bowel below the ligament of Treitz. **B,** The endoscope is withdrawn back into the stomach as the biopsy forceps are pushed outward through the end of the scope, holding the wire in place below the ligament of Treitz. Once the scope has been withdrawn back into the proximal stomach, the jejunal extension tube is passed over the wire until the distal end strikes the biopsy forceps at the end of the wire.

there is still a significant length of jejunal tube remaining outside the PEG. Although it is appropriate to open the biopsy forceps and release the wire at this point, the added length of the jejunal tube outside the PEG as the jejunal tube is pushed down and seated into position in the PEG often forms a loop in the stomach, and the procedure has to be repeated.

Trans-Percutaneous Endoscopic Gastrostomy Gastroscopy Technique

The trans-PEG gastroscopy technique may be performed with a small-caliber gastroscope if the patient's original PEG is 28-Fr in diameter. The technique can be performed through a PEG tube of smaller diameter, but a bronchoscope or ureteroscope may need to be substituted. The key to success with any of these small endoscopes is to stiffen the instrument by placing a biopsy forceps or a stiff guidewire down through the operating channel. Failure to do so causes excessive looping or curling in the stomach and possible inability to transcend the pylorus. In this simple technique, the endoscope is passed through the PEG, down through the pylorus, and through the third and fourth portion of the duodenum. It is difficult to get beyond the ligament of Treitz with this endoscope alone, but passing the wire out through the end of the endoscope once it is positioned in the distal duodenum may allow passage of the wire into the proximal jejunum below the ligament of Treitz. The endoscope is withdrawn, and the jejunal tube is placed over the guidewire (**Fig. 23.14**).

Securing the Percutaneous Endoscopic Gastrojejunostomy

The most frustrating aspect of the PEGJ procedure is that the jejunal tube frequently migrates back into the stomach. Two techniques may help prevent this migration. One is to use a rotatable hemoclip (Olympus America, Melville, NY) device to clip a suture affixed to the distal end of the feeding tube to the intestinal mucosa. Although this technique is easy to perform, the hemoclip holds the suture reliably in place only

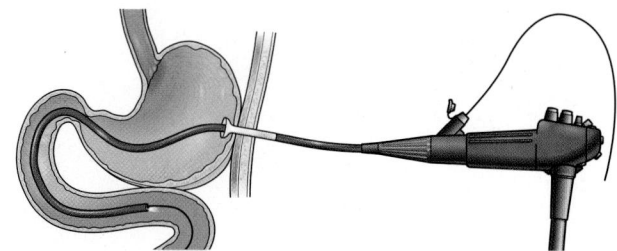

Fig. 23.14 Trans-percutaneous endoscopic gastrostomy (PEG) gastroscope percutaneous endoscopic gastrojejunostomy (PEGJ) technique. After first stiffening the small-caliber, 5.5-mm gastroscope with a biopsy forceps, the endoscope is passed through the PEG down to the distal duodenum and proximal jejunum. After removing the biopsy forceps, a single-stranded guidewire is passed out through the end of the endoscope, it is hoped beyond the ligament of Treitz. After the scope is withdrawn, the jejunal extension tube is passed over the wire.

for 7 to 10 days. A second technique is shown in **Fig. 23.15**, in which an anchor is created with a 1-cm segment from some other piece of tubing. A Salem sump, Foley catheter, or some other feeding tube may be used to create the 1-cm anchor. A 20-cm length of suture is affixed to the distal end of the feeding tube and secured to the anchor. The anchor is placed over the guidewire ahead of the jejunal feeding tube in the final step of the PEGJ procedure as the jejunal tube is passed over the wire into position in the small bowel (see **Fig. 23.15**).

At the completion of the PEGJ procedure by any of these methods, it is important that the operator confirms the proper position endoscopically. If the jejunal tube forms a loop up toward the gastroesophageal junction or forms a loop upon itself, the procedure may need to be repeated to achieve deeper positioning into the small bowel (**Fig. 23.16**). The natural action of this loop is to displace the tube upward toward the fundus, out from the small bowel. Proper positioning instead should have the appearance that the jejunal tube passes from the PEG directly toward the pylorus and down into the small bowel (see **Fig. 23.15**).

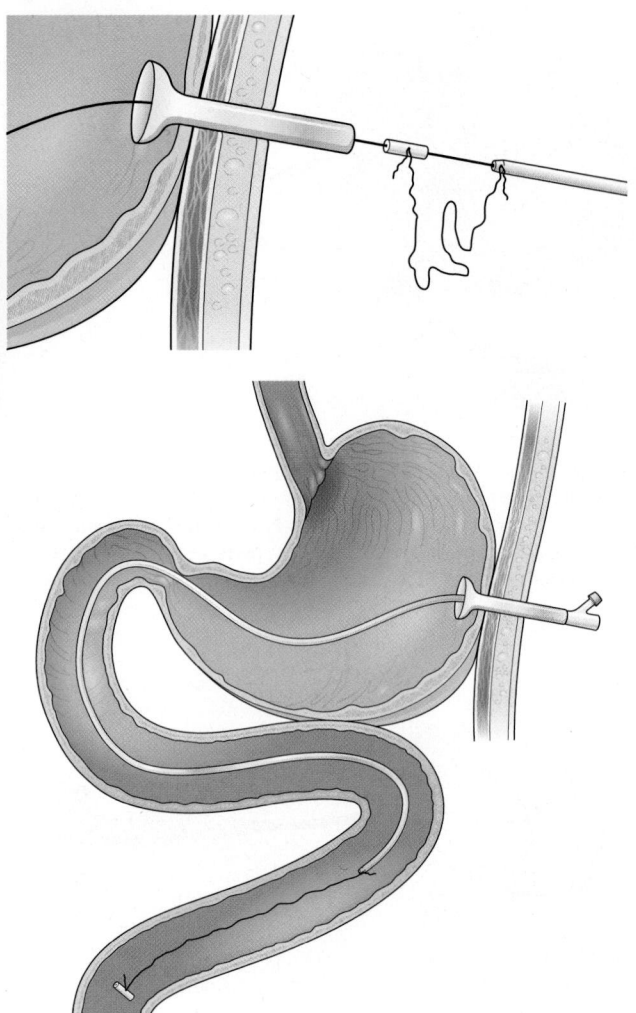

Fig. 23.15 Creation of a percutaneous endoscopic gastrojejunostomy (PEGJ) anchor. A single 1-cm section of tubing is created from any tube that is roughly the same diameter as the feeding tube, which is attached to the distal end of the feeding tube via a 20-cm silk suture. The anchor segment is preloaded on the guidewire ahead of the feeding tube and passed down into position in the distal duodenum and proximal jejunum. After removal of the wire, it is hoped that the anchor passes distally and helps hold the distal tip of the jejunal extension tube in place. This figure shows proper positioning of the jejunal extension tube, in which the tube passes directly from the PEG to the pylorus and on into the small bowel.

Direct Percutaneous Endoscopic Jejunostomy

Although DPEJ may be the most technically demanding procedure for enteral access, it provides probably the most reliable semipermanent access for a patient who has had difficulty with gastroparesis, nausea, vomiting, and previous intolerance to gastric feeding. Similar to an initial PEG placement, antibiotic prophylaxis is required for the DPEJ technique (as are the recommendations for patients receiving antiplatelet or anticoagulant therapy). Although the DPEJ technique is very similar to the Ponsky pull or Sachs-Vine push technique for PEG, many important differences exist. First, a much larger area of the abdomen from the costal margins bilaterally down to the iliac crests on both sides may need to be prepared because translumination may occur at more unusual sites any-

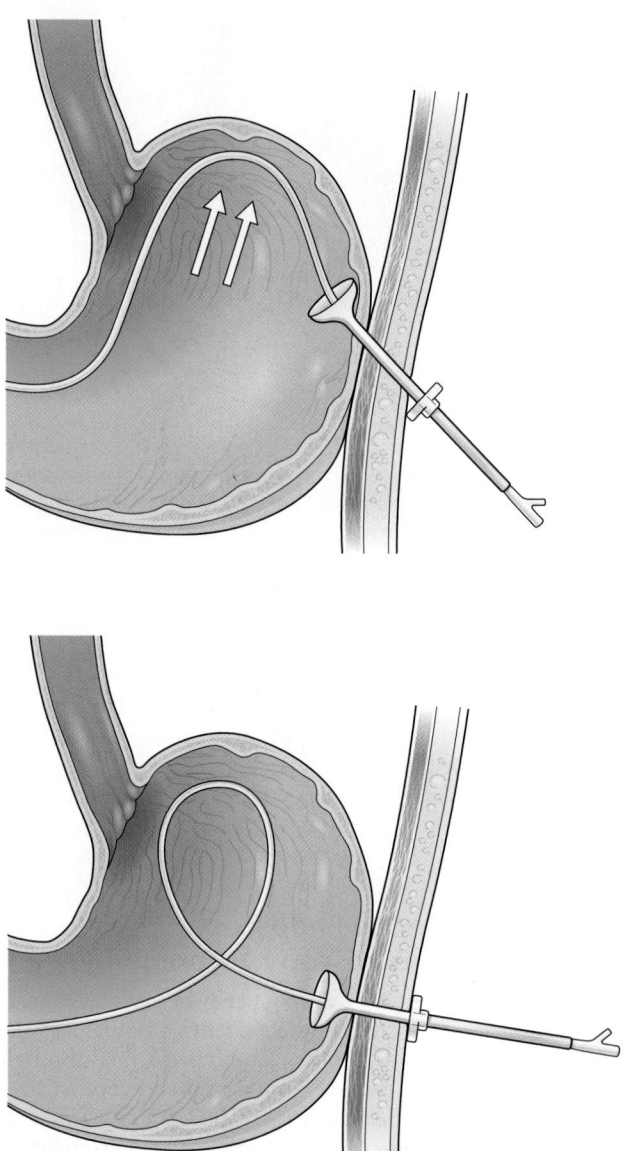

Fig. 23.16 Inappropriate position of the jejunal extension tube after percutaneous endoscopic gastrojejunostomy (PEGJ) conversion. Poor placement is shown in both figures: Although the tip of the jejunal tube is well down past the stomach, the tube passes toward the gastroesophageal junction first before passing down to the pylorus. If the tube is left in this position after placement, this angle serves to displace the tip of the jejunal tube back into the stomach. The *lower figure* also shows improper positioning of the jejunal extension tube, in which a loop of the tube is formed. Again, if left in place, this loop will serve to displace the tip of the jejunal tube back into the stomach.

where over the abdomen. If the patient has had previous partial gastrectomy and rerouting of the GI tract, the DPEJ may end up being placed significantly to the right of the midline.

The DPEJ is a two-person procedure, requiring an assistant at the level of the skin and a skilled endoscopist. The endoscopist should anticipate taking much longer (30 minutes and sometimes longer) to transluminate and to finger palpate a site. It is most appropriate to use a 21-gauge to 23-gauge spinal needle as a sounding needle in attempts to intubate the small bowel. The endoscopist should anticipate many more needle

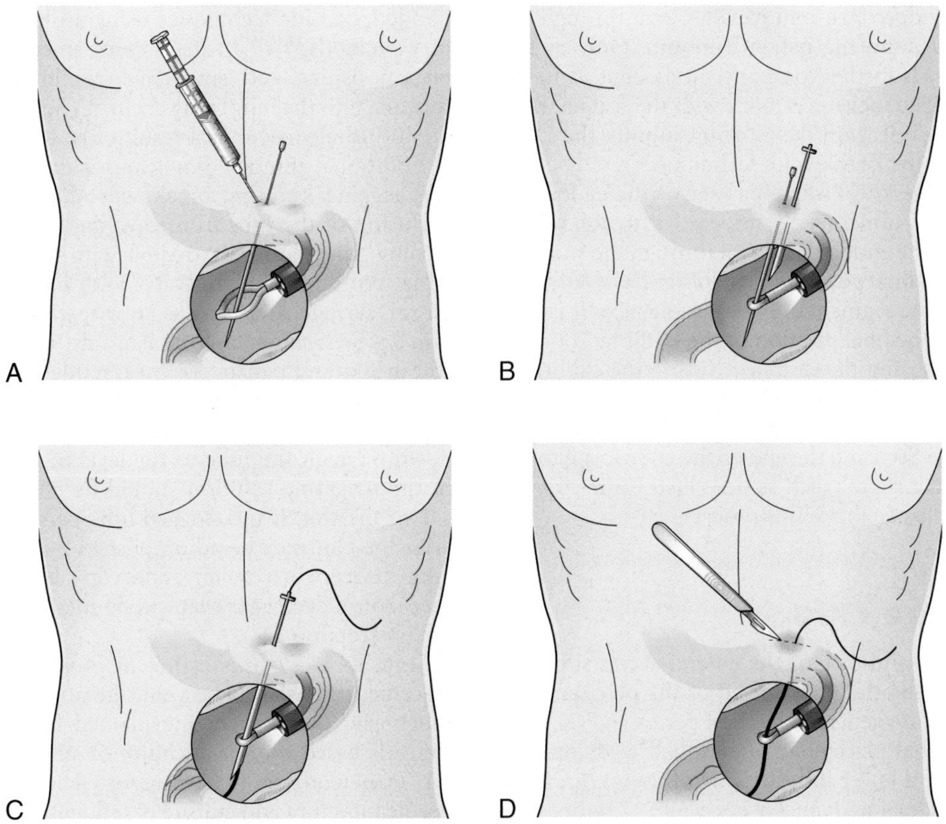

Fig. 23.17 Direct percutaneous endoscopic jejunostomy (DPEJ) technique. **A,** After quick initial skin anesthesia, a 23-gauge sounding needle is passed into the small bowel and grasped with a snare passed through the operating channel of the endoscope positioned in the small bowel. **B,** While holding the sounding needle in place with the snare, the trocar is passed at the same angle into the small bowel. The snare is opened, the sounding needle is withdrawn, and the snare is transferred to the trocar. **C,** A guidewire is passed through the trocar, the snare is opened enough to fall back onto the wire, and the trocar is removed. **D,** Only after the wire has been grabbed firmly by the snare should the skin incision be made over the guidewire. Once the wire has been withdrawn out through the mouth, the final placement is made using the Ponsky pull technique.

sticks with the spinal gauge needle compared with the PEG technique. The Ponsky pull technique may be better suited for DPEJ. The plastic leader on the Sachs-Vine push technique may not be long enough to reach the small bowel site. Most importantly, a tube should be selected with a small enteral bolster. A large balloon bolster may cause partial obstruction of the small bowel. A 15-Fr pediatric PEG tube with a flat enteral bolster, available commercially, is ideal for this procedure.

In passing the endoscope through the stomach and into the small bowel, it is important to pay attention to landmarks so that the endoscopist knows when the tip of the endoscope is below the ligament of Treitz. In a patient with Billroth II anatomy, it is important to document the efferent limb for DPEJ placement. The pediatric colonoscope is the instrument of choice in patients with intact anatomy or a "virgin abdomen." A more flexible gastroscope may be better suited for a patient with a partial gastrectomy and a Billroth II reanastomosis. In patients with an intact stomach, the colonoscope may need to be passed its entire length into the small bowel and withdrawn back to the proximal duodenum several times before a site can be identified by transillumination and finger palpation. Site selection is facilitated by starting to look for a site immediately beyond the ligament of Treitz and passing into each successive length of bowel (moving distally) if unsuccessful.

At the beginning of the procedure, the assistant at the skin should have the anesthetic needle and syringe in one hand and the sounding needle in the other hand. As the assistant observes translumination, a quick brief injection of the local anesthetic is followed by a quick abrupt puncture with the sounding needle. Care should be taken not to pass the sounding needle more proximally into the shaft of the endoscope. The endoscopist should place a snare through the instrument and out into the lumen, anticipating passage of the sounding needle into the lumen of the small bowel (**Fig. 23.17A**). Once the small bowel is intubated, the sounding needle is grasped firmly with the snare and held in place by the endoscopist. The assistant at the skin takes the trocar and passes alongside the sounding needle in the same axis to achieve intubation in the small bowel (**Fig. 23.17B**). Glucagon may be given intravenously at this point to maintain a hypotonic bowel.

A commercial model of a DPEJ device has combined the sounding needle and trocar together as one piece, making this section of the DPEJ technique a one-step procedure. After the trocar is passed into the lumen of the small bowel, the snare is released from the sounding needle and repositioned on the trocar. The sounding needle is withdrawn and removed. Still holding the bowel in place with the snare affixed to the trocar, a wire is passed through the trocar into the small bowel, and the snare is slipped off the trocar, grabbing the wire within the lumen of the small bowel (**Fig. 23.17C**). The wire is fed through the trocar as the endoscopist removes the wire through the stomach, esophagus, and the patient's mouth. Only at this point (**Fig. 23.17D**) is further local anesthesia applied in the area of the wire, and an incision is made with the scalpel. With the wire protruding out from the patient's mouth, the DPEJ tube is placed using the Ponsky pull technique.

Compared with the PEG (where passage of the endoscope after placement is optional), it is imperative to follow the enteral bolster with the endoscope down through the stomach and small bowel into final position. The bolster has a tendency to pop down from one segment of bowel to the next. It is very difficult to confirm the final position of the DPEJ by "blinded feel" alone, by measuring the distances (using the calibrated markings on the tube) between the skin and the enteral bolster, or by palpating the enteral bolster transabdominally with tension on the tube. Securing the end of the endoscope to the enteral bolster with a snare (such as described earlier for the PEG procedure) helps facilitate this process.

Postprocedure Care

Patient management and care of the enteral access site after placement is essentially the same for all of the percutaneous techniques. Patients are generally held nil per os (NPO) for 3 to 4 hours after initial placement, after which feeds may be initiated. Starting at a lower infusion rate of 25 mL/hr, feeds may be advanced as tolerated quickly every 6 to 12 hours such that goal infusion rate is obtained within 24 to 48 hours. For the first 7 to 10 days, a mild cleansing agent should be used once per day to clean the access site. Use of hydrogen peroxide washes or scented soaps that contain an alcohol base should be avoided because they have a drying desiccating effect on the tissue. Bandage dressings should be changed daily over this initial period. The external bolster should be moved back 4 days after initial placement to allow 0.5 to 1 cm of play between the skin and bolster. After 7 to 10 days, the frequency of dressing changes may be decreased.

Endoscopic Nasoenteric Tube Complications

The most common complication of the ENET procedure is postinsertion displacement. Tubes placed intentionally in the small bowel may be displaced back into the stomach in 3.7% to 7.0% of cases.[12] Inadvertent removal of the nasoenteric tube completely occurs in 21% to 41% of patients.[13,14] Inadvertent removal does not always occur in a setting with the typical profile of a patient with altered mental status. Most cases of inadvertent removal involve patients with normal mental status, occurring as a result of routine nursing duties (e.g., arising from bed, transport out of the unit, physical therapy) when there has been failure to secure the tube by proper methods.[13] Securing the distal end of the nasoenteric feeding tube by using a hemoclip (securing a suture on the tip of the tube to the intestinal mucosa) does not prevent displacement of the tube manually by the patient. Securing the proximal end with a nasal bridle or some kind of bandage clipping device (securing the proximal end to the skin) is needed. Displacement of nasoenteric tubes on initial placement occurs in 0.3% to 15% of cases (mean 3% to 4%), but this is related more to

blinded, bedside techniques using aspirate pH and auscultatory methods.[12,14,15] In these cases, pneumothorax, bronchopleural fistula, and empyema (resulting from infusion of formula into the lung) may occur.[12] These latter complications do not usually occur as a result of endoscopic placement.

Additional minor complications include epistaxis; persistent gagging; knotting, breaking, and kinking of the tube; and occlusion of the tube from clogging of the formula. Clogged feeding tubes are best treated with a pancreatin (Viokase) tablet crushed in warm water with bicarbonate, placed in a 10-mL syringe, and used as an irrigating solution. This solution has been shown in formal testing to be superior to various soft drinks and papain (or meat tenderizer).[16] If the clot fails to clear with this irrigating solution alone, an endoscopic retrograde cholangiopancreatography catheter should be placed down through the tube to the level of the clot, and infusion of the irrigating solution should be delivered directly at the site of the clot. If the clogged tube persists, further efforts to clear the clot may be accomplished by a mechanical declogging device, such as an endoscopy brush or spiral-shaped mechanical declogger that can be rotated or screwed through the obstruction.

Sinusitis is a complication of prolonged nasoenteric tube placement and should be a consideration in patients with such tubes who develop an unexplained fever. The incidence of sinusitis based on opacification of sinuses on radiograph or CT scan tends to be overreported at approximately 25%; needle puncture and culture of effluent from the sinuses more accurately places the incidence at approximately 11.4%.[17] Esophageal stricture is a theoretical complication of longstanding nasoenteric tubes, but the incidence is unclear and is probably underreported. A long-standing nasal bridle, in place for greater than 1 to 2 months' duration, may erode through the nasal septum.

Percutaneous Endoscopic Gastrostomy Complications

Reports from the literature of overall complications related to PEG placement indicate that this minimally invasive procedure has low morbidity and negligible mortality.[18,19] Two large series showed that the incidence of minor complications ranged from 4.9% to 13%, with major complications ranging from 1.3% to 3%.[18,19] Mortality in these two large series was 0.2% to 1.0%.[18,19] Two more recent large series duplicated these results, showing that the rate of minor complications ranged from 10.3% to 10.7%, with major complications ranging from 1.0% to 2.4%.[20,21] There was no mortality in these more recent series. Minor complications described in these reports include peristomal wound infections, tube disintegration, clogging, leakage, prolonged ileus, late inadvertent extubation, subcostal neuralgia, laceration of the left lobe of the liver, and delayed closure after removal. Major complications reported include aspiration, peritonitis, premature removal, tumor implantation at the PEG site, buried bumper syndrome, gastrocolocutaneous fistula, necrotizing fasciitis, and hemorrhage.[18–21]

A benign pneumoperitoneum occurs in 40% of cases after routine PEG placement.[22] In the absence of peritoneal signs (e.g., rebound tenderness), this finding is innocuous and does not preclude feeding within 4 hours of tube placement. Pneumoperitoneum may or may not be accompanied by a large air-filled distended stomach, which can be decompressed easily by uncapping the newly placed PEG tube.[23] Prolonged ileus after PEG placement was described in 1% of patients in one large series.[21]

The incidence of aspiration after PEG placement is difficult to determine because of varying definitions (witnessed aspiration event vs. new infiltrate on chest radiograph vs. aspiration of gastric contents labeled with a radioisotope or fluoroscopic colorimetric microsphere). The risk of aspiration immediately related to the procedure of PEG placement has been reported to be less than 1% of cases[18,24] and is thought to be related to oversedation, overinflation of the stomach, and performance of the procedure in the supine position. Aspiration as a long-term complication of PEG placement has been reported in 18% of cases.[25] In one small prospective study, patients randomly assigned to PEG placement had lower gastroesophageal reflux (as measured by 24-hour pH monitoring) compared with patients randomly assigned to nasogastric feeding.[26]

Risk for aspiration over the long-term is related to patient age (>70 years), reduced level of consciousness, history of neuromuscular disease, delayed gastric emptying, endotracheal intubation, trauma to the abdomen or pelvis, bolus versus continuous feeds, and nursing care.[27,28] Risk for aspiration increases fourfold when patients are moved from the ICU (low patient-to-nurse ratio) out to the medical or surgical floor (high patient-to-nurse ratio).[27] These studies reporting aspiration after PEG placement do not usually differentiate aspiration of contaminated oropharyngeal secretions from regurgitation and aspiration of contaminated gastric contents. Three studies suggest that the aspiration of contaminated oropharyngeal secretions compared with aspiration of bacteria-laden gastric contents is at least an equivalent if not greater factor in colonizing the trachea and upper respiratory tree.[29–31] Poor oral health has been well defined as an additional risk factor for aspiration in patients receiving tube feeding.[32]

Buried bumper syndrome is an underreported complication ranging from ulceration underneath the enteral bolster to total erosion of the PEG tube out through the gastric and abdominal wall. It most often occurs as a result of excessive tension between the external and enteral bolster; additional predisposing factors include smaller, stiffer enteral bolsters (made from silicone compared with polyurethane), presence of malnutrition or poor wound healing, or a significant weight gain in response to feeding.[24] Buried bumper syndrome may manifest simply as increased leakage around the PEG, infection at the PEG site, immobility of the catheter, resistance to infusion, or abdominal pain occurring with infusion of formula.[23,24,33,34] Various techniques are described in the literature to manage this complication. Usually the PEG tube has to be removed either by pulling it back into the stomach and out through the mouth or by pulling it out through the abdominal wall. In patients in whom the PEG tube has not been used for several weeks to months, the enteral bolster may be completely buried within the gastric and abdominal wall. In this situation, a needle-knife thermocoagulation catheter may be required to cut down to the bolster to facilitate removal.[33]

Gastrocolocutaneous fistulas may occur because of inadvertent puncture of an overlying loop of bowel at the time of initial placement or as a delayed complication occurring because of migration or erosion of the tube over time into the colon.[24,35] Insufficient translumination, inadequate gastric insufflation at the time of initial placement, and previous abdominal surgery in which a loop of bowel may be tacked down by scar tissue all are risk factors increasing the likelihood for this complication.[23,24] Gastrocolocutaneous fistula may manifest acutely with peritonitis, infection, fasciitis, or obstruction to flow of infusion of the formula. More often, it occurs chronically, manifesting after several months with either stool appearing around the PEG tube or insidious diarrhea in which the stool has the appearance of formula identical to that infused into the PEG. Frequently, this complication is not identified until the tube is removed and stool appears at the ostomy site. This complication is managed by first documenting the fistula with radiographic contrast studies. It is managed easily by removing the PEG, placing a bandage over the defect, and allowing the site to heal. Operative takedown is required only if the fistula fails to close.[23,24]

PEG site infection is one of the most common complications of PEG placement. Risk for developing PEG site infection is related to patient factors (e.g., diabetes, obesity, malnutrition, or long-term use of steroids), factors involving technique (pull or push type PEGs vs. introducer PEGs, small incisions, and lack of antibiotic prophylaxis), and nursing care (excessive traction on the bolsters). The incidence of wound infection around the PEG site ranges from 5.4% to 17.0%,[25,36,37] but most (>70%) are minor in degree.[38] Antibiotic prophylaxis at the time of initial placement is an important measure to reduce the incidence of this complication. In an older study, a single dose of antibiotic prophylaxis at the time of placement reduced the incidence of PEG site infection from 32% down to 7% ($P < .05$).[39] In a more recent study, a single dose of one or two antibiotics at the time of placement reduced the incidence of PEG site infection significantly from 13.2% to 0.5% compared with controls receiving no antibiotic prophylaxis ($P < .01$).[38] Patients already receiving concurrent antibiotics do not need additional prophylaxis at the time of PEG placement.[40] If infection develops around the PEG site, usually intravenous antibiotics and local wound care are sufficient to correct the complication. Surgical incision and drainage is rarely required. Peritonitis occurs less frequently in 0.4% to 1.5% of cases[18,24,35,41] and is differentiated from simple PEG site infection by the development of peritoneal signs and rebound tenderness. Prompt broad-spectrum intravenous antibiotics are usually sufficient. In the presence of peritonitis, however, contrast studies should be performed to rule out the presence of a leak. If there is leakage into the peritoneum, surgical intervention is required.[24]

Hemorrhage is a rare complication involving less than 2.5% of cases.[24,35] Various etiologic factors may contribute to this complication, including direct puncture of a blood vessel or traumatic tearing of the esophagus or stomach on initial placement, concomitant peptic ulcer disease, development of gastric ulcer underneath the enteral bolster, or erosion of the posterior gastric wall opposite from the enteral bolster of the PEG tube.[24,35] Management involves urgent endoscopy to document the source and appropriate steps to achieve hemostasis.

Leakage around the PEG site is reported in only 1% to 2% of cases,[21,41] but this probably represents underreporting of the incidence of this complication. Etiologic factors include corrosive agents (vitamin C [ascorbic acid] infused with formula, increased gastric acid arising from stop orders for prescribed acid-reducing agents, and continued hydrogen peroxide washes of the site after initial placement), cutaneous fungal infection around the site, development of granulation tissue, side-torsion on the tube creating ulceration on one wall of the tract, absence of an external bolster (allowing to-and-fro motion of the PEG tube through the tract), buried bumper syndrome, and PEG site infection. Management depends on defining the exacerbating factors, which can usually be ascertained by careful examination of the PEG site. Initial physical examination should rule out PEG site infection, confirm there is no fixation of the tube (suggesting buried bumper syndrome), and ensure there is no ulceration of the tract indicating side-torsion. The patient's list of medications should be reviewed, a proton pump inhibitor should be added if this agent has not been ordered, ascorbic acid should be stopped, and consideration should be given to providing an antifungal cream or zinc oxide to the site. Side-torsion creating ulceration in the tract may require stabilization of the PEG tube with a vertical clamp (which prevents side-to-side motion). Granulation tissue around the PEG site may be treated with silver nitrate sticks. Options for cases in which there is no external bolster include replacing the PEG tube with a commercial replacement PEG set that contains an external bolster and creating a homemade external bolster from the funneled end of a Foley catheter. PEG site infection should be treated, as should existence of the buried bumper syndrome according to previously described methods. In more severe cases, the tract may be damaged to the point that diverting the stream of infused formula down into the small bowel (by converting the PEG to a PEGJ) or completely removing the PEG tube and placing a nasoenteric aspirate or feed tube to allow the site to heal may be required.

Accidental extubation of the PEG tube occurs in 1.6% to 4.4% of cases; half of these cases occur prematurely before complete maturation of the PEG site.[20,25,35,37,42] Normally, the PEG site should mature over 7 to 10 days, at which point the gastric wall becomes fused to the anterior abdominal wall. Maturation of the PEG tract may be delayed 3 to 4 weeks in the presence of long-term steroid use, malnutrition, or ascites. Management is simple as long as no peritonitis is present.[35] A nasogastric tube can be placed for decompression, a broad-spectrum antibiotic should be started, and the PEG may be replaced within 7 to 10 days. Surgical intervention is required only if peritonitis develops.[35] Once the PEG tract is mature, simple bedside replacement with a PEG tube (or endoscopic placement if the site closes down) may be sufficient. Less common complications of PEG placement include tumor implantation at the PEG site, development of a broncho-esophageal fistula, migration of the enteral balloon bolster causing gastric outlet obstruction at the level of the pylorus, reversible apnea, subcostal neuralgia, and development of a gastroileocutaneous fistula.[20,43–47]

Percutaneous Endoscopic Gastrojejunostomy and Direct Percutaneous Endoscopic Jejunostomy Complications

Patients requiring placement of a PEGJ are at risk for all of the complications previously described for placement of a routine PEG tube. The most common additional problem encountered with PEGJ tubes is inadvertent migration of the jejunal tube from the small bowel back into the stomach, which occurs in 27% to 42% of cases.[48–50] Numerous factors contribute to this complication including a large dilated atonic stomach, failure to cut the PEG tube down to a shortened length, insufficient length of the jejunal tube, placement of the initial PEG high in the stomach, surgical PEG placement (in which the PEG tube is tunneled pointing toward the gastroesophageal junction), and recurrent nausea and vomiting. Steps that can be taken at the time of initial placement to reduce this complication include positioning the PEG tube immediately above and to the right of the umbilicus so that the entrance is in the gastric antrum, cutting the PEG tube down to approximately 10 cm in length, selecting a jejunal tube with the greatest length, and ensuring there is no loop in the stomach as the jejunal tube passes from the PEG to the pylorus. As mentioned earlier in the section on technique of PEGJ placement, securing the distal end to the intestinal mucosa with a hemoclip or placement of an anchor device may help hold the jejunal tube in place for a brief time.

Complications arising from DPEJ placement differ very little from the complications encountered with routine PEG placement. Of note, a jejunocolocutaneous fistula may occur. Intermittent small bowel obstruction may occur when a larger, balloon-type enteral bolster is selected for the procedure. Volvulus leading to necrotic bowel has been described with DPEJ.[51]

Conclusion

Multidisciplinary nutrition teams across the United States are pressured to obtain early enteral access because most of the literature shows that early use of the gut and maintenance of gut integrity significantly improve patient outcome. These teams rely on a skilled endoscopist to obtain enteral access, monitor enteral tube feeding, and help troubleshoot problems when the issue of intolerance arises. When short-term naso-enteric feeding is required or more long-term percutaneous access is needed, various techniques exist for almost any patient situation. Under each category of access, the endoscopist should learn one main technique well and then experiment enough with all of the techniques to know which one suits him or her best. Proper choice of instrument, correct accessory devices, and selection of the appropriate technique for the needs of the individual patient should optimize the chances for success and minimize the risk of complications when performing endoscopic procedures to obtain enteral access.

References

The complete reference list is available online at www.expertconsult.com.

Acute Colonic Pseudo-obstruction

Robert J. Ponec and Michael B. Kimmey

Introduction

Acute colonic pseudo-obstruction (ACPO) is a disorder characterized by massive dilation of the colon in the absence of mechanical obstruction. This severe motility disturbance, also known as Ogilvie's syndrome,[1] usually develops in hospitalized patients and is associated with various medical and surgical conditions. The tension on the colon wall resulting from the extreme dilation can lead to ischemic necrosis and perforation, especially in the cecum. The rate of spontaneous perforation has been reported to be 3% to 15% with an attendant 40% to 50% mortality rate.[2–5] Despite the potential risk of perforation, approximately 75% of patients with ACPO recover over an average of 3 to 5 days when treated with a variety of conservative measures.[3,4] During the sometimes prolonged recovery phase, however, ACPO contributes greatly to patients' discomfort and immobilization and may delay institution of enteral nutrition.

The risk of perforation and the morbidity of the long recovery led to a search for effective and safe therapies, not only to prevent perforation but also to speed resolution. Very few controlled trials have evaluated the standard therapies used for ACPO. Nonetheless, conservative management strategies such as nasogastric suction and measures to correct precipitating factors have been the mainstay of treatment.

For the minority (about 25%) of patients who fail to respond to conservative therapy and for patients who have severe, prolonged colonic dilation risking perforation, more active interventions are instituted. In the past, surgical cecostomy and hemicolectomy were the main options in severe or refractory cases. Subsequently, colonoscopy and various radiologic procedures were reported to help decompress the colon.[5–10] More recently, medications such as neostigmine have been shown to be effective.[11] The timing and combination of conservative and more active interventions must be individualized according to the severity of ACPO and the patient's comorbidities.

Epidemiology

ACPO is relatively uncommon. It can be triggered by various acute medical and surgical illnesses. Typically, rapid-onset abdominal distension begins within a few days of the onset of the underlying illness.[2] Because ACPO is uncommon, one must look at reviews that examine several years of reported cases to be able to draw conclusions about the epidemiology of the condition. Numerous case reports and reviews describe specific triggers. However, each proposed underlying condition seems to be associated with the development of ACPO in only a very small percentage of cases. ACPO has been reported after various surgeries, including orthopedic, urologic, gynecologic, neurologic, and organ transplants.[3,4,12–21,22] It is seen in obstetrics after vaginal deliveries and cesarean sections.[3,23,24] Trauma and burn patients sometimes develop ACPO.[3,4,12,25] Various medical illnesses are known to cause ACPO, including sepsis, respiratory failure, mechanical ventilation, renal failure, myocardial infarction, vascular emergencies, sickle cell crisis, and cancer.[3,4,12,26–37] Many medications can precipitate ACPO, especially narcotic analgesics and any medication that decreases peristalsis, such as tricyclic antidepressants or anticholinergic drugs.[5,7,38–40] **Table 24.1** lists these associated conditions. Although the connection between any of these causes and ACPO is most likely through a disturbance in the auto-

Table 24-1 **Conditions Associated with Acute Colonic Pseudo-obstruction**

Surgical	Obstetric	Trauma	Medical Illnesses	Medications
Orthopedic	Normal delivery	Fractures	Sepsis	Narcotic analgesics
Urologic	Cesarean section	Burns	Neurologic disorders	Tricyclic antidepressants
Gynecologic			Cancer	Anesthetic agents
Abdominal			Chemotherapy	Antiparkinsonian drugs
Transplant			Radiation therapy	Anticholinergics
			Hypothyroidism	
			Myocardial infarction	
			Stroke	
			Respiratory failure, mechanical ventilation	
			Renal failure	
			Electrolyte imbalance (potassium, magnesium, calcium, phosphorus)	
			Viral infections (herpes, varicella zoster)	

nomic innervation of the bowel, other variables, such as patient age; comorbidities; and factors such as immobility, medications, and electrolyte imbalances, are thought to help precipitate the onset in an individual patient.[2]

In one review of 351 ACPO cases from 1948–1980, 88% followed surgery, trauma, or acute medical illnesses.[3] The remaining 12% were classified as idiopathic. This review reported a 15% perforation rate, with a 45% mortality in patients with colonic perforation. This high mortality was attributed in part to the fact that these patients already had serious underlying medical or surgical problems.

In another review of 400 patients from 1970–1985, 95% of the cases had identifiable underlying medical, surgical, or obstetric conditions[4]; this left only 5% to be categorized as idiopathic. ACPO usually developed within 5 days of onset of the underlying condition. The median patient age was about 60 years, and the male-to-female ratio was 1.5:1. Perforation rate was 20%, and mortality in patients with perforation was about 40%. Overall, mortality in the group was 15%. Mortality rate was affected by age, cecal diameter, length of dilation of colon, presence of ischemia in bowel wall, and patient comorbidities. One important observation in this review was that patients with cecal diameter 8 to 25 cm usually had viable colon without significant ischemia. Cecal size alone is not the only factor in the risk of perforation. Other variables, such as the acuity of the onset and the duration of distention, were also potentially important factors.

Pathogenesis

In 1948, Ogilvie[1] first described massive colonic distention in two patients who had the onset of abdominal distention over a few weeks, rather than the more acute presentation that we currently refer to as Ogilvie's syndrome. Ironically, by today's criteria, neither would be categorized as ACPO. Both patients were ultimately found to have widespread intraabdominal malignancy with retroperitoneal involvement of nerve plexuses, leading Ogilvie to speculate that disruption of the autonomic innervation of the colon was the underlying cause of the disorder.[1]

Despite the variety of possible triggers of ACPO, the presentation is remarkably consistent. Generally, patients develop severe abdominal distention within 5 days of the onset of the medical or surgical insult. The intestinal dilation is usually most pronounced in the colon, especially proximal to the splenic flexure. On x-ray examination, the appearance is very similar to that of a patient who actually has an obstruction near the upper left colon, leading to the term *pseudo-obstruction*. These facts led to the hypothesis that the final common pathway of the development of the disease is an acute cessation of effective colonic motility resulting from a disruption of the autonomic supply of the left side of the colon. One hypothesis was that excess sympathetic stimulation of the colon was inhibiting contraction. This hypothesis seemed to be supported by the observation that this distention occurred in any sort of severe physical stress. In addition, epidural anesthesia to decrease sympathetic output has been reported to be beneficial treatment for ACPO.[41] However, when guanethidine was used to block sympathetic tone, there was very little effect on colonic function in ACPO patients.[42]

The leading current theory about the pathogenesis of ACPO is that a decrease in parasympathetic stimulus to the colon is more important than an excess of sympathetic input.[43] In the study of guanethidine mentioned previously, patients first were given guanethidine and then were treated with neostigmine to block acetylcholinesterase. Patients had a prompt return of colonic contraction only after the neostigmine, leading to the idea that a loss of parasympathetic tone is important in the development of ACPO. Some authors speculate that the parasympathetic deficiency is most pronounced in the left colon because of disruption of supply from the sacral plexus; this may explain why the left colon is contracted and aperistaltic in ACPO. Since these pioneering studies, the one medical treatment that has had the most consistent success in treatment of ACPO has been the use of neostigmine to cause a sudden increase in acetylcholine concentration at parasympathetic nerve synapses and an increase in colon peristalsis.

Other factors that likely contribute to the pathogenesis of ACPO are chronic underlying bowel motility disorders and constipation, patient immobility, electrolyte imbalance, medications such as narcotics, and mechanical ventilation. These other factors may contribute to the autonomic imbalance, directly suppress muscular function of the colon, or simply increase the amount of gas that is entering the digestive tract. At least 50% of patients with ACPO have significant electrolyte abnormalities, especially low potassium, magnesium, and calcium.[4] Secretory diarrhea (with high potassium and low sodium concentration in the stool) can occur in ACPO. This is thought to be due to the effect of autonomic nervous system disturbance and of colonic distension on the activity of the apical (BK) potassium channels in the colonic mucosa.[44]

The most feared complication of ACPO is colon perforation. When perforation occurs, it is usually in the right colon, especially the cecum. The pathophysiology relates to high wall tension in the cecum leading to ischemic necrosis and wall disruption. The right colon, which naturally has a thinner wall and larger diameter than the left side, has the highest wall tension when the colon is distended. This occurrence is described well by Laplace's law: $T = P \times R/2d$, where T is wall tension, P is pressure in colon lumen, R is radius of the colon, and d represents the thickness of the colonic wall. This equation helps to explain how small changes in colonic radius in the setting of severe distention of the thin-walled cecum can lead to relatively large changes in wall tension and increase the risk of perforation.

Usually the perforation risk is not very high in patients with cecal diameter less than 12 cm. Paradoxically, studies have shown that patients with ACPO and cecal diameter greater than 25 cm can recover without incident. Other variables, such as elasticity of the muscle wall, adequacy of blood supply, and time course of distention must be important as well in determining whether the colon remains viable. Some studies indicate an association between the duration of ACPO and perforation risk and indicate that patients with persistence of distention for more than 5 days have higher perforation rates.[45]

Clinical Features

ACPO is seen mainly in patients who are hospitalized for an acute medical, surgical, obstetric, or traumatic event. The condition progresses at a variable rate, usually over 2 to 7 days. The nearly universal symptom is progressive abdominal distention. The reported frequency of other symptoms is quite varied. Abdominal pain (10% to 80%), nausea (10% to 60%), vomiting (10% to 60%), diarrhea (30% to 40%), constipation (40% to 50%), and respiratory compromise resulting from distention all have been reported.[3-5,7] Patients with ischemia and perforation are much more likely to have abdominal pain and fever.

Physical examination findings include a markedly distended abdomen that is usually tympanitic to percussion. Bowel sounds are often present. Although some tenderness has been noted in 60% of patients in some reports, significant tenderness or guarding should raise suspicion for perforation.

Laboratory abnormalities include an elevated white blood cell count in up to 25% of patients without perforation and in almost 100% of patients with perforation.[4] Abnormalities in electrolytes such as potassium, calcium, magnesium, and phosphorus and abnormalities in thyroid function are not caused by ACPO but are thought to contribute to colonic dysfunction. These laboratory values should be checked and corrected, if abnormal.

Abdominal x-ray films show colonic distention, usually most pronounced in the cecum, ascending, and transverse colon. In contrast to patients with severe obstipation, the colon is distended primarily with gas, not stool. There is often an apparent "cutoff" near the splenic flexure with a collapsed left colon. The location of the cutoff varies. In one review, the cutoff was at the splenic flexure in 56% of patients, at the hepatic flexure in 18%, and at the descending or sigmoid colon in 27%. Although the small bowel is said usually to have less dilation in ACPO, one report indicated 80% of patients had some small bowel dilation. Air-fluid levels have been reported in 40%. X-ray evidence of gas in the bowel wall or free intraperitoneal air is indicative of colonic perforation. Radiographic water-soluble contrast enemas are often needed to rule out a true mechanical obstruction. As discussed in the treatment section, the use of water-soluble contrast material has been reported to have a therapeutic effect in some patients.[46]

Differential Diagnosis

Two major considerations in the differential diagnosis of ACPO are mechanical bowel obstruction and toxic megacolon resulting from an enteric infection or inflammatory bowel disease (IBD). In addition, patients with chronic colonic pseudo-obstruction are sometimes first diagnosed when they are hospitalized for other reasons, making it important to establish first that the condition is truly acute and not chronic.

Mechanical colon obstruction from causes such as colon cancer, sigmoid volvulus, and diverticulitis must be confidently ruled out before considering specific therapies for ACPO. Often the fact that patients with ACPO continue to have watery bowel movements is helpful to indicate that a complete obstruction is unlikely. In some cases, the presence of some gas in the rectum or throughout the entire colon also helps to rule out obstruction. Nonetheless, these parameters are not totally reliable. Either a water-soluble contrast enema or a colonoscopy may be required to rule out mechanical obstruction.

Toxic megacolon resulting from infections such as *Clostridium difficile* should be considered in patients who have been exposed to antibiotics or prolonged care in a hospital or nursing facility, where they may have contracted the infection. Generally, such patients had severe diarrhea before the onset of the abdominal distention. Other colonic infections leading to toxic megacolon have been reported, particularly in immunosuppressed patients. In some cases, these patients seem to have a presentation indistinguishable from classic ACPO. However, when the colonic distention is due to infection, patients usually have an elevated white blood cell count; thickening of bowel wall on x-ray films; and endoscopic evidence of severe colonic erythema, edema, ulceration, or pseudomembranes on flexible sigmoidoscopy. Stool studies for enteric pathogens and *C. difficile* toxin are important in this setting.[47]

Similarly, toxic megacolon resulting from IBD can usually be differentiated from ACPO by a review of clinical history, laboratory results, x-ray films, and findings on sigmoidoscopy.[48] Patients with IBD should have had a history of diarrhea (often bloody) and abdominal cramps before the development of colonic distention. Blood test results usually show leukocytosis. Abdominal x-ray films often show bowel wall edema. Sigmoidoscopy should show changes consistent with IBD. Lastly, the presence of chronic pseudo-obstruction can often be excluded by a careful review of the patient's history, old records, and prior abdominal radiographs when available.

Treatment

Because ACPO is uncommon, there have been few controlled trials of the treatments that are currently considered the standard of care. Most data are from reviews, observational studies, and case presentations. Therapy is generally divided into conservative measures and active interventions. Because at least 75% of patients with ACPO experience resolution with a combination of conservative measures, these are generally tried first for at least 24 to 48 hours in most patients before more active interventions are considered.[49] The reported success from these measures ranges from 33% to 100%.[25–27]

The following sections describe conservative therapy, medication therapy, colonoscopy, and surgical approaches for ACPO. These treatments are often combined. Conservative measures are typically continued when more active interventions are added. The order and combination of these measures must be individualized to a patient's clinical presentation and course. There have been a number of excellent recent reviews on the topic of treatment of ACPO.[50–56] **Fig. 24.1** outlines a proposed treatment algorithm for most patients with ACPO, modified from the American Society for Gastrointestinal Endoscopy practice guideline on treatment of this condition.[49]

Conservative Therapy

Conservative measures for treatment of ACPO include most, if not all, of the following, depending on individual circumstances.[38] The patient is made nil per os (NPO), and nasogastric suction is used to prevent more gas from entering the gastrointestinal tract. Patients are mobilized as much as possible. If the patient is bed-bound, the patient's position should be changed often from side to side and, when possible, into the prone and knee-to-chest position. A search for contributing factors should be done with correction of as many as possible. One should withdraw medications that interfere with colonic motility, such as narcotic analgesics, anticholinergics, and calcium channel blockers. Electrolyte imbalance (especially potassium, calcium, magnesium, and phosphorus) should be corrected. Regular rectal examinations every 6 hours have been advocated as a way to encourage passage of colonic gas. Placement of a rectal tube is more often used for this purpose. Gentle tap water enemas are controversial but are advocated by some authors as a way to liquefy remaining stool. A water-soluble contrast enema, which can liquefy stool, is commonly performed to exclude mechanical obstruction. Some authors have reported a stimulant effect on motility that sometimes speeds recovery.[46] Prophylactic antibiotics have not been studied and are not common practice. If a patient has a fever or elevated white blood cell count, broad-spectrum antibiotics can be considered while a careful evaluation is under way for signs of colonic ischemia, perforation, or other infections.

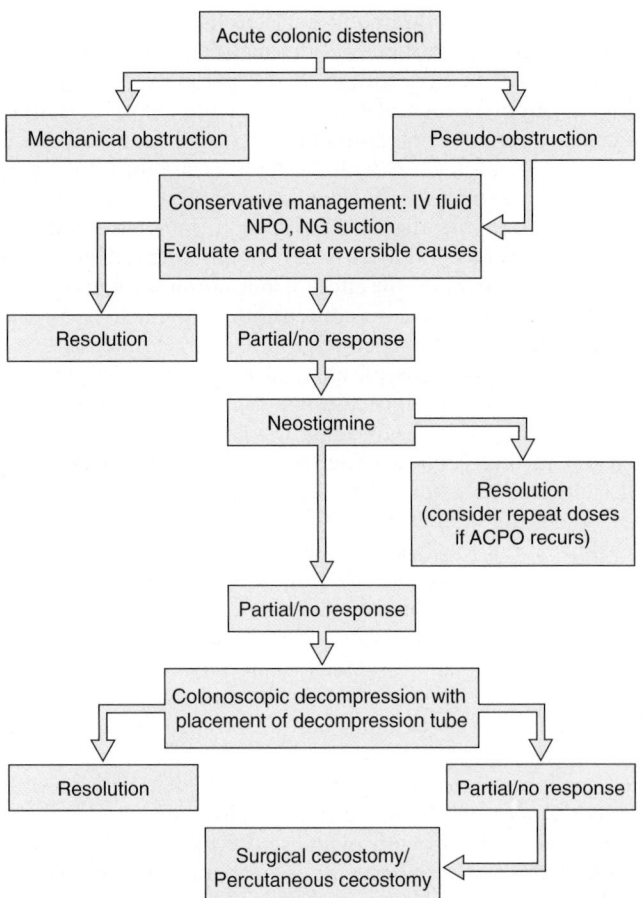

Fig. 24.1 Suggested algorithm for the management of acute colonic pseudo-obstruction (ACPO). This algorithm has been adapted from the Practice Guideline published by the American Society for Gastrointestinal Endoscopy. IV, intravenous; NG, nasogastric; NPO, nil per os. *(From Eisen GM, Baron TH, Dominitz JA, et al: Acute colonic pseudo-obstruction.* Gastrointest Endosc *56:789–792, 2002.)*

Conservative measures are continued for 24 to 48 hours before more active intervention is initiated. This recommendation is not based on controlled data but rather on the observation that patients whose severe colon dilation (>12 cm) persists for 4 to 5 days have a higher risk of ischemia and perforation.[4]

Although conservative therapy is generally successful, return of colon function in responders takes an average of 5 days. During this time, patients are contending with the consequences of ACPO, including distention, pain, delay in institution of enteral nutrition, compromised respiratory status, and delay in ambulation that can lead to other morbidities such as thromboembolism, atelectasis, and pneumonia These facts have led to a search for a safe and effective treatment not only for patients who are refractory to conservative measures but also to provide a more prompt resolution early in the course of the illness. Numerous active interventions have been reported to be useful for ACPO, including medications such as neostigmine,[11] colonoscopy with or without placement of a decompression tube,[57–63] meglumine diatrizoate (Gastrografin) enema,[46] radiologic procedures such as placement of a transanal decompression tube,[10] cecostomy, and surgical resection of part of the colon.

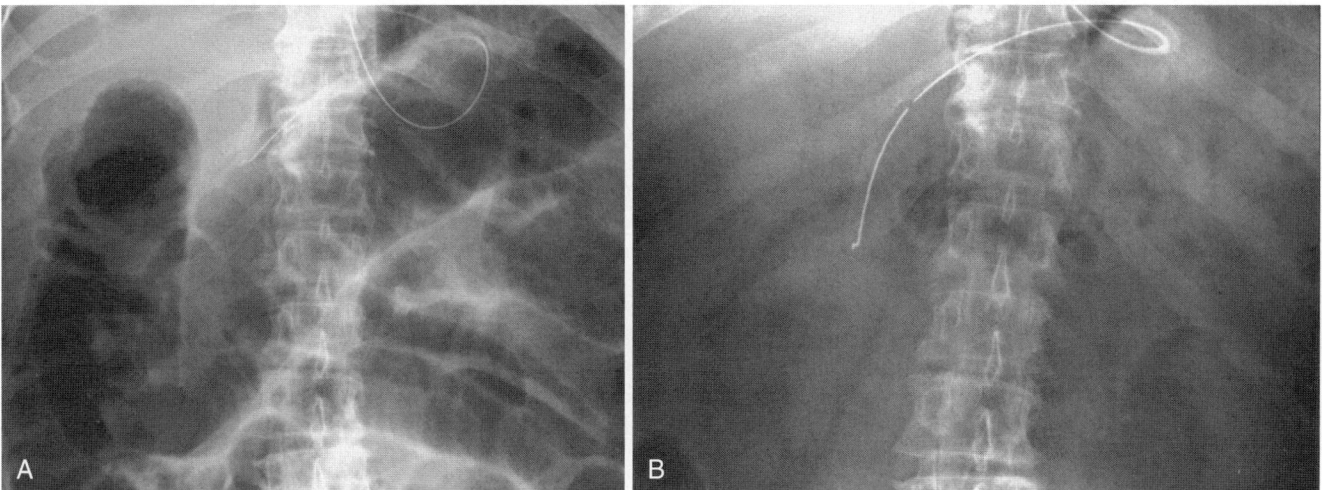

Fig. 24.2 A, Dilated transverse colon and hepatic flexure in a patient with acute colonic pseudo-obstruction (ACPO). A nasogastric tube is present in the stomach. **B,** Colonic gas is no longer present 3 hours after administration of neostigmine. The nasogastric tube remains in place. *(From Ponec RJ, Saunders MD, Kimmey MB: Neostigmine for the treatment of acute colonic pseudo-obstruction.* N Engl J Med *341:137–141, 1999. Copyright © 1999 Massachusetts Medical Society. All rights reserved.)*

Medical Therapy

Colonic decompression has been shown to be effective and has become the mainstay of treatment. Medications that stimulate colon motility have become popular. The most promising medication so far for treatment of ACPO is neostigmine, an inhibitor of acetylcholinesterase. Neostigmine causes a transient but significant increase in acetylcholine concentration, resulting in a pronounced increase in cholinergic stimulus throughout the body, including in the colon. The leading theory about the pathogenesis of ACPO is that there is an autonomic imbalance, with an increase in sympathetic tone and a decrease in the parasympathetic stimulus to the colon. Both of these changes are thought to have a negative impact on colon motility. This theory led to studies of drugs that either decrease sympathetic tone or increase parasympathetic tone as means to restore colon function.

In the 1960s, Neely and Catchpole[64] studied the effects of guanethidine (a sympathetic antagonist) and neostigmine (Prostigmine) (a cholinergic drug) on small bowel motility and found that these medications seemed to restore peristalsis. In 1992, Hutchinson and Griffiths[42] treated 11 ACPO patients first with guanethidine and then with neostigmine. They found that 8 of 11 patients had prompt return of bowel motility but only after the neostigmine infusion. In 1995, Stephenson and coworkers[16] presented results of a study showing that 11 of 12 ACPO patients treated with 2.5 mg of intravenous neostigmine had prompt resolution of their condition. These observations were confirmed by subsequent studies, including prompt clinical resolution in 75% of ACPO cases as presented by Turefano-Fuentes and coworkers[65] in 1997 and in 26 of 28 cases treated by Trevisani and colleagues,[66] whose results were published in 2000. Physiologic studies on neostigmine indicate that its indirect effect on muscarinic receptors in the bowel wall, presumably through increased local acetylcholine concentrations, results in increased colonic tone and increased coordinated colonic propulsion.[67]

Because ACPO often resolves with conservative therapy alone, controlled trials of neostigmine and other therapies are important. The only controlled trial published to date was performed at the University of Washington[11] and was published in 1999. The trial comprised 21 patients with ACPO (refractory to at least 24 hours of conservative measures and with a cecal diameter >10 cm) who were randomly assigned to receive either 2.0 mg of neostigmine or saline by a 3-minute intravenous infusion administered by a physician blinded to the treatment allocation. The responses recorded included immediate passage of flatus and stool; the amount of decrease in the measured abdominal girth; and the change in the diameters of the cecum, ascending, and transverse colon on abdominal x-ray films obtained 3 hours later (**Fig. 24.2**). Of the 11 patients randomly assigned to neostigmine, 10 had prompt resolution with substantial responses in all of the measured endpoints. The one nonresponder subsequently had a response when an open-label neostigmine dose was given 3 hours later. The median time to passage of flatus was 4 minutes (range 3 to 30 minutes). None of the patients given placebo responded, despite the continuation of conservative measures in all patients. Seven patients from the placebo group were treated with open-label neostigmine 3 hours later, and all had a prompt response. Since this publication, several uncontrolled studies have also reported similar results with usually about 80% to 90% of patients showing a prompt response to the drug. Sustained response after a single dose of neostigmine was similar in these other studies as well, usually about 60 to 70%.[68–75] Some studies have shown success with repeated doses of the drug for patients with partial responses and recurrences.[16]

Studies have been done on factors that predict response to neostigmine. One retrospective review showed an 89% initial response and a 61% sustained response to a single dose of neostigmine. They found that narcotic medication use decreased not only the spontaneous resolution rate but also the response rate to neostigmine. Ambulatory patients had higher response rates as well. Interestingly, colon diameter and duration of ACPO before treatment did not influence response rate.[71] Another study (prospective) enrolled 27 patients and found that electrolyte abnormalities and use of antimotility drugs were associated with poor response to neostigmine.[72]

Side effects of neostigmine include abdominal pain, nausea, vomiting, sweating, excess salivation, bronchospasm, and symptomatic bradycardia. Patients at risk for bradycardia, such as patients with preexisting bradyarrhythmias and patients receiving β blockers, are at potentially higher risk of complications from neostigmine, as are patients with severe bronchospasm. Some caution in patient selection is needed. Nonetheless, neostigmine can be used in most patients with ACPO when proper monitoring and precautions are in place. Patients should be kept supine on a pad or bed pan for the first 30 minutes after neostigmine and should be monitored by continuous electrocardiogram and frequent, intermittent blood pressure determinations. Transient bradycardia can occur but usually resolves quickly without treatment because of the short half-life of neostigmine. Atropine should be immediately available but should be given only if bradycardia is severe, prolonged, or associated with significant hypotension or persistent symptoms. Although neostigmine is partly cleared by plasma cholinesterase, about one-half of the clearance occurs in the kidneys; patients with renal failure have a prolonged half-life of neostigmine. In anephric patients, the elimination half-life is about 180 minutes compared with 80 minutes seen in patients with normal renal function.[76]

Glycopyrrolate, a selective anticholinergic agent, has been proposed as a way to decrease neostigmine side effects like bradycardia and bronchoconstriction. Since it has less effect on the bowel, glycopyrrolate might not interfere with the stimulatory effect of neostigmine in restoring colonic contraction. Although there has not been an organized study on this combined neostigmine/glycopyrrolate administration specifically in ACPO, one controlled study in spinal cord injury patients showed that the combination was as effective as neostigmine alone in prompting colon evacuation. Also, bradycardia and bronchoconstriction were not seen when the drugs were given together.[77] Because it seems to be rapidly effective in most patients with ACPO and has a low side-effect profile compared with other active therapies such as colonoscopy or surgery, neostigmine appears early in the suggested treatment algorithm.[47,78,79] Although mainly studied in adult patients, there have been case reports of successful use in pediatric patients as well.[37,80] Most studies indicate that as long as conservative measures are continued, the recurrence rate of ACPO after neostigmine is low.[11] Nonetheless, repeat doses can be tried in case of recurrence before one resorts to more invasive techniques. Because the elimination half-life is 80 minutes, retreatment is not advisable at intervals less than every 3 hours.

Since there is the issue of recurrence of colonic distension after neostigmine, as well as after colonoscopic decompression, efforts have been made to reduce recurrence. One controlled study showed that, after successful decompression with either neostigmine or colonoscopy (with decompression tube placement), the administration of polyethylene glycol solution twice daily (orally or per NG mixed with water) for 7 days reduced the recurrence rate for colonic distension (0/15 in PEG group versus 5/15 in placebo group).[81]

Although slower infusion of neostigmine has not been studied in ACPO, neostigmine drip over 24 hours at 0.4 to 0.8 mg per hour has been shown to be very effective in critically ill ICU patients with ileus. Eleven out of thirteen patients in the neostigmine group recovered bowel motility and passed stools while none of the eleven in the placebo group did.

Interestingly, these authors did not observe neostigmine side effects of bradycardia or bronchospasm.[82]

Other medical therapies have been reported, including prokinetics such as metoclopramide,[83] erythromycin,[84,85] and cisapride.[86] Most reports on these other agents have been anecdotes of one or two patients. The published reports on use of metoclopramide have been disappointing. Some reports have questioned the wisdom of applying a prokinetic such as metoclopramide out of concern that its main stimulus is on emptying the upper gut; this theoretically may deliver even more gas to the colon without adequate stimulus of the colon itself and worsen the distention there. Since the use of opioid medications has been associated with ACPO and also with failure to respond to conservative and neostigmine therapy, there may theoretically be some benefit to use of peripheral opioid receptor blockers like methylnaltrexone. However, the results of studies on the use of this and other peripheral opioid receptor antagonists like alvmivopan have been quite mixed.[87–89]

Colonoscopy

Colonoscopy is useful in treating ACPO in many ways. First, it is used to suction the extra gas and decompress the colon directly. Colonoscopy is also used rule out mechanical obstruction and to check for signs of colonic mucosal ischemia and necrosis. Lastly, it can be used to place a guidewire into the proximal colon over which a decompression tube can be placed. The reported rate of intubation proximal to the hepatic flexure in the setting of ACPO is at least 70%.[5]

Although there are no controlled trials proving its efficacy, colonoscopic decompression has been central in the therapy of ACPO patients who fail conservative measures. Its successful use was first reported in 1977 by Kukor and Dent.[6] Since then, numerous uncontrolled studies have reported initial clinical success with colonoscopy in about 70% of cases.[7,8,17,26] Nonetheless, a high recurrence rate of 40% may lead to repeated colonoscopy to maintain the response–sometimes two or more additional procedures.[5,7,57,90] Several authors have reported a lower recurrence rate if a decompression tube is left in place, especially if it is proximal to the hepatic flexure.[58–60] One institution compared the recurrence rate of colonoscopy with decompression tube placement with historical controls of colonoscopy alone and found recurrence rates of 0% versus 45%.[61] Some authors have criticized uncontrolled studies on colonoscopic decompression because they have not had control groups of conservative therapy alone (which may have differed over time) and have a referral bias of studying only patients specifically referred for the purpose of colonoscopic decompression.[5,62]

A summary of expert consensus on several aspects of therapeutic colonoscopy for ACPO follows.[63] Colonoscopy in ACPO patients is technically difficult (performed in the unprepared colon of seriously ill patients) and carries an increased perforation risk of 1% to 3%.[7,62] It should be performed only by expert endoscopists. Preparatory enemas are not needed because the stool remaining in the colon is usually already liquefied. In addition, enemas may increase the risk of perforation in patients with ACPO. Air insufflation must be kept to a minimum. Insufflation with carbon dioxide is preferable. As each new dilated segment is entered with the colonoscope, it should be decompressed. The mucosa should

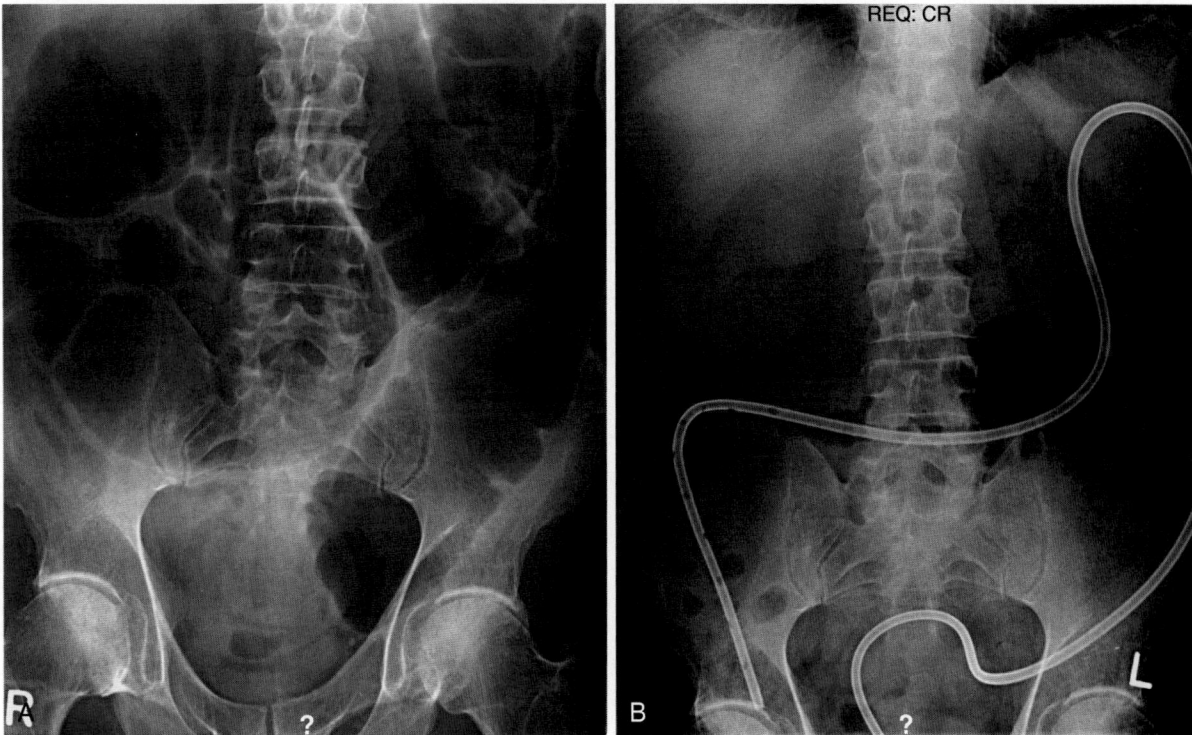

REQ: CR

Fig. 24.3 A, Plain abdominal radiograph from a patient with acute colonic pseudo-obstruction (ACPO). **B,** Radiograph after colonoscopy and place-ment of a 14-Fr colonic decompression tube reveals a significant reduction in colonic gas. *(From Nietsch H, Kimmey MB: Acute colonic pseudo-obstruction. In Waye J, Rex DK, Williams CB, editors:* Colonoscopy: Principles and practice, *London, 2004, Blackwell Science, pp 596–602.)*

periodically be washed to examine for ischemic changes: dusk-iness to frank cyanosis, mucosal hemorrhage, and ulceration. Cecal intubation is desired. One should try to advance the colonoscope beyond the hepatic flexure. Fluoroscopy is useful to help determine the position of the colonoscope tip and should be used regularly.

Traditionally, it has been recommended that if mucosal ischemia is found, the colonoscope should be withdrawn, and the patient should be sent for urgent surgical resection, usually of the right colon, which is most often involved. More recently, successful treatment with conservative measures and tube decompression has been reported even in patients with endo-scopic evidence of ischemia without necrosis (e.g., deep ulcer-ation, exudate, black mucosa).[91] Colonoscopic decompression can be attempted when the mucosal appearance noticeably improves promptly with decompression or if changes of ery-thema, mucosal hemorrhage, and scant shallow ulceration are present.

A tube for decompression should be placed at the initial colonoscopy. Various techniques have been described. The most popular and most effective to date is the placement of a guidewire through the colonoscope when the colonoscope tip is in the cecum or at least proximal to the hepatic flexure. The colonoscope is withdrawn over the wire, and the wire is used to guide a decompression tube into position. Fluoroscopy should be used to monitor the position of the colonoscope insertion tube, allowing straightening of the insertion tube during withdrawal and avoiding the problems of coiling of the tube and distal migration of the tip all the way back to the left colon during placement. A final position of the tube with the tip proximal to the splenic flexure can be satisfactory.

Commercially available decompression kits use a 0.035-inch wire, an inner stiffening catheter, and outer drainage catheters that range from 7-Fr to 14-Fr in diameter. Other authors suggest using stiffer wires and larger tubes, such as a modified 18-Fr Levin or nasogastric tube. The tube is taped securely to the buttock, placed on low intermittent suction, and flushed with water (50 to 150 mL) at least every 6 hours to decrease clogging. Endoscopic approach to ACPO was reviewed by Saunders in 2007[53] and was also outlined in 2010 in the ASGE guideline.[56] In the algorithm, a key point is that one starts with "acute colonic distention." First, ischemia, perforation, and cecal volvulus need to be excluded. Then, mechanical obstruc-tion (from tumor, benign stricture, sigmoid volvulus, etc.) is treated with endoscopic techniques or surgery, or at least ruled out with appropriate imaging. Finally, one starts down the part of the algorithm to treat ACPO only after all of these other possibilities are convincingly ruled out.

Daily abdominal x-ray films should be performed along with measurements of abdominal girth after colonoscopy and tube placement. The diameter of the colon in the cecum, ascending colon, and transverse colon should be tracked, and one should be vigilant for signs of free intraperitoneal air. Although there is sometimes a dramatic decrease in colonic dilatation immediately after decompression, more commonly the colonic dilatation decreases gradually (**Fig. 24.3**). One study showed that the mean change in cecal diameter 4 hours and 1 day after colonoscopic decompression was only about 2 cm.[92] One should be patient, especially with a tube in good position and one that irrigates easily.

One report describes an alternative method for advancing a transanal decompression tube into the proximal colon using a steerable tricomponent coaxial catheter under fluoroscopic guidance.[10] Successful placement proximal to the hepatic flexure and decompression was seen in four consecutive patients. Percutaneous endoscopic cecostomy[93] can be performed in patients with refractory or recurring colonic distention. The technique is virtually identical to the placement of a percutaneous endoscopic gastrostomy. Acute and delayed complications, including peritonitis, are reported to be an issue with percutaneous cecostomy.[94]

Surgery

Surgery is reserved for patients with ACPO who fail medical and colonoscopic therapy or for patients with advanced ischemia or evidence of colonic perforation. Retrospective studies have shown that surgery is associated with higher morbidity and mortality than other therapies. This finding probably reflects the fact that the patients selected for surgery had more severe ACPO and more serious underlying conditions, although the extra morbidity of general anesthesia and an abdominal operation in such patients undoubtedly also has a significant impact.

For patients without peritoneal signs, tube cecostomy is advocated. For patients with peritoneal signs, a more extensive exploration is recommended with the surgical findings guiding the type of intervention.[2] In patients with a viable cecum, a tube cecostomy can still be done. If there is significant ischemia or perforation, however, colonic resection is advised with the decision whether to do a primary anastomosis versus an ileostomy and mucous fistula depending on the patient's condition and the degree of peritoneal contamination. Cecostomy has a high success rate in terms of decompression of the right colon.

In addition to the more traditional open surgical approach and placement of a Foley catheter or similar drain into the cecum, there are other variations of the technique. One is to perform laparoscopy first to check cecal viability and then to use the laparoscope to help place a cecostomy tube. T-fasteners are used to hold the cecal wall up against the abdominal wall.[95] Some authors argue that with the availability and effectiveness of neostigmine and colonoscopy, surgery should be reserved for patients who have signs of perforation or peritonitis. Surgery for decompression in refractory cases should be infrequent.[96]

Other methods of placing cecal tubes have been reported.[97] Radiologic methods have used fluoroscopy or computed tomography (CT) scan to guide placement of T-fasteners and drainage tubes into the cecum.[9,98–100] Local operative complications and the morbidity of anesthesia and open abdominal surgery in patients who are generally already very ill make surgery a last resort for treatment of ACPO; this is especially true given the fact that conservative measures, medical therapies, and colonoscopy can successfully treat nearly all cases.

Future Trends

The major challenges in studying therapy for ACPO are that it is an uncommon condition that most often occurs in seriously ill hospitalized patients. It causes perforation in about 3%. Prospective, controlled studies designed to prove a difference in hard endpoints such as perforation and death are not likely to be forthcoming. However, controlled trials that track intermediate endpoints such as colon diameter and resolution of the distention are possible.

Most cases of ACPO resolve with conservative therapy, but the time to resolution can be many days, making spontaneous resolution still a significantly morbid event. Emphasis should be placed on finding therapies that speed resolution safely and with minimal dependence on invasive procedures. Future studies of ACPO fall into three categories: prevention, medication therapies, and interventional therapies.

Because ACPO can occur as the result of nearly any severe medical condition or postoperatively, it is hard to imagine how to prevent it completely. Nonetheless, certain situations are especially associated with ACPO, such as severe trauma, major orthopedic procedures, and pelvic surgeries. Although this has not been systematically studied, it is logical to hypothesize that early, prophylactic application of some of the measures described previously in the section on conservative therapy might prevent some of the cases.

Medication therapies are likely to be the biggest area of future research in ACPO. Safer prokinetic agents could be applied earlier and more liberally. Many authors have speculated that neostigmine might be rendered easier and safer to use if patients were concomitantly treated with another agent to block some of the unwanted systemic cholinergic side effects, without lessening the therapeutic benefit of the neostigmine. Glycopyrrolate, an acetylcholine receptor antagonist, has been proposed for this purpose. Some physiologic measurements have shown that patients who were pretreated with glycopyrrolate still have a significant increase in colonic motility after neostigmine administration.[101] Whether this combination would be as successful as neostigmine alone remains to be proven. The use of intravenous or oral medications to prevent recurrence is another potential area for future study. One hypothesis is that bowel-selective prokinetic agents might be used to decrease the high recurrence rate that is often seen in patients who have had successful initial decompressive therapy. If successful, such medicines could also be used in prophylaxis in high-risk situations, such as trauma patients. Lastly, although colonoscopy already has a high success rate, improvements in minimally invasive endoscopic techniques would be of further benefit.

References

The complete reference list is available online at www.expertconsult.com.

Diagnosis and Staging of Esophageal Carcinoma

Ian D. Penman and Nicholas I. Church

Video related to this chapter's topics can be found online at expertconsult.com.

Introduction

The incidence of esophageal carcinoma is increasing in many countries, and the disease remains highly lethal because most patients present with advanced disease. Squamous cell carcinoma (SCC) and adenocarcinoma are the most common subtypes, whereas verrucous carcinoma (a variant of SCC) and small cell carcinoma occur rarely. Nonepithelial tumors of the esophagus are discussed in Chapter 29. Diagnosis of early SCC and its precursors is discussed in Chapter 30. Diagnosis and surveillance of Barrett's esophagus is described in Chapter 26. The use of emerging endoscopic technologies in the diagnosis and assessment of early esophageal neoplasia is discussed in Chapter 27.

Epidemiology

Carcinoma of the esophagus ranked as the eighth most common carcinoma worldwide in 1990 and accounts for 7% of gastrointestinal (GI) malignancies.[1] Most patients in the Western world present after the age of 65 years. Approximately 13,900 people in the United States are affected annually with an overall age-adjusted incidence of 4.5 per 100,000, ranging from 2.1 per 100,000 in women to 7.7 per 100,000 in men.[2,3] Overall 5-year survival has improved in recent years to 14%, which is still low. There are significant epidemiologic differences between the two main carcinoma subtypes, and these are considered separately.

Squamous Cell Carcinoma

SCC can arise anywhere in the esophagus with an approximately equal distribution throughout (**Fig. 25.1**). Globally, SCC is more common than adenocarcinoma with an overall incidence of 2.5 to 5.0 per 100,000 for men and 1.5 to 2.5 per 100,000 for women.[4] There are, however, striking geographic variations in incidence. High-risk areas include the Transkei region of South Africa and the so-called "Asian esophageal cancer belt" comprising eastern Turkey, India, northern Iran, and northern China, where the incidence is greater than 100 per 100,000 population.[5] In the United States, African American men have the highest incidence of any ethnic group (16.8 per 100,000), and men are generally affected two to three times more often than women,[6] although the incidence is similar in the two groups in high-risk areas of the world. The disease is most prevalent among lower socioeconomic groups.

Variations in incidence have been attributed to numerous etiologic factors, including environmental exposure, dietary habits, infection, radiation exposure, and associated high-risk conditions. The most important risk factors for SCC (in the Western world) are tobacco and alcohol use,[7,8] the risk being greatest in individuals who both smoke and drink. Many carcinogens, including nitrosamines and polycyclic hydrocarbons, exist in both tobacco smoke and alcohol, and the risk may be compounded in alcohol abusers by concomitant nutritional and immunologic deficiencies.[5]

Numerous *high-risk* conditions have been described. Achalasia may predispose to SCC in association with chronic stasis of food and debris in the dilated esophagus, with an incidence of SCC of up to 9% after 15 to 20 years.[5] Lye strictures of the esophagus are associated with a 1000-fold increased risk of SCC compared with controls, with patients often presenting 40 to 50 years after lye ingestion. Up to 16% of patients with Plummer-Vinson syndrome (iron deficiency anemia, dysphagia, and postcricoid webs in elderly women) may develop pharyngeal or esophageal carcinoma.[9] Long-standing celiac disease is rarely associated with esophageal and pharyngeal SCC in addition to enteropathy-associated T-cell lymphoma and adenocarcinoma.[10] Tylosis is a rare autosomal dominant disease consisting of palmar and plantar hyperkeratosis along with thickening and fissuring of the skin. Up to 95% of patients develop esophageal SCC by age 65 years.[11] Patients with SCC of the head and neck have been reported to develop synchronous esophageal carcinoma in up to 8% of cases[12] with tobacco and alcohol as common risk factors for both.

Adenocarcinoma

Adenocarcinomas arise in the distal esophagus and at the esophagogastric (EG) junction (**Fig. 25.2**). Tumors at the EG junction and gastric cardia were previously considered as primary gastric carcinomas invading the distal esophagus. These tumors have been reclassified (**Fig. 25.3**) as type 1 when they arise from the distal esophagus, type 2 when the origin is the gastric cardia, and type 3 when they are subcardial.[13] Although this classification should allow more accurate characterization of tumors at the EG junction into primary esophageal or primary gastric types, changes in terminology and classification over time must be borne in mind when interpreting data from relevant studies.

Current evidence suggests that type 1 (and possibly type 2) carcinomas of the EG junction have a similar clinical course to distal esophageal tumors and should be staged as for esophageal carcinoma.[14] Epidemiologic differences between esophageal adenocarcinoma and type 3 adenocarcinoma of the EG junction suggest that these diseases are separate entities,[15] and type 3 tumors are usually staged according to criteria for gastric cancer.

In contrast to SCC, the incidence of esophageal adenocarcinoma has been increasing in many parts of the developed world since the 1970s, a consistent finding across the United States, Europe, and Australasia.[16-18] The most rapid increases

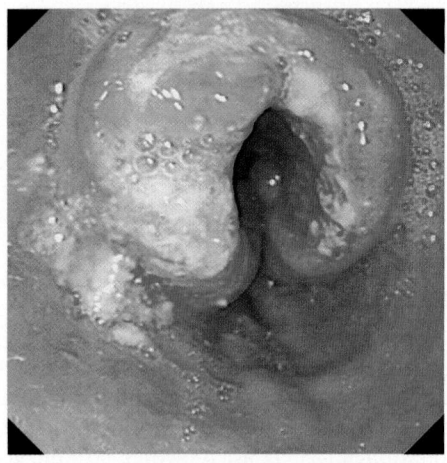

Fig. 25.1 Endoscopy in a patient with progressive dysphagia shows crescentic stenosing squamous cell carcinoma (SCC) in the midesophagus.

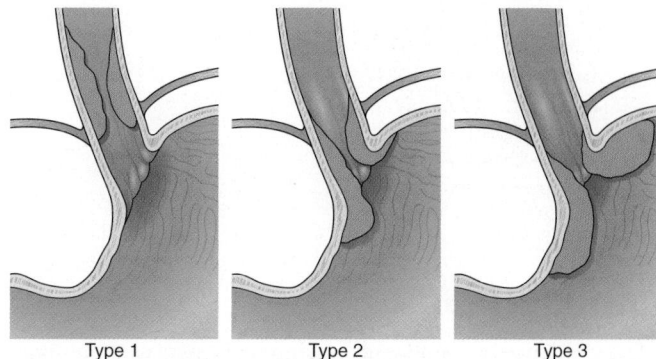

Type 1   Type 2   Type 3

Fig. 25.3 Schematic illustration of the proposed classification of carcinomas arising from the esophagogastric (EG) junction. Type 1 carcinomas are classified as esophageal in origin, as are type 2 tumors, although this is still debated. Type 3 carcinomas are classified as primary gastric in origin. *(From Siewert JR, Stein HJ: Carcinoma of the cardia: Carcinoma of the gastroesophageal junction—classification, pathology and extent of resection. Dis Esoph 9:173–182, 1996.)*

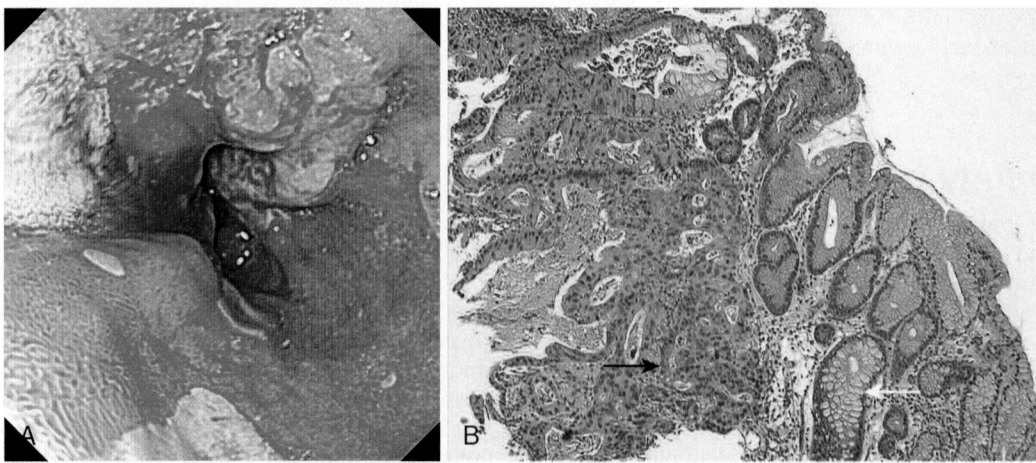

Fig. 25.2 A, Endoscopy reveals bulky polypoid distal carcinoma arising on a background of Barrett's esophagus. **B,** Biopsy specimen shows intestinal metaplasia with goblet cells *(open arrow)* and features of adenocarcinoma *(closed arrow)*.

have been reported in the United States at 10% per year,[19] especially in white men, and adenocarcinoma is now more common than SCC.[16] Current incidence in the developed world is approximately 4.0 per 100,000 population, varying from less than 1.0 in Eastern Europe to 5.0 to 8.7 per 100,000 in Great Britain.[3,4] Similar trends have not been observed to date in Asian populations.[20]

The predominant risk factors for adenocarcinoma are gastroesophageal reflux (GER) and Barrett's esophagus. In contrast to SCC, lower socioeconomic status and tobacco and alcohol use are not strongly associated with increased incidence,[21] although smoking has been found to be a risk factor in some studies.[22,23] Chronic GER predisposes to Barrett's esophagus[24] but was also associated independently with the development of adenocarcinoma in a large study of Swedish patients.[25] In this population, the development of adenocarcinoma correlated with duration, frequency, and severity of GER. Obesity has also been implicated as an independent risk factor in the development of adenocarcinoma, perhaps because of an influence on GER. A meta-analysis of eight studies reported an odds ratio for esophageal adenocarcinoma of 1.52 (95% confidence interval 1.147 to 2.009) in patients with a body mass index of 25 to 30 kg/m^2, increasing to 2.78 (95% confidence interval 1.850 to 4.164) in patients whose BMI was greater than 30 kg/m^2.[26] There are wide variations in the reported relative risk of cancer development in Barrett's esophagus, but it is estimated to be approximately 0.5% per year (i.e., 1 in 200 patient-years).[24,27] There is a weak correlation between length of the Barrett's segment and malignant potential.[28]

Clinical Features

The esophagus lacks a serosal covering, and early tumor growth causes asymptomatic dilation of the smooth muscle. In most patients, dysphagia results only when the lumen has narrowed to 50% to 75% of its normal circumference. By this time, local or nodal spread has often occurred, and the tumor is incurable. Cancers can manifest early with dysphagia, but this is uncommon. Dysphagia may be present for several months before medical advice is sought, and subjective localization of the site of obstruction is a poor indicator of the actual site of disease in the esophagus.[29] Symptoms are commonly gradual in onset, with progressive difficulty swallowing solids and then liquids. In rare cases, EG junction tumors infiltrating the submucosa affect motility and result in "pseudoachalasia" with no obvious endoscopic mucosal abnormality and clinical features similar to achalasia.

Anorexia and weight loss, which often precede the onset of dysphagia, are common, and odynophagia may occur with ulcerated tumors. Persistent retrosternal pain, unrelated to swallowing, and back pain are sinister symptoms suggesting mediastinal invasion.[29] Cough worsened by swallowing or recurrent pneumonia suggests esophagobronchial fistulization. This complication occurs in 5% to 10% of patients and is associated with poor outcome resulting in a median survival time of 1.5 to 4 months.[30] Hematemesis is uncommon.[31] Exsanguination resulting from aortoesophageal fistula is rare. Tumor involvement of the left recurrent laryngeal nerve results in hoarseness.

Physical examination may reveal evidence of weight loss and dehydration. Examination of the neck may detect cervical or supraclavicular lymphadenopathy. The oral cavity and pharynx should be carefully inspected in patients with SCC for evidence of synchronous head and neck malignancy. Signs of pneumonia may result from aspiration or fistula into airways. Hepatomegaly or jaundice from liver involvement indicates incurable disease.

Esophageal carcinoma progresses through direct extension, lymphatic spread, or hematogenous metastasis or a combination of these. Lack of a serosal covering facilitates direct extension and invasion of structures in the neck or chest. Early lymphatic spread via rich interconnecting lymphatic networks in the esophageal submucosa is common. Tumors at any site may involve nodes in the neck or the mediastinum, although proximal lesions metastasize more commonly to cervical nodes, and distal lesions metastasize to abdominal nodes.[32] Depth of invasion is a major determinant of lymph node metastasis. Disease confined to the mucosa is associated with nodal involvement in less than 5% of cases,[33] whereas penetration into the submucosa is associated with a 15% to 50% risk of metastases.[34,35] Hematogenous spread occurs to the lungs, liver, adrenals, kidneys, pancreas, peritoneum, bones, and brain.

Diagnosis

Esophagogastroduodenoscopy
Indications and Contraindications

Dysphagia is the cardinal symptom of esophageal carcinoma and the main indication for endoscopy in this disease. Other indications for endoscopy include persistent dyspepsia or reflux symptoms or the onset of new symptoms in patients older than 45 years. Odynophagia, retrosternal chest pain, nausea and vomiting, anorexia, and iron deficiency anemia are other indications. Screening for esophageal cancer by endoscopy is not indicated except perhaps in high-risk patient groups as described previously.

Flexible videoendoscopy with biopsy is the "gold standard" investigation for the diagnosis of esophageal carcinoma (see **Figs. 25.1 and 25.2**). Endoscopy is more sensitive and specific than double-contrast barium for the diagnosis of upper GI cancer,[36] and when biopsy and cytology are combined, the accuracy of endoscopy for diagnosis approaches 100%.[37] Rigid esophagoscopy is rarely necessary and is no longer recommended on the grounds of safety and cost-effectiveness.[38] In rare patients with pseudoachalasia and repeated negative mucosal biopsy results, endoscopic ultrasound (EUS) with or without fine needle aspiration (FNA) biopsy from within the esophageal wall may provide supportive evidence for malignancy and a tissue diagnosis.[39]

Contrast radiography has little, if any, role in the diagnosis or staging of esophageal cancer, although radiography retains a role in the evaluation of suspected perforation or fistulization. Contrast studies may also be useful when there is complete obstruction and when tortuous, complex strictures prevent passage of the endoscope. In these situations, a radiologic "road map" can facilitate dilation and subsequent completion of endoscopy or stent insertion.

There are few contraindications to endoscopy, and these are general contraindications to upper endoscopy. Patients who are very frail and terminally ill at presentation are unlikely to benefit. Coagulopathy, sepsis, dehydration, or severe metabolic abnormalities need to be corrected before endoscopy is performed. Severe cardiorespiratory disease is a relative contraindication.

Equipment

Good-quality videoendoscopes are essential. For assessment of dysplasia or early neoplasia, high-resolution instruments with magnification and instruments with enhanced imaging techniques (e.g., autofluorescence, narrow band imaging, or confocal endomicroscopy) can provide additional useful information.[40] Biopsy forceps and cytology brushes are essential, and either balloon or Savary bougie dilators (see Chapter 17) should be available if dilation is necessary to facilitate endoscope passage and completion of the procedure.

Anatomy

Clear understanding of EG anatomy and the use of precise measurements and terminology are vital when diagnosing and reporting the location and nature of esophageal malignancies to facilitate accurate staging and treatment planning. SCCs, esophageal adenocarcinomas, and cancers of the EG junction all may require different management strategies, and the endoscopy report should be as accurate and informative as possible. Key information includes the following:

1. Tumor location and length—the proximal and distal extent of the tumor (in centimeters from the incisors) must be noted.
2. Presence and extent of any associated Barrett's esophagus (using the Prague criteria [see Chapter 26]).

3. Presence and size of any associated hiatal hernia.
4. Position of the tumor relative to the EG junction, defined as the point where the gastric folds converge in the dilated esophagus. Tumors of the EG junction should be classified, if possible, as follows: *type 1*, primarily esophageal but extend down to or across the EG junction; *type 2*, arising at the cardia and straddling the EG junction more or less equally; *type 3*, primarily gastric arising in subcardia but extending up to or across the EG junction.
5. For SCC lesions, the presence of synchronous "satellite" lesions by careful inspection of the entire esophageal mucosa, including the hypopharynx, larynx, and oral cavity. The use of chromoendoscopy with Lugol's iodine may aid detection of early lesions elsewhere in the esophagus (see Chapter 30).
6. Morphology and size of small, early lesions using the Paris classification (**Fig. 25.4**).

Early lesions may appear as minor irregularities of the mucosa; areas of erythema; or depressed, raised, or ulcerated areas (**Figs. 25.5 and 25.6**; see also **Figs. 25.1 through 25.4**). A high index of suspicion is required, and biopsy specimens should be obtained of any tissue with these abnormalities. A more recent study has suggested that characterization of early lesions in Barrett's segments according to the Paris classification may offer useful information to aid decisions regarding the likelihood of submucosal invasion and the suitability for endoscopic mucosal resection (EMR) (see **Figs. 25.4 and 25.6C**). Elevated lesions (type 0-I) are associated with a higher prevalence of submucosal involvement, and ulcerated or depressed lesions (type 0-III) are technically unsuitable for

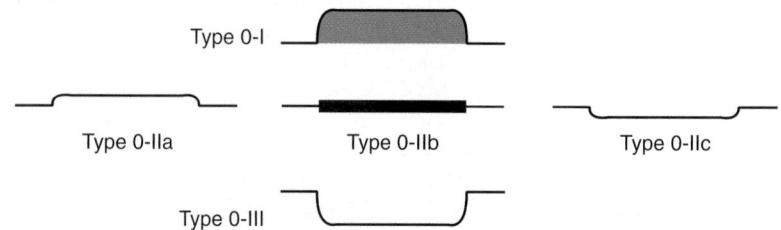

Fig. 25.4 Paris classification of early gastrointestinal (GI) neoplasia. Type 0-I lesions are elevated above the surface mucosa by more than half the height of the cups of closed biopsy forceps. Type 0-II lesions are flat but may be minimally elevated (0-IIa), flat (0-IIb), or depressed (0-IIc). Type 0-III lesions are ulcerated and depressed. Any combination of these features may coexist.

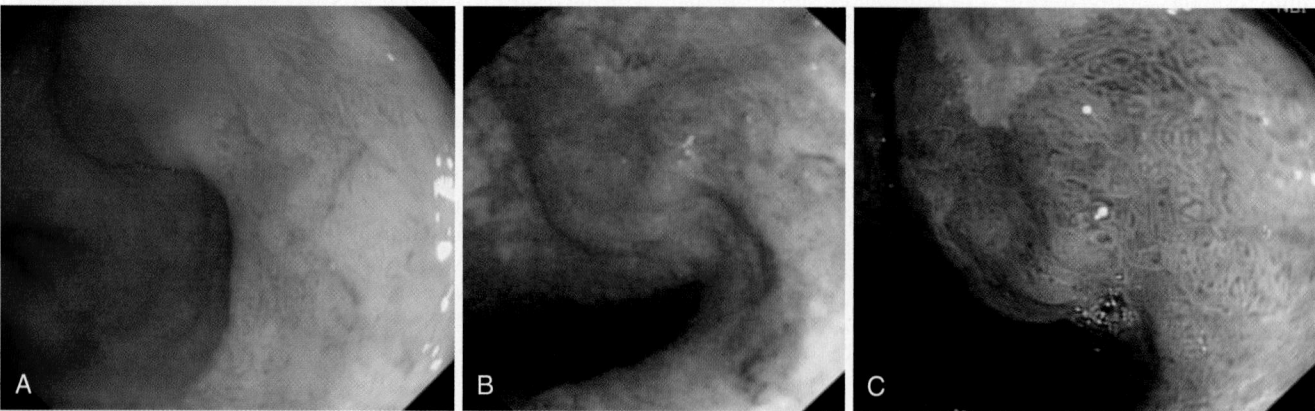

Fig. 25.5 Early esophageal adenocarcinoma (Paris type 0-Ia). **A**, White light image. **B**, Autofluorescence shows lesion as purplish discoloration. **C**, Narrow band imaging reveals irregular surface crypt pattern. The lesion was resected endoscopically and staged as T1m3.

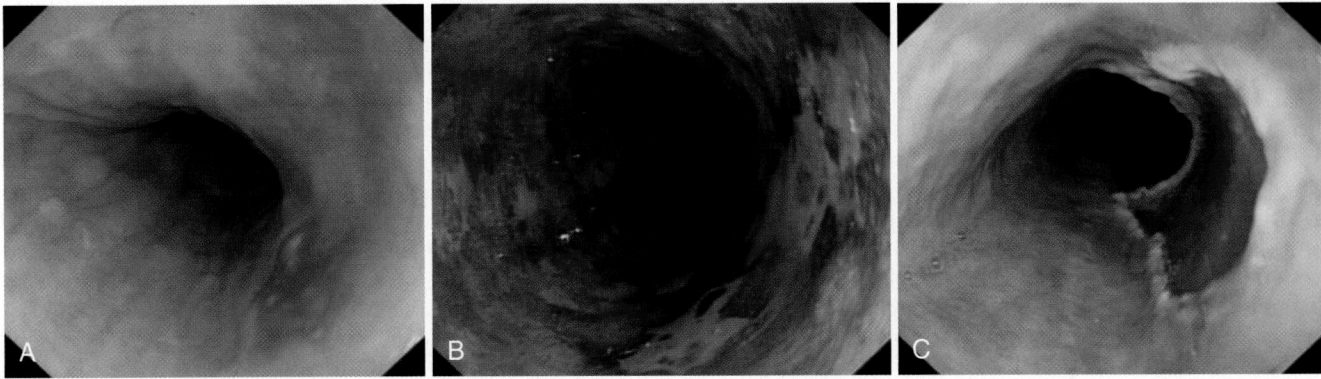

Fig. 25.6 Early esophageal squamous cell carcinoma (SCC) before (**A**) and after (**B**) staining with Lugol's iodine. **A**, Before staining, the mucosa appeared reddened and irregular. **C**, After staining with Lugol's iodine, the true extent of the lesion is apparent. Histology confirmed intramucosal carcinoma (T1m1).

EMR.[41] This study also showed that most early cancers in Barrett's esophagus were flat lesions that were difficult to visualize. Dye staining of the mucosa improves the detection rate and is discussed subsequently. More advanced lesions are usually obvious polypoid or ulcerating masses. Stenosis of the esophageal lumen may be present because of tumor bulk or involvement of the muscular layers. A tightly closed distal esophageal sphincter with normal mucosal appearance and resistance to the passage of the endoscope suggests pseudoachalasia.

Procedure

1. Diagnostic endoscopy is performed with the patient in the left lateral position using topical pharyngeal anesthesia or conscious sedation.
2. Intravenous sedation improves patient tolerance of prolonged procedures and allows esophageal dilation to be performed if necessary. Care must be exercised, however, to avoid oversedation and the attendant risks, especially pulmonary aspiration of food and secretions lying above a stenotic tumor.
3. The mouth, pharynx, and larynx should be carefully inspected, particularly in patients with a history of tobacco and alcohol use and patients in whom SCC may be present.
4. The entire esophagus should be visualized, and the endoscope should be retroflexed in the stomach to examine the EG junction and gastric cardia. In patients with Barrett's esophagus, particular care should be taken in the examination of the mucosa between the 12 o'clock and the 3 o'clock position because 48% of all dysplastic and neoplastic lesions occur in this area.[41]
5. Any suspicious lesions should be carefully inspected and documented.
6. To complete the procedure, the remainder of the stomach and the duodenum are examined.

Chromoendoscopy

The diagnosis of early carcinoma may be difficult in view of the subtle nature of the lesion. Chromoendoscopy involves the use of agents that enhance the distinction between diseased and normal mucosa, either by filling surface crevices or by differential uptake by diseased epithelium (vital staining). Many chromoendoscopy agents have been studied in the detection of esophageal carcinoma; Lugol's iodine and methylene blue have been most widely studied.

Lugol's iodine reacts with glycogen in squamous epithelial cells to produce a uniform dark brown coloration. Inflamed, dysplastic, and malignant cells are glycogen-depleted and consequently appear minimally stained or unstained.[42,43] Using a standard washing catheter inserted through the biopsy channel of the endoscope, 1% to 3% Lugol's iodine is sprayed onto the mucosa. Most highly dysplastic or malignant lesions remain unstained (see **Fig. 25.6**), and clinical trials have shown that biopsy of these areas enhances detection of high-grade dysplasia and early carcinoma.[44,45] The technique is simple and does not require specialized equipment or additional staff; it is described in more detail in Chapter 30.

Methylene blue is a vital stain taken up by the cytoplasm of absorptive cells. These include goblet cells present in Barrett's epithelium, in addition to normal cells of the colon and small intestine.[46] Methylene blue staining was first shown to stain selectively areas of specialized intestinal metaplasia in Barrett's esophagus in 1996.[47] Neoplastic change is associated with a reduction in goblet cell numbers, an increasing nuclear-to-cytoplasm ratio, and reduced absorption of methylene blue. Increasing grades of dysplasia may appear as heterogeneous or unstained areas, allowing targeted rather than random biopsy specimens to be taken.[48,49] However, the emergence of electronic chromoendoscopy in the setting of Barrett's esophagus has eclipsed methylene blue dye staining.

Biopsy and Cytology

Biopsy samples are obtained using forceps inserted via the biopsy channel of the endoscope. The cup volume of standard forceps is 12.4 mm^3. The cup volume of the larger jumbo forceps is 30.4 mm^3 allowing larger biopsy samples to be taken, but an endoscope with a 3.7-mm channel is required. A nonendoscopic balloon device for obtaining esophageal cytology has been developed in China mainly for use in screening high-risk populations.[50]

Jumbo forceps may provide better tissue samples for detection of high-grade dysplasia or early carcinoma in Barrett's esophagus.[51] Biopsy specimens are taken from the edge of ulcerated lesions to avoid necrotic tissue, and at least six samples are required to confirm the diagnosis in 100% of patients.[52] Larger biopsy specimens can also be obtained by a "turn and suction" technique, in which the forceps are inserted, opened, and withdrawn until flush with the endoscope tip. The tip is turned onto the esophageal wall or lesion while suctioning air from the lumen; this draws tissue into the forceps, which are closed and withdrawn in the usual way.[53]

Brush cytology alone may detect malignancy and in some studies has been shown to improve the diagnostic yield when combined with standard biopsy.[38,54] For best results, brushing should be performed before biopsy to minimize contamination with blood. Samples are obtained by passing the brush catheter into the lumen and drawing the brush across the lesion several times until minor mucosal bleeding is noted. Smears are made on slides and fixed in alcohol before staining using Papanicolaou's technique.

Use of Esophageal Dilation

In 20% to 40% of cases, a malignant stricture prevents the passage of a standard adult endoscope.[55] This situation may prevent both a complete examination and the performance of an adequate biopsy from within the main body of the tumor, but a cytology brush passed into the stricture may be a useful adjunct to obtain the biopsy sample from the proximal end of the lesion.[56] Dilation facilitates biopsy, relieves symptoms, and enables subsequent staging with EUS. Biopsy immediately after dilation is safe[57]; for dilation of malignant strictures, the complications of hemorrhage and perforation occur in 2.5% to 10% of patients.[58,59] Dilation provides only short-term palliation of malignant dysphagia, however, with the effects lasting days or at the most a couple of weeks. The issue of dilation before EUS staging is discussed later (see also Chapter 17).

Postprocedure Care

Most patients recover quickly after diagnostic upper endoscopy. Topical anesthesia wears off after 30 to 60 minutes, and patients can eat and drink normally after this time if a supervised test of swallowing with sterile water is successful. Standard nursing care for sedated patients applies. Patients who have undergone dilation should have nothing by mouth until reviewed and can resume fluids and then a soft diet when deemed well. Patients with chest or back pain, tachycardia, vomiting, or distress after dilation should have nothing by mouth and be urgently evaluated for possible perforation by erect chest x-ray and water-soluble contrast radiography or computed tomography (CT) scan. Before leaving the endoscopy unit, patients should be told of the likely diagnosis and how and when biopsy results will be communicated. They should also be given a clear explanation of the likely next steps (e.g., staging CT scan and EUS).

Staging of Esophageal Carcinoma

Prognosis depends on tumor stage at diagnosis. Patients with early disease (T1N0M0; stage I) have 5-year survival rates greater than 90% with surgery alone, but prognosis worsens with advancing stage at diagnosis; patients with stage IV disease have 5-year survival rates of less than 5%. In patients without nodal involvement at surgery (N0), 5-year survival is approximately 40% to 60%, but 5-year survival is only 5% to 17% in patients with nodal involvement (N1). Patients undergoing surgery alone for T3N1 disease have 5-year survival rates of 8% to 10%,[60,61] underlining the reality that although these tumors may be technically resectable, they are rarely curable. Accurate staging is essential in determining prognosis and in identifying patients for whom surgery alone is likely to be curative and patients with advanced disease for whom surgery has little to offer and for whom medical therapy or palliation should be the goal of therapy.

The benefits of neoadjuvant therapy have not yet been conclusively shown.[62–64] A full discussion of the relative benefits of neoadjuvant therapy is beyond the scope of this chapter; however, given its increasing use and the considerable morbidity associated with it, it is imperative that patients undergo accurate staging to guide stage-specific therapy with the hope of improving survival. These strategies vary according to local practice and must be understood by clinicians staging such patients. In addition, to obtain clinically useful and important information from future trials of neoadjuvant therapy, it is essential that study groups are well matched, and highly accurate staging is crucial in this regard.

Staging System

Tumors are staged using the tumor, nodes, and metastases (TNM) staging system developed by the International Union against Cancer (UICC) and American Joint Committee on Cancer (AJCC).[65] This system, revised in the seventh edition (TNM-7) in 2009, describes the anatomic extent of cancer at the time of diagnosis and before therapy and allows a classification of the stages of cancer for estimation of prognosis and comparison of the results of different treatments. The definition of TNM for all esophageal cancer subtypes and stage groupings are detailed in **Table 25.1**, based on the depth of invasion of the tumor into the esophageal wall or beyond, the presence or absence of regional lymph node involvement, the number of involved lymph nodes, and identification of distant metastasis.

For the purposes of staging, the esophagus is arbitrarily divided into several regions because clinical behavior and treatments may vary with the different anatomic segments. These segments are as follows:

> Cervical esophagus (cricoid cartilage to thoracic inlet)
> Intrathoracic esophagus (upper portion from the thoracic inlet to the tracheal bifurcation and midthoracic portion from the bifurcation to just above the EG junction)
> Lower thoracic and abdominal esophagus (including the EG junction)
> EG junction

For the UICC TNM-7 classification of malignant tumors,[65] a tumor with an epicenter within 5 cm of the EG junction and extending into the esophagus is staged as esophageal; a tumor with an epicenter in the stomach that is greater than 5 cm from the EG junction or is less than 5 cm from the junction but does not involve the esophagus is staged according to the gastric system.

Controversy exists over how best to classify patients with involvement of distant lymph nodes. In TNM-7, regardless of the site of the primary tumor, regional lymph nodes are nodes

Table 25.1 TNM Classification and Stage Grouping of Esophageal Carcinoma (Seventh Edition, 2009)

TNM CLASSIFICATION OF ESOPHAGEAL CARCINOMA

Primary Tumor (T)

TX	Primary tumor cannot be assessed
T0	No evidence of primary tumor
Tis	Carcinoma in situ
T1	Tumor invades lamina propria, muscularis mucosae, or submucosa
	T1a—Tumor invades lamina propria and muscularis mucosae
	T1b—tumor invades submucosa
T2	Tumor invades muscularis propria
T3	Tumor invades adventitia
T4	Tumor invades adjacent structures
	T4a—tumor invades pleura, pericardium, or diaphragm
	T4b—tumor invades other structures (e.g., aorta, vertebral body, trachea)

Regional Lymph Nodes (N)

NX	Regional lymph nodes cannot be assessed
N0	No regional lymph node metastases
N1	1–2 lymph node metastases
N2	3–6 lymph node metastases
N3	≥7 lymph node metastases

Distant Metastases (M)

MX	Distant metastases cannot be assessed
M0	No distant metastases
M1	Distant metastases

STAGE GROUPING OF ESOPHAGEAL CARCINOMA

Stage	T	N	M
0	Tis	N0	M0
IA	T1	N0	M0
IB	T2	N0	M0
IIA	T3	N0	M0
IIB	T1, T2	N1	M0
IIIA	T4a	N0	M0
	T3	N1	M0
	T1, T2	N2	M0
IIIB	T3	N2	M0
IIIC	T4a	N1, N2	M0
	T4b	Any N	M0
	Any T	N3	M0
IV	Any T	Any N	M1

From Sobin L, Gospodarowicz M, Wittekind C: International Union Against Cancer (UICC). TNM classification of malignant tumours, ed 7, Oxford, 2009, Wiley-Blackwell.

in the esophageal drainage area, and this includes nodes in the celiac axis and paraesophageal neck nodes but not supraclavicular nodes. TNM-7 also takes account of newer data, including a more recent study from the United Kingdom proposing a new N stage classification based on number of involved nodes and location (one or both sides of the diaphragm) as a more powerful predictor of prognosis.[66] In TNM-7, the presence of one or two involved regional nodes is classified as N1 disease, the presence of three to six involved nodes is classified as N2 disease, and the presence of seven or more nodes is classified as N3 disease. Further studies corroborating this approach are necessary; however, the presence of a high nodal burden or involved nodes in two compartments is associated with a poor prognosis.

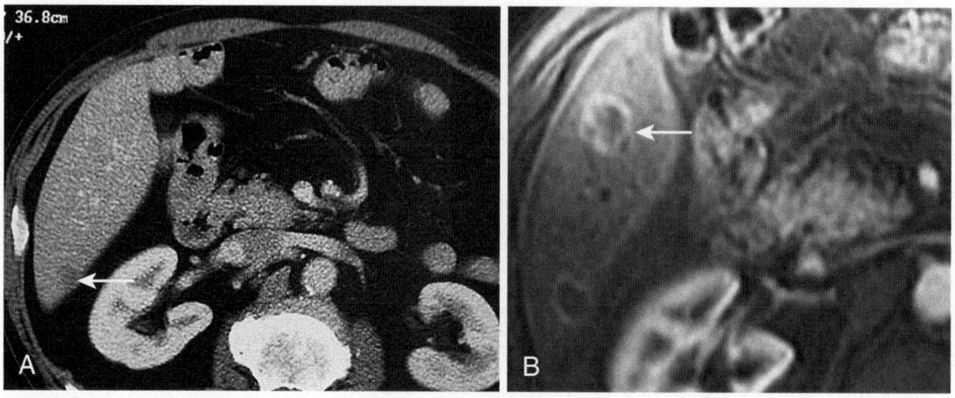

Fig. 25.7 A, Contrast-enhanced computed tomography (CT) scan shows possible lesion in right lobe of the liver (*arrow*). **B,** Subsequent gadolinium-enhanced magnetic resonance imaging (MRI) shows lesion more clearly and a separate metastatic lesion (*arrow*). *(Courtesy of Dr. C.L. Kay.)*

For T staging, the latest classification has minor changes. The T4 category is split into T4a (invasion of pleura, pericardium, or diaphragm) and T4b (invasion of other structures, such as aorta, vertebral body, or trachea), with the latter group being deemed unresectable.

Pretreatment staging should be performed in conjunction with a detailed assessment of the patient's fitness for major interventions such as surgery or chemoradiotherapy. Full staging is inappropriate in frail patients with significant comorbidity who are candidates for palliation only. Staging should begin with a careful history and physical examination to detect cervical lymphadenopathy or hepatomegaly and to assess general fitness and the severity of comorbid disease, in particular, cardiorespiratory problems. Detailed cardiac and respiratory investigations are used as appropriate on an individual basis, and these investigations can be performed in parallel with staging investigations. Documenting American Society of Anesthesiology status and assessing performance status (e.g., World Health Organization or Karnofsky score) may be clinically useful and are essential for patients entering study protocols.

The principal techniques used for staging esophageal cancer are CT, EUS, and often laparoscopy with or without laparoscopic ultrasound. Other techniques less frequently used include positron emission tomography (PET), video-assisted thoracoscopy, and transcutaneous ultrasound scanning of the neck. In clinical practice, when a diagnosis of esophageal carcinoma is made, staging in patients fit for radical therapy usually begins with noninvasive investigations to detect possible metastases, the finding of which obviates the need for further procedures such as EUS. The assessment of distant metastases (M) is described before tumor (T) and nodal (N) staging.

Assessment of Distant Metastases (M)

Distant metastases are present in approximately 20% of patients at diagnosis[61,67] and most commonly involve nonregional abdominal or supraclavicular lymph nodes. CT scanning is widely available and noninvasive and is the mainstay of initial staging in esophageal cancer. Its role in T and N staging is discussed later; for distant metastasis, CT has overall sensitivity of 52% (33% to 71%), overall specificity of 91% (86% to 96%), and accuracy of 63% to 90%.[68,69] Sensitivity for

detecting solid organ metastasis greater than 1 cm in size is approximately 80% but significantly less for smaller lesions (**Fig. 25.7**).

Diminutive liver lesions are assessed better by laparoscopy, which can also assess peritoneal involvement more accurately than CT (sensitivity 95% vs. 21% for CT).[70] Because of its noninvasive nature, relatively low cost, and availability, however, CT remains the primary modality for assessment of metastatic disease.

[18]F-Fluorodeoxyglucose-enhanced PET in combination with CT (CT/PET) may be superior to CT alone, but its routine use in the staging of esophageal cancer is unclear. Data suggest that PET may be superior to CT for detection of distant (e.g., celiac axis) lymph nodes (**Fig. 25.8**), but it is inaccurate for staging regional nodal disease. Limited spatial resolution impairs the ability to differentiate nodal involvement from the high signal in the adjacent primary tumor (see **Fig. 25.8**), and the presence of reactive inflammatory nodes can lead to false-positive results. Sensitivity for detection of regional nodes is also significantly less than that of EUS (30% to 40% vs. approximately 80%). PET may upstage a few patients owing to its greater sensitivity for distant metastases compared with CT alone,[68,71] but data on its utility in esophageal carcinoma are conflicting, and its use is decided on a case-by-case basis in many centers.

Because EUS is able to visualize only the GI wall layers and structures immediately adjacent to the gut wall, it is not primarily used to perform M staging, but it can provide useful M stage information in some patients without evidence of distant metastasis on CT. Small (<1 cm) metastases in the left lobe of the liver can be detected and are often amenable to EUS-guided FNA for tissue confirmation.[72] EUS is also highly sensitive for assessing the celiac axis for nodal involvement (**Fig. 25.9**). The excellent sensitivity and the potential for near 100% specificity with EUS-guided FNA have been shown in several studies.[69,73-79] In one retrospective study, high-quality thin-slice helical CT detected only 53% of celiac lymph nodes that were proven to be involved by EUS-guided FNA.[80] Of 48 patients, 12 who were thought to have resectable lesions by helical CT had either metastatic lymph node involvement or T4 disease by EUS-guided FNA. EUS can play a complementary role to CT in improving the accuracy of staging. EUS assesses morphologic features in addition to size and offers the potential for cytologic proof of malignancy through EUS-FNA

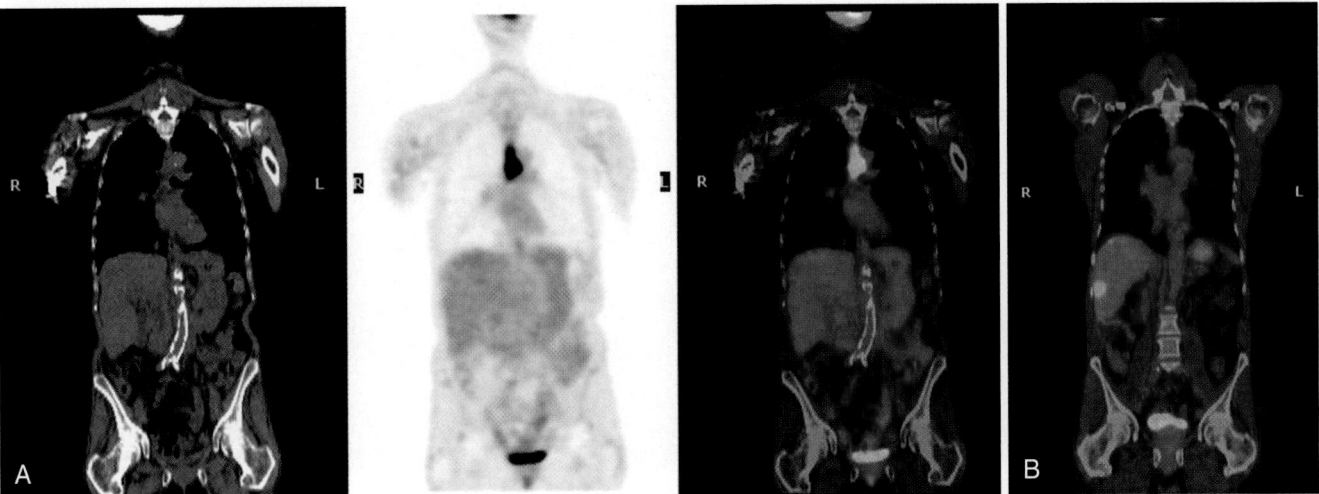

Fig. 25.8 Positron emission tomography (PET) scan. **A,** Primary tumor can be seen as positive uptake over the mediastinum *(central panel)*, and fused computed tomography (CT)/PET image *(right-hand panel)* provides more accurate localization. **B,** Fused CT/PET in a different patient shows two hepatic metastases, seen as yellow PET-avid signal.

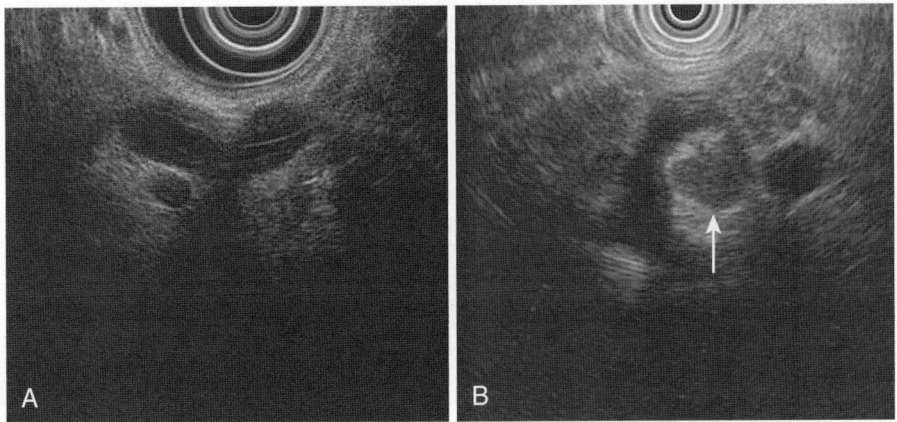

Fig. 25.9 Endoscopic ultrasound (EUS) imaging of celiac axis. **A,** Celiac trunk is traced from its origin at the aorta to its bifurcation into splenic and hepatic arteries (the "whale's tail"). **B,** Celiac lymph nodes are detected within 2 cm of the origin of the celiac trunk *(arrow)*. Nodes identified here are virtually always malignant, but fine needle aspiration (FNA) for cytologic confirmation of malignancy is important because this upstages patients (M1a or M1b; stage IV) and usually precludes surgical resection.

cytology. EUS may allow detection of low-volume ascites not visible on other imaging modalities. A study from the United Kingdom found that EUS detected low-volume ascites in 6.5% of 802 patients with EG cancer.[81] Of these, only half had operable disease at laparoscopy, and only half of the patients undergoing laparotomy achieved R0 resection—that is, 76% of patients with low-volume ascites at EUS had incurable disease.

Regional Lymph Node Staging (N)

Early spread to locoregional nodes is common because of the rich supply of interconnecting submucosal lymphatic channels; this applies equally to SCC and adenocarcinoma. The prevalence of nodal involvement increases with increasing T stage such that less than 5% of patients with T1m tumors have nodal involvement, increasing to approximately 25% in T1sm tumors, 60% in T2 tumors, and more than 80% in T3 or T4 tumors. Although the presence of peritumoral nodes does not prevent successful tumor resection, it has a major negative impact on prognosis, and cure rates after surgery are only 5%

to 10%.[82,83] In a study of 94 patients, the prognosis of patients with N1 disease was equally poor regardless of the T stage of the tumor, highlighting the overriding importance of accurate detection of nodal involvement so that such patients can be considered for neoadjuvant therapy.[84] In addition to the presence of nodes, the number detected is prognostically important; patients with three or more involved regional nodes fare particularly poorly.[82–85]

EUS not only assesses lymph node size but also assesses morphologic features, such as shape, margin, and internal echo features. Normal or reactive nodes in the mediastinum are usually flat or triangular in shape with indistinct borders and an echogenic center, whereas malignant involvement is suggested by a size of greater than 10 mm, round shape, distinct outer border, and hypoechoic echo features (**Fig. 25.10**).[86,87] Although the presence of all of these features is 80% accurate for malignant involvement, this occurs in only 25% to 40% of malignant nodes. Overall, the sensitivity of EUS for detecting nodal involvement is 85%, increasing to 97% with EUS-guided FNA,[88] and accuracy is approximately

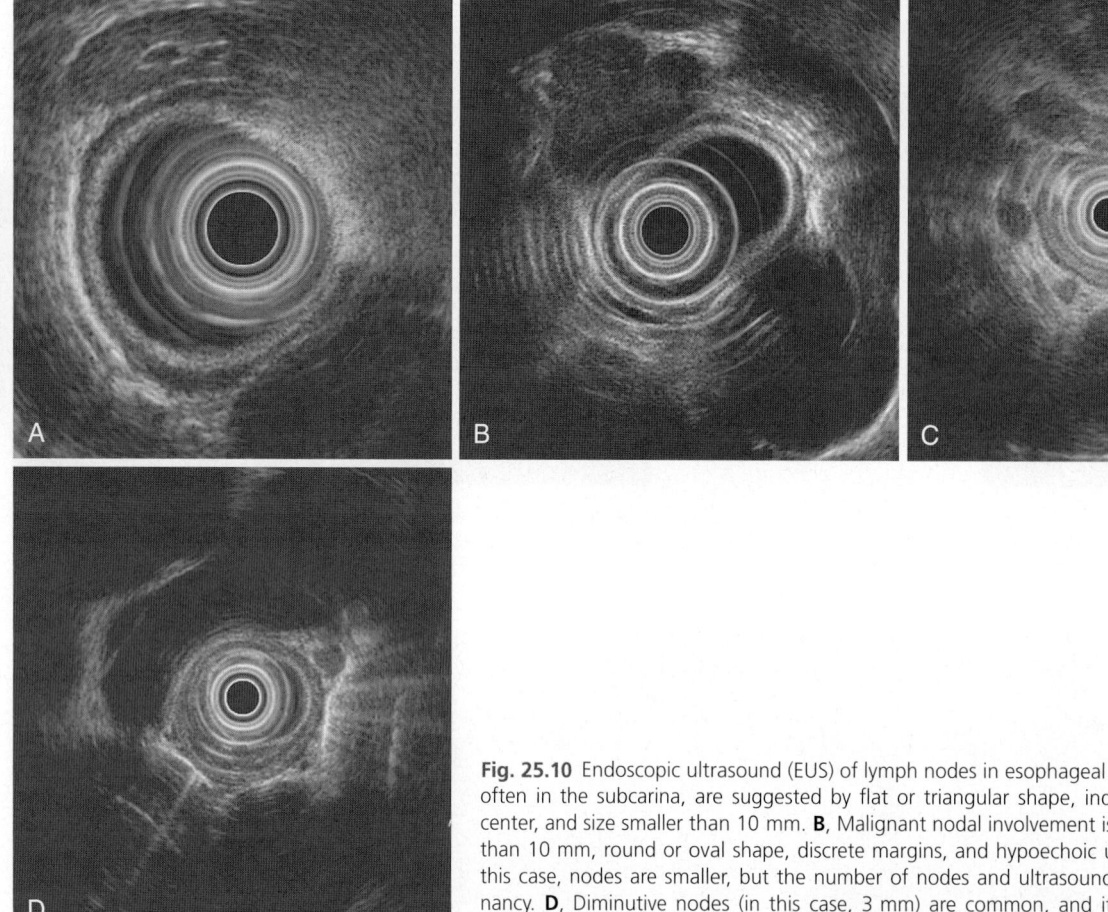

Fig. 25.10 Endoscopic ultrasound (EUS) of lymph nodes in esophageal cancer. **A,** Benign nodes, often in the subcarina, are suggested by flat or triangular shape, indistinct margin, echo-rich center, and size smaller than 10 mm. **B,** Malignant nodal involvement is suggested by size larger than 10 mm, round or oval shape, discrete margins, and hypoechoic ultrasound features. **C,** In this case, nodes are smaller, but the number of nodes and ultrasound features suggest malignancy. **D,** Diminutive nodes (in this case, 3 mm) are common, and it is usually impossible to predict whether there is malignant involvement or not at this size.

65% to 70%,[69,79,88] the latter declining with increasing distance from the primary tumor site. The number of nodes detected at EUS correlates well with the number detected histologically and with prognosis in SCC; it is valuable to document these carefully at EUS.[82] In a multivariate analysis, the detection of malignant-looking nodes by EUS was a statistically significant predictor of poor prognosis with a median survival of 13.5 months compared with more than 25 months in patients without nodes.[83]

As is the case with CT, size remains a problem despite the ability of EUS to visualize lymph nodes 2 to 3 mm in size. The addition of EUS-guided FNA can improve the accuracy of lymph node staging, and the overall accuracy of EUS-guided FNA for detecting malignant involvement in periintestinal lymph nodes is high (85% to 93%).[88–90] In one retrospective study, the accuracy improved from 70% to 93% with the addition of FNA; this was the result of an improvement in both sensitivity and, to a lesser extent, specificity.[91] Although safe, the addition of FNA prolongs procedure time, and performance of FNA may be impossible without traversing the primary tumor, risking contamination of the sample and obtaining false-positive results. However, FNA is useful if the information gained would upstage the patient and affect subsequent management. As discussed previously, FNA is particularly relevant in the assessment of distal nodal involvement, especially at the celiac axis, where conclusive cytologic proof of involvement usually results in a change in management to a nonsurgical approach in most cases.

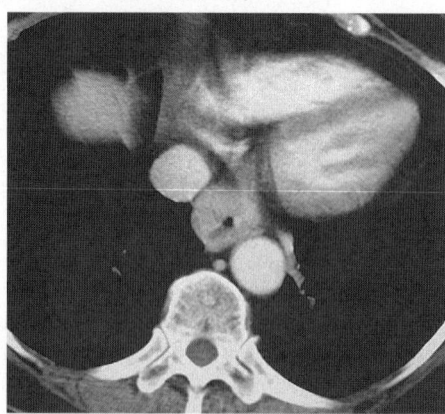

Fig. 25.11 Typical helical computed tomography (CT) image in esophageal cancer shows a bulky tumor in close proximity to the descending aorta, but detailed T staging is difficult. *(Courtesy of Dr. C.L. Kay.)*

Tumor Stage (T)

CT is incapable of showing individual wall layers, invasion of which forms the basis of assessment of T stage. Esophageal carcinomas are usually seen on CT as areas of either focal wall thickening or circumferential irregular thickening of the esophageal wall (**Fig. 25.11**). Proximal and distal extent of the tumor can also be difficult to measure, and it is often difficult to assess tumors of the EG junction accurately, unless the stomach is adequately distended. The presence of a hiatal hernia can also lead to overstaging. Although invasion of the periesophageal fat may suggest T3 disease, and T4 involvement may be suggested by such features as anterior bowing of the posterior wall of the trachea or loss of the triangular fat pad between the esophagus, aorta, and spine, these features lack sufficient accuracy to be reliable. Sometimes clear T4 disease can be seen on CT, but the main value of CT lies in assessment of visceral metastatic disease and possibly involvement of nonregional lymph nodes. It is also useful in radiotherapy planning and measurement of initial tumor bulk for subsequent assessment of response to chemoradiotherapy or chemotherapy protocols.

The ability of EUS to image the intestinal wall as a series of concentric layers makes it ideally suited to T staging, especially in the esophagus (**Figs. 25.12 and 25.13**). Multiple studies over the years have repeatedly shown the accuracy of EUS for assessment of T stage in esophageal carcinoma, and quoted overall accuracy rates are approximately 80% to 85%.[69,73–81] In a meta-analysis, the sensitivity and specificity of EUS for T1 disease were 81.6% and 99.4%; the corresponding results for T4 stage were 92.4% and 97.4%.[88] However, accuracy varies within each T stage and is generally best for T3 and T4 tumors

(**Fig. 25.14**). Accuracy has generally been reported to be poorest for T2 tumors, for which it ranges from 65% to 73%[69,80] possibly because of difficulty detecting microscopic invasion beyond the muscularis propria.

EUS is the only technique currently available for assessing patients with superficial (T1) tumors because these are rarely evident on CT (**Figs. 25.15 and 25.16**). Staging T1 tumors is especially important with the increasing use of local endoscopic therapies such as EMR, photodynamic therapy, or radiofrequency ablation as less invasive alternatives to surgical resection. Tumors confined to the mucosa (T1a) or perhaps the superficial one-third of the submucosa (T1b, T1sm1) may be suitable for EMR.[91,92] The accuracy of EUS for T1 disease has been reported to be approximately 85%. High-frequency ultrasound catheter probes may be useful in this setting with greater accuracy reported in some studies,[93,94] but imaging with these miniprobes can be technically challenging. Data from Japanese groups suggest that ultra-high-frequency catheter probes (30 MHz) can accurately distinguish superficial submucosal involvement (T1sm1) from deeper involvement (T1sm2 or T1sm3), but experience in Western countries is less encouraging, and results are not as good as the results obtained

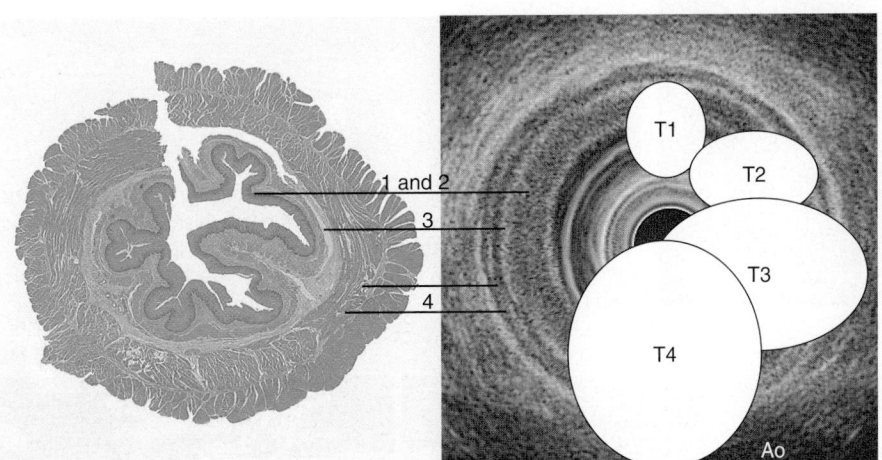

Fig. 25.12 Illustration of esophageal wall layers as seen by endoscopic ultrasound (EUS) with histologic correlation and T staging of esophageal cancer. T1 lesions invade but do not penetrate the submucosa, T2 lesions penetrate into but not beyond the muscularis, T3 lesions penetrate through the muscularis (esophagus lacks a true serosal covering), and T4 lesions invade adjacent structures (e.g., aorta [Ao], trachea, pericardium).

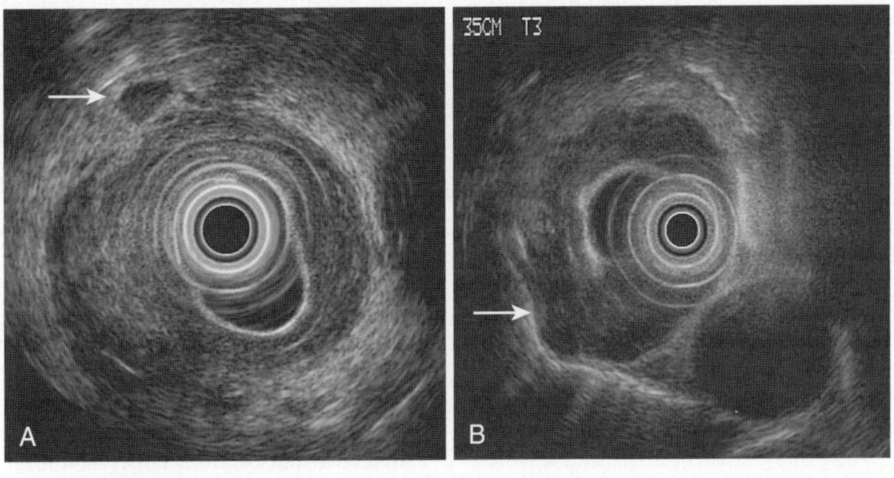

Fig. 25.13 Endoscopic ultrasound (EUS) images of T3 carcinomas. **A**, Bulky tumor extending beyond the muscularis is visible along with a 5-mm peritumoral lymph node (*arrow*). **B**, Bulky tumor abuts the pleura (*arrow*).

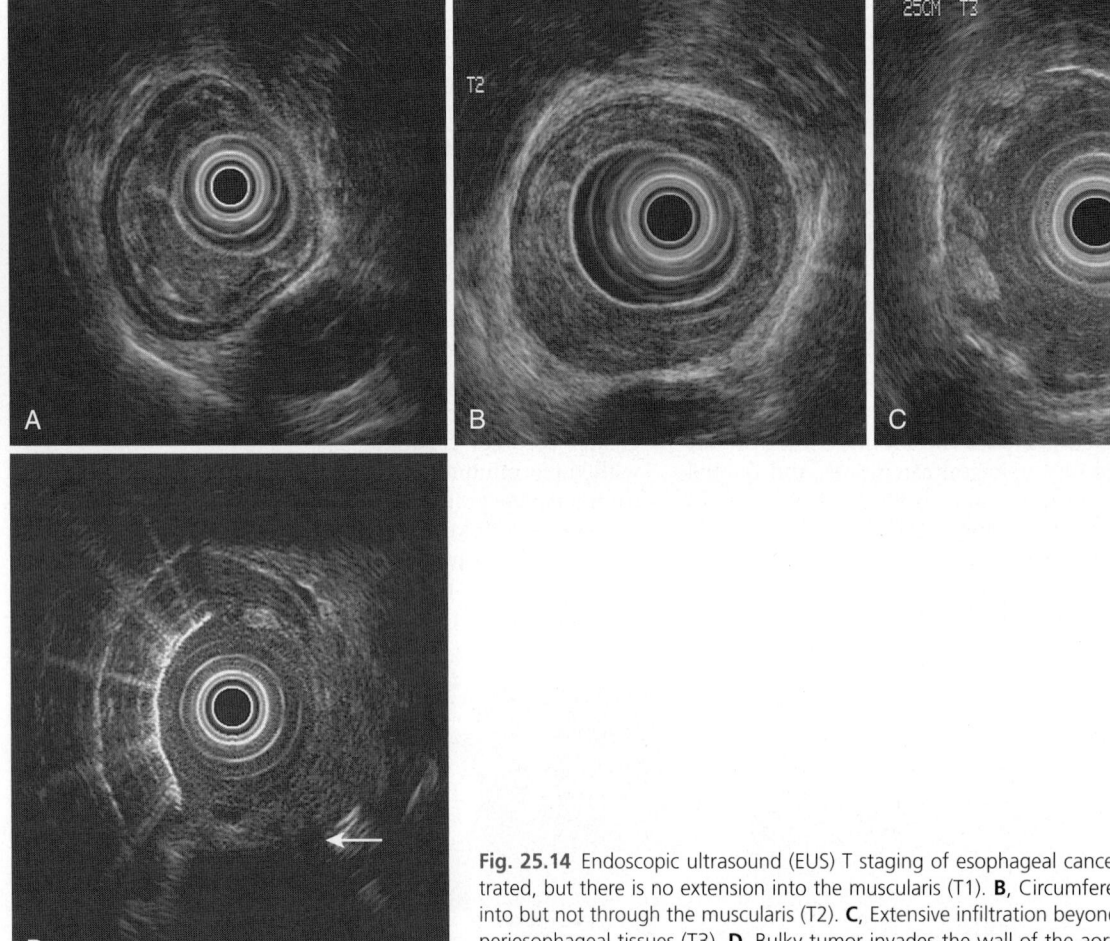

Fig. 25.14 Endoscopic ultrasound (EUS) T staging of esophageal cancer. **A,** Submucosa is infiltrated, but there is no extension into the muscularis (T1). **B,** Circumferential tumor has invaded into but not through the muscularis (T2). **C,** Extensive infiltration beyond the muscularis into the periesophageal tissues (T3). **D,** Bulky tumor invades the wall of the aorta with loss of the echo-rich plane of separation between tumor and aorta *(arrow)* (T4).

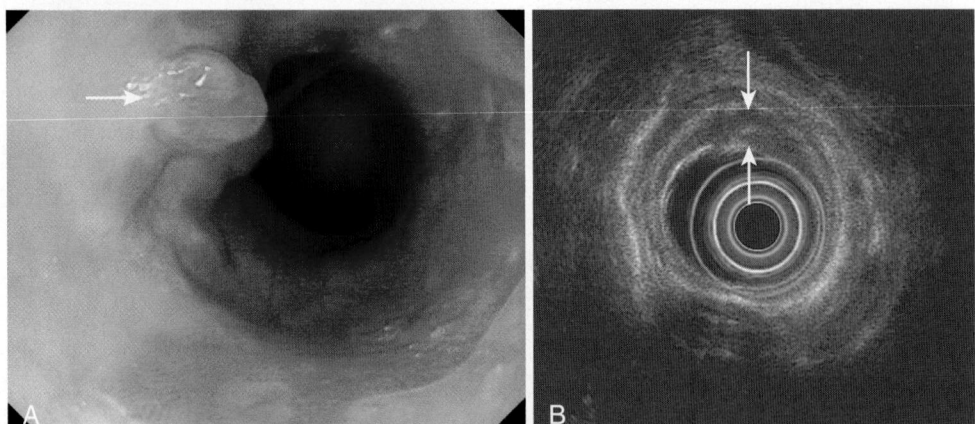

Fig. 25.15 A, Endoscopy shows extensive Barrett's esophagus with squamous islands but also a superficial type 0-I adenocarcinoma *(arrow)*. **B,** Endoscopic ultrasound (EUS) shows lesion involving the submucosa *(arrows)*. The lesion was staged as T1sm,N0 which was confirmed at surgery.

by high-resolution endoscopy alone or diagnostic EMR (see **Fig. 25.5**).[95,96] Greater availability and more simplified techniques for EMR have largely restricted the role of EUS in early tumors to looking for locoregional lymph nodes that have not been detected on CT.

At the opposite extreme, 20% to 30% of patients with esophageal cancer have esophageal stenosis of such severity

that it is impossible to traverse the stricture with a standard echoendoscope.[55,97–99] Failure to do so and to complete the procedure is associated with significant understaging; however, early studies of EUS reported unacceptably high rates of esophageal perforation, either resulting from the procedure itself or with prior dilation to 16 to 17 mm.[55] Since these reports, echoendoscope technology has advanced significantly,

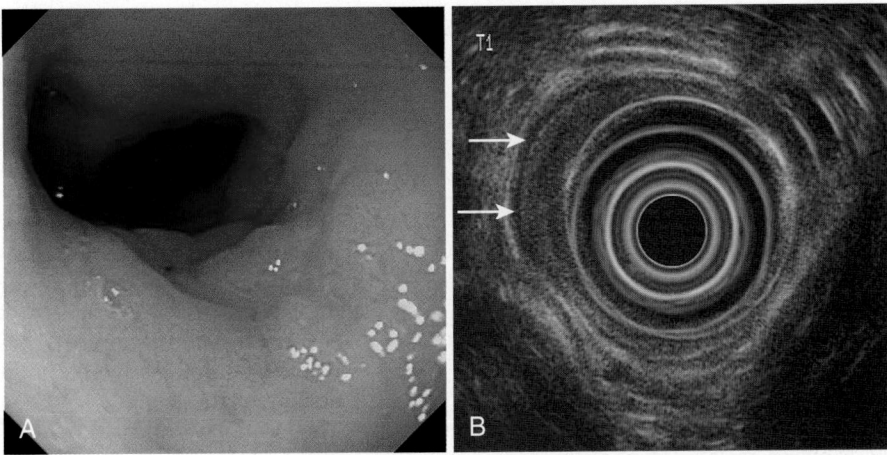

Fig. 25.16 A, Endoscopic view of an elevated and centrally depressed early adenocarcinoma (type 0-IIa+c) arising on a background of Barrett's esophagus. **B**, Endoscopic ultrasound (EUS) shows the lesion involves the submucosa (third layer) but without any involvement of the muscularis propria (fourth layer, *arrows*).

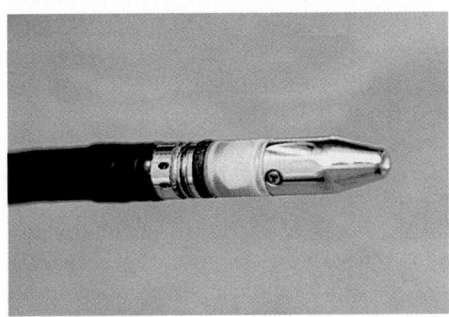

Fig. 25.17 Nonoptical 8-mm esophagoprobe (Olympus MH-908) for use in patients with tight, stenosing carcinomas.

and modern instruments are slimmer, have less bulky ultrasonic transducers at the tip and better video optics, and are rarely associated with esophageal perforation. In a large study of 132 patients, 32% required dilation up to 14 to 16 mm to complete the procedure in almost all patients, and only one perforation occurred.[100] In this study, dilation allowed detection of advanced disease (either T4 or M1a) in 19% of patients undergoing dilation.

If the information gained from completing the EUS procedure is likely to affect patient management, careful dilation should be undertaken, in stages if necessary, to allow completion of the procedure. An alternative is the use of the 7.8-mm esophagoprobe (Olympus MH-908) (**Fig. 25.17**). This conical-tipped instrument lacks endoscopic optics and is passed through strictures over a monorail guidewire placed endoscopically. With this instrument, it is possible to pass all but the tightest stenoses with no or minimal dilation. Several studies have shown the equivalent accuracy of this instrument compared with standard echoendoscopes with a reported T staging accuracy of 89%.[97,99] Catheter ultrasound probes have also been used with some success but are not routinely recommended in this situation because of the lack of penetration and suboptimal nodal imaging. If nodes in the celiac axis are detected by these methods, FNA may be necessary, and this is one argument in favor of the use of dilation and a standard echoendoscope in preference to other methods.

Accurate staging of tumors of the EG junction is a challenge for all imaging techniques, especially for type III lesions. Although EUS has been shown to be superior to CT for both T and N staging of type II tumors, neither EUS nor CT was very accurate for type III cancers with both understaging and overstaging occurring.[101] This poor accuracy may relate to the change of direction and oblique course of the intraabdominal esophagus, and this needs to be kept in mind when staging tumors in this location.

Endoscopic Ultrasound Staging of Esophageal Carcinoma
Indications and Contraindications
EUS is indicated in patients without clear evidence of metastatic disease on CT or other imaging techniques and who are fit for radical therapy. Exact mapping of tumor extent may be helpful in assisting radiotherapy planning in patients undergoing palliative radiotherapy. EUS is of little value in frail patients or patients with metastatic disease who are being considered for palliation only. Contraindications are the same as for EGD.

Equipment
EUS staging can be performed to the same degree of accuracy with either radial or linear echoendoscopes, although radial imaging is perhaps simpler and quicker to perform. Stenotic tumors require dilation to 15 to 16 mm beforehand to allow the tumor to be traversed safely. Alternatively, the nonoptical Olympus MH-908 instrument or catheter probes can be used to obtain some staging information. Appropriate needles must be available in the event FNA becomes necessary.

Anatomy
The key anatomic landmarks to understand and visualize are as follows:

Left lobe of liver
Celiac axis

Splenic and hepatic artery
Left gastric artery
Diaphragmatic hiatus
Pleura and pericardium
Prevertebral fascia
Inferior pulmonary veins
Carina and trachea
Lymph node stations

Procedure

1. EUS staging of esophageal cancer is usually performed under conscious sedation with the patient in the left lateral position.
2. Careful EGD is performed immediately before EUS (see earlier). EGD allows an assessment of the degree of luminal stenosis and a reasonable idea of the likely ability to traverse the stricture with a standard echoendoscope.
3. Dilation can be performed if necessary, or a guidewire can be placed for subsequent passage of the esophagoprobe.
4. EUS staging by either radial or linear methods is usually performed in a distal-to-proximal direction. The echoendoscope is inserted to the duodenal cap, and as much of the right lobe of the liver as possible is examined before withdrawing to the mid-body of the stomach.
5. Air is suctioned out, and the balloon is inflated to provide adequate acoustic coupling. The splenic artery and vein are identified posterior to the gastric wall, and the splenic artery can be traced back to its origin at the bifurcation of the celiac trunk as it arises from aorta. This bifurcation into the hepatic artery and splenic artery is often visible as a "Y" shape, sometimes referred to as the "whale's tail" (see **Fig. 25.9**). This area is examined thoroughly for the presence of lymph nodes at or within 2 cm of the celiac axis. Repeated efforts should be made to visualize this area thoroughly because of the prognostic implications of involved nodes at this site and their impact on patient management.
6. Purposeful withdrawal of the echoendoscope allows visualization of the left gastric artery territory and the lesser curve for lymph nodes.
7. At this level, the left lobe of the liver is usually seen and should be examined carefully for small metastases that may not have been apparent on CT.
8. The proximal gastric wall layers should be examined for evidence of tumor involvement. The endoscope is withdrawn through the EG junction into the distal esophagus, and the wall layers should be examined with care. The presence of a hiatal hernia can cause imaging difficulties because of overlapping gastric folds and the presence of air within the hernia sac. Attempts should be made to distend the layers by inflating the balloon and instilling water through the accessory channel of the instrument to improve image quality.
9. It is often necessary to deflate the balloon slightly when withdrawing through the EG junction into the mediastinum and if there is any resistance when withdrawing proximally through the tumor itself.

10. The tumor is examined carefully to determine the proximal and distal extent of involvement and to assess the T stage. Care must be taken to avoid overstaging from tangential imaging, and particular attention should be paid to the presence or absence of a hyperechoic plane of separation between the tumor and adjacent structures, such as the mediastinal pleura, aorta, pericardium, prevertebral fascia, pulmonary vessels, and main airways.
11. The mediastinum should be carefully assessed from the level of the diaphragm to above the top of the aortic arch, and the number, size, echo characteristics, and location of any lymph nodes should be carefully documented.
12. The location of nodes should be described according to the TNM regional lymph node stations.
13. FNA of identified lymph nodes should be considered if this would have an impact on management. Nonregional lymph nodes distant from the tumor are more important targets for FNA than nodes adjacent to the tumor, some of which may be impossible to access for FNA without traversing the primary tumor itself, risking contamination of the sample and a false-positive result.
14. Results of EUS should be carefully documented descriptively and according to T, N, and, if applicable, M stage.
15. Results should be discussed in conjunction with the endoscopic findings and results of other staging investigations at a multidisciplinary team meeting where all information can be integrated and inform the discussion about subsequent management.

Postprocedure Care

Postprocedure care is as described earlier for patients undergoing EGD.

Other Staging Techniques

Although CT and EUS are the mainstays of esophageal cancer staging, other modalities have an important role to play in certain patients. Patients with distal esophageal tumors or tumors of the EG junction may have significant intraabdominal disease (tumor extending down the lesser curve, lymphadenopathy, or peritoneal deposits), and careful laparoscopy with or without laparoscopic ultrasound has been shown to be useful in such cases. Several studies have shown the ability of laparoscopy to upstage a significant percentage of patients and reduce open-closed laparotomy rates.[68,70] Few studies have compared the information provided by a combined approach of CT, EUS, and laparoscopy, but this approach may improve further the detection of patients with unresectable tumors.

Although not widely available, video-assisted thoracoscopy is a sensitive and accurate means of detecting mediastinal lymph node involvement and assessing T4 involvement, especially of the airways. Few studies have directly compared this form of minimally invasive staging with CT and, in particular, EUS. Video-assisted thoracoscopy is significantly more invasive than EUS, has a small but significant complication rate, and requires general anesthesia. Finally, patients with SCC may have clinically undetectable involvement of supraclavicular lymph nodes, and several studies have shown the ability of ultrasound of the neck with FNA biopsy to detect these nodes with high sensitivity and specificity.[102,103] The exact place of cervical ultrasound in the staging algorithm of thoracic esophageal carcinoma remains to be defined, but it is a simple, safe, and relatively inexpensive procedure and one that merits consideration in patients with disease at this location.

Outcomes and Evidence

Results of studies of EUS in staging of esophageal carcinoma have been described previously. As multidetector CT and CT/PET technologies continue to evolve, studies comparing EUS with these techniques need to be reevaluated and studied further. There are other questions concerning the role of EUS in esophageal carcinoma.

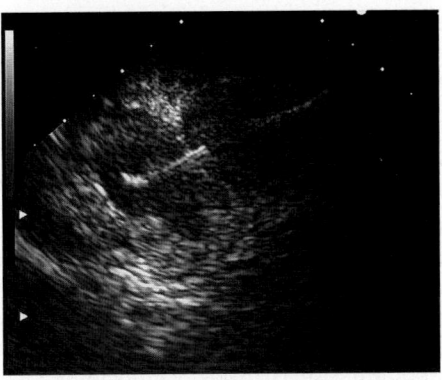

Fig. 25.18 The addition of endoscopic ultrasound–guided fine needle aspiration (EUS-FNA) of lymph nodes increases staging accuracy. In this case, two lymph nodes are seen, and FNA confirmed adenocarcinoma (N1).

Do Endoscopic Ultrasound Findings Correlate with Prognosis?

In recent years, numerous studies have assessed the prognostic value of EUS findings in patients with esophageal cancer. The presence of celiac axis lymphadenopathy (especially when proven by EUS-guided FNA) is associated with a poor prognosis regardless of whether or not patients undergo surgical resection.[104–106] In a multivariate analysis of 203 patients, the presence of malignant-looking regional lymph nodes was also a statistically significant predictor of survival.[83] In another study, median survival was only 8 months in patients with EUS features of malignant lymph node involvement compared with more than 28 months in patients with no EUS evidence or nodal involvement.[107] In a large Japanese study of 339 patients, the number of lymph nodes identified by EUS and transcutaneous ultrasound correlated well with prognosis. In this study, 5-year survival rates for patients with zero, one to three, four to seven, and eight or more detected nodes were 53.3%, 33.8%, 17%, and 0%.[82]

Two retrospective studies also identified T4 stage by EUS as a marker of poor survival regardless of subsequent therapy and showed that survival in these patients was not improved by surgery.[108,109] The findings of celiac lymph node, regional nodal, or T4 involvement at EUS not only influences management but also provides useful prognostic information. The more recent suggestion that staging should be modified to take account of node number and location in combination needs to be thoroughly tested in prospective studies.[66]

Can the Accuracy of Nodal Staging Be Improved?

Given the important prognostic implications of nodal involvement and the potential impact this may have in selecting patients for neoadjuvant therapy, it is essential to improve on the modest accuracy of EUS imaging alone. EUS-guided FNA of identified nodes (**Fig. 25.18**) is logical to improve specificity and accuracy; however, despite numerous reports of its performance, there have been relatively few randomized, prospective studies comparing EUS imaging alone with EUS-guided FNA of nodes in esophageal cancer.

One retrospective study assessed the impact of EUS-guided FNA in 64 patients.[91] The addition of FNA increased the accuracy of nodal staging to 93% largely by increasing the sensitiv-

ity and, to a lesser degree, specificity. The benefits were not as great for celiac nodes probably because enlarged lymph nodes at this location in esophageal cancer are rarely benign and reactive, a finding confirmed in other studies. The data available from these studies show that EUS-guided FNA reduces the rate of both false-positive and false-negative results, and the routine use of FNA sampling of detected nodes in all cases has been advocated by some authors. A meta-analysis of the performance of EUS in T and N staging of esophageal cancer supports this suggestion.[88] Studies from the Mayo Clinic have sounded a note of caution, however, showing that it is possible to obtain false-positive lymph node cytology at EUS-guided FNA as a result of contamination by suction of tumor cells shed into the GI tract lumen into the endoscope accessory channel and by traversing abnormal tissue to reach nodes.[110]

Does Endoscopic Ultrasound Have an Impact on Clinical Outcome?

Although EUS is the most accurate locoregional staging modality, a major impact of EUS staging on patient management and outcomes has not been shown, and properly designed outcome studies in this area are relatively few. A prospective study from the United Kingdom examined the effect of EUS on the management of 100 consecutive cases of esophageal carcinomas and carcinomas of the EG junction.[111] Three specialist surgeons were asked in a blinded fashion to select a management plan after reviewing full staging information before EUS and again after EUS. The additional EUS information led to a significant change in treatment plan in 16%, 18%, and 32% of cases among the three surgeons. Giovannini and coworkers[112] reported that EUS showed distant lymphadenopathy in 40 of 198 patients (20%) with esophageal cancer. FNA was performed with a sensitivity of 97% and a specificity of 100%, and the findings led to a change in treatment in 77.5% of this subgroup of patients (i.e., 16% of all patients). In a prospective study of 108 patients, EUS detected nodal or metastatic involvement in 16.5% of patients, in whom FNA was positive in 86%. When interpreted on an "intention to biopsy" basis, EUS-guided FNA was relevant to only 8.3% of the entire study population, and the overall impact was 13% in terms of changing the therapeutic strategy.[113] Further large studies of this type are needed, as are carefully designed economic studies to bolster the decision-modeling analyses that have already suggested the cost-effectiveness of an EUS-based strategy for staging esophageal cancer.

Is Endoscopic Ultrasound Useful for Restaging after Neoadjuvant Therapy?

Initial studies evaluating the accuracy of EUS restaging after neoadjuvant chemoradiotherapy were disappointing and highlighted the inability to differentiate residual tumor from inflammatory or fibrotic changes.[114-116] However, these studies reported T and N stage accuracy rates and were not surprisingly disappointing. Alternatively, documenting a reduction in maximal tumor cross-sectional area by EUS may be a promising means of predicting response to therapy. Several small studies have reported that a 50% or greater reduction in cross-sectional area is relatively accurate at predicting response.[117,118] In one study, EUS correctly predicted a tumor response to chemoradiation in 20 of 23 patients (87%) who had pathologic tumor regression, and overall the positive predictive value of EUS for pathologic regression was 80%.[119] Meta-analyses of available evidence found that EUS and PET were both reasonably accurate for restaging and superior to CT with maximum joint values for sensitivity and specificity of 85% to 86% compared with 54% for CT.[120] Whether or not the use of three-dimensional EUS imaging to estimate tumor volumes would be valuable in assessing responses to neoadjuvant therapy is unknown at the present time. As for nodal involvement, case reports have suggested the potential of EUS-guided FNA to document nodal downstaging after therapy, but the utility of this approach remains largely unexplored.[121]

Future Trends

Detection of esophageal cancer at an earlier stage is the most likely means by which significant improvements in survival would be achieved, and new imaging techniques in endoscopy are constantly being developed to achieve this.[40] Many of these techniques are now available, and the next few years are likely to see further developments and clarification of which (if any) will translate into routine practice.

EUS technology also continues to evolve with improvements in instrument design, software processing, and better biopsy needles. Other imaging modalities, such as multidetector CT and CT/PET are improving rapidly as well, and further carefully designed and adequately powered, prospective studies are necessary to define the optimal staging strategy for these patients.

References

The complete reference list is available online at www.expertconsult.com.

Diagnosis and Surveillance of Barrett's Esophagus

Gary W. Falk

Introduction

Barrett's esophagus is an acquired condition resulting from severe esophageal mucosal injury. It is unclear why some patients with gastroesophageal reflux disease (GERD) develop Barrett's esophagus whereas others do not. The diagnosis of Barrett's esophagus is established if the squamocolumnar junction is displaced proximal to the esophagogastric (EG) junction, and intestinal metaplasia is detected by biopsy, although controversy now exists regarding the need for intestinal metaplasia for the diagnosis. Diagnostic inconsistencies are a problem in Barrett's esophagus, especially in distinguishing short-segment Barrett's esophagus from intestinal metaplasia of the gastric cardia. Barrett's esophagus would be of little importance if not for its well-recognized association with adenocarcinoma of the esophagus. The incidence of esophageal adenocarcinoma continues to increase, and the 5-year survival rate for this cancer remains very poor. The overall disease burden of esophageal cancer remains low, however, and cancer risk for an individual patient with Barrett's esophagus is low.

Current strategies for improved survival in patients with esophageal adenocarcinoma focus on cancer detection at an early and potentially curable stage. Early detection can be accomplished either by screening more patients for Barrett's esophagus or with endoscopic surveillance of patients with known Barrett's esophagus. However, current screening and surveillance strategies are inherently expensive, inefficient, and of unproven benefit. New techniques to improve the efficiency of cancer surveillance continue to evolve and hold promise to change clinical practice in the future. Treatment options include aggressive acid suppression, antireflux surgery, chemoprevention, and ablation therapy, but there is still no clear consensus on the optimal treatment for patients with Barrett's esophagus.

Epidemiology

The incidence of Barrett's esophagus has increased markedly since the 1970s. This increase was previously thought to be due to the increased use of diagnostic upper endoscopy combined with the change in the definition of Barrett's esophagus to include shorter segments of columnar-lined epithelium.[1] However, more recent data from the Netherlands suggest that the incidence of Barrett's esophagus has increased from 14.3 per 100,000 person-years in 1997 to 23.1 per 100,000 person-years in 2002 in the general population independent of the number of upper endoscopies (**Fig. 26.1**).[2]

It is estimated that Barrett's esophagus is found in approximately 5% to 15% of patients undergoing endoscopy for symptoms of GERD.[3] A more recent study of a high-risk patient population (chronic GERD, white race, age >50 years) undergoing endoscopy for symptoms of GERD found

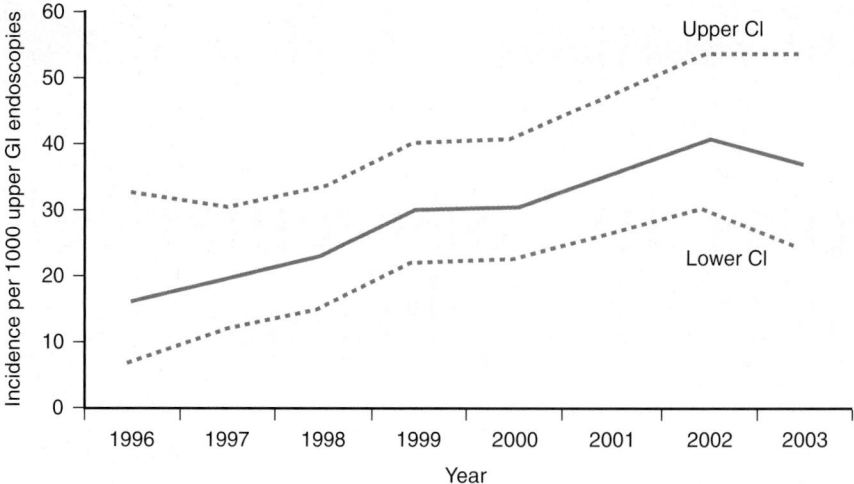

Fig. 26.1 Incidence of Barrett's esophagus per 1000 upper gastrointestinal (GI) endoscopies over calendar time, with upper and lower confidence intervals (CI) in the Netherlands. *(From van Soest EM, Dieleman JP, Siersema PD, et al: Increasing incidence of Barrett's oesophagus in the general population. Gut 54:1062–1066, 2005.)*

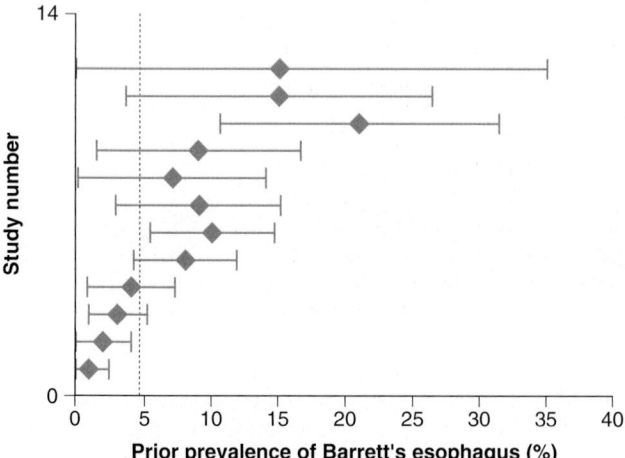

Fig. 26.2 Prior prevalence (point estimate with 95% confidence interval) of Barrett's esophagus among patients undergoing resection for incident esophageal adenocarcinoma in 12 studies. *Vertical line* gives the summary estimate of 4.7%. *(From Dulai GS, Guha S, Kahn KL, et al: Preoperative prevalence of Barrett's esophagus in esophageal adenocarcinoma: A systematic review. Gastroenterology 122:26–33, 2002.)*

of age.[12,13] The prevalence of Barrett's esophagus increases until a plateau is reached between the seventh and ninth decades.[10,14] Various risk factors have been identified for the presence of Barrett's esophagus, including frequent and long-standing reflux episodes, smoking, male gender, older age, and central obesity.[15–19] Body mass index itself does not seem to be a risk factor for Barrett's esophagus but rather the central obesity characteristic of male pattern obesity.[17,18]

Pathogenesis

Barrett's esophagus is an acquired condition resulting from severe esophageal mucosal injury. It is unclear, however, why some patients with GERD develop Barrett's esophagus whereas others do not. Animal studies suggest that the development of Barrett's esophagus requires injury to the esophageal mucosa accompanied by an abnormal environment of epithelial repair.[20] Epidemiologic data suggest that once injury occurs, Barrett's esophagus develops to its full extent fairly rapidly with little subsequent change in length.[10] The mechanism whereby injury triggers metaplasia and why this occurs in some but not all individuals is unknown. The cell of origin of columnar metaplasia is unclear. Candidates include dedifferentiation of squamous epithelium into columnar epithelium or stimulation of stem cells originating from the basal layer of the esophageal epithelium, esophageal submucosal glands, or bone marrow.[21–23] The transcription factor CDX2, which can be induced by both acid and bile salts, seems to play a role in promoting the columnar epithelial differentiation pathway.[24]

Barrett's esophagus is clearly associated with severe GERD. Compared with patients with erosive and nonerosive GERD without Barrett's esophagus, patients with Barrett's esophagus typically have greater esophageal acid exposure based on 24-hour pH monitoring.[25,26] Part of the increase in acid exposure in patients with Barrett's esophagus may be related to the almost uniform presence of a hiatal hernia, which is typically longer and associated with larger defects in the hiatus in patients with Barrett's esophagus than in controls or patients with esophagitis alone.[27,28] In addition, patients with Barrett's

Barrett's esophagus in 13.2% of the subjects.[3] Population-based studies suggest that the prevalence of Barrett's esophagus is approximately 1.3% to 1.6%.[4,5] Most of these patients in the general population have short-segment Barrett's esophagus, and approximately 45% have no reflux symptoms.

The prevalence of long-segment Barrett's esophagus (≥3 cm of intestinal metaplasia) is approximately 5%, whereas the prevalence of short-segment Barrett's esophagus (<3 cm of intestinal metaplasia) is approximately 6% to 12% in patients undergoing endoscopy in various settings.[6–8] It is estimated that only 5% of patients undergoing resection for esophageal adenocarcinoma have a prior diagnosis of Barrett's esophagus (**Fig. 26.2**).[9]

Barrett's esophagus is predominantly a disease of middle-aged white men.[10,11] However, approximately 25% of patients with Barrett's esophagus are women or younger than 50 years esophagus have a lower basal lower esophageal sphincter pressure compared with GERD patients without Barrett's esophagus.[26] Reflux of duodenal contents is also increased in patients with Barrett's esophagus compared with GERD patients without Barrett's esophagus.[29] Patients with short-segment Barrett's esophagus tend to have pathophysiologic abnormalities intermediate to the abnormalities of patients with long-segment Barrett's esophagus and normal controls.[30,31] Esophageal pH monitoring studies suggest a correlation between the length of Barrett's mucosa and the duration of esophageal acid exposure.[31]

Clinical Features

Patients with Barrett's esophagus are difficult to distinguish clinically from patients with GERD uncomplicated by a columnar-lined esophagus.[32] However, some observational studies suggest that features such as the development of reflux symptoms at an earlier age, increased duration of reflux symptoms, increased severity of nocturnal reflux symptoms, and increased complications of GERD (e.g., esophagitis, ulceration, stricture, bleeding) may distinguish patients with Barrett's esophagus from GERD patients without Barrett's esophagus.[16] Similar clinical risk factors have been identified for esophageal adenocarcinoma.[33] Identification of patients with Barrett's esophagus may be hampered by the paradox that patients with Barrett's esophagus have an impaired sensitivity to esophageal acid perfusion compared with patients with uncomplicated GERD.[34] Many patients with Barrett's esophagus are elderly, however, and this observation may be related to an age-related decrease in acid sensitivity.[35] A subset of patients with Barrett's esophagus may have an inherited predisposition; studies have reported families with multiple affected relatives over successive generations.[36–38] These reports suggest an autosomal dominant pattern of inheritance in certain patients with Barrett's esophagus.

Pathology

The columnar-lined esophagus is characterized by a mosaic of three different types of columnar epithelium above the lower esophageal sphincter zone: fundic-type epithelium, characterized by parietal and chief cells similar to the native gastric fundus; cardiac-type mucosa, characterized by mucous glands and no parietal cells; and specialized columnar epithelium, characterized by a villiform surface and alcian blue–staining

intestinal-type goblet cells.[39] At the present time, the diagnosis of Barrett's esophagus is established if the squamocolumnar junction is displaced proximal to the EG junction and intestinal metaplasia, characterized by acid mucin–containing goblet cells is detected by biopsy (**Fig. 26.3**). The requirement of intestinal metaplasia for the diagnosis of Barrett's esophagus has come under question more recently, however, as described later. In most cases, goblet cells are easily identified on routine hematoxylin and eosin preparations, and special stains such as alcian blue or periodic acid–Schiff (PAS) are unnecessary. However, alcian blue and PAS stain can help avoid overinterpretation of pseudogoblet cells characterized by distended surface foveolar-type cells that stain for PAS but do not contain alcian blue–positive acid mucins (**Fig. 26.4**).[40]

It is well recognized that pathologic interpretation of Barrett's esophagus specimens is problematic in the community and in academic centers. In a community study, intestinal metaplasia without dysplasia was recognized correctly by only 35% of pathologists, and gastric metaplasia without intestinal metaplasia was identified as Barrett's esophagus in 38% of the cases.[41] Pathologic interpretation is also problematic for expert gastrointestinal (GI) pathologists; interobserver reproducibility is substantial at the ends of the spectrum of Barrett's esophagus—negative for dysplasia and high-grade dysplasia and carcinoma but not especially good for low-grade dysplasia or indefinite for dysplasia.[42] There are also problems with interobserver agreement among pathologists in distinguishing high-grade dysplasia from intramucosal cancer, even when evaluating esophagectomy specimens.[43,44]

Factors that contribute to some of the problems in pathologic interpretation include experience of the pathologist, quality of the slides, and size of the specimens.[45] In an effort to improve pathologic interpretation, current practice guide-

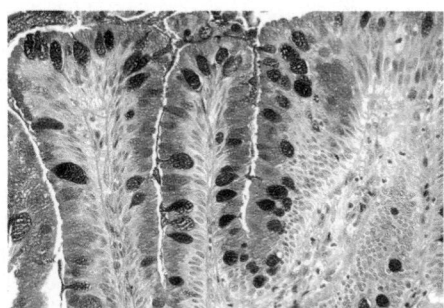

Fig. 26.3 Histologic appearance of specialized columnar epithelium, characterized by a villiform appearance, and goblet cells staining positive with periodic acid–Schiff staining. *(Courtesy of John Goldblum, M.D.)*

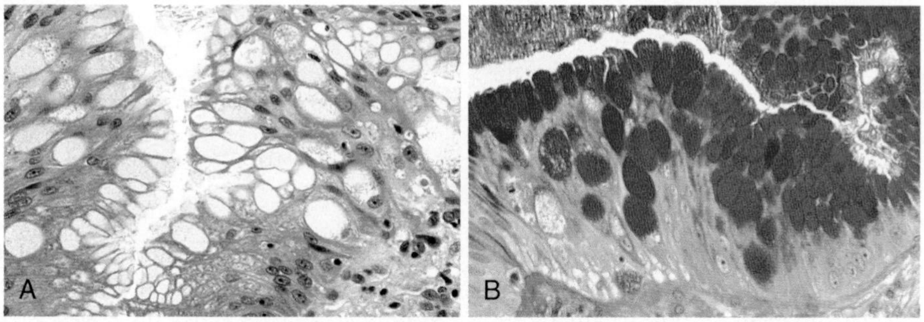

Fig. 26.4 Columnar epithelium with pseudogoblet cells characterized by distended gastric surface foveolar-type cells **(A)** that stain for periodic acid–Schiff but do not contain alcian blue–positive acid mucins **(B)**. *(Courtesy of John Goldblum, M.D.)*

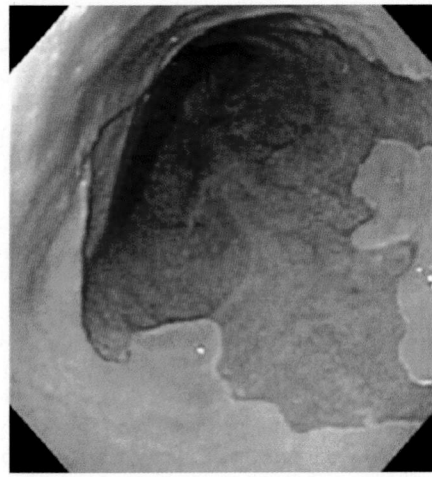

Fig. 26.5 Endoscopic appearance of a long segment of Barrett's esophagus.

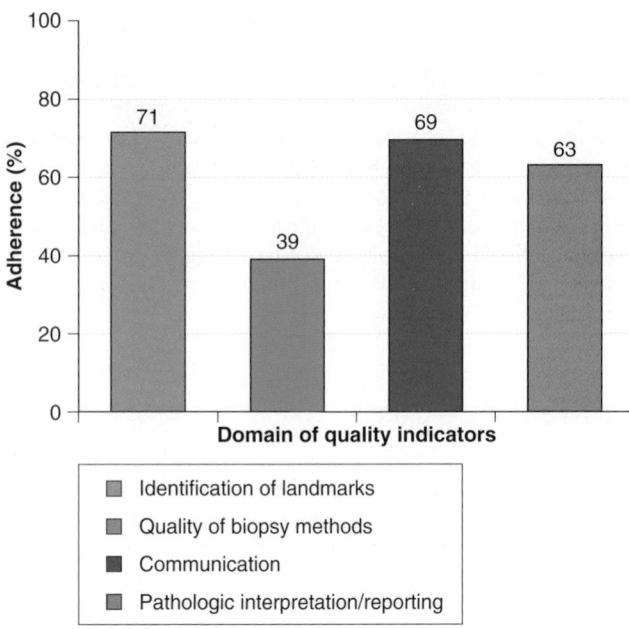

Fig. 26.6 Problems in quality of care of Barrett's esophagus—mean proportion of cases adhering to accepted standards in four different domains of care. *(From Ofman JJ, Shaheen NJ, Desai AA, et al: The quality of care in Barrett's esophagus: Endoscopist and pathologist practices. Am J Gastroenterol 96:876–881, 2001.)*

lines now recommend endoscopic mucosal resection (EMR) of any nodularity in the Barrett's segment before making final treatment decisions.[46,47] More recent data support such an approach. Mino-Kenudson and colleagues[45] found that interobserver agreement for Barrett's esophagus–associated neoplasia on EMR specimens was higher than that for mucosal biopsy specimens, especially in distinguishing intramucosal cancer from submucosal cancer.

Differential Diagnosis

The diagnosis of Barrett's esophagus has clear implications for patients. Patients are subject to surveillance endoscopy at regular intervals; worry about cancer risk, which they typically overestimate; face higher life insurance premiums; and are provided with conflicting information on how best to treat their condition.[48,49] It is crucial to diagnose Barrett's esophagus as accurately as possible given the downstream effects of such a diagnosis.

Barrett's esophagus is defined as a metaplastic change in the lining of the tubular esophagus. Endoscopically, this metaplastic change is characterized by displacement of the squamocolumnar junction proximal to the EG junction defined by the proximal margin of gastric folds (**Fig. 26.5**). At the time of endoscopy, landmarks should be carefully identified, including the diaphragmatic pinch, the EG junction as best defined by the proximal margin of the gastric folds seen on partial insufflation of the esophagus, and level of the squamocolumnar junction. It is commonly accepted that the proximal margin of the gastric folds is the most useful landmark for the junction of the stomach and the esophagus.[50] However, the precise junction of the esophagus and the stomach may be difficult to determine endoscopically because of the presence of a hiatal hernia, the presence of inflammation, and the dynamic nature of the EG junction, all of which may make targeting of biopsy specimens problematic.

Endoscopists identify landmarks necessary for the diagnosis of the columnar-lined esophagus inconsistently (**Fig. 26.6**)[51]; this leads to inconsistencies in defining the length of the columnar-lined esophagus.[52] The Prague classification scheme should help improve the description of the columnar-lined

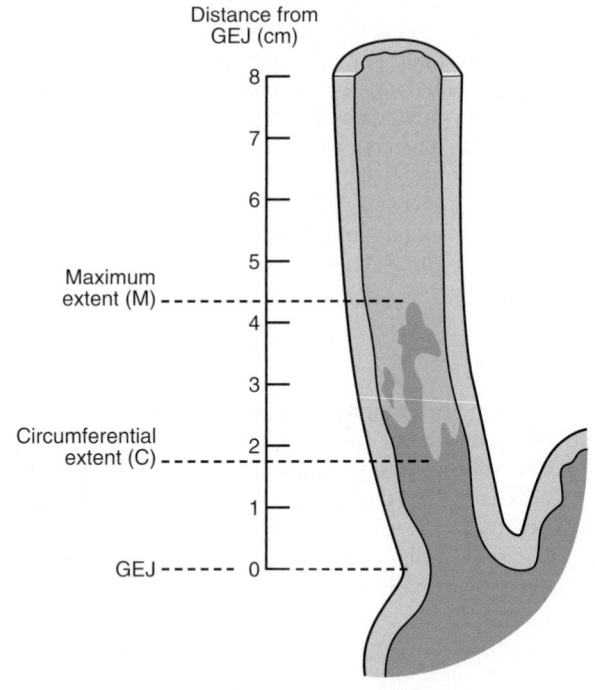

Fig. 26.7 Schematic representation of the Prague classification for Barrett's esophagus classified as a C2M4. Note that *C* is the circumferential extent of metaplasia, which extends up 2 cm, whereas *M* is the maximal extent of metaplasia, which extends up 4 cm from the gastroesophageal junction *(GEJ)*.

esophagus.[53] This classification scheme describes the circumferential extent (*C* value) and maximum extent (*M* value) of columnar mucosa above the proximal margin of the gastric folds (**Fig. 26.7**). The Prague classification does not include columnar islands, however. Reliability coefficients for both

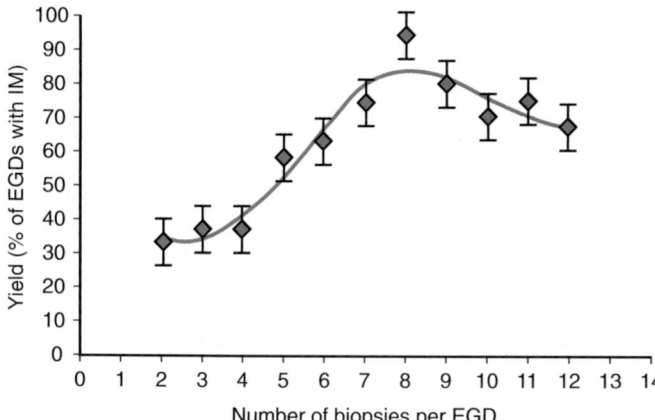

Fig. 26.8 Yield of endoscopy for detection of intestinal metaplasia compared with number of biopsy specimens per endoscopy. The optimal number of biopsy specimens to detect intestinal metaplasia is a minimum of eight. *(From Harrison R, Perry I, Haddadin W, et al: Detection of intestinal metaplasia in Barrett's esophagus: An observational comparator study suggests the need for a minimum of eight biopsies. Am J Gastroenterol 102:1154–1161, 2007.)*

criteria are excellent for segments greater than 1 cm in length. Recognition of less than 1 cm of columnar metaplasia even with this scoring system is still problematic, pointing out the difficulties in measuring such short segments.

If the squamocolumnar junction is above the level of the EG junction, as defined by the proximal margin of the gastric folds using partial insufflation, biopsy specimens should be obtained for confirmation of columnar metaplasia. There is ongoing debate regarding the presence of intestinal metaplasia for the diagnosis of Barrett's esophagus.[54] The professional societies of North America all require intestinal metaplasia for the diagnosis of Barrett's esophagus, whereas the British Society of Gastroenterology and a global consensus group do not require the presence of intestinal metaplasia for the diagnosis.[46,55-57] More recent evidence suggests that non–goblet cell columnar metaplasia shows DNA content abnormalities indicative of neoplastic risk similar to neoplasias encountered in intestinal metaplasia.[58] The issue of intestinal metaplasia versus columnar metaplasia as a diagnostic criterion remains unsettled at the present time.

There is no agreement at the present time on the appropriate number of biopsy specimens to obtain to detect intestinal metaplasia. Detection of intestinal metaplasia seems to be related to many factors, including location of biopsies, length of columnar-lined segment, number of biopsy specimens obtained, male gender, and increasing age.[59,60] Intestinal metaplasia is more commonly found in biopsy specimens obtained in the proximal portion of the columnar-lined esophagus where goblet cell density is also greater.[61] More recent work suggests that the detection of intestinal metaplasia increases with increasing number of biopsy specimens per endoscopy: Four biopsy specimens had a yield of 34.7%, whereas eight biopsy specimens had a yield of 94% for intestinal metaplasia (**Fig. 26.8**).[62] Taking more than eight biopsy specimens does not seem to enhance the yield of intestinal metaplasia.

It may be difficult to determine endoscopically where the esophagus ends and the stomach begins for the reasons outlined earlier. It is impossible to distinguish reliably columnar metaplasia of the distal esophagus from columnar metaplasia of the stomach. A biopsy specimen of the squamocolumnar

junction should not be routinely obtained in clinical practice if it is at the level of the EG junction. Intestinal metaplasia may be seen in the cardia of normal individuals and in patients with chronic reflux disease. The prevalence of intestinal metaplasia at a normal-appearing EG junction varies from 5% to 36%.[63] In contrast to Barrett's esophagus, there is no clear gender predominance in patients with intestinal metaplasia of the EG junction and cardia because this condition is more common in older patients who are often infected with *Helicobacter pylori* and have evidence of gastritis or intestinal metaplasia or both elsewhere in the stomach.[8,64] A subset of these patients may have GERD, however, and it is unclear if this condition is a sequela of aging, *H. pylori* infection, GERD, or some combination of these factors.

Short-segment Barrett's esophagus is clearly associated with some risk of developing dysplasia and esophageal cancer, which is not substantially lower than the risk in patients with long-segment Barrett's esophagus. Dysplasia and carcinoma have been reported in patients with intestinal metaplasia of the EG junction or cardia, but the magnitude of that risk seems to be less than the risk of short-segment Barrett's esophagus.[65] A reliable biomarker to distinguish between intestinal metaplasia of the cardia versus intestinal metaplasia of the esophagus would be beneficial. Techniques such as the Das-1 antibody and cytokeratin immunohistochemical staining patterns do not reliably distinguish between these two entities.[66] However, some features such as mucosal and submucosal esophageal glands, squamous epithelium overlying columnar crypts with intestinal metaplasia, and hybrid glands characterized by intestinal metaplasia confined to the superficial aspect of cardia-type mucus glands are more often associated with the columnar-lined esophagus than intestinal metaplasia of the cardia.[67] Precise targeting of biopsy specimens above the proximal margin of the gastric folds and communication of this information to pathologists are crucial from a quality perspective.

Barrett's Esophagus and Esophageal Adenocarcinoma

Barrett's esophagus is a clearly recognized risk factor for the development of esophageal adenocarcinoma compared with the general population.[68] Studies show that the incidence of this cancer has increased by approximately sixfold between 1975 and 2001, a rate greater than that of any other cancer in the United States during that time.[69] This increase has been accompanied by an increase in mortality rates from 2 to 15 deaths per 1 million during that same time period.[69] Similar findings are occurring elsewhere in the Western world. However, the overall burden of esophageal adenocarcinoma remains relatively low. It was estimated that there would be 16,470 new cases of esophageal cancer (not all of which would be adenocarcinoma) in the United States in 2009.[70]

Despite the alarming increase in the incidence of esophageal adenocarcinoma, the precise incidence of adenocarcinoma in patients with Barrett's esophagus is uncertain, with rates varying from approximately 1 in 52 to 1 in 694 years of follow-up.[71] It is estimated that the risk of developing cancer in a patient with Barrett's esophagus is approximately 0.5% to 0.7% annually with no clear evidence of geographic variation.[71,72] Evolving epidemiologic data suggest that despite the alarming increase in the incidence of esophageal adenocarcinoma, most patients with Barrett's esophagus never develop esophageal cancer and die of causes other than cancer.[73–75] The survival of patients with Barrett's esophagus is similar to survival of the general population.[74]

The reason for the increase in the incidence of esophageal adenocarcinoma is unknown. Barrett's esophagus is clearly a risk factor for adenocarcinoma of the esophagus. Various epidemiologic factors have been identified that either increase or decrease the risk for the development of esophageal adenocarcinoma. The well-accepted risk factors for the development of esophageal adenocarcinoma include increasing age; male gender; white ethnicity; obesity, especially male pattern central obesity; and smoking.[76–79] Protective factors include aspirin and nonsteroidal antiinflammatory drug (NSAID) ingestion and a diet high in fruits and vegetables.[80–82] Factors of uncertain significance include family history, infection with *H. pylori*, alcohol consumption, antireflux therapy (surgical or pharmacologic), and dietary supplements.[79]

Cancer Biology

Compelling evidence exists for a dysplasia-carcinoma sequence in Barrett's esophagus whereby nondysplastic columnar epithelium progresses to low-grade dysplasia, high-grade dysplasia, and finally to carcinoma. Foci of carcinoma typically appear adjacent to dysplasia.[83] The time course for this progression is highly variable, and most patients never progress to dysplasia.

It is hypothesized that cancer develops in a subset of patients who have acquired genomic instability in Barrett's epithelium.[84] This genomic instability predisposes to the development of abnormal clones of cells that accumulate progressively more genetic errors, which include numerical and structural chromosomal rearrangements, gene mutations, loss of normal cell cycle control, and increased cell proliferation rates.[85,86] Among the most frequently described molecular changes that precede the development of adenocarcinoma in Barrett's esophagus are alterations in p53 (mutation, deletion, or loss of heterozygosity [LOH]) and p16 (mutation, deletion, promoter hypermethylation, or LOH) and aneuploidy.[87–90] However, there is no clearly predictable sequence of genetic abnormalities that leads to the development of cancer. Upregulation of cyclooxygenase-2 (COX-2) expression also occurs in the metaplasia-dysplasia-carcinoma sequence.[91,92] Increased COX-2 expression is associated with increased cellular proliferation and decreased apoptosis in vitro, and administration of selective COX-2 inhibitors can decrease cell growth and increase apoptosis in esophageal adenocarcinoma cell lines.[93] This finding may have implications for chemoprevention strategies under investigation.

Screening and Surveillance Strategies for Barrett's Esophagus

Esophageal adenocarcinoma is a lethal disease with a 5-year survival of approximately 12% to 14%.[94,95] Survival depends on the stage, and early spread before the onset of symptoms is characteristic of this tumor. Early invasive cancer may be classified as intramucosal when neoplastic cells penetrate through the basement membrane to the lamina propria or muscularis mucosa and submucosal when neoplastic cells infiltrate into the submucosa. The prognosis for these two lesions is very different because the risk of lymph node metastasis is approximately 0% to 7% for intramucosal cancer but increases to 5% to 50% for submucosal cancer.[96–99] Lymph node metastases are a clear prognostic factor for decreased survival.[100] Approximately 95% of esophageal adenocarcinomas are diagnosed in patients without a prior diagnosis of Barrett's esophagus.[9] The best hope for improved survival of patients with esophageal adenocarcinoma is detection of cancer at an early and potentially curable stage.

Screening

One potential strategy to decrease the mortality rate of esophageal adenocarcinoma further is to identify more patients at risk, such as patients with Barrett's esophagus. Population-based studies suggest that in patients with newly diagnosed esophageal adenocarcinoma, a prior endoscopy and diagnosis of Barrett's esophagus was associated with both early stage cancer and improved survival.[101] Only a few patients with esophageal adenocarcinoma have undergone prior endoscopy, however.[102] Current professional society practice guidelines equivocate on screening patients with chronic GERD symptoms for Barrett's esophagus.[46,47,56] The 2009 American Cancer Society cancer screening guidelines does not include any recommendation for screening of either esophageal cancer or Barrett's esophagus.[103]

Endoscopy with biopsy is still the only validated technique to diagnose Barrett's esophagus. It has clear limitations as a screening tool, however, including cost, risk, and complexity. If screening with endoscopy and biopsy were applied to the estimated 20% of the population with regular GERD symptoms, the cost implications would be staggering.[104] Unsedated upper endoscopy using small-caliber instruments still has the potential to change the economics of endoscopic screening because this technique may decrease sedation-related complications and costs. Unsedated small-caliber endoscopy detects Barrett's esophagus and dysplasia with sensitivity comparable to conventional endoscopy.[105] Although both procedures are well tolerated by patients, a major hurdle for unsedated endoscopy is patient resistance to undergoing a test without sedation. It is uncertain if endoscopy without sedation would meet with patient acceptance given the cultural preference for sedation in the United States. Otherwise, there are still no validated alternative techniques to screen for Barrett's esophagus that overcome the cost and risks associated with conventional upper endoscopy.

There has been considerable interest in esophageal capsule endoscopy as a screening alternative to conventional upper endoscopy. Studies to date show a sensitivity of 60% to 79% and a specificity of 75% to 100% compared with conventional upper endoscopy.[106–108] Modeling studies suggest that capsule endoscopy is not a cost-effective alternative to conventional endoscopy either.[109] Adoption of esophageal capsule endoscopy as a screening alternative to upper endoscopy is unlikely in the near future.

After a normal initial upper endoscopy, some clinicians wonder if a repeat screening upper endoscopy should be undertaken in symptomatic GERD patients at a later date. Several studies have addressed this point with consistent

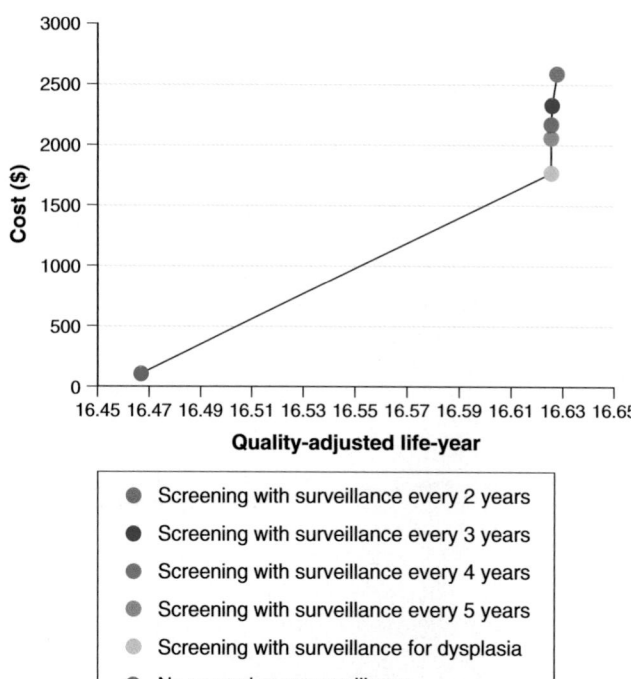

Fig. 26.9 Cost and benefit of screening and surveillance for Barrett's esophagus in a hypothetical 50-year-old white man with symptoms of gastroesophageal reflux disease (GERD) compared with no screening or surveillance. *(From Inadomi JM, Sampliner R, Lagergren J, et al: Screening and surveillance for Barrett esophagus in high risk groups: A cost-utility analysis. Ann Intern Med 138:176–186, 2003.)*

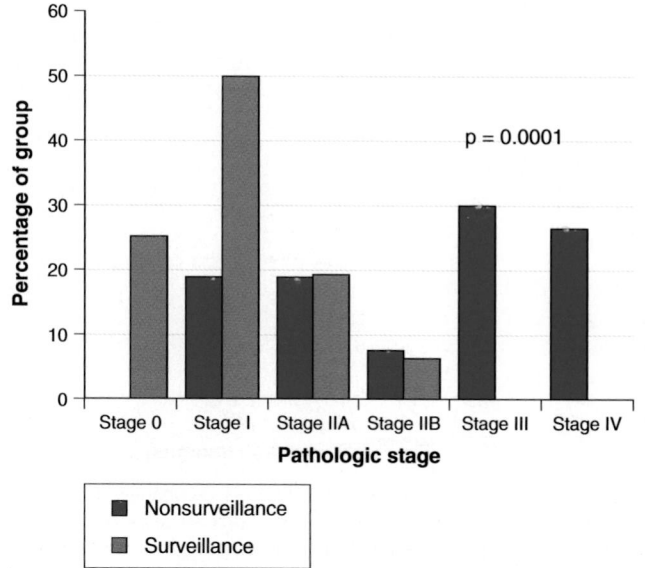

Fig. 26.10 Improved pathologic stage at diagnosis of esophageal adenocarcinoma for patients diagnosed during endoscopic surveillance compared with patients diagnosed without prior surveillance. *(From Van Sandick JW, Lanschot JJ, Kuiken BW, et al: Impact of endoscopic biopsy surveillance of Barrett's esophagus on pathological stage and clinical outcome of Barrett's carcinoma. Gut 43:216–222, 1998.)*

results. In patients with nonerosive reflux disease at the index endoscopy, Barrett's esophagus is rarely found if the repeat endoscopy is performed within 5 years.[110,111] Barrett's esophagus may be present in 9% to 12% of patients with erosive esophagitis at the time of index endoscopy, and higher grades of esophagitis are associated with a higher case finding rate of Barrett's esophagus on repeat endoscopy.[112,113] Screening for Barrett's esophagus in GERD patients should take place only after initial therapy with a proton pump inhibitor (PPI). A negative endoscopy at baseline makes it highly unlikely to find Barrett's esophagus if endoscopy is repeated.

There are still no data from randomized controlled trials or observational studies to evaluate the strategy of screening. A decision analysis model by Inadomi and colleagues[114] examined screening of 50-year-old white men with chronic GERD symptoms for Barrett's esophagus and found that one-time screening is probably cost-effective if subsequent surveillance is limited to patients with dysplasia on initial examination (**Fig. 26.9**). This strategy would result in a cost of $10,440 per quality-adjusted life year saved compared with a strategy of no screening or surveillance. Other modeling studies support screening in patients with chronic GERD symptoms as well but only if the following conditions are met: patients at high risk for Barrett's esophagus, high-grade dysplasia, or adenocarcinoma; high sensitivity and specificity of endoscopy with biopsy; and little or no reduction in quality of life with esophagectomy.[115,116] Any variation of these ideal conditions quickly made this strategy cost-ineffective.

There is clearly a need to develop either a better profile of patients at high risk for Barrett's esophagus and high-grade

dysplasia or a far less expensive tool to provide mass population screening. A simple questionnaire and nomogram has been described in an effort to predict Barrett's esophagus in patients with GERD symptoms.[117] The sensitivity of this questionnaire for predicting Barrett's esophagus was 77% with a specificity of only 63%. Although clearly cost saving, this questionnaire would miss patients with Barrett's esophagus with GERD symptoms and not account for individuals without any symptoms of GERD.

Screening strategies need to consider the following options: limiting screening to high-risk patients only; offering mass endoscopic screening to all adults older than 50 years as part of a periodic health appraisal preventive strategy; or doing nothing until clinical trials provide the evidence to support such a strategy. Problems inherent in showing the utility of a screening program such as healthy volunteer bias, lead time bias, and length time bias all need to be addressed.

Surveillance

Current practice guidelines recommend endoscopic surveillance of patients with Barrett's esophagus in an attempt to detect cancer at an early and potentially curable stage.[46,47,55,56] Numerous observational studies suggest that patients with Barrett's esophagus in whom adenocarcinoma was detected in a surveillance program have their cancers detected at an earlier stage (**Fig. 26.10**), with markedly improved 5-year survival compared with similar patients not undergoing routine endoscopic surveillance (**Fig. 26.11**).[102,118–121] Nodal involvement is far less likely in patients undergoing surveillance compared with patients not undergoing surveillance.[120] Because survival in esophageal cancer is stage-dependent, these studies suggest that survival may be enhanced by endoscopic surveillance. Several decision-analysis models support the concept of endoscopic surveillance.[114,122,123] The model of Provenzale and

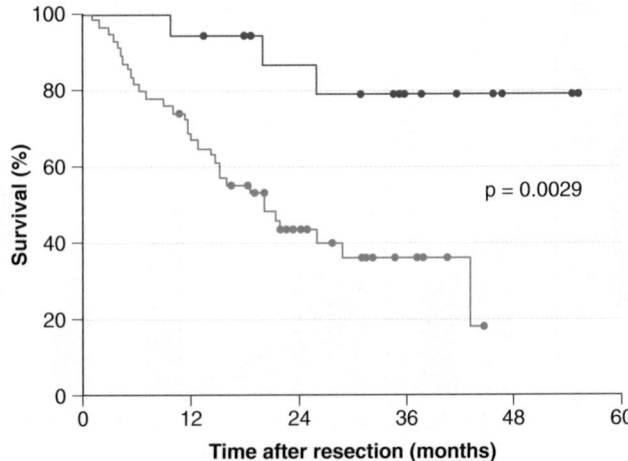

Fig. 26.11 Improved postoperative survival in esophageal adenocarcinoma for patients diagnosed during endoscopic surveillance compared with patients diagnosed without prior surveillance. *(From Van Sandick JW, Lanschot JJ, Kuiken BW, et al: Impact of endoscopic biopsy surveillance of Barrett's esophagus on pathological stage and clinical outcome of Barrett's carcinoma.* Gut *43:216–222, 1998.)*

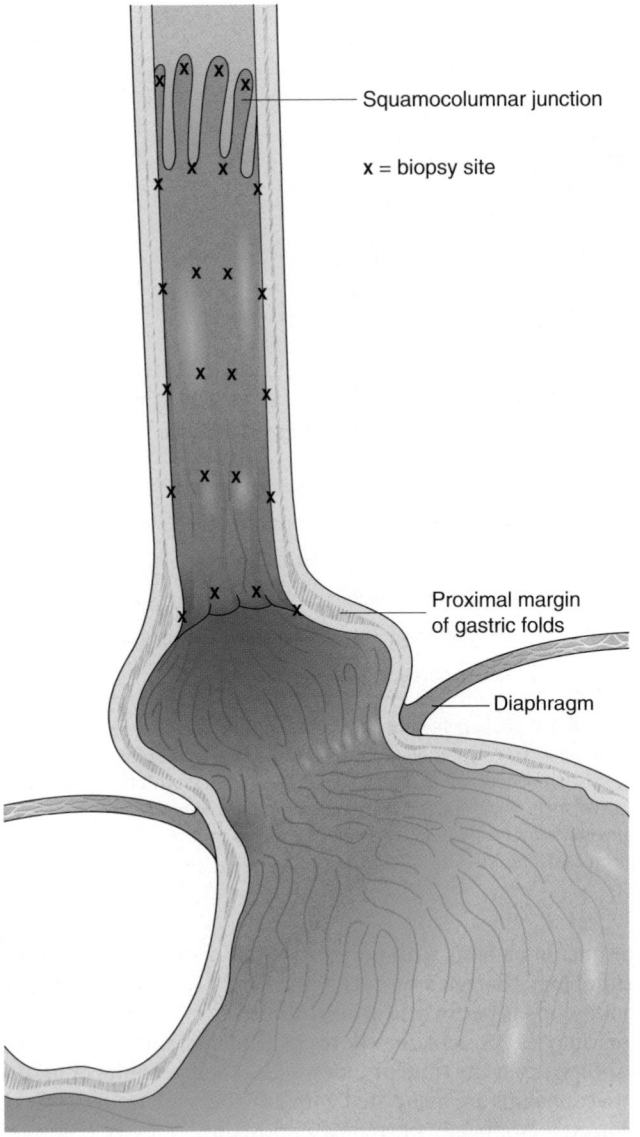

Fig. 26.12 Technique of endoscopic surveillance. Landmarks including the diaphragm, proximal margin of gastric folds, and squamocolumnar junction should be identified first. Four-quadrant biopsy specimens should be obtained every 2 cm in the involved segment. *(From Falk GW: Endoscopic surveillance of Barrett's esophagus.* Tech Gastrointest Endosc *2:186–193, 2000.)*

coworkers[122] suggests that surveillance every 5 years is the most effective strategy to increase length and quality of life, whereas the model of Inadomi and colleagues[114] suggests that surveillance should be limited only to individuals with dysplasia at the time of initial endoscopy.

Other authors argue that because most patients with Barrett's esophagus do not die of esophageal cancer, the benefit for surveillance remains uncertain, and endoscopic surveillance is not warranted until substantiated by prospective studies.[124] Design flaws such as selection bias, healthy volunteer bias, lead time bias, and length time bias are inherent in the observational studies that support endoscopic surveillance. The resources encumbered by vigorous endoscopic surveillance are considerable. Despite the concern regarding the esophageal cancer "epidemic," the overall burden of disease is limited in the Western world compared with other malignancies such as colon cancer. A randomized controlled trial of surveillance versus no surveillance in Barrett's esophagus has not been performed and is not likely to be performed in the future.

Candidates for Endoscopic Surveillance

Patients with documented Barrett's esophagus are candidates for surveillance. Before entering into a surveillance program, patients should be advised about risks and benefits, including the limitations of surveillance endoscopy and the importance of adhering to appropriate surveillance intervals.[47,56,125] Other considerations include age, likelihood of survival over the next 5 years, and ability to tolerate either endoscopic or surgical interventions for early esophageal adenocarcinoma.

Surveillance Techniques

The aim of surveillance is to detect dysplasia. The description of dysplasia should use a standard five-tier system: (1) negative for dysplasia, (2) indefinite for dysplasia, (3) low-grade dysplasia, (4) high-grade dysplasia, and (5) carcinoma.[42] Active inflammation makes it more difficult to distinguish

dysplasia from reparative changes. It is essential that surveillance endoscopy is performed only after any active inflammation related to GERD is controlled with antisecretory therapy. The presence of ongoing erosive esophagitis is a contraindication to performing surveillance biopsies.

Current guidelines suggest obtaining systematic four-quadrant biopsy specimens at 2-cm intervals along the entire length of the Barrett's segment after inflammation related to GERD is controlled with antisecretory therapy (**Fig. 26.12**).[46,47,55,56] A systematic biopsy protocol clearly detects more dysplasia and early cancer compared with ad hoc random biopsies.[126,127] Extensive biopsies of subtle mucosal abnormalities, no matter how trivial, such as ulceration, erosion, plaque, nodule, stricture, or other luminal irregularity in the Barrett's segment, should also be performed because there is an association of such lesions with underlying cancer.[128] Current guidelines also recommend, however, that patients with

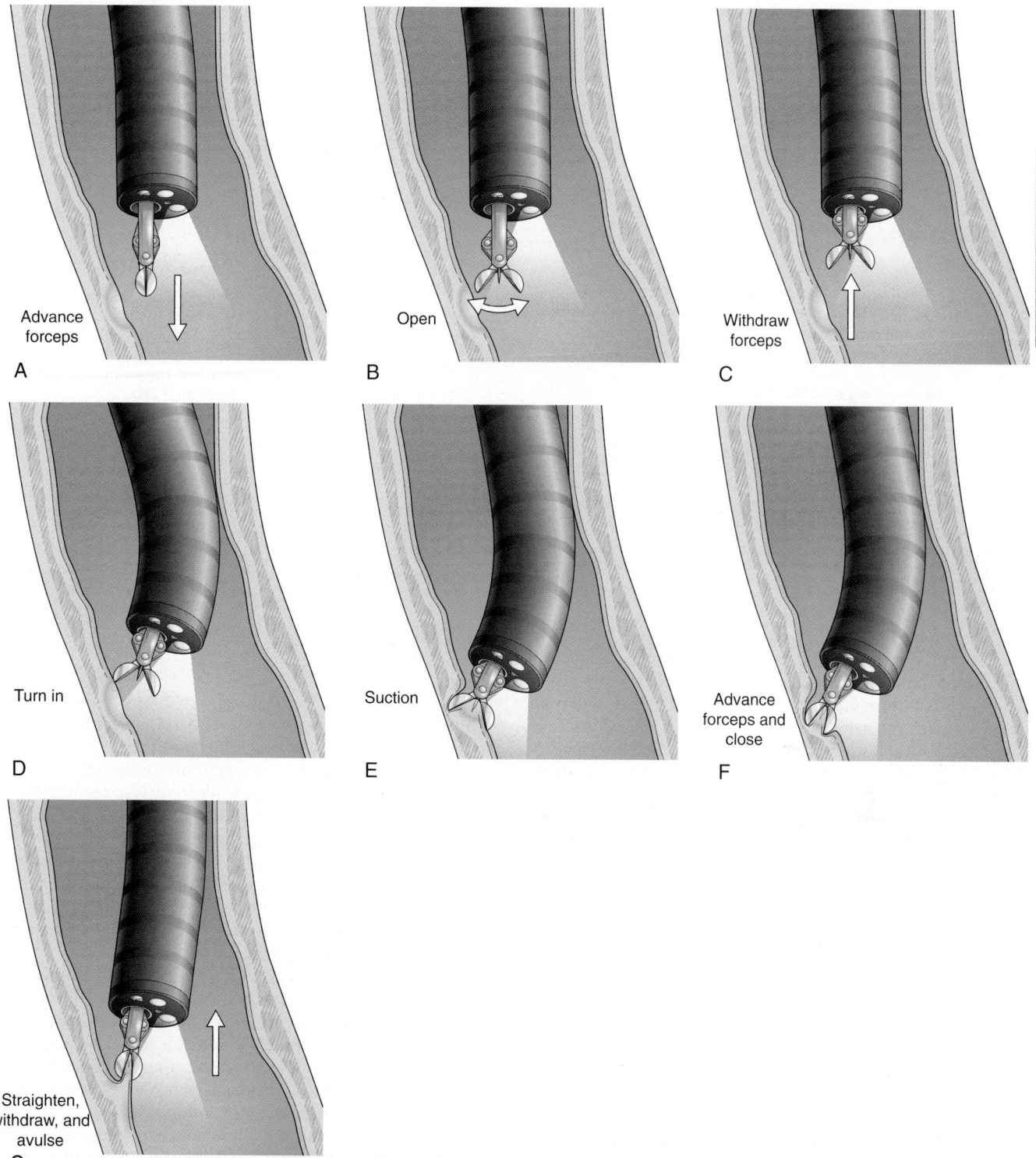

Fig. 26.13 Turn and suction technique of obtaining biopsy specimens in Barrett's esophagus. The biopsy forceps is advanced in the lumen (**A**), opened (**B**), and drawn back into the endoscope until it is flush with the endoscope tip (**C**). The endoscope is turned into the esophageal wall (**D**), after which suction is applied (**E**). The biopsy forceps is advanced slightly and closed (**F**), after which the endoscope is straightened followed by withdrawal of the forceps to avulse a mucosal sample (**G**). *(From Levine DS, Reid BJ: Endoscopic biopsy technique for acquiring larger mucosal samples.* Gastrointest Endosc *37:332–337, 1991.)*

mucosal abnormalities, especially in the setting of high-grade dysplasia, should undergo EMR.[46,47] Studies suggest that EMR changes the diagnosis in approximately 50% of patients, given the larger tissue sample available for review by the pathologist.[129] The "turn and suction" technique (**Fig. 26.13**) allows

acquisition of biopsy specimens that are significantly larger than the specimens obtained by the traditional techniques of advancing an open biopsy forceps into the lumen and then closing it to obtain the biopsy sample.[130] The safety of systematic endoscopic biopsy protocols has been shown.[131]

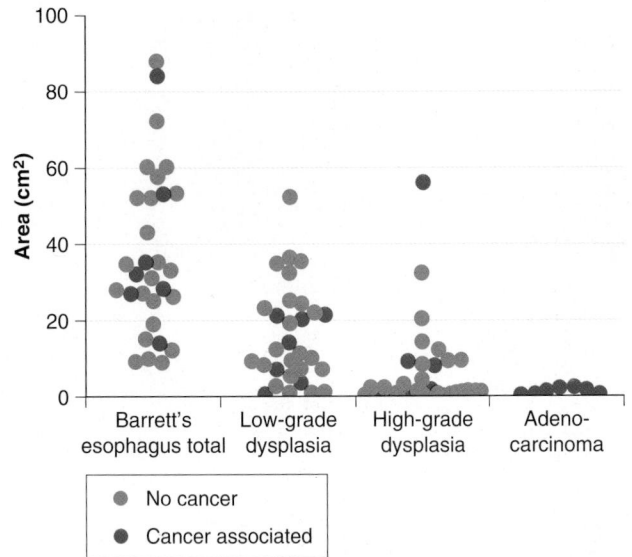

Fig. 26.14 Surface area involved with Barrett's esophagus, low-grade dysplasia, high-grade dysplasia, and adenocarcinoma in 30 patients without obvious carcinoma undergoing resection for high-grade dysplasia or superficial adenocarcinoma. *(From Cameron AJ, Carpenter HA: Barrett's esophagus, high-grade dysplasia and early adenocarcinoma. Am J Gastroenterol 92:586–591, 1997.)*

Table 26.1 2008 American College of Gastroenterology Practice Guidelines for Endoscopic Surveillance of Barrett's Esophagus

Dysplasia Grade	Interval
None	Every 3 yr after two endoscopies are negative within 1 yr
Low-grade	Expert GI pathologist confirmation
	Repeat endoscopy within 6 mo to ensure no higher grade of dysplasia
	Every year until no dysplasia on two consecutive endoscopies
High-grade	Expert GI pathologist confirmation
	If Barrett's segment flat—redo endoscopy and biopsies within 3 mo
	If mucosal abnormality—endoscopic mucosal resection
	Counsel patient with options
	Intensive surveillance
	Endoscopic therapy
	Esophagectomy

GI, gastrointestinal.
Adapted from Wang KK, Sampliner RE: Updated guidelines 2008 for the diagnosis, surveillance, and therapy of Barrett's esophagus. Am J Gastroenterol 103:788–797, 2008.

The rationale for such a comprehensive biopsy program comes from observations that high-grade dysplasia and early carcinoma in Barrett's esophagus often occur in the absence of endoscopic abnormalities and from the focal nature of dysplasia. Systematic esophagectomy mapping studies show just how focal dysplasia and superficial cancer may be. In 30 esophagectomy specimens from patients undergoing surgery for either high-grade dysplasia or early invasive adenocarcinoma with no endoscopic evidence of cancer, the median surface area of total Barrett's esophagus was found to be 32 cm^2; low-grade dysplasia, 13 cm^2; high-grade dysplasia, 1.3 cm^2; and adenocarcinoma, 1.1 cm^2 (**Fig. 26.14**).[132] The three smallest cancers had surface areas of 0.02 cm^2, 0.3 cm^2, and 0.4 cm^2.

Because of the focal nature of dysplasia and cancer, some experts recommend that endoscopic surveillance should use a large particle (jumbo) forceps to obtain biopsy specimens.[133] However, other authors have found that jumbo forceps biopsies still miss cancer in patients with high-grade dysplasia if the biopsies are performed at both 1-cm and 2-cm intervals.[134] This technique requires passage of a therapeutic endoscope, and the generalizability of this technique to clinical practice is problematic. Large-capacity forceps are available for passage through standard diameter endoscopes, which should render this issue less important than in the past. The extensive use of EMR has changed biopsy sampling considerably. Current guidelines suggest that available evidence does not support the routine use of the jumbo biopsy forceps.[47]

Surveillance Intervals

Surveillance intervals, determined by the presence and grade of dysplasia, are based on the limited understanding of the biology of esophageal adenocarcinoma. The most recently published recommendations from the American College of Gastroenterology are shown in **Table 26.1**. These intervals are arbitrary, however; they have never been subject to a clinical trial and likely never will be. Guidelines from various professional societies are not in agreement on surveillance intervals or techniques. The American College of Gastroenterology[46] and the American Society for Gastrointestinal Endoscopy[55] both recommend surveillance every 3 years as adequate in patients without dysplasia after two negative examinations. The American Gastroenterological Association[47] recommends extending the surveillance interval up to 5 years, whereas the British Society of Gastroenterology[56] recommends continued surveillance at 2-year intervals in this setting.

If low-grade dysplasia is found, the diagnosis should first be confirmed by an expert GI pathologist owing to the marked interobserver variability in interpretation of these biopsy specimens. Data suggest that if there is a consensus diagnosis by two or three expert GI pathologists, the risk of progression is greater than if there is no such agreement.[135] These patients should receive aggressive antisecretory therapy for reflux disease with a PPI to decrease the chances of regeneration that make pathologic interpretation of this category so difficult. A repeat endoscopy should be performed within 6 months of the initial diagnosis. If low-grade dysplasia is confirmed, annual surveillance is recommended when low-grade dysplasia is present until two examinations in a row are negative.[46] There is no agreement on the biopsy protocol to use, although a protocol of four-quadrant biopsy specimens at 1-cm intervals as would be used for high-grade dysplasia makes sense. EMR should be performed if any mucosal abnormality is present in these patients.

If high-grade dysplasia is found, the diagnosis should first be confirmed by an experienced GI pathologist as well. If the segment is flat and without any mucosal abnormalities, the endoscopic biopsy protocol should be repeated within 3 months to exclude an unsuspected carcinoma using careful inspection with high-quality white light endoscopy.[46] It is still unclear how much enhanced imaging techniques add to careful inspection with high-resolution or high-definition white light endoscopy (see later). The presence of any mucosal abnormality warrants EMR in an effort to maximize staging accuracy.

If high-grade dysplasia is confirmed, there is no consensus on the appropriate management of these patients. Options include continued surveillance, endoscopic therapy, or esophagectomy. Although continued surveillance has been compared with endoscopic approaches in randomized controlled trials, esophagectomy has not been compared with endoscopic ablative therapy in any randomized controlled trials.[136] Observational studies suggest, however, that survival and cancer-free survival are comparable in patients treated either surgically or endoscopically for high-grade dysplasia.[137] If continued surveillance is chosen, one proposed option is surveillance at 3-month intervals for 1 year.[138] If there is no high-grade dysplasia on two consecutive endoscopies for the first year, endoscopy frequency is lengthened to every 6 months for the second year and then to annually thereafter as long as high-grade dysplasia is not encountered again. If high-grade dysplasia persists, continued short-interval endoscopy is warranted.

The extent of high-grade dysplasia is thought by some authors to be a risk factor for the subsequent development of adenocarcinoma.[139] However, there are currently no uniform criteria for defining the extent of high-grade dysplasia, and there are conflicting data on the clinical significance of extent of high-grade dysplasia in biopsy specimens and risk for unsuspected carcinoma.[139,140] Mucosal abnormalities in patients with multifocal high-grade dysplasia may also be a risk factor for adenocarcinoma.[141,142] High-grade dysplasia remains a worrisome lesion, although progression to carcinoma may take many years and is not inevitable. The ultimate approach to a patient with high-grade dysplasia should consider factors such as available surgical and endoscopic expertise; age of the patient; length of Barrett's epithelium that would require biopsy to eliminate sampling error; compliance with endoscopic surveillance; future need for multiple surveillance endoscopies; and suspicious lesions such as plaques, nodules, and strictures.

Limitations of Surveillance

As currently practiced, endoscopic surveillance of Barrett's esophagus has numerous shortcomings. Dysplasia and early adenocarcinoma are endoscopically indistinguishable from intestinal metaplasia without dysplasia. The distribution of dysplasia and cancer is highly variable, and even the most thorough biopsy surveillance program has the potential for sampling error. There are considerable interobserver variability and quality control problems in the interpretation of dysplasia in both community and academic settings. Current surveillance programs are expensive and time-consuming. Survey data indicate that although surveillance is widely practiced, there is considerable variability in the technique and interval of surveillance because practice guidelines are not widely followed in the community (**Fig. 26.15**).[143–146] However, education programs can enhance compliance with guidelines.[145]

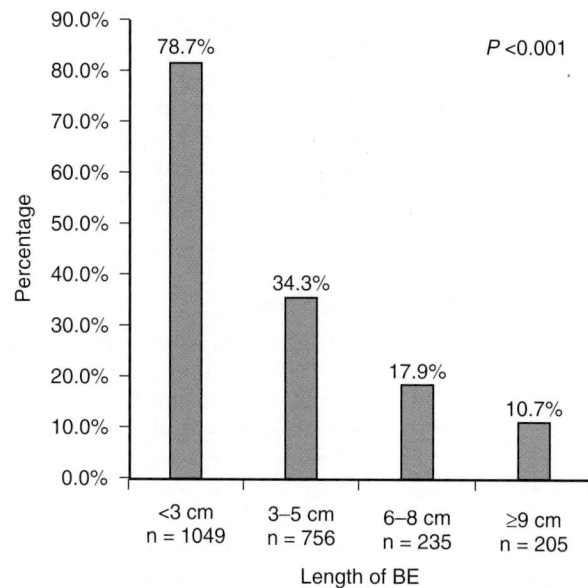

Fig. 26.15 Adherence to Seattle biopsy protocol in the community setting by length of Barrett's esophagus. *(From Abrams JA, Kapel RC, Lindberg GM, et al: Adherence to biopsy guidelines for Barrett's esophagus surveillance in the community setting in the United States. Clin Gastroenterol Hepatol 7:736–742, 2009.)*

Currently, all patients with Barrett's esophagus are managed in a similar fashion unless dysplasia is present. Most patients do not have dysplasia, however, and never develop cancer. It is necessary to make surveillance techniques more effective by sampling larger areas of Barrett's mucosa, targeting biopsies to areas with a higher probability of harboring dysplasia, or developing risk stratification tools to allow clinicians to concentrate efforts on individuals at greatest risk, while decreasing the frequency and intensity of surveillance in individuals at lower risk.

Potential Strategies to Enhance Surveillance

Chromoendoscopy

Methylene blue is a vital stain that selectively diffuses into the cytoplasm of absorptive epithelium of the small intestine and colon. The presence of staining in the esophagus indicates the presence of intestinal metaplasia.[147] Some studies have suggested that methylene blue chromoendoscopy increases the efficiency of detecting dysplasia; fewer biopsies are required, and more patients are identified with dysplasia compared with four-quadrant biopsy specimens obtained at 2-cm intervals.[148] However, other studies were unable to detect any differences in detection of dysplasia between methylene blue–directed biopsies compared with a standard biopsy protocol.[149] Chromoendoscopy is appealing because it is simple, inexpensive, and safe. However, there is no agreement on application technique in terms of the concentration, volume, and "dwell time" of various reagents, and interpretation of staining is subjective. Methylene blue chromoendoscopy also adds additional procedure time. A meta-analysis found that methylene blue chromoendoscopy resulted in no incremental yield compared with random biopsies for the detection of intestinal metaplasia, high-grade dysplasia, or early cancer.[150]

Acetic acid has also been used as a chromoendoscopy technique. Application of 3% acetic acid in 100 patients with Barrett's esophagus showed a normal uniform pattern in 85 patients, none of whom had dysplasia, and an abnormal irregular pattern in 15, of whom 87% had dysplasia.[151] Other authors showed that acetic acid–enhanced endoscopy improves image quality but does not increase the detection rate of dysplasia or adenocarcinoma.[152]

Optical Contrast Endoscopy

Various optical imaging enhancements have been developed to enable detailed inspection of the mucosal and vascular surface patterns. Narrow band imaging involves the placement of optical filters that narrow the band width of white light to blue light. This technique allows for detailed imaging of the mucosal and vascular surface patterns in Barrett's esophagus without the need for chromoendoscopy. Two postprocessing software driven systems are available to accomplish similar visualization (iScan System and FICE). Almost all of the published literature to date has examined narrow band imaging.[153]

Studies of narrow band imaging with optical zoom found that irregular mucosal and vascular patterns were highly predictive of early neoplasia.[154,155] A tandem endoscopy study that compared standard resolution white light endoscopy with narrow band imaging combined with high-definition white light endoscopy found the latter to be superior to conventional white light endoscopy for the detection of early neoplasia and required fewer biopsy specimens to accomplish this.[156] Other studies suggest that although narrow band imaging improves overall image quality, it does not lead to enhanced detection of early neoplasia compared with high-resolution white light endoscopy.[152,157]

A more recent systematic review found that narrow band imaging has a sensitivity of 77% to 100% and a specificity of 79% to 94% for the detection of intestinal metaplasia.[158] The sensitivity for the detection of high-grade dysplasia or cancer is 77% to 100% with a specificity of 58% to 100%. There are many unresolved issues regarding narrow band imaging, however, including multiple classification schemes for the mucosal and vascular patterns, image interpretation based on still images instead of real-time endoscopy, the use of optical versus electronic zoom, and the use of study populations enriched with early neoplasia in tertiary care centers. Despite these limitations, narrow band imaging is a promising technique for distinguishing intestinal metaplasia from gastric columnar metaplasia and early neoplasia from nonneoplastic tissue. It also may be useful for detecting residual columnar epithelium after ablative therapies. All classification schemes concentrate on regular versus irregular mucosal and vascular patterns.

Spectroscopy

Initial work with laser-induced fluorescence spectroscopy in a group of 36 patients had a sensitivity of 100% for high-grade dysplasia and a specificity of 70% for no dysplasia, but all six patients with low-grade dysplasia were classified as benign by laser-induced fluorescence spectroscopy.[159] A spectroscopic probe that combined the techniques of fluorescence, reflectance, and light scattering spectroscopy in 16 patients with

Barrett's esophagus had a sensitivity and specificity of 100% for separating high-grade dysplasia from low-grade dysplasia and no dysplasia and a sensitivity of 93% with a specificity of 100% for separating any dysplasia from no dysplasia.[160] Elastic scattering spectroscopy has also shown promise.[161] However, spectroscopic techniques, as currently configured, require a "point and shoot" method of touching the mucosa with the probe followed by biopsy. To be clinically helpful, these techniques need to image a larger field by "spraying light" followed by targeted biopsies of abnormal optical regions.

Optical Coherence Tomography

Optical coherence tomography uses infrared light to produce high-resolution images of mucosal tissue in vivo. Current technology is limited to a "touch and image" technique and is unable to sample large areas rapidly. Data to date suggest that the accuracy of current systems is insufficient for clinical application.[162]

Autofluorescence Endoscopy

Autofluorescence endoscopy is an imaging technique with the potential to examine a large surface area of GI mucosa rapidly to detect small areas of dysplasia or cancer. Autofluorescence endoscopy is based on the principle that normal, metaplastic, and dysplastic tissues have different autofluorescence colors visible to the naked eye. It involves illumination of tissue of interest with short-wavelength light, which leads to excitation of endogenous substances known as fluorophores and emission of fluorescence light of longer wavelengths.[163]

Early work with autofluorescence endoscopy involved fiberoptic technology. Despite some promising preliminary studies, a randomized crossover trial of fiberoptic autofluorescence endoscopy versus white light video endoscopy in Barrett's esophagus found no difference in the detection rates for high-grade dysplasia or adenocarcinoma between the two techniques.[164] Fiberoptic autofluorescence endoscopy was limited by poor image quality and poor maneuverability of the bulky imaging platform, making this technique of limited clinical value.

Although fiberoptic autofluorescence endoscopy seems to provide no advantage over conventional white light imaging, video-based technology, especially when combined with narrow band imaging, offers potential for enhancing endoscopic surveillance of Barrett's esophagus. Kara and associates[165] found that video-based autofluorescence endoscopy increased the detection of high-grade dysplasia and early carcinoma lesions that were not seen with high-resolution white light video endoscopy. When used as a standalone technique, however, autofluorescence endoscopy was still associated with a high number of false-positive areas of abnormal fluorescence. In this study, 28 of 81 regions (35%) of abnormal fluorescence were associated with no dysplasia.

In an effort to decrease the high false-positive rates found with autofluorescence endoscopy when used as a standalone technique, the Amsterdam group subsequently combined autofluorescence endoscopy with narrow band imaging and optical zoom technology in a series of studies. This technique uses autofluorescence videoendoscopy as a "red flag" technique to identify suspicious areas of Barrett's mucosa, followed by narrow band imaging combined with magnification endoscopy to examine the vascular and mucosal patterns of these suspicious lesions.

The combination of high-resolution white light, narrow band imaging, and autofluorescence in one endoscope is known as trimodal imaging. In one study, the combination of the three techniques decreased the false-positive rate from 40% to 10%, whereas in a second study, the false-positive rate was decreased from 81% to 26%, and the detection rate of intramucosal carcinoma or high-grade dysplasia lesions was increased compared with high-resolution white light endoscopy alone.[166,167] Taken together, these studies show the promise of autofluorescence endoscopy when combined with narrow band imaging and high-resolution white light endoscopy for surveillance of Barrett's esophagus. For this technology to have future clinical application, image quality still needs to be improved, and the false-positive rate needs to be decreased further.

Confocal Laser Endomicroscopy

Confocal laser endomicroscopy is a new endoscopic imaging technique that allows for subsurface imaging and in vivo histologic assessment of the mucosal layer during standard white light endoscopy.[168] It is a potentially ideal small field imaging technique that optimally should be used with a "red flag" method to target image acquisition. The goal of endomicroscopy is to distinguish neoplastic from nonneoplastic tissue and provide the potential for decreased number of biopsies. Two different platforms are available: an endoscope-based device that is integrated into the distal tip of the endoscope and a probe-based device that can be inserted through a standard endoscope. Both devices require administration of fluorescein, an intravenous fluorescence agent.

Several studies have examined confocal laser endomicroscopy in Barrett's esophagus. Using a scope-based device, a confocal Barrett's esophagus classification scheme involving cellular and vascular architecture was developed to predict histopathology in the columnar-lined segment. The sensitivity and specificity for the prediction of nondysplastic Barrett's epithelium were 98% and 94% and for Barrett's esophagus–associated neoplasia were 93% and 98%. The κ value for interobserver agreement was .843.[169] A similar pilot study of probe-based confocal laser microscopy yielded a sensitivity of 75% to 89% and specificity of 75% to 91%.[170] More recent work also suggests that confocal endomicroscopy with the scope-based technique improves the diagnostic yield of endoscopically inapparent neoplasia compared with standard white light endoscopy and surveillance biopsies.[171]

Risk Stratification

Numerous clinical and biologic markers may define patients at increased risk for the development of adenocarcinoma. Clinical risk factors for the development of high-grade dysplasia or adenocarcinoma include gender, ethnicity, age, dysplasia, hiatal hernia size, length of Barrett's segment, body mass index, and smoking.[79] Although esophageal cancer develops in both short and long segments of Barrett's esophagus, segment length does not seem to be a strong risk factor for the development of cancer.[71,172]

Dysplasia is still the best available marker of cancer risk. Dysplasia is recognized adjacent to and distant from Barrett's esophagus–associated adenocarcinoma in resection specimens from patients with Barrett's esophagus. Patients with Barrett's esophagus progress through a phenotypic sequence of no dysplasia, low-grade dysplasia, high-grade dysplasia, and adenocarcinoma, although the time course is highly variable, and this stepwise sequence is not preordained.[120,173] Some patients may progress directly to cancer without prior detection of dysplasia of any grade.[174] Dysplasia is the only factor at the present time that is useful in clinical practice for identifying patients at increased risk for the development of esophageal adenocarcinoma.

The natural history of low-grade dysplasia is poorly understood. First, the diagnosis is often transient[175,176]; this may be due in part to the high degree of interobserver variability in establishing this diagnosis and the variable biopsy protocols by which these patients are followed, resulting in issues related to tissue sampling. Although most patients with low-grade dysplasia do not progress to adenocarcinoma or high-grade dysplasia, a subset of these patients do progress to a higher grade lesion. More recent studies suggest an intermediate risk of progression to cancer with a weighted average incidence rate of 1.69% per year.[177] Factors associated with progression to cancer include consensus agreement among two or more pathologists and extent of low-grade dysplasia.[135,178]

High-grade dysplasia in Barrett's esophagus is a well-recognized risk factor for the development of adenocarcinoma.[138,139,179] Unsuspected carcinoma is detected at esophagectomy in approximately 40% of patients with high-grade dysplasia (range 0% to 73%).[180] More recent studies using EMR before esophagectomy suggest that finding unsuspected cancer is reduced considerably to approximately 13%.[137] Several studies have improved understanding of the natural history of high-grade dysplasia. Buttar and colleagues[139] followed 100 patients with high-grade dysplasia with continued endoscopic surveillance and found cancer at 1 year and 3 years in 38% and 56% of individuals with diffuse high-grade dysplasia and 7% and 14% of individuals with focal high-grade dysplasia. Reid and associates[179] followed 76 patients for 5 years and encountered cancer in 59%. Schnell and colleagues[138] found cancer in 5% of 79 patients during the first year of surveillance and in 16% of the remaining patients followed for a mean of 7 years (20% of the total group developed cancer). Other studies have reported regression of high-grade dysplasia over time as well.[138,181] A more recent meta-analysis found that the incidence of adenocarcinoma in patients with high-grade dysplasia was approximately 6.58% annually.[182] Mucosal abnormalities in patients with multifocal high-grade dysplasia may also be a risk factor for adenocarcinoma.[139,183] Although progression to carcinoma may take many years and is not inevitable, high-grade dysplasia remains a worrisome lesion.

Dysplasia is an imperfect marker of increased cancer risk. It is typically indistinguishable endoscopically and often focal in nature, making targeting of biopsies problematic. There is considerable interobserver variability in the grading of dysplasia in both community and academic settings, and the ability of pathologists to distinguish between intramucosal carcinoma and high-grade dysplasia is problematic even in esophagectomy specimens as described previously. A less subjective marker for cancer risk that could supplement or replace the current dysplasia grading system is needed.

Biomarkers of Increased Risk

Numerous molecular markers may define patients at increased risk for the development of esophageal adenocarcinoma. Among the most frequently described molecular changes that precede the development of adenocarcinoma in Barrett's esophagus are alterations in p53 (mutation, deletion, or LOH)[87,88,184,185] and p16 (mutation, deletion, promoter hypermethylation, or LOH)[89,90,186] and aneuploidy by flow cytometry.[187,188] Neoplastic progression in Barrett's esophagus is accompanied by flow cytometric abnormalities such as aneuploidy or increased G2/tetraploid DNA contents, and these abnormalities may precede the development of high-grade dysplasia or adenocarcinoma. The potential importance of flow cytometry as a prognostic biomarker was illustrated in work by Reid and colleagues,[189] who found that for patients with no flow cytometric abnormalities at baseline and with histology that showed no dysplasia, indefinite dysplasia, or low-grade dysplasia, the 5-year incidence of cancer was 0%. In contrast, aneuploidy, increased 4N fractions, or high-grade dysplasia was detected in each of the 35 patients who went on to develop cancer within 5 years.

Mutations of p53 and 17p LOH have been reported in 92% and 100% of esophageal adenocarcinomas.[190] Both abnormalities have been detected in Barrett's epithelium before the development of carcinoma. Reid and colleagues[88] found that the prevalence of 17p (p53) LOH at baseline increased from 6% in patients negative for dysplasia to 20% in patients with low-grade dysplasia and to 57% in patients with high-grade dysplasia. More importantly, the 3-year incidence of cancer was 38% for individuals with 17p (p53) LOH compared with 3.3% for individuals with two 17p alleles. However, techniques to detect p53 mutations and 17p LOH are labor-intensive and have not achieved widespread acceptance in clinical practice to date. Similarly, p16 LOH and inactivation of the p16 gene by promoter region hypermethylation have been reported frequently in esophageal adenocarcinoma.[90] 9p LOH is commonly encountered in premalignant Barrett's epithelium and can be detected over large regions of the Barrett's mucosa.[90] It is hypothesized that clonal expansion occurs in conjunction with p16 abnormalities creating a field in which other genetic lesions leading to esophageal adenocarcinoma can arise.

Epigenetic changes in the form of hypomethylation and hypermethylation and alteration to histone complexes have also been implicated in the progression of Barrett's esophagus to adenocarcinoma. Hypermethylation of p16, RUNX3, and HPP1 all are independently associated with an increased risk of progression of Barrett's esophagus to high-grade dysplasia or esophageal adenocarcinoma.[191]

Given the complexity and diversity of alterations observed to date in the metaplasia-dysplasia-carcinoma sequence, a panel of biomarkers may be required for risk stratification. Two studies examined the use of biomarkers with promising results. The combination of 17p LOH, 9p LOH, and DNA content abnormality has been shown to predict 10-year adenocarcinoma risk better than any single biomarker alone. Patients with a combination of these abnormalities had a markedly increased risk of developing cancer compared with patients with no baseline abnormalities (relative risk 38.7, 95% confidence interval 10.8 to 138.5). In patients with no abnormalities of any of these biomarkers at baseline, 12% developed adenocarcinoma at 10 years. In contrast, patients with the combination of 17p LOH, 9p LOH, and DNA content abnormality had a cumulative incidence of adenocarcinoma of 79% over the same period.[192] A risk stratification model using a methylation index constructed from the methylation values for p16, HPP1, and RUNX3 also showed potential for prediction of progression to high-grade dysplasia or adenocarcinoma.[193] Although these studies show the potential for biomarkers to predict risk of esophageal adenocarcinoma, none of these biomarkers have been validated in large-scale clinical trials to date and are not yet useful for clinical decision making.

Treatment

Medical Therapy

Because Barrett's esophagus has the most severe pathophysiologic abnormalities of GERD, PPIs are the cornerstone of medical therapy for Barrett's esophagus. Studies show that PPIs consistently result in symptom relief and heal esophagitis in patients with Barrett's esophagus.[194–196] However, even at high doses, PPIs result in either no regression of the Barrett's segment or modest regression that is of uncertain clinical importance.[197–199] PPIs typically increase squamous islands in the Barrett's segment, but biopsy specimens taken from such islands often show underlying intestinal metaplasia.[200]

Alleviation of reflux symptoms in Barrett's esophagus is not equivalent to normalization of esophageal acid exposure, despite the use of high-dose PPI therapy. Persistent abnormal acid exposure is encountered in approximately 25% of patients with Barrett's esophagus despite use of twice-daily PPIs.[201,202] The importance of complete control of esophageal acid exposure in patients with Barrett's esophagus is unknown. Some studies provide support, however, for the concept of aggressive acid suppression in these patients. Normalization of intraesophageal acid exposure in patients with Barrett's esophagus decreases cellular proliferation rates and increases cellular differentiation rates over 6 months, whereas inability to normalize intraesophageal acid exposure results in no difference in proliferation or differentiation rates.[203] However, this change is not accompanied by any effect on apoptosis or COX-2 levels.[204]

A more recent Veterans Administration cohort study suggested that PPI therapy, especially long duration use, was associated with a decreased risk for the development of dysplasia.[205] However, most of the cases of dysplasia were low-grade—a lesion with an intermediate and highly variable risk for development of cancer. Similar observational data on reduction of dysplasia risk with administration of PPIs have been obtained in Australia.[206] However, there are no randomized controlled trials that have examined the issue of dysplasia or cancer prevention and administration of PPIs as standalone therapy.

Antireflux Surgery

Antireflux surgery effectively alleviates GERD symptoms in patients with Barrett's esophagus.[207–209] A randomized controlled trial that was completed more recently found that the outcome of laparoscopic antireflux surgery was similar in GERD patients with and without Barrett's esophagus and comparable to use of esomeprazole, although antireflux surgery afforded better intraesophageal acid control.[210] The indications for surgery in patients with Barrett's esophagus are the same as the indications for GERD patients without Barrett's esophagus.

Some authors have hypothesized that antireflux surgery provides protection from progression of Barrett's esophagus to adenocarcinoma.[211] However, two lines of evidence suggest that antireflux surgery does not protect patients from developing esophageal adenocarcinoma. A large population-based cohort study of GERD patients from Sweden who underwent antireflux surgery found that surgery did not protect against the development of esophageal adenocarcinoma.[212] The standardized incidence ratio of esophageal adenocarcinoma in the surgically treated group was 14.1 (95% confidence interval 8.0 to 22.8) compared with 6.3 (95% confidence interval 4.5 to 8.7) in the medically treated group.

A Veterans Administration cohort study also found no attenuation of the risk for developing esophageal adenocarcinoma in GERD patients treated surgically compared with patients treated medically (0.072%/yr vs. 0.04%/yr).[213] Similar findings are seen in patients with Barrett's esophagus. A meta-analysis of surgical versus medical therapy of Barrett's esophagus found no difference in the risk of esophageal adenocarcinoma between the two groups.[214] A subsequent systematic review by Chang and coworkers[215] found no difference in the incidence of esophageal adenocarcinoma in medically treated versus surgically treated patients and found that any evidence suggesting otherwise was driven by uncontrolled case series. The best available evidence suggests that antireflux surgery does not decrease cancer risk in patients with GERD or Barrett's esophagus.

Chemoprevention

Chemoprevention is pharmacologic intervention for either the prevention of cancer or the treatment of identifiable precancerous lesions.[216] Various chemoprevention agents have been proposed for patients with Barrett's esophagus, including PPIs, celecoxib, aspirin, lyophilized black raspberries, antioxidants, green tea, retinoids, ursodeoxycholic acid, statins, and curcumin.[217–219]

Most attention at the present time is directed toward the use of aspirin and NSAIDs. Observational studies suggest that NSAIDs, including aspirin, may play a protective role against esophageal adenocarcinoma by inhibiting COX-1 and COX-2 enzymes, which regulate prostaglandin E_2 production.[80,81,220,221] Animal studies also suggest that administration of selective and nonselective cyclooxygenase inhibitors decreases the development of esophageal adenocarcinoma in experimentally induced Barrett's esophagus.[222] One possible mechanism that is involved in reflux-associated carcinogenesis in Barrett's esophagus is COX-2 activation and high levels of prostaglandin E_2 production induced by acid and bile salts. A systematic review suggested that the protective effect of aspirin and NSAIDs was greater with more regular use, an observation supported in a cohort study as well.[80,81]

A single clinical trial examined the effect of celecoxib at a dose of 200 mg twice daily given for 48 weeks in patients with low-grade and high-grade dysplasia on change in proportion of biopsy samples with dysplasia between patients treated with celecoxib compared with a placebo.[223] No differences were found between the two groups. A small crossover study showed

that high-dose PPI therapy in conjunction with aspirin at a dose of 325 mg daily can decrease mucosal prostaglandin E_2 content in mucosal biopsy specimens from patients with Barrett's esophagus.[224] These findings led to a large randomized clinical trial in the United Kingdom (ASPECT) and a smaller clinical trial in the United States in an effort to examine the potential for chemoprevention with aspirin in conjunction with a PPI as a clinical strategy in patients with Barrett's esophagus. However, it is premature to administer aspirin or NSAIDs routinely to these patients until more data become available.

Endoscopic Therapy

Given the above-described limitations of conventional medical and surgical therapy, various mucosal ablative techniques have been studied, including thermal ablation, photodynamic therapy, and EMR. The theory of mucosal ablation therapy is that reinjury of the metaplastic epithelium followed by the regeneration of normal squamous epithelium from a pluripotential stem cell in an environment of decreased acidity may decrease or eliminate the risk of developing esophageal adenocarcinoma.

The overall goals of ablation therapy of Barrett's esophagus are to eliminate columnar epithelium completely, eliminate cancer or risk of progression to cancer, and possibly decrease the need for surveillance endoscopy. Ideally, ablation techniques should be inexpensive, safe, and easy to apply and require a limited number of sessions to achieve the desired results. It is essential for techniques to provide a uniform application to the esophagus; this requires compensating for movement related to respiration and esophageal motility. Methods such as the centering balloon used for photodynamic therapy or the balloon-based radiofrequency devices that isolate esophageal segments during the application of the ablation technique are appealing.

Each of the endoscopic techniques is able to eliminate much or all of the Barrett's epithelium while the esophagus remains in situ, and the risks of surgery for high-grade dysplasia or cancer are avoided. More recent data with these techniques are encouraging, showing low morbidity and mortality and excellent 5-year survival.[225] Each of these techniques has disadvantages as well, however, including the need for continued meticulous surveillance, the potential for "at-risk" mucosa remaining after therapy, and diagnostic uncertainty. The decision to perform endoscopic therapy in patients with Barrett's esophagus is complex. Many factors enter into the decision-making process, including grade of dysplasia, characteristics of the lesion in question, patient characteristics, and institutional factors including expertise in pathology, surgery, and interventional endoscopy.

Thermal Ablation Techniques

Thermal ablation of Barrett's esophagus can be accomplished by various techniques, including laser, multipolar electrocoagulation, heater probe, argon plasma coagulation, radiofrequency ablation, and cryotherapy. Randomized controlled trials have been conducted to compare various thermal ablation techniques with each other. These clinical trials have highlighted the difficulty in obtaining complete endoscopic and histologic ablation with argon plasma coagulation and multipolar electrocoagulation.[226–228] Studies of these techniques routinely found incomplete macroscopic regression of the Barrett's segment and buried intestinal metaplasia beneath the neosquamous epithelium, which led to reports of subsquamous cancers developing in patients with previously nondysplastic Barrett's epithelium.[229–231] Consequently, techniques such as multipolar electrocoagulation, heater probe, and argon plasma coagulation all seem to have fallen by the wayside.

The reasons that these techniques likely have no long-term future include difficulty in obtaining uniform ablation, cost, side effects, and persistent endoscopically evident or microscopic columnar epithelium after therapy. The only conceivable place at the present time for techniques such as multipolar electrocoagulation and argon plasma coagulation is for small islands and areas of residual Barrett's esophagus after treatment with another, more effective modality. Current thermal techniques still in use include radiofrequency ablation and cryotherapy. All thermal techniques have one important disadvantage: complete pathologic confirmation of the index lesion can never be obtained, leaving both the physician and the patient uncertain as to the results of the treatment.

Radiofrequency Ablation

Radiofrequency ablation involves the application of high-power radiofrequency energy using bipolar electrodes, causing rapid heating of the tissue with ablation to a depth of approximately 0.5 mm. Studies on radiofrequency ablation have involved a stepwise progression from animal studies; to human studies before esophagectomy; to human dosimetry studies, single-center studies, multicenter nonrandomized studies, and multicenter randomized controlled trials.[232–234] This process also led to modifications in the radiofrequency ablation technique to include both a 360-degree balloon-based device and a focal ablation device.

Radiofrequency ablation has been studied for nondysplastic and dysplastic Barrett's esophagus. Sharma and colleagues[234] described their 12-month results with circumferential radiofrequency ablation of nondysplastic Barrett's epithelium in 70 patients; complete elimination of intestinal metaplasia was achieved without any buried glands in 69% of subjects. Buried intestinal metaplasia was not encountered in any of the biopsy specimens. Subsequently, longer term follow-up for up to 30 months after additional focal radiofrequency ablation showed complete elimination of metaplasia in 97% of patients at 30 months.[235] No buried intestinal metaplasia was encountered in any of the biopsy specimens at 12 months and 30 months. Adverse events were believed to be minor and were encountered in 15.1% after the circumferential ablation phase of the study and 2.6% after the focal ablation phase of the study. Any postablation symptoms resolved within 4 days of the procedure.

A randomized sham control study evaluated radiofrequency ablation for low-grade dysplasia and high-grade dysplasia.[236] This study showed complete resolution of high-grade dysplasia in 81% of the treatment group compared with 19% of the sham group and complete resolution of low-grade dysplasia in 91% of the treatment group compared with 23% of the sham group using a combination of the circumferential and focal probes at 1-year follow-up (**Fig. 26.16**). Among patients with high-grade dysplasia, progression to cancer occurred in

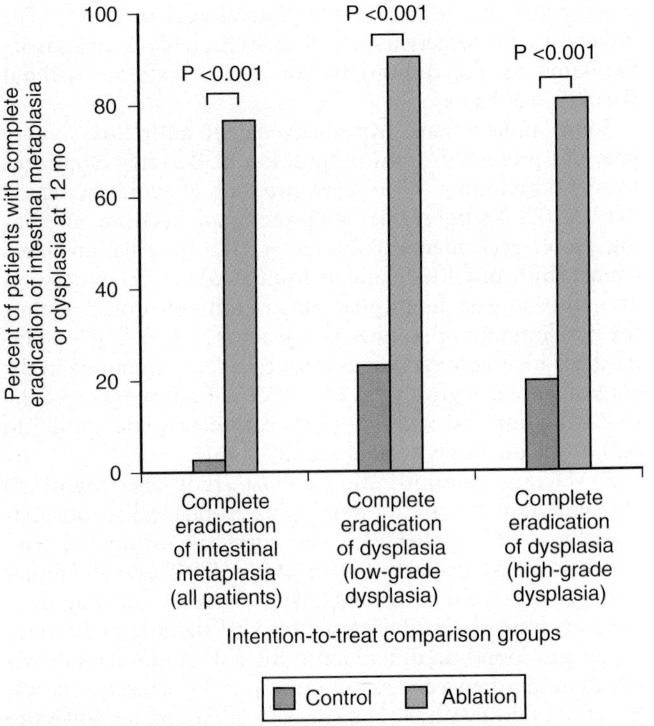

Fig. 26.16 Complete histologic eradication of intestinal metaplasia and complete eradication of dysplasia in the subgroups with low-grade dysplasia and in the subgroup with high-grade dysplasia at 12 months after radiofrequency ablation. *(From Shaheen NJ, Sharma P, Overholt BF, et al: Radiofrequency ablation in Barrett's esophagus with dysplasia. N Engl J Med 360:2277–2288, 2009.)*

2.4% of the treatment group compared with 19% of the sham group. Complete elimination of intestinal metaplasia occurred in 77% of the treatment group compared with 2% of the sham group. Adverse events were encountered in 3 of 298 treatments including bleeding and chest pain; 6% developed strictures that were easily dilated.

Taken together with other data on radiofrequency ablation, it is known that a combination of circumferential and focal probes provides optimal results, that this technique can be safely combined with EMR, that preexisting genetic abnormalities resolve, and that buried intestinal metaplasia seems to be rare.[237] This method does not completely eliminate cancer risk or progression of low-grade dysplasia to high-grade dysplasia. As with other ablative techniques except for EMR, radiofrequency ablation does not allow tissue confirmation of efficacy, leaving some uncertainty for each patient. Only a few patients have been studied to date, and long-term results beyond 2.5 years are still unknown.

Cryotherapy

Cryotherapy freezes the gut mucosa to induce cell death. There are two techniques: carbon dioxide and liquid nitrogen. However, very limited data are available regarding efficacy in Barrett's esophagus, and there are no randomized controlled trials to date. Johnston and colleagues[238] treated 11 patients with liquid nitrogen, with complete endoscopic and histologic reversal in 7 of 11 patients at 6 months. A case series reported 26 patients with high-grade dysplasia treated with liquid nitrogen, of which 32% were free of dysplasia at 12 months of follow-up.[239] The concern with this technique, besides lack of published data to date, is the uneven application inherent in spraying of the cryogen rather than direct balloon-based application to isolated segments of the esophagus.

Photodynamic Therapy

Photodynamic therapy is a process in which a light-sensitive drug concentrates in neoplastic tissue. The drug is activated by laser light of an appropriate wavelength directed at the abnormal tissue producing a cytotoxic substance, singlet oxygen, which selectively damages neoplastic tissue. Photodynamic therapy in Barrett's esophagus has involved various agents, including porfimer sodium, hematoporphyrin derivative, and 5-aminolevulinic acid. Each of these compounds is characterized by a different depth of tissue destruction and duration of cutaneous photosensitivity. Only porfimer sodium is available in the United States.

A randomized controlled study evaluated photodynamic therapy with porfimer sodium compared with a strategy of continued surveillance for patients with high-grade dysplasia.[240] At 2 years, complete ablation of high-grade dysplasia occurred in 77% of patients in the photodynamic therapy group compared with 39% of patients in the surveillance group with progression to cancer in 13% in the photodynamic therapy group and 28% in the surveillance group. Complete elimination of all intestinal metaplasia and dysplasia occurred in 52% of the photodynamic therapy group and 7% of the surveillance group. Complications were common—strictures in 36% and photosensitivity in 69%. At 5 years, the probability of complete ablation of high-grade dysplasia after photodynamic therapy was 48%, and progression to cancer occurred in 15%.[241] At the Mayo Clinic, patients with high-grade dysplasia treated with photodynamic therapy with or without concomitant EMR had long-term survival comparable to patients treated with esophagectomy and low rates of cancer-associated death.[242]

Photodynamic therapy has the advantages of leaving the esophagus in situ, evidence from randomized controlled trials that it is superior to continued surveillance and evidence from cohort studies that survival is comparable to esophagectomy. Disadvantages include the considerable capital expense of the equipment required, high rate of strictures, prolonged photosensitivity, lack of tissue confirmation, and problems in attaining complete ablation of intestinal metaplasia. Persistent genetic abnormalities have been noted in residual dysplastic and nondysplastic epithelium after photodynamic therapy with reports of subsequent redevelopment of high-grade dysplasia.[243-246]

Endoscopic Mucosal Resection

EMR is a therapeutic option for patients with either high-grade dysplasia or intramucosal carcinoma in the setting of appropriate risk stratification. As described earlier, EMR permits accurate histologic staging of neoplasia arising in Barrett's epithelium compared with esophageal resection specimens. Negative margins on EMR specimens correlate well with absence of residual disease at the time of surgery, but submucosal involvement is associated with both residual disease at the time of surgery and lymph node metastases.[247]

As emphasized by the Wiesbaden group, EMR for superficial cancer with curative intent should be attempted only for lesions with the following criteria: lesion diameter less than 20 mm and macroscopically type I (polypoid), IIa (flat and slightly elevated), IIb (flat and level), or IIc (flat, depressed, and <10 mm); well or moderately differentiated histologic grade; lesions limited to the mucosa proven by histology of the resected specimens; and no invasion of lymph vessels or veins. The issue of submucosal cancer limited to the superficial layer is an evolving area of debate.

The pioneering work of the Wiesbaden group with EMR in 100 patients with high-grade intraepithelial neoplasia or intramucosal carcinoma resulted in complete local remission in 99 after a mean of 1.47 EMRs with no strictures and only minor bleeding in 11 patients.[248] However, there were 11 metachronous lesions in 11 patients for a recurrence rate of 11%, characterized by local recurrence in 6 and disease at a different location in 5. There were two deaths in the series: One patient with CREST (calcinosis, Raynaud's phenomenon, esophageal dysmotility, scleroderma, and telangiectases) died of pneumonia, and one patient died of carcinoma of the oral cavity. The 5-year life-table survival of these patients was 98%.

It is important to emphasize some key methodologic aspects of the work of the Wiesbaden group. Before entry into the study, patients with confirmed adenocarcinoma were meticulously staged with the following techniques: high-resolution white light endoscopy, methylene blue chromoendoscopy, biopsy specimens of all macroscopically visible lesions and unstained areas on chromoendoscopy, four-quadrant biopsy specimens every 1 to 2 cm of the Barrett's segment, and endoscopic ultrasound. All patients with proven adenocarcinoma underwent chest radiography, computed tomography scan of the abdomen and chest, and ultrasound of the abdomen. There was no standard approach to residual Barrett's epithelium, although 49 patients underwent thermal ablation with either argon plasma coagulation for short-segment Barrett's esophagus or aminolevulinic acid photodynamic therapy for long-segment Barrett's esophagus. Follow-up examinations were rigorous and involved four-quadrant biopsy specimens and biopsy specimens of any visual lesions at 1 month, 2 months, 3 months, 6 months, 9 months, and 12 months followed by every 6 months for 5 years along with endoscopic ultrasound and computed tomography scans at every other visit. Residual or metachronous disease, defined as high-grade epithelial neoplasia or early cancer after complete local remission, was treated by EMR. Although the work by Ell and associates[248] makes a very strong case for the safety of EMR in superficial adenocarcinoma of the esophagus meeting low-risk criteria, their work also points out the problem of at-risk mucosa that remains after therapy because recurrent or metachronous lesions were found in 11% of patients.

Studies to date suggest that circumferential EMR results in complete remission of high-grade dysplasia and intramucosal adenocarcinoma in 75% to 100% of patients.[249-253] A single-center series of circumferential EMR by Chennat and colleagues[254] showed complete elimination of all Barrett's epithelium, dysplasia, and early cancer in 31 of 32 patients at a mean follow-up of 23 months with a stricture rate of 37% and no bleeding or perforation. Complication rates vary in other series, but early bleeding, occasional perforation, and late strictures remain issues.

EMR has the advantages of leaving the esophagus in situ, tissue confirmation of disease, and evidence from cohort studies regarding excellent long-term survival. Disadvantages include need for continued and high-frequency meticulous surveillance and at-risk mucosa remaining. The role of circumferential EMR is evolving but is still hampered by high stricture rates.

Combination Therapy

More recent studies indicate that complete ablation of Barrett's esophagus with EMR in combination with radiofrequency ablation is feasible. The Amsterdam group described the technique of circumferential and focal radiofrequency ablation in a few patients with Barrett's esophagus with residual dysplasia after EMR of visible lesions.[255,256] Gondrie and colleagues[255] found complete absence of Barrett's epithelium, dysplasia, cancer, and buried intestinal metaplasia in all 12 patients treated by EMR of all visible lesions followed by radiofrequency ablation of the residual Barrett's esophagus segment at a median follow-up of 14 months. Other investigators have described excellent long-term results with combinations of EMR and photodynamic therapy.[242,257]

Comparisons with Surgical Therapy

Although there are no randomized controlled trials that have compared endoscopic with surgical approaches for the management of high-grade dysplasia and superficial carcinoma, numerous observational studies suggest that long-term survival of the two techniques is comparable.[242,257-259] Studies extending over 5 years are available on EMR, photodynamic therapy, and a combination of the two showing long-term survival comparable to esophageal surgery for high-grade dysplasia or intramucosal adenocarcinoma and low rates of cancer-associated death. A population-based study of patients with early esophageal cancer found comparable long-term survival for patients managed with endoscopic therapy compared with patients treated with surgical resection.[258] Although the 5-year survival is comparable between the two treatment modalities, cancer develops during follow-up in approximately 6% to 12% of patients treated endoscopically.

Unresolved Issues in Endoscopic Therapy

There are many unresolved issues in ablation therapy. Assuming equal endoscopic skills, it is important to know which endoscopic therapy should be applied to a given patient. Should EMR be limited to focal lesions only? What is the length threshold for circumferential EMR? Who should receive thermal techniques, and what parameters should be used to determine which patient should get which combination techniques? What factors predict if a patient will respond to a given therapy? Possible variables include segment length, hiatal hernia size, adequacy of acid suppression, and biomarkers. One study to date has evaluated biomarkers to predict response to photodynamic therapy. Prasad and coworkers[260] found that p16 loss, detected by fluorescence in situ hybridization of cytology specimens obtained before photodynamic therapy for high-grade dysplasia or intramucosal carcinoma, predicted a lesser response to photodynamic therapy. A multivariate analysis by Pech and associates,[261] based on the long-term results of the Wiesbaden group's approach to patients with high-grade intraepithelial neoplasia and intramucosal adenocarcinoma with EMR with or without photodynamic therapy, identified the following as risk factors for disease recurrence after ablation therapy: long-segment Barrett's esophagus, multifocal neoplasia, piecemeal resection, and no ablative therapy of the residual Barrett's segment after a complete response by EMR.

Although early data with radiofrequency ablation are promising, it is difficult to conceive of any technique reliably eliminating all subsquamous intestinal metaplasia. Biomarker abnormalities persist in this subsquamous epithelium, and it is still unknown what degree of subsquamous columnar epithelium, if any, can be tolerated after ablation. Studies in a few patients with buried intestinal metaplasia after photodynamic therapy found that buried Barrett's epithelium had reduced crypt proliferation and near-normal DNA content compared with Barrett's epithelium before treatment, raising the question of the neoplastic potential of the buried Barrett's epithelium.[262] Better techniques of detecting buried columnar epithelium are needed.

Several reports suggest that the cardia behaves in unexpected and potentially undesirable ways after ablation therapy. Nodules with high-grade dysplasia or cancer may develop months to years after therapy.[263,264] The reason for this development is unknown. Although squamous epithelium may develop below the EG junction after ablation, it is unclear what the natural history of that metaplastic mucosa is.[265] Not only can problems develop at the cardia, but also techniques such as radiofrequency ablation are difficult to apply to the cardia, even with the focal probe, owing to positioning and the anatomic alterations in the setting of a large hiatal hernia.

As shown by the studies cited earlier for EMR, photodynamic therapy after EMR, and radiofrequency ablation, cancer may still develop in a small subset of these patients after endoscopic therapy. The emerging concept of EMR of visible lesions combined with either circumferential EMR or thermal injury treatment of the remaining at-risk mucosa is now taking hold.

Finally, despite the ready availability of various ablation techniques, it is difficult to justify a decision to perform ablation for all patients with Barrett's esophagus without dysplasia at this time for the following reasons: (1) Cancer risk for an individual patient is low, (2) the need for surveillance is unchanged, (3) all of the techniques involve considerable financial cost, and (4) adverse events still occur. In regard to any treatment of patients with nondysplastic Barrett's epithelium, even if one assumes a risk reduction of 50% for the development of cancer, from an estimated 0.50% per year to 0.25% per year, the number needed to treat to prevent 1 cancer in nondysplastic Barrett's epithelium would be approximately 400 patients.[266]

Conclusions and Future Trends

Barrett's esophagus is a complication of severe GERD and is associated with an increased risk of esophageal adenocarcinoma. Management of patients with Barrett's esophagus should continue to focus on relieving symptoms of GERD and carefully performed endoscopic surveillance at appropriate intervals. However, many questions remain unanswered about

Barrett's esophagus. What predisposes only a small subset of patients with GERD to develop Barrett's esophagus, and how does it develop? Is there a simple way to distinguish reliably between short-segment Barrett's esophagus and intestinal metaplasia of the cardia? How can pathologic consistency in interpretation of biopsy specimens from these patients be improved? Would screening GERD patients for Barrett's esophagus be an effective strategy? Would small-caliber endoscopes be accepted and effective? Could an alternative to endoscopy be developed? Would improvements in endoscopic technology make a difference in surveillance programs? Is there an alternative to current time-consuming endoscopic surveillance techniques? In particular, which biomarkers of increased risk would help stratify patients by individual risk? If biomarkers are validated, could testing be done at an affordable price? Finally, would any treatment—be it acid suppression, antireflux surgery, chemoprevention, or ablation—have any effect on the natural history of this disease? Answers to these and other questions are eagerly awaited.

References

The complete reference list is available online at www.expertconsult.com.

Endoscopic Treatment of Superficial Esophageal Cancers

Kenneth K. Wang

Video related to this chapter's topics can be found online at expertconsult.com.

Introduction

Endoscopic therapy of gastrointestinal (GI) neoplasms has been a goal of therapeutic endoscopists since the inception of the field. Initial techniques included argon plasma coagulation (APC) and thermal laser therapy. Technologic improvements in cancer staging have allowed endoscopists to determine tumor depth precisely and assess the risk of regional metastasis accurately, which allows endoscopic therapy to become a reality. In addition, techniques have been developed that permit resection of even greater amounts of mucosa, and endoscopic imaging techniques have been developed to assess the presence of early cancers with the potential to avoid the need for additional histologic confirmation. Finally, residual mucosa that could become neoplastic can be treated with ablative therapies that can be applied with less morbidity than previously. Endoscopic methods to treat neoplasia have become an important tool for the gastroenterologist with outcomes similar to open surgical techniques.

Biology of Early Esophageal Cancer

To treat esophageal cancer that most often develops in Barrett's esophagus in Western countries, it is important to develop an understanding of the biology of the problem. Barrett's esophagus is a very heterogeneous tissue with metaplastic epithelium that overlies generally altered subepithelial components such as activated fibroblasts in the mucosa and increased populations of lymphocytes in the submucosa. The literature regarding early esophageal carcinoma has primarily concerned the pathogenesis of squamous cell carcinoma, which previously was the predominant form of cancer in the United States and still is predominant in Asia and has clearly been associated with alcohol and tobacco usage. Most early esophageal cancers found in the United States at the present time are adenocarcinomas associated with Barrett's esophagus.

In contrast to Asia, where the high incidence of esophageal cancer has led to screening programs, esophageal cancer in the West has primarily been found when patients become symptomatic. Although it has been established that older white men with reflux symptoms are at greatest risk of esophageal adenocarcinoma and Barrett's esophagus, the high prevalence of Barrett's esophagus in patients without symptoms makes screening for this condition in only symptomatic patients problematic.[1,2] Surveillance endoscopy finds patients with earlier staged malignancies that are suitable for endoscopic therapies.[3]

Cancers related to Barrett's esophagus apparently arise from chronically inflamed areas of the mucosa. The mechanism of carcinogenesis seems to be related to inflammation producing increased levels of prostaglandin E_2, which is an inflammatory mediator that can cause increased cell proliferation.[4] Cell proliferation has been used as a marker of neoplasia and is an early event in cancer development. Increased cell proliferation drives the cell cycle, and progression to cancer in Barrett's esophagus usually involves the loss of cell cycle checkpoint gene products such as p16. The loss of p16 function through either promoter inactivation via hypermethylation or loss of heterozygosity occurs early in carcinogenesis and is found almost universally in dysplastic Barrett's mucosa.[5] This loss of cell cycle control leads to further acceleration of the cell cycle, which allows further genetic events to occur including loss of p53, which is well recognized to be an important tumor suppressor gene that is also involved in promoting apoptosis of cells that have accumulated genetic defects.[6] The loss of p53, which is important for elimination of cells with chromosomal abnormalities, and the increase in proliferation of cells caused by the loss of p16 lead to further chromosomal instability, which is manifested by the appearance of aneuploidy, or abnormal amounts of DNA.[7] These large-scale changes of chromosomal loss are related to the degree of histologic changes of dysplasia in the tissue with minimal DNA loss in nondysplastic tissue, moderate loss in low-grade dysplasia, and large degrees of loss in patients with high-grade dysplasia or cancer.

The important aspect of the biology of Barrett's esophagus to the endoscopist is that these genetic changes do not always correlate with histologic changes, especially when ablative therapies have been applied. Ablative therapy has the ability to decrease histologic changes of dysplasia, while allowing genetic abnormalities to persist.[8] These persistent genetic abnormalities over time lead to recurrence of dysplasia and cancer. These findings suggest that histologically benign Barrett's esophagus after ablative therapy may be precancerous, and long-term control of the neoplastic risk in Barrett's esophagus may involve elimination of any of the tissue with genetic abnormalities.

These findings were verified by data from a randomized prospective study of photodynamic therapy for Barrett's esophagus with high-grade dysplasia. In this study of 208 patients randomly assigned to either photodynamic therapy in combination with omeprazole or omeprazole alone, patients in whom complete elimination of Barrett's mucosa was achieved did not progress to cancer, whereas patients with any residual Barrett's mucosa did have a significant chance of developing cancer.[9] The complete elimination of the intestinal metaplasia may be difficult even with newer therapies such as radiofrequency ablation; in a randomized trial of patients with low-grade and high-grade dysplasia, the dysplasia could be eliminated in greater than 90% of patients, but the intestinal metaplasia remained in 77%.[10]

Staging of Early Esophageal Cancer

Endoscopic treatment of early esophageal cancer must involve careful and accurate staging of the malignancy. Previously, early esophageal cancer was primarily defined endoscopically on the basis of size. An example of an early cancer in Barrett's esophagus is shown in **Fig. 27.1**. Cancers that were 2 cm or less in diameter were generally thought to be early cancers.[11] This definition was inaccurate because visualization of local lymph nodes and assessment of the depth of tumor invasion were impossible without surgical resection during this time period. However, surgical resections have shown physicians that early mucosally based cancers above the muscularis mucosae are rarely associated with metastatic disease. In a survey of European centers that performed 253 esophagectomies for early squamous cell carcinomas, it was found that patients with disease confined to the epithelium had a survival rate of 92.8%.[12] With penetration into the submucosa, the 5-year survival rate decreased to 72.8%. The overall mortality rate for esophagectomy for early cancers in this series was

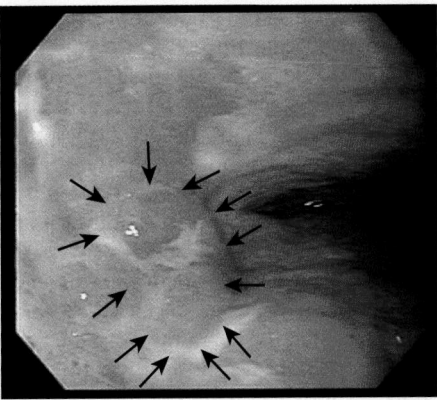

Fig. 27.1 Endoscopic view of early esophageal cancer is outlined by *arrows* in the setting of chronically inflamed mucosa in Barrett's esophagus.

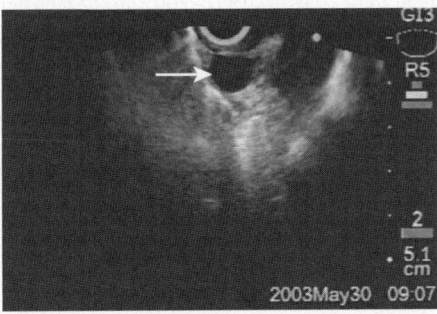

Fig. 27.2 Endoscopic ultrasound (EUS) (linear array instrument) shows suspicious periesophageal lymph node *(arrow)* located between the pleural reflection on the left and the aorta on the right. The lymph node is hypoechoic and rounded, both of which are features of a malignant node.

9.1%. Similar results for squamous cell carcinomas were reported from Japan, where there was increased chance of metastasis if squamous cell carcinoma was found to penetrate beyond the muscularis mucosae.[13]

The advent of endoscopic ultrasound (EUS) has affected the need for surgical resection to define the depth of cancer invasion accurately. EUS can be performed with either dedicated echoendoscopes or high-frequency ultrasound probes. The echoendoscopes allow the endoscopist to visualize at 7.5- to 12-MHz frequencies, which permits examination of the periesophageal lymph nodes (N1 stage), celiac lymph nodes (M1a stage), nodes of the lesser curve of the stomach (N1 stage), most of the liver (M1b stage), and pleural or vascular involvement (T4 stage) by the tumor. An example of a periesophageal lymph node on EUS is shown in **Fig. 27.2**. A lymph node is suspicious on EUS if it is hypoechoic, rounded, in proximity to the tumor, and more than 1 cm in diameter. If suspicious lymph nodes are found, they should be sampled by fine needle aspiration performed using a linear array instrument.

For mucosally based lesions, ultrasound probes are more desirable because they can image at 20 to 30 MHz allowing the endoscopist to image at the resolution needed to resolve the muscularis mucosae to a greater extent. In addition, the use of probes allows visualization using water filling the esophagus, which is necessary to view small mucosal cancers without the artifact caused by the compression by a balloon that is traditionally used with echoendoscopes. Ultrasound probes cannot image deep into the tissue to visualize lymph nodes, however, so to stage an early cancer accurately, both probes and echoendoscopes are needed.[14] Despite the use of careful ultrasound examination, lymph nodes can be missed or inaccessible because of Barrett's mucosa that is in the field of view. It is believed that false-positive findings can be caused by contamination with epithelial cells.[15]

Small case series have been performed of patients with Barrett's esophagus and early cancers staged by EUS before esophagectomy. At one center, the technique was 100% sensitive for detection of submucosal invasion but was only 90% specific for invasion in a group of 22 patients.[16] Inflammatory changes are virtually impossible to differentiate from early cancer invasion by EUS techniques. Overall, EUS seems to have a tendency to overstage the depth of tumor invasion. A retrospective review of the experience of a single center with EUS staging of esophageal cancer from 1991–2001 in 222 patients found that the accuracy of EUS in tumor staging was only 54%, and the accuracy of EUS in lymph node staging was 65%.[17] These results did not seem to be related to a "learning curve" in EUS interpretation because the accuracy in the first half of the time period studied was similar to the accuracy in the second half of the study period. More recent publications emphasize that although EUS may not be as accurate as previously hoped in staging, the information provided from having a negative evaluation for lymph nodes or for resectability was nonetheless valuable.[14]

Endoscopic mucosal resection (EMR) has been used to help define the depth of cancer penetration and as a primary treatment for early cancer in Barrett's esophagus. EMR involves the use of a friction fitted cap that attaches to the tip of a standard endoscope. This technique was pioneered in Japan, where EMR has become the standard of care for early mucosal esophageal cancers. A survey of more than 145 Japanese hospitals found that 76% used EMR for the treatment of early esophageal cancers.[18]

The cap technique is the predominant technique used in the United States because of its commercial availability. The cap is available in the two styles shown in **Fig. 27.3**; one is completely level, whereas the other has the lip of the cap at an oblique angle. The cap also varies in terms of the consistency of the material from which it is made. Generally, hard plastic caps are favored when there is a need to try to suction more scarred tissue, whereas soft caps are more useful when passing the caps through the upper pharynx. The oblique cap is favored in resection of larger pieces of tissue, whereas the straight cap seems to be more favored when precision is required in the amount of tissue necessary for resection.

The technique of EMR is performed in a similar fashion. For early esophageal cancers, it is critical that the endoscopist is able to obtain adequate lifting of the lesion to be removed using an injection of a saline-epinephrine solution. Depending on the visibility of the lesion, the borders may need to be marked using a cautery device such as a multipolar coagulator before injection to ensure that the area to be removed can be visualized after injection. The area of carcinoma has usually been previously established by biopsy, and the area is lifted by positioning an injection needle proximal to the lesion. Generally, it is not advisable to inject into the lesion because it is theoretically possible to disseminate cancer cells into the submucosa. The sequence of an injection with adequate lifting of the target lesion is shown in **Fig. 27.4**.

Once the target cancer is lifted by the injection, the lesion should be removed with mucosal resection. If removal is not accomplished within a few hours, inflammation induced by the injection may cause the cancer to become adherent to the

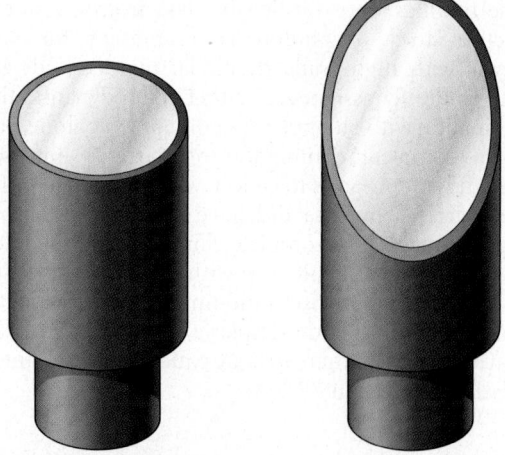

Fig. 27.3 Endoscopic mucosal resection (EMR) cap comes in a straight resection style *(left)* and an angled resection tip *(right)*.

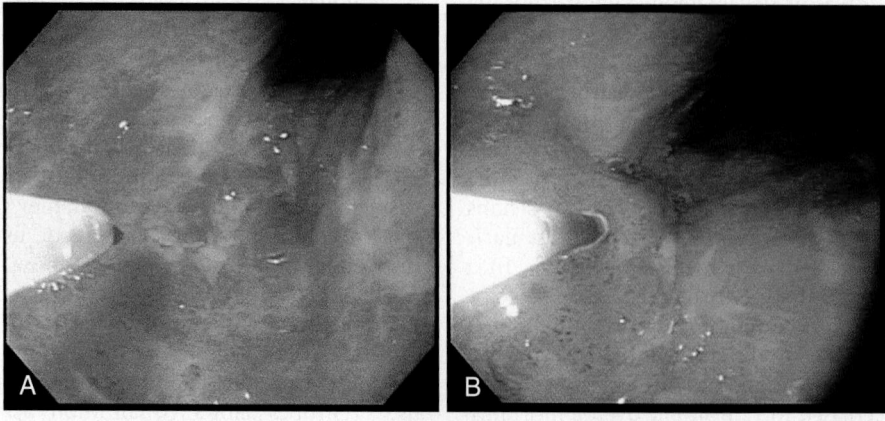

Fig. 27.4 A, Injection needle poised over the target mucosa. **B,** Injection in process with the lifting of the mucosa with the fluid.

submucosa or muscularis propria, which would make resection difficult if not impossible. The mucosal resection component of this technique is similar to a standard polypectomy except that suction is needed to create the pseudopolyp for mucosal removal. The endoscope with the resection cap attached is advanced into the stomach. It is generally recommended that the snare be positioned in the antrum of the stomach because the mucosa there is smoother and allows easier deflection of the snare around the diameter of the cap. Individuals experienced in this technique can position the snare using mucosa from the esophagus or proximal stomach, although this can be challenging.

The sequence of positioning a snare around the lip of a mucosal resection cap is shown in **Fig. 27.5**. This is often the most difficult portion of the mucosal resection because if the snare is not properly formed, suctioning the tissue into the cap can result in dislodgment of the snare and improper tissue resection. In addition, the snare is easily deformed and can be twisted during the process of forming the loop around the lip of the resection cap resulting in the need for a new crescent snare. When the snare is positioned, it is important that the technician assisting with the snare not move it because even slight disruptions in the position of the snare can cause it to dislodge.

The tissue resection is completed by suctioning the tissue into the cap as shown in **Fig. 27.6**. To accomplish a wider resection, more tissue must be suctioned into the cap similar to what is done in variceal band ligation. The submucosa is often resected with the mucosa during EMR. When sufficient tissue is suctioned into the cap, the snare is closed, and cautery is applied until the tissue is transected. This process takes several more seconds than with polypectomy because the amount of tissue to be resected is much greater. The average diameter of resected mucosa is about 1 cm when assessed by the pathologist, and the defect left behind by the resection is often about 2 to 3 cm in diameter. The resection and the residual ulcer are also shown in **Fig. 27.6**. Because tumors are often larger than the size of a single EMR, a second resection can be performed directly adjacent to the first resection; care must be taken not to suction the muscularis propria exposed at the site of the first resection into the cap. Multiple resections in the same area should be attempted only by endoscopists familiar with the mucosal resection technique.

EMR can be used for diagnosis of unusual-appearing lesions within Barrett's esophagus. In our experience, regions of nodularity or mucosal irregularity have a significantly higher incidence of carcinoma being present. A study of agreement among expert pathologists on distinguishing intramu-

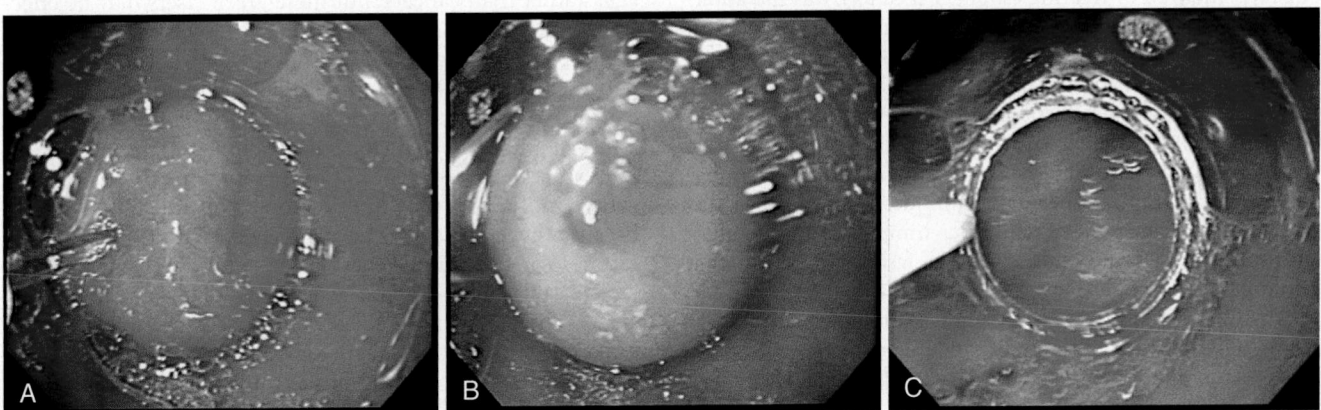

Fig. 27.5 A, The snare is carefully advanced out while the mucosa is suctioned into the cap. The mucosa is used to deflect a point on the tip of the snare toward the lip of the resection cap. **B,** Once the snare is deflected to the side of the cap and the point of the snare is safely embedded onto the lip of the cap, the snare can be advanced allowing the loop to be formed around the lip of the cap. **C,** The snare is properly positioned around the lip of the mucosal resection cap.

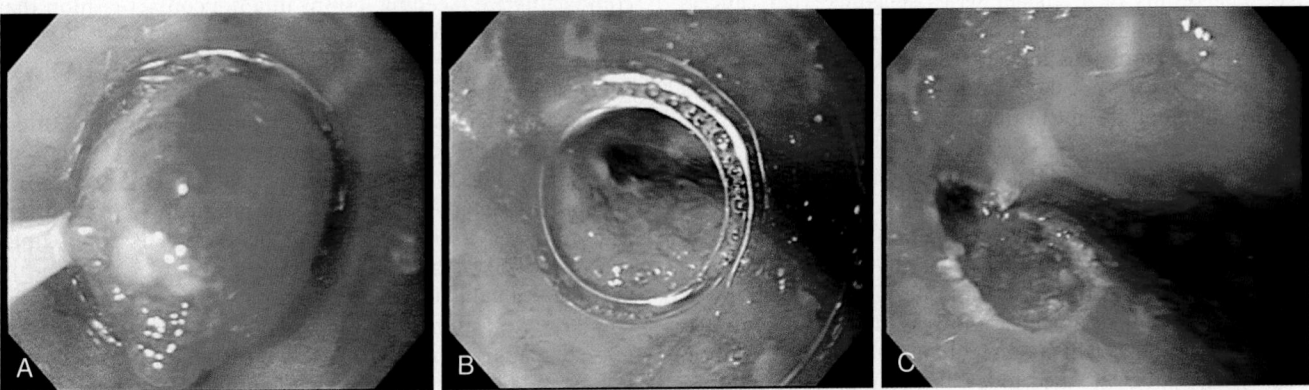

Fig. 27.6 A, The targeted cancer is suctioned into the cap, and the snare is closed. **B,** The defect created by the endoscopic mucosal resection (EMR) is shown. There is obvious residual cancer, calling for a second resection adjacent to the first resection. **C,** A second EMR is performed next to the first and removes the residual tumor.

cosal carcinoma versus high-grade dysplasia found only moderate agreement with a κ score of less than .6 even when the pathologists could agree to standard definitions.[19] It was thought that limited tissue from pinch biopsies often obscured the pathologist's ability to determine invasion. Using EMR, our group found that the diagnosis of adenocarcinoma increased by 40% in a group of 25 patients with Barrett's esophagus because EMR furnishes larger specimens.[20] EMR is also an excellent tool for staging esophageal carcinoma as has been shown in Japan.[21] It has been established that if the tumor can be found to be m1 or m2 stage (confined to the lamina propria), the tumor can be safely resected with only rare incidence of metastasis. Metastasis was found in 6% of patients who had cancers that penetrated to the muscularis mucosae or superficially into the submucosa. The technique of EMR gives the endoscopist similar tools to evaluate cancer curability as surgeons have had in the past—the ability to obtain histology and pathologic depth of staging.

Methods of Endoscopic Treatment of Esophageal Cancer

Thermal Lasers

An early method of treating esophageal cancer was the application of thermal energy. These techniques originated from therapies developed for palliation of esophageal cancer, which involved the application of laser or intensive thermal energy to create a new lumen through obstructing cancers. Because 80% to 90% of esophageal cancers manifest as obstructive disease, this was naturally the starting point of most esophageal cancer therapies. Thermal techniques were ideal for this application because they could offer immediate tumor ablation and allowed the endoscopist to fashion a lumen that could pass food easily. However, laser therapies were found to be costly and required several applications to achieve long-term palliation in contrast to expandable metal stents.[22]

Laser therapy was used as primary treatment of superficial cancers of the esophagus and stomach. The choice of lasers has varied, with the initial choice being neodymium:yttrium-aluminum-garnet (Nd:YAG), which produces infrared laser light (1063 nm) that can penetrate 2 cm through tissue. This therapy was used in the 1980s with relative success against predominately superficial squamous cell esophageal carcinomas. The results of a smaller series suggested that cancers could be eliminated in 73% of 33 patients with superficial cancers of the esophagus and gastric cardia with most patients followed for at least 2 years.[23] The treatment could be repeated 6 times, although the mean frequency of retreatment was 2.6 times.

The problem with this type of therapy was that the results often depended on the endoscopist's skill and experience with the laser. In addition, the determination of the superficial nature of the tumor was solely based on the endoscopic appearance. During this early time period, the methods of assessing depth of tumor invasion were limited to computed tomography scans, which were of much poorer resolution than what can be obtained today. In addition, assessment of cure was limited to biopsies of the treated sites because assessment of regional lymph nodes and evidence of submucosal disease was impossible without surgical resection.

More recent studies using Nd:YAG laser therapy in combination with multipolar coagulation have involved very small numbers of patients. One study enrolled only six patients over 7 years and found that the treatment failed in one patient and left residual Barrett's mucosa in three others.[24] Three Nd:YAG sessions and three multipolar coagulation treatment sessions were required on average to treat each patient. Although this form of therapy could be effective, it requires multiple endoscopic treatment sessions and can fail. One case report in the literature suggests that with Nd:YAG therapy, failure could occur underneath normal-appearing squamous tissue and may be difficult to detect.[25]

Other laser therapies that have been employed to treat superficial cancers include potassium titanyl phosphate:yttrium-aluminum-garnet (KTP:YAG) and argon lasers because they have a more limited depth of penetration than Nd:YAG lasers. These lasers all operate in the visible green light region (532 nm) spectrum and penetrate tissue to a depth of only about 2 mm. These lasers have been advocated for the treatment of vascular lesions because of their limited depth of penetration and their intense absorption by hemoglobin. Several more recent series have reported that these lasers can be used to treat Barrett's esophagus because they offer the safety of superficial therapy. These lasers have been used more for ablation of dysplastic lesions in Barrett's esophagus rather than cancers, but these green lasers may be effective for some very superficial cancers. One case series found that KTP:YAG laser was able to destroy early cancers in two patients, although this required multiple treatments and had evidence of intestinal epithelium under squamous mucosa in 2 in 10 patients treated (for Barrett's mucosa).[26]

Despite these reports of laser therapy for early esophageal cancer, most endoscopy units no longer operate thermal lasers because their indications have largely been replaced by newer technologies. The use of thermal lasers for dysphagia has been largely supplanted by the availability of expandable metal stents. The use of thermal lasers for vascular lesions has been replaced by multipolar coagulation and APC. It is unlikely that thermal lasers will be used in the future for the treatment of superficial cancers because their availability and expertise level is decreasing in the GI endoscopy community.

Argon Plasma Coagulation

APC was originally developed as a hemostatic device that could cauterize bleeding lesions in a noncontact fashion that were awkward to reach with traditional probes. APC has the ability to treat superficially and has been thought to represent decreased risks of perforation. Mucosal ablative therapy for Barrett's esophagus has been investigated by several investigators who reported good to excellent results.[27–35] The technique is shown in **Fig. 27.7**. The primary goal of APC is to apply a current to the target lesion without producing a perforation. The argon gas is released under pressure. The endoscopist must be vigilant against allowing the tip of the probe to become embedded into the mucosa during treatment; this could result in submucosa air or, worse, a perforation. For this reason, coagulation performed with the argon plasma coagulator should be done only while the probe is being withdrawn toward the endoscope; this should ensure that the tip of the probe is not embedded in the mucosa. Settings for treating adenocarcinoma should be in the higher power ranges; 80 to

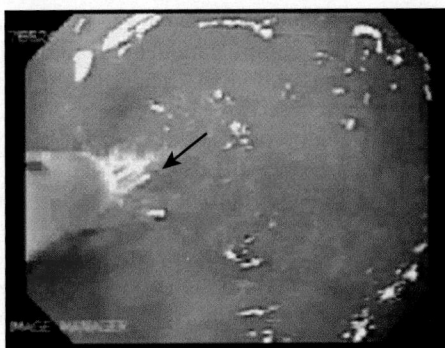

Fig. 27.7 Argon plasma coagulation (APC) is used to cauterize the mucosa by conduction of the electrical charge *(arrow)* along a stream of ionized argon gas. The current can reach areas that are not directly in line with the argon probe.

90 W has been cited in the literature. Higher output powers seem to be associated with improved outcomes in Barrett's esophagus with high-grade dysplasia, although complications such as perforation and strictures are also seen at these dosages.[33,36,37]

Treatment of intraepithelial carcinoma in Barrett's esophagus has been reported in a limited series of patients. In one series of only three intraepithelial cancers, treatment with APC was ineffective and resulted in invasive disease.[37] This cancer also failed treatment with subsequent photodynamic therapy. Similar results were observed in another small series of three patients with early esophageal cancers who were treated with APC, with one recurrence noted that was subsequently treated with photodynamic therapy.[38] In the Asian literature, early squamous cell carcinomas and high-grade dysplasia were treated with the APC with good results.[39,40] In one series, 29 patients with early squamous carcinomas and 42 patients with high-grade dysplasia were first treated with EMR with any residual treated with APC.[40] The early results seem promising with only three of the cancers (10%) found to recur after 4 months. Esophageal strictures were found in four of the cases after EMR of most of the diameter of the esophagus. Overall, it seems that although APC is well tolerated with few described complications, its efficacy in elimination of early esophageal cancer is limited with significant (33%) failure rates in small numbers of Barrett's esophagus–related cancers and lower failure rates (10%) in superficial squamous cell carcinomas. This finding is not surprising given the decreased depth of injury associated with this treatment.

Endoscopic Mucosal Resection for Early Cancers

Since its inception in Japan, EMR has been used to treat early esophageal and gastric cancers.[41] The technique was performed by Japanese surgeons who had excellent endoscopic skills and anatomic understanding of cancer surgery. Initial resections were performed with an overtube that was used to anchor tissue. A standard endoscope was placed within the lumen of the overtube and used to remove the tissue with a snare from the endoscope or one that was preformed around the overtube. The large ulcers that these procedures produced were worrisome, but these ulcers all were found to heal within 2 months.[42] The most commonly used of these devices was the

Makuuchi tube, which had been used in 152 cases of superficial esophageal cancer in 1992.[43] These pioneers of mucosal resection established that vascular invasion or metastasis was extremely rare when cancers were either intraepithelial or confined to the upper two-thirds of the mucosa. Only when cancers penetrated into the bottom one-third of the mucosa did vascular invasion or lymph nodes become apparent in 25% of the patients. In their hands, patients with intraepithelial disease had 5-year survivals approaching 100%. However, once the cancers penetrated into the submucosa, the 5-year survival rate decreased to about 55% to 59%.

Initially, mucosal resection was recommended only for esophageal cancers that were less than 2 cm in size and occupied less than one-third of the circumference of the esophagus in patients who were not ideal surgical candidates.[44] In one study that correlated the lymph node metastasis to depth of cancer invasion, the presence of lymph node metastasis was found to be zero if the lesion was confined to the mucosa, 10% if the muscularis mucosae became invaded, and 43% if the submucosa was invaded.[45] Over time, recommendations concerning treatment of early esophageal cancers were altered because about one-quarter of all esophageal cancers were classified as early stage owing to intensive screening programs.[46] By the late 1990s, a survey of Japanese institutions found that EMR was favored as the treatment of choice for all esophageal cancers confined to the upper two-thirds of the mucosa.[47] All patients with mucosally confined disease survived, but disease that penetrated to the submucosa had a significantly worse prognosis than disease that remained mucosal.

EMR techniques in the United States are similar to the above-described techniques. There are other methods of performing EMR, such as using a two-channeled therapeutic endoscope. One channel is used to place a snare around the lesion, and a forceps is passed through the other channel to grasp the lesion and tent it toward the endoscope; this positions the tissue within the snare for removal. In addition, another technique that is simple to use is an endoscopic variceal band ligator that can create a pseudopolyp. The lesion is lifted with a saline and epinephrine solution as with the other techniques followed by banding of the lesion with a variceal band ligation kit. The band ligator creates a pseudopolyp that can be removed with a small snare. Although this is a simple technique, multiple esophageal intubations are required to accomplish all of the steps, and the cost of the variceal ligation device is typically more than that of the mucosal resection caps discussed earlier. In addition, the variceal band technique requires the snare to be performed as soon as possible after placement of the band because if there is a large amount of mucosa present, the band starts to slip and fall off of the mucosa. In contrast to a varix, there is no vein for the band to constrict, so depending on the density of the tissue, the band may not stay on the lesion at all. All of these techniques are designed to elevate a region of relatively flat mucosa. No specific technique has been established to be better than any other in terms of tissue removal, although the larger sized mucosal resection caps seem to resect larger pieces of tissue.

The results of using EMR for the treatment of adenocarcinoma within Barrett's esophagus have been limited to a few series. In most cases, EMR is used as a staging or treatment technique, and additional therapy is applied to remove the remainder of the dysplastic tissue. In a large retrospective comparison study, EMR combined with photodynamic therapy was compared with surgical treatment in a series in 178 patients with T1a cancers. Cumulative survival in the endoscopically treated patients was 17% versus 20% in the surgical patients.[48] Cancer-related deaths occurred in both groups (<2%). In a series from Germany, 100 patients with early esophageal adenocarcinoma were managed with EMR with a 99% local response rate but with an 11% rate of metachronous or recurrent cancer rate.[49] It has been found that endoscopically favorable lesions are lesions that are polypoid, elevated, or flat, which are characteristics that occur in most patients.[50] The results of these series have led to recommendations about which lesions can be approached with EMR (**Table 27.1**).

Endoscopic Submucosal Dissection

Endoscopic submucosal dissection has been popularized in Asia as a method for complete excision of neoplastic lesions. A disadvantage of EMR has been the presence of neoplastic tissue remaining at the margins of resection, which generally indicates that neoplastic tissue remains in the tissue despite the use of cautery.[51] These findings have led to an attempt to perform en bloc resections using endoscopic mucosal dissection techniques to try to define areas of tissue that require large resections. In particular in Japan, large superficial gastric cancers have been approached in this fashion.[52] Retrospective studies comparing EMR with endoscopic submucosal dissection in terms of esophageal cancer have found that endoscopic submucosal dissection increases the ability to cure early cancer from 71% to 97% in squamous cell carcinoma.[53] This difference was not apparent if the cancers were less than 1.5 cm in diameter, which is probably the limit of resection using EMR cap techniques. Similar findings have been described with gastric cancers approached with either EMR or endoscopic submucosal dissection with 1.5 cm being the a priori cutoff between the two techniques with similar complications and success rates of cancer removal.[54] Even cancers of the esophagogastric junction can be resected with reasonable success rates using these techniques, although this resection is more technically difficult.[55]

More recent studies have compared EMR and endoscopic submucosal dissection in animal models and found that endoscopic submucosal dissection, particularly with a water jet assistance, can achieve resection faster than traditional EMR.[56] The first steps in endoscopic submucosal dissection are to mark the area to be resected, usually by using cautery, to ensure that the complete lesion and at least a 3-mm margin are resected (**Fig. 27.8**).

A submucosal bleb is formed similar to with EMR except that usually a solution that is designed to persist is used, such as sodium carboxymethylcellulose, sodium hydroxypropyl methylcellulose, sodium hyaluronate, hypertonic dextrose solution, hypertonic saline, glycerol, or fibrinogen. The goal is to allow dissection in the submucosal plane, which can be very difficult depending on the technique used. The devices available for endoscopic submucosal dissection vary greatly, and it would not be prudent for any endoscopist to master all of these. However, several of these "knives" can be applied by a skilled endoscopist with appropriate training so long as certain principles are followed. Japanese experts perform the entire dissection with a single knife. However, the knives vary in their applicability, and some are best suited for certain portions of the procedure (**Fig. 27.9**).

The lesions are generally circumscribed with a knife to free the lesion completely from the rest of the normal mucosa. Sharp-edged knives, such as the needle knife or IT knife, have an advantage to allow easier application through the tissue. The cut is made carefully to avoid penetrating the entire wall, and once the defect is made, knives similar to the IT knife have an advantage by not having a sharp tip to penetrate through the muscularis layer. The submucosal dissection is performed using a small dissection cap to lift the mucosa and cut the fibrous tissue that is underneath. This is the most challenging portion of the dissection and requires careful control. The

Table 27.1 Characteristics of Esophageal Cancers Amenable to Endoscopic Mucosal Resection	
Characteristic	**Favorable Outcome**
Size	<2 cm
Depth of penetration	No penetration of muscularis mucosa
Grade of cancer	Well-differentiated cancer
Appearance	Polypoid, elevated, or flat

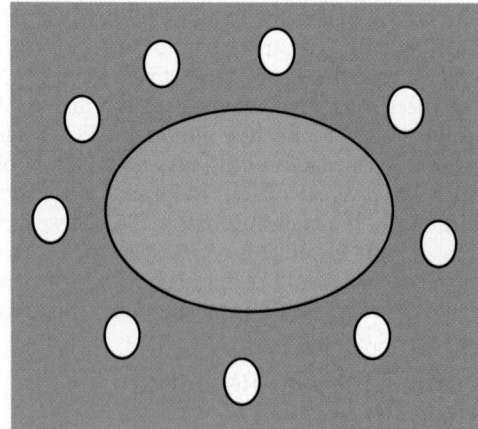

Fig. 27.8 The area of the tumor is surrounded by cautery marks approximately 3 mm from the nearest visible area of tumor.

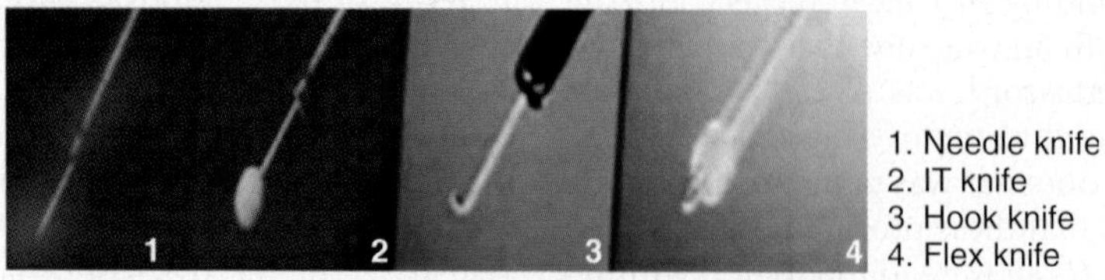

1. Needle knife
2. IT knife
3. Hook knife
4. Flex knife

Fig. 27.9 Endoscopic submucosal dissection devices. These devices are able to resect tissue and have been approved in the United States.

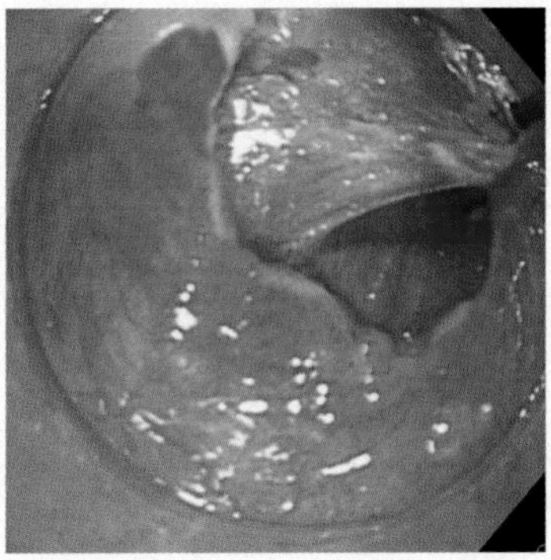

Fig. 27.10 Hook knife that has been used to retract a large bundle of fibrous tissue that now can be separated using a cautery current.

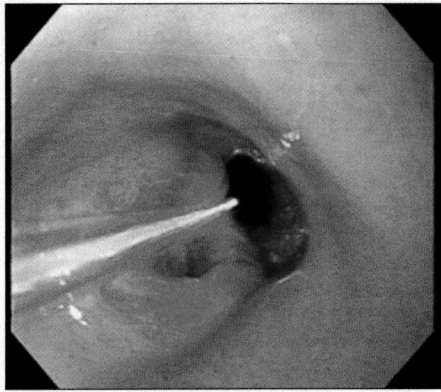

Fig. 27.11 The cylindrical diffusing fiber is placed on an ulcerated cancer in the esophagus. Based on its appearance, this type of tumor would not respond well to mucosal resection.

hook knife has an advantage because the knife can "hook" the fibrous tissue from underneath the mucosa, and the cutting can be done more in the endoscopic field of vision (**Fig. 27.10**). The dissection is a substantial undertaking, although a typical lesion can be removed in 1 to 2 hours by an experienced endoscopist.

Photodynamic Therapy for Early Esophageal Cancer

Photodynamic therapy has been investigated since its origins in 1961 as a treatment for cancer.[57] The therapy has traditionally involved the use of a combination of a drug termed a photosensitizer and light of a specific wavelength that is required to activate the drug. The typical practice is to administer the drug days or hours before light delivery to allow the photosensitizer to concentrate into the neoplastic tissue. Light from a laser is applied to the mucosa, which causes general tissue destruction and cell death.

Current photosensitizers are derivatives of porphyrin compounds that are generally given intravenously. The normal tissue generally excretes the photosensitizer sooner than the neoplastic tissue; this is the reason that the current commercially available photosensitizer, porfimer sodium (Photofrin II) is given 48 hours before photoradiation. These photosensitizers can be activated by red light of 630 nm wavelength. Other wavelengths of light can activate these porphyrin compounds, but red light is selected because it can penetrate the tissue significantly better than shorter wavelengths and can avoid absorption by hemoglobin. Lasers generally deliver the light because it is necessary to channel the light energy through an endoscope. The laser light must be "coupled" into a fiber, which requires the coherence and concentration of laser light sources to accomplish. Older laser systems used dye lasers, which basically took light of a short wavelength (e.g., an argon laser [532 nm]) and converted it into the longer red light. These systems are still available and can produce powers of 7 W. Because the dye lasers required combining two laser systems, there were problems with laser alignment and in the energy requirements of these laser systems. They required special electrical outlets and water cooling systems. Newer solid state diode lasers can be operated on ordinary room current and are air cooled. They are much smaller, which makes their transport much simpler. The current system incorporates a power output meter into the system so that the

laser can tune its output to what is needed rather than require the endoscopist to calibrate the system.

Photoradiation is usually performed by placing an optical fiber through the biopsy channel of the endoscope. The tip of this optical fiber has a cylindrical diffusing fiber that can be placed in the lumen of the esophagus. Generally, in the case of an early tumor, the fiber is pressed against the tumor as shown in **Fig. 27.11**. Treatment parameters for photodynamic therapy for Barrett's esophagus with a cancer using porfimer sodium involve a drug dosage of 2 mg/kg body weight. The drug is given 48 hours before photodynamic therapy. Red light is delivered through a diffusing fiber at a power output of 400 mW/cm fiber for a total energy of around 300 J/cm fiber. If there is no endoscopically apparent disease and mucosal resection has completely removed the lesion, a smaller dose of light such as 200 J/cm fiber can be used to treat the remaining Barrett's mucosa.

Patients can experience numerous complications. After injection of the drug, cutaneous photosensitivity can occur and persist for 30 to 90 days. After photoradiation, patients can experience severe chest pain within 24 hours. This pain can require narcotic administration to achieve pain relief. Transdermal administration of narcotics usually is preferred because patients have odynophagia from the therapy. Dehydration occurs because of the inability to obtain adequate fluid intake and may require intravenous fluids to resolve. Nausea occurs in the first 1 to 3 days after photoradiation and can require administration of antiemetics. Rare side effects include injury of organs that are located near the esophagus, resulting in atrial fibrillation or pleural effusions.[58,59] Esophageal strictures are a major problem because they occur in about one-third of patients treated. These strictures are often quite fibrotic and require multiple dilations to large diameters to resolve the constriction.

Results of photodynamic therapy for the treatment of esophageal cancer are shown in **Table 27.2**.[11,59–66] The overall results are quite impressive if only the early cancers are considered. Significant (23%) 5-year survivals were reported in patients who had advanced stage esophageal cancer. Most of the series involved similar photosensitizers, such as hematoporphyrin derivative or porfimer sodium II, although a few involved temoporfin, which is unavailable in the United States and is believed to have a deeper depth of penetration than porfimer

Table 27.2 Results of Photodynamic Therapy for Esophageal Cancer

Reference	No. Patients	Tumor Type	Tumor Stage	Drug	Success
Jin et al[60]	207	Cardia tumors (59%)	All advanced	HpD	23% 5-yr survival
Sibille et al[11]	123	Squamous cell carcinoma (85%); adenocarcinoma (15%)	"Early"	HpD	74% 5-yr disease-free survival
McCaughan et al[61]	77	Adenocarcinoma and squamous cell carcinoma	Stage I-IV	Porfimer sodium (Photofrin II)	Stage I patients, 62% 5-yr survival
Grosjean et al[62]	31	Squamous cell carcinomas	87% microscopic cancer	Temoporfin	83% microscopic cancers complete response at 15 mo
Gossner et al[63]	22	Adenocarcinoma	T1 and T2	ALA	77% complete response at 9 mo
Tan et al[64]	12	Adenocarcinoma	2 T0; 10 T1-2	ALA	17%
Panjehpour et al[65]	13	Adenocarcinoma	12 T1; 1 T2	Porfimer sodium	77%
Pacifico and Wang[66]	23	Adenocarcinoma	23 T0-T1	HpD and porfimer sodium	84%
Wolfsen et al[59]	14	Adenocarcinoma	T0-T1	Porfimer sodium	93%

ALA, aminolevulinic acid; HpD, hematoporphyrin derivative.

sodium. Among the series using porphyrin compounds, the survival rates range from 62% to 93% with a median response of about 75%. An important factor illustrated best by the study by Sibille and colleagues[11] is that although disease-free survival was excellent, overall survival over 5 years was only 25%, indicating that these are medically ill patients who have severe comorbidities. These results are very good considering that most of the series contain patients with more invasive disease with penetration of the submucosa and even the muscularis propria. Complications that have been reported in these series are similar to the complications discussed earlier with strictures occurring in about one-third of the patients.

These results indicate that endoscopic therapy for early cancers may be a viable alternative to traditional esophagectomy. An algorithm for consideration when evaluating patients with esophageal cancer is shown in **Fig. 27.12**. If a patient has early stage cancer, endoscopic therapy should be considered as a possible option.

The options for endoscopic treatment for early esophageal cancer consist primarily of using EMR alone or in combination with a mucosal ablative therapy such as photodynamic therapy or a thermal ablative technique such as radiofrequency ablation. Photodynamic therapy alone seems to have a reasonable number of reports regarding efficacy, but the use of EMR would decrease the uncertainty about staging this tumor. The decision whether endoscopic therapy is a viable alternative to surgical treatment depends on further studies in which these modalities are prospectively studied. The benefit of surgical cure versus the risk of surgical complications would need to be weighed.

Combinational Therapy

Endoscopic therapy of superficial neoplasms currently involves the use of multiple treatment modalities. One major issue is

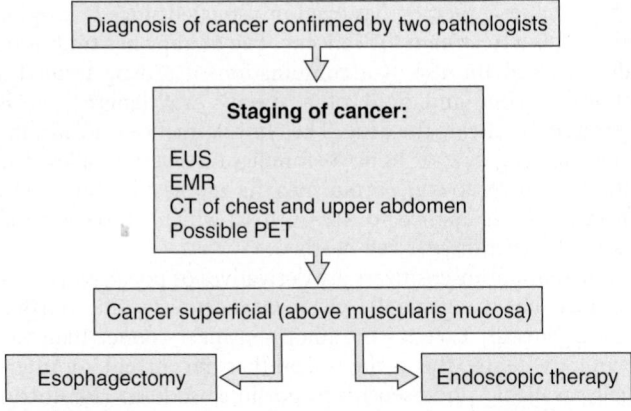

Fig. 27.12 Management of early esophageal cancer. CT, computed tomography; EMR, endoscopic mucosal resection; EUS, endoscopic ultrasound; PET, positron emission tomography.

the treatment of the primary lesion and careful staging regarding depth of penetration. This staging is usually done using an EMR or submucosal dissection technique depending on the size of the lesion. There is a clinical problem that the removal of a lesion is done without actually knowing if the depth of penetration precludes endoscopic treatment. Generally, lesions that penetrate deeply cannot be separated from the submucosa and cannot be lifted with injection for removal. Lesions that penetrate into the submucosa on EUS and can still be lifted and removed may be downstaged by histology. Performance of an EMR for depth staging would preclude an endoscopic submucosal dissection at a later point because of all the scarring produced. If the lesion is resected but there is still residual tumor present at the margins, another procedure is indicated after allowing for the area to heal, and another resection can be performed at the edge of a prior mucosal resection. Endoscopic submucosal dissection is difficult under these circumstances because the mucosal dissection is much more difficult.

If the resection is complete, the cancer should be inspected for depth of invasion, and cancers that penetrate beyond the muscularis mucosae should be considered for some other type of therapy. Cancers that infiltrate a duplicated muscularis mucosae are at increased risk of metastasis.[67] However, cancers that infiltrate the lymphovascular system also seem to be at a high risk of metastasis if they already invade the submucosa.[68]

Once the primary tumor is removed, a decision must be made about elimination of any preneoplastic tissue present. This decision is usually determined by the overall health of the patient, the anticipated survival, and the ability of the patient to tolerate ablation. There is a concern that techniques such as EMR and endoscopic submucosal dissection increase risk of stricture formation after ablative therapy, although this has not been shown in a prospective fashion. In techniques such as radiofrequency ablation, the sizing balloon used to determine the treatment balloon size can be difficult to use because there is some fibrosis within the tissue. This difficulty can be addressed by direct observation of the sizing balloon to ensure there is no slippage or by downsizing the balloon to the next smaller size.

Complete elimination of all preneoplastic mucosa can be difficult in situations such as squamous cell carcinomas. In these cases, careful observation and elimination of new neoplastic lesions is probably needed. Overall success of endoscopic therapies is excellent, and more recent data show that endoscopic therapy compares favorably with surgical therapy in terms of survival in adenocarcinoma in Barrett's esophagus, although there is a 12% recurrence rate.[48] The success of endoscopic therapy in early squamous cell carcinoma is also excellent.

Acknowledgments

The author would like to acknowledge the support of NIH grants CA85992-01 and R01CA097048-01.

References

The complete reference list is available online at www.expertconsult.com.

Chapter 28

Endoscopic Palliation of Malignant Dysphagia and Esophageal Fistulas

Marjolein Y. V. Homs and Peter D. Siersema

Video related to this chapter's topics can be found online at expertconsult.com.

Introduction

Annually, cancer of the esophagus and gastroesophageal junction (GEJ) is diagnosed worldwide in more than 500,000 patients, which makes it the eighth most common malignancy and sixth most common cause of cancer mortality.[1] It is difficult to determine the true incidence because cancer of the GEJ is classified sometimes as gastric cancer and sometimes as esophageal cancer. In clinical practice, this distinction is unimportant because the curative and palliative options for treatment are the same for both adenocarcinoma of the esophagus and adenocarcinoma of the GEJ.

Overall, cancer of the esophagus and GEJ has a poor prognosis with a 5-year survival rate of less than 20% in the Western world.[2] This poor prognosis is at least partly due to the fact that more than 50% of patients with carcinoma of the esophagus or GEJ already have inoperable disease at presentation.[3] Most of these patients require palliative treatment to relieve progressive dysphagia or to treat associated problems such as the presence of a fistula.

This chapter focuses on the epidemiology and pathogenesis of inoperable cancer of the esophagus and GEJ. Clinical features and pathologic characteristics of these tumors are also reviewed. Endoscopic methods for palliation of dysphagia and treatment of esophagorespiratory fistulas are discussed. Future developments for treatment of malignant dysphagia are discussed at the end of this chapter.

Epidemiology

Squamous Cell Carcinoma

The incidence of squamous cell carcinoma (SCC) varies from country to country; also, it may occur more often in certain regions within a country. About two-thirds of new cases of SCC are detected in China (47%) and Central Asia (19%); this is known as the Central Asia Esophageal Cancer Belt. The incidence of SCC in this area ranges from 19 per 100,000 in Azerbaijan to 340 per 100,000 in northern China. Other areas of relatively high risk are southern and eastern Africa, south central Asia, and (in men only) Japan. The incidence of SCC in Western Europe and the United States is much lower (i.e., 53 to 86 per 100,000). In Western countries, SCC of the esophagus is mainly found in older people with the highest incidence between 50 and 70 years of age. Esophageal cancer is more common in men in most areas—the sex ratio is 7:1 in Eastern Europe—although in the high-risk areas of Asia and Africa, the sex ratio is much closer to unity.[1] The distribution between men and women is 3:1 to 4:1.[3]

Adenocarcinoma

Until about 1970, more than 90% of esophageal cancers were SCCs. However, population-based studies have shown a large increase in the incidence of adenocarcinoma of the esopha-

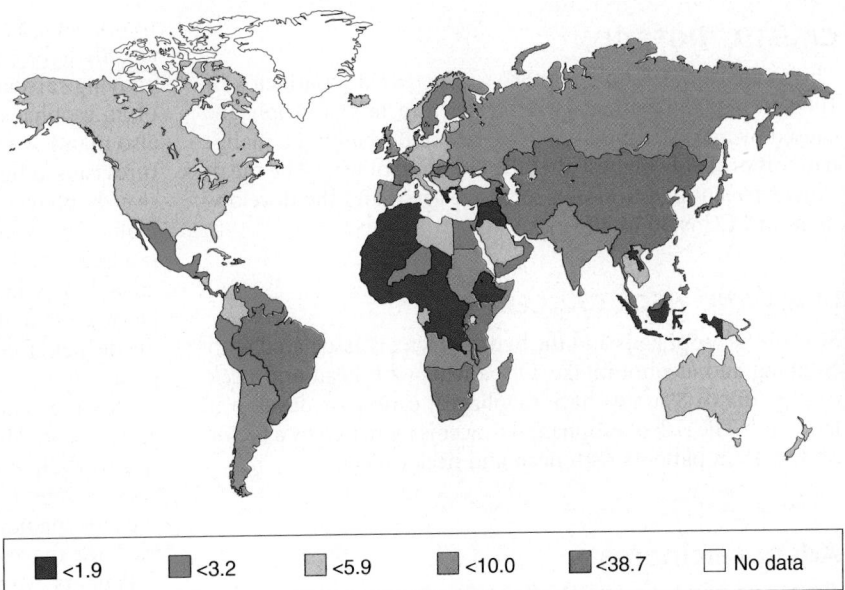

Fig. 28.1 Incidence of esophageal cancer: age-standardized rate (world) for men (all ages). *(From Parkin DM, Bray FI, Devesa SS: Cancer burden in the year 2000: The global picture. Eur J Cancer 37:4–66, 2001.).*

■ <1.9   ■ <3.2   ■ <5.9   ■ <10.0   ■ <38.7   □ No data

gus and GEJ over the last 30 years in North America and Western Europe, especially among white men but also in white women to a lesser degree.[4,5] In men, the incidence of adenocarcinoma of the esophagus and GEJ has surpassed SCC.[6] In the United States, the annual rates of esophageal adenocarcinoma per 100,000 population are 7.8% for white men and 6.5% for women, increasing from 0.7 during 1974–1976 to 3.2 during 1992–1994, an increase of more than 350%.[5] The same trend, although occurring less rapidly, has been reported in other areas, including Australia, New Zealand, and Western Europe.[7]

It is generally believed that the increase in esophageal adenocarcinoma is related to an increase in the incidence of Barrett's esophagus. In a report from The Netherlands, van Soestal and colleagues[8] found that the incidence of new diagnoses of Barrett's esophagus increased from 14.3 per 100,000 person-years in 1997 to 23.1 per 100,000 person-years in 2002. The number of upper gastrointestinal endoscopies decreased from 7.2 per 1000 person-years to 5.7 per 1000 person-years over the same time period. The rate of detection of Barrett's esophagus increased over the same years from 1.4 to 42.7 (16.5 if only cases with histologic confirmation were included) per 1000 endoscopic procedures.

Multiple reports confirm that adenocarcinoma of the esophagus and GEJ occurs more frequently in white men. The distribution between men and women is 4:1. Most patients with esophageal adenocarcinoma are older individuals with a peak incidence around age 65 years.[9] The worldwide distribution of esophageal cancer (for men) is shown in **Fig. 28.1**.

Pathogenesis

Squamous Cell Carcinoma
Smoking and Alcohol

The most important risk factors for SCC in Western Europe and the United States are smoking and alcohol intake. Risk of SCC is increased by a factor of 5 for moderate smokers and a factor of 10 for heavy smokers. It has been shown that alcohol

intake and smoking are independent risk factors for the development of esophageal SCC.[10]

Food

In Hong Kong, a correlation has been established between the use of pickled vegetables and the development of SCC. This correlation was found to be caused by herbs that were used for these vegetables, which were often contaminated with toxic fungi.[11]

Other Factors

Prior radiation therapy has been associated with an increased risk of SCC. A study showed that patients who underwent radiation therapy for breast cancer more than 10 years ago had an increased risk of developing SCC in the esophagus.[12]

Hot drinks, particularly tea in certain areas in Asia, such as the Golestan province in northern Iran, are associated with an increased risk of developing SCC. The suggested mechanism is chronic irritation of the esophageal mucosa caused by the hot drinks.[13]

The role played by human papillomavirus (HPV) is unclear. In South Africa, where the incidence of SCC is high, HPV DNA was detected in more than 50% of cancers.[14] In contrast, in the Netherlands, the presence of HPV in SCC is rare.[15]

Disorders Associated with Increased Risk of Squamous Cell Carcinoma
ACHALASIA

In a cohort study from Sweden, in which 1062 patients with achalasia were followed, the risk of SCC was increased by a factor of 16 after a follow-up of 9864 patient-years.[16] Because most tumors were detected at an advanced stage, a curative resection was possible in only a few patients. Nonetheless, follow-up with endoscopic surveillance in patients with long-standing achalasia has been suggested. It needs to be determined whether this approach is cost-effective.

CAUSTIC INGESTION

The incidence of esophageal SCC is increased by a factor of 1000 to 3000 in patients with a stricture in the esophagus caused by a caustic ingestion. The risk of developing a malignancy is probably highest after the ingestion of lye.[17] The mean time between ingestion of a corrosive agent and the development of SCC is 30 to 40 years.

HEAD AND NECK CANCER

SCC of the esophagus and the hypopharynx is associated with smoking and alcohol intake. Of patients with head and neck cancer, 1% to 8% also have esophageal cancer or develop it later on.[18] The risk of esophageal cancer is increased by a factor of 3 to 10 in patients with head and neck cancer.

Adenocarcinoma

Gastroesophageal Reflux Disease

Lagergren and coworkers[19] found a direct association between reflux and adenocarcinomas, rather than the presumed sequence of reflux disease leading to Barrett's esophagus and this condition leading to adenocarcinoma. The esophageal adenocarcinoma risk was 7.7 times increased in individuals with heartburn and acid reflux occurring at least once a week. For people with severe symptoms for 20 years or longer, the risk was 43.5 times increased for esophageal adenocarcinoma but only 4.4 times increased for adenocarcinoma of the gastric cardia. There was no correlation with SCC.

Barrett's Esophagus

Barrett's esophagus is a disorder of the distal esophagus in which the squamous epithelium is replaced by metaplastic columnar epithelium. Barrett's esophagus is a complication of long-standing gastroesophageal reflux disease.[20] A causal relationship between Barrett's esophagus and the development of esophageal adenocarcinoma has been established.

In older reports, the risk of esophageal adenocarcinoma in long-segment Barrett's esophagus was 30 to 52 times greater than the normal population. Cancer was diagnosed at a median rate of about 1 per 100 patient-years of follow-up. These reports were often based on a short period of follow-up, however, with the possibility of including prevalent cancers as incidence cases, and may have overestimated the cancer risk. More recent reports with longer follow-up times found 1 cancer per 180 to 2200 patient-years of follow-up.[21] The prevalence of Barrett's esophagus in consecutive patients undergoing endoscopy for any clinical indication ranges from 0.3% to 2%.[22] Several studies have shown that Barrett's esophagus is a disorder of white patients and is mainly found in Western Europe. The distribution between men and women is 2.5 to 4:1.[9]

Clinical Features

Local effects of esophageal carcinoma include dysphagia, odynophagia, coughing, regurgitation, vomiting, or a vague discomfort in the back of the throat. At the time of diagnosis, tumor length is mostly more than 4 cm, and patients often already have 6 weeks to 4 months of dysphagia with accompanying substantial weight loss.[23] Dysphagia is not diagnostic of an esophageal malignancy because nonmalignant diseases also manifest with dysphagia such as achalasia or peptic strictures caused by reflux esophagitis. In cases of rapidly progressive dysphagia and weight loss, however, the suspicion of a malignant tumor of the esophagus or GEJ is high. Dysphagia is a late symptom of an esophageal malignancy. Only when a mass lesion has come to a critical size does it impair the passage of food. At this time, the tumor has usually invaded the deeper layers of the esophageal wall, making the prognosis poor.

Odynophagia is seen in nearly 50% of patients with esophageal cancer. The pain associated with this tumor is usually steady, dull, and substernal and occasionally radiates to the back. Severe or persistent pain is a poor prognostic sign and suggests mediastinal extension of the tumor; pain radiating to the back suggests perineural compression of spinal nerves.

Patients with esophageal cancer may develop iron deficiency anemia. Bleeding from the tumor is usually a slow, occult process. Sometimes patients experience frank hemorrhage. Rarely, when the tumor invades the aorta or another major vessel, a patient may experience exsanguination, which is a frequent cause of death.[23]

Physical examination is usually not helpful for a diagnosis at an early stage. When present, weight loss, lymphadenopathy, and hepatomegaly are signs of an advanced stage of disease. Lymphadenopathy can be detected in the cervical, supraclavicular, and axillary node areas, in order of decreasing frequency. Auscultation and percussion may reveal findings of tracheoesophageal fistula, pneumonia, pleural effusions, or a cavitary lung abscess.

There is no evidence that the presentation of esophageal cancer has changed with the increase in the incidence of adenocarcinoma of the esophagus and GEJ in Western countries; however, more than 50% of patients present with inoperable disease. Reasons for inoperable cancer include the presence of distant metastatic disease in 65%, locally advanced cancer in 20%, or severe comorbidity precluding the possibility of surgery in 15% of patients.

Pathology

Squamous Cell Carcinoma

Of SCCs, 24% occur in the upper third, 47% occur in the middle third, and 29% occur in the lower third of the esophagus.[24] It has been shown that SCC develops from low-grade or high-grade dysplasia to intraepithelial carcinoma and finally invasive esophageal carcinoma. Endoscopic follow-up in 327 Chinese patients with high-grade dysplasia showed that SCC was diagnosed at a median rate of 4 cases per 100 patient-years of follow-up.[25] In the Western world, less than 10% of patients with SCC are diagnosed at an early stage.[24]

Adenocarcinoma

Adenocarcinomas of the esophagus and GEJ are located in the distal esophagus and proximal stomach. There is also clear evidence for a dysplasia-carcinoma sequence in Barrett's

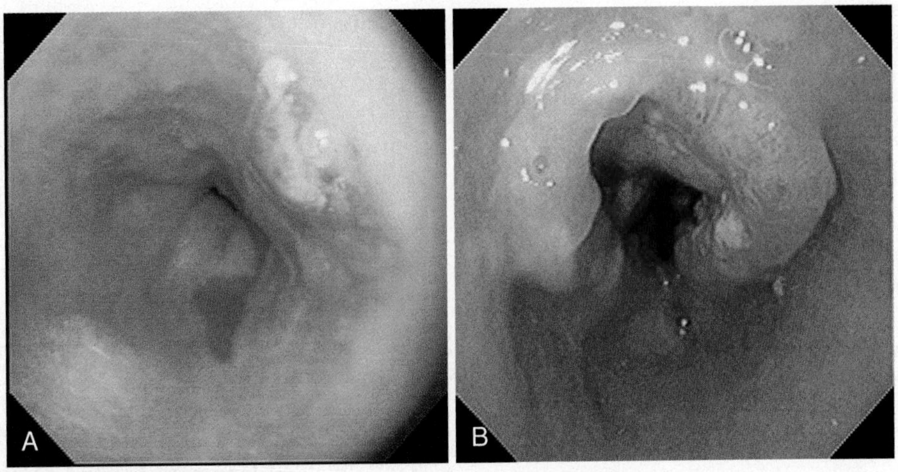

Fig. 28.2 Endoscopic view of early (**A**) and advanced (**B**) esophageal cancer.

esophagus, whereby Barrett's esophagus without dysplasia progresses to low-grade dysplasia, high-grade dysplasia, and ultimately carcinoma.[26] During a mean follow-up of 3 to 5.2 years, progression from Barrett's esophagus without dysplasia to low-grade dysplasia occurred in 12% to 18% of patients, and progression from low-grade to high-grade dysplasia or adenocarcinoma occurred in 10% to 25% of patients.[27,28] Progression from high-grade dysplasia to carcinoma occurs in 17% to 66% of patients over 0.75 to 9 years.[29,30] The distribution of the grade of dysplasia in transversal studies of patients with Barrett's esophagus is 80% no dysplasia, 18% low-grade dysplasia, and 2% high-grade dysplasia or adenocarcinoma.[31,32]

Given the dismal prognosis among patients with symptomatic esophageal cancer, guidelines from the American College of Gastroenterology[33] recommend endoscopic surveillance of patients with Barrett's esophagus in an attempt to prevent death from adenocarcinoma. Retrospective studies have found that patients whose esophageal adenocarcinoma was detected in a surveillance program presented at an earlier stage and had better 5-year survival rates than patients without surveillance who presented with cancer.[34] A more recent study showed that less than 5% of patients who presented with esophageal adenocarcinoma actually underwent endoscopic surveillance.[35]

Esophageal cancer grows by intraesophageal spread, direct extension, and lymphatic and hematogenous metastases. The tumor typically invades adjacent structures, and lymph node metastases range from 40% to 70%. Because esophageal lymph node flow is bidirectional, sites of nodal metastases are many. Distant metastases, particularly to liver, lung, and bone, are present in 25% to 30% of patients at diagnosis.[36]

Early esophageal carcinomas are usually slightly elevated, coarse, or polypoid with denuded epithelium at endoscopy (**Fig. 28.2A**). The gross appearance of SCCs and adenocarcinomas is practically indistinguishable. Adenocarcinoma of the esophagus, especially in its early stage, can be distinguished from SCC by the presence of Barrett's esophagus. If esophageal adenocarcinoma is advanced, however, it is often impossible to detect Barrett's esophagus because the tumor has presumably overgrown its precursor. The macroscopic features of advanced esophageal cancers can be ulcerative, stenotic, polypoid, or a combination of these (**Fig. 28.2B**).

Differential Diagnosis

The differential diagnosis of esophageal carcinoma includes peptic stricture, Schatzki ring, corrosive stricture, postradiation stricture, and achalasia. Rarely, one should consider bronchogenic carcinoma invading the esophagus or metastatic cancer in the mediastinum compressing or invading the esophagus.

Patients with a peptic stricture usually have a long history of pyrosis; however, substantial weight loss is uncommon. Endoscopy reveals a smooth lining of the stricture with inflammation and scar tissue on histologic examination. Peptic strictures are not as common in the Western world probably because of the widespread use of proton pump inhibitors (PPIs). A Schatzki ring is characterized by the presence of a ringlike stricture at the GEJ. If a Schatzki ring is causing symptoms of odynophagia or dysphagia, it is often associated with gastroesophageal reflux disease or a hiatal hernia or both. The occurrence of symptoms is usually intermittent. A stricture that is the result of a prior corrosive insult is usually short and irregular, and sometimes multiple strictures are present in the esophagus. Patients with postradiation strictures have a history of previous radiation therapy. These strictures are erosive but otherwise often regular, and telangiectasias are found in the esophageal mucosa. Dysphagia is intermittent and nonprogressive in patients with achalasia. In most patients with achalasia, the esophagus is elongated and dilated.

Treatment

The preferred treatment for esophageal cancer is surgical resection. Resection of the esophagus with a gastric pull-up or a colonic interposition is an invasive procedure, however, with significant morbidity and mortality.[36] A discussion of the different surgical techniques, long-term results, and complications after surgery is beyond the scope of this chapter. In the past decade, endoscopic methods have been developed to remove early cancers in the esophagus nonsurgically. Indications and contraindications for endoscopic treatment of early esophageal cancer are discussed in Chapter 27.

In patients with inoperable esophageal cancer resulting from locally advanced or metastatic disease or with severe

Table 28.1 Palliative Modalities for Esophageal Carcinoma

NONENDOSCOPIC TECHNIQUES

Surgery
External beam radiation therapy
Chemotherapy
Chemoradiation therapy
Intraluminal radiation therapy (brachytherapy)

ENDOSCOPIC TECHNIQUES

Stent placement
  Self-expanding metal stents
  Self-expanding plastic stents
Dilation (repeat)
Photodynamic therapy
Argon plasma coagulation
Cryoablation therapy
Nutritional support
  Nasoenteric feeding tube
  Percutaneous endoscopic gastrostomy

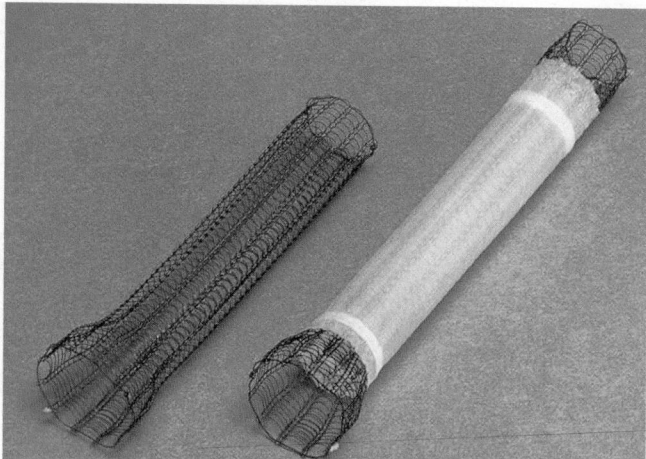

Fig. 28.3 Uncovered *(left)* and covered *(right)* versions of the Ultraflex stent.

comorbidity, restoration of the ability to eat is one of the main treatment goals. Because most of these patients live no longer than 6 to 12 months, the aim of palliative treatment is to relieve dysphagia rapidly with minimal or no hospital stay, to maintain swallowing during life, and to avoid serious complications. Treatment of incurable esophageal cancer should be individualized and based on tumor stage, medical condition and performance status of the patient, and the patient's personal wishes. In addition, the available expertise and equipment and the results of prospective, randomized studies should be taken into consideration.

Various palliative techniques are currently available (**Table 28.1**). The main options can be divided into nonendoscopic modalities, of which chemoradiation therapy is most commonly used, and endoscopic procedures, of which placement of a self-expanding metal stent to relieve obstruction resulting from a malignant stricture in the esophagus is the most frequently used technique. Some of the endoscopic procedures for palliation of malignant dysphagia are discussed.

Self-Expanding Metal Stents

Placement of a self-expanding metal or plastic stent is a frequently used method for palliation of malignant dysphagia. Since 1990, more than 130 studies have been published on the outcome of metal stent placement for palliation of malignant dysphagia and esophageal fistulas.[37–39]

Metal Stents versus Rigid Plastic Endoprosthetics

Metal stents have several advantages over previously used prosthetic tubes. They can be inserted with minimal dilation because the diameter of the delivery catheters is only 7 to 11 mm. After placement of a metal stent, the stent expands gradually, which potentially decreases the occurrence of subsequent procedure-related complications. The larger lumen achieved (16 to 24 mm) and the flexibility of metal stents should improve the quality of swallowing compared with prosthetic tubes. An advantage of prosthetic tubes is low cost compared with expensive metal stents.

Several randomized trials have compared metal stents with prosthetic tubes.[40–45] These studies have shown that placement of a metal stent is associated with fewer procedure-related complications than placement of a prosthetic tube.[41,42,44,45] In one study, metal stents were also more effective in improving dysphagia.[43] Studies on cost-effectiveness have shown that, despite the high initial purchase cost, metal stents were more cost-effective than prosthetic tubes because of a shorter hospital stay for procedures for stent-related complications.[40,41,43,46]

Covered versus Uncovered Metal Stents

A disadvantage of the first-generation metal stents, which were not covered by a membrane, was that tumor ingrowth through the wire mesh of the stent led to recurrent dysphagia in 20% to 30% of patients. Stents were subsequently developed with a membrane to prevent tumor ingrowth. Covered metal stents are now the most commonly used type to avoid ingrowth of tumor through the metal mesh. It has been suggested that covered metal stents are more likely to migrate than bare metal stents, especially in the region of the distal esophagus and gastric cardia. This increased risk of migration could be caused by insufficient anchoring of the stent cover to the esophageal wall.

In a prospective randomized trial by Vakil and coworkers,[47] covered and uncovered Ultraflex (Boston Scientific, Natick, MA) stents were compared in 62 patients with obstructing tumors at the GEJ (**Figs. 28.3 and 28.4**). Tumor ingrowth or overgrowth was significantly more common in the uncovered stent group (9 of 30 [30%]) than in the covered stent group (1 of 32 [3%]). Stent migration was not different between the two treatment groups (uncovered stent, 2 of 30 [7%], vs. covered stent, 4 of 32 [12%]). Covered stents apparently give better long-term palliation of malignant dysphagia than uncovered stents.

Currently Available Covered Metal Stents

Special stent characteristics are needed for the effective palliation of tumors of the distal esophagus and the gastric cardia. The ideal stent would have the following characteristics:

1. It would have a large internal diameter to ensure the passage of a normal diet.
2. It would be flexible and nontraumatic while still achieving full expansion.
3. It would not migrate, yet could be repositioned or removed if necessary.

An ideal stent does not exist. However, all available covered metal stents meet some of these criteria (**Table 28.2**).

The Ultraflex stent consists of a knitted nitinol wire tube, and the covered version has a polyurethane layer that covers the midsection of the stent extending to within 1.5 cm of either end of the stent (see **Figs. 28.3 and 28.4**). The stent has

a proximal flare with two sizes: 28 mm (distal diameter 23 mm) and 23 mm (distal diameter 18 mm). The Ultraflex stent has an easy-to-use delivery system of the stent and can be deployed gradually from the proximal to the distal end or vice versa. The degree of shortening after stent placement is 30% to 40%. The radial force of the Ultraflex stent is the lowest among currently available metal stents. Partial obstruction of the stent can occur in stents that are sharply angulated after passing across the GEJ.

The Polyflex stent (Boston Scientific) is a silicone device with an encapsulated monofilament braid made of polyester. The meshes are completely covered by a silicone layer with a smooth inner surface and a more structured outer surface (see **Fig. 28.4**). The edges of the monofilaments are protected with silicone to avoid impaction or tissue damage at the proximal and distal ends. The stent has a proximal flare of 25 mm, 23 mm, and 21 mm and body diameter of 21 mm, 18 mm, and 16 mm. It is available in three lengths: 9 cm, 12 cm, and 15 cm. The stent needs to be loaded in the introducer sheath before placement. This introduction device has a diameter of 14 mm, 13 mm, and 12 mm. This is the largest stent system compared with other systems and the system is rigid; investigators have suggested that the relatively high occurrence of perforations after Polyflex stent placement is at least partly due to these characteristics.[48] In addition, the stent is less suitable for angulated strictures because the distal dilator is short. The inappropriate forced transmission of such an introduction sheath may complicate its passage across angulated strictures. Finally, because the stent has only a mesh on the outside and no other antimigration properties, it is associated with an increased risk of stent migration.[48] The Polyflex stent is more frequently used for benign strictures in the esophagus than for malignant strictures.[49]

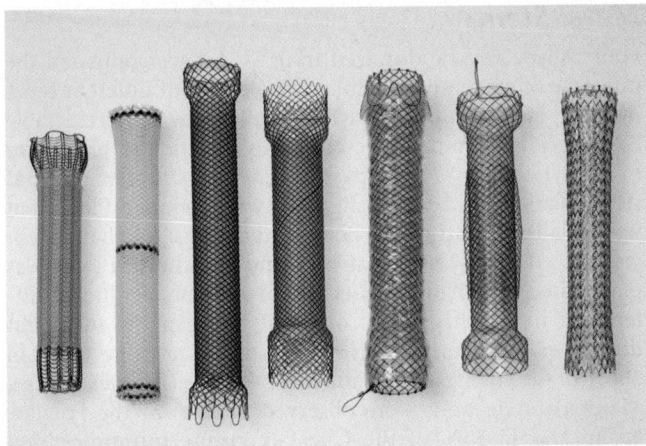

Fig. 28.4 Currently available covered metal stents, from *left to right:* Ultraflex stent, Polyflex stent, Wallflex stent, Evolution stent, SX-Ella stent, Niti-S stent, and Alimaxx-E stent. As can be seen, some of these stents are fully covered, whereas others are only partially covered.

Table 28.2 Characteristics of Presently Available Types of Metal Stents

Stent Type	Covering	Length (cm)	Diameter (mm)	Release System	Radial Force	Degree of Shortening	Flexibility	Stent Material	Manufacturer
Ultraflex	Partial	10, 12, 15	18, 22	Proximal/ distal	Low	30%-40%	High	Nitinol/ polyurethane	Boston Scientific, Watertown, MA
Polyflex	Full	9, 12, 15	16, 18, 21	Distal	High	0%	Low	Polyester/ silicone	Boston Scientific, Watertown, MA
Wallflex	Partial	10, 12, 15	18, 23	Distal	High to strong	30%-40%	Moderate	Nitinol/ silicone	Boston Scientific, Watertown, MA
Evolution	Partial	8, 10, 12.5, 15	20	Distal	Moderate	10%-20%	Moderate	Nitinol/ silicone	Cook Medical, Limerick, Ireland
SX-Ella	Full	8.5, 11, 13.5	20	Distal	High	10%-20%	Low	Nitinol/ polyethylene	Ella, Hradec Kralove, Czech Republic
Niti-S	Full	6, 8, 10, 12, 15	18	Proximal/ distal	Moderate	10%	Moderate	Nitinol/ polyurethane	Taewoong, Pusan, South Korea
Alimaxx-E	Full	7, 10, 12	18, 22	Distal	Low	0%	Moderate to high	Nitinol/ polyurethane	Merit, South Jordan, UT

The Wallflex stent (Boston Scientific) consists of a wire braided construction and is partially covered with nitinol extending to within 1.5 cm of either end of the stent (see **Fig. 28.4**). The stent has a proximal and distal flare with two sizes: 28 mm (body diameter 23 mm) and 23 mm (body diameter 18 mm). The degree of shortening after Wallflex stent placement is considerable (i.e., 30% to 40%). The radial force of the Wallflex stent is one of the highest among currently available metal stents. Clinical experience is limited to one prospective follow-up study showing favorable results with the partially covered Wallflex stent.[50]

The Evolution stent (Cook, Limerick, Ireland) is constructed of a single woven nitinol wire. The stent has an internal and external silicone coating and uncoated flanges on both ends (see **Fig. 28.4**). The body diameter of the stent is 20 mm, and the flange diameter is 25 mm on both ends. The stent is available in four lengths: 8 cm, 10 cm, 12.5 cm, and 15 cm. The stent slightly foreshortens because of its design. A pistol-grip delivery system handle allows step-by-step stent deployment or recapturing. Initial studies have shown that this stent type is safe and effective in treating malignant esophageal strictures.[51]

The SX-Ella stent (Ella, Hradec Kralove, Czech Republic) is made of nitinol and a single braided wire. To decrease the risk of migration, the SX-Ella stent has a flip-flop type of antimigration ring that is circumferentially attached to the proximal stent portion (see **Fig. 28.4**). This ring functions as a circular hook that prevents migration; however, the ring is flexible and everts when the traction force is too strong. The stent flares to 25 mm at its proximal and distal ends with a body diameter of 20 mm. It is available in lengths of 85 mm, 110 mm, and 135 mm. Initial studies showed that the antimigration ring did not reduce stent migration, but the stent was associated with an increased risk of hemorrhage. In addition to hemorrhage, severe pain and fistula formation at the upper end of the SX-Ella stent were frequently observed. In normal circumstances, stents exert some pressure on the tumor and the normal mucosa of the esophagus to fixate the stent to the esophageal wall to reduce migration risk. In case of the SX-Ella stent, this effect may be more pronounced because of the pressure effect of the antimigration ring, particularly when it is flipping in and out for its antimigration effect.[52]

The Niti-S stent (Taewoong, Pusan, South Korea) has a double-layer configuration over its entire length, consisting of an inner polyurethane layer and an outer uncovered nitinol wire (see **Fig. 28.4**). This double layer was designed to reduce the risk of stent migration. The stent flares to 26 mm at its proximal and distal ends and has a body diameter of 18 mm. It is available in five lengths: 6 cm, 8 cm, 10 cm, 12 cm, and 15 cm. It has both a proximal and a distal release system.[48,53]

The Alimaxx-E stent (Merit, South Jordan, UT) is also made of nitinol, and it is fully covered with polyurethane to resist tissue ingrowth (see **Fig. 28.4**). This stent has a proximal flare of 27 mm and 23 mm, a luminal diameter of 22 mm and 18 mm, and a distal flare of 25 mm and 21 mm. The outward force of the stent is most pronounced at the body. The stent also has a pistol type of release system, similar to the Evolution stent (see earlier). In the initial versions of this stent, it could be introduced over a guidewire (Alimaxx-E GW system) but also under direct vision using a delivery system in which the delivery catheter fitted over a small-caliber endoscope (Alimaxx-E DV system). The latter system featured a window at the end of the introduction sheath to view stent deployment. The size of the introduction catheter of the Alimaxx-E DV was 30 Fr, whereas the size of the introduction catheter of the Alimaxx-E GW was 22 Fr. Because the DV system was difficult to manipulate owing to its size and stiffness, and perforations were noted with this system, this system was withdrawn from the market. Another issue was that the initial version of the Alimaxx-E stent had 20 antimigration struts to prevent stent migration; this was increased to 45 antimigration struts, however, because the migration rate was more than 30% with the original stent design.[54]

Comparison of Different Types of Metal Stents

Four prospective randomized trials[48,55–57] have compared the outcome of currently available stent designs of different types of metal stents. In one study, 101 patients with unresectable esophageal carcinoma were randomly assigned to placement of a Polyflex ($n = 47$) or a partially covered Ultraflex ($n = 54$) stent.[55] Patients with GEJ malignancy were excluded. Placement was equally successful with both stent designs: A Polyflex stent was placed in 46 (98%) patients, and an Ultraflex stent was placed in 54 (100%) patients. There were no significant differences in dysphagia improvement between the two stent designs (after 1 week improvement by at least one grade in 100% of the Polyflex group and in 94% of the Ultraflex group). Major complications were observed in 48% of the Polyflex group and in 33% of the Ultraflex group. Intraprocedural perforation occurred in one Polyflex patient and one Ultraflex patient. Two Polyflex patients had postprocedural hemorrhage. Recurrent dysphagia occurred in 20 (44%) patients with a Polyflex stent and 18 (33%) patients with an Ultraflex stent because of tumor overgrowth, stent migration, hyperplastic granulomatous reaction, or food bolus impaction. Multivariate analysis showed a significantly higher complication rate with Polyflex stents than with Ultraflex stents (odds ratio 2.3, 95% confidence interval 1.2 to 4.4). Median survival was similar: 134 days with Polyflex stents and 122 days with Ultraflex stents. The authors concluded that palliation of dysphagia was not different between the two stents. Significantly more complications, especially late stent migration, were observed in the Polyflex group.

In another prospective study, 125 patients with dysphagia from inoperable carcinoma of the esophagus or gastric cardia were randomly assigned to placement of an Ultraflex stent ($n = 42$), Polyflex stent ($n = 41$), or Niti-S stent ($n = 42$).[48] Stent placement was technically successful in all patients with an Ultraflex stent, in 34 of 41 (83%) patients with a Polyflex stent, and in 40 of 42 (95%) patients treated with a Niti-S stent ($P = .008$). The dysphagia score improved in all patients. There were no differences in major complications among the three stent types. Recurrent dysphagia, caused by tissue ingrowth or overgrowth, migration, or food obstruction, was significantly different between patients with an Ultraflex stent and patients with a Polyflex stent or Niti-S stent (22 [52%] vs. 15 [37%] vs. 13 [31%]; $P = .03$). Stent migration occurred more frequently with Polyflex stents, whereas tissue ingrowth or overgrowth was seen more frequently with partially covered Ultraflex stents and, to a lesser degree, Niti-S stents. No differences were found in survival (median survival Ultraflex stent, 132 days, vs. Polyflex stent, 102 days, vs. Niti-S stent, 159 days) among the three stent types. It was concluded that all three stents were safe and offered adequate palliation of dysphagia from esophageal or gastric cardia cancer. Nonetheless, Polyflex stents seemed the least preferable stent type in this patient group because placement of this device is technically demanding and associated with a high rate of stent migrations.

In a prospective trial, 100 patients were randomly assigned to one of three types of covered metal stents: the Ultraflex stent, the Flamingo Wallstent, and the Z-stent.[56] There were no significant differences in dysphagia improvement and the occurrence of complications or recurrent dysphagia, although there was a trend toward more complications with the Z-stent (Ultraflex stent, 8 of 34 [24%]; Flamingo Wallstent, 6 of 33 [18%]; and Z-stent, 12 of 33 [36%]; $P = .23$). In another prospective trial, the Ultraflex stent and the Flamingo Wallstent were compared in patients with distal esophageal cancer.[57] The two stent types were equally effective in the palliation of dysphagia in this patient group, and the complication rate associated with their use was comparable (Ultraflex stent, 7 of 31 [23%], and Flamingo Wallstent, 5 of 22 [23%]).

From these data, it can be concluded that there are only minor differences between the most commonly used stent types. The choice of stent in patients with a malignant stricture in the esophagus or gastric cardia should be determined by the location and the anatomy of the malignant stricture on the one hand and the specific characteristics of the stent on the other hand (**Table 28.3**; see **Table 28.2**). Based on the currently available results, caution is needed when using Polyflex stents (migration, robust introduction device), SX-Ella stents (complications owing to the antimigration ring), or Alimaxx-E stents (migration) for this indication.

Metal Stents for Tumors of the Gastroesophageal Junction

Because the incidence of adenocarcinoma of the distal esophagus is increasing rapidly,[4,5] the deployment of metal stents across the GEJ is likely to increase. However, stent placement for tumors of the distal esophagus and GEJ constitutes a particular problem. Compared with stents placed for more proximally located esophageal tumors, these procedures provide inferior palliation and have higher complication rates.[58] Migration is more likely with stents placed across the GEJ than with stents placed for more proximally located tumors because the distal part of the stent projects freely into the fundus of the stomach, and this part cannot fix itself to the wall.

How can migration of stents be prevented? Following are some considerations:

1. The design of the stent plays a role in reducing stent migration. Most currently available metal stents are covered from the inside, which exposes the mesh of the stent to the outer part of the stent; this may help embed the stent into the esophageal wall.
2. Another factor in reducing stent migration is stent diameter. Large-diameter stents have been introduced for the prevention of migration but may be associated with more complications. Verschuur and colleagues[59] evaluated 338 prospectively followed patients with dysphagia from obstructing esophageal or gastric cardia cancer who were treated with either a small-diameter ($n = 265$) or a large-diameter ($n = 73$) stent. Three different stent types were used in the study. All patients underwent stent placement for an inoperable malignant obstruction of the esophagus or gastric cardia or recurrent dysphagia after prior radiation. Improvement in dysphagia was similar between patients with a small-diameter or a large-diameter stent. The occurrence of major complications, such as hemorrhage, perforation, fistula, and fever, was increased only in patients with a large-diameter Z-stent compared with patients treated with a small-diameter Z-stent (4 [40%] vs. 16 [20%]; adjusted hazard ratio 5.03), and complications were not increased in patients with a large-diameter Ultraflex stent or Flamingo Wallstent. Dysphagia from stent migration, tissue overgrowth, and food bolus obstruction recurred more frequently in patients with a small-diameter stent than in patients with a large-diameter stent (Ultraflex stent, 54 [42%] vs. 3 [13%], adjusted hazard ratio 0.16; Z-stent, 21 [27%] vs. 1 [10%], adjusted hazard ratio 0.97; and Flamingo Wallstent, 21 [37%] vs. 6 [15%], adjusted hazard ratio 0.40). The investigators concluded that large-diameter stents reduce the risk of recurrent dysphagia from stent

Table 28.3 Summary of Occurrence of Complications and Recurrent Dysphagia with Currently Available Stent Types Based on Two Randomized Controlled Trials* and Case Series†

	Ultraflex	Polyflex	Wallflex	Evolution	SX-Ella	Niti-S	Alimaxx-E
Total complications	=	=	=	=	↑↑	=	=
Major complications					++		
Minor complications							
Recurrent dysphagia	↑	↑↑	↑	↑	=	=	↑↑↑
Migration		++					++
Tissue ingrowth/overgrowth	+		+	+			
Food obstruction	+						

*See references 41 and 47.
†See references 40 and 42–46.

migration, tissue overgrowth, or food obstruction. However, increasing the diameter in some stent types may increase the risk of stent-related complications to the esophagus.

3. If the stent is only partially covered, stent migration may also be reduced. Fully covered stent designs are associated with a higher risk of migration. Partially covered stents have the advantage that the uncovered stent end can embed into the esophageal wall. An issue with partially covered stents is nontumoral tissue ingrowth through the uncovered stent part, a cause of recurrent dysphagia after stent placement. This ingrowth has increasingly been recognized over the years as an important cause of recurrent dysphagia with partially covered stents. Mayoral and associates[60] were the first to report this complication in 2000. They found granulation tissue, reactive hyperplasia, and fibrosis, mostly at the proximal end but also on the distal end of the stent, in 32% of their patients after a mean interval of 154 days after stent placement. They suggested that the type of metal used in the stent (nitinol) might have played a causative role in the formation of nontumoral tissue growth at both stent ends. However, nontumoral tissue overgrowth can also be seen with nonmetal, fully covered Polyflex stents. In our experience, the formation of nontumoral, hyperplastic tissue ingrowth or overgrowth is related to both the radial force and size of the stent and the duration of stent placement, with a prolonged stent placement increasing this risk.

4. An increased incidence of bleeding has also been reported for stents placed across the GEJ. This bleeding could be the result of two factors. First, the lower end of the stent may erode the posterior wall of the stomach, resulting in ulceration and subsequent bleeding. Second, a stent that passes the GEJ cannot remain straight because of the normal anatomic angle between the esophagus and the gastric cardia. Consequently, the asymmetric lateral force exerted by the proximal part of the stent on the esophagus above the tumor results in an increased rate of pressure-related complications, such as ulceration and subsequent bleeding. This angulation of the stent may also explain the finding that the improvement in quality of swallowing is inferior with stents across the GEJ compared with more proximally placed stents. Finally, patients with a stent crossing the GEJ often experience symptoms of reflux.

5. Stents placed across the GEJ are also associated with an increased risk of gastroesophageal reflux. Patients with a stent in this position are usually advised to use high-dose PPIs to inhibit gastric acid secretion, to sleep in an upright position, and to avoid late-night meals and snacks. To overcome the problem of gastroesophageal reflux, stents with an antireflux valve have been introduced (**Table 28.4**).[61–72] The first results with a plastic tube with an antireflux mechanism were published in 1984.[61] Over the past few years, several other design metal stents with an antireflux mechanism have been developed.[62–72] In most cases, the cover of the stent at the distal end is extended beyond the lower metal cage to form a windsock-type valve (**Fig. 28.5**). The first results with this design were reported in a study

comprising 18 patients. The authors concluded on the basis of symptoms and barium studies that the antireflux stent was effective in the treatment of malignant dysphagia and prevented major gastroesophageal reflux.[71]

Five randomized trials comparing an antireflux stent with a standard stent have been published with conflicting results (see **Table 28.4**).[65,67–69,72] In the only study in which the standard stent was combined with a PPI, no differences in reflux symptoms were noted. It still remains to be established whether stents with an antireflux mechanism are able to prevent the reflux of gastric fluid into the esophagus; this should be established in randomized trials measuring symptoms but also using objective measures such as pH/impedance measurement to demonstrate effectiveness.

Currently available evidence suggests that it is probably best to use partially covered stents with a larger diameter for tumors at the distal esophagus and cardia. As stated above, stent migration, especially if placed across the GEJ, can be reduced by using a stent of a greater diameter or partially covered stent design. However, when partially covered stents are used, nontumoral tissue ingrowth is an issue. Further studies are needed to establish the balance between the advantages of less stent migration and the possible increased risk of complications associated with large-diameter stents. Stents across the GEJ should not be placed too distally to minimize the risk of ulceration of the gastric wall or blocking food passage through the stent. Finally, the addition of an antireflux valve may be effective in decreasing gastroesophageal reflux in patients needing stents that extend into the gastric cavity; however, further studies are needed to establish the clinical value of this effect.

Stent Placement Procedure

Placement of metal stents is usually done with the patient under sedation (see Video). The first step is to inspect the tumor for its characteristics (severity of stenosis, length, extension into the stomach) (**Fig. 28.6A**). When fluoroscopy is used, the proximal and distal margins of the stricture are demarcated endoscopically by skin markers, tissue clips, or intramucosal injection of a radiopaque contrast agent (**Fig. 28.6B**). Injection of the lipid-soluble contrast agent lipiodol results in a persistent mark. Accurate placement of the Ultraflex stent is also possible under endoscopic guidance without the aid of fluoroscopy. An external marker is applied at the level of the proximal radiopaque marker on the stent, allowing the stent to be placed under direct endoscopic visualization.[73] In addition, some stents have markers on the introduction system that reliably aid in stent placement. The distance on the introduction catheter at the level of the incisors corresponds with the upper end of the stent. This technique is at present possible only with the Ultraflex stent and the SX-Ella stent. Finally, metal stents also can be placed under fluoroscopic guidance only, without the use of endoscopy.[74]

In many institutions, a stenotic malignant stricture is dilated to a diameter of 9 to 10 mm before stent placement to measure stricture length and to place a guidewire accurately. Dilation may increase the risk of perforation, however. For that reason, it is recommended to use a small-caliber endoscope or, alternatively, contrast media and fluoroscopy to delineate characteristics and length of the malignant stricture and to place the

Table 28.4 Gastroesophageal Reflux (Symptoms) after Placement of an Antireflux Stent for Palliation of Malignant Dysphagia: Summary of Published Studies

Reference	Intervention	No. Patients (%)			Objective Measurement	Results	Best Antireflux Effect with
		Total	Reflux	PPI			
RANDOMIZED TRIALS							
Sabharwal, 2008[72]	FerX-Ella stent (antireflux)	22	3 (14)	No	None		No difference found
	Ultraflex	26	2 (8)	Standard			
Wenger et al, 2006[69]	Dua antireflux stent	19	2 (5)	No			No difference found
	Z-stent	22	2 (9)	No			
Shim et al, 2005[68]	cSEMS	12	5 (42)	No	24-hr pH monitoring	60.44*	Modified antireflux stent
	Dostent (antireflux)	12	4 (33)	No		105.29*	
	Modified antireflux stent	12	0 (0)	No		12*	
Homs et al, 2004[67]	FerX-Ella stent (antireflux)	15	3 (13)	No	24-hr pH monitoring	23%[†]	Standard stent
	FerX-Ella stent (standard)	15	2 (13)	No		10%[†]	
Laasch, 2002[65]	Flamingo stent	25	24 (96)	19 (79)	None		Dua antireflux stent
	Dua antireflux stent	25	19 (76)	1 (4)			
COMPARATIVE STUDIES							
Power et al, 2007[70]	Ultraflex stent	25			24-hr pH monitoring	27.6*	Hanarostent (antireflux)
	Hanarostent (antireflux)	24				2.1*	
Osugi et al, 2002[66]	Ultraflex stent	7	3 (25)	No	24-hr pH monitoring	37.8%[†]	Antireflux stent
	Antireflux stent	5	0 (0)	No		2.9%[†]	
PROSPECTIVE STUDIES							
Schoppmeyer et al, 2007[71]	Z-stent (antireflux)	18	4 (22)	9 (50)	None		
Dua et al, 2001[64]	Z-stent (antireflux)	11	2 (18)	2 (18)	24-hr pH monitoring	1%[†]	
Do et al, 2001[63]	Antireflux stent	17	0	No	Barium study	7 no reflux; 10 minimal reflux	
Kocher, 1998[62]	ELLA-CS stent (antireflux)	18	2 (11)	No	Barium study	4 patients minor reflux	
Valbuena, 1984[61]	Plastic antireflux stent	40	0	No	Barium study	8 no reflux	

*Demeester score.
[†]Total acid.
PPI, proton pump inhibitor.

guidewire. There is no consensus on whether one or more dilation sessions preceding stent placement reduce this risk of perforation. The next step is to place a stiff guidewire, such as a 0.038-inch Savary guidewire, across the stricture into the stomach and withdraw the endoscope.

A premounted stent or a stent that has been advanced into the introduction system is advanced over the guidewire and deployed. It is reasonable to confirm endoscopically that the upper end of the stent is in place proximal to the upper tumor margin. However, the endoscope should be passed through the stent only if no friction with the endoscope is felt to avoid dislodgment of the stent (**Fig. 28.6C**).

Except for the Polyflex stent and the Alimaxx-E stent, all stents shorten to some extent. Both the Ultraflex stent and the Wallstent shorten during expansion (see **Table 28.2**), which must be taken into consideration when positioning the introduction system. To prevent migration of the stent on release from the introduction system, the system should not be advanced too far distally. An advantage of the Wallflex stent and the Evolution stent is that they can be recaptured (if not expanded >50%) by advancing the constraining sheath and repositioning the entire stent. The stent should be 2 to 4 cm longer than the stricture to allow for a 1- to 2-cm extension above and below the proximal and distal tumor margins.

For stents placed across the GEJ, stent length is guided by the rule that the proximal covered portion of the stent should lie at least 1 to 2 cm above the tumor margin, whereas the distal covered portion should not overlap the tumor margin by more than 1 cm, to prevent ulceration of the posterior wall of the stomach by the distal end of the stent. All currently available stents, whether fully expanded, partially expanded, unexpanded, or migrated after release from the introduction system, can be repositioned or removed by pulling at the upper rim of the stents or at the lasso attached inside the proximal flange of most stents, causing the radial diameter of the stent to decrease. Stent expansion can best be confirmed fluoroscopically, by a chest radiograph, or by barium swallow.

Currently, stent placement is typically an outpatient procedure. Placement of a metal stent takes about 15 to 20 minutes in experienced hands.

Variations and Unusual Situations

FISTULA FORMATION

Progressive esophageal carcinoma can infiltrate into surrounding tissue with subsequent development of a fistula, most commonly between the esophagus and the respiratory tract (i.e., the trachea or bronchi) and occasionally between the aorta, the mediastinum, or pleura. In a series of 1943 patients with esophageal cancer, it was found that 5% of patients developed a fistula over time. In the same publication, it was reported that 0.2% of 5714 patients with bronchogenic carcinoma developed an esophagorespiratory fistula.[75] Fistulas may also develop secondary to radiation or laser therapy or

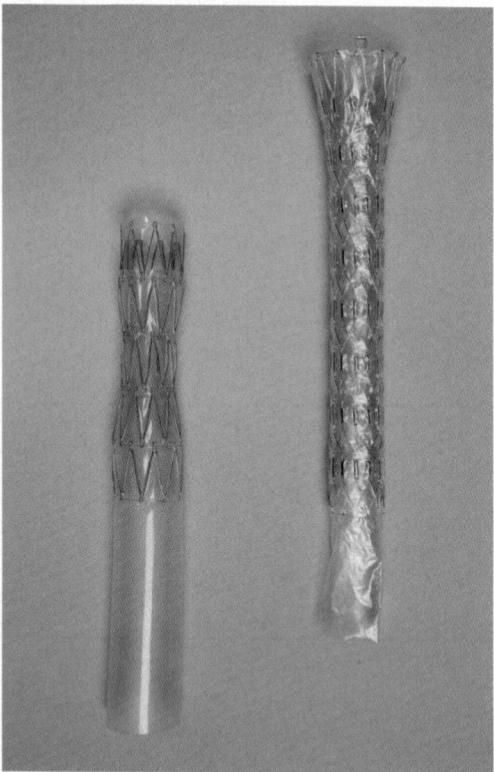

Fig. 28.5 Two types of windsock-type antireflux valves for the prevention of gastroesophageal reflux: Z-stent *(left)* and FerX-Ella stent *(right).*

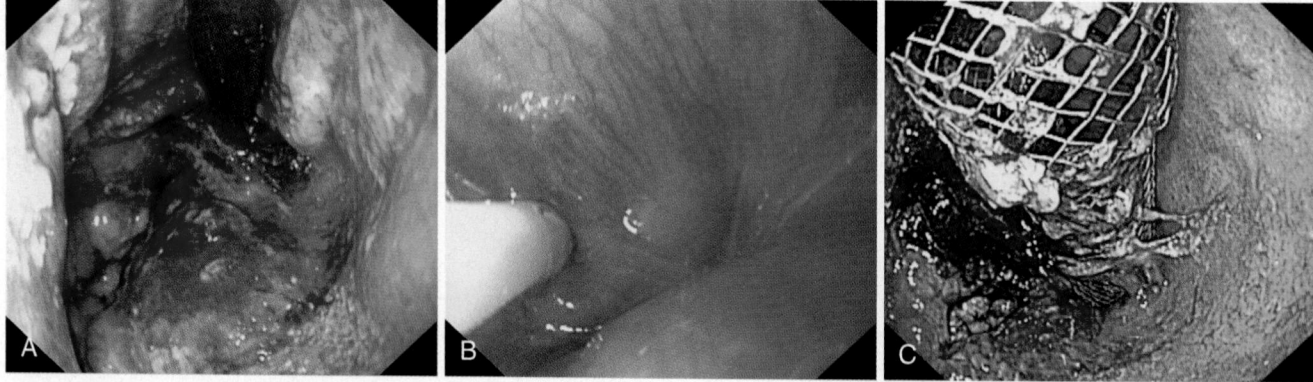

Fig. 28.6 The first step of esophageal stent placement is to identify the upper and lower ends of the tumor. **A**, A patient with a gastric cardia tumor is shown in retroversion. The proximal and distal margins of the tumor are demarcated by the intramucosal injection of the lipid-soluble contrast agent lipiodol. **B**, The upper end of a gastric cardia tumor (at the esophagogastric junction) is injected. **C**, Stent expansion and position can be confirmed endoscopically under direct vision.

both. Finally, pressure necrosis caused by the proximal edge of a previously placed metal stent sporadically results in the development of a fistula. Treatment of a fistula should be expeditious because fistula formation is a life-threatening complication, which in the case of esophagorespiratory fistulas can result in serious pulmonary infections from aspiration pneumonia.

Esophagorespiratory Fistulas

A history of repeated coughing associated with drinking, eating, or both in combination with worsening dysphagia and dyspnea is highly suggestive of an esophagorespiratory fistula. The fistula can be diagnosed radiographically or endoscopically. Curative resection is usually impossible because of the concomitant presence of an advanced tumor stage; palliative surgery (including a combination of cervical esophagostomy and feeding gastrostomy or a bypass operation) is associated with a mortality rate of up to 50%.[76]

Until the early 1990s, cuffed prosthetic tubes were used to seal esophagorespiratory fistulas.[77] These devices were effective in 60% to 90% of patients. However, cuffed endoprostheses were associated with a complication rate that was comparable to conventional prosthetic tubes. An additional disadvantage of these devices was that the cuff of the tube migrated through the lumen of the fistula into the bronchial lumen in 25% of patients, causing acute respiratory distress.[78]

At the present time, endoscopic placement of a covered self-expanding metal stent is the treatment of choice for an esophagorespiratory fistula (**Figs. 28.7 and 28.8**). Several retrospective and prospective series have been published reporting the outcome of endoscopic placement of a covered metal stent for this indication (**Table 28.5**).[79–89] In most of these publications, complete sealing of the fistula was established in

more than 90% of patients with no clear difference between the presently available covered metal stents. Dysphagia scores improved significantly in most patients. The complication rate (early and late complications) ranged from 10% to 30%, whereas recurrent dysphagia was mainly the result of tumor overgrowth or stent migration. The median survival was poor and ranged from 35 to 148 days, which likely reflects the advanced tumor stage in most of these patients.

Symptoms from esophagorespiratory fistulas can be treated successfully with one of the presently available covered metal stents. Although studies have not been performed, it can be anticipated that the quality of life in patients with an esophagorespiratory fistula will be improved with this treatment.

Parallel Stent Placement

In some patients with esophageal cancers that infiltrate into the trachea, dysphagia and dyspnea may develop simultaneously. In some cases, placement of a metal stent in the esophagus to seal a fistula can result in obstruction of the trachea and acute dyspnea. In these circumstances, it is important to consider the placement of a stent in the trachea or bronchi or both in combination with an esophageal stent. Tracheobronchial stents that are placed in the trachea used to be uncovered[90] but presently at least partially or fully embed themselves in the mucosa of the respiratory tract.[91] These stents are uncovered because this decreases the risk that the stent will migrate distally leading to acute respiratory distress. Another indication for parallel stent placement is a tracheoesophageal fistula near the upper esophageal sphincter. Esophageal stents alone are not always effective in sealing the fistula at this location. Placement of a covered stent in the proximal part of the trachea in addition to a proximal esophageal stent may be considered.[79] Complications occur more commonly with parallel stent placement. Fatal complications such as perforation

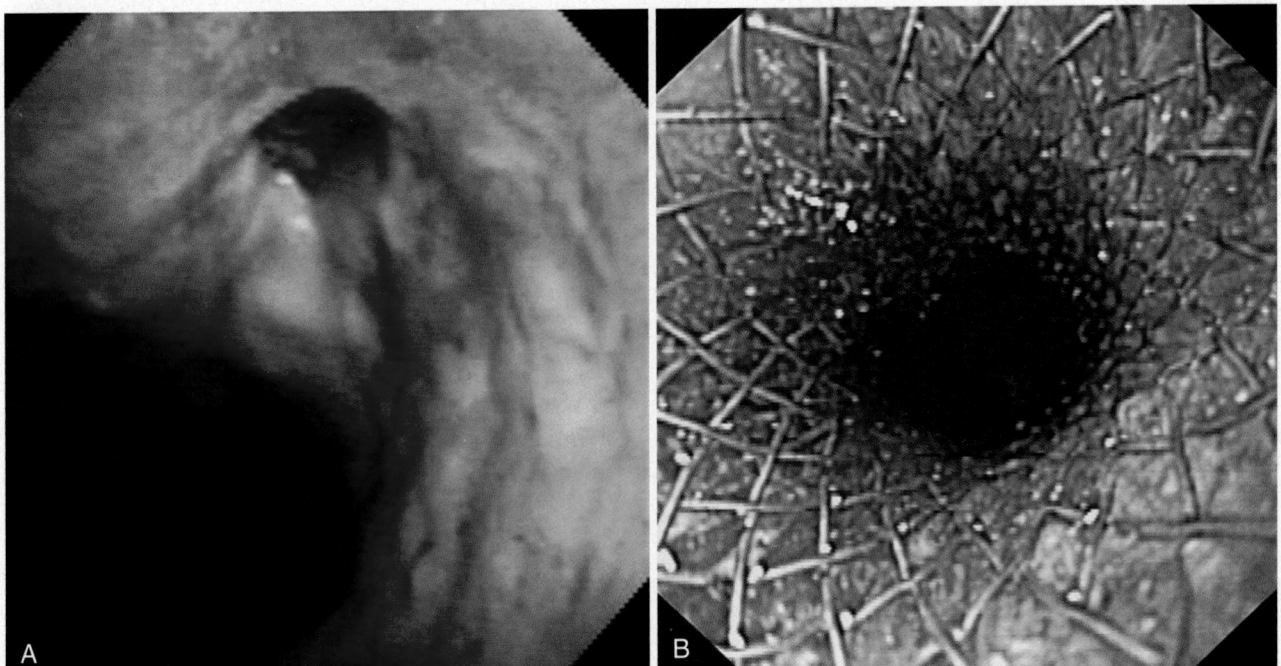

Fig. 28.7 A, Endoscopic view with a small-caliber endoscope of an esophagorespiratory fistula in the midesophagus caused by metastatic bronchogenic carcinoma. **B,** Partially covered Ultraflex stent was placed to seal the fistula (picture taken with a normal-caliber endoscope).

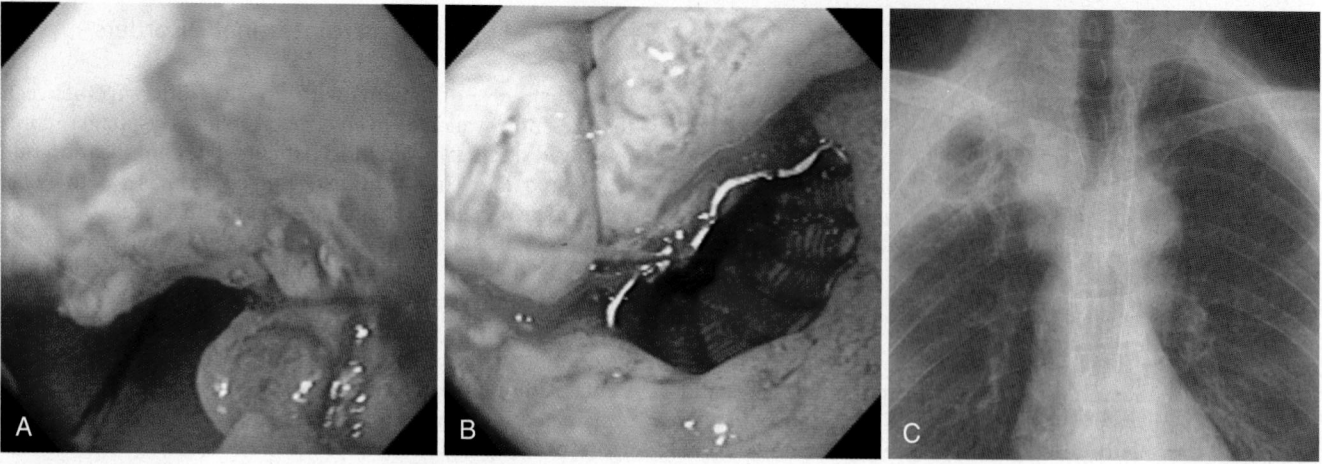

Fig. 28.8 A, Endoscopic view of squamous cell carcinoma in the proximal esophagus just below the upper esophageal sphincter. **B,** Ultraflex stent was placed just below the upper esophageal sphincter. **C,** Chest radiograph shows Ultraflex stent in the proximal esophagus.

Table 28.5 Studies Reporting the Outcome of Placement of a Covered Metal Stent for Esophagorespiratory Fistulas: Summary of Published Studies

Reference	No. Patients	Stent Type	Complete Sealing	Dysphagia Improvement	Early Major Complications	Late Major Complications	Recurrent Dysphagia	Median Survival
Do et al, 1993[79]	8	Z-stent	8/8 (100%)	? → 1.3	0	1/8 (13%)	0	Mean ~10 wk
Bethge et al, 1995[80]	6	Wallstent	6/6 (100%)	4 → 1.2	1/6 (17%)	1/6 (17%)	0	64 days
Kozarek et al, 1996[81]*	11	Z-stent	8/11 (73%)	?	?	?	?	?
Morgan et al, 1997[82]	39	Wallstent (n = 36)	37/39 (95%)	3 → 1	6/39 (15%)	5/39 (13%)	4/39 (10%)	81 days
		Z-stent (n = 3)	(10 patients, 2 stents)					
Nelson et al, 1997[83]	8	Wallstent	7/8 (88%)	5 → 3.2 (1–6 scale)	0	?	5/8 (63%)	59 days
Low et al, 1998[84]	13 (plastic)	Cook/ Atkinson (n = 13)	10/13 (77%)	3.2 → 0.2	7/13 (54%)	?	3/13 (23%)	1.1 mo
	12 (metal)	Wallstent/ Z-stent (n = 12)	11/12 (92%)	2.5 → 0.8	2/12 (17%)	?	5/12 (42%)	3.1 mo
May et al, 1998[85]	11	Z-stent	10/11 (91%)	3 → 0.6	0	1/11 (9%)	1/11 (9%)	121 days
Raijman et al, 1998[86]	13	Wallstent	13/13 (100%)	?	?	?	?	?
Dumonceau et al, 1999[87]	17	Wallstent/ Z-stent (n = 5)	1/5 (20%)	2 → 0	2/17 (12%)	1/17 (6%)	6/17 (35%)	98 days
		Ultraflex (n = 12)	12/12 (100%)	3.1 → 0.6	?	?	?	146 days
Siersema et al, 2001[88]	16	Z-stent (n = 11)	16/16 (100%)	?	1/16 (6%)	2/16 (13%)	6/16 (38%)	58 days
		Ultraflex (n = 5)	(2 patients, 2 stents)					
Abadal et al, 2001[89]	15	Z-stent (n = 4)	14/15 (93%)	3.4 → ?	0	2/15 (13%)	3/15 (20%)	148 days
		Wallstent (n = 9)						
		Ultraflex (n = 2)						

*Publication on metal stent placement for malignant dysphagia and fistulas; outcome data of fistulas were not separately presented.

and bleeding have been described, caused by tissue necrosis resulting from the high radial force exercised by both stents.[92]

PROXIMAL ESOPHAGEAL CARCINOMA

Endoscopic intubation has traditionally been contraindicated for malignancies within a few centimeters below the upper esophageal sphincter because of the risk of foreign body sensation, tracheal compression, and proximal migration of the prosthesis into the hypopharynx. However, positive results have been reported in studies on palliation of proximal lesions with metal stents.[59,88,93–96] The results are summarized in **Table 28.6**. The largest study comes from our institution. We evaluated 104 patients with dysphagia from a malignant stricture close to the upper esophageal sphincter.[96] Patients had primary esophageal carcinoma ($n = 66$) or recurrent cancer after gastric tube interposition ($n = 38$) within 8 cm distal of the upper esophageal sphincter. A tracheoesophageal fistula was also present in 24 (23%) patients. The mean distance from the upper esophageal sphincter to the upper tumor margin was 4.9 ± 2.6 cm and to the upper stent margin was 3.1 ± 2.3 cm.

The procedure was technically successful in 100 of 104 (96%) patients. Fistula sealing was achieved in 19 of 24 (79%) patients. After 4 weeks, dysphagia had improved from a median score of 3 (liquids only) to 1 (some difficulties with solids). Total complications were seen in 34 of 104 (33%) patients. Of these, major complications (aspiration pneumonia [$n = 9$], hemorrhage [$n = 8$], fistula [$n = 7$], and perforation [$n = 2$]) occurred in 22 (21%) patients; pain after stent

Table 28.6 Placement of a Metal Stent for Proximal Esophageal Carcinoma: Summary of Published Studies

Reference	No. Patients	Stent Type	Dysphagia Improvement	Complications (Early and Late) and Recurrent Dysphagia
Bethge et al, 1997[93]	8	Ultraflex ($n = 2$)	$3.5 \rightarrow 1.6$	1/8 distal stent migration
		Wallstent ($n = 6$)		1/8 tumor overgrowth
				2/8 fistula formation
Conio et al, 1999[94]	6	Ultraflex	$3.5 \rightarrow 0.8$	3/6 insufficient expansion of stent
				1/6 cervical pain
				4/6 tumor overgrowth
Macdonald et al, 2000[95]	22	Metal stent	$3 \rightarrow 2$	2/22 technical failure
				4/22 foreign body sensation
Siersema et al, 2001[88]	10	Ultraflex ($n = 6$)	$3.6 \rightarrow 1.9$	1/10 insufficient expansion of stent
		Z-stent ($n = 4$)		1/10 perforation
				1/10 aspiration pneumonia
				2/10 tumor overgrowth
Profili et al, 2002[96]	10	Ultraflex	$3.6 \rightarrow 1.5$	2/10 interference with swallowing
				1/10 too distally placed stent
				1/10 food impaction
				1/10 stent twisting
				4/10 tumor ingrowth
Verschuur et al[97]	104	Ultraflex ($n = 50$)		*Major complications* (21%)
		Z-stent ($n = 28$)		9/102 aspiration pneumonia
		Flamingo Wallstent ($n = 15$)		8/102 hemorrhage
		Other ($n = 11$)*		2/102 perforation
				Minor complications (15%)
				16/102 some pain after stent placement
				Recurrent dysphagia (28%)
				10/102 tissue ingrowth or overgrowth
				7/102 food bolus obstruction
				3/102 stent migration
				11/102 other reasons
				8/102 globus sensation (8%)

*Some patients had more than one stent placed.

placement was observed in 16 (15%) patients. Recurrent dysphagia occurred in 29 (28%) patients. Eight (8%) patients complained of globus sensation; however, stent removal was not indicated in any of the patients. It was concluded that stent placement is safe and effective in patients with a malignant stricture close to the upper esophageal sphincter.

Stent characteristics are an important consideration in the treatment of cancers that are located in the cervical esophagus. First, in our opinion, metal stents should not shorten or minimally shorten to ensure exact placement just below the upper esophageal sphincter. Second, the stent should be covered to prevent tumor ingrowth and to seal any coexisting fistula. Finally, the stent should have a body diameter of 18 mm or less, and, most important, the stent should be flexible to avoid globus sensation and tracheal compression. Although such a stent is unavailable, the Ultraflex stent and the Alimaxx-E are probably the stent types that are most preferable in this situation (see **Fig. 28.8**). Other methods for the palliation of malignant strictures near the upper esophageal sphincter include radiation therapy with or without chemotherapy if the patient is fit enough to undergo a more intensive treatment or laser treatment. In case of failure of these treatments or a poor general condition of the patient, a nasoduodenal feeding tube and placement of a percutaneous endoscopic gastrostomy (PEG) are the safest options.

EXTRINSIC COMPRESSION

A specific problem is dysphagia caused by extraesophageal malignancies that compress the esophagus. The origins of these malignancies are diverse, ranging from bronchogenic carcinoma to metastatic breast cancer, although most are caused by pulmonary malignancies. These patients are mostly unsuitable for curative therapy and need rapid relief of dysphagia to improve nutritional status. Palliative treatment options include radiation therapy, chemotherapy, combined chemoradiation, and metal stent placement. The effect of radiation therapy or chemotherapy is often too slow in these patients with only a short life expectancy.

The experience with metal stents for palliation of dysphagia resulting from extrinsic compression is limited (**Table 28.7**).[98-101] In a nonrandomized study, the safety and efficacy of stents for extrinsic compression (n = 24) were compared with stents for primary esophageal malignancies (n = 21).[100] Dysphagia scores improved significantly in both groups; however, the improvement was significantly greater in patients with primary esophageal tumors (P = .012). The frequency of complications was comparable between both groups. Two other studies described the results of metal stent placement for extrinsic compression in 13 patients and 17 patients.[98,101] These studies both concluded that dysphagia caused by extraesophageal malignancies can safely and effectively be treated with metal stents. In addition, there is no evidence that uncovered metal stents give better results than covered stents (**Figs. 28.9 and 28.10**). A characteristic of extrinsic compression is that the lesion is often irregular and noncircumferential. Because these tumors are often solid, stent deployment sometimes may take more than 24 to 48 hours. In addition, there is no tumor tissue in the esophageal lumen to fix the stent. Despite these unfavorable tumor characteristics, stent migration rate in these studies was comparable to that of stents for primary esophageal carcinoma. With regard to stent

choice, there is a preference for flexible stent types, such as the Ultraflex stent and Alimaxx-E stent, which both tend to adjust to the asymmetric anatomy of the esophagus in case of extrinsic compression.

RECURRENT DYSPHAGIA AFTER PREVIOUS SURGERY

Surgery is generally considered to offer the best chance for cure in patients with esophageal carcinoma; however, locoregional or systemic tumor recurrence occurs often in these patients. A few studies have been published in which metal stents were used to improve dysphagia resulting from tumor recurrence after esophagectomy.[88,102-104] In our institution, 21 patients with recurrent tumor after esophagectomy were treated; the tumor was located in 10 patients in the proximal part of the gastric tube interposition (including the anastomosis) and in 11 patients in the midportion or distal portion of the interposition. In most of these patients, a large-diameter metal stent was used to cover the dilated lumen of the neo-esophagus effectively (see **Fig. 28.10**). Dysphagia improved from a mean of 3.2 (able to drink fluids only) to 1.5 (dysphagia for some solids), and median survival was 63 days. Major complications occurred in 4 of 21 (19%) patients, consisting of bleeding (n = 2), fistula formation (n = 1), and severe pain (n = 1). Recurrent dysphagia occurred in 8 of 21 (38%) patients and was due to tumor overgrowth.[88] In case of recurrent cancer in a gastric tube interposition, it is preferred to use a large-diameter stent because the lumen above the stricture is often dilated owing to the gastric tube.

Dysphagia caused by recurrent tumor after partial or total gastrectomy presents specific problems because there is often complete luminal obstruction or sharp angulation of the luminal axis or both. We treated 10 patients with recurrent carcinoma after partial (n = 4) or total (n = 6) gastrectomy with a small-diameter Ultraflex stent or Z-stent. Dysphagia improved substantially, and median survival was 64 days. Complications occurred in 5 of 10 patients and consisted of perforation (n = 1), bleeding (n = 1), and pain (n = 3).[88] Pain after stent placement generally is a problem following stent placement in a stenotic gastrojejunostomy. For that reason, we prefer stents with a low to moderate radial force (i.e., Ultraflex, Alimaxx-E, Niti-S, or Evolution). Although experience is limited, metal stent placement can be used for palliation of dysphagia from tumor recurrence after esophagectomy or gastrectomy.

EFFECT OF PRIOR RADIATION AND CHEMOTHERAPY ON OUTCOME OF STENT PLACEMENT

It has been suggested that prior radiation or chemotherapy or both increase the risk of complications after placement of a self-expanding metal stent in patients with inoperable cancer of the esophagus and GEJ; however, this relationship is controversial. Nine studies addressed this question.[44,102,105-111] Four studies showed an increased risk for the development of complications after prior chemoradiation therapy,[44,102,105-110] and five studies did not find such a relationship.[106-109,111] The results of these studies are summarized in **Table 28.8**. In a study with 200 prospectively followed patients from our institution, it

Table 28.7 Metal Stent Placement for Palliation of Dysphagia Caused by Extrinsic Compression of Extraesophageal Malignancies: Summary of Published Studies

Reference	No Patients	Tumor	Stent Type	Mean Dysphagia Improvement	Early Complications	Late Complications	Mean Survival
De Gregorio et al, 1996[98]	13	Lung (n = 9)	Cov. Z-stent	3.2 → 0.6	4/13	2/13	2.2 mo
		Breast (n = 2)			Chest pain (n = 3)	Migration (n = 1)	
		Laryngeal (n = 1)			Migration (n = 1)	Benign stricture (n = 1)	
		Colon (n = 1)					
Kozarek et al, 1997[99]*	10	Lung (n = 6)	Cov. Z-stent	?	?	?	?
		Mesothelioma (n = 1)					
		Lymphoma (n = 1)					
		Mediastinal metastases (n = 2)					
Bethge et al, 1998[100]	24	Lung (n = 8)	Uncov. Wallstent (n = 21)	3.5 → 1.6	2/24	7/24	3 mo
		Recurrent gastric cancer (n = 10)	Uncov. Ultraflex (n = 2)		Migration (n = 1)	Fistula (n = 1)	
		Breast (n = 3)	Part. cov. Ultraflex (n = 1)		Stridor (n = 1)	Tumor ingrowth (n = 3)	
		Recurrent laryngeal cancer (n = 2)				Food bolus impaction (n = 3)	
		Thyroid (n = 1)					
Gupta et al, 1999[101]	17	Lung (n = 12)	Uncov. (n = 13)				
		Breast (n = 1)	Cov. (n = 6)				
		Larynx (n = 1)	(19 stents placed in 17 patients)	3.1 → 1.3	7/17	4/17	2.1 mo
		Melanoma (n = 1)			Pneumonia (n = 1)	Tumor overgrowth (n = 2)	
		Renal cell carcinoma (n = 1)			Migration during placement (n = 1)	Food bolus impaction (n = 2)	
		Unknown (n = 1)			Chest pain (n = 5)		

*Part of a larger patient group; no separate data are given.
Cov., covered; Part. cov., partially covered; Uncov., uncovered.

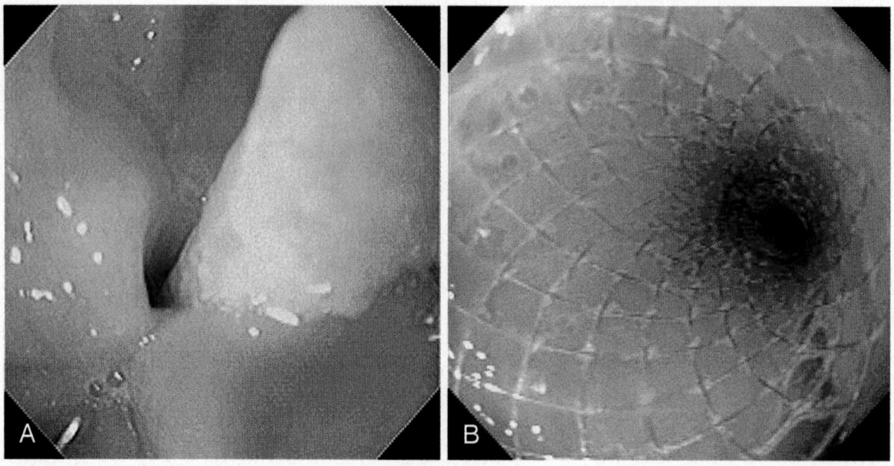

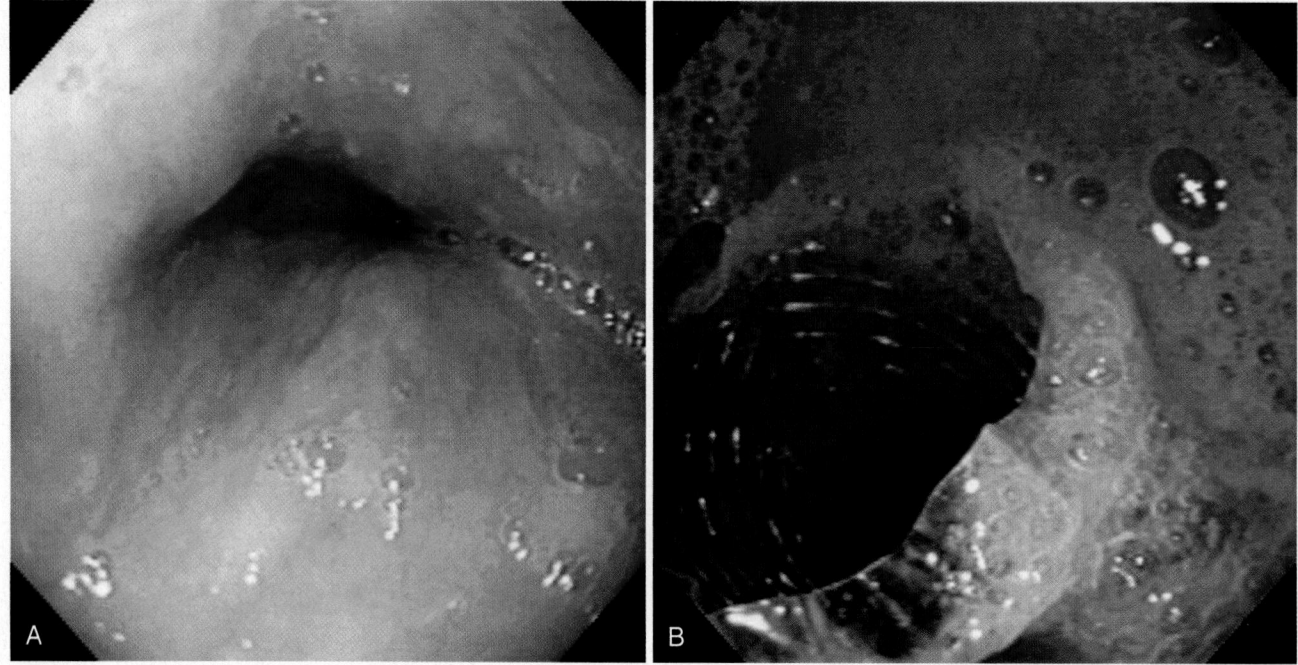

Fig. 28.9 **A**, Endoscopic view of extrinsic compression in the midesophagus resulting from metastatic breast cancer. **B**, A stent was placed. The stent has not completely deployed at 1 day after stent placement.

Fig. 28.10 **A**, Endoscopic view of extrinsic compression in the proximal esophagus after resection with gastric tube formation resulting from metastatic esophageal cancer. **B**, A large-diameter stent was placed.

was concluded that the incidence of complications and the outcome after placement of a self-expanding metal stent for carcinoma of the esophagus and GEJ were not affected by prior radiation or chemotherapy or both. Only retrosternal pain occurred more frequently in patients who had undergone prior chemoradiation.[111] Stent placement in patients with prior radiation or chemotherapy or both is probably as safe as in patients who have not undergone prior treatment; however, patients should be informed that there is an increased risk of chest pain after stent placement.

Limitations and Success Rate

The technical success rate for placement of metal stents is close to 100%. Limitations to successful placement include severe pain during placement; extensive tumor growth in the stomach;

failure of the stent to release from the introduction system, as can occur with Ultraflex stents; and immediate stent migration because the stent has been placed too deeply. Almost all patients experience improvement of dysphagia, and this is sustained unless and until a specific complication arises. The dysphagia grade usually improves from a mean of 3 (able to drink liquids only) to a mean of 1 (able to eat most solid foods), with no difference in effectiveness between the different available stent types (see **Table 28.2**), including the Ultraflex, the Wallstent, and the Z-stent. Some patients with advanced cancer at the distal esophagus or gastric cardia do not experience relief of dysphagia after technically successful stent placement because of other (unidentified) sites of intestinal obstruction, often peritoneal carcinomatosis, or gastric paresis resulting from neural involvement by the tumor. These patients usually require feeding through a nasoenteral tube or, preferably, a PEG.

Table 28.8 Effect of Prior Radiation or Chemotherapy (RTCT) on the Outcome of Stent Placement: Summary of Published Studies

Reference	No. Patients with and without Prior RTCT	Type of Study	Type of Stent	Life-Threatening Complications (Prior RTCT vs. No Treatment)
INCREASED RISK				
Kinsman et al, 1996[105]	Prior RTCT (n = 22)	Retrospective	Z-stent	8/22 (36%) vs. 1/37 (3%)
	No treatment (n = 37)			
Bethge et al, 1996[102]	Prior RTCT (n = 13)	Prospective	Wallstent	3/17 (18%)
	Prior surgery (n = 4)			
	No controls			
Siersema, 1998[44]	Prior RTCT (n = 28)	Prospective	Prosthetic tubes (n = 38)	12/28 (43%) vs. 8/47 (17%)*
	No treatment (n = 47)		Z-stent (n = 37)	
Muto et al, 2001[110]	Prior RTCT (n = 13)	Retrospective	Ultraflex (n = 9)	7/13 (54%)
	No controls		Wallstent (n = 2)	
			Z-stent (n = 2)	
NO DIFFERENCE				
Kozarek et al, 1996[106]	Prior RTCT (n = 27)	Retrospective	Z-stent (n = 26)	1/27 (4%) vs. 1/11 (9%)
	No treatment (n = 11)		Wallstent (n = 10)	
			Esophacoil/Ultraflex (n = 2)	
Nelson et al, 1997[107]	Prior RTCT (n = 6)	Retrospective	Wallstent	0/6 (0%)
	No/other treatment (n = 15)			
Raijman et al, 1997[108]	Prior RTCT (n = 39)	Retrospective	Wallstent	3/39 (8%) vs. 2/21 (10%)
	No treatment (n = 21)			
Bartelsman et al, 2000[109]	Prior RTCT (n = 54)	Retrospective	Song stent	No relationship (not further specified)
	No treatment (n = 99)			
Homs et al, 2004[111]	Prior RTCT (n = 49)	Prospective	Z-stent (n = 70)	14/49 (29%) vs. 31/151 (21%)†
	No treatment (n = 151)		Wallstent (n = 71)	
			Ultraflex (n = 59)	

*Device-related complications, most complications from prosthetic tubes (8/12 and 6/8).
†Stent-related complications.

Complications and Recurrent Dysphagia

Procedure-related complications after metal stent placement mainly consist of perforation, aspiration pneumonia, fever, bleeding, and severe pain and occur in 5% to 15% of patients. Delayed complications and recurrent dysphagia after stent placement include hemorrhage, fistula formation, gastroesophageal reflux, stent migration, tumor overgrowth or ingrowth, and food bolus obstruction and occur in 30% to 45% of patients. Minor complications are mild retrosternal pain and gastroesophageal reflux, which are reported by 10% to 20% of patients.

PERFORATION

Perforation is occasionally noted during or occurs after stent placement, sometimes owing to preceding dilation of an obstructing tumor to facilitate placement of the stent.

Perforation is treated conservatively including nasoduodenal tube feeding, keeping the patient nil per mouth, and antibiotics. Placement of a stent is the best option, which was already the original indication for the procedure. In some cases, a second stent to seal the perforation might be necessary. To start feeding shortly after the procedure, a contrast (water-based) swallow should be performed after stent placement to determine effective sealing of the perforation.

FEVER

Fever that occurs without evidence of aspiration pneumonia or perforation is most likely to be caused by a mechanical effect of the stent on the tumor, possibly by releasing toxic products from the tumor. Patients usually recover uneventfully after prophylactic treatment with antibiotics for 1 to 3 days. It is important to rule out another cause of fever, such as aspiration pneumonia or perforation.

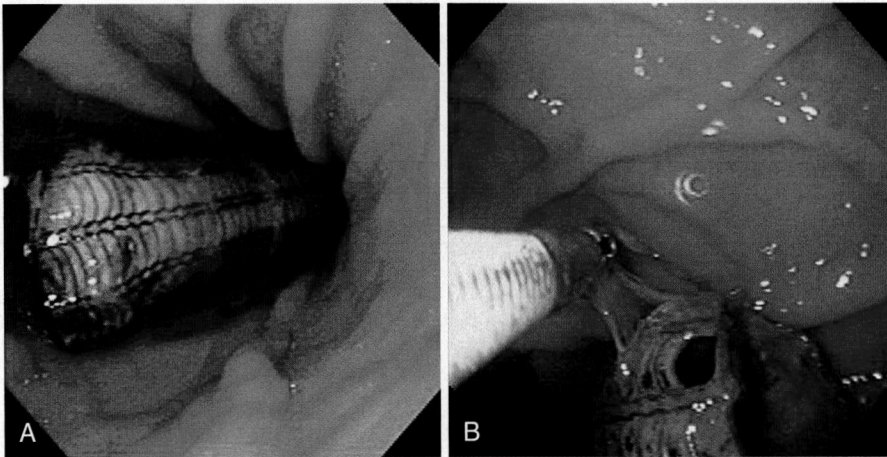

Fig. 28.11 Migration of an Ultraflex stent that occurred 2 months after placement. **A**, Migrated Ultraflex stent in the stomach. **B**, The lasso inside the proximal flange of the Ultraflex stent was grasped with a forceps. Subsequently, the stent was repositioned in the distal esophagus.

HEMORRHAGE

Hemorrhage, including hematemesis and melena, mostly occurs as a late complication of stent placement. It is often unclear whether bleeding is due to the stent placement or progression of the disease. In our experience, the latter is often the cause of the hemorrhage. During endoscopy, the precise source of blood loss is often not discovered. Treatment consists of blood transfusions in case of severe hemorrhage in combination with a short course of external beam radiation therapy (e.g., five sessions of 4 Gy).

RETROSTERNAL PAIN

Transient retrosternal pain is a frequently reported complication after stent placement, particularly after prior radiation or chemotherapy or both. Golder and coworkers[112] recorded the daily opioid analgesic requirements of 52 patients from 3 days before until 7 days after stent placement. Of patients, 26 (50%) needed opioid analgesia for chest pain within 48 hours of the procedure compared with 11 (21.2%) before stent placement. This difference was statistically significant ($P < .001$). In other studies, figures ranging from 5% to 50% for chest pain after stent placement have been reported.* In our experience, mild retrosternal pain after stent placement can be treated effectively with acetaminophen or a nonsteroidal anti-inflammatory drug. Rarely, new opioid analgesics are indicated for a few days to a maximum of 14 days. Severe pain after stent placement occurs in 1% to 2% of patients. In these patients, removal of the stent is sometimes indicated to relieve the pain.

GASTROESOPHAGEAL REFLUX

Gastroesophageal reflux is a common problem, occurring in 10% to 20% of patients with distally located tumors where the distal end of the stent is placed through the lower esophageal sphincter.† The management of gastroesophageal reflux has already been discussed in the section on metal stents for tumors of the GEJ. As a preventive measure, PPIs are pre-

scribed to many patients with a stent passing the lower esophageal sphincter. Metal stents with an antireflux mechanism have been developed to prevent gastroesophageal reflux. At the distal end of the stent, the cover of the stent is extended beyond the lower metal cage to form a windsock-type valve (see **Fig. 28.5**).

STENT MIGRATION

Stent migration is a common complication with reported incidence rates ranging from 5% to 15%.* The most frequently used method for reintervention after stent migration is placement of a second stent. In certain cases, repositioning of a distally migrated stent is possible with the use of a forceps or a snare[116] or by placing the endoscope in a retroflexed position.[117,118] We do not recommend using the latter technique because esophageal perforation may occur. In addition, this method may result in damage to the endoscope.[118] If repeated episodes of stent migration occur in the same patient, other palliative treatments, such as brachytherapy, photodynamic therapy (PDT), argon plasma coagulation therapy, cryoablation therapy, or laser therapy, need to be considered.

Based on our own experience and that of others,[115] retrieval after migration is often not indicated because perforation or obstruction of the digestive tract is uncommon. If a migrated stent causes obstruction of the pylorus or symptoms of pain or if successful placement of a second stent is impossible, the stent should be removed. Several methods of stent retrieval have been described. In case of an Ultraflex stent with a lasso at the proximal end, this can be done by collapsing the stent with a grasping forceps using the lasso suture attached to the proximal flange of the stent (**Fig. 28.11**). The most frequently used described method is by decreasing the diameter of the stent with a polypectomy snare at 2 to 5 cm from the proximal end of the stent.[109,120] Other investigators have used a biopsy forceps in combination with a snare, which requires passage of a double-channel therapeutic endoscope.[121] Apart from a snare, one can use Endoloops, which may have a greater constriction force than a polypectomy snare.[122]

---

*References 48, 56, 57, 59, 97, 112.
†References 48, 56, 57, 59, 97, 113, 114.

---

*References 48, 56, 59, 113–115.

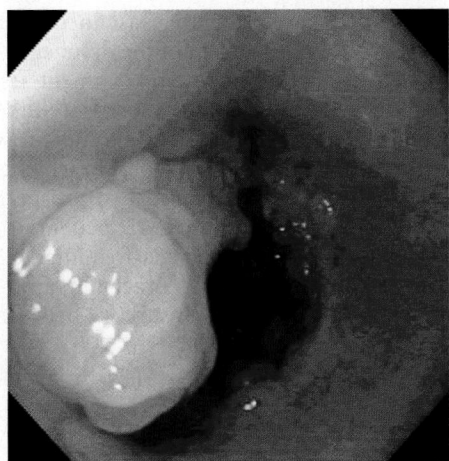

Fig. 28.12 Endoscopic view of tumor overgrowth at the proximal end of the stent.

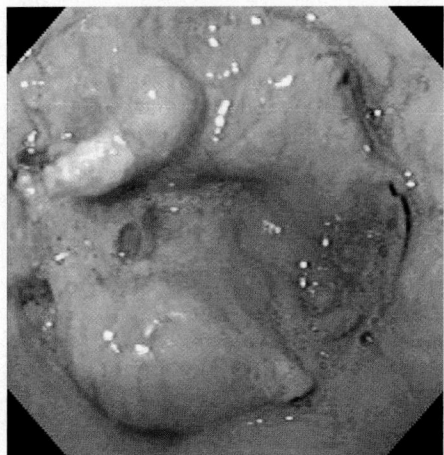

Fig. 28.14 Endoscopic view of food bolus obstruction in the lumen of the stent.

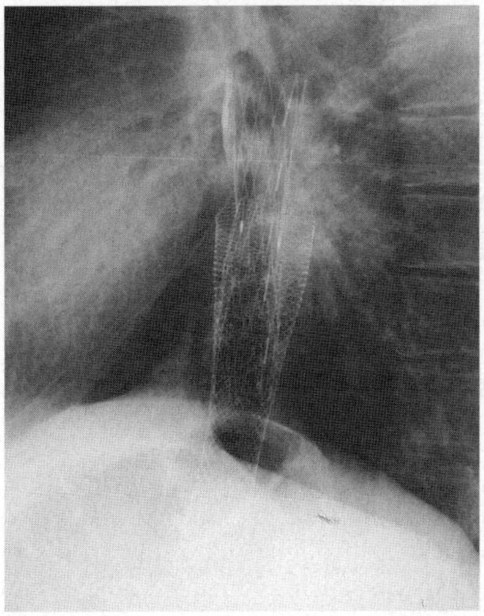

Fig. 28.13 Plain radiograph of the abdomen showing a stent in the distal esophagus and proximal stomach placed for inoperable carcinoma of the gastric cardia. After 3 months, a second stent was placed for tumor overgrowth at the proximal end of the stent.

TUMOR INGROWTH OR OVERGROWTH

Tumor ingrowth or overgrowth is often the result of progression of the malignancy rather than a failure or a complication of the stent. It affects both ends of the stent at a similar rate and is seen in 10% to 20% of patients after a mean period of 2 to 4 months after stent placement (**Fig. 28.12**).* Tumor ingrowth or overgrowth can be reduced by inserting a stent that is, after expansion, approximately 2 to 4 cm longer than the malignant stricture to allow for a 1- to 2-cm extension above the proximal and below the distal end of the tumor.

The most frequently used method to treat tumor overgrowth is placement of a second stent. In addition, laser therapy or argon plasma coagulation can be used to debulk the tumor. In case of placement of a second stent, the stent is placed proximal or distal to the previously placed stent with a part of the second stent overlapping the primary stent (**Fig. 28.13**).

In our experience, another important cause of recurrent dysphagia is nonmalignant obstructive tissue, such as granulation tissue, reactive hyperplasia, and fibrosis at the proximal or distal end of the stent. The pathogenesis of nonmalignant tissue ingrowth or overgrowth has already been discussed in the section on metal stents for tumors of the GEJ, and nonmalignant tissue ingrowth or overgrowth is an unlikely event. Mayoral and colleagues[60] reported this cause of recurrent dysphagia in more than 30% of their patients at a mean interval of 22 weeks after stent placement. We observed the development of this nonmalignant tissue in many patients undergoing endoscopy for reasons other than recurrent dysphagia. It was predominantly found at the proximal end of the stent but did not seem to cause dysphagia. It can also be treated by placing a second, partially overlapping stent.

OTHER CAUSES OF RECURRENT DYSPHAGIA

Food bolus obstruction is common with reported rates of 5% to 15% (**Fig. 28.14**).* It can be treated successfully by endoscopic stent clearance. However, care should be taken to prevent the stent from migrating while doing this. Prevention of food bolus obstruction can be achieved by providing eating instruction, including chewing the food thoroughly and drinking carbonated drinks during and after a meal.

Laser Therapy
Thermal Therapy

Treatment of obstructing esophageal cancer with the high-power neodymium:yttrium-aluminum-garnet (Nd:YAG) laser was first described in 1982.[123] Over the years, the procedure has become an accepted and effective method for palliation of malignant dysphagia. Early investigators used an anterograde technique; a retrograde approach with initial dilation is preferred at the present time.[124] Tumors that are relatively short (<6 cm), nonangulated, exophytic, noncircumferential, and located in the midesophagus or distal esophagus are most amenable to laser ablation. Laser treatment is unsafe for

*References 48, 56, 57, 59, 97, 113, 114.

*References 48, 56, 57, 59, 97, 113, 114.

submucosal tumors, tumors causing extrinsic compression, and angulated tumors, whereas circumferential tumors are vulnerable to stricture formation. In various studies, technical success was around 90%, and functional success was approximately 70%.[125–129] Depending on the length of follow-up, recurrent dysphagia occurs in 40% to 60% of patients 4 to 10 weeks after initial treatment. Patients are usually reassessed at 4- to 6-week intervals. Complications include perforation, fistula formation, hemorrhage, and sepsis in 5% to 10% of patients.

Photodynamic Therapy

PDT involves the local destruction of tumor tissue by light of a specific wavelength activating a previously administered photosensitizer that is retained in malignant tissue. Porphyrin compounds, such as porfimer sodium (Photofrin), have been the most commonly used photosensitizers for the palliation of malignant dysphagia. As opposed to the thermal destruction induced by the Nd:YAG laser, the damage by PDT is initiated by a photochemical effect. PDT may be useful for long tumors, for tumors that are narrow or angulated, and for flat infiltrating tumors. The costs of PDT are high because of the high costs of a special laser unit and the costs of the photosensitizer Photofrin.[130]

The most frequent complication of PDT is prolonged skin photosensitivity. Patients must avoid direct sunlight for at least 6 weeks after treatment. Major complications, including perforation, fistula formation, and strictures, have been reported in 30% of patients. Other side effects include fever, chest pain, and pleural effusion, probably secondary to a transient, local inflammation, but these side effects are usually mild.[131–135]

Clinical experience with PDT for palliation of malignant dysphagia is limited to a few centers worldwide. One or two treatment sessions are usually required for an adequate tumor response. PDT is considered technically easier and less operator-dependent than Nd:YAG laser ablation. Two randomized trials compared PDT with Nd:YAG laser therapy.[134,135] Lightdale and coworkers[134] found equivalent improvements in dysphagia score with a trend toward an improved response with PDT in patients with tumors located in the upper third or lower third of the esophagus, in patients with long (>10 cm) tumors, and in patients who had prior chemotherapy or radiation therapy or both. Complications were similar in both treatment groups, but side effects (i.e., skin photosensitivity, nausea, and transient fever) occurred more often after PDT. Heier and colleagues[135] found an improved performance status and a longer duration of response (84 days vs. 57 days) after PDT compared with laser therapy, with similar functional results and complication rates. Because of the high costs of the treatment, the side effects, and the necessity of repeated treatments every 8 weeks, PDT as a sole treatment is not an optimal treatment for palliation of malignant dysphagia.

Laser Therapy in Combination with Brachytherapy

It has been suggested that thermal laser therapy in combination with brachytherapy (intraluminal radiotherapy) should be able to increase the long-term effectiveness of laser therapy. First, laser therapy should be applied to reduce the tumor bulk, followed by a single treatment of brachytherapy with a maximum dose of 10 Gy, leading to a sustained effect of laser therapy with a better improvement of the dysphagia score and a reduction in the need for repeated treatment sessions. In four nonrandomized studies, laser therapy (Nd:YAG) plus brachytherapy was studied prospectively and proved to be safe and effective.[136–139] Laser therapy plus brachytherapy was compared with laser therapy alone in two prospective, randomized trials in 39 patients and 22 patients.[140,141] Both studies showed a prolonged dysphagia-free interval after the combination of laser therapy and brachytherapy; however, this did not result in a difference in survival between the two treatment groups.

Laser Therapy versus Stent Placement

Two nonrandomized studies[142,143] and two randomized trials compared laser treatment with stent placement.[129,144] Both nonrandomized trials concluded that laser therapy was a safer treatment than stent placement with a similar effectiveness. Dallal and coworkers[129] compared laser treatment (mostly Nd:YAG) with metal stents in 65 patients with esophageal carcinoma in a randomized trial. Median survival was longer for the laser group, but relief of dysphagia was disappointing in both groups with similar complication rates and costs. Adam and colleagues[144] randomly assigned 60 patients to laser therapy, uncovered stent placement, or covered stent placement and concluded that stent placement was more effective for the palliation of malignant dysphagia.

Other Endoscopic Methods
Dilation (Repeat)

Dilation can relieve dysphagia temporarily, but it provides palliation often for only a few days to 2 weeks. It is frequently used to allow access through the tumor for different forms of palliative treatments, such as metal stent placement or laser therapy. Dilation is a simple and cheap modality; however, complications, including perforation and hemorrhage, are common.[145–147]

Some authors advocate dilation of the malignant stricture gradually over several sessions before stent placement to reduce the risk of complications.[42,147] The most commonly used dilators are polyvinyl wire-guided bougies, including tapered dilators (Savary), rubber dilators (Maloney), and through-the-scope hydrostatic balloons. There is as yet no study comparing these dilators in patients with malignant strictures. Because dilation as a sole therapy must be repeated at frequent intervals, it should be performed only in extremely ill patients with a very short life span.

Ablative Therapies

Ablative therapies, such as PDT, argon plasma coagulation, and cryoablation therapy, can be used as an alternative to nonendoscopic techniques or stent placement. In most cases, ablative therapies are used as an initial treatment before radiation therapy, chemotherapy or a combination of these because it takes some weeks before an effect of these treatments is actually seen. Alternatively, argon plasma coagulation is sometimes used to treat tissue overgrowth after stent placement. A disadvantage of ablative methods is that their effect lasts only for a few weeks because tumor regrowth occurs in most cases.

Chemical Injection Therapy

Chemical injection therapy for the treatment of malignant dysphagia is an inexpensive alternative requiring no special equipment. Ethanol or polidocanol in aliquots of 0.5 to 1 mL is injected into the tumor, leading to tumor necrosis within several days after therapy. Exophytic tumors are most amenable to injection therapy, whereas firm and fibrotic tumors (after radiation therapy) prove difficult to inject. Studies on injection therapy for malignant dysphagia are limited.[148–151] Dysphagia score improved from 3 (liquids only) to 1 (some difficulties with solid foods). Complications are rare; only fistula formation ($n = 2$), perforation ($n = 1$), and mediastinitis ($n = 1$) have been reported.[149,150] Generally, two sessions were necessary to obtain a maximum effect, and retreatment was necessary at 4- to 5-week intervals. A comparative study in 34 patients between injection therapy with polidocanol and Nd:YAG laser therapy concluded that both techniques were safe and equally effectively for the palliation of malignant dysphagia.[149]

Nutritional Support

In case of failure of different palliative therapies or if other palliative modalities are technically impossible, nutritional support to maintain an adequate calorie intake should be considered. The overall condition and the prognosis of the patient are important factors to take into consideration before nutritional support is offered to the patient. Placement of a nasoenteral feeding tube is the easiest and least invasive feeding method; however, for patients with a longer life expectancy, placement of a PEG or percutaneous endoscopic jejunostomy is preferred. Rarely, central venous alimentation is indicated for maintaining or restoring an adequate nutritional status.[152]

Placement of a PEG using the classic pull method through a preexisting esophageal stent or in the presence of a malignant tumor can be problematic. In these cases, PEG placement without endoscopy using a nasogastric tube with gastric insufflation, fluoroscopic monitoring, and a direct percutaneous catheter insertion technique (push method) should be considered.[153] Adler and coworkers[154] described the results of nine patients undergoing classic PEG placement after stent placement and reported a good functional result and only one stent migration following PEG placement (11%).

Quality of Life

To evaluate the effectiveness of a palliative treatment modality, it is important not only to assess functional outcome and complications but also to assess the outcome from the perspective of patients, particularly quality of life. The aim of palliative treatment of esophageal cancer is to relieve dysphagia with minimal morbidity and mortality and maximum quality of life.[155] Data on quality of life after palliative treatment for esophageal carcinoma are scarce. Validated measures that can be used to assess quality of life before and after treatment are the oncology-specific European Organization for Research and Treatment of Cancer (EORTC) QLQ-C30 questionnaire[156] and the esophageal carcinoma–specific EORTC OES-24 or OES-18 questionnaires.[157]

O'Hanlon and colleagues[158] investigated quality of life at 6 and 16 weeks after treatment in 43 patients undergoing intubation or radiation therapy. Although the dysphagia score improved significantly after treatment, none of the other parameters assessed were significantly improved at 16 weeks after treatment. Barr and Krasner[125] assessed quality of life after palliative Nd:YAG laser treatment for malignant dysphagia in 40 patients at monthly intervals. The linear-analogue self-assessment questionnaire, assessing 25 items on physical condition, psychological effects, and social interactions and a physician's assessment using a quality-of-life index consisting of a structured interview on specific items were performed. The patient's swallowing ability, the items on the linear-analogue self-assessment questionnaire, and the quality-of-life index all were improved at some time after laser therapy. Blazeby and colleagues[159] assessed quality of life in 37 patients after palliative treatment (intubation [$n = 30$] or palliative radiation or chemotherapy [$n = 7$]) and compared this with patients undergoing surgery for esophageal cancer using the EORTC QLQ C-30 questionnaire at 3-month intervals. Patients with palliative treatment reported worse baseline quality-of-life scores compared with patients undergoing surgery. However, following palliative treatment, most aspects of quality of life from the EORTC QLQ-C30 were maintained until death.

Our group investigated generic and disease-specific health-related quality of life (HRQoL) after palliative treatment (i.e., placement of a covered Ultraflex stent [$n = 108$] or single-dose [12 Gy] brachytherapy [$n = 101$]).[160] Longitudinal data on disease-specific (dysphagia score, EORTC OES-23, visual analogue pain scale) and generic (EORTC QLQ-C30, Euroqol [EQ]-5D) HRQoL were obtained by monthly home visits by a specially trained research nurse. Dysphagia improved more rapidly after stent placement than after brachytherapy, but long-term relief of dysphagia was better after brachytherapy. For generic HRQoL, there was an overall significant difference in favor of brachytherapy on four out of five functional scales of the EORTC QLQ-C30 (role, emotional, cognitive, and social). Generic HRQoL deteriorated over time on all functional scales of the EORTC QLQ C-30 and EQ-5D, in particular, physical and role functioning (on average -23 and -24 on a 100-point scale during 0.5 year of follow-up). This decline was more pronounced in the stent group. Major improvements were seen on the dysphagia and eating scales of the EORTC OES-23, in contrast to other scales of this disease-specific measure, which remained almost stable during follow-up. Reported levels of chest or abdominal pain remained stable during follow-up in both treatment groups, and general pain levels increased to a minor extent. It was concluded that the effects of single-dose brachytherapy on HRQoL compared favorably with the effects of stent placement for the palliation of esophageal cancer.

These studies indicate that more data are necessary on quality of life after palliative treatments and that comparisons between different palliative treatments are needed. Future studies on palliative care for esophageal cancer should at least include generic HRQoL scales because these were more responsive in measuring patients' functioning and well-being during follow-up than disease-specific HRQoL scales. The EORTC OES-24 questionnaire addresses issues that are relevant to patients undergoing palliative treatment for esophageal carcinoma and is probably a worthwhile tool in combination with the EORTC QLQ-C30 questionnaire and the dysphagia score for assessing quality of life after palliative treatment for malignant dysphagia.

Future Trends

Endoscopic treatments presently available for the palliation of malignant dysphagia are, as yet, not optimal in achieving fast and sustained dysphagia relief with minimal morbidity and mortality. Metal stents are reasonably effective in improving dysphagia; however, the complication rate and number of reinterventions necessary for recurrent dysphagia are still too high. Dilation and ablative therapies are short-lasting and are not without any complications. The disadvantage of laser treatment is the need for retreatment every 4 to 6 weeks, and expertise and expensive equipment are needed to perform the procedure.

It is anticipated that combination therapies might increase the efficacy of treatments, but these therapies are likely to increase the length of initial hospital stay or the frequency of hospital visits or both. Randomized controlled trials are warranted to compare different treatment modalities or to compare combination modalities with monotherapies, with special reference to dysphagia relief, complications, quality of life after treatment, and costs.

New types of stents are being developed and include biodegradable stents, stents with a radioactive coating, and drug-eluting stents. Biodegradable stents have been developed for benign stenoses[9,161]; however, a possible application could be the initial treatment of dysphagia in patients undergoing palliative chemotherapy. Because results of chemotherapy for this indication are improving,[162] stent migration is more likely to occur in patients with a good response to chemotherapy.

Other developments for malignant esophageal strictures include the incorporation of beta-emitting agents[163] and cytotoxic agents in esophageal stents, which may prevent recurrent tumor overgrowth at both ends of the stent.

References

The complete reference list is available online at www.expertconsult.com.

Nonepithelial Tumors of the Esophagus and Stomach

Nicholas Nickl

Video related to this chapter's topics can be found online at expertconsult.com.

Introduction

Neoplasms of nonepithelial origin, although uncommon, are lesions that a busy gastrointestinal (GI) endoscopist can expect to encounter with some regularity. Although the number of such pathologic entities is manageably small, the spectrum of clinical behavior manifested by these lesions spans from trivial to life-threatening. The difficulty in managing patients with such lesions is that the tumor originates from within the GI tract wall and often appears as a mass beneath otherwise normal mucosa. Encountering such a seemingly innocent façade behind which lurks a range of ominous possibilities, the GI endoscopist is challenged to use new diagnostic tools appropriately to direct the patient's care.

Epidemiology

The clinical starting point for patients with lesions of nonepithelial origin is the discovery of a mass impinging on the GI tract mucosa from beneath—the so-called submucosal tumor (**Fig. 29.1**). In its classic form, a discrete tumorous appearance is present with overlying mucosa that, although most commonly bland, may be erythematous, pale, dimpled, or ulcerated. Lesions are often initially identified at esophago-gastroduodenoscopy (EGD), but the patient may also be

referred to an endoscopist for evaluation of an abnormal radiograph (e.g., barium-contrast examination).

Applied literally, the term *submucosal* would imply the presence of an intramural mass originating in the submucosal layer of the GI wall. However, the term has come to be used for a range of lesions that create a similar appearance, including intramural and extramural structures. Such submucosal tumors may include both neoplastic and nonneoplastic masses, and even mucosal neoplasms have been reported to exhibit a submucosal appearance.[1] Examples of nonepithelial lesions in all four categories are listed in **Table 29.1**. This discussion centers on neoplasms that primarily originate from nonepithelial GI tract cell lines, but all types of pathology must be considered when developing a management plan.

Depending on the clinical circumstances and type of tumor, the lesion may cause symptoms such as bleeding, obstruction, or pain. However, such lesions commonly are serendipitously found during evaluation for a different, unrelated problem. Because most such lesions are asymptomatic, epidemiologic data are skewed by the nature of their discovery incidental to a different, usually unrelated condition. In one study of 15,104 EGD reports, submucosal tumors were identified in 0.36%.[2] Because most in this series were life-threatening tumors, the study database likely underreported less serious lesions. Many such lesions turn out to be normal extramural organs. Allgayer[3] found that among 30 patients referred for submucosal tumors, normal extramural structures were present in 14 (47%). Motoo and coworkers[4] also reported normal organs in 16 of 19 submucosal tumors, as did Caletti and colleagues[5] in 10 of 25 tumors; organs identified include the spleen, liver, splenic vessels, and pancreas.

Because submucosal tumors are often left in situ, the pathologic distribution among tumors is unknown. It is reported that 1% to 3% of resected gastric tumors are stromal cell tumors[6]; it can be inferred that the actual incidence, when including tumors that were not resected, is considerably higher. In a small prospective study,[7] among 45 submucosal tumors, most were found to have a benign appearance that required no follow-up. From these available data, it may be cautiously concluded that submucosal tumors are found in less than 1% of routine upper endoscopy examinations, half of such lesions are found to be normal extramural structures, most remaining lesions are benign, and stromal cell tumors constitute most such neoplasms.

Clinical Features

Lumps and bumps of all sorts are regularly encountered in endoscopic examinations; the decision regarding which to evaluate further depends on the endoscopic appearance, the clinical circumstances, and the inclination of the endoscopist. Because few standardized guidelines exist to direct such decisions, great variation in practice exists. Symptoms attributed to the mass nearly always drive further investigation, but our own endoscopic ultrasound (EUS) study of a subset of such lesions found that nearly 90% were asymptomatic.[8] GI bleeding may be seen in many submucosal lesions, most commonly in the form of slow blood loss causing iron deficiency anemia. The surface of the tumor may be ulcerated in such cases (**Fig. 29.2**). Malignant tumors may be more prone to ulceration and bleeding[9]; this might be taken as a sign of a potentially malignant form that compels definitive treatment. However, benign lesions may also cause severe bleeding,[10] and occasionally rapid hemorrhage may occur.[11] Less often, GI tract obstruction may be caused by such masses,[12] especially if the lesion is located in a narrow area such as the esophagogastric junction or pylorus; intussusception caused by such masses has been reported.[13] Pain may be a presenting complaint, especially if the submucosal tumor is neoplastic or malignant.[14]

Because most lesions are incidentally found during endoscopic examination for another problem, the clinical features of submucosal masses are primarily those that, in the

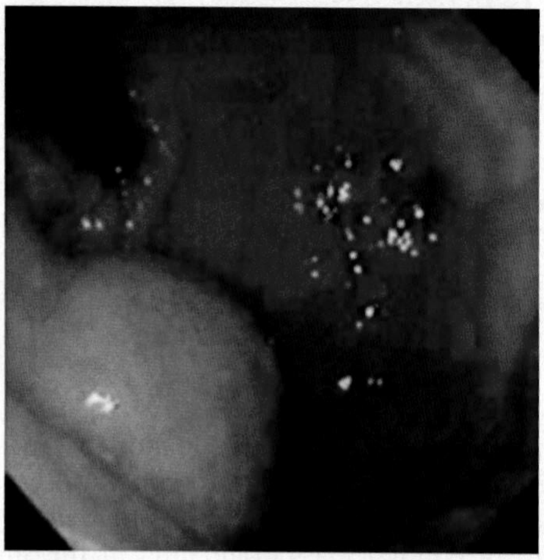

Fig. 29.1 Endoscopic view of medium-sized submucosal tumor (retroflexed view).

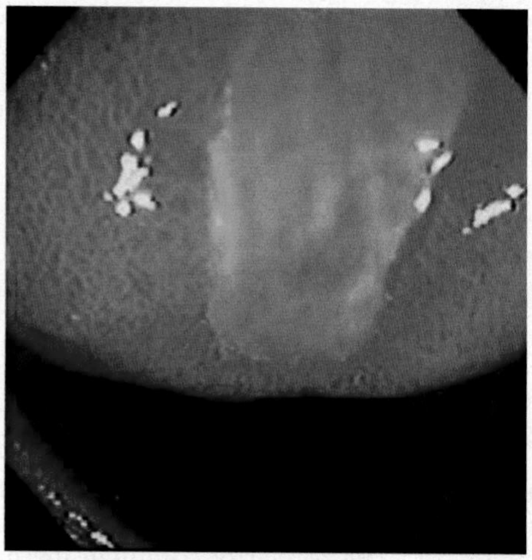

Fig. 29.2 Endoscopic view of duodenal lipoma with ulceration at tip.

Table 29.1 Types of Masses Causing Esophageal and Gastric Submucosal Tumors

	Neoplastic Masses	**Nonneoplastic Masses**
Intramural masses	Stromal cell tumor	Varices
	Lipoma	Duplication cyst
	Granular cell tumor	Inflammatory granuloma
	Lymphoma	Foreign body (e.g., surgical suture or clip)
	Fibrovascular polyp	Pancreatic rest
	Hemangioma/hemangiosarcoma	
	Lymphangioma/lymphangiosarcoma	
	Metastatic neoplasm	
Extramural masses	Primary neoplasm of adjacent organs (benign and malignant)	Benign lymph node
	Metastatic lymph node	Inflammatory mass of adjacent organs (e.g., pancreas, spleen)
		Organomegaly (e.g., spleen, liver)

endoscopist's opinion, compel further evaluation. Large size has been proposed as an ominous finding,[15] and lesions with an ulcerated or irregular (lumpy) surface often undergo additional testing or treatment. Patients with submucosal tumors who have a prior history of malignancy should receive further evaluation to exclude metastatic disease. Finally, patients with submucosal lesions that change appearance on serial examination are usually directed by an alert clinician to further testing.

Pathology

Extramural masses compose half of suspected submucosal tumors and include normal organs, nonneoplastic masses, and extramural neoplasms. Normal liver, spleen, pancreas, gallbladder, colon, and kidney all have been reported to appear as suspected submucosal tumors.[3-5] Vascular structures often produce the appearance of a discrete tumor, including normal vessels of the spleen[16] and abnormal vessels such as varices and aneurysms.[17] Neoplasms and nonneoplastic masses involving these same organs can also produce this appearance, as can such masses involving the peritoneum, mediastinum, and the lymph nodes adjacent to the upper GI tract. The various malignancies, cysts, and inflammatory masses of these structures need no further elaboration here because a large variety of such findings have been noted in the case report literature.

Masses that arise within the wall of the esophagus and stomach require further discussion, particularly because many are peculiar to the GI tract. Most neoplasms in this category are mesenchymal tumors, meaning that they arise from cells of mesodermal origin. Most such neoplasms are clinically benign, although, as shown subsequently, tumor histology may not provide reliable clues to malignant behavior. A large variety of such neoplasms have been described (**Table 29.2**), but most are exceedingly rare. The tumors most likely to be encountered in the esophagus and stomach in a routine clinical setting are discussed here.

Gastrointestinal Stromal Tumor

Most mesenchymal GI tumors are pale, firm, spherical, or ovoid structures embedded in the wall of the affected organ. The microscopic appearance of musclelike eosinophilic, spindle-shaped cells in uniform sheets and the proximity of the tumors to the muscular wall layers led early observers to believe that these tumors were of myogenic origin[18]—hence the name leiomyoma and its variations (e.g., leiomyosarcoma, leiomyoblastoma). However, it later became clear that these neoplasms not only are not of obvious myogenic origin but also often lack any specific markers of differentiation whatsoever.[19] Immunohistochemical analyses showed variable expression of smooth muscle features such as desmin and actin and neural proteins such as S-100.[20] For the sake of clarity, these lesions came to be referred to as gastrointestinal stromal tumors (GISTs), an acknowledgment that they originate in mesenchymal stroma.

A significant breakthrough occurred with the discovery that most GI stromal tumors stain positive for a specific membrane protein, designated CD117,[21] and subsequently identified as KIT, a tyrosine kinase receptor.[22] Tyrosine kinases are a class of transmembrane receptors that mediate various cellular growth functions. The extracellular portion of KIT binds stem

Table 29.2 Classification of Gastrointestinal Mesenchymal Tumors

Tumor Type	Examples
Stromal tumors	Smooth muscle tumors (leiomyoma, leiomyosarcoma), glomus tumors, leiomyomatosis, pleomorphic sarcoma
Neural tumors	Neuroma/neurofibroma, paraganglioma, ganglioneuromatosis
Endothelial and vascular tumors	Hemangioma, hemangiosarcoma, Kaposi's sarcoma, lymphangioma
Lipocytic tumors	Lipoma, liposarcoma, lipohyperplasia (ileocecal valve), lipomatosis (colon)
Granular cell tumor	Granular cell tumor
Inflammatory fibroid polyp	Inflammatory fibroid polyp
Fibrohistiocytic tumors	Fibrovascular polyp, fibrous histiocytoma, desmoid tumors (mesentery), fibroepithelial polyp
Striated muscle tumors	Rhabdomyosarcoma

Data from Lewin K, Riddel RH, Weinstein WM: Mesenchymal tumors. In: Gastrointestinal pathology and its clinical implications, New York, 1992, Igaku-Shoin, pp 284–341.

cell factor, causing a conformational change. The receptor subsequently forms a dimer with another activated KIT receptor, and the intracellular region of the resulting dimer triggers various cell signaling cascades.[23] Among these are proliferation pathways such as mitogen-activated protein kinase (MAPK) and signal transducers and activators of transcription (STAT) proteins as well as antiapoptotic mediators such as AKT (protein kinase B).[24] KIT and some other tyrosine kinases are important regulators of cell growth and proliferation.

Abnormal cell growth is a fundamental element of cancer physiology, and hyperfunction of the KIT receptor can lead to neoplasia. In this case, numerous gain-of-function mutations in the KIT gene have been described.[25] These acquired (or, rarely, inherited) mutations produce KIT receptors that are capable of initiating the aforementioned intracellular growth cascades without activation by stem cell factor. The resulting dysregulated growth seems to be an important initial step to tumorigenesis. This concept is supported by the observation that nearly all GISTs express KIT. It has further been observed that the interstitial cells of Cajal (ICC) share some phenotypic and ultrastructural similarities with GIST and normally express the KIT receptor; this observation has led to the current hypothesis that GISTs arise from ICC[26] or from ICC precursor cells. Finally, it has been noted that this gain-of-function mutation is not found in true leiomyomas.[27] Some pathologists have suggested that CD117 positivity is required to confirm a diagnosis of GIST.[28] It is now known, however, that a few otherwise obvious GISTs do not express KIT. Many of these tumors have been identified as expressing platelet-derived growth factor receptor α (PDGFRα), another distinct tyrosine kinase receptor that also mediates many of the same growth and antiapoptotic proliferation pathways.[29] Several gain-of-function mutations have been reported in the PDGFRα gene, and the resulting tumors are otherwise indistinguishable from GISTs that are KIT-positive.

There also remains a small subset of GISTs that express neither KIT nor PDGFRα; presumably other pathophysiologic pathways exist to account for these. Most benign and malignant GISTs express KIT or PDGFRα. It is postulated that the gene mutation is the first step in GIST formation, but that other factors not fully understood are necessary for progression to overt malignant behavior.

Nearly all upper GI tumors of this type occur in the stomach, but duodenal lesions have been described.[30] Most esophageal stromal tumors lack the CD117 protein and may be true leiomyomas.[28] The endoscopic appearance is a dome-shaped, firm submucosal mass; central umbilication or frank ulceration is common, and there may be a lobulated or irregular appearance. The tumors are most often solitary except in the case of specific disease entities such as Carney's triad (GIST, pulmonary chondroma, and extraadrenal paraganglioma). Germline KIT mutation kindreds have been described,[31] however, in which case multiple GISTs are seen. Giant sizes of greater than 10 cm have been noted, but most tumors are less than 3 cm.

Pathologically, the tumor usually consists of uniform pale tissue, although hemorrhagic and necrotic areas may be seen. Microscopically, the cells are spindle-shaped with uniform nuclei and general cytologic uniformity. Some cell groups may show epithelioid configurations (closely packed polygonal cells), and there may be nuclear pleomorphism. It has been observed more recently that the histologic pattern is sometimes related to the nature of the underlying genetic abnormality; KIT mutations at exon 13 or 17 more often show spindle-cell morphology,[32] whereas PDGFRα GISTs often exhibit epithelioid histology.[33] Ultrastructural cellular abnormalities have also been linked to specific gene mutations.[34] However, malignant behavior has not been associated with specific mutation patterns.

It has long been known that malignant behavior in GISTs is difficult to predict given the relatively bland cytology and slow growth of these neoplasms. It has been reported that even small, benign-appearing stromal tumors have been known to metastasize.[35] This discovery led to considerable confusion about the appropriate criteria to categorize these tumors as benign or malignant. Older pathologic scoring systems relied on numerous histologic features[19] and were plagued with problems. More recent attention has focused on the size of the tumor and the number of mitoses observed (mitotic index), at least in part because these are easily quantifiable findings. In one study of 100 cases, tumors with more than 5 mitoses per 10 high-power fields (HPFs) were significantly more likely to metastasize, although 40% of malignant lesions in that study had fewer mitoses.[36] In another study, multivariate analysis of various clinical and pathologic features in 122 specimens showed that more than 10 mitoses/50 HPFs correlated with poor outcome, whereas site, epithelioid histology, and tumor size were not independently predictive.[37]

Attempts to correlate tumor marker status such as CD117 positivity with malignant behavior have produced generally confusing or negative results,[38] as have studies of specific KIT mutations[27,39] and other tumor markers.[40,41] Older GIST scoring systems have been abandoned following a National Institutes of Health (NIH) consensus conference, which

Table 29.3 National Institutes of Health Criteria for Malignant Risk in Gastrointestinal Stromal Tumors

Risk Level	Size (cm)	Mitoses/50 HPF
Very low risk	<2	<5
Low risk	2–5	<5
Intermediate risk	<5	6–10
	5–10	<5
High risk	>5	>5
	>10	Any
	Any	>10

HPF, high-power field.

Data from Berman JJ, O'Leary TH: Gastrointestinal stromal tumor workshop. Hum Pathol 32:578–582, 2001; Toquet C, Le Neel JC, Guillou L, et al: Elevated (> or = 10%) MIB-1 proliferative index correlates with poor outcome in gastric stromal tumor patients: A study of 35 cases. Dig Dis Sci 47:2247–2253, 2002; Hedenbro JL, Ekelund M, Wetterberg P: Endoscopic diagnosis of submucosal gastric lesions: The results after routine endoscopy. Surg Endosc 5:20–30, 1991.

defined malignancy risk based on size and mitotic index alone.[42,43] The NIH criteria divide tumors into four categories of malignant risk (**Table 29.3**), an acknowledgment that even the most innocent lesion poses a slight but definite risk of malignant behavior.

If all such neoplasms entail malignant risk, prudence might dictate that they should always be resected. However, more recent data suggest that GISTs are more common than previously thought. Up to 10% of resection and autopsy specimens contain such tumors,[44] and microscopic GISTs (also called seedling GISTs, minimal GISTs, or GIST tumorlets) can be seen in 35% of some patient groups.[45,46] These incidental and microscopic GISTs display the same KIT and PDGFRα mutations as their larger counterparts. The finding that synchronous GISTs from the same patient regularly show different gene mutations (and are independent sporadic GISTs) confuses the picture further.[47] GISTs that were earlier classified as metastatic or recurrent may have been distinct neoplastic events. If it turns out that most small and asymptomatic GISTs stay that way, a conservative approach may be the most prudent.

A second breakthrough in GISTs has been the development of tyrosine kinase inhibitors such as imatinib mesylate that are effective in reducing the KIT enzyme activity and that are useful for tumor treatment. Imatinib targets the specific abnormal enzyme activity in the neoplasm and does not rely on generalized cytotoxicity for its effect. In an open label study of 147 patients with unresectable malignant GISTs, an overall response rate of 38% was seen.[48] Among responders, results are often dramatic (**Fig. 29.3**). The recognition of the malignant potential of GIST, combined with the availability of effective treatment even for unresectable disease, has compelled new thinking in the accurate diagnosis of this neoplasm.

Glomus Tumors

Glomus tumors are paragangliomas that generally occur in the skin; a morphologically similar lesion has long been known in the stomach[49] and is usually classified with GISTs.

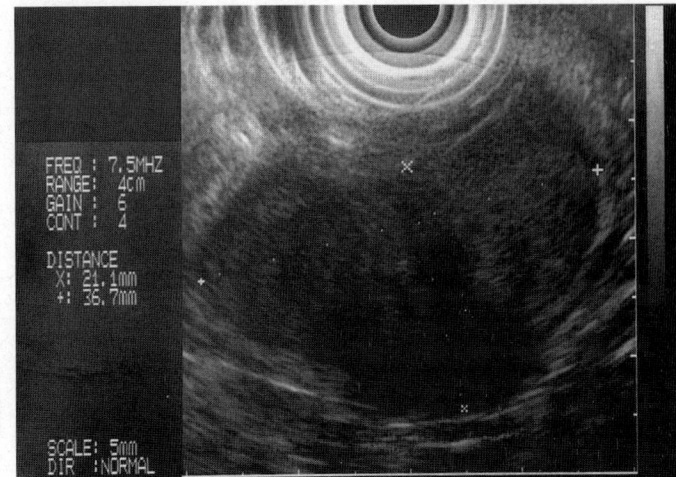

Fig. 29.3 Endoscopic ultrasound (EUS) of malignant gastrointestinal stromal tumor (GIST) treated with imatinib methylate. This large tumor initially measured 21 mm by 37 mm (main image) and decreased to 7 mm by 17 mm (inset) after 11 months of treatment.

They are typically located in the antrum and are generally small, although they can range up to 5 cm.[50] An immunohistochemical study of 32 cases showed that all examined glomus tumors were negative for desmin, S-100, and KIT,[51] suggesting a different histogenesis from leiomyomas, neuromas, and GISTs. In this same study, one patient died of metastatic disease, suggesting a malignancy risk that is low but not zero.

Neural Tumors

Technically, most tumors that appear to be of neural origin continue to be classified as stromal tumors, although the more recent revolution in GIST understanding brought about by the discovery of CD117 mutations has led to confusing terminology in some cases including neural tumors. Many experts consider stromal tumors that are positive for S-100 and negative for CD117 to be of neural origin.

Neural tumors may represent glial cell proliferation, sometimes in combination with other neural elements. Neuroma, neurofibroma, and schwannoma are largely interchangeable terms, although some pathologists observe differences among these lesions. When ganglion cells are present, the term *ganglioneuroma* is often applied. They seem to arise from ganglion cells in either the myenteric plexus or submucosal plexus.

Neuroma and Neurofibroma

Neuroma and neurofibroma are well-circumscribed, nonencapsulated tumors arising from either the submucosa or the muscularis propria layer. Except in the case of von Recklinghausen's neurofibromatosis, they are usually solitary nodules. They consist of bland spindle-shaped cells and are often classified as neuromas (as opposed to GISTs) if neural markers are identified on immunohistochemical stain.

Gangliocytic Paraganglioma

Gangliocytic paragangliomas are rare tumors that range from 0.5 to 4 cm in size and are found in the periampullary duodenum. They may be present in either the submucosa or the muscularis propria layers and consist of a combination of ganglion cells and epithelioid cells; they usually also contain a component resembling carcinoid tumor.

Immunocytochemically, somatostatin is usually present, and other neuropeptides may also be seen. They are always benign but may be locally infiltrative.

Endothelial and Vascular Tumors

Cavernous hemangiomas are vascular neoplasms that rarely occur in the GI tract and even more rarely in the upper tract. They appear as sessile red or blue nodules and can be difficult to distinguish from vascular ectasias (which are not neoplastic). A malignant counterpart, hemangiosarcoma, is exceedingly rare but has been described in nearly all parts of the GI tract.[52] Lymphatic tumors are also exceedingly rare in the GI tract, primarily being reported in the duodenum. They are described as having a smooth, sessile, polypoid translucent appearance endoscopically.[53] Histologically, they are mucosal or submucosal and contain hamartomatous rather than true neoplastic elements[52]; they are always benign.

Lipocytic Tumors: Lipoma and Liposarcoma

Submucosal lipomas are usually harmless neoplasms arising from submucosal adipocytes. They are most common in the colon but may appear in any part of the GI tract, particularly the gastric antrum.[54] The typical endoscopic appearance is a pale yellowish, soft submucosal tumor; usually a solitary lesion is seen. The overlying mucosa can sometimes be tented up with a biopsy forceps, and the lesion deforms easily when pushed with the forceps. Histologically, such tumors are encapsulated and consist of typical benign mature lipocytes. When they contain a large number of blood vessels, they are sometimes called angiolipomas. It is rarely necessary to evaluate them further or remove them unless they cause bleeding or obstruction. They are normally small, but giant lipomas have been described[55] that can cause obstruction or intussusception.[56] The clinically aggressive malignant form, liposarcoma, is exceedingly rare.[57]

Granular Cell Tumor

The esophagus is the most common site of granular cell tumors, but they may be found throughout the GI tract. They are most often located in the submucosa and often have a polypoid shape. Multiple tumors are common. They may be of Schwann cell origin and consist of masses of histiocytelike cells containing periodic acid–Schiff–positive cytoplasmic granules. A literature review of 117 cases found dysphagia as the most common symptom in roughly half of patients; three-fourths were smaller than 2 cm.[58] It is uncertain that there is a malignant form of the neoplasm; the same review found that in four locally invasive cases distant metastases were not noted. They generally appear as yellowish, plaquelike, round or oval lesions less than 2 cm across.[59] The overlying squamous epithelium of the esophagus may show pseudoepitheliomatous hyperplasia.[60] If this is misinterpreted as metaplastic mucosal transformation, confusion may lead to additional investigations in search of an epithelial neoplasm.

Inflammatory Fibroid Polyp

Inflammatory fibroid polyps are uncommon tumors that can occur anywhere in the GI tract; the stomach is the most common site,[19] but they have been described elsewhere.[61] Pathologically, they consist of nonencapsulated myxoid stroma that includes blood vessels, inflammatory cells, and invariably eosinophils. The eosinophilic infiltrate had previously led to the (now discarded) designation of this tumor as localized eosinophilic gastroenteritis. They are often small, but giant tumors have been described that can cause (as usual) bleeding, obstruction, or intussusception.[62] Current theories of their pathogenesis focus on myofibroblasts or fibroblasts,[63] but the cell of origin is unknown. They tend to originate in the muscle layers of the GI tract wall, beginning as an intramural bulge but later assuming a polypoid shape; there may often be a significant extramural (subserosal) extension. There seems to be no malignant potential.

Fibrous (Fibrovascular) Polyp

Fibrous polyps are esophageal tumors that can grow to an enormous size. They occur predominantly in male patients, usually originate in the upper esophagus, and often assume a polypoid shape.[64] Tumors greater than 15 cm have been described[65] and can cause dysphagia, globus, bleeding, and asphyxiation from laryngeal impaction.

Although these tumors may have ulcerated overlying mucosa, the sheer size of the lesion may make it difficult to identify endoscopically.[66] Histologically, a large variety of cytologic elements are seen, including spindle cells, lipocytes, mononuclear inflammatory cells, and vascular connective tissue. However, because some typical characteristics of inflammatory fibroid polyps are lacking and because of differing epidemiology and location, these lesions are classified separately from inflammatory fibroid polyps and should not be confused with them (despite the similar names). They are of uncertain histogenesis but do not seem to possess malignant potential. Nevertheless, because fatal outcomes have been described arising from the mechanical size of these tumors, removal is considered prudent.

Metastatic Tumors

Intramural metastases to the GI tract are less common than compression or invasion from extramural cancer. In a study of gastric mural metastases, the most common primary sites were lung, breast, and esophagus, but malignant melanoma was the most frequent tumor to metastasize to the stomach. Half appeared endoscopically as submucosal tumors, and the rest were ulcerated or fungating; one-third showed multiple lesions.[67]

Cystic Tumors

Various cystic intramural lesions may manifest as submucosal tumors. In an individual patient, it may be unclear until EUS is performed that these tumors are cystic. However, it is worth collectively listing lesions (some of which have already been discussed) that can assume such an appearance. Small lymphatic ectasias are a common endoscopic finding,[52] particularly in the duodenum, and represent cystic structures less than 5 mm in size; they are not neoplasms. Duplication cysts are another nonneoplastic intramural cyst that may be seen as a submucosal tumor. These are very rarely encountered lesions in the upper GI tract[68,69] and are due to embryonic epithelial nodules that fail to regress. Brunner's gland hamartomas and heterotopic pancreas have also been described as having a cystic appearance.[70] Among neoplastic cysts, lymphangiomas[71] and hemangiomas[72] (and hemangiosarcomas) assume a cystic appearance. In addition, any malignant neoplasm with central necrosis may appear as a cystic intramural lesion.

Differential Diagnosis

As has been shown, submucosal tumors may represent the full spectrum of symptoms and pathology from innocent to critical. Various diagnostic tools are available to sort out the possibilities.

Conventional Endoscopy, Computed Tomography, and Transabdominal Ultrasound

Confronted with a submucosal tumor, the alert endoscopist should not permit the presence of mucosa between the endoscopic camera and the mass to preclude preliminary conclusions about the nature of the unseen tumor. Despite the multitude of possibilities already discussed, a short list of half a dozen lesions covers nearly everything likely to be found in all but the largest referral centers. Each has distinctive clinical and endoscopic features (**Table 29.4**) to provide an adequate preliminary assessment, which can be used to direct further management.

Routine endoscopic pinch biopsies are often performed but rarely yield diagnostic material, even when large size (jumbo) pinch forceps are used.[73] Other efforts to obtain tissue during routine endoscopy have been described, including standard fine needle aspiration (FNA) needles,[74] a special guillotine aspiration biopsy needle,[75] and mucosal stripping after forceps biopsy[76]; these show variable success but have not yet gained widespread acceptance.

Conventional computed tomography (CT) has traditionally been unhelpful in evaluating intramural tumors because of their small size, but new CT methods show promise. Multidetector high-resolution CT scanners can identify most tumors larger than 1 cm, although further characterization may be difficult.[77] Three-dimensional computerized reconstruction

Table 29.4 Endoscopic Appearance of Typical Upper Gastrointestinal Submucosal Tumors

Clinical Characteristics	Most Likely Tumor
Lower esophagus: <2 cm, plaquelike, firm, yellowish, sometimes multiple	Granular cell tumor
Upper esophagus: firm, large, polypoid	Fibrous (fibrovascular) polyp
Stomach: ovoid, firm, any size, single lesion	GIST
Stomach: <1 cm, firm, dimpled	Heterotopic pancreas
Any organ: translucent, soft	Lymphangioma
Any organ: soft, yellowish, soft, compressible, any size, single lesion	Lipoma

GIST, gastrointestinal stromal tumor.

Table 29.5 Important Endoscopic Ultrasound Features in Intramural Masses

Attribute	Attribute Values
Location	Organ (e.g., stomach) and position (e.g., greater curve)
Size	Measured (in three dimensions if possible)
Background echogenicity	Hypoechoic, hyperechoic, or anechoic
Focal echogenicity	Hypoechoic foci, hyperechoic foci, both, or neither
Shape/margin shape	Round, oval; smooth margins, irregular margins
Margin definition	Well-defined margins, poorly defined margins
Position/origin relative to wall layers	Involves mucosa, submucosa, muscularis propria
Tumor extension or invasion	T stage relative to site organ

techniques are also able to detect intramural tumors reliably and may provide useful images.[78] Ongoing improvements in CT resolution may yet result in clinically important images, but current conventional technology is not generally worthwhile.

Conventional transabdominal ultrasound has likewise been unhelpful in this setting, but similar to CT useful progress is being reported. High-resolution transabdominal ultrasound, using transducer frequencies of 5 MHz or 7.5 MHz and a water-filled stomach, provides remarkable imaging of tumors 10 mm in size and their relationship to the five-layer GI tract wall.[79] Although unsuitable for obese patients or many anatomic tumor locations, this technique could potentially replace many EUS examinations of such tumors.

Endoscopic Ultrasound

High-resolution scanning from an intraluminal position makes EUS ideally suited for evaluation of submucosal tumors and for complete characterization of intramural masses that are identified. Extramural impression from normal and abnormal structures can be reliably shown, and intramural masses can be readily characterized. The ability to relate intramural tumors to the five-layer wall structure of the GI tract permits conclusions about the origin of the lesion (and its probable histology) and, where appropriate, the degree of local invasion (T stage). **Table 29.5** lists some important features that can be derived from EUS and that are usually helpful diagnosing the lesion and directing further management.

Several studies have documented the ability of EUS to characterize such lesions accurately. Yasuda and coworkers[80] reported their experience with 308 patients, including 210 submucosal tumors. Characteristic echo features of benign and malignant stromal tumors, varices, cysts, lipomas, lymphoma, and aberrant pancreas were described. Rösch and colleagues[81] described the appearance of 102 submucosal lesions collected in a multicenter German study group. Characterizing the accuracy of EUS for this purpose is difficult and depends on the question being asked. The ability of EUS to measure tumor size accurately has been documented,[82] as has reliability in identifying extramural structures. However, distinguishing among different classes of lesions (e.g., cystic, fatty, stromal) or pathologic entities (e.g., stromal tumor, car-

cinoid) is hampered by the fact that pathologic confirmation is not uniformly available in these research subject groups. Rösch and coworkers[81] reported sensitivity and specificity figures of 64% to 92% and 80% to 100%, for various types of pathologic distinctions being examined.

These and other authors have characterized the typical appearance of several intramural lesions. Lipomas (**Fig. 29.4**) are brightly echogenic structures with uniform echotexture and well-demarcated margins, and they are generally associated with the submucosal layer (layer three). They are easily deformed by compression from the transducer tip. Because they are virtually always benign, identifying continuity of the muscularis propria layer behind the tumor is helpful in confirming the diagnosis. Varices (**Fig. 29.5**) are also easy to recognize as anechoic vermiform structures. They are nearly always in groups, and extramural varices can usually be seen. When a variceal structure is seen in isolation, a hemangioma or lymphangioma should be considered because these may have a similar appearance. Cysts such as duplication cysts also have an anechoic internal structure (**Fig. 29.6**), although debris may be seen as hyperechoic foci within the cyst structure. Aberrant pancreas (**Fig. 29.7**) is usually suspected by the endoscopic appearance, and the EUS structure of a hypoechoic lesion associated with the submucosal layer is confirmatory. Internal echogenic spots are often observed with this lesion.

The most frequent finding is of a hypoechoic intramural structure (**Figs. 29.8 and 29.9**). Various tumors, mostly neoplasms, can have this appearance, including GISTs, carcinoids, granular cell tumors, lymphomas, and metastatic tumors. These lesions all show generally hypoechoic (ground-glass) background echotexture, often containing hyperechoic foci or hypoechoic and anechoic foci (or both hyperechoic and hypoechoic foci). The tumor margins are typically well defined and smooth, and the overall shape is round or oval. Despite the similarities, some EUS clues may help to distinguish among these lesions. Granular cell tumors, usually located in the esophagus, are typically seen within the third (submucosal) echo layer and are generally smaller than 2 cm (see **Fig. 29.8A**). Carcinoid tumors are most common in the mucosal

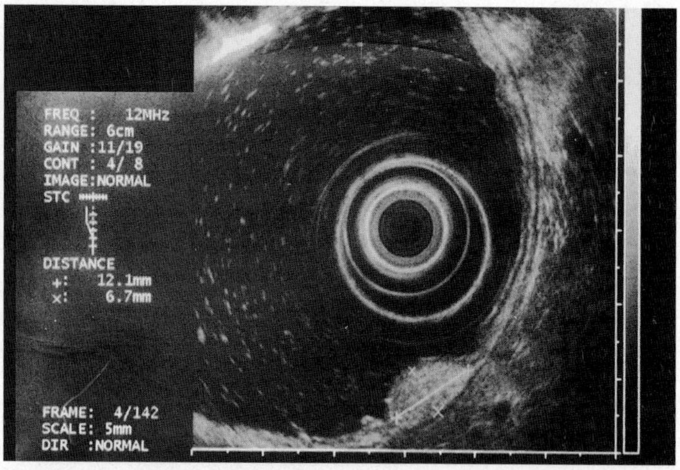

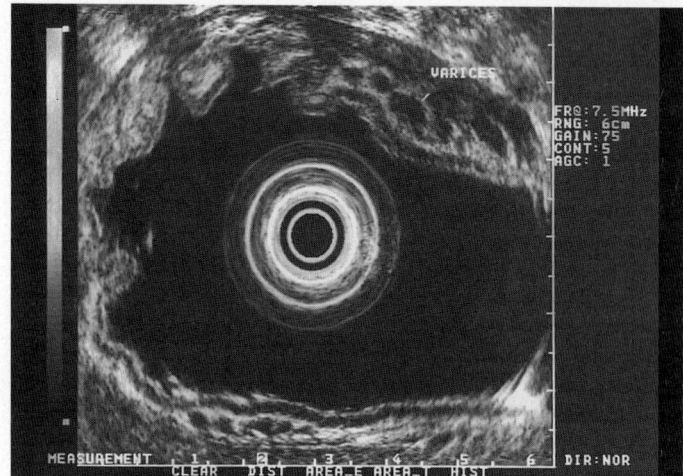

Fig. 29.4 Endoscopic ultrasound (EUS) of gastric lipoma. Note uniform hyperechoic echogenicity and submucosal position with intact muscularis propria layer.

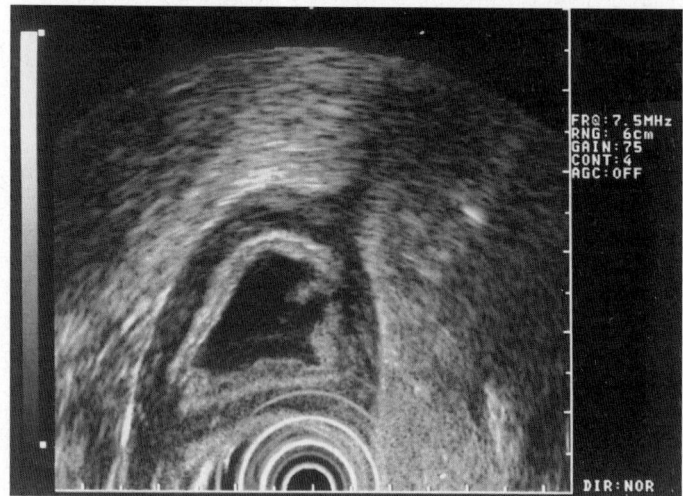

Fig. 29.5 Endoscopic ultrasound (EUS) of gastric varices. Note multiple anechoic serpiginous structures; on real-time images, the continuous nature of these structures is obvious.

Fig. 29.6 Endoscopic ultrasound (EUS) of gastric duplication cyst. The cyst wall contains a multilayer echo similar to the normal wall structure.

and submucosal layers (see **Fig. 29.8B**), as are lymphomas (see **Fig. 29.8C**), whereas metastatic tumors (see **Fig. 29.8D**) may occupy any layer in any organ.

Stromal tumors (see **Fig. 29.9**) are typically located in the muscularis propria layer and indistinguishably blend into it. Their most innocent appearance is of rounded, well-circumscribed, smooth tumors of 1 to 2 cm with uniform echogenicity (see **Fig. 29.9A**). Other EUS features may be seen, however, and significant effort has been expended to determine whether those features can distinguish benign from malignant behavior. Giant size (see **Fig. 29.9B**) and irregular or knobby margins (see **Fig. 29.9C**) have been imputed to predict malignancy, as have internal foci that are hyperechoic or hypoechoic (see **Fig. 29.9D**).

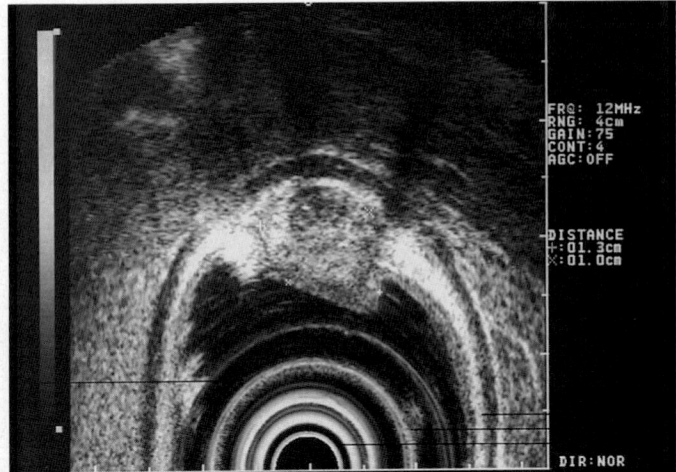

Fig. 29.7 Endoscopic ultrasound (EUS) of ectopic pancreas. Note heterogeneous structure located in the mucosal layer and submucosal layer.

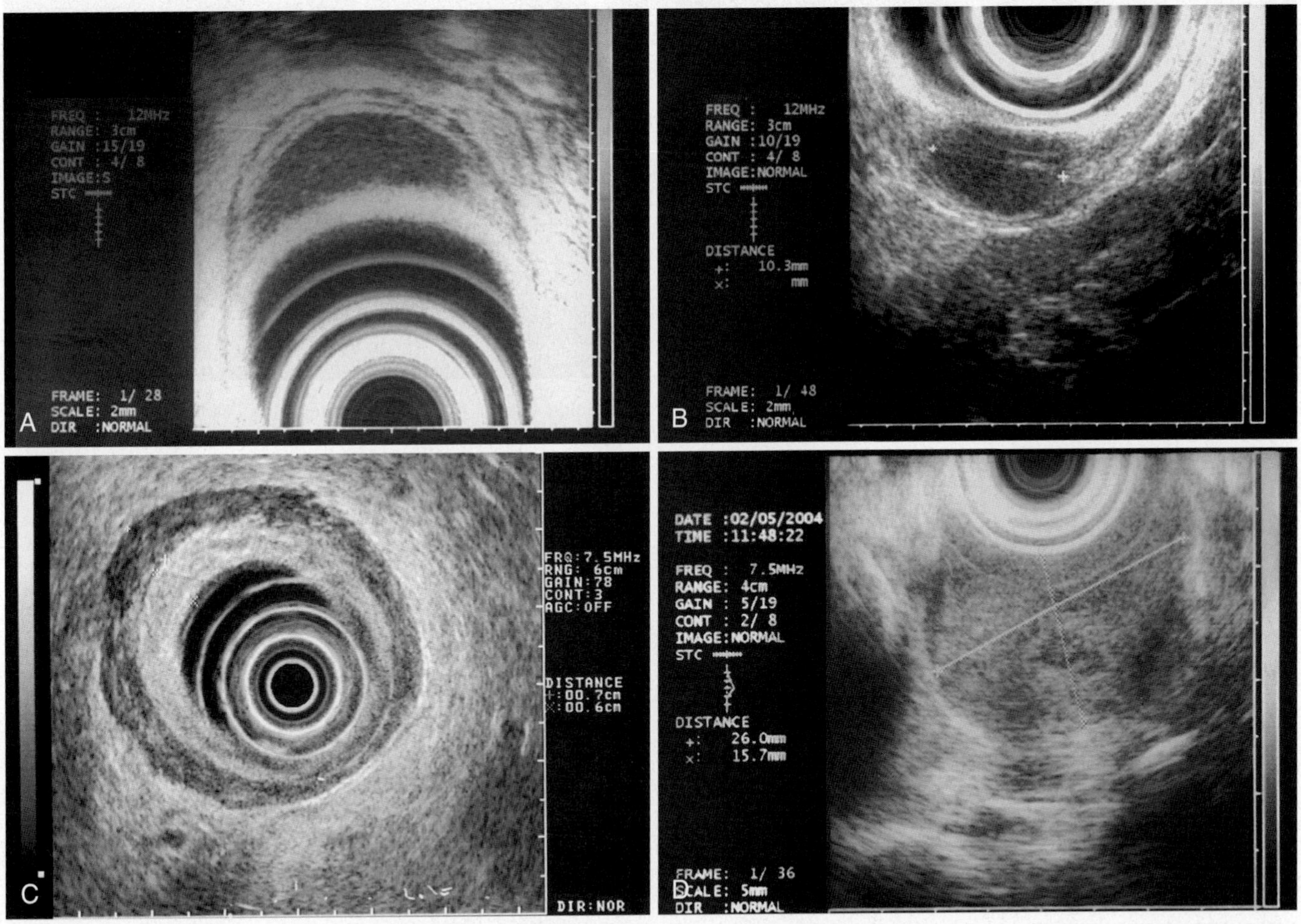

Fig. 29.8 Endoscopic ultrasound (EUS) appearance of intraepithelial neoplasms. **A,** Granular cell tumor of the esophagus, seen as a hypoechoic structure located within the submucosal layer (note intact muscularis propria layer). **B,** Carcinoid tumor of the duodenum, a hypoechoic tumor in the submucosa. **C,** Infiltrating lymphoma causing thickening of both the third and the fourth echo layers. **D,** Large metastatic tumor that mostly replaces the entire wall locally.

Early proposals that all these features were ominous[83] have been investigated further with mixed results. Tsai and coworkers[84] showed a correlation of each of these features with malignant histology, but no single factor or combination of factors yielded satisfactory diagnostic accuracy. Chak and colleagues[85] showed sensitivity figures of 80% to 100% for malignancy in a

retrospective videotape study using these factors, but there was only fair to moderate intraobserver agreement for the factors themselves, especially for hyperechoic and hypoechoic foci; specificity was 80%. A multicenter prospective study, the largest prospective series to date (198 tumors), attempted to validate these criteria further and found that tumor size, surface

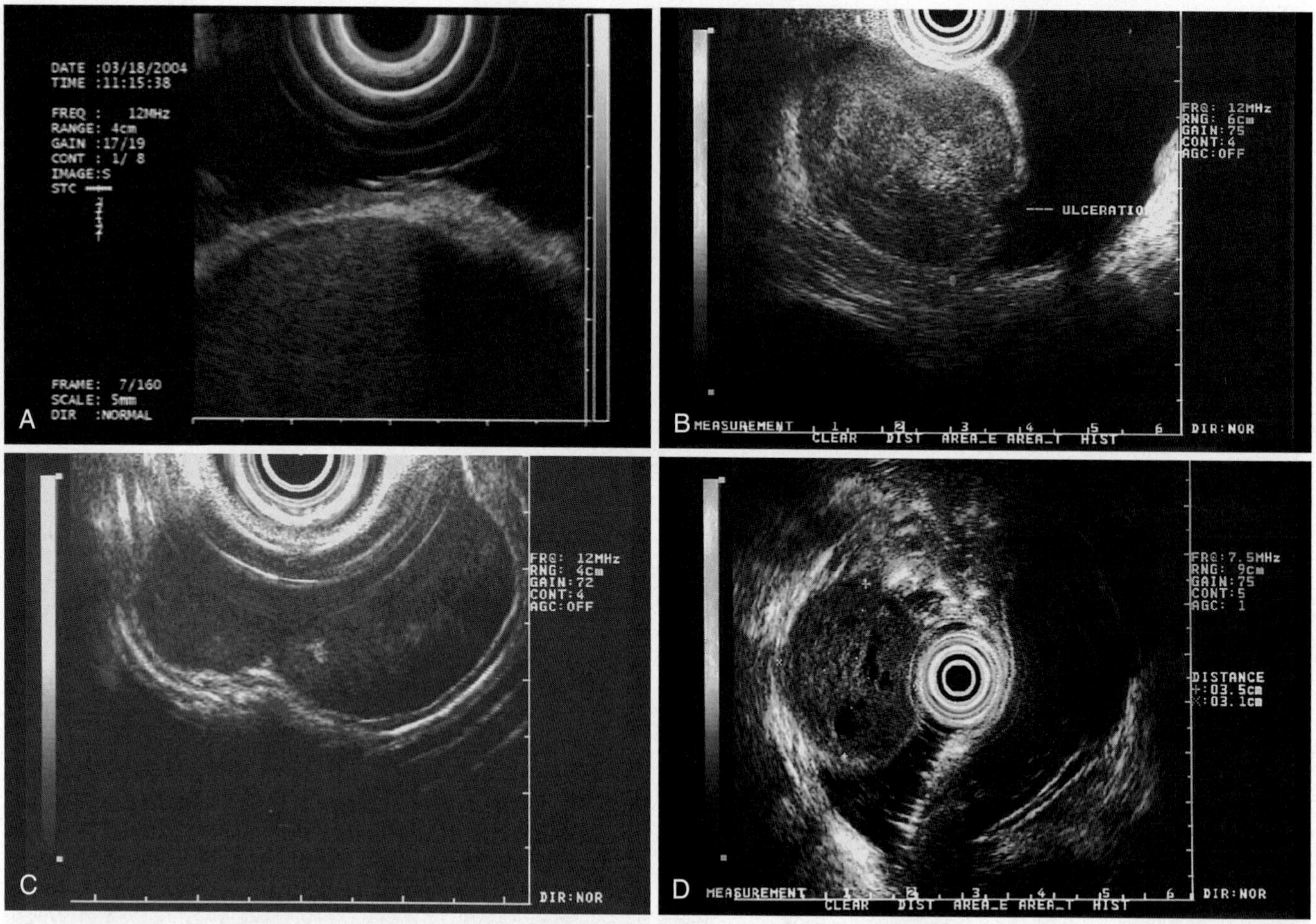

Fig. 29.9 Endoscopic ultrasound (EUS) appearance of gastrointestinal stromal tumors (GISTs). **A,** Benign-appearing GIST. Note small size, layer four (muscularis propria) location, and smooth and well-defined margins. **B,** Large gastric GIST greater than 3 cm with surface ulceration and hyperechoic internal foci. **C,** GIST with multilobed irregular margins and hyperechoic foci. **D,** Hypoechoic (anechoic) foci within large GIST.

ulceration, nonoval shape, and irregular or indistinct margins were associated with malignancy, whereas hyperechoic and hypoechoic internal foci were not correlated.[8] The authors also reported that serial surveillance of initially innocent lesions by repeat EUS provided a very low yield of additional malignant neoplasms. Reviewing the literature on the subject collectively, most experts agree that size greater than 3 cm and irregular or indistinct margins are worrisome features.

Fine Needle Aspiration Biopsy

Given the ambiguous predictive value of EUS morphology in identifying tissue histology or predicting malignant behavior when considering hypoechoic intramural tumors, efforts to obtain diagnostic tissue assume greater importance. Transcutaneous sampling under CT or ultrasound guidance is possible for some lesions and can yield diagnostic material in up to three-fourths of lesions.[86] Likewise, endoscopic FNA by direct puncture or under EUS guidance yields adequate diagnostic material in up to 90%[74] and, when combined with immunohistochemical stains, can distinguish GIST from leiomyoma.[87] Although such specimens are usually adequate to distinguish other neoplasms from GISTs, they are unable to distinguish reliably benign from malignant GISTs. The fact that the cellularity is insufficient to obtain a mitotic index is

a major obstacle, but the addition of immunohistochemical stains in biopsy specimens, including c-KIT and Ki-67, improves the diagnostic accuracy of stromal tumors[88] and can strongly suggest malignant risk. A more recent modeling study suggested that biopsy can improve clinical management of hypoechoic tumors,[89] lending support to the routine performance of needle biopsy of hypoechoic tumors, with immunostaining when appropriate.

Treatment

Ultimately, treatment for intramural tumors is reduced to two choices: leave it in place or take it out. New diagnostic and therapeutic options make the decision easier. The use of EUS appearance combined with FNA biopsy specimens and immunostaining provides important information to direct the choice. Similarly, new options for removing the tumors have emerged to supplant or replace the traditional choice of open laparotomy or thoracotomy.

Indications and Contraindications

Several clear-cut indications have emerged to direct resection of intramural tumors. Most obvious is the presence of symptoms that are caused by the lesion, such as bleeding, obstruction, or intussusception. Beyond this, lesions that are malignant or pose a significant risk of becoming malignant require resection, whereas clearly benign tumors, such as granular cell tumors and lipomas, pose no meaningful malignant risk and may be safely left in situ. Because GISTs compose most intramural tumors, it remains to identify which hypoechoic lesions are GISTs and how high the malignant risk is for a given GIST. For this reason, EUS combined with FNA biopsy and immunostaining is emerging as the diagnostic procedure of choice. In a more recent study, 71% of resected hypoechoic tumors were GISTs; 12% of these were malignant GISTs, and another 41% were GISTs of indeterminate malignant potential.[8] Given what seems to be a significant malignant risk among such tumors, criteria to direct resection should have high sensitivity, even at the expense of low specificity. It seems reasonable to perform resection of hypoechoic tumors with size greater than 3 cm, irregular or indistinct margins, ulceration, or nonoval shape. Rapid growth on serial examination, although not a validated criterion, is nevertheless a sufficiently alarming finding also to direct removal of the tumor.

Preoperative History and Considerations

In selecting patients with GISTs who should be directed to surgical resection, it is important to maintain perspective on the actual level of malignant risk compared with the surgical risk. Despite the suggestion that the proportion of GISTs containing a meaningful malignant risk may approach 50%, the fact is that most GISTs, if left alone, remain benign and asymptomatic. Among patients with an average surgical risk, it is reasonable to maintain a low threshold for resection of tumors with alarming EUS or histologic features. However, for patients with advanced age or significant comorbidities that render surgical resection risky, a higher threshold is warranted. In such patients, a more diligent search for immunohistochemical markers of malignancy, such as MIB-1 or KI-67, would be prudent in directing surgery.

Description of Techniques

Some submucosal tumors are appropriate for endoscopic removal. Numerous reports document success in removal of tumors of the mucosa or submucosa, including lipomas, inflammatory fibroid polyps, carcinoids,[90] and granular cell tumors.[91] Stromal cell tumors that do not involve the muscularis propria can also be successfully removed endoscopically.[92] Generally, a snare or inject/snare technique is described. Bleeding is the most common complication and may require transfusion, endoscopic therapy,[90] or surgery.[93] Despite the reported success of this technique, the number of tumors appropriate for endoscopic removal is limited. The most problematic intramural tumors are tumors that show EUS features of GIST; because most of these involve the muscularis propria, they are unsuitable for endoscopic treatment. Endoscopic removal is likely to remain of limited applicability for this condition.

Advances in minimally invasive surgery have made laparoscopic removal possible for many such tumors. Several small case series describe successful laparoscopic removal of GISTs in various gastric sites,[94,95] including the posterior wall of the stomach.[96] Tumors up to 7 cm in size can be removed.[97] Surgical techniques described include tumor enucleation, wedge resection, and partial gastrectomy. A combined endoscopic and laparoscopic approach may be required when the tumor cannot be readily identified from the serosal surface.[98] In these small series, few complications are reported,[94] but conversion to open resection may be required.[96] A more recent retrospective study comparing open and laparoscopic resection of GISTs found a shorter mean hospital stay for the latter (3.8 days vs. 6.2 days) but otherwise comparable technical and safety outcomes,[99] and a smaller prospective study found a similar decrease in hospital stay but also noted hospital costs to be 31% less in the laparoscopy group.[100] It has been emphasized that such resections require a high degree of technical skill in laparoscopic surgery.[99] As experience widens, it is likely that laparoscopic resection will become the procedure of choice in the near future for GISTs requiring removal; the convenience and patient acceptance of this method may lead to decreased resistance to resection of GISTs of equivocal malignant potential. Natural orifice endoscopic surgery would be expected to offer a resection method well suited to mesenchymal tumors of all sorts including GISTs but has not been described for this purpose to date.

Future Trends

An alert reader perusing the literature on the subject must be struck by the extremely variable quality of the data available. It cannot be otherwise: All the lesions discussed here range from "uncommon" to "never in my lifetime," and even the largest of case series rarely contains more than a few dozen subjects. Developing a management algorithm—or even a reasonable plan for a single patient—based on such scant data is a hazardous undertaking.

Despite the dearth of clinical material, great strides have been made. The advance in the understanding of stromal tumors by the discovery of KIT and its dovetailing with other known oncogenic markers has provided great insight into the histogenesis and growth mechanism of these neoplasms and has pioneered treatment agents, such as imatinib, of novel therapeutic action. Extending this work will provide exciting new insights and therapies, and the "Grail" of GISTs—a reliable test of benign versus malignant behavior—may be right around the corner. Another revolution has been in the development of laparoscopic surgical approaches to these tumors. The ability to remove intramural masses safely and reliably in what may soon become an outpatient procedure enormously increases the management options. However, the pressure on GI endoscopists to establish efficacy and cost efficiency in endoscopic management is also substantially increased. Multiple endoscopic evaluations and serial surveillance of submucosal lesions, by either EGD or EUS, makes little sense when the tumor can be easily and conveniently dispensed with altogether.

A more recent modeling suggests that the GI endoscopist who cannot establish definitive patient management in an average of 1.7 EUS examinations is wasting the patient's time and money.[8] This suggestion leads to what is, from the GI endoscopist's perspective, a critical need. Clinical studies that

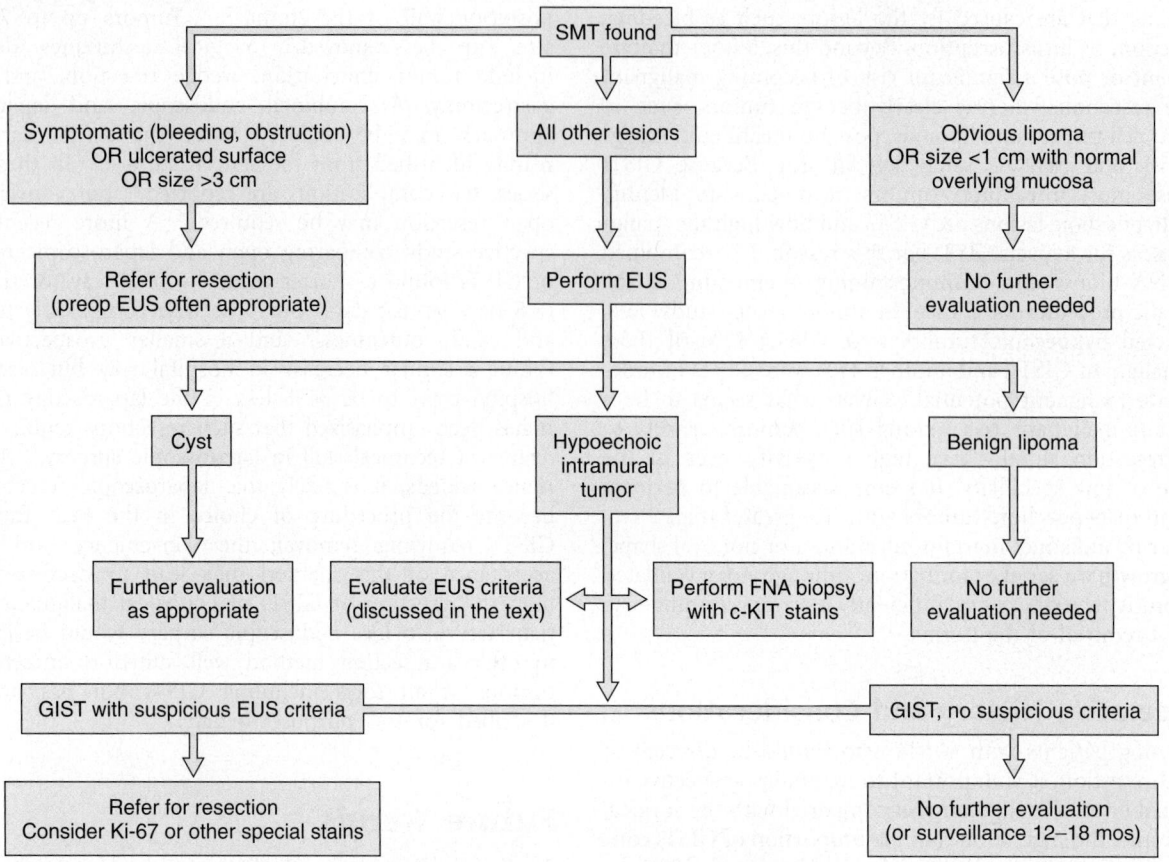

EUS, endoscopic ultrasonography; FNA, fine needle aspiration; GIST, gastrointestinal stromal tumor.

Fig. 29.10 Provisional treatment algorithm.

reliably define submucosal tumors that require further investigation and that establish the performance characteristics of EUS and other diagnostic modalities would permit the endoscopist to direct further management of submucosal tumors safely and reliably. A provisional treatment algorithm ("fools rush in …") is proposed here (**Fig. 29.10**), but substantial work remains to be done to validate the steps that would translate this provisional algorithm into a reliable management tool.

References

The complete reference list is available online at www.expertconsult.com.

Screening for Esophageal Squamous Cell Carcinoma and Its Precursor Lesions

Sanford M. Dawsey and David E. Fleischer

Video related to this chapter's topics can be found online at expertconsult.com.

Introduction

Esophageal cancer is the sixth leading cause of cancer death worldwide.[1] In 2002, it was estimated that there were 462,000 new esophageal cancer cases and 386,000 deaths caused by esophageal cancer, only 25,000 fewer deaths than were caused by breast cancer.[1] About 80% of esophageal cancer cases occur in developing countries.[1] In the United States, esophageal cancer is the ninth leading cause of cancer death; an estimated 16,470 new cases and 14,530 deaths occurred as a result of esophageal cancer in 2009.[2]

One striking characteristic of esophageal cancer throughout the world is its great geographic variation in incidence, with 10-fold differences reported over distances of a few hundred kilometers.[3] Worldwide, the highest risk populations are found in two geographic belts: one in central Asia from the Caspian Sea to north central China and one from eastern to southern Africa (**Fig. 30.1**).[4] Age-adjusted incidence rates over 100 cases per 100,000 inhabitants per year have been reported from some areas in these regions.[3,5,6] Populations with intermediate risk are found in southern South America (in southern Brazil, Uruguay, Paraguay, and northern Argentina) and in northwestern France.[5] People throughout most of the world are considered to be at low risk, with incidence rates less than 10 per 100,000 inhabitants per year.[5] In the Surveillance Epidemiology and End Results (SEER) cancer registries in the United States, the age-adjusted incidence of EC per 100,000 population per year in 2002–2006 was 7.9 in white men, 1.9 in white women, 9.3 in black men, and 3.0 in black women.[7]

In low-risk countries such as the United States, the male-to-female ratio of cases is usually about 3 : 1 to 4 : 1,[7] but in the highest risk populations, this ratio approaches or even falls below 1 : 1.[3,6]

Throughout most of the world, most esophageal cancer cases are esophageal squamous cell carcinomas (ESCCs).[5] In Western countries, the incidence of ESCC has been gradually declining, and the incidence of esophageal adenocarcinoma has been rapidly increasing over the last 30 years,[5,8] so that now greater than 50% of esophageal cancer cases in the United States are esophageal adenocarcinoma.[5,7]

In most low-risk countries, cigarette smoking and alcohol consumption are the dominant risk factors for ESCC.[9–11] In the United States, greater than 90% of ESCC cases can be attributed to these two exposures alone.[12] Additional contributing risk factors include a low dietary intake of fruits and vegetables and factors related to low socioeconomic status.[13–16] A few host medical conditions have also been associated with increased risk of ESCC in low-risk populations, including previous or concurrent squamous cell carcinoma of the head and neck region, achalasia, tylosis, caustic esophageal strictures, and Plummer-Vinson syndrome.[17]

In most high-risk populations, tobacco and alcohol are not major risk factors for ESCC. Tobacco consumption in these groups is typically low, both in terms of the prevalence of smoking and in the amount of tobacco consumed by smokers, and alcohol consumption is even lower.[18–20] In addition, in the highest risk areas, where there are nearly as many ESCC cases in women as in men, virtually none of the women smoke or

INCIDENCE OF ESOPHAGUS CANCER - MEN

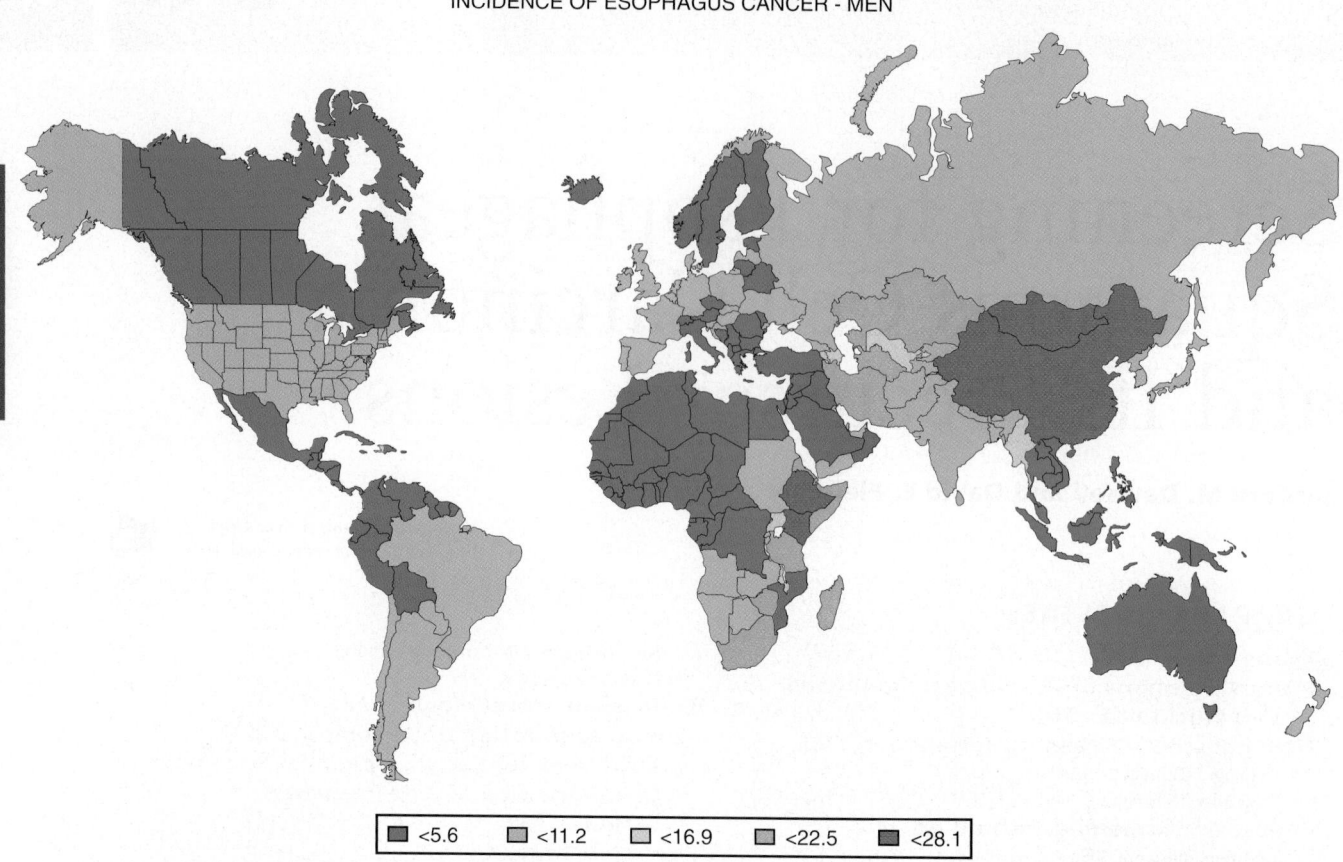

| ■ <5.6 | □ <11.2 | □ <16.9 | ■ <22.5 | ■ <28.1 |

Fig. 30.1 Worldwide incidence of esophageal cancer in men, 2002. *(Data from Ferlay J, Bray F, Pisani P, et al: GLOBOCAN 2002: Cancer incidence, mortality and prevalence worldwide: IARC cancer base No. 5. version 2.0, Lyon, 2004, IARC Press.)*

drink.[18–20] These high-risk groups may be exposed to some of the major tobacco carcinogens, however, such as polycyclic aromatic hydrocarbons (PAHs), nitrosamines, and acetaldehyde, in other ways. Studies have documented high levels of PAH exposure in Linxian, a county in the high-risk region in north central China[21]; in northeastern Iran[22]; and in southern Brazil.[23] The source of these exposures is unknown; in Linxian, it may be related to ingestion of ambient soot particles released from heating and cooking with soft coal in unvented stoves,[24,25] and in Brazil, it may be caused by drinking the beverage maté.[23,26] Nontobacco exposure to nitrosamines and acetaldehyde has also been suggested in Linxian[27,28] and in northeastern Iran[29] possibly secondary to changes in oral bacteria that accompany poor oral hygiene and tooth loss. Other risk factors reported in high-risk areas include diets low in fruits and vegetables[20,30,31]; low levels of certain micronutrients, especially selenium and zinc[32,33]; low socioeconomic status[34]; exposure to fungal toxins such as fumonisins[35]; and drinking hot liquids.[30,36,37]

One of the most consistent risk factors for ESCC in high-risk populations is family history,[20,38,39] and preliminary molecular studies support a role for genetic susceptibility in the etiology of ESCC in these areas. Studies have shown high frequencies of loss of heterozygosity (LOH),[40] characteristic patterns of gene expression,[41] and significant differences in both LOH and gene expression by family history[41,42] in tumors from north central China, but no major susceptibility gene for ESCC has yet been identified.

Both cell types of esophageal cancer have a very poor prognosis. In SEER data for 1999–2005, the overall 5-year relative (disease-specific) survival for EC patients was 16.4%.[7] This survival rate is improved from 4.7% in 1975–1979,[43] but it is still the third lowest survival rate (after pancreas and liver) among major cancers. In developing countries, the 5-year survival rates are usually less than 10%.[5]

The main reason for poor survival in esophageal cancer is that most tumors are asymptomatic and go undetected until they have spread beyond the esophageal wall. The esophagus is a distensible organ—it distends to let food pass—so most patients do not complain of dysphagia or other symptoms until the tumor significantly obstructs the lumen, and by that time it has usually invaded through the wall or metastasized or both. Significant reduction in esophageal cancer mortality both in low-risk and in high-risk populations requires the development of successful new strategies for screening asymptomatic high-risk individuals that can lead to diagnosis and treatment of more cases at earlier, more curable stages of the disease.

Five components needed for a successful early detection and treatment program for esophageal cancer are as follows:

1. Identification of clinically important precursor lesions, which would be the targets for screening and treatment
2. Accurate, cost-effective primary screening tests that can detect precursor and early invasive lesions and are acceptable to asymptomatic high-risk individuals

3. Reliable techniques for endoscopic localization of precursor and early invasive lesions so that diagnostic biopsies and focal therapy can be accurately targeted
4. Reliable techniques for accurate staging of early invasive lesions so that patients can be triaged to the most appropriate treatment
5. A spectrum of curative therapies for precursor and early invasive lesions that is acceptable to asymptomatic people

Table 30.1 summarizes these components for ESCC and our understanding of the current techniques available for each component. Techniques that are possible but are not yet established are followed by a question mark. Because the subject of this chapter is screening, we discuss only the first three of these components. Staging and endoscopic therapy are discussed in other chapters of this text.

Precursor Lesions of Esophageal Squamous Cell Carcinoma

In low-risk countries, squamous dysplasia (including carcinoma in situ) is accepted as the histologic precursor of ESCC because it is the established precursor in other organs lined by squamous epithelium, such as the cervix, and because it is often found adjacent to invasive cancer in esophagectomy specimens.[44] In high-risk populations, squamous dysplasia is also accepted as a precursor of ESCC,[45-49] but other histologic lesions, such as chronic esophagitis, atrophy, and basal cell hyperplasia, have also been proposed as precursors, based primarily on differences in the prevalence of these lesions in high-risk and low-risk groups.[46,49,50] These ecologic comparisons have not always been consistent, however.[51] In the only two prospective studies, in which patients who underwent biopsy were followed over time, only squamous dysplasia was

significantly associated with the later development of ESCC,[45,47,48] and increasing grades of dysplasia were associated with increasing risk.[45,48] In the larger of these prospective studies, members of our group followed 682 adults from Linxian who underwent endoscopy without initial evidence of invasive cancer for up to 13.5 years and compared the cumulative incidence and relative risk of developing ESCC among patients with different initial biopsy diagnoses (**Fig. 30.2** and **Table 30.2**).

Table 30.1 Components Needed for Successful Early Detection and Treatment Program for Esophageal Squamous Cell Carcinoma

Component	Current State of the Art
Identification of precursor lesion	Squamous dysplasia
Primary screen	Endoscopy
	Cytology?
	Molecular?
Endoscopic localization	Iodine staining
	Narrow band imaging?
	Magnification endoscopy?
Staging	Endoscopic morphology?
	Endoscopic ultrasound?
Therapy	
High-grade lesions	Endoscopic mucosal resection
	Focal ablation
	Esophagectomy
Low-grade lesions	Chemoprevention?

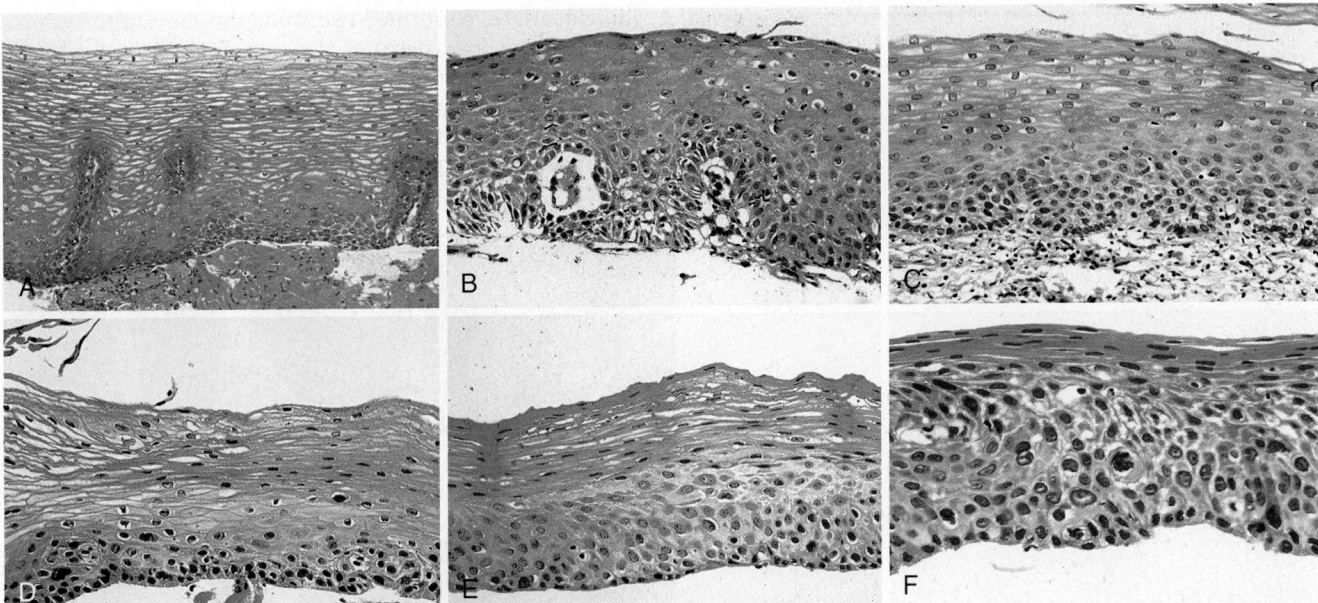

Fig. 30.2 Histologic categories used in endoscopic studies in Linxian, China. **A,** Normal. **B,** Esophagitis. The epithelium is infiltrated by polymorphonuclear leukocytes. **C,** Basal cell hyperplasia. The basal zone is greater than 15% of the epithelial thickness, without cellular atypia. **D,** Mild squamous dysplasia. There is cellular atypia, confined to the lower third of the epithelium. **E,** Moderate squamous dysplasia. There is cellular atypia involving the lower two-thirds of the epithelium. **F,** Severe squamous dysplasia. The cellular atypia involves all thirds of the epithelium, without invasion of the lamina propria.

We believe that squamous dysplasia is the only confirmed, clinically relevant precursor lesion of ESCC in high-risk and low-risk populations. More recent consensus conferences and World Health Organization guidelines prefer to use the term *intraepithelial neoplasia* rather than *dysplasia* throughout the gastrointestinal (GI) tract, and they prefer to subdivide these lesions into two grades: low-grade intraepithelial neoplasia and high-grade intraepithelial neoplasia.[52,53] In the squamous lesions of the esophagus, the guidelines suggest that high-grade intraepithelial neoplasia should include severe dysplasia and carcinoma in situ.[52] The above-described data suggest, however, that there are three quite different levels of risk that are identifiable by histologic examination, and both moderate and severe dysplasia need to be targeted for screening and treatment.

Nonendoscopic Screening Techniques

Cytologic Techniques

The most common nonendoscopic screening technique for early detection of esophageal cancer is esophageal balloon cytology screening in high-risk populations. Two principal types of cytologic samplers have been used in these screenings: an inflatable balloon sampler first developed in China[54–57] and an encapsulated sponge sampler first developed in Japan (**Fig. 30.3**).[58–61] In the balloon technique, a deflated balloon covered by a cloth net or rubber ribbing is swallowed into the stomach, inflated, and withdrawn, collecting exfoliated cells and scraping the mucosal surface of the esophagus. At the upper esophageal sphincter, the balloon is deflated and removed. In the sponge technique, a polyurethane mesh is compressed inside a gelatin capsule and attached to a string or a thin plastic stylet. The capsule is swallowed into the stomach, where the gelatin dissolves, and the mesh expands. The mesh is pulled up the esophagus by the string, collecting exfoliated and scraped mucosal cells. In both methods, the collected cells are processed and stained for cytology and read for cellular abnormalities. Several studies of both of these methods have reported high sensitivities for detecting ESCC in symptomatic patients, but there are few data on their accuracy for detecting squamous dysplasia or for detecting ESCC in asymptomatic individuals, who would be the target group for any population screening effort.

To investigate further the potential of nonendoscopic esophageal cytology for screening asymptomatic high-risk individuals, we performed two studies in Linxian to evaluate the screening characteristics of two commonly used Chinese balloons, a new American balloon, and an American-made encapsulated sponge. In this study, asymptomatic adults were examined by the cytology samplers, followed by Lugol's iodine chromoendoscopy of all participants. The cytology slides were

Table 30.2 Incidence and Relative Risk of Esophageal Squamous Cell Carcinoma (ESCC) during 13.5 Years of Follow-up, by Initial Histology, in an Endoscopy Cohort from Linxian, China

Initial Diagnosis	No. Patients	Cumulative ESCC Incidence (%)	Relative Risk (95% CI)
Normal	375	8.3	1.0 (reference)
Acanthosis	77	7.8	0.9 (0.4–2.2)
Esophagitis	33	6.1	0.8 (0.2–3.2)
Basal cell hyperplasia	40	15.0	1.9 (0.8–4.5)
Mild dysplasia	76	23.7	2.9 (1.6–5.2)
Moderate dysplasia	30	50.0	9.8 (5.3–18.3)
Severe dysplasia	39	74.4	30.8 (15.3–52.3)
Dysplasia NOS*	12	58.3	12.7 (5.5–29.6)
Total	682	16.7	NA

*Dysplasia not otherwise specified, not graded owing to small size or poor orientation of biopsy specimen.

CI, confidence interval; NA, not applicable.

Adapted from Wang GQ, Abnet CC, Shen Q, et al: Histological precursors of oesophageal squamous cell carcinoma: Results from a 13 year prospective follow up study in a high risk population. Gut 54:187–192, 2005.

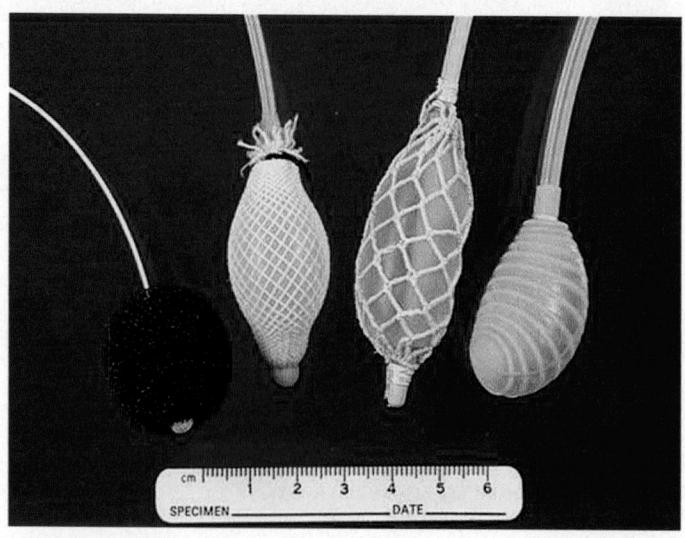

Fig. 30.3 Sponge and balloon cytologic samplers used in Japan and China.

Table 30.3 Screening Characteristics of Esophageal Balloon Cytology Samplers for Identifying Patients with Biopsy-Proven Esophageal Squamous Dysplasia in Linxian, China

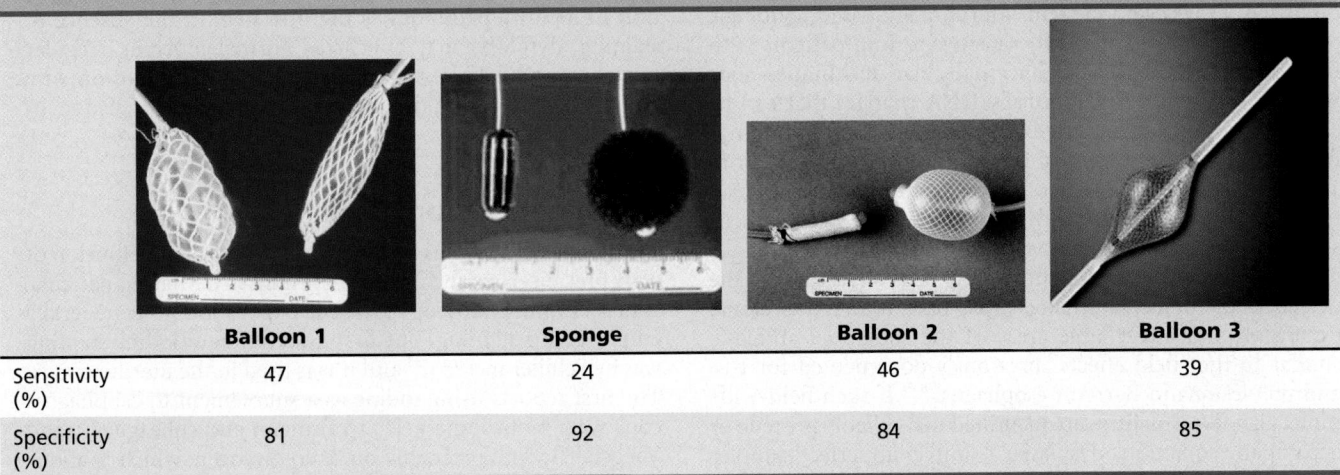

	Balloon 1	Sponge	Balloon 2	Balloon 3
Sensitivity (%)	47	24	46	39
Specificity (%)	81	92	84	85

read using the Bethesda System, the standard Western cytologic criteria for diagnosing cervical and vaginal smears, and the cytologic diagnoses were compared with the "gold standard" biopsy diagnoses. In the first study,[62] 439 patients were examined by both a Chinese balloon and the encapsulated sponge, in random order, and in the second study,[63] 359 patients were examined by the second Chinese balloon, and 381 patients were examined by the American balloon. The results of these studies were not encouraging: None of the samplers achieved a sensitivity of 50% for identifying biopsy-proven squamous dysplasia or cancer (**Table 30.3**). The most important problem with this screening technique appears to be two kinds of sampling error: blind sampling of a large organ and missing small lesions and morphologic evaluation of only a small percentage of the collected cells.

Molecular Techniques

Molecular markers have several attributes that make them potentially useful for primary screening in an early detection and treatment program for ESCC and its precursor lesions. Molecular changes occur early in the neoplastic process (earlier than morphologic changes). Changes sometimes can be detected in clinical samples such as blood or stool that can be collected noninvasively. Molecular changes in DNA (e.g., hypermethylation, LOH, and mutations) can be amplified by polymerase chain reaction, so rare events can be found in complex clinical samples. Some molecular changes undergo clonal expansion, so they are present over a much larger field of tissue than the discrete foci of morphologic dysplasia, which should make them easier to detect when mucosal sampling is incomplete. Finally, measurement of molecular changes is more objective and less variable than cytologic or histologic identification of dysplasia.

Blood or one of its components would be an ideal clinical sample for primary screening purposes. Possible serologic approaches to screening include looking for tumor-specific DNA, RNA, or proteins that are secreted into the circulation or are released during tumor cell death and looking for autoantibodies produced by the host in response to tumor antigens. A few authors have looked for tumor-specific hypermethylated genes in the serum or plasma of patients with ESCC and have found them to be present in a few cases.[64,65] Hibi and colleagues[64] found hypermethylated p16 in tumor tissue in 31 (82%) of 38 ESCCs and found this same marker in the serum of 7 (23%) of the 31 patients with positive tumors. Kawakami and associates[65] found hypermethylated APC in tumor tissue from 16 (50%) of 32 ESCCs and in the corresponding serum from 2 (12%) of the 16 tumor-positive patients. In the latter study, detection of hypermethylated APC in the plasma of esophageal adenocarcinomas was significantly associated with tumor stage (1 of 26 [4%] positive in stage I-II tumors; 12 of 26 [46%] positive in stage III-IV tumors); this should probably also be true of ESCCs. Although the proportion of tumors showing some hypermethylation increases when multiple genes are evaluated,[66] it still seems unlikely that many intraepithelial precursor lesions or stage I ESCCs would shed altered DNA into the serum or plasma that can be detected by such evaluations. Preliminary serologic studies looking for tumor-associated RNA[67] and proteins[68] have also been performed. Another possible serologic screening approach that has shown promise for detection of early squamous cell carcinomas of the lung and the head and neck region is identification of host autoantibodies generated against tumor-specific antigens.[69–71]

Stool is another clinical sample that could potentially contain information about the esophagus and could be collected noninvasively. Several authors have shown that neoplasia-specific DNA mutations can be detected in stool from patients with colorectal adenomas and adenocarcinomas,[72,73] and the sensitivity of these assays can be increased by testing panels of markers[73a] and by employing more sensitive new technologies.[74] There are also two reports of detection of other, more proximal aerodigestive malignancies, including esophageal carcinomas, by measuring high-molecular-weight or "long" DNA (DNA from nonapoptotic cells, which are more commonly sloughed from neoplasms)[75] or tumor-specific DNA mutations[76] in stool. Detection of esophageal precursor lesions or early invasive ESCCs by these methods may be unlikely, but it should still be evaluated.

At least for the near future, nonendoscopic molecular screening for early ESCC and its precursor lesions may still need to depend on evaluation of esophageal cell samples. As discussed previously, current morphology-based cytologic techniques are not sufficiently sensitive to find patients with focal squamous dysplasia, but molecular techniques may improve this sensitivity, especially DNA changes that can be amplified. One study reported promoter methylation findings for eight genes in esophageal balloon cytology samples from 147 patients with endoscopic biopsy diagnoses ranging from normal to severe squamous dysplasia and showed a 50% sensitivity and 68% specificity for identifying patients with high-grade dysplasia.[77] The most promising possibility may be the detection of molecular changes that have undergone clonal expansion and affect large areas of the squamous mucosa, similar to the "field effects" previously documented for p16 and p53 lesions in Barrett's esophagus.[78,79] If such field-wide molecular abnormalities are identified that reliably precede or accompany squamous dysplasia, a simple, imperfect sampler that is acceptable to patients, such as an encapsulated sponge, may be able to identify accurately or rule out the presence of an abnormal field, which may be sufficient to triage patients appropriately to endoscopy.

Endoscopic Screening Techniques

Various different endoscopes have been used to screen for early ESCC and its precursor lesions. These endoscopes may differ in size, resolution, and magnification characteristics. Ultrathin endoscopes measuring less than 6 mm (with a biopsy channel) may be used. A trial with a 3.1-mm stand-alone battery-powered fiberoptic esophagoscope (which did not have a biopsy channel) showed that it was feasible and accurate in detecting esophageal pathology.[80] Typically, instruments with diameters of 9 mm are employed. Standard resolution and magnification instruments suffice, but advantages of higher resolution and magnification have been described.[81] Conventional videoendoscopes are equipped with CCD chips of 100k to 300k pixels, meaning that each image is built up from 100,000 to 300,000 individual pixels. This technical feature, pixel density, determines the resolution. Newer instruments with CCDs having 600,000 to 1 million pixels are now commercially available and are referred to as high-resolution instruments. The feature of high resolution is distinct from high magnification, which can be accomplished by either optical magnification or electronic magnification. With optical magnification, a mechanical system that can move a lens at the tip of the endoscope along the longitudinal axis of the endoscope creates the ability for the endoscopist to adjust the focal distance of the device to allow for close viewing of mucosal details. Depending on which endoscope and which optical magnification system is used, the image can be enlarged 75 to 115 times. With optical magnification, image resolution can be preserved during the magnification process. With an electronic magnification technique, the actual magnification is performed by the videoprocessor. An area in the center of the endoscopic images magnifies only the pixels in the target area, which are used to generate the enlarged image. It is often more difficult to preserve image resolution in this method. Features of high resolution and high magnification can be combined. Most of the published literature regarding endoscopic screening describes the use of standard endoscopes.

When screening is performed endoscopically, visual inspection to identify pathology is the first step. In the absence of staining, dysplasia may appear as normal mucosa, irregular mucosa, a small white patch, a focal red area, an erosion, or a plaque. Early ESCC is usually seen as an erosion, a plaque, or a nodule (**Fig. 30.4**).[82]

Chromoendoscopy

Chromoendoscopy has been shown to assist with definition of early precancerous and cancerous lesions in numerous patients. When chromoendoscopy is used, Lugol's iodine is generally employed for staining. The first description of iodine staining was by Schiller in 1933,[83] and it was used in the uterine cervix. The first reports using iodine as a supplement to esophagoscopy were by Brodmerkel,[84] Nothmann and colleagues,[85] and Voegeli.[86] Iodine reversibly binds to glycogen, which is abundant in normal nonkeratinized squamous epithelial cells. Iodine staining causes a brown color change in normal esophageal mucosa. Inflamed, dysplastic, or cancerous cells are relatively depleted of glycogen and do not take up as much of the dye. Foci of glycogenic acanthosis have more than the usual amount of glycogen and appear overstained. Lugol's iodine can be used to identify abnormal mucosal areas (unstained lesions), including esophagitis, dysplasia, and ESCC (**Fig. 30.5**). It also can be valuable in delineating the margins of these lesions, which is particularly relevant if endoscopic mucosal resection or an ablative treatment is contemplated.

In a typical procedure, the patient is placed in the left lateral decubitus position. Sedation may or may not be used. Often a "Cetacaine-type" medication is sprayed onto the throat, or a "Dicaine-type" slurry is drunk. If sedation is used, typically a benzodiazepine with or without a narcotic is given. The esophageal mucosa must be assessed in its entirety, so evaluation must begin as soon as the instrument passes the upper esophageal sphincter. The endoscopist searches for mucosal abnormalities as described previously (see **Fig. 30.4**).

If the initial endoscopy without staining is to be followed by chromoendoscopy, biopsies are deferred until after the staining. Various concentrations of Lugol's iodine have been employed, but in most cases the concentration is between 1% and 2%. The formula of the iodine stain that we use (12 g iodine + 24 g potassium iodide dissolved in 1000 mL of water) was taken from the work of Endo and Ide.[87] This formula is slightly stronger than Lugol's original solution (1 g iodine + 2 g potassium iodide in water to 100 g). The formula we use has been called 1.2% Lugol's by some authors, referring to its elemental iodine content, and 3% Lugol's by other authors, referring to the total (iodine + potassium iodide) iodine content. For this reason, it is important to specify the formula that is used.

Some investigators advocate pretreatment with a water rinse or a mucolytic agent to remove mucus from esophageal mucosa.[88] It has not been our practice to do so.

The dye is delivered through a spray catheter passed via the biopsy channel of the endoscope. Specifically designed spray catheters can be used (e.g., Olympus PW-5L spray catheter; Olympus America, Inc., Melville, NJ) or endoscopic retrograde cholangiopancreatography catheters. Typically, spraying begins distally, at the squamocolumnar junction, and as the

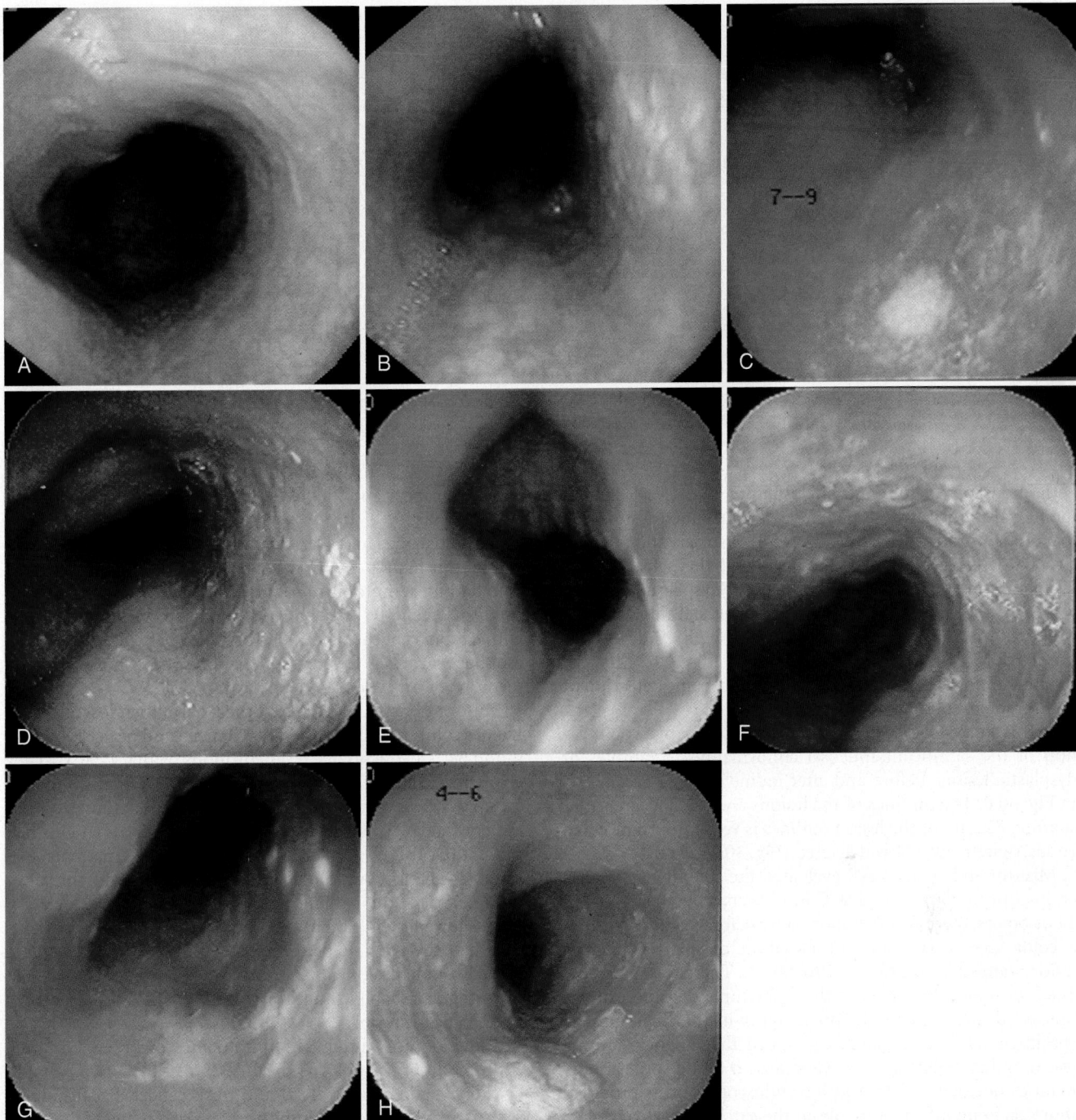

Fig. 30.4 Endoscopic categories used in the studies in Linxian, China. **A,** Normal mucosa. **B,** Irregular mucosa, seen focally at 3 o'clock position. **C,** Small white patch, at 6 o'clock position. **D,** Focal red area, at 3 o'clock position. **E,** Small punched-out erosion, at 3 o'clock position. **F,** Large broad-based erosion, at 11 to 4 o'clock position. **G,** Plaque, at 2 to 6 o'clock position. **H,** Nodules, at 4 o'clock position and 5 to 7 o'clock positions.

endoscope is withdrawn proximally, it is rotated so that the dye covers the entire mucosal surface. One should be careful not to withdraw proximally all the way to the upper sphincter, to avoid inadvertently spraying proximal to the sphincter. Generally, 20 to 25 mL of Lugol's solution is sprayed. If the entire surface is not covered, further spraying is necessary. The normal mucosa becomes brown in appearance. The dye begins to fade in 5 to 8 minutes, so biopsy specimens should be taken as quickly as possible. If unstained lesions are seen, directed

biopsy specimens are taken. If there are no unstained areas, biopsy specimens should be taken in a systematic way. At the end of the examination, the stomach should be carefully suctioned to remove as much of the iodine solution as possible.

Our group evaluated the utility of mucosal iodine staining to improve endoscopic visualization of dysplasia and ESCC in the high-risk population of Linxian, China.[89] In our mucosal staining study, 225 patients with evidence of dysplasia or carcinoma found on previous balloon cytology were evaluated

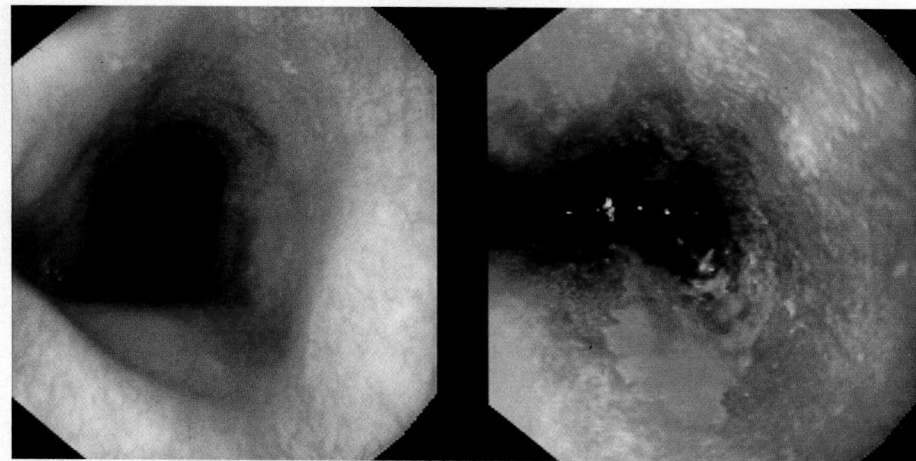

Fig. 30.5 Detection of squamous dysplasia by iodine chromoendoscopy. Before staining, all of the mucosa appears normal. After staining, the normal mucosa stains brown, but an abnormal area at the 6 o'clock position remains unstained. Biopsy specimens of this unstained lesion showed mild dysplasia.

with endoscopy before and after staining with 1.2% Lugol's iodine solution. In these patients, 253 unstained lesions, 94 foci of high-grade (moderate or severe) dysplasia and 20 invasive ESCCs were found. Before staining, the sensitivity of visible lesions for identifying high-grade dysplasia or ESCC was 62%, and the specificity was 79%. After staining, the sensitivity of unstained lesions for identifying high-grade dysplasia or ESCC was 96%, and the specificity was 63%. Mucosal iodine staining significantly improved endoscopic detection of high-grade dysplasia and ESCC.

In this study, Lugol's staining also greatly improved delineation of the significant mucosal abnormalities. Examples of dysplastic lesions before and after iodine staining are shown in **Fig. 30.6**. The outlines of the lesions are much clearer after staining. Clarity of the lesion outlines is very important when endoscopic treatment is delivered (**Fig. 30.7**).[90]

Misumi and colleagues[88] evaluated the role of Lugol's dye endoscopy in diagnosing ESCC in 17 lesions in 10 patients. In 14 instances, there was an abnormality before staining—either a color change (redness) or elevation or depression. The lesions ranged in size from 0.7 to 4.0 cm. There was good correlation in all cases between the endoscopic detection of the unstained area and the lesion margins in the final surgical specimen. The investigators concluded that Lugol's staining was useful in diagnosing ESCC because it found some abnormalities not detected by routine endoscopy, and it provided more accurate information about the extent of the cancer.

Freitag and coworkers[91] studied patients at risk for squamous cell carcinoma in southern Brazil, where esophageal cancer is the fourth most frequent neoplasm in men and the eighth most common neoplasm in women. When Lugol's solution was applied in this high-risk group, if unstained lesions were found, there was an 80% sensitivity and 63% specificity for the detection of dysplasia.

Shiozaki and associates[92] used Lugol's iodine to screen asymptomatic patients with head and neck cancer for esophageal cancer. Of 178 screened patients, 9 (5%) had one or more esophageal cancers identified. Of the 13 cancers found, 8 were early stage disease, with no lymph node metastases. Only 4 of the 13 lesions were seen at routine endoscopy. The investigators concluded that Lugol's chromoendoscopy should be considered in asymptomatic patients with a history of head

and neck cancer and in any other patient populations at high risk for ESCC.

Ina and colleagues[93] also evaluated the utility of Lugol's staining in male patients with oral or oropharyngeal cancer who had no symptoms of esophageal disease. Lugol's dye was used to screen 101 patients with oral cancer and 26 patients with oropharyngeal cancer. Of these 127 patients, 8 (6%) had esophageal cancer; in 5 of the 8 patients, no abnormality was seen on routine endoscopy or barium swallow.

Muto and associates[94] performed chromoendoscopy with Lugol's solution in 389 patients with head and neck cancer and found 54 (14%) who had a synchronous primary ESCC. They characterized the staining pattern in the 389 patients into four groups. Type I patients had normal brown staining; type II patients had 10 or fewer unstained areas; type III patients had more than 10 unstained areas; and type IV patients had irregular-shaped, multiform unstained lesions. In the latter group, 55% of the patients had ESCC. Muto and associates[94] also followed their patients for more than 1 year, and patients who had the type IV pattern were more likely to develop a metachronous lesion during that time. They concluded that the irregular-shaped, multiform lesions likely represented a "field cancerization."

Using iodine staining, Hashimoto and coworkers[95] found 8 cases of dysplasia (7%) and 10 cases of ESCC (8%) in 118 Brazilian patients with head and neck cancer. Because most reports using Lugol's staining in high-risk patients are from Asia, this Brazilian study lends support to its utility in any patient population at risk throughout the world.

In addition to patients with head and neck cancer, alcoholics are another group at high risk for developing esophageal squamous cancer. Yokoyama and colleagues[96] studied a cohort of 629 male alcoholics by endoscopy with iodine staining. Unstained lesions were observed in 162 patients (26%), and 36 unstained lesions in 21 patients (3%) were superficial ESCC. Because these lesions were superficial, endoscopic mucosal resection could be performed in 17 patients. In a similar group of 255 alcoholic Japanese patients, Ban and associates[97] found unstained lesions in 22% and cancer in 4%.

In southern Brazil, Fagundes and colleagues[98] studied 190 patients who were at risk for esophageal cancer because of increased consumption of alcohol or the beverage maté (a hot

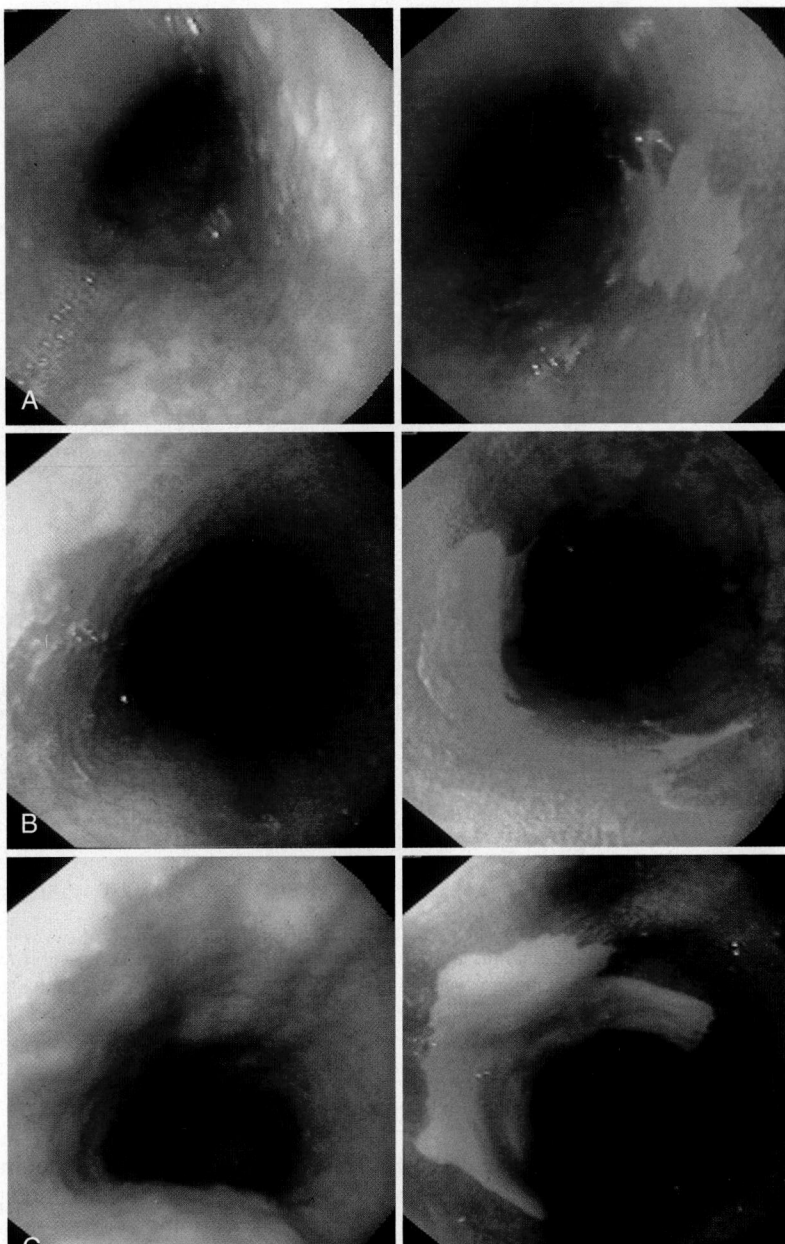

Fig. 30.6 Improved delineation of squamous dysplasia by iodine chromoendoscopy. **A,** Before staining, irregular mucosa is seen at the 3 o'clock position. After staining, the outline of the lesion is much more distinct. Biopsy specimens showed moderate dysplasia. **B,** Before staining, a large broad-based erosion is seen at the 7 to 10 o'clock position. After staining, the borders of this lesion are clearer, and a second lesion is identified at the 5 o'clock position. Biopsy specimens of both lesions showed severe dysplasia. **C,** Before staining, the mucosa appears normal. After staining, a large unstained lesion with sharp borders is seen. Biopsy specimens showed severe dysplasia.

infusion of herbs). Unstained lesions were present in 23 of these asymptomatic patients, of which 6 showed dysplasia. In some patients with a normally stained midesophagus, there was also evidence of dysplasia, but the likelihood of finding dysplasia was eightfold higher in areas that were unstained. The investigators concluded that iodine chromoendoscopy improves the detection of dysplasia and should be added to conventional upper GI endoscopies in patients in selected populations at high risk for squamous cell carcinoma.

Strader and colleagues (D. Strader, personal communication, January 1, 2004)[99] screened 98 alcoholic American veterans with endoscopy and iodine staining; 28 (29%) had unstained lesions, but no foci of dysplasia or cancer were found. Screening in this study began at age 40, which may have been too young in this population. Meyer and associates[100] prospectively compared the diagnostic accuracy of videoendoscopy with and without Lugol's staining for the detection of esophageal cancer in 158 alcoholic and smoking patients in France. Before staining, 12 patients had 14 endoscopically identifiable dysplastic or cancerous lesions. After staining, these numbers increased to 13 patients with 17 lesions. The unstained areas were significantly larger than the mucosal abnormalities seen before staining.

In an attempt to understand staining patterns with Lugol's iodine better, Mori and colleagues[101] applied iodine staining to 24 ESCC specimens resected by subtotal esophagectomy. They divided the staining patterns into four groups: type I, hyperstaining; type II, normal brown staining; type III, less intense staining; and type IV, unstained. Most type IV lesions were invasive carcinomas, carcinomas in situ, or severe dysplasia. Moderate to mild dysplasia or atrophy appeared as type III staining. The investigators also showed that there was good

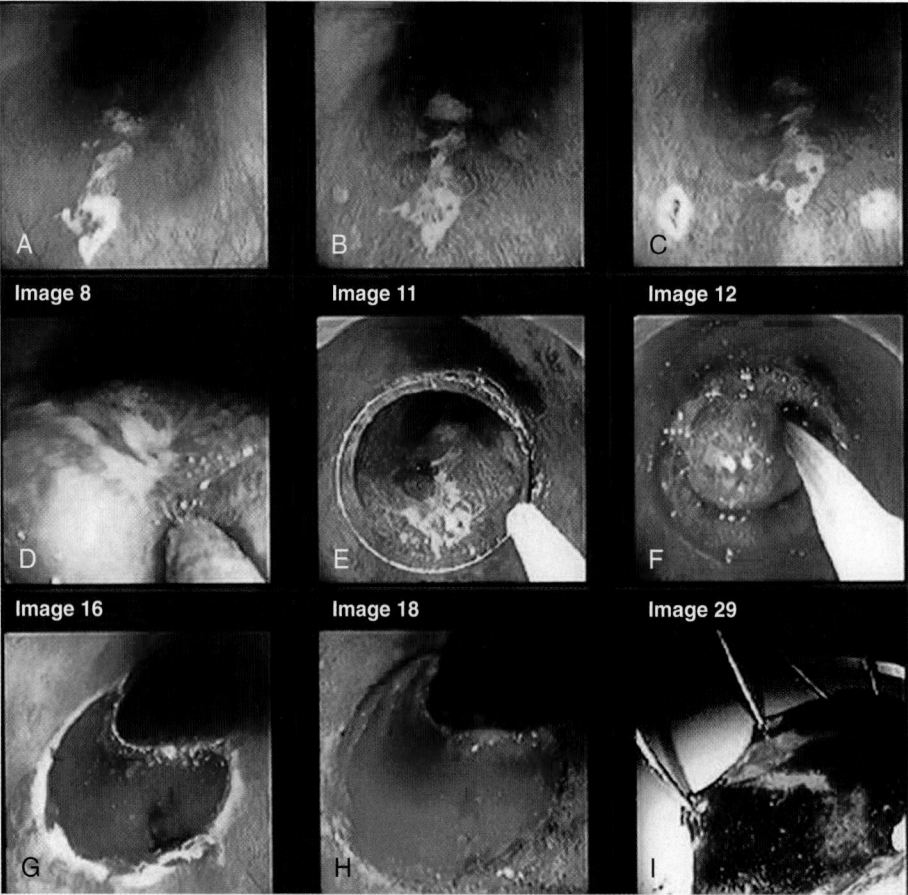

Fig. 30.7 Use of chromoendoscopy for endoscopic mucosal resection. **A,** Dysplastic lesion before staining. **B,** Immediately after staining with Lugol's iodine. **C,** Stain is fading 5 minutes later; two cautery marks are in place. **D,** Injection with saline. **E,** Lesion seen through the cap on the tip of the endoscope for snare technique removal. **F,** Snare now closed around lesion. **G,** Esophageal defect seen after endomucosal resection. **H,** Repeat stain with iodine to assess for residual pathology. **I,** Resected specimen.

correlation between the histologic tumor margin and the absence of staining.

Table 30.4 summarizes the detection of significant lesions before and after iodine staining in the above-described studies. In these patients, who had various degrees of risk for developing ESCC, 39% of the lesions were detected only after staining with iodine. This finding underscores our belief that mucosal iodine staining improves endoscopic detection and delineation of high-grade squamous dysplasia and ESCC.

Although Lugol's iodine is generally regarded as safe when sprayed onto esophageal mucosa to facilitate early detection of squamous cell carcinoma, some side effects have been reported.[102,103] Mucosal irritation can be manifested by retrosternal pain, discomfort, or nausea. Free iodine, one of the components of Lugol's, causes these side effects, and the risk of complication is greater with increasing concentrations of iodine.

Sodium thiosulfate (STS), a water-soluble neutral chemical, can be used as an intravenous antidote for cyanide, iodine, arsenic, or heavy metal intoxication. STS spray was first reported as being effective for reducing symptoms caused by staining with iodine solutions in 1993.[103,104] Kondo and coworkers[105] compared the utility of 5% STS with no treatment and with aluminum magnesium hydroxide gel (Maalox) in 120 patients after spraying the esophagus with 3% Lugol's

iodine. STS was most effective in reducing adverse symptoms, and the authors recommended its routine use after staining with iodine.

Although the largest experience using dyes to assist with screening for ESCC and its precursor lesions is with Lugol's iodine, there are also some reports using toluidine blue (also called tolonium chloride). Toluidine blue stains cellular nuclei, and this property makes it useful for identifying malignant tissue, which has an increased DNA content and a higher nuclear-to-cytoplasmic ratio. The mucosa of a normal esophagus does not stain with toluidine blue (**Fig. 30.8**).

When toluidine blue is used, a proteolytic enzyme (e.g., proteinase) in water is frequently used.[87] It may be ingested by mouth or sprayed on the mucosal surface. Toluidine blue is delivered as a 2% solution through a spray catheter in a manner identical to Lugol's iodine.

Seitz and colleagues[106] screened 100 patients with a history of alcohol and tobacco abuse using toluidine blue. Two carcinomas and 15 cases of dysplasia were detected. Two studies have looked at the use of toluidine blue dye spraying in patients with head and neck cancers. Hix and Wilson[107] found a 17% prevalence of ESCC in 18 asymptomatic patients with a history of head and neck malignancy. Contini and colleagues[108] found three esophageal neoplasms, two of which were not seen on routine endoscopy. Additional cases of

Table 30.4 **Detection of Squamous Dysplasia and Esophageal Squamous Cell Carcinoma (ESCC) in Studies Using Iodine Chromoendoscopy**

Reference	Population	No. Lesions	No. Seen before Stain	No. Seen after Stain	% Seen Only after Stain
Misumi et al[88]	Known ESCC	17	14	17	18
Shiozaki et al[92]	HN CA	13	4	13	69
Ina et al[93]	HN CA	8	3	8	63
Hashimoto et al[95]	HN CA	18	8	18	56
Yokoyama et al[96]	ETOH	36	12	36	67
Meyer et al[100]	ETOH	17	14	17	18
Fagundes et al[98]	ETOH	23	12	23	48
Mori et al[101]	Resected ESCC	32	26	32	19
Dawsey et al[89]	Asymptomatic high risk	114	70	109	34
Freitag et al[91]	Asymptomatic high risk	64	20	44	39
Total		342	183	317	39

HN CA, head and neck cancer patients; ETOH, alcoholics.

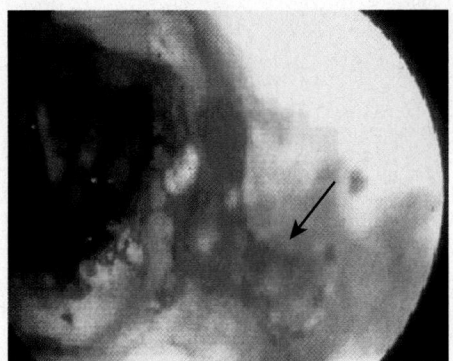

Fig. 30.8 Toluidine blue chromoendoscopy.

leukoplakia and esophagitis were also identified. To date, no complications have been reported with toluidine blue. Because the dye is absorbed through the GI tract and excreted in the urine, caution should be observed in cases with decreased renal function.

New Techniques for Screening without Chromoendoscopy

Various new adjunct techniques have been combined with standard endoscopy to determine if they can improve the diagnosis of neoplastic esophageal lesions and assist with staging and therapy. These "high-tech" approaches have attempted to improve on the "low-tech" method of chromoendoscopy, which has been extremely valuable and has withstood the test of time. Some more promising newer methods are (1) narrow band imaging (NBI) and multiband imaging, (2) autofluorescence, (3) endoscopic ultrasound (EUS), (4) optical coherence tomography, (5) endocytoscopy, and (6) confocal laser microscopy.[109]

NBI is a technique that uses optical filters instead of dyes. In NBI, the depth of light penetration in tissue depends on its wavelength. The shorter the wavelength, the more superficial

the penetration. In the visible light spectrum, blue penetrates most superficially and is the most valuable for mucosal imaging. Red light penetrates more deeply and is more appropriate for submucosal imaging. With NBI, the intensity of the blue light improves, which gives better definition to mucosal patterns and to blood vessels, particularly because blue light is preferentially absorbed by hemoglobin. Several endoscopic images with NBI are shown in **Fig. 30.9**. There has been considerable investigation with the use of NBI for Barrett's esophagus. Hamamoto and associates[110] were the first to use NBI for Barrett's esophagus. Kuraoka and colleagues[111] reported on the use of NBI and screening for early esophageal cancer in a group of patients who were at high risk because of heavy alcohol intake and previous head and neck cancers. They found a sensitivity, specificity, and positive predictive value of 100%, 59%, and 10%. Katada and coworkers[112] studied NBI for detecting metachronous superficial pharyngeal squamous cell carcinomas.

Multiband imaging, initially known as Fujinon Intelligent Chromoendoscopy (FICE), uses certain dedicated wavelengths similar to NBI. However, in contrast to NBI, which uses optical filters to narrow the bandwidth, FICE takes an ordinary endoscopic image from the videoprocessor and processes the photons in a way that allows virtual images to be constructed with a choice of different wavelengths (**Fig. 30.10**). Pasha and coworkers[113] reported on the use of FICE for studying the colonic mucosa. Many exquisite photographs showing high-resolution endoscopy plus NBI are contained in a text edited by Cohen.[114]

In standard endoscopy, incident light reacts with the tissue, and the reflected light is captured by the endoscope and processor. In addition to the standard imaging that occurs, there are other tissue interactions, one of which is autofluorescence. With autofluorescence, an incoherent violet-blue light is used as the source of excitation. The optical signals that result depend on the structure and molecular composition of the tissues being excited. Because neoplasia changes the composition of the tissue, it is theoretically possible to distinguish between normal tissue, dysplasia, and neoplasia (**Fig. 30.11**). The Erlangen group has contributed considerably

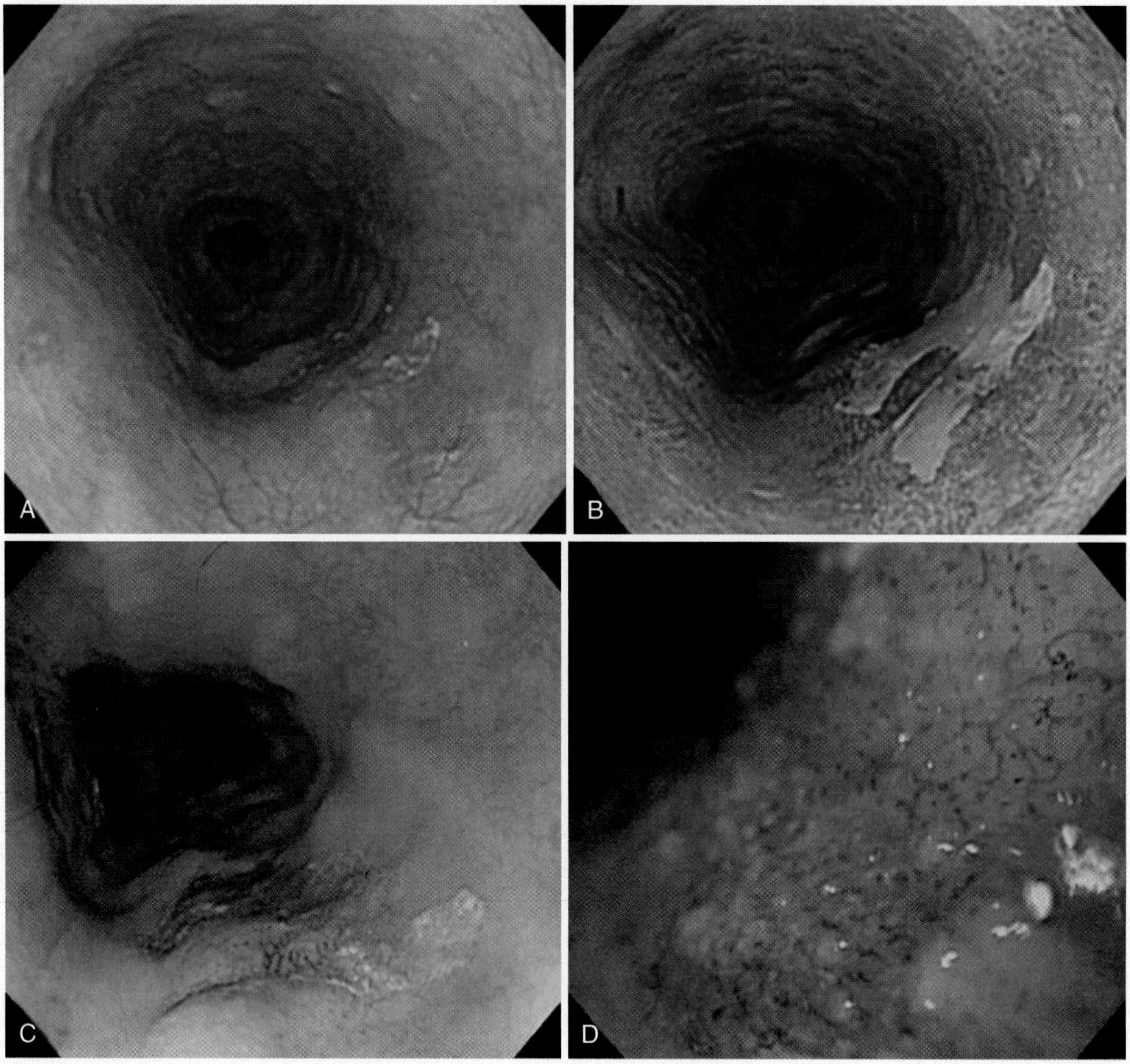

Fig. 30.9 Detection of early squamous cell carcinoma with narrow band imaging (NBI). **A,** Small flat erosion is observed at the 5 o'clock position. With white light it is difficult to see. **B,** With Lugol's iodine, it shows the lesion more distinctly. Biopsy specimen showed squamous cell carcinoma. **C,** Using NBI, the lesion is seen as a brown spot, and the contour is more easily appreciated. **D,** Intraepithelial papillary capillary loops (IPCLs) are noted. *(Photographs courtesy of Dr. Jonathan Cohen.)*

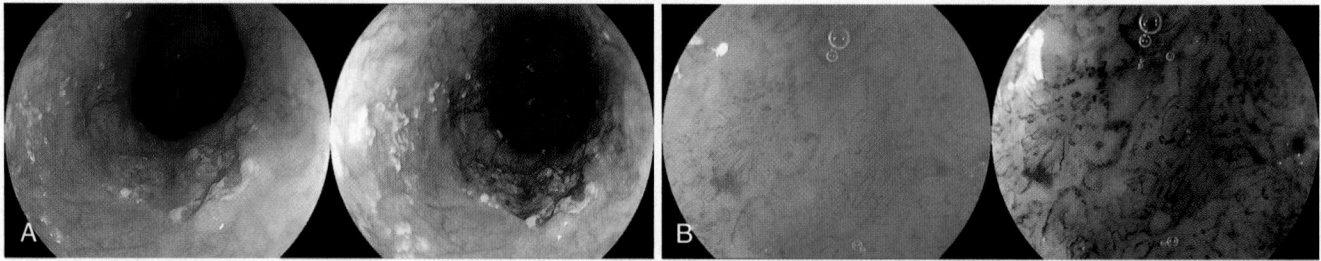

Fig. 30.10 Fujinon Intelligent Chromoendoscopy (FICE). **A,** Esophageal cancer is seen with white light endoscopy and with FICE. **B,** Magnified view shows intraepithelial papillary capillary loops (IPCLs) with white light and with FICE. *(Photographs courtesy of Jason Ylizarde, Fujinon, Inc.)*

in this area. Mayinger and colleagues[115] used 129 endogenous fluorescence spectra in evaluating nine patients with squamous cell carcinoma and four patients with adenocarcinoma. Malignant and benign spectra were differentiated with the aid of a mathematical algorithm; by using this algorithm, the investigators had a sensitivity of 97% and a specificity of 95%

for the diagnosis of esophageal carcinoma. A commercially available endoscope by Olympus allows for the detection of autofluorescence.

EUS has made a significant impact on staging cancers of the digestive tract including esophageal cancer. To date, however, it has had limited utility for detecting dysplasia or defining the exact level of mucosal or submucosal penetration by early esophageal cancer. A study by May and colleagues[116] looked at the accuracy of staging early esophageal cancer using high-resolution endoscopy and high-resolution EUS. The study was carried out in 100 patients using a 20-MHz miniprobe. Overall, rates of accuracy were 79% using EUS staging for mucosal lesions, but for submucosal tumors the overall accuracy for EUS was only 48%.

Optical coherence tomography is a method analogous to high-resolution EUS, but it employs light waves instead of sound waves. It has a high resolution, but the sampling depth is limited to 1 to 2 mm. It has been studied in assessing Barrett's esophagus, but it has not been formally studied in ESSC.

The "Holy Grail" for endoscopy has been defined as an imaging system that would allow for an optical biopsy, which is a real-time image that would be equivalent to histopathologic sections. Advances have been made in this area using the principles of light contact microscopy. Endocytoscopy

(Olympus, Tokyo, Japan) uses a system by which a 3.2-mm probe is passed through the accessory channel of an endoscope. Kumagai and coworkers[117] studied 12 patients with superficial esophageal cancer. They sprayed the esophageal mucosal surface with 1% methylene blue and studied the targeted mucosa. In normal esophageal mucosa, the nuclei showed regular staining and a low nucleus-to-cytoplasm ratio. In contrast, in esophageal cancer, there were irregularities in cell distribution and a high nucleus-to-cytoplasm ratio. Inoue and associates[118] studied endocytoscopy in patients who had already undergone chromoendoscopy and NBI. They reported an overall accuracy for differentiating nonmalignant from malignant pathology in 82% of patients.

Confocal laser microscopy is a technology in which laser illumination is combined with an optical technique that allows different illumination detection systems to be focused in the same plane; it is referred to as confocal. The tissue can be scanned at various depths. Currently two companies have products in this area (EC383FK; Pentax, Tokyo, Japan, and Cellvizio; Mauna Kea Technologies, Paris, France). Both systems permit simultaneous endoscopic and endomicroscopic examination, permitting in vivo histologic examination of the mucosa with high resolution. With confocal laser microscopy, a fluorescein dye is injected intravenously; about 30 seconds later, there is a color change in the GI mucosa. Magnification is up to 1000 times. The observation range is 475 to 600 μm, the lateral resolution is approximately 1 μm, and the vertical resolution is 3 to 7 μm.

Several authors have reported on their experience using confocal laser and endomicroscopy for imaging of early squamous cell cancer.[119–121] The authors were able to show differences in both the cellular structure and the vascular structure, including a demonstration of intrapapillary capillary loops (IPCLs). The confocal images were compared with standard histology. The cancer tissues exhibited more irregular cellular arrangements, increased diameter of IPCLs, and irregularly shaped IPCLs. This technology is promising but is still in its early stages of development. Confocal images are shown in **Fig. 30.12**. It is hoped that these "high-tech" developments will contribute to meaningful advances in the management of a large number of patients.

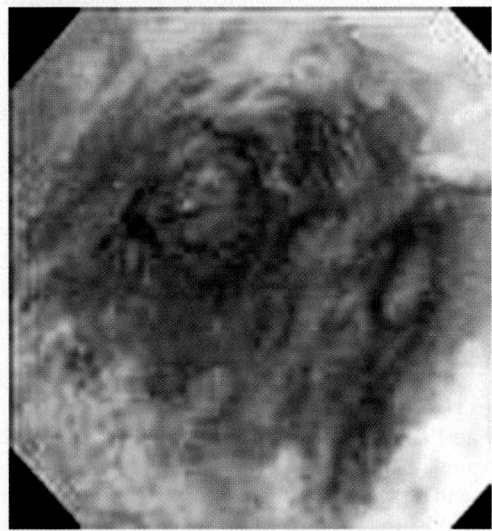

Fig. 30.11 Autofluorescence imaging. The purple area of autofluorescence seen at the 2 to 6 o'clock position highlights an area of esophageal cancer. Normal nonneoplastic areas are seen in green.

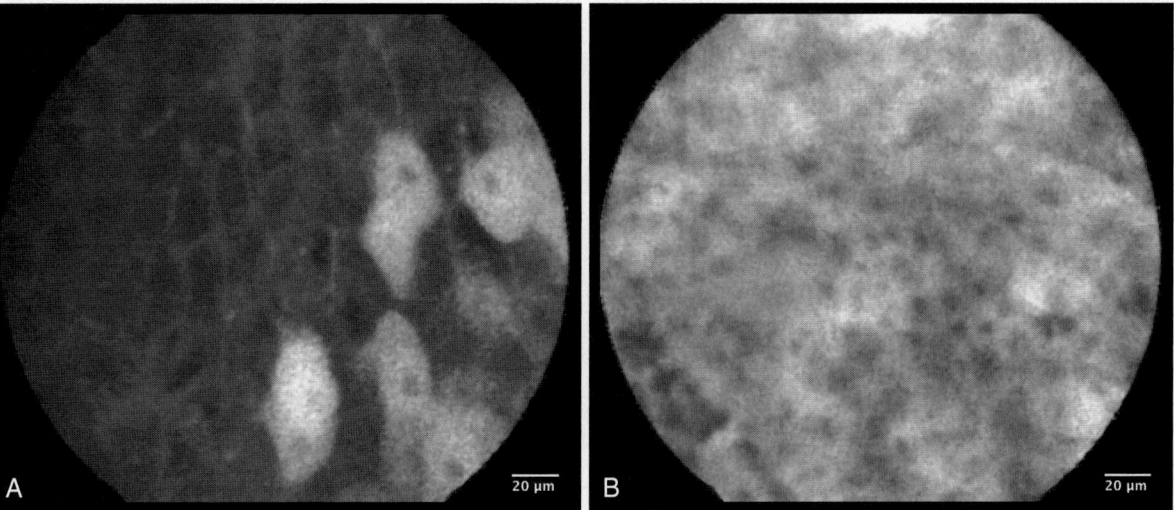

Fig. 30.12 Confocal laser microscopy. **A,** Confocal image of normal squamous epithelium shows normal cellular structure. **B,** Image of esophageal cancer shows disorganized cells with enlarged and hyperchromatic nuclei. *(Photographs courtesy of Dr. Cuong Nguyen and Dr. Ananya Das.)*

Endoscopic Morphology

Several classification systems have been used for defining the morphologic appearance of early GI cancer. The lack of standardization has led to confusion, and two separate literatures have evolved in the "East" and the "West" concerning the macroscopic appearance of superficial neoplastic lesions. This development discouraged international collaboration. A meeting was held in Paris in 2002 with leaders from the East and the West and terms were agreed on; this is referred to as the Paris classification of superficial neoplastic lesions of the GI tract.[122] A follow-up meeting was held in Osaka in 2003. A description of this classification follows.

Neoplastic lesions of the esophagus are called superficial when their endoscopic appearance suggests that invasion is limited to the mucosa or submucosa, and these types of lesions are considered to be type 0 (for increasingly deeper lesions, the classification goes to higher numbers I, II, III, and IV). Type 0 is divided into three categories: 0-I, protruding; 0-II, nonprotruding and nonexcavated; and 0-III, excavated. Type 0-II is subdivided further into slightly elevated (IIa), completely flat (IIb), and slightly depressed (IIc). **Table 30.5** and **Fig. 30.13** summarize this classification.

Table 30.5 Morphologic Classification of Type 0 Esophageal Lesions with a Superficial Appearance at Endoscopy

Morphologic Appearance	Type
Protruding	
Pedunculated	0-Ip
Sessile	0-Is
Nonprotruding and nonexcavated	
Slightly elevated	0-IIa
Completely flat	0-IIb
Depressed	0-IIc
Excavated	0-III

Clinical Application of Screening and Treatment for Early Esophageal Squamous Cell Carcinoma and Its Precursor Lesions

When either squamous cell carcinoma or adenocarcinoma of the esophagus is discovered after symptoms have begun, the prognosis is very poor, with a 5-year survival of less than 15%. In addition, the quality of life of patients who are diagnosed with esophageal cancer at a late stage is poor because in addition to the primary disease and the treatments for it, the social stigma of difficulty eating adds an additional burden to the last months of a patient's life. Both with screening programs for adenocarcinoma that focus on patients with Barrett's esophagus and with screening programs for patients with squamous cell carcinoma in high-risk categories, the goal is early diagnosis so that treatment can be carried out at a curable stage.

In the United States and Europe, where adenocarcinoma is common and Barrett's esophagus has been identified as the precursor lesion, screening for Barrett's esophagus and surveillance for progression in patients who have Barrett's esophagus have led to the application of several new therapies. When localized elevated endoscopic abnormalities are found in patients with Barrett's esophagus, endoscopic mucosal resection is a valuable treatment. If the lesion is superficial and fully removed, consideration can be given to other endoscopic therapies that eradicate larger segments of Barrett's tissues. A study by Shaheen and colleagues[123] showed in a randomized sham-controlled trial that radiofrequency ablation was beneficial for patients with low-grade or high-grade glandular dysplasia. There has also been interest in pursuing similar endoscopic therapy for patients with early esophageal cancer.

Pouw and colleagues[124] more recently described successful radiofrequency ablation for widespread early squamous cell carcinoma in a single case. A collaborative international effort has begun in China to study radiofrequency ablation for high-grade squamous intraepithelial neoplasia and early ESCC (G. Wang, personal communication, January 15, 2009). Chinese

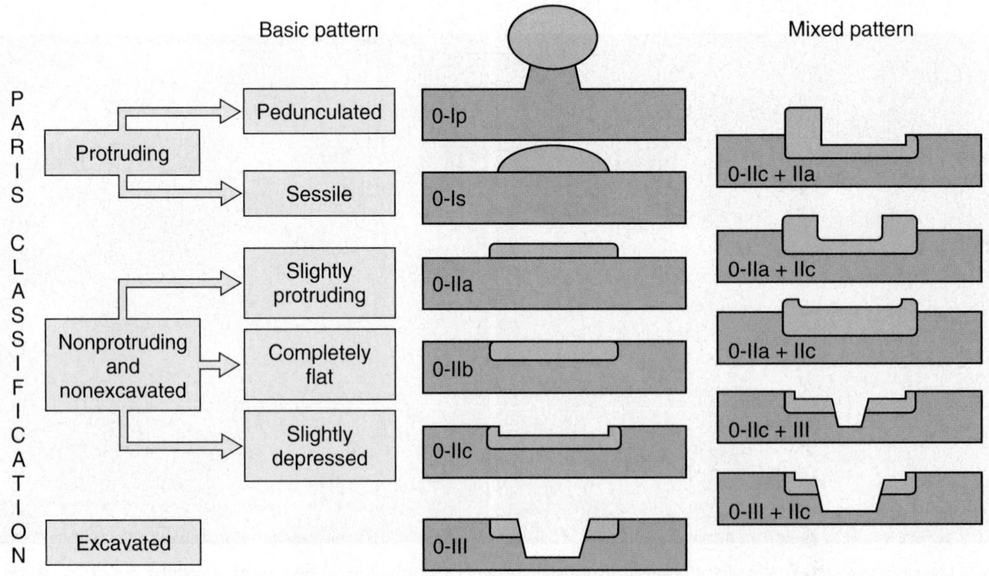

Fig. 30.13 Paris classification of superficial neoplastic lesions in the digestive tract.

investigators from the Cancer Institute, Chinese Academy of Medical Sciences and Feicheng Medical Center, are collaborating with American and Dutch physicians to evaluate this treatment technique in patients with moderate or severe dysplasia or invasive squamous cell carcinoma limited to the lamina propria (T1m2). To be eligible, the esophageal mucosa must be flat, without nodules or ulceration (type 0-IIb), and patients can have no signs of metastasis on EUS or CT. The primary endpoint will be the percentage of subjects who are completely free of dysplasia or cancer at 12 months after the first ablation procedure. If such endoscopic techniques are shown to be effective for treatment of early neoplastic lesions in such high-risk populations, primary screening for early ESCC and its precursor lesions would be even more valuable.

Summary

To reduce the mortality of ESCC, practical and accurate screening procedures for high-risk asymptomatic individuals need to be developed. The feasibility, acceptability, and cost-effectiveness of specific screening techniques would vary among different populations, so all screening programs would need to be tailored to local conditions. Finding the relatively few affected patients, such as the 7000 people who develop ESCC in the United States each year, at a T0-T1 stage would

be a challenge and probably would require screening large numbers of risk-stratified individuals in primary care settings.

Chromoendoscopy with Lugol's iodine solution is an excellent technique for confirming and localizing squamous dysplasia and early ESCC, and it is probably a practical method for screening patients at very high risk, such as patients with previous head and neck cancer, but it is impractical for primary screening in most other high-risk groups. New adjunctive endoscopic techniques are being studied to determine if they might affect screening in a way that improves on chromoendoscopy. Although there is great promise, their utility beyond that of chromoendoscopy has yet to be established. The main purpose of nonendoscopic screening is to identify accurately which patients should be triaged to endoscopy. In most settings, current cytologic techniques are not sensitive enough to perform this triage function successfully. New molecular techniques, alone or combined with cytology, may significantly improve the accuracy and practicality of nonendoscopic primary screening, which may offer new hope for early detection and treatment of this disease.

References

The complete reference list is available online at www.expertconsult.com.

Chapter 31

Extraintestinal Endosonography (including Celiac Block)

Adam J. Goodman and Frank G. Gress

Video related to this chapter's topics can be found online at expertconsult.com.

Introduction

The use of endoscopic ultrasound (EUS) has grown over the last 25 years, and it is now a well-established diagnostic method for the assessment of a range of gastrointestinal (GI) disorders, including the evaluation and staging of many types of endoluminal cancers. The role that EUS currently occupies in detection of disorders outside the limits of the GI tract was not considered several years ago.

This chapter discusses EUS applications relating to extraintestinal structures, organs, and lesions. The objectives of this chapter are to review the utility of EUS for evaluating the mediastinum in both benign and malignant disease processes, including the detection of mediastinal lymph node metastases in lung cancer. Mass lesions in the paragastric and retroperitoneal organs (excluding the bile duct, gallbladder, and pancreas) are reviewed, including detection of lesions of the adrenal gland, liver, and kidneys. Ascites and pleural fluid are examined along with unusual extraintestinal lesions. In addition, the EUS-guided technique of celiac plexus block (CPB) for chronic pancreatitis and celiac plexus neurolysis (CPN) for managing malignant pain are reviewed.

Lung Cancer

Lung cancer is the leading cause of cancer death in the United States in men and women and has an overall 5-year survival rate of 15%.[1,2] Treatment decisions are based on the location and extent of the tumor. The presence of extrapulmonary metastasis is crucial because patients without mediastinal involvement are potential candidates for resection. The distinction between non–small cell lung cancer (NSCLC), which accounts for 80% of tumors, and small cell lung cancer (SCLC), which accounts for 20% of tumors, is important because of the more aggressive nature of SCLC. SCLC is usually classified as limited or extensive disease, although the criteria for these two categories remain controversial.[3–5] Although the TNM (primary tumor, regional nodes, metastases) staging system traditionally has not been used in staging SCLC, it is expected to be included in the forthcoming seventh edition of the TNM classification of malignant tumors.[6–9] Metastatic disease is detected in 80% of SCLC cases at the time of diagnosis and tends to spread quickly so that surgery is considered less often in SCLC compared with NSCLC. Although highly responsive to radiotherapy and chemotherapy, SCLC usually recurs within 2 years.

In comparison, half of NSCLC cases are localized or locally advanced and can be treated by surgery, the cornerstone of therapy for NSCLC, or with adjuvant therapy with or without resection.[10–12] NSCLC, which includes adenocarcinoma, squamous cell cancer, and large cell cancer, continues to be staged using the 2002 International Staging System, which is unchanged from the 1997 revision (**Box 31.1**).[12–14] This section focuses on EUS applications in the diagnosis and staging of NSCLC, although much of what is covered can be applied to SCLC.

Staging and Staging Modalities

Mediastinal lymph node metastases are present in nearly half of all patients with NSCLC. Accurate staging of NSCLC is crucial in determining treatment options because the detection of mediastinal lymph node metastasis preoperatively has therapeutic implications. In the absence of distant metastasis, the documentation of mediastinal metastasis is probably the most common deterrent to cure.[15–26] The TNM staging system used for lung cancer (see **Box 31.1**) designates ipsilateral peribronchial, intrapulmonary, or ipsilateral hilar lymph nodes as N1 disease and ipsilateral mediastinal and subcarinal lymph node involvement as N2 disease. Although N2 disease is potentially resectable, most patients with N2 disease receive multimodality treatment. Contralateral lymph node involvement of mediastinal or hilar nodes or either ipsilateral or contralateral scalene or supraclavicular lymph nodes is designated N3 disease, which precludes resection (**Table 31.1** and **Fig. 31.1**, and see **Box 31.1**).[12–14,26,27]

Various techniques are currently available to diagnose and stage lung cancer, including plain radiography, computed tomography (CT), magnetic resonance imaging (MRI), positron emission tomography (PET), endobronchial ultrasound (EBUS), and EUS. CT scan of the chest is the current standard by which mediastinal lymphadenopathy is detected. Generally, lymph nodes larger than or equal to 1 cm on chest CT scan are considered abnormal. A review of previously published studies reveals an accuracy of CT staging of the mediastinum of 52% to 88%.[28–38] This variation has been attributed to the wide range of correlation of lymph node size to the presence of malignant involvement. Although the general trend is increased risk for metastasis correlating with increasing lymph node size, lymph node size is not an accurate criterion for assessing risk. Problems associated with size as a criterion include the inability to differentiate inflammatory or reactive lymph nodes from malignant involvement. In one study, 37% of mediastinal lymph nodes that ranged in size from 2 to 4 cm were benign,[38] and 40% of enlarged nodes in another series were not cancerous.[39] Similarly, normal-sized lymph nodes can contain foci of cancer. McKenna and colleagues[40] found no correlation between the presence of mediastinal nodal metastases and nodal size. Metastases may be found in 21% of normal-sized nodes.[41]

MRI may be slightly superior to CT in the detection of mediastinal disease,[42] and PET has been shown to be superior to CT for staging for the mediastinum.[43,44] PET does not rely on an arbitrary cutoff of size to diagnose malignant nodes but detects the increased glycolytic rate in metabolically active tumors. In a meta-analysis, PET had a sensitivity of 79% and

Box 31.1 International Staging System for Lung Cancer, 1997 Revision

Primary Tumor (T)

Tx: Primary tumor cannot be assessed

T0: No evidence of primary tumor

Tis: Carcinoma in situ

T1: Tumor <3 cm without bronchoscopic evidence of invasion more proximal than the lobar bronchus (not the main bronchus unless superficial tumor of any size with invasion limited to the bronchial wall, which may extend proximal to the main bronchus)

T2: Tumor >3 cm or any size with any of the following:
    Involves the main bronchus (at least 2 cm distal to the carina)
    Invades visceral pleura
    Associated with atelectasis or obstructive pneumonitis that extends to the hilar region but does not involve the entire lung

T3: Tumor of any size that invades any of the following:
    Chest wall, diaphragm, mediastinal pleura, or parietal pericardium or tumor in the main bronchus <2 cm distal to the carina (without involvement of the carina)
    Atelectasis or obstructive pneumonitis of the entire lung

T4: Tumor of any size that invades any of the following:
    Mediastinum, heart, great vessels, trachea, esophagus, vertebral body, or carina
    Separate tumor nodules in the same lobe
    Malignant pleural effusion

Nodal Involvement (N)

Nx: Regional lymph nodes cannot be assessed

N0: No regional lymph nodes metastasis

N1: Metastasis to ipsilateral peribronchial or ipsilateral hilar lymph nodes, or both, and intrapulmonary nodes including involvement by direct extension of primary tumor

N2: Metastasis to ipsilateral mediastinal or subcarinal lymph nodes, or both

N3: Metastasis to contralateral mediastinal, contralateral hilar, ipsilateral or contralateral scalene, or supraclavicular lymph nodes

Metastasis (M)

Mx: Distant metastasis cannot be assessed

M0: No distant metastasis

M1: Distant metastasis present (includes separate tumor nodules in a different lobe)

Stage Grouping

Occult carcinoma: TxN0M0
Stage 0: TisN0M0
Stage IA: T1N0M0
Stage IB: T2N0M0
Stage IIA: T1N1M0
Stage IIB: T2N1M0, T3N0M0
Stage IIIA: T1N2M0, T2N2M0, T3N1M0, T3N2M0
Stage IIIB: Any T N3 M0, T4 Any N M0
Stage IV: Any T any N M1

Data from Greene FL, Page DL, Fleming ID, et al, editors: AJCC (American Joint Committee on Cancer) cancer staging manual, ed 6, New York, 2002, Springer-Verlag, pp 167–174; and Mountain CF: Revisions in the International System for Staging Lung Cancer. Chest 111:1710–1717, 1997.

Table 31.1 **Lymph Node Map Definitions**	
Nodal Station	**Anatomic Landmarks**
N2 NODES: **ALL N2 NODES LIE WITHIN THE MEDIASTINAL PLEURAL ENVELOPE**	
1. Highest mediastinal nodes	Nodes lying above horizontal line at the upper rim of the brachiocephalic (left innominate) vein where it ascends to the left, crossing in front of the trachea at its midline
2. Upper paratracheal nodes	Nodes lying above horizontal line drawn tangential to the upper margin of the aortic arch and below the inferior boundary of the No. 1 nodes
3. Prevascular and retrotracheal nodes	Prevascular and retrotracheal nodes may be designated 3A and 3B; midline nodes are considered to be ipsilateral
4. Lower paratracheal nodes	Lower paratracheal nodes on the right lie to the right of the midline of the trachea between horizontal line drawn tangential to the upper margin of the aortic arch and line extending across the right main bronchus at the upper margin of the upper lobe bronchus and contained within the mediastinal pleural envelope; lower paratracheal nodes on the left lie to the left of the midline of the trachea between horizontal line drawn tangential to the upper margin of the aortic arch and line extending across the left main bronchus at the level of the upper margin of the left upper lobe bronchus, medial to the ligamentum arteriosum and contained within the mediastinal pleural envelope.
	Researchers may wish to designate the lower paratracheal nodes as No. 4s (superior) and No. 4i (inferior) subsets for study purposes; No. 4s nodes may be defined by a horizontal line extending across the trachea and drawn tangential to the cephalic border of the azygos vein; No. 4i nodes may be defined by the lower boundary of No. 4s and the lower boundary of No. 4 as described previously
5. Subaortic (aortopulmonary window)	Subaortic nodes are lateral to the ligamentum arteriosum or the aorta or left pulmonary artery and proximal to the first branch of the left pulmonary artery and lie within the mediastinal pleural envelope
6. Paraaortic nodes (ascending aorta or phrenic)	Nodes lying anterior and lateral to ascending aorta and the aortic arch or the innominate artery, beneath line tangential to the upper margin of the aortic arch
7. Subcarinal nodes	Nodes lying caudal to the carina of the trachea but not associated with the lower lobe bronchi or arteries within the lung
8. Paraesophageal nodes (below carina)	Nodes lying adjacent to the wall of the esophagus and to the right or left of the midline, excluding subcarinal nodes
9. Pulmonary ligament nodes	Nodes lying within the pulmonary ligament, including nodes in the posterior wall and lower part of the inferior pulmonary vein
N1 NODES: **ALL N1 NODES LIE DISTAL TO THE MEDIASTINAL PLEURAL REFLECTION AND WITHIN THE VISCERAL PLEURA**	
10. Hilar nodes	Proximal lobar nodes, distal to the mediastinal pleural reflection and the nodes adjacent to the bronchus intermedius on the right; radiographically, hilar shadow may be created by enlargement of both hilar and interlobar nodes
11. Interlobar nodes	Nodes lying between the lobar bronchi
12. Lobar nodes	Nodes adjacent to the distal lobar bronchi
13. Segmental nodes	Nodes adjacent to the segmental bronchi
14. Subsegmental nodes	Nodes around the subsegmental bronchi

From Mountain CF, Dresler CM: Regional lymph node classification for lung cancer staging. Chest *11:1718–1723, 1997.*

a specificity of 91% compared with CT, which had sensitivity and specificity of 60% and 77%, for the detection of mediastinal disease.[43] In another meta-analysis by Toloza and colleagues,[44] the performance characteristics of CT, PET, and EUS for staging the mediastinum in NSCLC were compared. PET was more accurate than CT or EUS for detecting mediastinal metastases with a sensitivity of 84% and a specificity of 89% for PET compared with CT (sensitivity 57% and specificity 82%) and EUS (sensitivity 78% and specificity 71%). However, PET is limited for small lesions (≤1 cm), has false-negative results in tumors with low metabolic activity, and has false-positive results in benign lesions such as granulomatous disease. Although PET has a relatively high sensitivity, because of the importance and implications of staging, specificity is still too low, and pathologic staging is still generally sought.[45-47]

Fritscher-Ravens and associates[48] performed a prospective comparison of CT, PET, and EUS for the detection of metastatic lymph nodes metastases in patients with lung cancer being considered for operative resection. After bronchoscopic evaluation, CT, PET, and EUS were performed to evaluate potential mediastinal involvement with bronchoscopic biopsy and cytology–proven (*n* = 25) or radiologically suspected (*n* = 8) lung cancer before surgery. Surgical histology was used as the "gold standard" and revealed NSCLC in 30 patients, neuroendocrine tumor in 1 patient, and benign disease in 2 patients. With respect to the correct prediction of mediastinal lymph node stage, the sensitivities of CT, PET, and EUS were 57%, 73%, and 94%; specificities were 74%, 83%, and 71%; and accuracies were 67%, 79%, and 82%. Results of PET could be improved when combined with CT (sensitivity 81%,

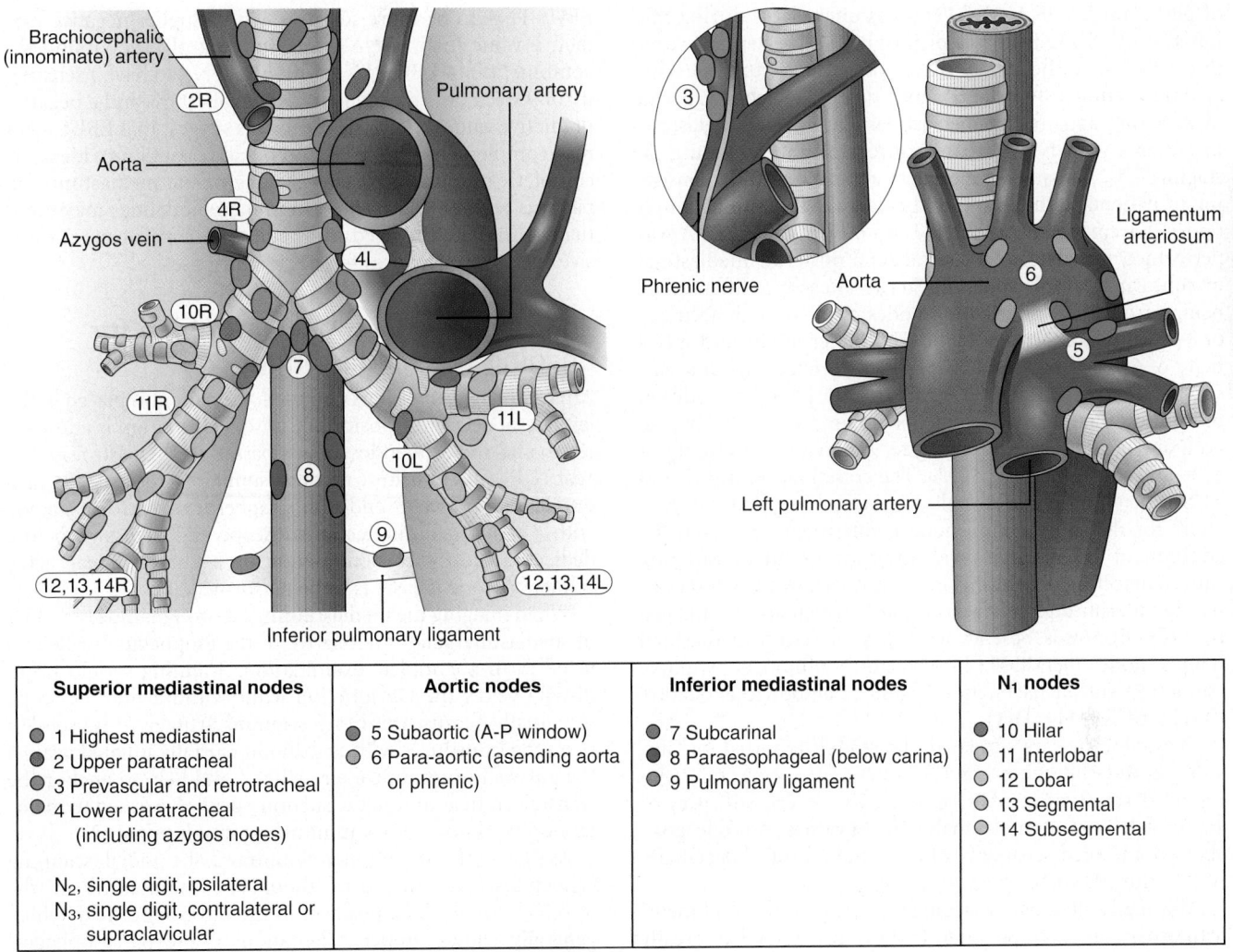

Brachiocephalic (innominate) artery

2R

Aorta

4R

Azygos vein

10R

11R

12,13,14R

7

8

9

10L

11L

12,13,14L

Inferior pulmonary ligament

Pulmonary artery

4L

3

Phrenic nerve

Aorta

6

5

Ligamentum arteriosum

Left pulmonary artery

Superior mediastinal nodes	Aortic nodes	Inferior mediastinal nodes	N₁ nodes
● 1 Highest mediastinal ● 2 Upper paratracheal ● 3 Prevascular and retrotracheal ● 4 Lower paratracheal (including azygos nodes) N_2, single digit, ipsilateral N_3, single digit, contralateral or supraclavicular	● 5 Subaortic (A-P window) ● 6 Para-aortic (asending aorta or phrenic)	● 7 Subcarinal ● 8 Paraesophageal (below carina) ● 9 Pulmonary ligament	● 10 Hilar ○ 11 Interlobar ○ 12 Lobar ○ 13 Segmental ○ 14 Subsegmental

Fig. 31.1 Lymph node stations. *(From Mountain CF, Dresler CM: Regional lymph node stations for lung cancer staging. Chest 111:1718–1723, 1997.)*

specificity 94%, accuracy 88%). The specificity of EUS (71%) was improved to 100% by fine needle aspiration (FNA) cytology. The authors concluded that no single imaging method alone was conclusive in evaluating potential mediastinal involvement. They also suggested that CT may be necessary to evaluate the pretracheal region and the rest of the thorax and that PET may be valuable to detect distant metastases.

Whenever enlarged lymph nodes are seen in the mediastinum on chest CT scan, standard practice is to perform a lymph node biopsy for more accurate staging. The traditional methods for performing a lymph node biopsy are via CT or bronchoscopy or both. Bronchoscopy with FNA is commonly used to evaluate suspicious paratracheal, hilar, and subcarinal lymph nodes seen on CT.[49–52] The role of bronchoscopy in the diagnosis and staging of NSCLC is well established and has a sensitivity of approximately 60%.[53–59] Bronchoscopy is unable to access the aortopulmonary window or the inferior mediastinal nodes, however. CT-guided biopsy of the mediastinum is limited by overlying vascular and bony structures. When the lymph node status is not determined with CT or bronchoscopy or both, mediastinoscopy and in some cases limited thoracotomy are performed to clarify the disease stage.[37,60–62] However, these procedures are more invasive and require

general anesthesia and inpatient recovery, increasing the time, cost, and risk of the staging process.[63]

Endoscopic Ultrasound

The advent of EUS has made it possible to image the GI tract and surrounding extraluminal structures such as the mediastinum with precise resolution. EUS has played an increasingly important role as an accurate and safe method for staging patients with NSCLC.[64–85] With the advent of transesophageal EUS-guided FNA, suspicious posterior mediastinal lymph nodes, including aortopulmonary window, subcarinal, and inferior (below carina) paraesophageal nodes, can be sampled. Tracheal air artifact generally precludes reliable assessment of the anterior mediastinum lesions, pretracheal nodes, and upper paratracheal nodes; however, the advent of EBUS technology seems to be minimizing this limitation. The use of EUS and EBUS technology can enhance the overall accuracy for detecting mediastinal lymph node metastasis.

The results of an early pilot study evaluating the role of EUS in 17 patients with lung cancer found EUS to be very accurate at detecting mediastinal lymphadenopathy with an overall accuracy of 71% versus 41% for CT.[83] However, the capability of performing EUS-guided FNA was unavailable during this initial study. Sampling of suspicious lymph is essential except in N1 nodes. In the 1990s, several prospective studies evaluated the accuracy of EUS, EUS-guided FNA, and chest CT scan in detecting and staging mediastinal lymph node metastasis in patients with NSCLC based on correlation with surgical staging.[69,70,75] Gress and colleagues[75] reported a study consisting of patients with NSCLC and enlarged mediastinal lymph nodes (>1 cm) seen on chest CT scan. EUS-guided FNA was performed for suspicious contralateral posterior mediastinal or subcarinal lymph nodes. EUS criteria used to differentiate benign from malignant lymph nodes resulted in an accuracy of 84% compared with 49% for CT. The sensitivity and specificity of CT was 64% and 35%, which compared with a sensitivity and specificity of 86% and 83% for EUS. The addition of transesophageal EUS–guided FNA improved the overall accuracy of lymph node staging to 96% with a sensitivity of 93% and a specificity of 100%. The combination of CT and EUS did not improve overall accuracy above that for EUS alone for detecting lymph node involvement. However, the addition of CT aided in evaluating the extent of the lung cancer, detecting distant metastasis not seen by EUS and evaluating anterior and pretracheal nodes, which are not imaged by EUS. EUS was best at accurately detecting mediastinal lymph node metastasis in the aortopulmonary window (station 5), subcarinal (station 7), and paraesophageal (station 8) regions (see **Fig. 31.1**).

These findings are similar to the studies reported by Giovannini and colleagues[73] and Silvestri and coworkers,[74] who reported sensitivities of 81% and 89% and specificities of 100% each. A recent meta-analysis by Micames and colleagus[67] showed a pooled sensitivity of 83% and a pooled specificity of 97% for EUS-FNA staging of NSCLC.

Although still not approaching the "gold standard" of mediastinoscopy and lymph node biopsy, EUS-FNA has greatly improved minimally invasive staging of NSCLC. As noted earlier, where EUS fails is in the anterior mediastinum where tracheal air artifact generally precludes reliable assessment of the anterior mediastinum lesions, pretracheal nodes, and upper paratracheal nodes. In an attempt to view the anterior mediastinum, radial EBUS was initially developed in the 1990s. There was limited use of the technology, however, because it was impossible to perform real-time guided FNA of lesions. In more recent years, convex, linear probe technology has been developed and now allows for real-time EBUS-guided transbronchial needle aspiration (TBNA). A systematic review of EBUS-TBNA showed that it was a safe and effective modality to aid in the staging of NSCLC with a sensitivity ranging from 85% to 100% without reported complications.[68] Gu and colleagues[69] performed a meta-analysis of studies aimed at measuring EBUS-TBNA accuracy and found a 93% sensitivity and 100% specificity in detecting mediastinal lymph node metastasis. Given the high sensitivity and specificity of both EUS-FNA and EBUS-FNA, many investigators have been seeking to perform a complete, "medical mediastinoscopy," with the hope of avoiding the more traditional, invasive staging, including mediastinoscopy, of NSCLC before operative intervention.

The largest study to date was performed by Wallace and colleagues,[70] who compared the use of TBNA, EUS-FNA, and EBUS-TBNA using pathologic confirmation of malignancy or benign disease as the diagnostic standard. This group found

EBUS-FNA to be more sensitive, with a higher negative predictive value than TBNA. More importantly, they found the combination of EBUS-FNA with EUS-FNA to have a sensitivity of 93%, a positive predictive value of 100%, and a negative predictive value of 97%. These results suggest that EBUS-FNA may complement EUS-FNA and possibly could provide near-complete, minimally invasive staging of the mediastinum in patients with NSCLC. These combined modalities may eventually eliminate the need for mediastinoscopy or other invasive surgical procedures for staging purposes.

Endoscopic Ultrasound Technique for Imaging the Mediastinum

After informed consent is obtained, the patient is placed in the left lateral decubitus position. Conscious sedation is administered, and the echoendoscope is passed to the gastroesophageal (GE) junction in a manner similar to the passage of a duodenoscope. Many endosonographers first perform staging with a radial scanning echoendoscope and then switch to a dedicated biopsy echoendoscope or a curved linear array echoendoscope if FNA is to be performed.

When imaging the mediastinum, a thorough understanding of mediastinal anatomy relative to the esophagus is essential to perform a complete examination. Scanning should begin distally below the GE junction while withdrawing the scope proximally because this limits scanning artifacts. It is useful to press the transducer with its balloon partially inflated against the gut wall to minimize air artifacts and help to anchor the transducer. In addition, the suction port is depressed to maintain optimal imaging by minimizing intraluminal air.

As the endosonographer withdraws the radial scanning echoendoscope, the aorta should be maintained in the 5 o'clock to 6 o'clock position in the ultrasound field, which generally allows proper orientation of the paraesophageal structures. The aorta is easily recognized as a circular anechoic structure, approximately 1.5 to 2 cm in diameter, with a relatively bright border resulting from back wall enhancement (a normal artifact seen in vessels). As the echoendoscope is withdrawn into the distal esophagus, the aorta, spine, left lobe of the liver, inferior vena cava, and heart can be seen. The spine is also easily identified in the 7 o'clock position next to the aorta and has irregular echo features with artifacts produced by poor penetration of echoes through bony structures. The left lobe of the liver appears at the 6 o'clock to 12-o'clock position, and often the hepatic veins and inferior vena cava can be seen as they course through the liver. Slightly more proximally, the beating of the heart is appreciated as the left atrium comes into view at the 12 o'clock position. The mitral valve leaflets can be seen as the valve opens from the left atrium into the left ventricle, and the pulmonary veins can be seen entering the left atrium. The left pulmonary artery arches posteriorly to the left of the ascending aorta and tends to be easier to view than the right pulmonary artery, which can be seen just below the carina. The left ventricle, right atrium, and right ventricle lie deep to the left atrium; it can be more difficult to visualize these structures completely. As the aorta moves toward the left, the spine and azygos vein are seen posteriorly. The aortic outflow tract can be appreciated as the endoscope is withdrawn further. The spine continues to be a useful landmark because it consistently appears as a hyperechoic structure located posteriorly throughout the chest.

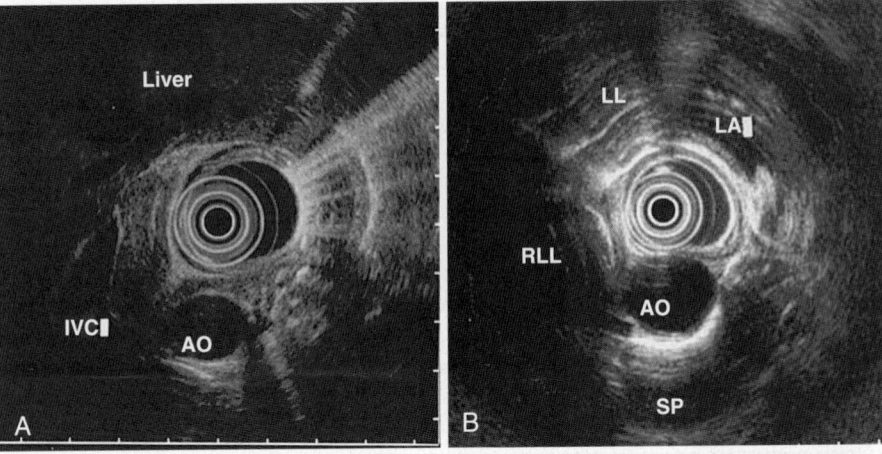

Fig. 31.2 A, Radial imaging at the distal esophagus showing the liver, inferior vena cava (IVC), and aorta (AO). The spine lies immediately deep to the aorta. **B,** Imaging slightly higher in the distal esophagus showing the right lower lobe of the lung (RLL), left lung (LL), aorta (AO), spine (SP), and a portion of the left atrium (LA).

Careful inspection of this area may reveal the thoracic duct adjacent to the aorta and spine.

The right lung appears as hyperechoic rings emanating from the 9 o'clock position, whereas the left lung appears at the 2 o'clock position. In the midesophagus, the right and left bronchi are easily demarcated by the hyperechoic rings (echogenic air) seen at the 11 o'clock and 1 o'clock positions. The two bronchi join together to form the trachea normally at 27 to 28 cm from the incisors. The azygos vein can be seen coming into position to the right of the aorta and moves anterior to the spine and toward the right lung. As the endoscope is withdrawn further, the azygos vein can be seen to move forward and extend anteriorly into the superior vena cava. The ascending aorta can be difficult to trace because this structure runs deep to the hilar structures (pulmonary vessels), and because of air within the bronchi and trachea, the ascending aorta is often not fully imaged. In the proximal esophagus, the aortic arch is identified on the left and moves rightward and anteriorly across the screen. In the cervical esophagus, above the level of the aortic arch, the carotid vessels and, occasionally, the thyroid gland can be seen (**Figs. 31.2, 31.3, and 31.4**).

Evaluation of the mediastinum using linear EUS requires rotation of the echoendoscope every few centimeters for a thorough evaluation. As in radial EUS, vascular structures provide the major landmarks for orientation, and the home base structure is the descending aorta, which is first located approximately 35 cm from the incisors. The echoendoscope is rotated initially clockwise (right) bringing structures anterior to the esophagus into view and then counterclockwise (left) bringing posterior structures into view. The left atrium is found by rotating the shaft of the scope 180 degrees in the distal esophagus to midesophagus until a large, echolucent structure is seen within which the mitral valve leaflets are located. By tipping the scope upward and with slight withdrawal, the subcarinal lymph node station is located immediately beneath the endoscope at approximately 27 cm between the left atrium and right pulmonary artery. The aortopulmonary window is located by following the descending aorta cephalad to the arch and pushing the endoscope in again about 2 cm. The endoscope is turned 90 degrees clockwise and

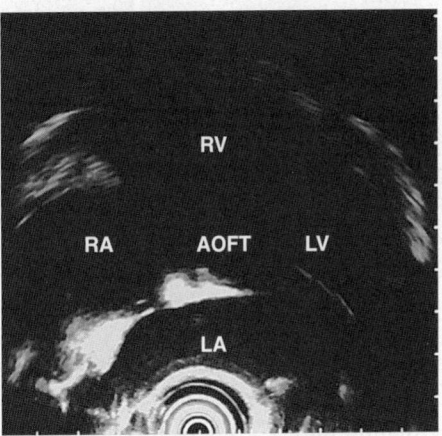

Fig. 31.3 Radial endoscopic ultrasound (EUS) from the distal esophagus. The left atrium (LA), right atrium (RA), right ventricle (RV), and left ventricle (LV) can be seen. The leaflets of the mitral valve and the base of the aortic outflow tract (AOFT) are also visible.

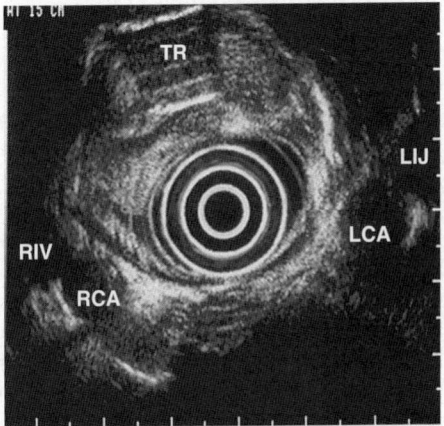

Fig. 31.4 Radial endoscopic ultrasound (EUS) from the most proximal aspect of the esophagus. The left common carotid artery (LCA), left internal jugular vein (LIJ), right internal jugular vein (RIV), right common carotid artery (RCA) are seen. In addition, the thyroid gland is seen on either side of the trachea (TR).

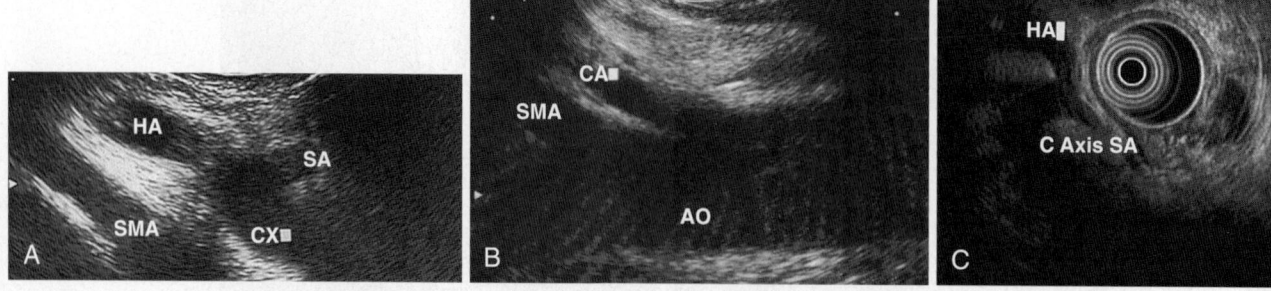

Fig. 31.5 **A,** Linear array imaging of the celiac axis is depicted showing the takeoff of the superior mesenteric artery (SMA) and celiac axis (CX) along with the hepatic artery (HA) and splenic artery (SA) branches. **B,** More typical linear images as seen from the proximal stomach. **C,** Radial imaging showing the celiac axis.

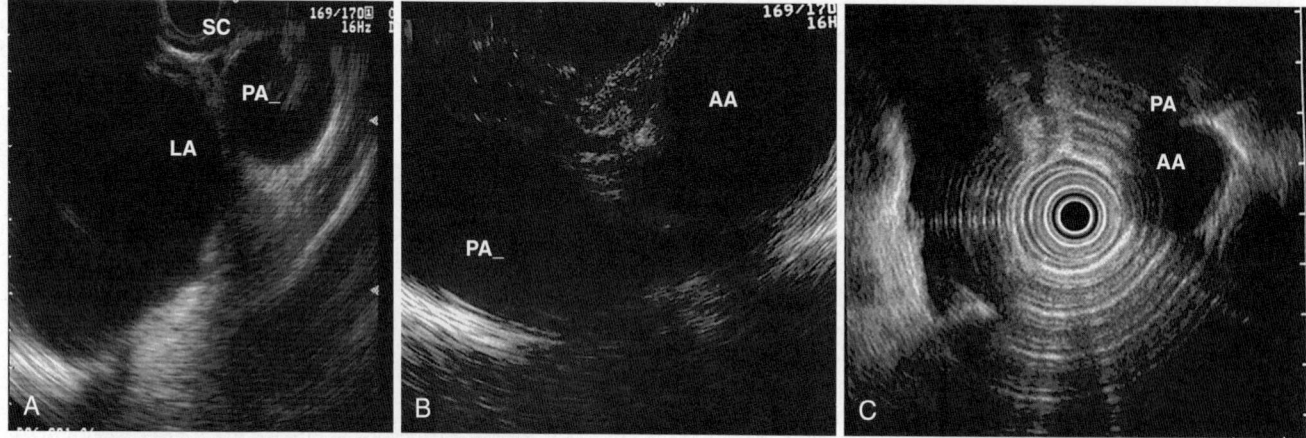

Fig. 31.6 **A,** Curved linear array view through the midesophagus of the subcarinal (SC) region. The left atrium (LA) is next to the right pulmonary artery (PA) with the ascending aorta lying deep to these structures. **B,** Linear array view through the midesophagus of the aortic arch (AA) and the pulmonary artery (PA)—the "AP window." **C,** Radial imaging of the area of the AP window.

tipped up slightly until a cross-sectional view of the aortic arch and the more distally located left pulmonary artery are seen. The area between these structures is known as the "AP window." Another potentially important area for FNA of lymph nodes is the celiac axis. This area is located by finding the abdominal aorta at the level of the GE junction and the takeoff of the celiac artery with the superior mesenteric artery just distal to this (**Figs. 31.5 through 31.8**).

Techniques for Staging Non–Small Cell Lung Cancer with Endoscopic Ultrasound

EUS is performed under conscious sedation in an outpatient setting with a radial scanning or linear array scanning echoendoscope. In experienced hands and with careful planning, EUS of the mediastinum can be performed quickly regardless of the type of EUS technology used. When FNA of mediastinal lymph nodes is performed, the procedure is slightly prolonged, depending on the availability of the cytopathologist.

The preparation of the patient is the same as for standard endoscopy. Prophylactic antibiotics are not administered unless recommended by the American Heart Association or the American Society of Gastrointestinal Endoscopy because EUS-guided FNA of mediastinal lesions is not associated with

significant bacteremia. However, prophylactic quinolone antibiotics are recommended for FNA of cystic mediastinal lesions, which is similar to the recommendations for pancreatic cystic lesions and perirectal lesions.[86–93] After informed consent is obtained and conscious sedation is administered (we have found propofol to be effective), the instrument is advanced into the stomach, and the celiac axis is imaged. The probe is slowly withdrawn to the GE junction and then cephalad using radial scanning images generally obtained with 7.5-MHz frequencies at each 1-cm interval while keeping the aorta at the 5 o'clock or 6 o'clock position. All mediastinal lymph nodes seen are "mapped" by location according to the American Thoracic Society classification scheme (see **Box 31.1**, **Table 31.1**, **Fig. 31.1**, and video on expertconsult.com).[12–14]

An objective determination is made as to whether the mediastinal lymphadenopathy detected by EUS is consistent with benign or malignant status according to previously reported studies using the same criteria.[82,87,94–100] EUS criteria used to diagnose malignant lymph nodes are round shape, sharp distinct borders, hypoechoic texture, and a short-axis diameter greater than 5 mm. Each of these parameters should be present for a lymph node to be considered as potentially malignant; however, FNA has significantly improved the sensitivity and specificity of detection of malignant lymph nodes.[73–75,84,85,87,100,101]

The liver and left adrenal gland are carefully inspected, and any ascites or pleural fluid that is unexpectedly detected is

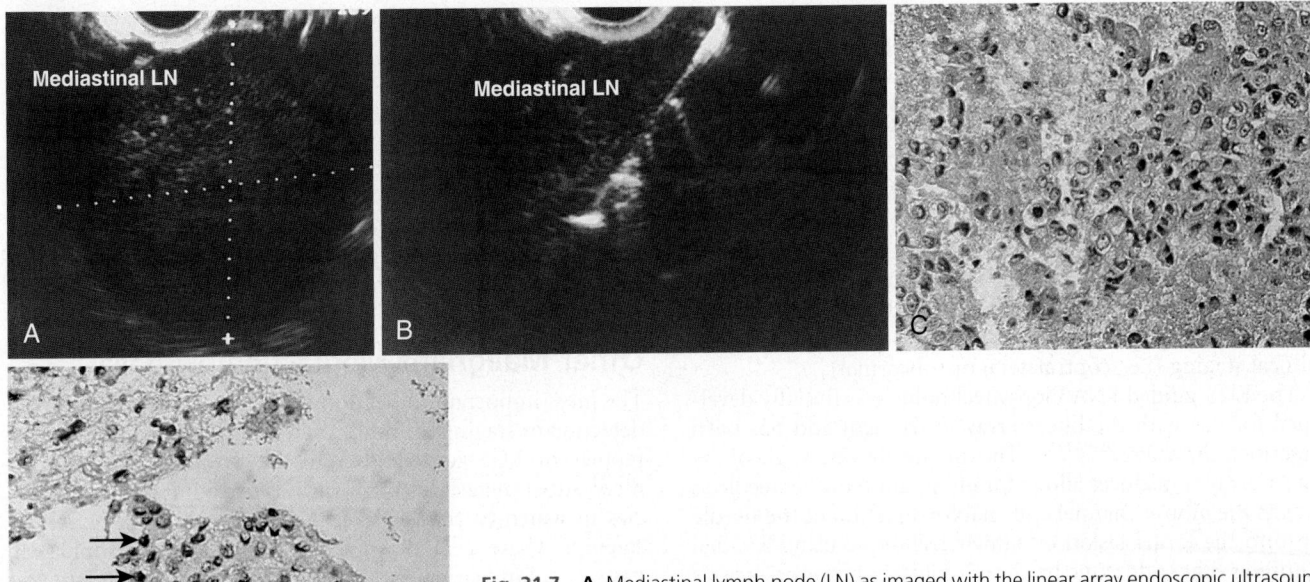

Fig. 31.7   **A,** Mediastinal lymph node (LN) as imaged with the linear array endoscopic ultrasound (EUS) system. **B,** The fine needle aspiration (FNA) needle is seen exiting the scope; the tip of the needle is seen to be in the center of the LN. **C,** High-power magnification of hematoxylin and eosin stain on cell block reveals metastatic adenocarcinoma. **D,** High-power magnification of immunoperoxidase stain on cell block. Tumor nuclei *(arrows)* are positive for TTF1 antibody consistent with non–small cell lung carcinoma.

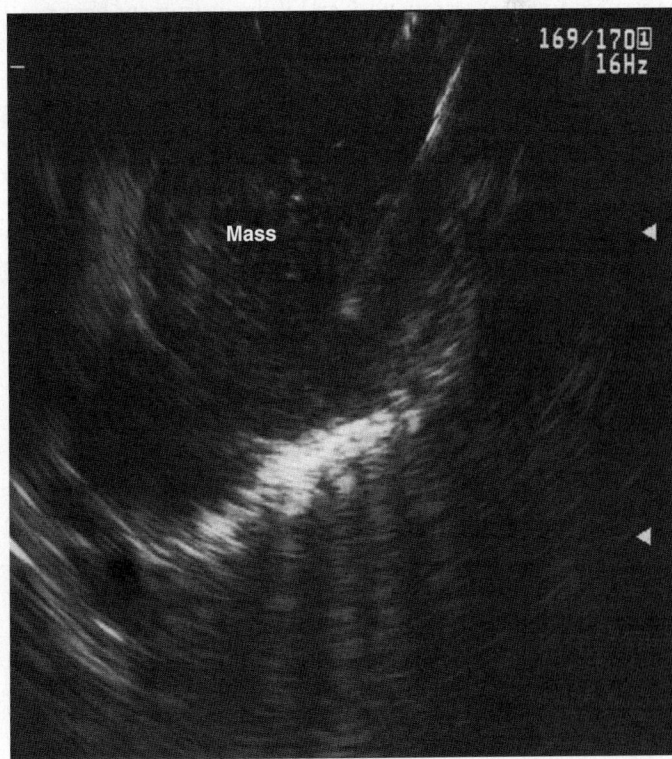

Fig. 31.8   Linear endoscopic ultrasound (EUS) reveals a hypoechoic mass within the mediastinum. EUS-guided fine needle aspiration (FNA) was performed and revealed metastatic non–small cell lung cancer (cytology favored a large cell neuroendocrine-type lesion).

inspected. If suspicious lymphadenopathy or other suspicious findings are seen that may represent metastatic disease, the linear echoendoscope is introduced (if not already in use), and EUS-guided FNA is performed. Many centers have successfully used only linear technology for diagnostic imaging and for obtaining needle aspiration cytologic samples, and this may become the modality of choice after gaining more experience with the technique.

Technique for Performing Endoscopic Ultrasound–Guided Fine Needle Aspiration

Mediastinal Lymph Nodes

EUS-guided FNA became available after the development of a specially designed needle catheter system consisting of a

4-cm, 23-gauge needle attached to a 180-cm long, 5-Fr aspiration catheter (Echo-Tip; Wilson-Cook Medical, Inc, Winston-Salem, NC) and the 22-gauge, 10-cm needle (GIP, Medi-Globe, Inc, Tempe, AZ). At the present time, several EUS catheter–FNA needle systems are available with various needle lengths (up to 14 cm) and gauges (19-gauge to 25-gauge) available. We routinely perform EUS-guided FNA on all posterior mediastinal lymph nodes that are suspicious for malignant involvement by clinical suspicion or EUS criteria or both. Many patients have more than one suspicious lymph node or finding. In our patients, we sample only the most suspicious lymph node or finding that would have the greatest impact on the clinical staging (i.e., contralateral or subcarinal).

The EUS-guided FNA biopsy technique was initially developed for use with the linear array instrument and has been described elsewhere.[95–97,102,103] The unique viewing angle of the linear array transducer allows for observation of the needle as it exits the biopsy channel and enables direction of the needle tip into the target lesion. A similar technique using a radial scanning echoendoscope has been reported; however, serious complications have been described via this technique, and it is not recommended.[94,103]

EUS-guided FNA involves the insertion of the FNA catheter device through the accessory channel of the echoendoscope followed by deployment of the needle under EUS guidance into the lymph node to be sampled. The handle mechanism is secured to the accessory port, and if the instrument has an elevator, the elevator should be fully released into the down position to allow easy passage of the needle. The elevator can be used during the biopsy to direct the needle gently into the lesion. Doppler is used to identify surrounding vascular structures. The FNA needle is slowly advanced toward the target lesion. With certain needles, it helps if the stylet is withdrawn a few millimeters (2 to 3 mm), and the needle and the stylet are then directed into the target. When the needle has entered the lesion, the stylet is advanced (to clear the needle) and then removed. The endosonographer or assistant applies suction to the catheter system using a 5-mL or 10-mL Luer-Lok syringe. Suction is followed by "in-and-out" movements of the catheter after firmly locking the needle-catheter system to the appropriate depth so that the needle is not advanced beyond a desired depth. Typically, we make 7 to 10 gradual in-and-out movements within the lesion. Before removing the needle, the negative pressure is released slowly, the needle is removed from the lesion, and subsequently the needle system is unscrewed from the echoendoscope. It has been suggested to perform EUS-guided FNA of lymph nodes without the use of suction because suction may result in a bloody sample that may be more difficult for the cytopathologist to examine.[100]

Preliminary cytology findings are obtained immediately during the FNA procedure by a cytopathologist or cytotechnologist present during the study. We recommend having a cytopathologist or cytotechnologist present during the EUS-guided FNA portion of the procedure because it can improve the efficiency of the technique. If a cytopathologist or cytotechnologist is unavailable, two to three passes should be taken by the endosonographer for lymph nodes (or liver metastases) and five to six passes should be taken for masses (similar to pancreatic masses) to ensure adequate cellularity in more than 90% of cases.[100,104] However, this approach is associated with a 10% reduction in definitive cytologic diagnoses, increased time and risk, and potentially the need for additional needles.[104]

The FNA sample obtained is prepared for reviewing using Diff-Quik stain (HARLECO; EMD Chemicals, Inc, Gibbstown, NJ) applied to the slide containing the deposited specimen or fixed with ethanol. Additional passes are made until a positive cytology or adequate tissue sample is obtained. When lymphoma is suspected, added material is collected if possible and placed in a preservative solution (GIBCO RPMI Media 1640; Life Technologies, Carlsbad, CA) for subsequent flow cytometry and immunocytochemistry as indicated.[105,106] If an infection is suspected, a culture media can be used.

Other Malignant Mediastinal Disease

The most important indication for mediastinal imaging is the detection or staging (or both) of lung cancer. There are several reports of EUS-guided FNA in the cytologic diagnosis of mediastinal metastases from various extrathoracic malignancies in which EUS has played a pivotal role in detection or staging. These include metastatic pancreatic, esophageal, gastric, colon, laryngeal, germ cell, renal cell, breast, and ovarian cancers.[76,77,79–83,107–110]

Most of the experience with EUS in patients with lymphoma has been in the setting of gastric lymphoma, although more recent studies support the use of EUS-FNA with flow cytometry for the diagnosis of mediastinal lymphoma as well.[80,111–113] In a study by Fritscher-Ravens and colleagues, 153 patients with mediastinal lymphadenopathy undergoing EUS-guided FNA, lymphadenopathy originating from the lung was present in greater than 80% of patients without a previous cancer diagnosis, whereas recurrence of extrathoracic sites was the major cause of mediastinal lymphadenopathy in patients with a previous malignancy.[80] Benign lesions and treatable second cancers were found in a significant minority of patients.

Devereaux and colleagues[110] retrospectively reviewed a large, single-center experience with EUS-guided FNA for the diagnosis of mediastinal mass or lymphadenopathy in the absence of known pulmonary malignancy. In this report, 49 patients were analyzed; a malignant process was diagnosed in 22 of 49 (45%), and a benign process was found in 24 of 49 (49%). These included four patients with previously undiagnosed lung cancer, whereas metastatic breast carcinoma was the most frequent (6 of 22 [27%]) lesion. EUS-guided FNA was diagnostic in 46 of 49 (94%) patients. Catalano and coworkers[107] reported a multicenter study of 62 patients in which FNA results were classified as benign or infectious, malignant pulmonary, and malignant mediastinal (lymphoma, metastatic malignancy); EUS-guided FNA was diagnostic in 90% of cases. Panelli and associates[115] reported a series of 33 patients with mediastinal masses, which represented 2.3% of 1447 upper EUS examinations over a 5-year period. EUS-guided FNA was performed in 25 of 33 (76%), of which 22 (67%) ultimately were determined to be malignant. Wiersema and coworkers[82] reported a series of 82 patients with mediastinal lymphadenopathy, and EUS-guided FNA after other nonsurgical techniques failed to provide a diagnosis or could not be used. The sensitivity and specificity of EUS-guided FNA were 96% and 100%. In addition, a meta-analysis identified 76 studies, 32 of which described EUS-guided FNA, which confirm a high sensitivity and specificity for EUS-guided FNA in the diagnosis of mediastinal lymphadenopathy.[116] These studies suggest that in the absence of

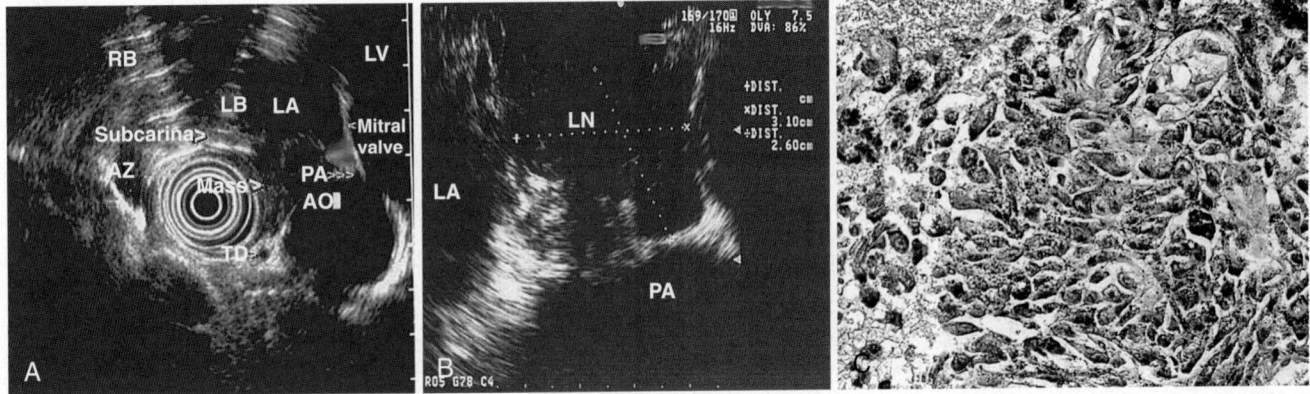

Fig. 31.9 A 71-year-old woman with a history of breast cancer and melanoma was found to have mediastinal lymphadenopathy on chest computed tomography (CT). **A,** Radial endoscopic ultrasound (EUS) revealed a subcarinal 3.1 cm × 2.6 cm necrotic-appearing lymph node versus mass. **B,** Linear array imaging depicting fine needle aspiration (FNA) of this lesion. **C,** High-power magnification of hematoxylin and eosin stain on cell block shows metastatic pigmented melanoma. AO, aorta; AZ, azygos vein; LA, left atrium; LB, left bronchi; LV, left ventricle; PA, pulmonary artery; RB, right bronchi; TD, thoracic duct.

accessible extrathoracic disease lesions or as an alternative, EUS-guided FNA is a useful technique for the cytodiagnosis of extrathoracic cancers that are metastatic to the mediastinum (**Fig. 31.9**).

Nonmalignant Mediastinal Disease

Although commonly present in patients with suspected or known pulmonary malignancy, mediastinal lymph nodes are also present in patients with benign diseases such as histoplasmosis, tuberculosis, and sarcoidosis.[80,110,117–121] In addition, benign cystic structures such as congenital foregut cysts account for approximately 20% of mediastinal masses.[93]

Wiersema and coworkers[117] described three patients with dysphagia from compression of the esophagus by mediastinal masses. EUS showed that the masses were enlarged lymph nodes with anechoic areas thought to represent caseating necrosis. The EUS-guided FNA finding of reactive lymphocytes along with a positive complement fixation titer was instrumental in making the diagnosis of mediastinal histoplasmosis. Savides and colleagues[119] described 11 patients with dysphagia who had a midesophageal submucosal mass or stricture. EUS findings consisted of large, matted posterior mediastinal lymph nodes in all patients. The diagnosis of histoplasmosis was supported by the EUS finding of lymph node calcifications in seven of these patients, symptomatic improvement in response to antifungal medication in all seven patients who were treated, and a mean follow-up of 20.5 months in which none of the patients developed signs of a malignancy.

EUS has been reported to be an accurate and simple method for the diagnosis of sarcoidosis, a systemic granulomatous disease with a predilection for the lung and mediastinal lymph nodes.[106,107,120–123] In most situations, the recommended procedure is a transbronchial biopsy, which has a diagnostic yield of 40% with one biopsy and 90% when four biopsy specimens are obtained.[122] If the transbronchial approach is unsuccessful, more invasive diagnostic procedures such as mediastinoscopy or lung biopsy may be used.

Several more recent reports have described the utility of EUS-guided FNA in the diagnosis of sarcoidosis manifesting with mediastinal lymphadenopathy.[106,107,120–122,124] Mishra and coworkers[120] described seven patients with mediastinal lymphadenopathy in which EUS helped confirm the diagnosis of sarcoidosis. Nodes were 1.8 to 6 cm in the long axis and were elongated and triangular and described as draping around the esophagus. In a retrospective review of 21 consecutive patients, Gress and colleagues[123] found EUS with FNA to have a sensitivity of 86% in diagnosing sarcoidosis in patients with mediastinal lymphadenopathy, but they failed to identify reliable EUS characteristics (shape, size, echogenicity, or homogenicity pattern) specific for the disease.

A study reporting the results of EUS-guided FNA evaluation in 19 patients with suspected sarcoidosis revealed enlarged mediastinal lymph nodes (mean size 2.4 cm) located subcarinally (n = 15), in the aortopulmonary window (n = 12), and in the lower posterior mediastinum (n = 5).[107] The nodes were described as isoechoic or hypoechoic, with "atypical" vessels in five cases. The aspirate obtained using EUS-guided FNA was adequate in all patients and contained blood in excess of normal in some, which was believed to be indicative of a high degree of vascularity. Cytology showed epithelioid cell granuloma formation, and cultures for mycobacteria were negative in all of the patients except one, in whom the final diagnosis was tuberculosis. The specificity and sensitivity of EUS-guided FNA in the diagnosis of sarcoidosis were 94% and 100%. Fritscher-Ravens and coworkers[80] found 2 patients with tuberculosis in 101 patients without a history of cancer who had EUS-guided FNA of mediastinal lymph nodes. This study highlights the need for acid-fast staining and culture to exclude tuberculosis in cases of noncaseating granulomas. In addition, there is potential for EUS-guided FNA in the cytologic diagnosis of intraabdominal and pancreatic sarcoidosis (**Figs. 31.10 and 31.11**).[122,123,125,126]

Approximately 4% of regional lymph nodes of carcinomas have noncaseating epithelioid granulomas so that a presumptive diagnosis of sarcoidosis or another granulomatous disease should be made only after careful exclusion of malignancy and close follow-up.[127] Detectable mediastinal lymph nodes may also be present in normal subjects and are often found in patients undergoing EUS examinations for various indications (**Fig. 31.12**).[82,128] It has been postulated that detectable mediastinal lymph nodes in asymptomatic individuals may be

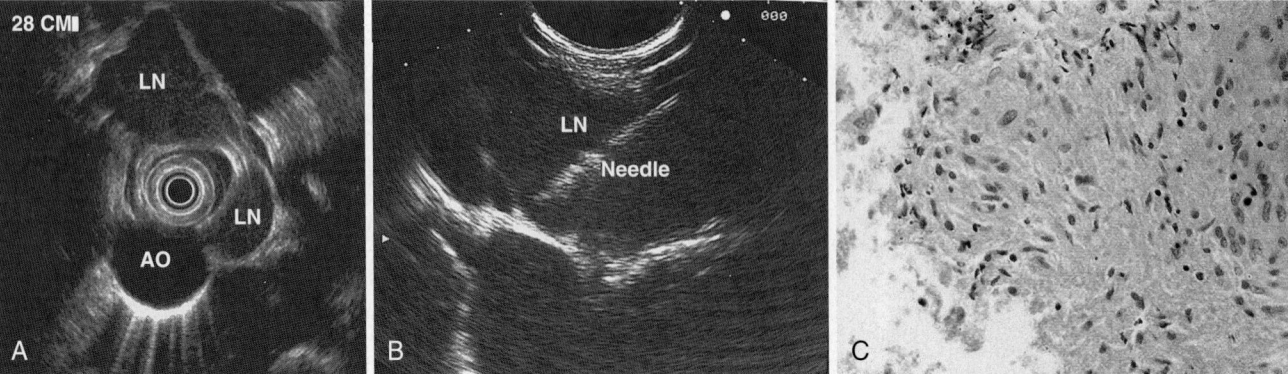

Fig. 31.10 **A,** Radial imaging of large hypoechoic, oblong, and teardrop-shaped mediastinal lymph nodes (measuring up to 3.7 cm × 3.4 cm) in a patient with fever and elevated angiotensin-converting enzyme level. **B,** Fine needle aspiration (FNA) performed with linear array echoendoscope. **C,** High-power magnification of hematoxylin and eosin stain on cell block reveals a noncaseating epithelioid granuloma consistent with sarcoidosis. Special stains (acid-fast bacilli, Gomori methenamine silver) to rule out tuberculosis and fungal infections were negative. AO, aorta; LN, lymph node.

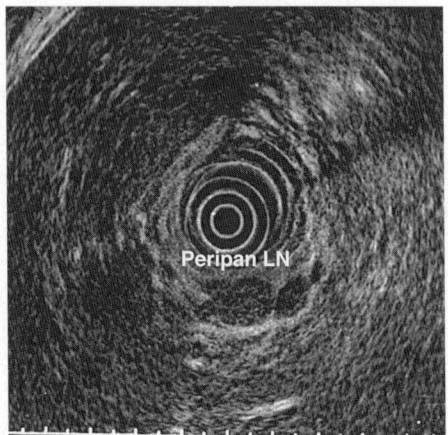

Fig. 31.11 Radial endoscopic ultrasound (EUS) from the body of the stomach in a patient with a history of sarcoidosis with peripancreatic lymphadenopathy that increased in size on serial transabdominal imaging. EUS revealed several hypoechoic lymph nodes. Fine needle aspiration (FNA) yielded tissue with prominent granulomatous inflammation thought to represent abdominal sarcoidosis.

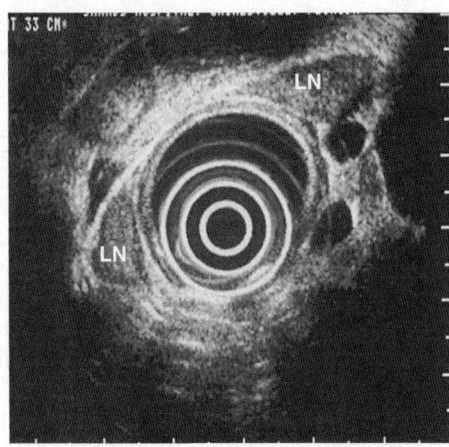

Fig. 31.12 Radial imaging of benign-appearing mediastinal lymph nodes.

related to prior histoplasmosis or other pulmonary infections.[119] Devereaux and colleagues,[110] in their retrospective study of 49 patients with mediastinal masses in the absence of known pulmonary malignancy, found a benign process in 24 of 49 (49%) including 8 patients with histoplasmosis, 1 patient with sarcoid, 2 patients with leiomyoma, 2 patients with duplication cyst, 1 patient with teratoma, and 10 patients with benign lymph node cytology on EUS-guided FNA.

EUS is often useful in distinguishing cystic lesions from solid lesions in the mediastinum, whereas chest CT scan can have limited utility in providing this distinction.[91,129–134] Wildi and coworkers[91] reported on a retrospective review of the results of EUS in 20 patients with suspected mediastinal cysts. The features used to classify cysts were as follows: Benign simple cysts appear as anechoic or hypoechoic smooth, spherical structures with well-defined thin walls; esophageal duplication cysts are adherent to the esophagus, whereas cysts originating from the airways are designated as bronchogenic cysts. Cysts that do not fall into either category are termed *nonspecific duplication cysts.* A layered wall structure supports the diagnosis of duplication cyst but is not mandatory. Simple

cysts include mesothelial cysts, lymphogenous cysts, and thoracic duct cysts. Simple cysts do not have a layered wall and do not have a connection to the airways or esophagus and are termed *nonspecific simple cysts.* When solid tissue is seen within the fluid, the cysts are considered complex (e.g., benign cystic teratoma, thymic cyst), and the diagnosis of a benign simple cyst is excluded.

In 19 of 20 patients reported by Wildi and coworkers,[91] definite diagnosis of a mediastinal cyst was established by EUS (12 anechoic, 6 hypoechoic, 1 anechoic with small echoic foci). In only 4 of 18 cases was CT (17 cases) or MRI (1 case) diagnostic of a cyst. In three cases with mixed echo features, EUS-guided FNA was performed with administration of prophylactic antibiotics. In a fourth case, without prior prophylactic administration of an antibiotic, FNA was performed in a solid-appearing duplication cyst misdiagnosed by EUS as extensive lymphadenopathy. Mediastinitis subsequently developed requiring thoracotomy, in which an infected bronchogenic cyst was diagnosed. The authors concluded that aspiration of cysts should be avoided in lesions with clearly anechoic features because of the risk of infection, whereas FNA should be considered for hypoechoic lesions (when a cyst cannot be clearly distinguished from a solid tumor), but prophylactic antibiotics should be administered (**Fig. 31.13**).

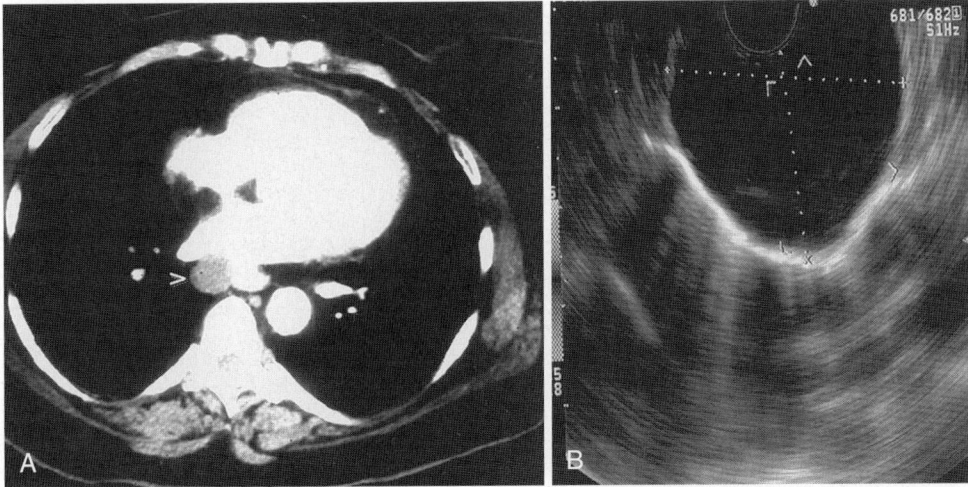

Fig. 31.13 **A,** Chest computed tomography (CT) shows an ill-defined soft tissue density adjacent to the midesophagus. **B,** Linear array imaging of this lesion reveals a paraesophageal duplication cyst.

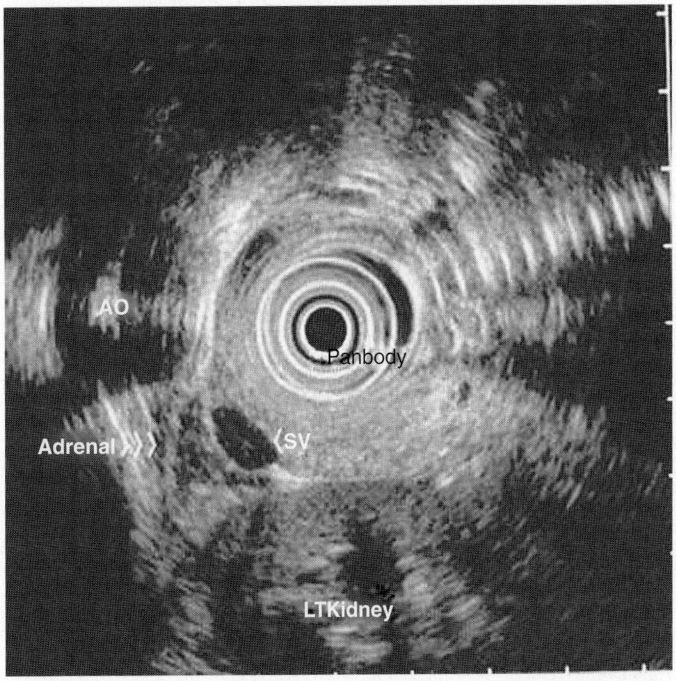

Fig. 31.14 Radial imaging from the body of the stomach showing the left adrenal gland, aorta (AO), splenic vein (SV), left (LT) kidney, and body of the pancreas (PANBODY).

Adrenal and Renal Lesions

EUS can provide early excellent images of the left adrenal gland. The right adrenal gland is also accessible by EUS, and its routine evaluation may be feasible, although it is more difficult to visualize than the left adrenal gland, and the procedure is not routinely performed.[135] The left adrenal gland is more difficult to view than the right gland when imaging with transabdominal ultrasound.[136–138]

When imaging the left adrenal gland, the echoendoscope is advanced into the proximal stomach, and the aorta is identified just below the GE junction. The splenic vein is imaged by advancing the transducer forward with a clockwise rotation. Following the splenic vein laterally, the splenic hilum is found by further clockwise rotation and slight withdrawal. The left kidney is imaged by advancing the scope from the splenic hilum with a slight counterclockwise rotation. The left adrenal gland lies just below the splenic vein, between the left kidney (superior and medial to the kidney) and the aorta. In a study by Chang and colleagues,[138] the average long-axis dimension of the adrenal gland was 2.5 cm, and the short-axis dimension was 0.8 cm. The adrenal gland as imaged on EUS is homogeneous and hypoechoic with two basic morphologic types: seagull shape and elliptical shape. Occasionally, the adrenal gland can appear as both shapes in the same patient with a slight change in the orientation of the EUS probe tip.[138] In some patients, the central region of the gland may appear more echogenic than the peripheral region (**Fig. 31.14**).

Incidental benign adrenal lesions, so-called adrenal incidentalomas, are commonly found on CT scans performed for various indications. Unless unequivocally benign, biopsy of these lesions should be performed in certain scenarios. CT

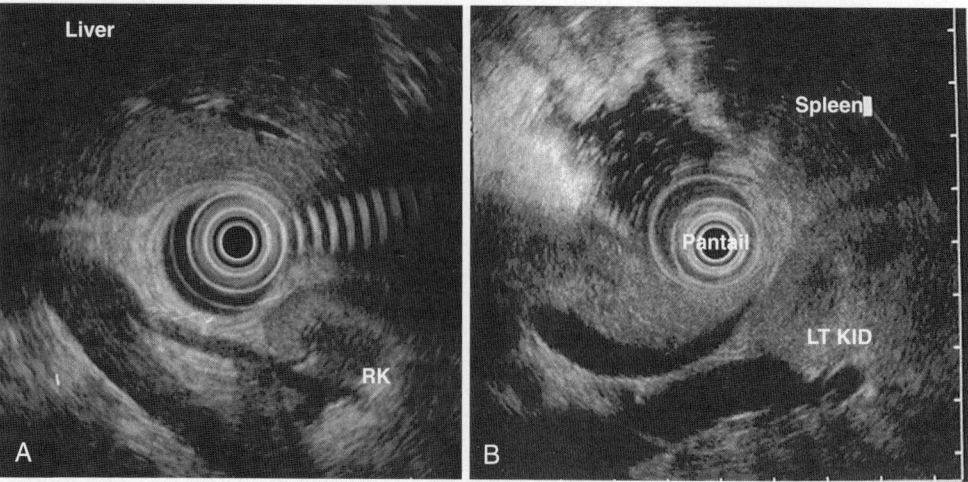

Fig. 31.15 **A,** Radial imaging from the duodenum shows excellent images of the right kidney in this patient with malrotation of the right kidney. The liver is seen in the upper portion of the image. **B,** Radial imaging from the body of the stomach shows the left (LT) kidney, spleen, body and tail of the pancreas (closest to the transducer) and above the splenic vein. The left renal vein is seen exiting the kidney.

scans performed in the staging work-up of lung cancer reveal that more than 16% of patients have adrenal masses on screening examination.[138-143] Metastasis to the adrenal glands as the cause of isolated mass lesions occurs in 32% to 93% of cases of NSCLC as determined by FNA cytology.[141,144] In autopsy series of NSCLC, adrenal metastases are found in 59% of cases.[145,146]

EUS-guided FNA may provide an alternative to percutaneous aspiration technology in the evaluation of adrenal lesions. EUS-guided biopsy of an adrenal mass has been reported in a patient in whom CT-guided FNA was unsuccessful.[147] Chang and associates[147] reported the identification of the left adrenal gland in 97% of 31 consecutive patients undergoing EUS for known pulmonary or GI malignancies. In one patient with a history of lobectomy for lung cancer, staged as T1N0, a follow-up CT scan showed interval enlargement of an adrenal mass from 2.5 cm to 4 cm. A previous CT-guided FNA was negative for malignancy. An EUS-guided FNA of the left adrenal gland was performed and revealed metastatic disease. A more recent case series also suggests that the right adrenal gland may be more accessible by EUS-guided FNA than previously believed.[135] Given the clinical impact of an adrenal metastasis, routine assessment of the left and possibly right adrenal glands in patients with lung cancer is recommended during the EUS evaluation.[147]

EUS of the right and left kidneys is possible because of the immediate approximation between the GI lumen and the kidneys. The right kidney can be imaged by placing the transducer in the second portion of the duodenum and rotating laterally. The left kidney can be imaged from the body of the stomach, posterior to the spleen, as described previously. The left kidney often is easier to show than the right kidney. The kidneys have a hyperechoic central medulla, a hypoechoic outer cortex, and a thin echogenic capsule (**Fig. 31.15**).

Approximately 85% of renal masses detected on CT are renal cell carcinomas, and 15% of CT-detected renal masses are benign lesions.[148,149] Biopsy of malignant-appearing masses that are resectable should not be routinely performed. Biopsy of a solitary renal mass is generally accepted in cases with a known primary extrarenal malignancy when the presence of

a metastasis would alter management.[148,150] Biopsy specimens of renal masses have traditionally been obtained under either transabdominal ultrasound or CT guidance with a sensitivity of 62% to 100% and a specificity of 0% to 100% in the diagnosis of renal cell carcinoma.[114,148] No data currently exist regarding the frequency with which renal masses are identified during upper EUS examinations. A few case reports exist showing the possibility of making a diagnosis of renal cell carcinoma using EUS-guided FNA[148,151]; however further experience is required before the establishment of EUS-guided FNA as a modality for performing renal biopsy.

Ascites and Pleural Fluid

The identification of malignant pleural effusion or malignant ascites is diagnostic of advanced disease in various malignancies. EUS seems to be more sensitive than CT in the detection of small amounts of ascites and pleural fluid. Drainage of pleural fluid or ascites at the time of EUS is possible and can be helpful if positive for malignancy. The technique of EUS-guided FNA of ascites or pleural fluid is similar to the technique applied to other lesions. Seeding of malignant cells into the fluid through the GI tract is a concern. The site of the needle penetration in the GI lumen must not be involved with tumor (**Fig. 31.16**).

Chang and associates[147] first reported the detection of malignant fluid via EUS-guided FNA of pleural effusion and ascites in patients with gastric cancer. In a larger retrospective study, these same investigators reported the utility of EUS for the detection of ascites and EUS-guided FNA in 571 consecutive patients who underwent upper EUS for various indications.[152] EUS detected ascites in 85 (15%) patients, whereas CT detected ascites in 14 (18%) of the 79 patients who underwent CT scanning before EUS. Of 85 patients, 31 underwent EUS-guided FNA paracentesis, and malignant ascites was diagnosed in 5 of these patients. More recently, investigators have been looking at whether detection of low-volume ascites by EUS is a good predictor of outcomes in esophageal cancer.[139,153] These studies have shown that patients with ascites detected only by EUS examination have a shorter

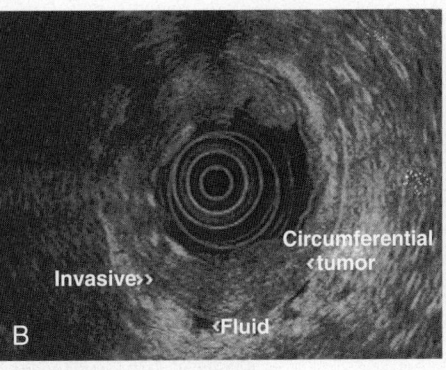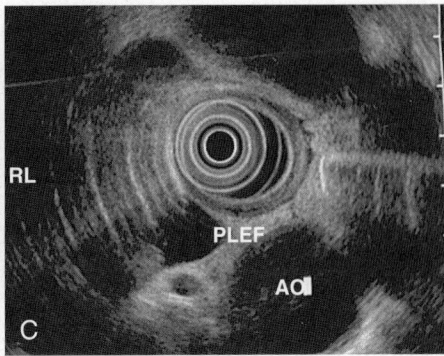

Fig. 31.16 **A,** Radial imaging of trace ascites in a patient with pancreatic cancer. The pancreatic mass is seen below the ascites. **B,** Ascites in a patient with linitis plastica. **C,** Pleural effusion (PLEF) seen adjacent to the right lung (RL). AO, aorta.

survival than patients without low-volume ascites. However, patients with ascites whose tumors were still deemed surgically resectable had the same survival rate as patients without ascites. These findings have been supported by similar studies that have described the clinical significance of peritoneal fluid detected by EUS.[154,155]

Liver Lesions

EUS provides very good imaging of the left lobe of the liver and a significant portion of the right lobe of the liver. The left lobe and hilum of the liver are examined from the gastric body and fundus. The tip of the echoendoscope is placed in the gastric antrum; then, slowly withdrawing the echoendoscope, the tip is deflected up and rightward. When the liver comes into view, the instrument is rotated to evaluate portions of the liver. The right lobe of the liver is best imaged from the duodenum but can also be seen from the antrum. Liver lesions near the second or third portion of the duodenum, peripheral lesions near the dome of the diaphragm, and lesions in the inferior portion of the right lobe of the liver can be difficult to visualize (see **Figs. 31.2 and 31.15**).[156]

CT-guided and ultrasound-guided FNA of liver lesions have been reported to have sensitivities of 83% to 93% for the detection of malignant disease.[138,140–143] Although EUS has not traditionally been used in evaluation of the liver, early experience suggests that EUS-guided FNA is comparable to CT-guided FNA in terms of safety and diagnostic utility for hepatic lesions.[156–161] Nguyen and associates[156] conducted a prospective study in which 574 consecutive patients with a history or suspicion of GI or pulmonary tumor who were undergoing upper EUS examinations underwent EUS evaluation of the liver. They found small focal liver lesions that were undetected with conventional CT. Of patients, 14 (2.4%) were found to have focal liver lesions (five right lobe, nine left lobe) and underwent EUS-guided FNA. The median largest diameter of the liver lesions was 1.1 cm (range 0.8 to 5.2 cm), and the mean number of passes per lesion was 2.0 (range 1 to 5 passes). Of the 15 liver lesions sampled via EUS-guided FNA, 15 were malignant and 1 was benign. Before EUS, CT depicted liver lesions in only 3 of 14 (21%) patients; in most patients, CT was performed within 2 months of the EUS procedure. In seven patients, the initial diagnosis of cancer was made by means of EUS-guided FNA of the liver. There were no immediate or late complications.

Rarely, percutaneous FNA of the liver has been associated with tumor seeding, intrahepatic hematoma, and hemorrhage.[162–166] As postulated by Nguyen and coworkers,[156] EUS-guided FNA has the possible advantage over the percutaneous route of shorter insertion length of the needle if the liver lesion is deep to the skin surface. With EUS-guided FNA, there is continuous visualization of the needle tip, which helps to minimize risk for bleeding when the procedure is performed in conjunction with color flow and Doppler ultrasound. tenBerge and colleagues[161] reported a multicenter study of 167 cases of EUS-guided FNA of the liver. Complications were reported in six (4%) cases, including death in one patient with an occluding biliary stent and biliary sepsis, bleeding (one case), fever (two cases), and pain (two cases). In 23 of 26 patients, EUS-guided FNA helped diagnose malignancy after nondiagnostic FNA with transabdominal ultrasound guidance. EUS was able to localize an unrecognized primary tumor in 17 of 33 (52%) cases after CT showed only liver metastases. This study highlighted the fact that adequate biliary drainage is recommended in the setting of cholangitis before or coincident with the FNA procedure. EUS-guided FNA of liver lesions seems to be safe and effective and may become a more useful diagnostic method for liver lesions.

Miscellaneous

The close proximity of the intestinal tract to abdominal organs raises the possibility of EUS-guided FNA of idiopathic abdominal masses. Catalano and coworkers[167] retrospectively evaluated the diagnostic accuracy of EUS-guided FNA of abdominal masses of unknown cause and its impact on subsequent evaluation. From five tertiary referral centers, 34 patients with idiopathic abdominal masses underwent EUS-guided FNA after evaluation including CT or transabdominal ultrasound, or both. CT showed an intraabdominal mass in all patients. Four patients had a history of intraabdominal cancer (two cervical, one ovarian, one colon), but these cancers were considered to be in remission. A final diagnosis for the mass lesions was established in all patients by various methods, including EUS-guided FNA, surgery, autopsy, or long-term follow-up. Abdominal masses were classified into three categories: infectious, benign or inflammatory, and malignant. EUS-guided FNA established a tissue diagnosis in 29 of 34 (85%) patients: infectious, 80% including abscess and infected pseudocyst; benign or inflammatory, 67% including hematoma or

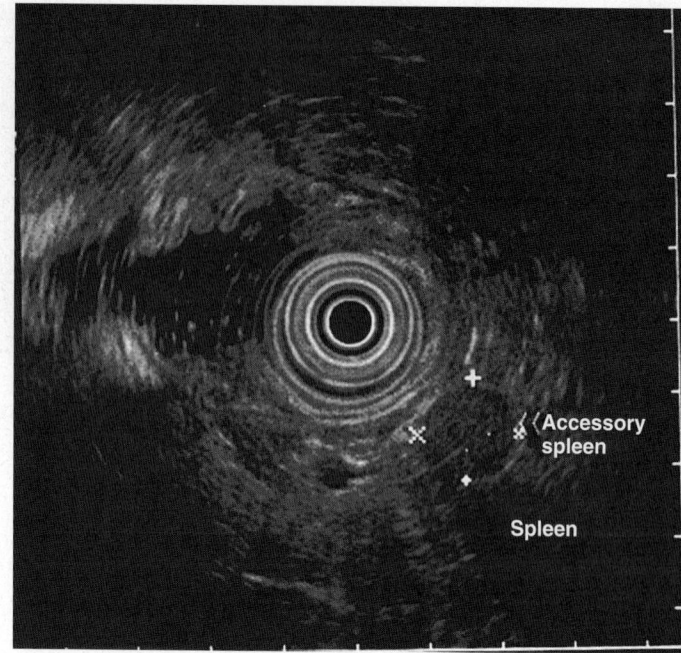

Fig. 31.17 Radial imaging from the stomach of an accessory spleen.

postsurgical inflammatory mass, leiomyoma, and sarcoidosis; and malignant, 91% including sarcoma, lymphoma, hepatoma, adenocarcinoma of unknown primary, ovarian cancer, transitional bladder carcinoma, uterine or cervical cancer, recurrent colon cancer, neuroendocrine tumor, paraganglionoma, metastatic lung cancer, and prostate cancer. EUS-guided FNA was instrumental in directing subsequent evaluation in 29 (85%) patients and therapy in 26 (77%). The number of fine needle passes needed for adequate tissue sampling was lower for nonmalignant (2.2 to 3.2 passes) versus malignant diseases (4.6 passes). A perirectal abscess developed in one patient and was treated successfully with antibiotics.

Cases using EUS-guided FNA to diagnose a schwannoma of the mediastinum[168] and a retroperitoneal neurilemoma have been described.[169] In addition, studies by Erickson and Tretjak[170] and Anand and colleagues[171] have helped show that EUS-guided FNA is an effective method with a high sensitivity and specificity for diagnosing and altering patient management of nonpancreatic lesions adjacent to the GI tract.

Accessory spleen may be a potential cause of misinterpretation on EUS. Barawi and colleagues[172] described the EUS features of accessory spleen in 10 (8 accessory spleen, 2 lobulated spleen) patients. The mean size of these lesions was 2.7 cm × 3.1 cm. Nine accessory spleens were round, and one was oval. All were located inferolateral to the pancreatic tail and medial to the spleen. All of these lesions had a sharp and regular outer margin and homogeneous echo texture; four were hypoechoic, and six were hyperechoic. CT scan may be helpful in confirming the presence of lobulated spleen and accessory spleen (**Fig. 31.17**).

Fritscher-Ravens and associates[173] described EUS-guided FNA of splenic lesions in 12 patients when other modalities were inconclusive (*n* = 5), not attempted because of small size (0.9 to 1.4 cm; *n* = 4), or considered dangerous (adjacent to the splenic hilum or located peripherally; *n* = 3). The lesions ranged in size from 0.8 to 4.2 cm (median 1.4 cm). A positive diagnosis was made in 10 of 12 patients (83%); cytology was inadequate in 1 patient. Bacteriology was positive for *Staphylococcus aureus*

and *Serratia* in one patient each and for *Mycobacterium tuberculosis* in two patients. Diagnoses included lymphoma, sarcoidosis, abscesses, tuberculosis, metastatic colon cancer, and infarction (in one patient). One patient experienced pain after the procedure, but no hematoma was shown on subsequent ultrasound examination. Since this study, other studies have been performed supporting the possibility that EUS-guided FNA of splenic masses is feasible and safe.[174,175]

Complications

EUS-guided FNA is a relatively safe procedure compared with CT-guided FNA, bronchoscopy with transbronchial FNA, mediastinoscopy, or open or exploratory procedures. Generally, when complications occur, these are usually mild and self-limited. In reports and more recent prospective studies that have addressed complications of EUS-guided FNA, rare complications included endoscope-induced perforations, febrile episodes (after FNA of pancreatic cystic lesions), hemorrhage, pancreatitis, and pneumoperitoneum; false-positive diagnoses have been described.[79,89,92,93,158,176–180] As alluded to previously, the role of prophylactic antibiotics for EUS-guided FNA is unclear. The general practice has been to administer antibiotics to any patient undergoing FNA of cystic pancreatic or perirectal lesions. Barawi and colleagues[86] studied 108 consecutive EUS-guided FNA cases that did not show bacteremia at 30 minutes and 60 minutes after the procedure. However, the study by Van de Mierop and colleagues[93] revealed a 19% incidence of bacteremia with EUS-guided FNA of solid lesions.

Endoscopic Ultrasound–Guided Celiac Plexus Block and Celiac Plexus Neurolysis

Pain resulting from pancreatic cancer and chronic pancreatitis is often difficult to manage. Many approaches have been used to treat these patients, including narcotic analgesia, antidepressants, pancreatic enzymes, octreotide, denervation procedures (most commonly CPB), and various palliative or decompression or drainage procedures.[180–192] The effectiveness of these therapies is not only highly variable but also often controversial, especially in the treatment of chronic pancreatitis. Opioid analgesics are probably used most often and can treat pain effectively, but they are associated with numerous side effects, including constipation, delirium, nausea, and the potential for addiction in patients with chronic pancreatitis.[193,194] Nonpharmacologic methods of pain control may improve quality of life and minimize drug-related side effects.[193]

The celiac plexus lies anterior to the aorta at the level of the celiac artery. Most of the sensory nerves returning from the pancreas and other intraabdominal viscera pass through the celiac ganglion and splanchnic nerves. Interruption of these fibers may lessen pain in pancreatic malignancies and in chronic pancreatitis.[195] CPB, a temporizing treatment, most commonly refers to injection of a steroid and long-acting local anesthetic into the celiac plexus to control pain associated with chronic pancreatitis. In contrast, CPN generally refers to injection of alcohol or phenol, a more permanent agent, into the celiac axis area.[195] This technique induces a chemical splanchnicectomy that ablates the nerve fibers that transmit pain and is used in patients with pancreatic cancer; however, neural regrowth may limit the effect.[195] In practice, the terms CPB and CPN are often interchangeable.

The efficacy of CPN for the treatment of cancer pain has been shown in numerous studies. The benefit seems to be similar independent of the method used with pain control in 70% to 90% of patients up to 3 months after the procedure.[196–201] CPB and CPN have traditionally been performed via various percutaneous (most common posterior route) and surgical approaches and most recently under endoscopic guidance.[202] Of the nonsurgical approaches, EUS offers the most direct access to the celiac plexus. Wiersema and coworkers[193,195,203] recognized the anatomic advantage that EUS provides in visualizing the celiac region and were successful in performing transgastric EUS-guided CPN with results similar to the more traditional approaches.

The timing of CPN relative to pain onset seems to predict response. In one study, CPN was more effective when the block was performed early after pain onset.[197] This result was postulated to be related to involvement of visceral and somatic nerves late in the disease and pain apparently deriving mainly from the celiac plexus early on.[195,197] More recently, it has been proposed that direct injection into the celiac ganglia, multiple injections in the area of the ganglia, or bilateral injections around the celiac ganglia are safe and may be more beneficial in providing sustained pain relief.[204–206] These studies are contradictory, however, and better prospective trials are needed to determine if these approaches make an improvement over the standard technique of EUS-guided CPB.

Studies suggest that CPB may have a role in the treatment of pain related to chronic pancreatitis.[207,208] In a study of 18 patients with chronic pancreatitis, reduction in pain was noted in 50% (5 of 10) of EUS-guided CPB compared with 25% (2 of 8) of CT-guided blocks.[207] The benefit persisted for 24 weeks in 30% of responders. A cost comparison showed a $200 saving for EUS-guided CPB compared with CT-guided CPB. Another report of 90 patients by the same investigators found a significant improvement in overall pain scores in 55%

at 4 weeks and 8 weeks of follow-up.[208] A persistent benefit beyond 24 weeks was observed in only 10% of patients. Pain relief was more likely in older patients (>45 years old) and patients who had not had previous surgery for chronic pancreatitis. Further studies are needed to clarify what role EUS-guided CBP will play in the management of painful chronic pancreatitis.

Technique for Performing Endoscopic Ultrasound–Guided Celiac Plexus Block and Celiac Plexus Neurolysis

This section focuses on endoscopic methods of EUS-guided CPB and CPN. Patients with inoperable pancreatic cancer and pain requiring narcotic analgesics are potential candidates for CPN. Selection of patients with pain related to chronic pancreatitis for CPB is less clear. Patients with pain refractory to high doses of narcotics may be appropriate candidates, although the response may be minimal.

The celiac artery is readily visualized with a curvilinear array EUS scope and provides the important landmark structure when performing EUS-guided CPB and CPN. For practical purposes, the celiac ganglia is located at the origin of the celiac artery, although its exact location has been described anywhere from 1 cm to 9 mm inferior to the artery takeoff (the right ganglion is most commonly 6 mm inferior and the left ganglion is most commonly 9 mm inferior to the celiac artery origin).[195,197] Although the celiac ganglia themselves can be visualized in some cases, the celiac axis is more routinely identified by its relative position to the artery. The proximity of the celiac ganglia to the posterior gastric wall ensures an accurate passage of the needle into the ganglia, minimizing the risk of complications and potentially increasing the effectiveness.

The patient is hydrated before the procedure with intravenous saline (500 to 1000 mL) and is placed in the left lateral decubitus position, and sedation is administered. Blood pressure, pulse oximetry, and electrocardiogram are continuously monitored. The linear array echoendoscope is advanced to just below the GE junction. A sagittal view of the aorta is obtained through the posterior gastric wall. The aorta is traced to the celiac trunk, the first large vessel emerging off the aorta, and the second branch is usually easily identified as the superior mesenteric artery. Identifying both the celiac artery and the superior mesenteric artery helps to confirm the correct location. Color flow Doppler should be used to exclude any intervening vessels.

After the stylet is removed from the 22-gauge FNA needle, the entire system is flushed with normal saline to remove any air because this can interfere with imaging. Using real-time imaging, the sterile FNA needle is inserted immediately lateral and anterior to the aorta at the level of the celiac trunk via a transgastric approach. A small amount (2 mL) of 0.9% saline is injected to clear the needle. An assistant aspirates a 10-mL syringe filled with 0.9% saline for approximately 10 seconds to confirm that the needle is not within any of the regional blood vessels.

Two techniques are available: one in which the injection is performed by rotating to each side of the celiac trunk and one in which the entire injection is performed just anterior and cranial to the celiac artery takeoff.[193,195] For CPB, 10 mL of preservative-free bupivacaine (0.25%; Abbott Laboratories, Abbott Park, IL) and 1 mL of triamcinolone (40 mg; Fujisawa USA, Deerfield, IL) are injected on both sides of the celiac trunk. The aspiration test is repeated before each steroid injection. A 3-mL saline flush is performed before needle withdrawal on each side. For CPN, 10 mL of bupivacaine (0.25%) is injected followed by 10 mL of dehydrated 98% absolute alcohol. Before alcohol injection, the 10-second aspiration test is repeated. The needle is flushed with 3 mL of saline before withdrawal of the needle. The procedure is repeated on the opposite side of the aorta. With alcohol injection, an echo-dense cloud is typically seen, but this is not usually seen with steroid injection.

For the alternative approach, a single-site injection at the base of the celiac artery takeoff is performed with the entire amount of the injectant—20 mL of bupivacaine (0.25%) and 20 mL of dehydrated alcohol in CPN and 20 mL of bupivacaine (0.25%) and 80 mg (2 mL) of triamcinolone in CPB. There are no studies comparing the two techniques, but it is believed that they have similar results. Anatomic variations may determine which technique is used.

The examination, performed on an outpatient basis, is usually completed in 30 minutes. Recovery time is usually 2 hours. Before discharge, orthostatic blood pressure changes should be checked, and patients should be counseled regarding potential complications (see video on expertconsult.com).

Complications

CPB and CPN are generally effective, safe, and well-tolerated procedures. The three most common complications are transient hypotension (20% to 40%), transient diarrhea (4% to 38%), and transient increase in pain (9%), which are expected in CPB performed via any route.[195,198,209] Interruption of the plexus can result in a sympathetic blockade.[210] Clinical manifestations of sympathetic blockade can include diarrhea and hypotension resulting from a relative unopposed visceral parasympathetic activity. Mesenteric vasodilation accounts for the hypotension, which resolves in approximately 2 days. Diarrhea and increase in baseline pain are also usually limited to 2 days. Less common complications include unilateral paresis or paraplegia, pneumothorax, loss of sphincter function, retroperitoneal bleeding, renal puncture, and prolonged gastroparesis.[193,195,198,199,209] In addition, cephalic spread of the neurolytic agent may result in involvement of the cardiac nerves and plexus.[211] Although not unique to EUS-guided CPN, EUS may decrease the incidence of complications because the needle does not traverse the paraspinal region or somatic nerves or traverse the diaphragm and pleural space.[180,193,195] Another benefit with EUS-guided CPN is the ability to perform the block as part of a single procedure that may include tumor staging and FNA.[212] Infectious complications are uncommon but potentially serious. In a series of 90 patients, only 1 patient developed an infectious complication (peripancreatic abscess), which resolved with a 2-week course of antibiotics.[208] The authors reasoned that there may have been a predisposition to infection owing to gastroduodenal colonization with bacteria because the patient was taking a proton pump inhibitor. They suggested that prophylactic antibiotics should be considered in patients who are receiving acid suppression. The bactericidal nature of ethanol seems to minimize this risk for infection, and some experts do not routinely use antibiotics in this setting, regardless of concurrent acid suppression.[193]

Conclusion

Over the last 2 decades, EUS has played an increasingly important role as an accurate and safe method for staging patients with NSCLC. EUS is now integrated into the evaluation of non-GI pathology, especially in the assessment of mediastinal pathology. EUS-guided FNA should be considered in patients in whom a previous attempt at lymph node FNA was unsuccessful using CT or bronchoscopy. Depending on the local expertise, EUS may be considered the primary procedure for biopsy of lesions arising from the posterior mediastinum, especially at levels 5 (aortopulmonic), 7 (subcarinal), or 8 (periesophageal) because these are most readily accessed by EUS. EBUS may also be considered where available to evaluate the lesions in the anterior mediastinum traditionally not visualized well with EUS alone. This consideration is of particular relevance for staging of NSCLC, in which contralateral mediastinal lymph node metastases preclude curative resection. Identification of ipsilateral mediastinal lymph node involvement may be helpful for identifying patients who could benefit from neoadjuvant therapy. Mediastinoscopy, thoracoscopy, or partial thoracotomy could be reserved for patients with enlarged anterior lymph nodes or patients with suspicious nodes not successfully sampled by CT, bronchoscopy, EBUS, or EUS. EUS-guided FNA has been shown to be a highly accurate modality for evaluating unknown mediastinal masses or lymph nodes including lymphoma, sarcoidosis, and histoplasmosis.

In patients with otherwise operable lung cancer, EUS-guided FNA may be a viable alternative to percutaneous aspiration biopsy of a left adrenal mass. EUS can detect small focal liver lesions and small pockets of ascites or pleural fluid that are not detected by CT. Findings of EUS-guided FNA can confirm a cytologic diagnosis of metastasis and establish a definitive M stage that may change clinical management. EUS-guided FNA of renal masses may be a safe means of confirming the presence or absence of malignancy and may preclude the need for CT-guided studies. EUS-guided FNA provides minimally invasive tissue sampling and may obviate the need for exploratory laparotomy in cases of abdominal masses of undetermined origin. EUS seems to be a safe and effective method for performing CPN. EUS-guided CPN may also allow a diagnostic, staging, and therapeutic procedure all in one setting. Studies suggest that EUS CPB may have a role in the treatment of pain related to chronic pancreatitis.

References

The complete reference list is available online at www.expertconsult.com.

Evaluation of Gastric Polyps and Thickened Gastric Folds

Alberto Herreros de Tejada and Irving Waxman

Video related to this chapter's topics can be found online at expertconsult.com.

Introduction

Gastric polyps are detected in 3% of upper endoscopic evaluations,[1] but the incidence is higher than in the past because of the increasing use of endoscopy for diagnosis and treatment of upper digestive tract diseases.[2] These polyps are usually asymptomatic and are often found incidentally on endoscopic or radiographic examination. They may occur sporadically or be associated with polyposis syndromes. Gastric polyps may be single or multiple in number and pedunculated or sessile in form. Depending on the type of polyp, variable sizes can be encountered ranging from millimeters to several centimeters in diameter. Generally, gastric polyps are usually small (diameter <1 cm), well circumscribed, clearly demarcated, and project above the level of surrounding mucosa. Because of its diagnostic accuracy and therapeutic ability, endoscopy is the examination of choice in the diagnosis and treatment of gastric polyps.

Gastric polyps can be divided into epithelial and nonepithelial lesions. This chapter reviews the various types of epithelial gastric polyps and discusses the endoscopic techniques of gastric polypectomy, surveillance, and management. Nonepithelial gastric tumors including submucosal tumors are discussed in Chapter 29, and the management of upper gastrointestinal (GI) hereditary polyposis syndromes is discussed in Chapter 34. This chapter concludes with a discussion of the evaluation of thickened gastric folds, differential diagnoses, and endoscopic techniques and management.

Epithelial Gastric Polyps

Epithelial gastric polyps are divided into nonneoplastic and neoplastic lesions. In contrast to colonic polyps, most gastric polyps are nonneoplastic (80%–90%), including fundic gland and hyperplastic polyps. Although hyperplastic polyps are not neoplastic, dysplasia or gastric adenocarcinoma, or both, may rarely develop within the lesion.[3] Neoplastic epithelial gastric polyps include adenomas and polypoid gastric carcinomas.

Fundic Gland Polyps

Fundic gland polyps (also known as Elster's glandular cysts and cystic hamartomatous epithelial polyps) constitute up to 77% of all gastric polyps and are observed in 3.2% of routine upper endoscopy procedures.[4] They are more common in women and patients with *Helicobacter pylori* infection.[5,6] The pathogenesis is unknown. These polyps usually occur sporadically but at increased frequency in patients with familial adenomatous polyposis (FAP) and patients receiving long-term proton pump inhibitor treatment.[6,7] Although fundic gland polyps are traditionally considered a condition with little or no malignant potential, some reports have shown a possible increased association of concomitant colorectal adenomas or carcinomas in patients with fundic gland polyps.[8,9] Dysplasia and adenomatous changes in fundic gland polyps have developed in 1% to 1.9% of sporadic cases[10] and in 25% to 44% of

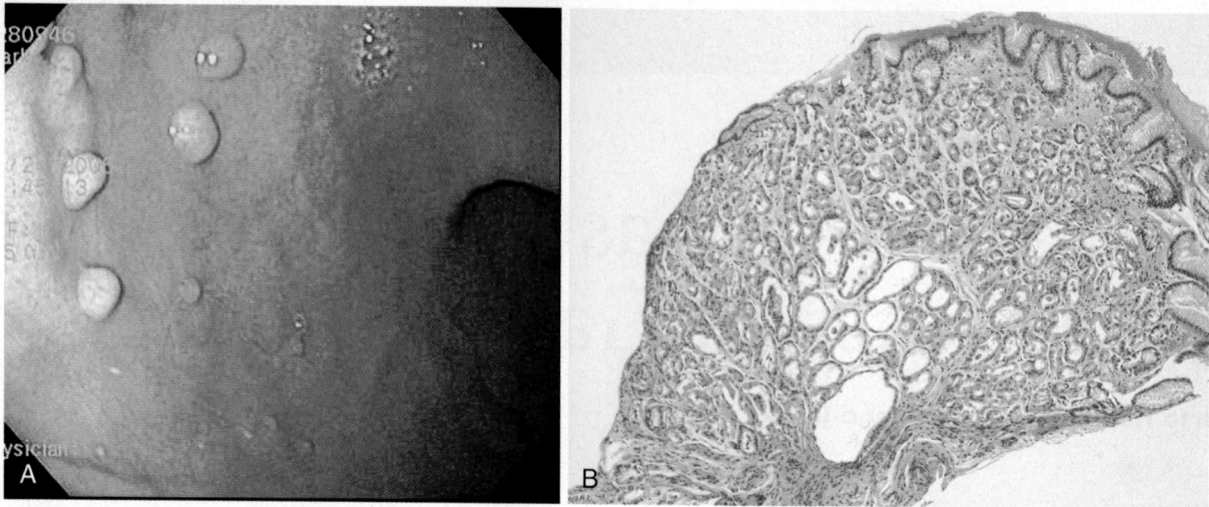

Fig. 32.1 A, Small fundic gland polyps in the gastric body. **B,** Microphotography of a fundic gland polyp (hematoxylin and eosin stain). *(Courtesy of Dr. Noffsinger.)*

patients with FAP.[9,11] In addition, reports have suggested malignant transformation of fundic gland polyps in patients with FAP, which may occur more often than previously believed.[11,12] Management of FAP syndrome is discussed in Chapter 34. The development of fundic gland polyps has also been associated with long-term proton pump inhibitor use,[13–15] but some studies have shown that a causal pathogenetic relationship is unlikely.[16,17]

Histologically, fundic gland polyps are characterized by dilated glands forming microcysts lined with fundic-type parietal and chief cells. Endoscopically, fundic gland polyps are usually found in the fundus or body of the stomach (**Fig. 32.1**). They may be found as a solitary lesion, but are often multiple in closely packed clusters, resembling small round grapes. These lesions are generally 2 to 3 mm in diameter, and because of their small size, they are sometimes hidden between folds. The mucosal surface typically is the normal surrounding mucosal color but also can be pale in coloration; visualization is best when the stomach is fully distended.

Hyperplastic Polyps

Hyperplastic polyps are another common polypoid lesion in the stomach, constituting 73% of all gastric polyps in some series.[18] The large variability in frequency is likely due to differing definitions of hyperplastic polyps. Men and women are equally affected, with predominance in adults older than 60 years. These polyps have previously been regarded as having no malignant potential; however, this is no longer thought to be true because of the increasing number of dysplastic changes or carcinoma found in gastric hyperplastic polyps.[3,19,20] Focal carcinomas occurred in 2.1% of gastric hyperplastic polyps in one large Japanese series.[21] In addition, within the same series, foci of dysplasia were seen in 4.0% of gastric hyperplastic polyps. The prevalence of true dysplasia arising from hyperplastic polyps is debated, with reported rates ranging from 1.9% to 19%.[22] In contrast to gastric fundic gland polyps that tend to arise from otherwise normal gastric mucosa, hyperplastic polyps have been associated with chronic gastritis, particularly with autoimmune

gastritis,[22–24] and *H. pylori* gastritis.[25] It has been shown more recently that *H. pylori* eradication leads to hyperplastic polyp disappearance[26,27]; this may provide an initial medical therapy before endoscopic removal.

The histology of gastric hyperplastic polyps differs from that of hyperplastic colorectal polyps in that gastric ones have submucosal edema with prominent foveolar hyperplasia and inflammation of the lamina propria. Endoscopically, hyperplastic polyps can be found throughout the stomach and range in size from small nodules of a few millimeters to a large mass of many centimeters that may be mistaken for carcinoma. They can be solitary or multiple and may be sessile or pedunculated with an associated stalk. If multiple polyps are found, the prevalence of associated atrophic gastritis may be 20% to 30%, and the polyps usually are more proximal in location.[22,28] The overlying mucosa may be normal in appearance, but the mucosa often has a reddish coloration in larger polyps (**Fig. 32.2**). Because of local trauma, larger hyperplastic polyps often have a friable, ulcerated whitish tip of granulation tissue and may be surrounded by atrophic or inflamed-appearing mucosa. There is no consensus regarding endoscopic removal and surveillance of hyperplastic gastric polyps. Details of management are discussed later.

Gastric Adenomatous Polyps

Adenomatous polyps of the stomach are less common than nonneoplastic epithelial lesions, constituting 7% to 10% of gastric polypoid lesions.[29,30] Gastric adenomas are true neoplasms and are premalignant lesions with an increasing risk of developing into adenocarcinoma depending on the size and structure. Up to 24% of gastric adenomas may harbor a focus of adenocarcinoma, especially if greater than 2 cm in diameter.[31] Malignancy can be found in lesions of any size, however. These lesions often arise in stomachs with a background of mucosal atrophy and are a marker for increased risk of adenocarcinoma elsewhere in the stomach.[30,32] Gastric adenomas have been associated with FAP but not as frequently as fundic gland polyps.

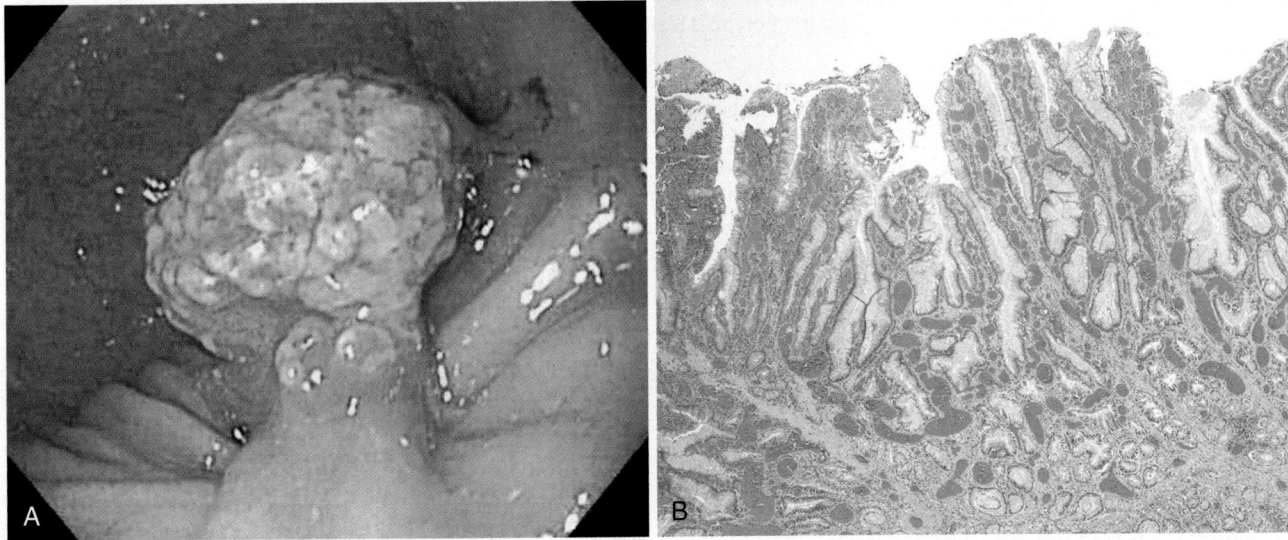

Fig. 32.2 **A,** Large hyperplastic polyp in the gastric antrum. **B,** Microphotography of hyperplastic polyp (hematoxylin and eosin stain). *(Courtesy of Dr. Noffsinger.)*

Histologically, gastric adenomas are characterized by columnar epithelium that is pseudostratified and shows elongated atypical nuclei and increased mitotic activity; they can be divided into tubular, villous, and tubulovillous types. Dysplasia and carcinomatous changes occur most often in villous and tubulovillous adenomas (28.5% to 40%).[33–36] Endoscopic evaluation of gastric adenomas should consist of a careful complete examination of the surrounding mucosa and biopsy of any suspicious lesion. These lesions can be found in any location of the stomach but seem to have a predilection for the antrum.[37] Gastric adenomas are generally larger than hyperplastic polyps, usually around 3 to 4 cm in diameter, but can also range in size from a few millimeters to several centimeters. The mucosal surface is usually smooth with a reddish coloration and often with a cerebriform mucosal pattern. The shape of gastric adenomas can vary, ranging from single, round, sessile projections to multilobulated lesions. Villous-type lesions are sometimes difficult to detect because of the flat, sessile, carpetlike appearance that can blend in with the surrounding rugae. Rarely, flat or depressed adenomas are encountered.[38]

Because of their malignant potential, the consensus is that all gastric adenomatous polyps need to be completely removed either endoscopically or by laparoscopic wedge resection. In addition, a thorough biopsy of the surrounding gastric mucosa should be performed. The recurrence rate of adenomatous polyps may be 16% after polypectomy.[39] Endoscopic techniques and management are discussed in more detail later.

Polypoid Gastric Carcinoma

Because of similar appearance, endoscopic determination of adenomatous gastric polyps versus genuine malignant lesions is extremely difficult without histologic confirmation. Synchronous or metachronous gastric cancers have been found in 11% of patients with adenomas.[34] Gastric adenocarcinomas may develop as polypoid lesions (Borrmann type A) and are differentiated into type I (protruded, polypoid type) and type IIa (superficial elevated type).[40]

Subepithelial Gastric Polyps

Subepithelial gastric polyps consist of a heterogeneous group of lesions that are usually small and difficult to differentiate between hyperplastic and adenomatous polyps. These nonepithelial lesions are usually covered by normal-appearing mucosa and have various causes, including carcinoid tumors, lipomas, aberrant pancreas (pancreatic rest, heterotopic pancreas), inflammatory fibroid polyps, and gastrointestinal stromal tumors (including leiomyomas, leiomyosarcomas, schwannomas, fibromas, and others). Chapter 29 contains a complete discussion of nonepithelial tumors of the stomach.

Endoscopic Techniques and Management

Gastric polyps are rarely symptomatic and often discovered incidentally. The first step in the management of a gastric polyp is to identify the tissue histology (**Fig. 32.3**). Because the histology of a gastric polyp cannot be reliably distinguished using a standard endoscope, biopsy or excision of gastric polypoid lesions found on upper endoscopy should be performed. This recommendation may change, however, as more studies using magnification or zoom endoscopy identify mucosal patterns that correlate with histology.[41,42] Although forceps biopsy is a simple method of obtaining tissue, it may provide inadequate tissue or sampling error. Studies have shown inconsistencies between histologic diagnosis made by forceps biopsy and a subsequent snare polypectomy specimen.[43,44] Muehldorfer and coworkers[45] conducted a prospective multicenter study comparing the diagnostic accuracy of forceps biopsy versus polypectomy in 222 gastric polyps greater than 5 mm (excluded fundic gland polyps). Relevant differences were found in 2.7% of cases in which there was failure to reveal foci of carcinoma on forceps biopsy in a group of hyperplastic polyps. Similarly, a study from Hungary showed significant disagreements in 27% of cases.[43] Endoscopic

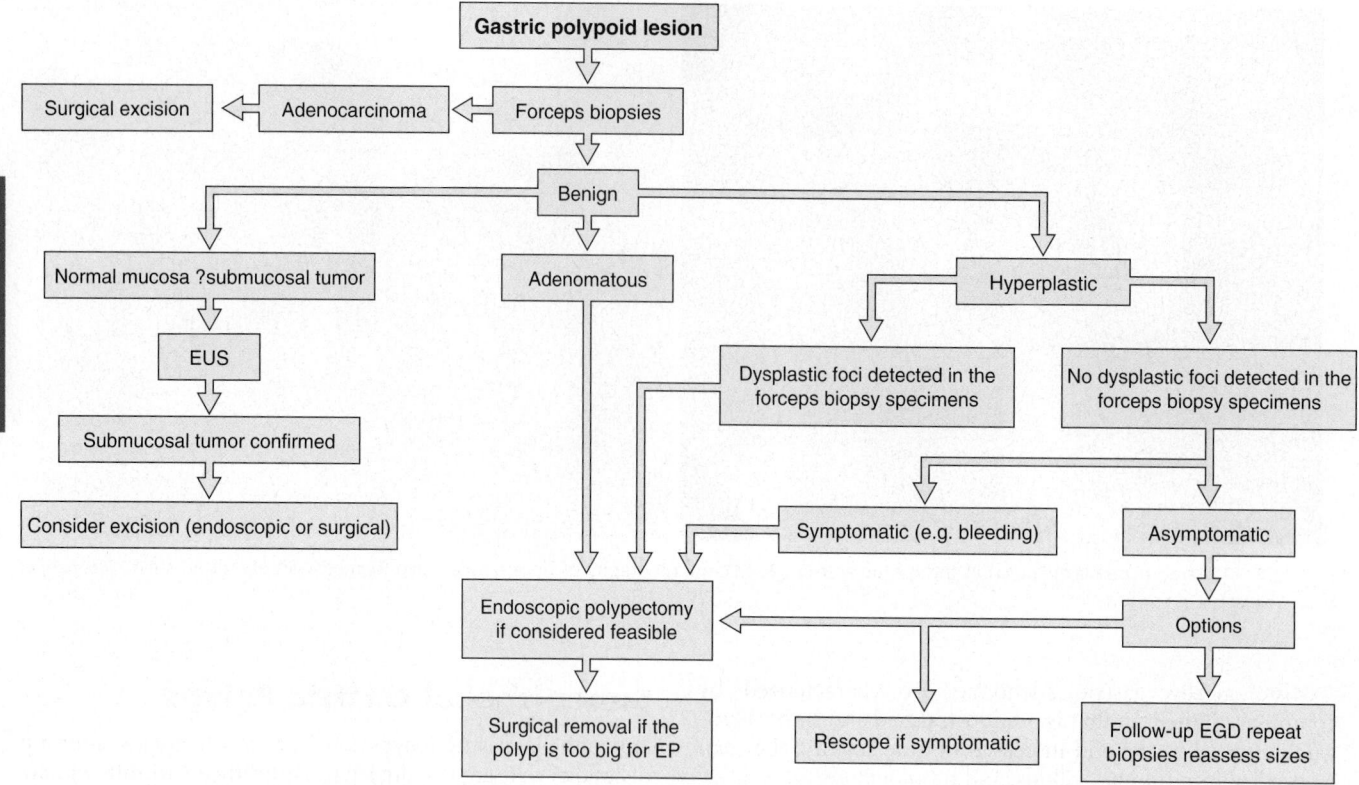

Fig. 32.3 Evaluation and management of a gastric polypoid lesion. *(Adapted from Lau CF, Hui PK, Mak KL, et al: Gastric polypoid lesions—illustrative cases and literature review. Am J Gastroenterol 93:2559–2564, 1998.)*

removal of all epithelial gastric polyps larger than 5 mm is encouraged by these authors.

If multiple gastric polyps are found, additional risk is presented to the patient if multiple snare excisions are performed. Although complete excision is preferred, this may not be technically feasible or practical; the risks and benefits should be individualized for each patient. In this scenario, resection could be delayed until forceps biopsy results are reviewed. Although gastric polyps that are multiple in number are usually of the same histologic type,[46] hyperplastic and adenomatous polyps can be found together.[35,39] One strategy to use when addressing multiple gastric polyps is to remove the larger polyps when feasible and safe by snare excision and perform multiple forceps biopsies of the smaller polyps. It is hoped that this approach would give a complete representation of the histology of the lesions encountered, while minimizing risk of a missed neoplasm. If one or more foci of dysplasia are detected in a biopsy specimen from a gastric hyperplastic polyp, the polyp should be removed, even if it is not symptomatic.

Controversy exists regarding the management of incidentally found gastric hyperplastic polyps with no focus of dysplasia on biopsy. Some authors recommend endoscopic removal of all hyperplastic polyps encountered because of the small risk of missing an area of dysplasia within the forceps biopsy.[34,43,44,47] Others propose endoscopically removing small polyps and periodic biopsy of hyperplastic polyps that are too large for safe complete polypectomy,[48] depending on the level of endoscopic expertise.

There is no consensus at the present time on the most appropriate frequency and duration of endoscopic follow-up of hyperplastic polyps.[49] Until well-designed, long-term prospective studies are available on the management of gastric polyps, the American Society for Gastrointestinal Endoscopy has developed general recommendations, as follows[50]:

1. Adenomatous gastric polyps are at increased risk for malignant transformation and should be resected completely. Hyperplastic polyps have a rare malignant potential. Endoscopy cannot differentiate histologic subtypes of polyps; biopsy or polypectomy is recommended when a polyp is encountered.
2. Polypoid defects of any size detected radiographically should be evaluated endoscopically, with biopsy or removal of the lesions.
3. Polyps should be endoscopically excised wherever feasible and clinically appropriate. If endoscopic polypectomy is impossible, a biopsy of the polyp should be performed, and if adenomatous or dysplastic tissue is detected, referral for surgical resection should be considered. If representative biopsy samples are obtained and the polyp is nondysplastic, no further intervention is necessary. If it is thought that endoscopic biopsy cannot sufficiently exclude the presence of dysplastic elements, referral for surgical resection is reasonable in polyps that cannot be removed endoscopically.
4. When multiple gastric polyps are encountered, biopsy of the largest polyps should be performed, or they should be excised, and representative biopsy specimens should be taken from some others. Further management should be based on histologic results.

5. Surveillance endoscopy 1 year after removing adenomatous gastric polyps is reasonable to assess recurrence at the prior excision site, new or previously missed polyps, and supervening early carcinoma. If the results of this examination are negative, repeat surveillance endoscopy should be repeated no more frequently than at 3-year to 5-year intervals. Follow-up after resection of polyps with high-grade dysplasia and early gastric cancer should be individualized.
6. No surveillance endoscopy is necessary after adequate sampling or removal of nondysplastic gastric polyps.

Endoscopic Techniques and Considerations

Gastric polypectomy, similar to all invasive procedures, carries a potential for injury to the patient. The patient should be aware of the added risks of possible complications before giving informed consent, especially if the diagnosis of gastric polyps is already known. Pedunculated polyps with thin stalks can be safely removed by snare cautery. For larger polyps on a thick pedicle, there is concern of a "feeder vessel" within the stalk. For pedunculated polyps greater than 1 cm in diameter, endoscopic resection can be assisted by using a grasping forceps through a snare technique, as described by Akahoshi and colleagues.[51] In this technique, using a dual channel endoscope, grasping forceps are inserted in one channel through the detachable snare loop previously inserted in the second channel. The detachable snare loop (Endoloop; Olympus America, Center Valley, PA) can provide extra hemostasis to reduce the risk of bleeding after polypectomy. Endoscopic resection using a detachable loop is a useful method of preventing polypectomy-related bleeding.[52]

Large gastric polyps that are sessile can be removed in piecemeal fashion, but if a transmural lesion is suspected, endoscopic ultrasound (EUS) and high-frequency miniprobes[53] can be useful in determining the depth of invasion. Early cancer polypoid lesions can be successfully removed with the use of endoscopic mucosal resection (EMR) and endoscopic submucosal dissection.[54] With the assistance of ultrasound, EMR is safe and effective for the management of selected submucosal lesions.[53] The approach to submucosal tumors and techniques of EMR are discussed in more detail in Chapter 29.

The incidence of hemorrhage from gastric polypectomy is about 7%.[55] For hemostasis, 2 to 4 mL of 1:10,000 epinephrine solution diluted with saline can be injected into the stalk before or after resection. Additional hemostasis can be provided by endoscopically deployed metallic clips (Hemoclip; Olympus America, Center Valley, PA) to provide mechanical compression to the target tissue. A retrospective study showed that the prophylactic use of hemoclips is associated with a low risk of bleeding (3.3%) after polypectomy of polyps 15 to 40 mm in diameter.[56] In addition, thermal hemostatic devices such as bipolar electrocautery or heater probe (Olympus America, Center Valley, PA) can deliver thermal energy to give additional hemostasis.

Resected polyps should be recovered and sent for pathologic examination, which is essential when the diagnosis is uncertain. Devices designed for polyp retrieval include grasping forceps, nets, baskets, and plastic traps.[57] The Roth retrieval net (United States Endoscopy Group, Inc., Mentor, OH) is a single-use device that comprises a net over a retractable loop that captures the polyp after polypectomy.

Thickened Folds

Thickened folds often present a diagnostic challenge to the endoscopist, particularly in the stomach. Standard endoscopic biopsies are often unrevealing and often contain only superficial mucosa despite tunneled deep biopsy specimens. Although obtaining specimens from deeper layers with a diathermic snare can increase the diagnostic yield, there is increased risk of hemorrhage or perforation.[58,59] In addition, the etiologies of thickened gastric folds are extremely varied, and thickened gastric folds are a common feature in both benign and malignant diseases. The more common and classic etiologies are discussed individually.

With the introduction of EUS, individual gut wall layers and accurate measurement of wall thickness is possible. Both high-frequency ultrasound probe sonography and dedicated echoendoscopes are useful for evaluation.[60,61] The gastric wall is considered thickened if greater than 3.6 mm and especially if greater than 4.0 mm. In normal gastric folds, there are five wall layers of the GI tract that are roughly proportional in size. The five EUS layers are: layer 1, the interface between the transducer or the fluid surrounding the transducer and the mucosa; layer 2, the deep mucosa and the muscularis mucosae; layer 3, the submucosa; layer 4, the muscularis propria; and layer 5, the serosa/adventitia. Different diseases show different levels of infiltration with regional thickening of distinct layers, which can refine potential diagnoses by EUS. Specific causes of thickened folds and their EUS features are listed in **Table 32.1**.

The initial EUS approach to thickened gastric folds should be to evaluate the layer thickness. When EUS abnormalities involve only the mucosal layer or layer 2, endoscopic biopsies are usually diagnostic.[62] If layers 2 and 3 are involved, deep or large forceps biopsies should be considered. Malignancy should be strongly suspected if layer 4 is involved or the muscularis propria is thickened, even if normal biopsy

Table 32.1 Diseases Considered in Evaluation with Endoscopic Ultrasound (EUS) of Thickened Folds and Layers Principally Involved

Etiology of Thickened Folds	EUS Wall Layer Involved
Gastric varices	2 and 3
Gastritis	2 and 3
Carcinoma and lymphoma	2–5
Hypertrophic gastric folds	2 and 3
Zollinger-Ellison syndrome	2 and 3
Ménétrier's disease	2 and 3
Gastritis cystica profunda	3
Hyperrugosity	2 and 3
Rectal ulcer and prolapse syndromes	2, 3, and 4

specimens are obtained.[62-64] Finally, many experts instill water into the lumen to improve image quality during EUS, although risk of aspiration should be carefully considered. An algorithm for the evaluation of thickened gastric folds is presented in **Fig. 32.4.**

Gastric Varices

Gastric varices are seen in the submucosal layer as distinct hypoechoic structures by EUS and are often described as wormlike. The mucosal and submucosal layers (layers 2 and 3) may be thickened in portal hypertension. Engorgement of larger vessels, such as the splenic and portal veins, perigastric collateral veins, and gastric perforating veins, may also be seen.[65] If gastric varices are identified or suspected, biopsies should not be done. Thickened gastric folds in the cardia or fundus should be evaluated by EUS if indicated.[66] The use of color Doppler EUS can verify blood flow and calculate blood flow volume and velocity, which can be monitored during therapy.[67] In addition, EUS has been used for local treatment with cyanoacrylate injection.[68]

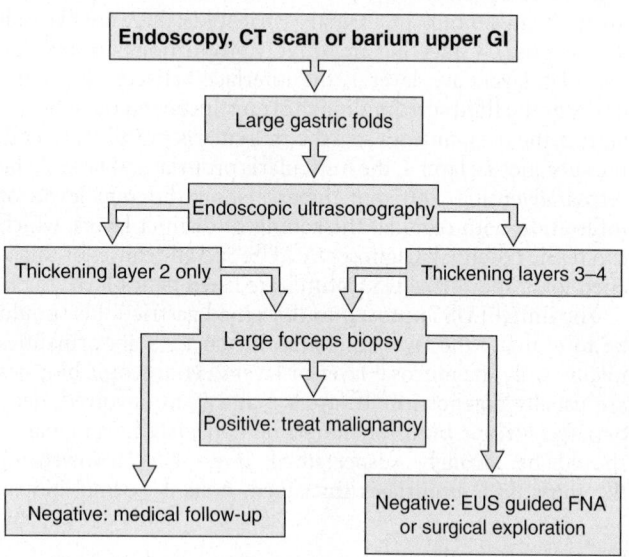

Fig. 32.4 Flow chart illustrating the work-up of large gastric folds. CT, computed tomography; EUS, endoscopic ultrasound; FNA, fine needle aspiration; GI, gastrointestinal.

Gastritis

Another cause of superficial wall layer thickening is gastritis, which involves the mucosa and submucosa (layers 2 and 3). Infectious etiologies are common, especially *H. pylori.*[69,70] Resolution of *H. pylori* gastritis–induced gastric fold thickening occurs after eradication of the organism.[70] Inflammatory conditions have also been implicated, particularly conditions resulting in granuloma formation such as sarcoidosis[71] and Crohn's disease.[72,73] Hirokawa and colleagues[73] described a "bamboo joint–like" endoscopic appearance characterized by swollen longitudinal folds traversed by erosive fissures in the stomach of 15 of 23 patients who had Crohn's disease. Mucosal nodularity or cobblestone mucosa with thickening of the antral folds in patients with Crohn's disease has also been described.[72] When infection or the inflammatory reaction is severe, involvement can sometimes include deeper wall layers as well, raising concern for malignancy.[74]

Ménétrier's Disease (Giant Hypertrophic Gastritis)

Ménétrier's disease is a rare condition whose origin seems to be related to an overexpression of transforming growth factor-α in the surface mucous cells in the body and fundus of the stomach.[75] It involves marked thickening of EUS layers 2 and 3 with histologic features of foveolar hyperplasia and atrophy of glands (**Fig. 32.5**). Erosions or ulceration may be present on the enlarged folds and may appear convoluted or cerebriform with a reddish coloration. These patients usually present with weight loss, diarrhea, and edema. Ménétrier's disease is characterized by (1) giant folds, especially in the fundus and body of the stomach; (2) hypoalbuminemia; and (3) histologic features of foveolar hyperplasia, atrophy of glands, and a marked overall increase in mucosal thickness. EUS differentiation of Ménétrier's disease and lymphoma may be difficult because both display similar echo patterns. Pinch biopsies are usually insufficient for diagnosis, whereas loop biopsy using a polypectomy snare over a fold yields better results for diagnosis. Submucosal saline injection technique can also be applied to help raise the lesion before removal.

Lymphoma and Carcinoma

Malignancy should always be considered when evaluating thickened gastric folds. As mentioned previously, involvement

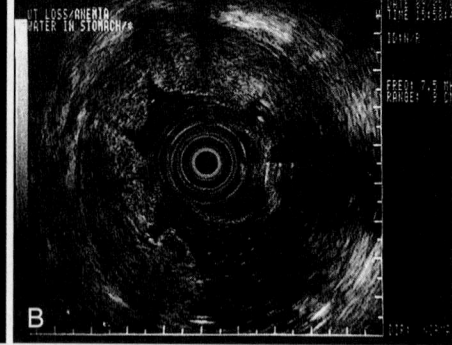

Fig. 32.5 A, Endoscopic images reveal gastric body thickened folds. Biopsy specimens are nondiagnostic. **B,** Endoscopic ultrasound (EUS) reveals marked expansion of acoustic layers 1, 2, and 3, consistent with Ménétrier's disease.

of the muscularis propria (EUS layer 4) should prompt concern for malignancy and consideration of surgical biopsy, even if aggressive endoscopic biopsy techniques are performed and return unremarkable. In these situations, the muscularis propria layer can be thickened fourfold to sixfold compared with controls.[64,76] Both lymphoma and carcinoma involve the deeper wall layers exclusively, without mucosal disease,[63] so this diagnosis could easily be missed on standard endoscopy. EUS-guided fine needle aspiration (FNA) or a surgical approach should be attempted for obtaining tissue diagnosis. Diffuse gastric cancers (linitis plastica, scirrhous carcinoma) are seen as diffuse hypoechoic wall thickening covered by normal-appearing mucosa but often with distorted layers and an irregular-appearing outer margin on EUS (**Fig. 32.6**). In contrast, in patients with hypertrophic gastritis only the mucosal layer is thickened.[76]

Lymphoma more often involves the superficial layers as well, particularly in mucosal-associated lymphoid tissue (MALT) lymphoma. The role of EUS in MALT lymphoma has received considerable attention, primarily because EUS can predict disease that may respond to *H. pylori* eradication as the sole means of therapy.[77] Complete remission rates of 100% have been described for patients with T1 stage low-grade MALT lymphoma (**Fig. 32.7**).[78] In addition, EUS surveillance helps detect persistent disease, recurrences, and the need for aggressive chemotherapy.[79] Miniature ultrasound probes have been advocated for initial staging and follow-up of MALT lymphoma because of better resolution of superficial lesions.[80,81]

Zollinger-Ellison Syndrome

Gastrinoma, or Zollinger-Ellison syndrome (ZES), is a rare condition that can be associated with thick gastric folds. It is estimated to occur in 0.1 to 3 patients per 1 million of the U.S. population, with a mean age of diagnosis of 50 years.[82] ZES should be suspected in patients with severe erosive esophagitis, multiple or refractory peptic ulcers, and ulcers in unusual locations and in patients with a family history of multiple endocrine neoplasia type I and related gastrinomas.[83] Ulcers in ZES are usually less than 1 cm in diameter, and approximately 75% of ulcers are located in the first portion of the duodenum. Histologically, ZES is characterized as hyperproliferation of enterochromaffinlike and parietal cells with glandular hyperplasia resulting from trophic effects of gastrin produced by a gastrinoma. EUS evaluation of thickened folds shows thickening of layers 2 and 3 in the body and fundus. EUS accuracy for gastrinomas is around 80%.[84] Tumor localization is done by somatostatin receptor scintigraphy, EUS, or both.

Miscellaneous

There are several rare miscellaneous causes of thickened gastric folds. Metastatic disease, particularly from breast cancer, may manifest as thickening and disruption of the wall layers.[85] Gastritis cystica profunda involves EUS layer 3 and appears as multiple small cysts, which are histologically benign. Malignant infiltration may also result in cystic changes in EUS layers 2 and 3; diagnosis must be based on adequate histologic analysis such as EMR specimens.[86]

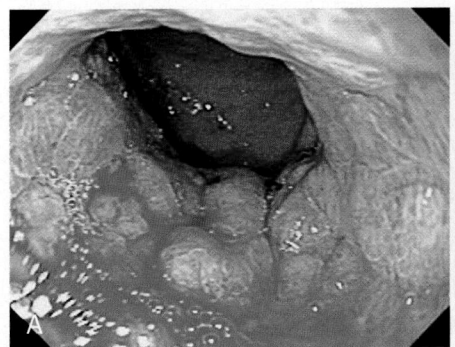 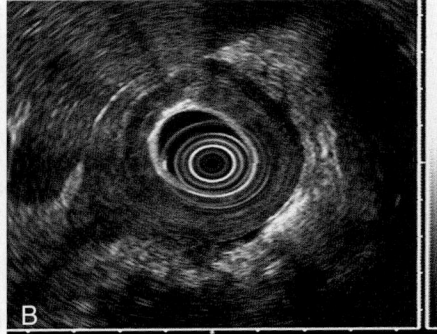 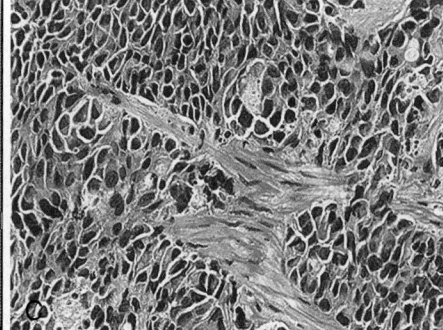

Fig. 32.6 **A,** Endoscopic images of thickened folds with negative standard biopsy specimens. **B,** Endoscopic ultrasound (EUS) reveals infiltration of layers 3 and 4 and transmural extension consistent with linitis plastica or lymphoma. **C,** EUS-guided Tru-cut biopsy specimen reveals adenocarcinoma.

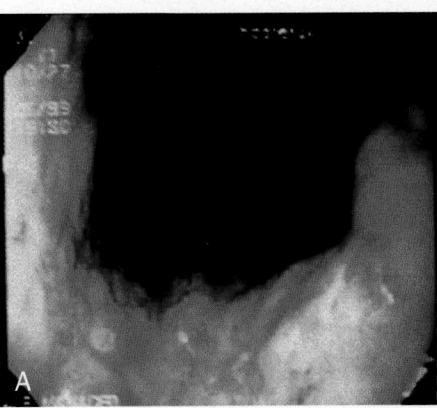 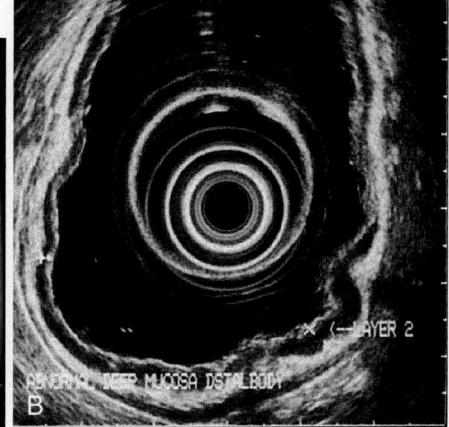

Fig. 32.7 **A,** Endoscopic images of severe antral gastritis with biopsy specimens consistent with a mucosal-associated lymphoid tissue (MALT) lymphoma. **B,** Endoscopic ultrasound (EUS) shows disease limited to layers 1 and 2 (superficial and deep mucosa) making it amenable to antibiotic therapy.

Conclusion

The evaluation of gastric polyps and thickened folds presents both technical and diagnostic challenges to the endoscopist. Obtaining adequate tissue to secure a diagnosis is crucial in evaluating new lesions. Guidelines for surveillance after polypectomy or monitoring thickened folds are not yet established. Clinical experience and numerous published studies have shown that EUS is an important tool for diagnosis and characterization of polypoid lesions and large gastric folds by examining individual layers of the gut wall. Nevertheless, histologic examination is still of paramount importance, and cutting-edge modalities such as EMR and endoscopic submucosal dissection can provide adequate specimens for final diagnosis and local staging.

References

The complete reference list is available online at www.expertconsult.com.

Endoscopic Therapy for Gastric Neoplasms

Chang Beom Ryu and Yang K. Chen

Video related to this chapter's topics can be found online at expertconsult.com.

Introduction

Gastrointestinal (GI) endoscopy has evolved at an amazing pace in the past decade. The scope of therapeutic endoscopy has increased dramatically mostly as a result of advances in technology. Such technologic breakthroughs have stimulated the proliferation of novel endoscopic techniques for diagnosing and treating GI diseases, including gastric neoplasms.

The development and clinical application of endoscopic ultrasound (EUS) have enabled GI specialists to evaluate previously inaccessible intramural gastric lesions and to determine the layer of origin. With the ability to determine, with almost pinpoint accuracy, the depth of gastric wall layer involvement and to exclude lymph node metastasis, the endoscopist can safely proceed to endoscopic removal of a gastric neoplasm. Introduction of new techniques such as endoscopic mucosal resection (EMR), endoscopic submucosal dissection (ESD), and thermal ablation techniques such as argon plasma coagulation (APC) have made it possible to remove or destroy certain types of gastric neoplasms safely and completely.[1-7]

A gastric tumor is defined as any mass lesion occurring in the wall of the stomach. Its metastatic potential defines the difference between benign and malignant neoplasms. Epithelial neoplasms include adenomas and carcinomas. Intramural lesions include gastric stromal cell tumors and lymphoma. **Box 33.1** shows the classification of gastric neoplasms. The primary emphasis of this chapter is on endoscopic therapy for early gastric cancer (EGC).

Gastric Cancer

Gastric cancer is still the world's second leading cause of cancer mortality after lung cancer, despite its worldwide decline in incidence and mortality. It has been estimated that 700,000 deaths per year from the disease occurred in 2002 accounting for more than 10% of all cancer deaths.[8,9] Adenocarcinoma accounts for approximately 90% of gastric cancers, with the remainder being due to non-Hodgkin's lymphoma (NHL) and leiomyosarcoma.

Epidemiology

The annual incidence of gastric cancer varies worldwide. There is a difference in the prevalence of gastric cancer between the East and the West (**Fig. 33.1**).[10] In Eastern Asian countries such as Japan and China and in many developing countries, gastric cancer is the most prevalent malignant neoplasm and the leading cause of cancer mortality.[11] **Fig. 33.2** shows the incidence of gastric cancer in Eastern Asia and the United States.[10] There is a high incidence of gastric cancer in the East, the former Soviet Union, some portions of Central and Eastern Europe, and Central America (e.g., Costa Rica) and South America (e.g., Chile). The lowest rates occur in the United States and in some parts of Africa.

The International Agency for Research on Cancer (IARC) data for 1996 reported an age-standardized incidence rate of 95.5/105 in Japanese men in Yamagata, Japan, and 7.5/105 in white men in the United States.[11] Most of the geographic variation is due to differences in the incidence of gastric cancer

Box 33.1 **Gastric Neoplasms**

Epithelial neoplasms
   Adenomas
   Carcinomas
     Primary
     Secondary
   Carcinoids
Lymphoma
Stromal tumors

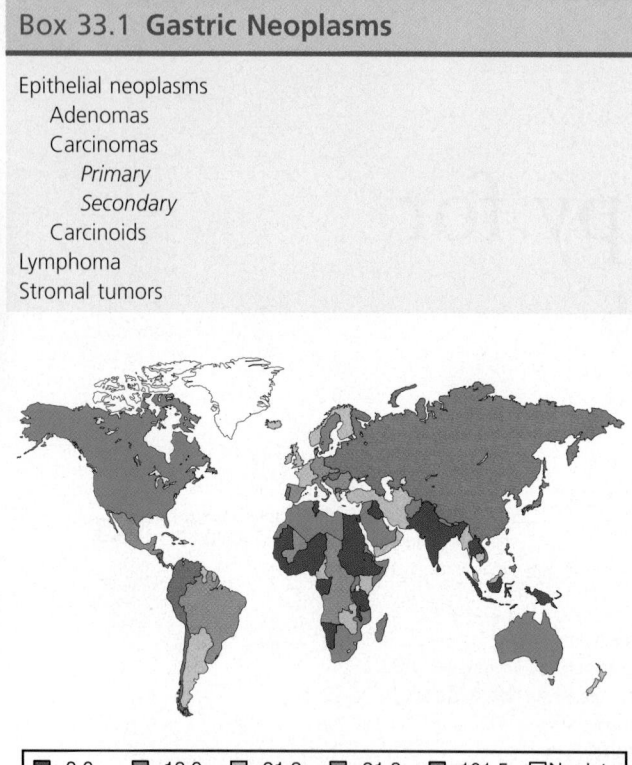

| ■<8.6 | ■<13.9 | □<21.2 | ■<31.8 | ■<101.5 | □No data |

Fig. 33.1 Worldwide incidence of gastric cancer. *(Redrawn from data from Ferlay J, Bray F, Pisani P, et al: GLOBOCAN 2002: Cancer incidence, mortality and prevalence worldwide IARC CancerBase, Lyon, France, 2004, IARC Press.)*

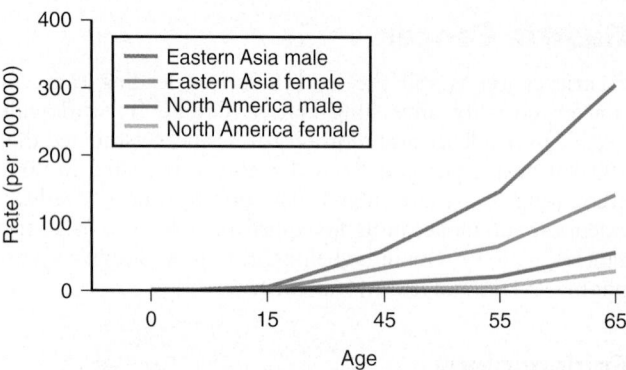

Fig. 33.2 Incidence of gastric cancer in East Asia and the United States according to gender and age.

not localized in the cardia (noncardia gastric cancer); cancer that is localized in the cardia has a more uniform distribution. Ethnic groups that migrate from a country with a high incidence to a country with a low incidence have an overall risk intermediate between that of their homeland and that of their new country. First-generation migrants tend to retain their high risk, whereas subsequent generations have risk levels approximating that of their host country.[12]

Both the incidence and the mortality rates for gastric cancer have declined sharply during the last several decades, particularly in the United States and in Western Europe. In the United States, gastric cancer is the 13th most common cancer and the 8th most common cause of cancer death. A steady decline in the incidence of noncardia gastric cancer has occurred since

1930 throughout the world.[13] The incidence of adenocarcinoma involving the cardia or the esophagogastric junction, or both, has increased in developed countries such as the United States.[14] The reasons for this trend are unknown.

There are variations in the overall incidence and mortality of noncardia gastric cancer between gender and ethnic groups. In the United States, the incidence is greater among Native Americans, Hispanic whites, and African Americans.[15] The ethnic distribution for cancer of the gastric cardia is also different, with a preponderance in American whites over African Americans.[11] The incidence of gastric cancer increases with age, with most patients 50 to 70 years of age. The incidence of gastric cancer in patients younger than 36 years has increased from 1.8% before 1970 to 4.2% after 1970, with most (62.5%) occurring in Hispanics. Noncardia gastric cancer is more common in men than women by a ratio of approximately 2:1. Gastric cancer located in the cardia has an even higher male-to-female ratio of up to 6:1 in U.S. whites.[16] **Figs. 33-3 and 33-4** summarize the trends in the incidence and mortality of gastric cancer in the United States during the years 1975–2006 according to gender and ethnicity.[17]

Pathogenesis

Gastric cancer has a poor prognosis with a 5-year survival of less than 5%. This poor prognosis is mostly due to the fact that four out of five patients present at an advanced stage.[18] Incidental diagnosis of gastric cancer has been reported to increase patient survival.[19,20]

Japan has the highest incidence of gastric cancer worldwide. However, the establishment of an aggressive mass screening policy has resulted in a remarkably high detection rate of EGC—40% to 66.4% of all gastric cancers diagnosed.[21,22] Consequently, the most extensive experience with treatment of EGC has come from Japan.

The Japanese Society of Gastrointestinal Endoscopy defines EGC as cancer confined to the mucosa or submucosa, with or without lymph node metastasis. This designation was based on the observation that this subgroup of patients has an excellent prognosis, with a 5-year survival of greater than 90% after gastrectomy and removal of both the primary and the secondary lymph nodes.[1,21] In the West, 10% to 20% of surgical resections for gastric carcinoma are for EGC[23]; in Japan, more than 50% of surgical specimens are classified as EGC.[24,25]

Helicobacter pylori

Since the bacterium *Helicobacter pylori* was first reported in 1983, a wealth of evidence has been gathered concerning its role in the etiology of gastric cancer.[26–28] In 1994, the IARC classified *H. pylori* as carcinogenic to humans. Evidence supporting an etiologic association between *H. pylori* and gastric cancer can be found in ecologic studies, case-control studies, and prospective cohort studies.[27,29–31] Meta-analyses of prospective studies suggest that the risk of gastric cancer is increased twofold to threefold in individuals with chronic *H. pylori* infection.[32,33] One prospective, nested case-control study found a significant association between prior *H. pylori* infection and gastric adenocarcinoma overall, but there was no association with cancer of the cardia.[34] Individuals without *H. pylori* colonization seem to have a minimal risk of gastric carcinoma.[35]

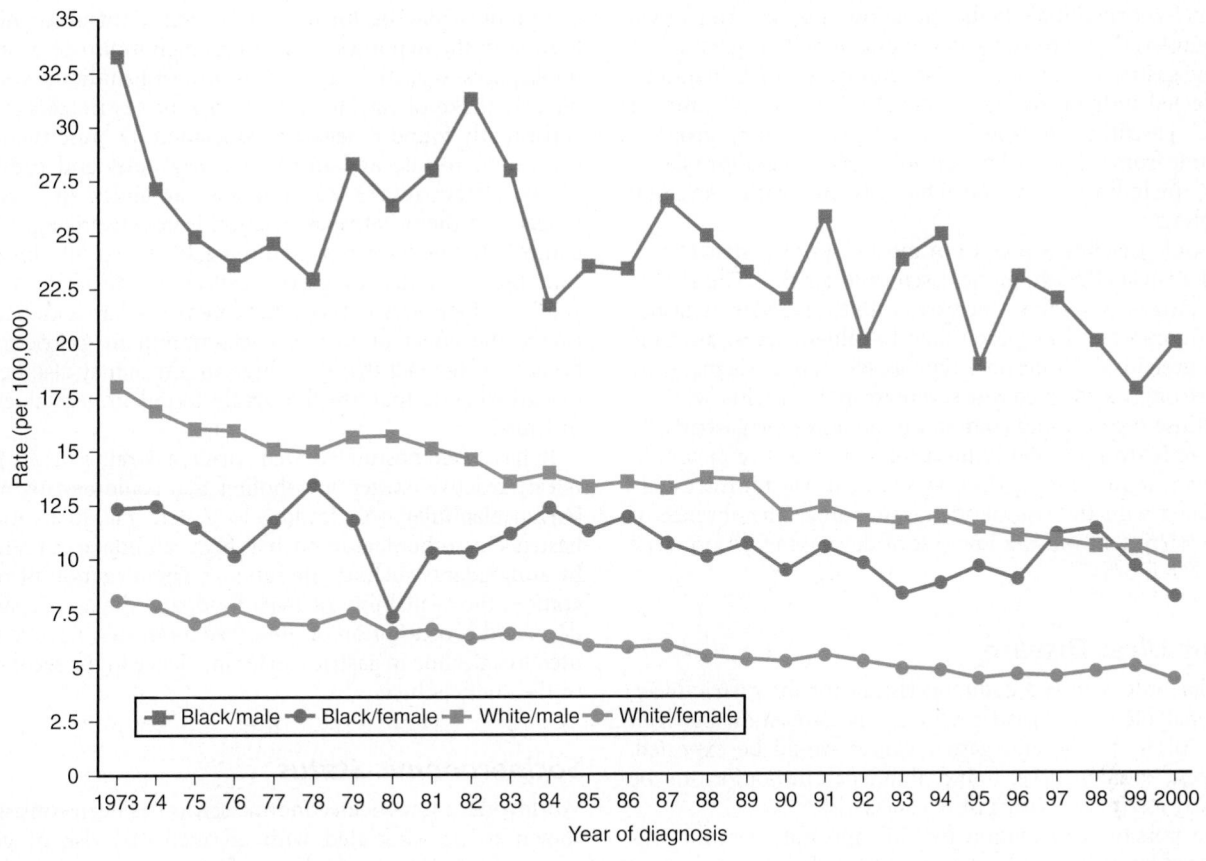

Fig. 33.3 Incidence of gastric cancer in the United States according to gender and race.

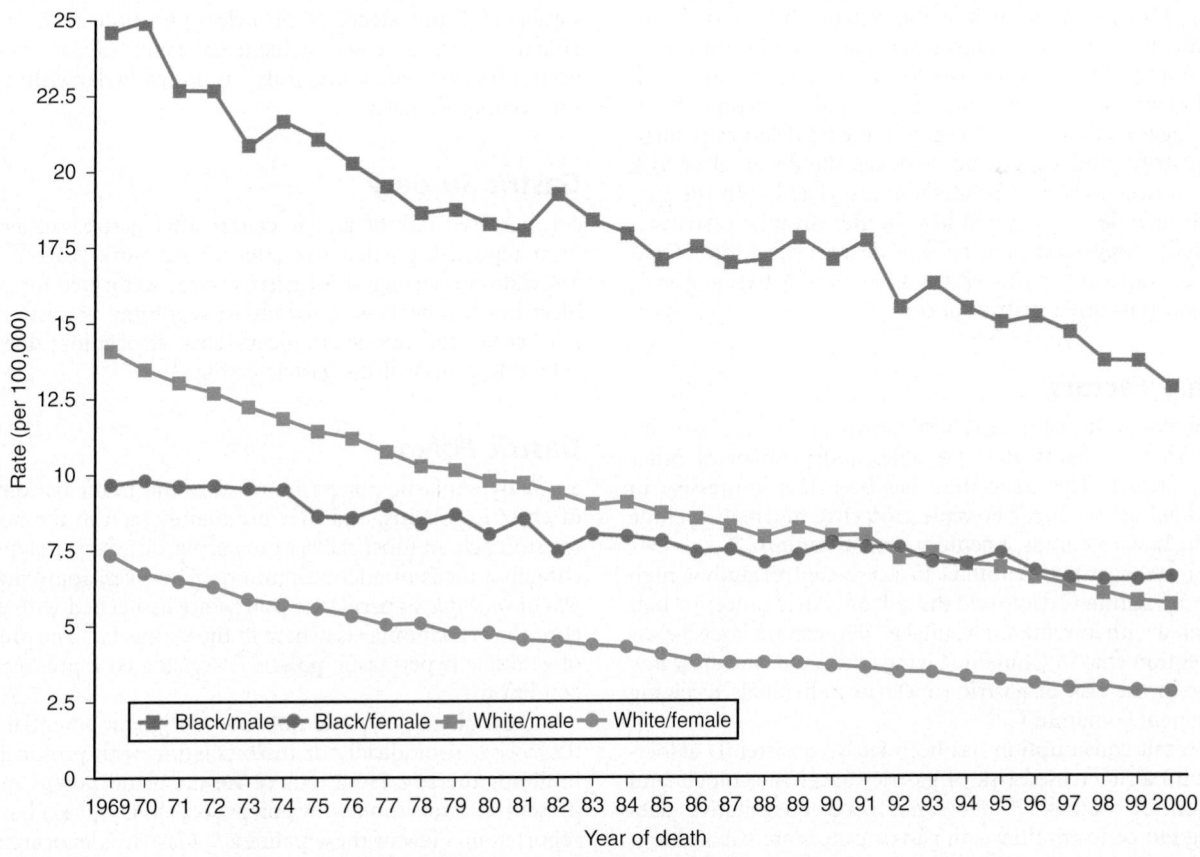

Fig. 33.4 Mortality of gastric cancer in the United States (1975–2006) according to gender and race.

H. pylori contributes to the causation of gastric cancer via mechanisms that involve the development and progression of chronic gastritis.[36] Infection causes chronic gastritis in almost all infected individuals and accounts for almost all cases of chronic gastritis.[37] *H. pylori*–induced gastritis may progress over time from superficial nonatrophic gastritis to more severe forms, including severe atrophic gastritis with intestinal metaplasia.

Chronic gastritis is present in most cases of gastric cancer and is associated with an increased cancer risk.[36] The risk of developing gastric cancer increases with the severity of gastritis, with reported risks greater than 10-fold for severe atrophic antral gastritis.[36,38] Intestinal-type gastric cancer seems to be more strongly associated with severe atrophic gastritis, whereas the diffuse type is more common in nonatrophic gastritis.[36]

There is strong evidence for a role for virulence factors in *H. pylori* carcinogenesis. The Cag A virulence factor is strongly associated with the risk of adenocarcinoma. The absence of Cag A carries, at most, a low risk of developing diffuse-type adenocarcinoma.[39]

Peptic Ulcer Disease

H. pylori infection is a common risk factor for gastric ulcer, duodenal ulcer, and gastric cancer. An association between peptic ulcer disease and gastric cancer would be expected. However, studies have found duodenal ulceration to be inversely associated with gastric cancer risk.[40]

One possible explanation for this apparent paradox was suggested by Parsonnet,[41] who argued that *H. pylori* infection can progress to gastric cancer or duodenal ulcer but seldom to both. Other factors, such as the genetic characteristics of the individual and the organism, may play a significant role in determining which disease would occur. The age at which infection was acquired may also influence the outcome. It has been suggested that infection early in life predisposes to atrophic gastritis and cancer but reduces duodenal ulcer risk owing to decreased acid production associated with the gastritis. If infection is acquired later in life, atrophic gastritis is less likely, and gastric cancer risk is decreased.[41] More recent evidence supports a moderate association between gastric ulcer and noncardia gastric cancer.[42,43]

Dietary Factors

Several observational studies have shown a protective association with fresh fruits and vegetables, independent of other dietary factors. The association has been less impressive in limited cohort studies.[44] Possible protective nutrients include vitamin E, carotenoids, selenium, and vitamin C.[44] The evidence is stronger for vitamin C. In a case-control study, a high intake of vitamin C decreased the risk of gastric cancer by half compared with low vitamin C intake.[45] However, a large 5-year intervention trial in China involving adults did not show any change in the risk of gastric cancer in individuals receiving supplemental vitamin C.[46]

High salt consumption has been fairly consistently associated with an increased risk of gastric cancer in ecologic and case-control studies.[47–49] However, good quantitative data linking salt consumption with gastric cancer are still lacking.

N-nitroso compounds have been shown to be carcinogenic in animal studies.[50] In the human stomach, these compounds may be formed from dietary nitrite or nitrate, leading to the hypothesis that a diet high in nitrite or nitrate predisposes to gastric cancer. Case-control studies examining dietary intake of nitrate and the risk of gastric cancer have consistently found a negative association. Because the major sources of nitrate and nitrite are vegetables and preserved meats, nitrate intake was probably an index of vegetable intake, and the negative association is not surprising.[44] Case-control studies have reported a weak, statistically insignificant increased risk of gastric cancer (relative risk 1.12 to 1.28) for high versus low nitrite intake.[51–54] It is difficult to isolate the effect of nitrate consumption in gastric cancer because of the fact that diets high in nitrite may also be high in antioxidants that are frequently found in vegetables and in fruits.[54]

It has been postulated that virulent strains of *H. pylori* release reactive oxygen metabolites that could destroy neighboring glandular cells leading to gastric glandular atrophy, hastened by other factors such as high salt intake but retarded by antioxidants such as vitamin C.[55] The invention of refrigeration, the availability of fresh food, and the accompanying decreased consumption of preserved foods may have contributed to a decline in gastric cancer incidence in the second half of the 20th century.

Socioeconomic Status

Worldwide, a low socioeconomic status has been consistently shown to be associated with an increased risk of gastric cancer.[16] The higher prevalence of gastric cancer among individuals with lower socioeconomic status is matched by a similar high prevalence of *H. pylori* infection in these individuals.[56,57] An increased incidence of cancer of the cardia has been observed predominantly in individuals with higher socioeconomic status.[14]

Gastric Surgery

An increased risk of gastric cancer after gastric surgery has been reported, particularly after 15 or more years.[58,59] The association is strongest for gastrectomy performed for gastric ulcer but less persuasive for either vagotomy or gastrectomy performed for duodenal ulcer. This association does not extend to cancer of the gastric cardia.[40]

Gastric Polyps

Single hyperplastic polyps are often found in the background of chronic gastritis, and they are mainly seen in the body of the stomach. At most, 0.3% of hyperplastic gastric polyps may contain a focus of adenocarcinoma. However, approximately 3% of *multiple* hyperplastic polyps are associated with a synchronous carcinoma elsewhere in the stomach.[60] The presence of *multiple* hyperplastic polyps is considered a precancerous condition.

Fundic gland polyps do not have malignant potential when they occur sporadically or in association with proton pump inhibitor therapy. Hundreds of fundic gland polyps may be present in association with polyposis coli. Dysplasia has been reported in a few of these patients.[61] Gastric adenocarcinoma associated with fundic gland polyposis in familial polyposis coli has been reported.[62]

Adenomatous polyps occur in the setting of intestinal metaplasia and associated chronic gastritis. Endoscopic features that increase the risk of malignant transformation include large size and a red, erosive surface color. A carcinoma may be contained in 40% of pyloric gland adenomas and generally 10% of tubular adenomas.[60,63] Approximately 11% of patients with adenomatous polyps have a synchronous or metachronous gastric adenocarcinoma.[63]

Genetic Factors

Genetic predisposition may play a role in the development of gastric cancer, with a twofold to fourfold increased risk in first-degree relatives. Similarly, patients who have hereditary lesions, such as Lynch syndrome II, have an increased risk of gastric cancer.[64,65]

Miscellaneous Factors

A higher risk for gastric cancer has been reported in patients with Ménétrier's disease, ataxia telangiectasia, and blood type group A.[66–68] Pernicious anemia and its association with autoimmune chronic gastritis increases the risk of developing gastric cancer by twofold to threefold, according to population-based studies.[69,70] Regular endoscopic surveillance in young patients with pernicious anemia has been advocated.[71]

Smoking may increase the incidence of premalignant gastric lesions and dysplasia; however a dose-response relationship has not been clearly shown.[72–74] No clear relationship between alcohol consumption and gastric cancer has been shown.[29,72,74]

Molecular Abnormalities

Abnormalities at the molecular level have been described in patients who develop gastric cancer. These include allelic deletions of the atrial premature complex (*APC*) gene, the migrating motor complex (*MCC*) gene, and the tumor-suppressor gene *TP53*. Allelic deletions of *TP53* can be found in 64% of gastric cancers. These deletions are common late events in gastric cancer.[75] In addition, mutations of the *APC* gene and loss of heterozygosity on chromosomes 1q, 5q, and 17p have been reported in gastric carcinoma.[76]

Loss of E-cadherin–dependent cell-cell adhesion secondary to mutation of beta-catenin has been found in gastric cancer.[77] Reduced expression of E-cadherin has been found to be significantly associated with recurrence of cancer and decreased survival.[78] Microsatellite instability has also been found in gastric carcinoma.[79] Higher expression of Sialyl-Tn has been associated with a poor prognosis in patients with gastric cancer.[80] Patients with overexpression of c-erbB protein have been found to have a poorer prognosis than patients without c-erbB expression in poorly differentiated gastric adenocarcinoma.[81] Germline truncating mutations in the E-cadherin gene (*CDH1*) have been found in several families with hereditary diffuse gastric cancer.[82,83]

Clinical Features
Early Gastric Cancer

Observational studies have shown that approximately 70% of patients with EGC have symptoms of dyspepsia but no anemia, dysphagia, or weight loss. It is uncommon to find gastric cancer at an early stage (<20% of diagnosed cases) in countries with a relatively low risk for the disease. In countries with high risk such as Japan, endoscopic screening has been practiced since the 1960s, and as a result, the incidence of EGC is 40% to 50%. In the absence of suggestive symptoms, detecting EGC requires a high index of suspicion and a low threshold for endoscopic examination, especially in patients belonging to relatively high-risk groups.

Advanced Gastric Cancer

Most patients with gastric adenocarcinoma present with advanced disease. Accompanying symptoms, such as weight loss, vomiting, anorexia, early satiety, abdominal pain, and anemia, may mimic peptic ulcer disease and other GI conditions. Typically, patients have been symptomatic for less than 12 months, and 40% of patients have been symptomatic for less than 3 months. Signs and symptoms are due to cancer invasion beyond the muscularis propria by direct extension or by distant metastasis. Liver and lungs are the most common sites of gastric cancer metastases (40%); bone and peritoneum are less frequent sites (10%). Occasionally, patients may present with a paraneoplastic syndrome, such as Trousseau's syndrome (thrombosis), acanthosis nigricans (pigmented skin lesion, classically of the axilla), or dermatomyositis.[84,85]

Pathology

Most primary gastric cancers are adenocarcinoma, with an occasional squamous or adenosquamous carcinoma. Other rare gastric cancers include parietal cell carcinoma, choriocarcinoma, and rhabdoid tumor. Cancer metastasizing to the stomach is uncommon, with lung cancer being the most frequent primary tumor. A few cases of gastric carcinosarcoma and spindle cell carcinoma have been reported.[86]

Histologically, gastric adenocarcinoma can be divided into two categories[87]: (1) intestinal type, a well-differentiated neoplastic lesion that forms glandlike structures that ulcerate frequently, and (2) diffuse type, characterized by infiltration and thickening of the gastric wall without the formation of a discrete mass. Approximately 16% of gastric cancers cannot be categorized or are of the mixed type.[86] The decline in incidence of gastric cancer has been predominantly in the distal stomach intestinal type, whereas a steady increase in the incidence of the proximal stomach diffuse type has been observed in the United States and in Europe.[88,89] There has been inconsistent classification of gastric cardia and distal esophageal cancer in the literature because many, if not most, of these represent distal spread from specialized intestinal metaplasia of the distal esophagus or the esophagogastric junction.

Intestinal Type

Grossly, intestinal adenocarcinoma is a well-demarcated neoplastic tumor that tends to be nodular, polypoid, or ulcerated. Histologically, intestinal adenocarcinoma is characterized by a well-formed glandular pattern, which may contain solid or papillary areas. The malignant cells are columnar or cuboidal, with a basally located nucleus.

Diffuse Type

Grossly, diffuse adenocarcinoma is more likely to have a plaquelike surface and ill-defined infiltrating growth. Histologically, the infiltrating growth is composed of individual cells or cords of cells, and a fibrous or mucoid stroma is present between the cells or cords of cells. Many cells of diffuse carcinoma contain mucin droplets that sometimes produce a signet-ring appearance. Most cases of linitis plastica are classified as diffuse carcinomas. Most diffuse carcinomas are poorly differentiated.

Histologic Typing

The histologic classification should be based on the predominant pattern of tumor.[90]

COMMON TYPES

Papillary adenocarcinoma (pap)
Tubular adenocarcinoma
    Well-differentiated type (tub 1)
    Moderately differentiated type (tub 2)
    Poorly differentiated adenocarcinoma
        Solid type (por 1)
        Nonsolid type (por 2)
    Signet-ring cell carcinoma (sig)
    Mucinous adenocarcinoma (muc)

Note 1: Undifferentiated carcinoma combined with a small adenocarcinoma component should be classified as poorly differentiated adenocarcinoma.

Note 2: In clinicopathologic or epidemiologic studies, papillary or tubular adenocarcinoma can be interpreted as differentiated or intestinal type, whereas "por" and "sig" can be regarded as the undifferentiated or diffuse type. Mucinous carcinoma can be interpreted as either intestinal or diffuse, depending on the other predominant elements (i.e., pap, tub, por, or sig).

SPECIAL TYPES

Adenosquamous carcinoma
Squamous cell carcinoma
Carcinoid tumor
Other tumors

Differential Diagnosis

Diagnosis of gastric cancer requires histologic confirmation. Gastric carcinoma can mimic peptic ulcer disease radiographically and endoscopically. It is mandatory to obtain a biopsy specimen in all gastric ulcers to establish the correct benign or malignant diagnosis. Radiographic or endoscopic detection of EGC can be very difficult, requiring recognition and tissue sampling of very subtle abnormalities, such as slight depressions or elevations, minor differences in color or texture, or changes in peristalsis.

Advanced cancer is more commonly encountered at the time of diagnosis. Of gastric cancers, 50% are located in the antrum, and one out of four is located in the body. The remaining tumors involve either the cardia or the entire stomach. Advanced carcinoma may be fungating, polypoid, flat (superficial), ulcerated, or diffusely infiltrating (linitis plastica). Ulcerating or fungating gastric cancers account for 60% to 70% of cases. Ulcerating types may mimic benign ulcers but are usually larger, with more heaped-up edges (rather than appearing "punched out") and a more irregular or "shaggy" ulcer base. Linitis plastica or "leather bottle" stomach constitutes 10% of cases; there is no luminal mass, but the stomach wall is diffusely infiltrated and usually markedly thickened.

Staging

Initial staging of gastric cancer should include spiral computed tomography (CT) of the abdomen to determine the presence or absence of metastatic disease. In the absence of metastasis, EUS is helpful for assessing resectability. Determination of surgical resectability for cure using EUS has been found to be 91% accurate.[91]

EGC is defined by the Japanese Society of Gastrointestinal Endoscopy as gastric cancer confined to the mucosa or submucosa, with or without lymph node metastasis. Patients with EGC have an excellent 5-year survival of greater than 90%.[1,92] The risk of lymph node metastasis is 3% for intramucosal lesions (T1m) and 20% if there is submucosal involvement.[93] Other independent risk factors for lymph node metastasis in EGC include lymphovascular invasion on histopathology, histologic ulceration, and tumor diameter more than 3 cm.[94] For T1m tumors less than 3 cm without evidence of lymphovascular invasion or histologic ulceration, the risk of lymph node metastasis is only 0.36%. Gotoda and colleagues[95] assessed the risk of lymph node metastasis of intramucosal cancer. None of the 1230 well-differentiated intramucosal cancers that were less than 30 mm in diameter regardless of ulceration findings were associated with metastases. None of the 929 lesions without ulceration were associated with nodal metastases regardless of tumor size. Similar to findings for intramucosal cancers, for submucosal lesions, there was a significant correlation between tumor size larger than 30 mm and lymphatic-vascular involvement with an increased risk of lymph node metastasis. None of the 145 differentiated adenocarcinomas less than 30 mm in diameter without lymphatic or venous permeation were associated with lymph node metastasis, provided that the lesion had invaded less than 500 μm into the submucosa.[95]

Treatment
Indications and Contraindications

The main indications for treatment can be classified according to the goal of the therapeutic intervention:

1. Curative—this involves the complete removal or destruction of the lesion.
2. Palliative—this involves the use of endoscopic techniques to improve the life of a patient in whom complete resection is impossible.

Preoperative History and Considerations

Appropriate patient selection and accurate diagnosis and staging are essential to ensure good outcomes from endoscopic therapy. Unnecessary risks should be avoided. Is the lesion amendable to surgical or endoscopic removal? Should endoscopic therapy be performed at the same time as the staging procedure or deferred to a subsequent intervention? Referral to a tertiary care center with extensive experience in cancer resection and therapeutic endoscopy should be considered. Overnight observation may be appropriate for patients undergoing high-risk endoscopic procedures and for patients who have significant comorbidities.

Gastroscopy

During gastroscopy, the stomach should be well distended to allow full inspection of the entire gastric lining. The intestinal type of gastric cancer is found mostly in the antropyloric region and along the lesser curvature. Biopsy specimens should be obtained of areas with discoloration (erythema or pallor), ulceration, nodularity, or protrusion or depression. A high index of suspicion is very important for the diagnosis of EGC.

A morphologic staging classification based on the macroscopic endoscopic appearance of EGC has been described by Japanese investigators, as follows[96]:

Type I—protruding more than 5 mm
Type IIa—slightly raised lesion
Type IIb—irregular but flat
Type IIc—flat but slightly depressed
Type III—excavating ulcerations

Types I, IIa, and IIc are considered to be endoscopically resectable. Certain adjuncts to morphologic staging also help to predict that a lesion is amendable to minimally invasive (endoscopic) therapy and is likely to have the same outcome as surgery: lesions less than 1 cm in size, absence of a scar or ulcer histologically and endoscopically (0.2% lymph metastasis), and a well-differentiated histology (<1% lymph metastasis).[1,92]

Narrow Band Imaging and Magnification Endoscopy

Diagnosis of gastric neoplasia using magnification endoscopy has been attempted in the past decades.[97] However, compared with the colonic surface, standardized systemic classification of the magnified gastric surface has not been established owing to diverse histology of gastric carcinomas; the existence of three different types of proper gastric mucosa; and various changes on mucosal structures by atrophy, chronic inflammation, metaplasia, and erosions. The narrow band imaging system provides very clear images of fine superficial structure and microvasculature of the gastric mucosa and has improved the endoscopic diagnosis of superficial gastric cancers. Nakayoshi and coworkers[98,99] reported that significant correlation between histopathology and microvascular pattern obtained with narrow band imaging magnification enables the sensitive diagnosis of superficial depressed gastric cancer, and the modality can assist in determining feasibility of EMR of gastric cancer.

Nakayoshi and coworkers[98] measured the correlation between the magnified images obtained with narrow band imaging and the histologic findings, especially with regard to the microvascular pattern; 165 cases of superficial depressed gastric carcinoma (109 well-differentiated adenocarcinomas and 56 poorly differentiated adenocarcinomas) were evaluated. Microvascular patterns on the mucosal surface were classified into two patterns: fine network pattern and corkscrew

pattern. The fine network pattern appears as a mesh, and abundant microvessels are well connected with one another. In contrast, the corkscrew pattern has isolated and tortuous microvessels and looks like a corkscrew. A fine network pattern was recognized in 72 cases (66.1%) of 109 well-differentiated adenocarcinomas (intestinal type). The corkscrew pattern was observed in 48 cases (85.7%) of 56 poorly differentiated adenocarcinomas (diffuse type). For the magnifying endoscopic diagnosis of superficial depressed gastric carcinoma, both the existence of irregular microvessels and the disappearance of fine superficial structure are essential.

Endoscopic Ultrasound and Endoscopic Ultrasound–Guided Fine Needle Aspiration Cytology

EUS is now established as the best local staging modality for esophageal, gastric, and rectal cancer with a T stage accuracy of about 90%.[100,101] Kelly and associates[91] reported that T staging by EUS was more accurate for gastric cancer than for esophageal cancer, although there was no difference for nodal staging. EUS has been shown to be the most accurate imaging modality for staging EGC,[101,102] with an accuracy of greater than 90% for assessing the depth of tumor invasion.[103,104]

Early-generation conventional echoendoscopes had limited image resolution for the gastric wall because of relatively low transducer frequencies of 7.5 to 12 MHz. Newer echoendoscopes provide a wider range of frequencies from 5 to 20 MHz. Higher frequencies allow more detailed assessment of superficial lesions.

Long-term disease-free survival in GI malignancies is a function of lymphatic and distant tumor spread. The linear-array echoendoscope has enabled the endoscopist to place a needle precisely under real-time EUS guidance and obtain tissue samples both from the primary tumor and from transluminal lesions such as lymph nodes and liver metastasis. Other imaging modalities, such as CT scan, are still necessary to exclude more distant metastases. The overall performance of EUS with fine needle aspiration (FNA) cytology for benign versus malignant lymph node involvement has been found to have a sensitivity of 92% (range 84% to 97%), specificity of 93% (range 75% to 100%), and accuracy of 92% (range 82% to 98%).[105] Disadvantages of dedicated echoendoscopes include inability to traverse critical stenoses and technical difficulty of evaluating superficial lesions in some areas of the stomach such as the cardia.

High-Frequency Ultrasound Probes

High-frequency ultrasound (HFUS) probes provide a higher range of frequencies (12 to 30 MHz), allowing the gut wall to be visualized in finer detail. These miniature probes can be passed through the operating channel of any standard gastroscope. Acoustic contact is ensured by filling a transparent plastic bag with water around the probe. At high frequencies, a nine-layer wall can be identified, with the muscularis mucosa as the fourth layer. We prefer a double-channel therapeutic gastroscope for catheter probe examination because of its larger working channel; the second channel can be used to immerse the gastric lesion in water for better acoustic contact and for introducing a second device when using the "cut and lift" endoscopic resection technique. It is sometimes technically easier to position a miniature probe at a small target lesion in the gastric fundus that could not be easily accessed with a conventional echoendoscope. However, HFUS probes do not have the depth of penetration to visualize regional lymph nodes or metastases for TNM (primary tumor, regional nodes, metastases) staging.

The miniature probe can also be used to evaluate a lesion after saline injection, to confirm complete separation of the lesion from the underlying muscularis propria layer of the gastric wall before EMR.[106] Inability to separate the lesion from the muscularis propria after saline injection is a predictor of unresectability and obviates the need for additional imaging to determine endoscopic resectability.

High-Frequency Ultrasound Staging of Early Gastric Cancer

A classification system for EGC has been developed based on depth of tumor penetration into the mucosa (m) and submucosa (sm), as defined by using HFUS probes. The superficial cancers are divided further into the upper, middle, and lower third of the layer involvement as m1, m2, m3, sm1, sm2, and sm3.[103]

An overall T staging accuracy of about 80% has been reported using HFUS in patients with EGC.[103,107,108] T staging accuracy is greater for Tm1 (92.1%) than for Tsm1 (62.8%) or T2 muscularis propria (42.9%).[109] The curative effect of EMR is excellent for intramucosal cancers (m1, m2, and probably

m3) but not for submucosal cancers (sm1 to sm3).[14] The ability to distinguish between m3 and sm1 lesions is crucial. Using a 20-MHz frequency probe, Yanai and colleagues[110] were able to distinguish EGC involving the mucosa from EGC involving the submucosa with an accuracy of 72.3%.

The usefulness of HFUS was evaluated in 33 patients referred for endoscopic management of superficial or submucosal neoplastic lesions.[111] The depth of invasion was accurately predicted by HFUS before EMR in 25 of 26 patients (96%). Of the nine gastric lesions removed, eight had HFUS before EMR. There was 100% agreement between the depth of invasion determined by HFUS and pathologic staging. Almost half of the resected lesions were gastroduodenal, including gastric adenocarcinoma, gastric and duodenal adenoma, gastric and duodenal carcinoid, pancreatic rest, fibrovascular submucosal polyp, ampullary adenoma, and duodenal lipoma. The diagnostic accuracy of HFUS probes for small gastric lesions (<4 cm) has been found by some researchers to be comparable to dedicated (standard) echoendoscopes.[112]

Description of Techniques
Endoscopic Mucosal Resection

EMR involves the lifting of a lesion from the deep muscle layer of the gut wall, either by injection or by suction of the lesion into a cap fitted to the tip of the endoscope, followed by snare removal of the lesion (**Fig. 33.5**). Complete removal of the lesion en bloc during a single therapeutic procedure is ideal,

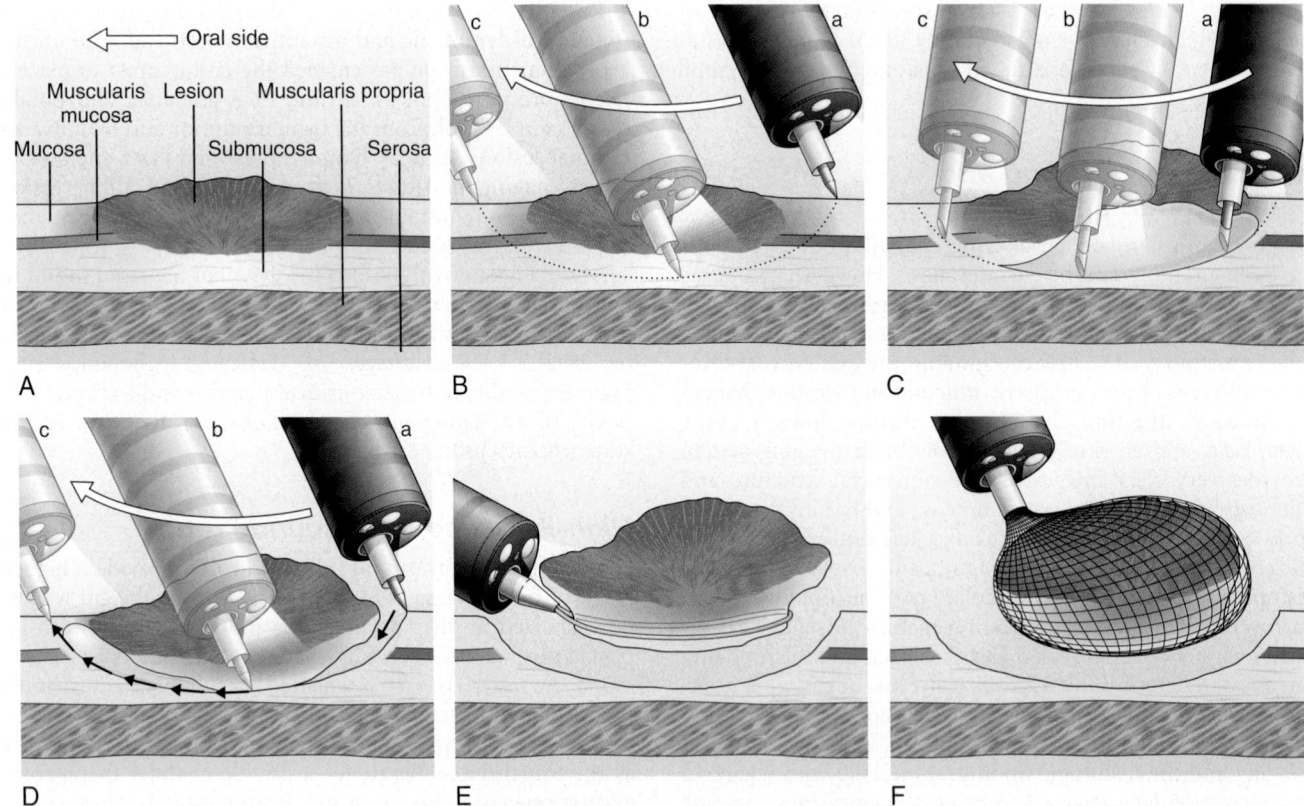

Fig. 33.5 En bloc endoscopic mucosal resection (EMR). **A,** Lesion involving the mucosal layer. **B,** Marking of incision around the lesion with a needle-knife from the distal to proximal edge. **C,** Submucosal injection of sodium hyaluronate below the lesion and around the lesion from the distal to proximal edge. **D,** Incision of marked area around the lesion with a needle-knife from the distal to proximal edge of lesion. **E,** Snare excision of entire lesion. **F,** Retrieval of lesion with Roth net.

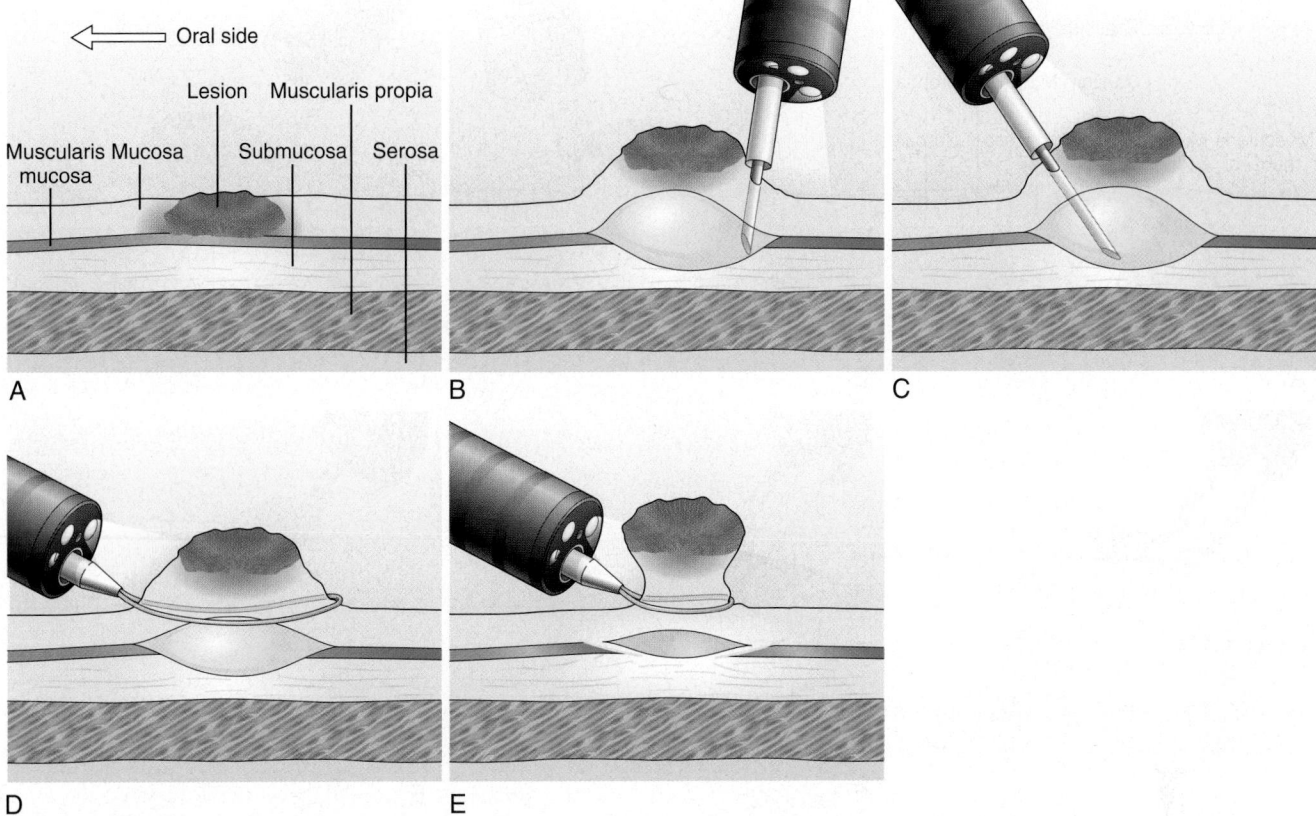

Fig. 33.6 Inject and cut. **A,** Lesion involving the mucosal layer. **B,** Submucosal injection at the distal edge of the lesion. **C,** Submucosal injection at the proximal edge of the lesion. **D,** Snaring of raised lesion. **E,** Tightening of snare and excision of raised lesion.

although large lesions may require piecemeal resection. The availability of the resected specimen for pathologic examination is a distinct advantage of EMR over ablation therapies. Because EUS and HFUS cannot reliably distinguish between tumor infiltration and inflammation that may be associated with a malignant lesion, EMR provides both curative benefit and final staging confirmation.

The following EMR techniques have been described[113–115]:

1. Inject and cut technique
2. Inject, lift, and cut technique
3. EMR with ligation
4. Cap-assisted EMR

Inject and Cut Technique

In the inject and cut technique, the lesion is lifted from the underlying muscularis propria by injecting a solution submucosally to produce a bleb beneath the lesion. The lesion is captured and resected by using an electrosurgical snare (**Fig. 33.6**). The required volume of submucosal injection varies according to the size of the lesion, provided that the bleb is sufficient to ensure a good lift of the entire lesion so that it can be safely captured and resected.

One technical caveat is to perform the initial injection at the periphery and distal margins of the lesion (farthest away from the tip of the endoscope), followed by injection at the lateral margins and at the periphery of the lesion closest to the endoscope. This injection sequence minimizes the problem of obscuring the endoscopic view of the distal margins of the

lesion yet to be injected. The submucosal bleb provides a *pseudostalk* for the snare and a protective cushion beneath the lesion, decreasing tissue resistance and minimizing electrocautery injury to the deeper wall layers.

Various solutions are available for injection. A hypertonic saline and epinephrine solution is widely used in the hopes of decreasing the risk of bleeding[116]; other solutions have been used to obtain a more durable lift of the lesion.[117] The use of hypertonic solutions except for glycerol has been questioned more recently because of concern about possible tissue damage. A study by Fujishiro and associates[118] concluded that a combination of hyaluronate and glycerol is the most favorable submucosal injection solution, taking into consideration tissue damage and lesion-lifting ability. Also, various snares and currents (e.g., blended, ERBE, Tübingen, Germany) are preferred by different endoscopists. To date, no randomized trials have been conducted to compare the safety and effectiveness of different types of snares and injectants.

The advantage of the inject and cut technique is its simplicity and the fact that it does not require additional equipment. A disadvantage is that most solutions used to lift the lesion dissipate very rapidly making it difficult sometimes to capture the lesion safely with the snare.

INJECT, LIFT, AND CUT TECHNIQUE (STRIP BIOPSY)

With the inject, lift, and cut technique, the submucosal injection is performed in the standard manner, as already described.

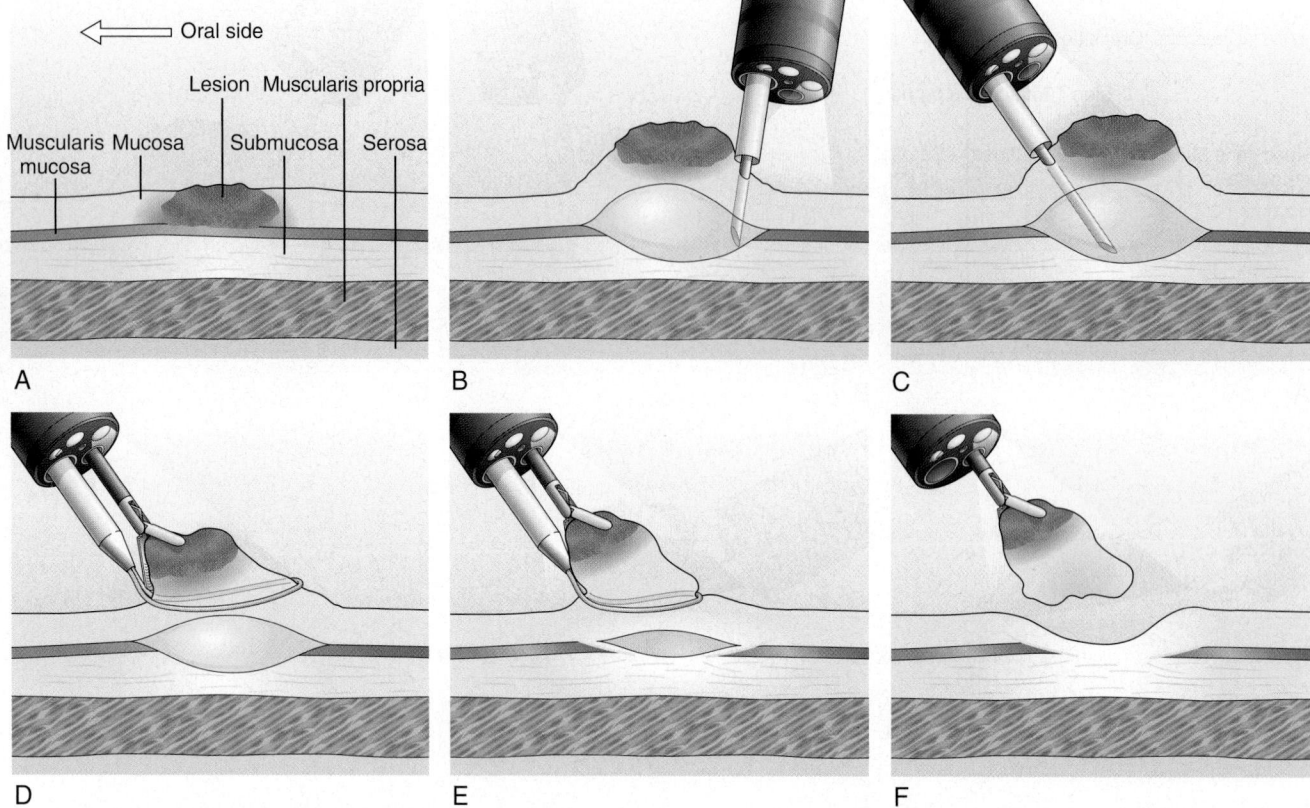

Fig. 33.7   Strip biopsy. **A,** Lesion involving the mucosal layer. **B,** Submucosal injection at the distal edge of the lesion with double-channel endoscope. **C,** Submucosal injection at the proximal edge of the lesion. **D,** Grasping forceps pulling the lesion into the open snare. **E,** Tightening of snare and excision of lesion. **F,** Mucosal defect created after removal of lesion.

A snare and grasping forceps are passed through the operating channels of a dual-channel endoscope. First, the grasping forceps is captured by the open snare, and the snare is closed over the forceps. Working as a unit, the forceps is used to grasp the lesion, the snare is opened, and the lesion is pulled through the open snare. The snare is closed over the lesion, and resection of the lesion is performed (**Fig. 33.7**).[119–121] This technique is more cumbersome than the inject and cut technique and requires a dual-channel endoscope and two assistants to perform EMR.

ENDOSCOPIC MUCOSAL RESECTION WITH LIGATION

In the EMR with ligation technique, the lesion is removed with or without previous submucosal injection (**Fig. 33.8**).[122–124] More recently, a conventional band ligation device (MBL; Wilson-Cook Medical, Inc, Winston-Salem, NC) was modified by widening the threading channel of the cranking device from 2 to 3.2 mm.[125] This device allows for the insertion of a 7-Fr catheter through the threading channel of the cranking device into the 3.7-mm working channel of the endoscope. Band ligation can be performed with the polypectomy snare still within the working channel without any increased friction during winding of the thread; this enables sequential banding and snare resection of esophageal mucosa without the need to change the endoscope.[125]

An advantage of this technique is that it requires only conventional devices and instruments. A disadvantage is subop-

timal visualization of the margins of the lesion when the variceal ligation device is loaded. No serious procedure-related complications have been reported.

CAP-ASSISTED ENDOSCOPIC MUCOSAL RESECTION

In cap-assisted EMR, a specially designed transparent plastic cap is used.[126,127] The plastic cap is fitted over the tip of the endoscope; various cap sizes are available. Submucosal injection of the lesion is performed in the standard manner. A crescent-shaped snare is prelooped into the groove of the rim of the specialized cap by gently suctioning normal mucosa into the cap and opening the snare to allow it to rest along the inside groove of the rim of the cap (SD-221L-25 or SD-7P-1; Olympus America, Inc). After prelooping the snare, the suction is turned off to release the normal mucosa. The cap is now used to suction the lesion while maintaining a constant medium to high vacuum. When the lesion is trapped completely inside the cap, the snare is closed over the lesion. After the lesion is tightly strangulated by the snare, the suction is turned off, and the lesion with the snare around it is allowed to leave the cap. Resection of the lesion is then performed with application of current. Gentle suction of the specimen into the cap allows safe and complete recovery of the specimen (**Fig. 33.9**). This technique is particularly useful for upper GI lesions.[127–129] Matsuzaki and colleagues[128] reported the use of a soft 18-mm diameter cap for en bloc resection of larger gastric

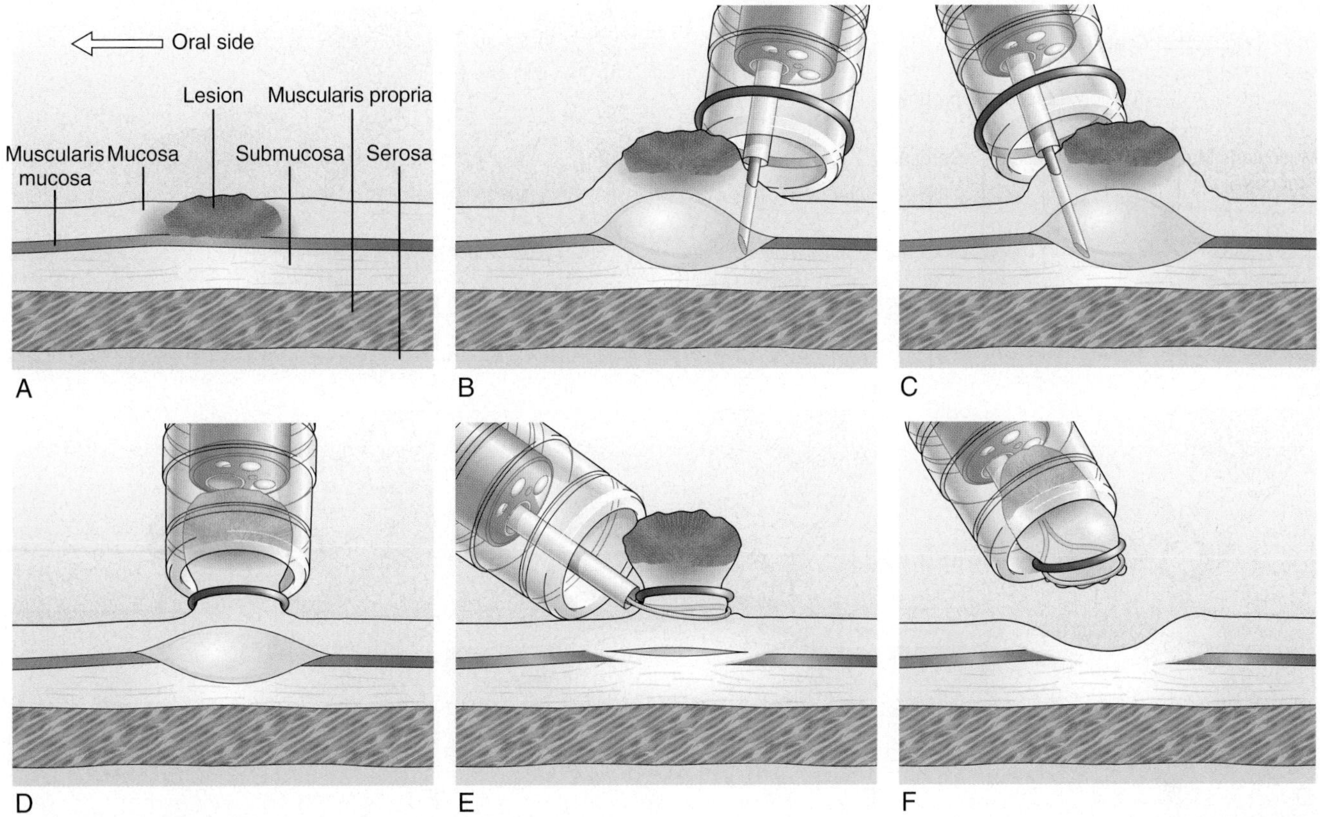

Fig. 33.8 Endoscopic mucosal resection (EMR) with ligation. **A,** Lesion involving the mucosal layer. **B,** Submucosal injection at the distal edge of the lesion. **C,** Submucosal injection at the proximal edge of the lesion. **D,** Suction of lesion into the hood and ligation with rubber band. **E,** Snaring and excision of the lesion below the rubber band. **F,** Mucosal defect created after removal of lesion.

lesions up to 1.4 times the size that can be removed with a standard cap.

For larger lesions greater than 3 cm, some endoscopists have used a more viscous material, sodium hyaluronate, for submucosal injection. A small-caliber tip transparent hood that accommodates a needle-knife or an insulated thermal knife with a ceramic cap is used to cut around the lesion on its entire circumference. The final step is the complete removal of the lesion using a large snare.[130,131]

ENDOSCOPIC SUBMUCOSAL DISSECTION

The concept and technique of ESD are markedly different from conventional EMR. The procedure begins by making circumferential markings all around the lesion at about a 5-mm distance, at 2-mm intervals. Injection of sodium hyaluronate or another solution to create a long-lasting submucosal fluid cushion between the lesion and the muscle layer is performed to prevent perforation during ESD (**Fig. 33.10**).[117]

Sodium hyaluronate is harmless to the injected tissue because of its isotonicity, but it needs to be diluted when used for ESD because of its high viscosity. Among different mixtures tested, a mixture of high-molecular-weight sodium hyaluronate with a sugar solution, with or without glycerin, seems to be the most cost-effective.[132] Adding indigo carmine dye (0.004%) to the mixture is optional. To minimize resistance to injection, a high-flow injection needle with a large inner lumen should be used. The solution is first injected just outside the marking spots, where a circumferential incision to isolate

the lesion to be resected from the normal mucosa is made using the electrosurgical knives selected for the procedure. For the insulated-tip (IT) knife, a small initial incision is made with a standard needle-knife to allow for its insertion into the submucosal layer. Several electrosurgical knives have been developed for ESD.

Needle-Knife

First used by Hirao and colleagues[116] in 1988, the needle-knife (KD-10Q-1; Olympus) has a fine tip and a small contact area, which allows a sharp incision. The cutting power required for mucosal incision (150 W) is so high that perforation is likely to occur unless the operator is highly skilled.

Insulated-Tip Knife

The IT knife (KD-610L; Olympus; **Fig. 33.11A**) is a needle-knife that is equipped with a ceramic ball at the top of the incising needle. The tip is blunted and insulated to prevent perforation; the knife was developed by Hosokawa and Yoshida[133] for safe performance of ESD. The IT knife is most frequently used for ESD of the stomach; special care should be taken when operating in the colon. The second-generation IT knife (ITKnife2; KD-611L; Olympus; **Fig. 33.11B**) has an additional electrode at the back of its insulating tip that makes cutting easier, especially in the lateral direction.

Hook Knife

The hook knife (KD-620LR; Olympus; **Fig. 33.11C**) is a needle-knife with 1 mm of the tip bent to form a right angle.

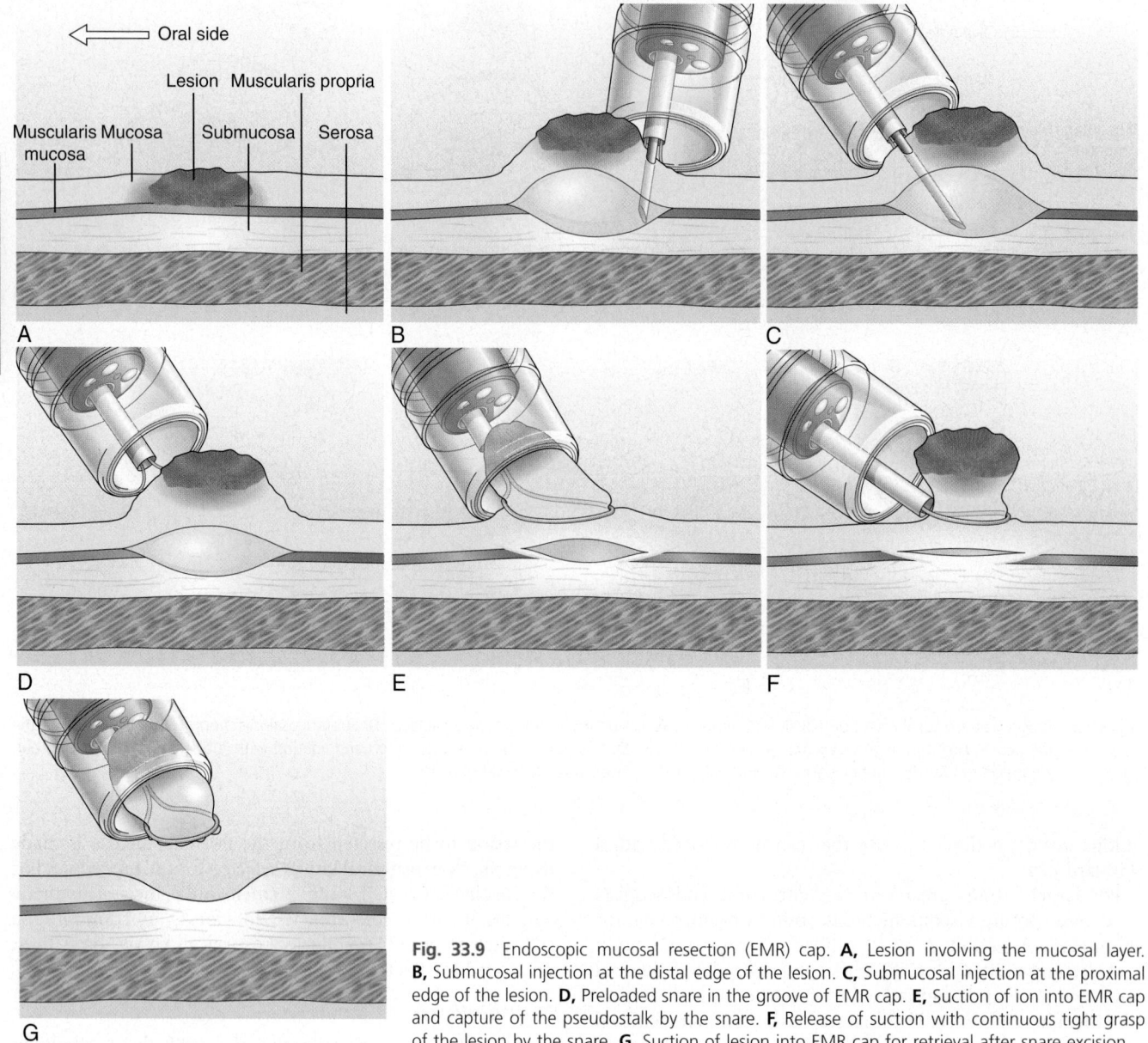

Fig. 33.9 Endoscopic mucosal resection (EMR) cap. **A,** Lesion involving the mucosal layer. **B,** Submucosal injection at the distal edge of the lesion. **C,** Submucosal injection at the proximal edge of the lesion. **D,** Preloaded snare in the groove of EMR cap. **E,** Suction of ion into EMR cap and capture of the pseudostalk by the snare. **F,** Release of suction with continuous tight grasp of the lesion by the snare. **G,** Suction of lesion into EMR cap for retrieval after snare excision.

Submucosal tissue can be hooked and pulled before incision, which improves safety. Safety can be enhanced further by the concomitant use of a transparent hood. This knife has a rotating function so that operators can select any direction for hooking. Because of its high maneuverability, the hook knife is a useful endo-knife for esophageal ESD.[134]

Flex Knife

The flex knife (KD-630L; Olympus; **Fig. 33.11D**) has a rounded tip with a twisted wire similar to a snare, with a length that can be adjusted according to circumstances. The outer sheath of the knife is soft and flexible with a thick tip that functions as a stopper. Because of all these characteristics, perforation is less likely to occur with this needle, which can be used independently on the location of the lesion.[135] A transparent hood for better visualization of the operating field is usually used.

Triangle-Tip Knife

The triangle-tip knife (KD-640L; Olympus; **Fig. 33.11E**) has a triangle-shaped conductive tip at the distal end, facilitating cutting of the mucosa. This knife can be used for any step in the ESD procedure: marking, precutting, incision, and dissection.

ESD Knife

The ESD knife (MTW, **Fig. 33.11F**) is a needle-knife that is equipped with a sapphire ball tip at the top of the incisioning needle. When the circumferential incision has been completed, additional solution is injected in the center of the lesion to lift up the mucosa adequately. Small lesions can be resected with an electrosurgical snare in the same way as with the standard polypectomy technique.[136] Larger lesions require a more complex procedure, however, in which the submucosa is directly dissected using the electrosurgical knife until exfoliation of the entire tumor en bloc is obtained.[131]

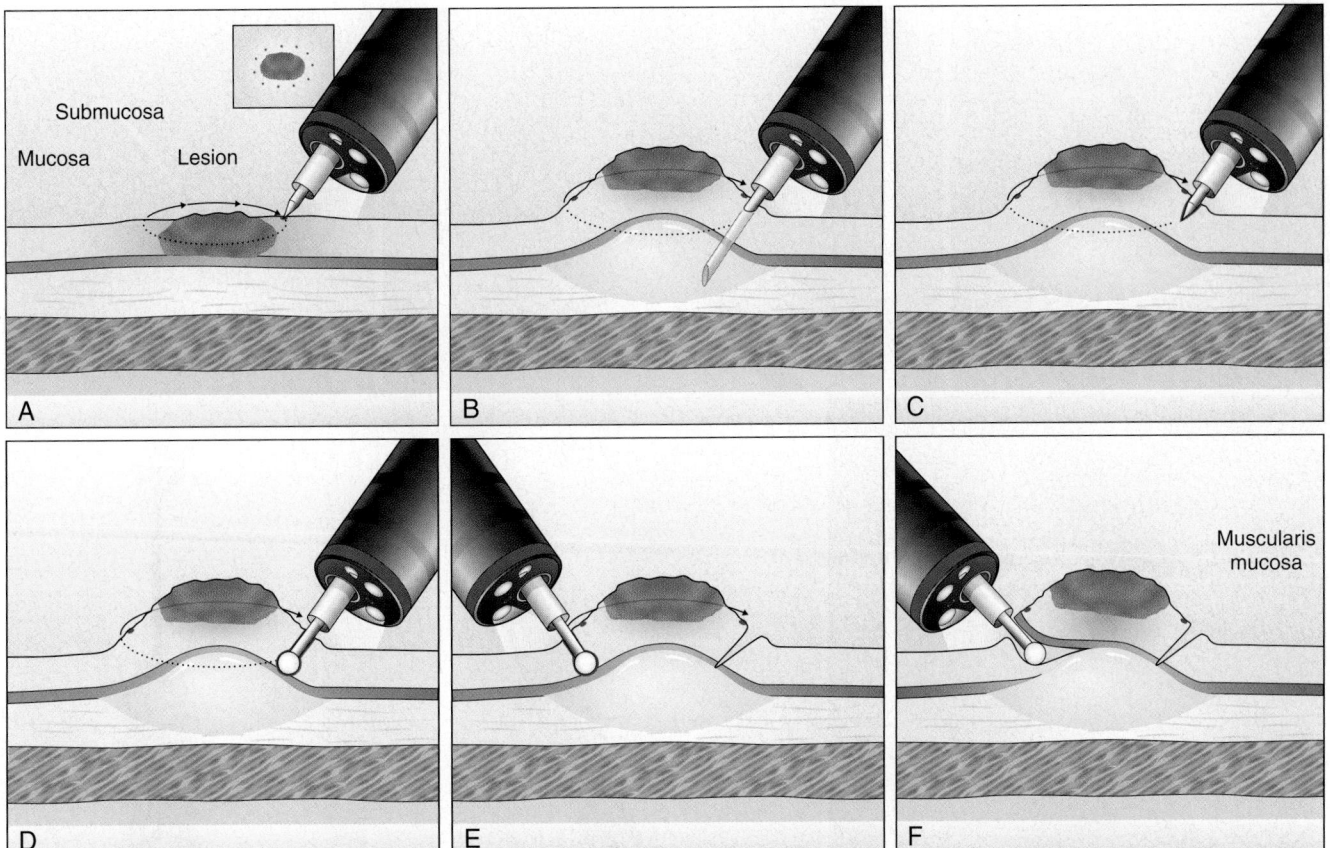

Fig. 33.10 Endoscopic submucosal dissection (ESD). **A,** Markings with knife or argon plasma coagulation (APC) probe around the edge of the lesions. **B,** Submucosal injection around the edge of the lesions. **C,** Incision hole with a needle-knife or hook knife. **D,** Margin cutting with insulated-tip (IT) knife at the incision hole. **E,** Circumferential margin cutting. **F,** Submucosal dissection with IT knife beneath the muscularis mucosa.

Hybrid Knife

The hybrid knife (ERBE; **Fig. 33.11G**) is a stainless steel tube that incorporates a microcapillary lumen with a diameter of 150 mm to provide a water jet function.[137] The flexible instrument has an outer diameter of 2.0 mm and a length of 2.2 mm and can be used with any standard endoscope. This flexible device allows injection, hydrodissection with preselected pressure (maximal water pressure 80 bar, adjustable from 0 to 80 bar), or dissection with any electrical current after usage of the saline-only solution without having to exchange the catheter. This novel device is the latest entry of clinically available ESP knives.

ENDOSCOPIC MUCOSAL RESECTION AND ENDOSCOPIC SUBMUCOSAL DISSECTION FOR EARLY GASTRIC CANCER

Endoscopic resection is now considered a curative procedure for EGC and has increasingly replaced surgical resection for this indication in Japan, although the technique is not universally accepted as a first-line treatment in the West. Endoscopic resection has also been used as a histologic staging technique to assess the depth of penetration in EGC to help determine the best definitive treatment.

Correct diagnosis of the depth of invasion and the absence of lymph node metastasis are crucial for achieving a cure with endoscopic therapy. The important endoscopic points to consider are the following:

1. The extension of the surface and the morphology of the lesion determine the procedure. EMR is not recommended for lesions greater than 2 cm in size. ESD is recommended for lesions without ulcer or scar up to 3 cm in size and lesions with ulcer or scar less than 2 cm in size.
2. The depth of invasion should be no deeper than the mucosa and sm1. This needs to be determined by EUS before endoscopic resection and should be corroborated by pathologic examination of the resected specimen.
3. High-grade dysplasia is the earliest stage of malignancy. A high degree of differentiation favors endoscopic treatment. Even though poorly differentiated lesions have a higher risk of distant spread, lesions less than 5 mm in size could be treated endoscopically.
4. Multifocal EGC can be treated endoscopically provided that the entire morphology is compatible with an intramucosal cancer.[138]
5. The degree of difficulty in performing endoscopic resection depends on the location in the stomach. Lesions in the posterior wall and lesser curvature technically are more difficult to remove.
6. The success or failure of curative endoscopic resection is assessed by clear lateral and vertical margins seen on pathology and by endoscopy and biopsy obtained during follow-up.

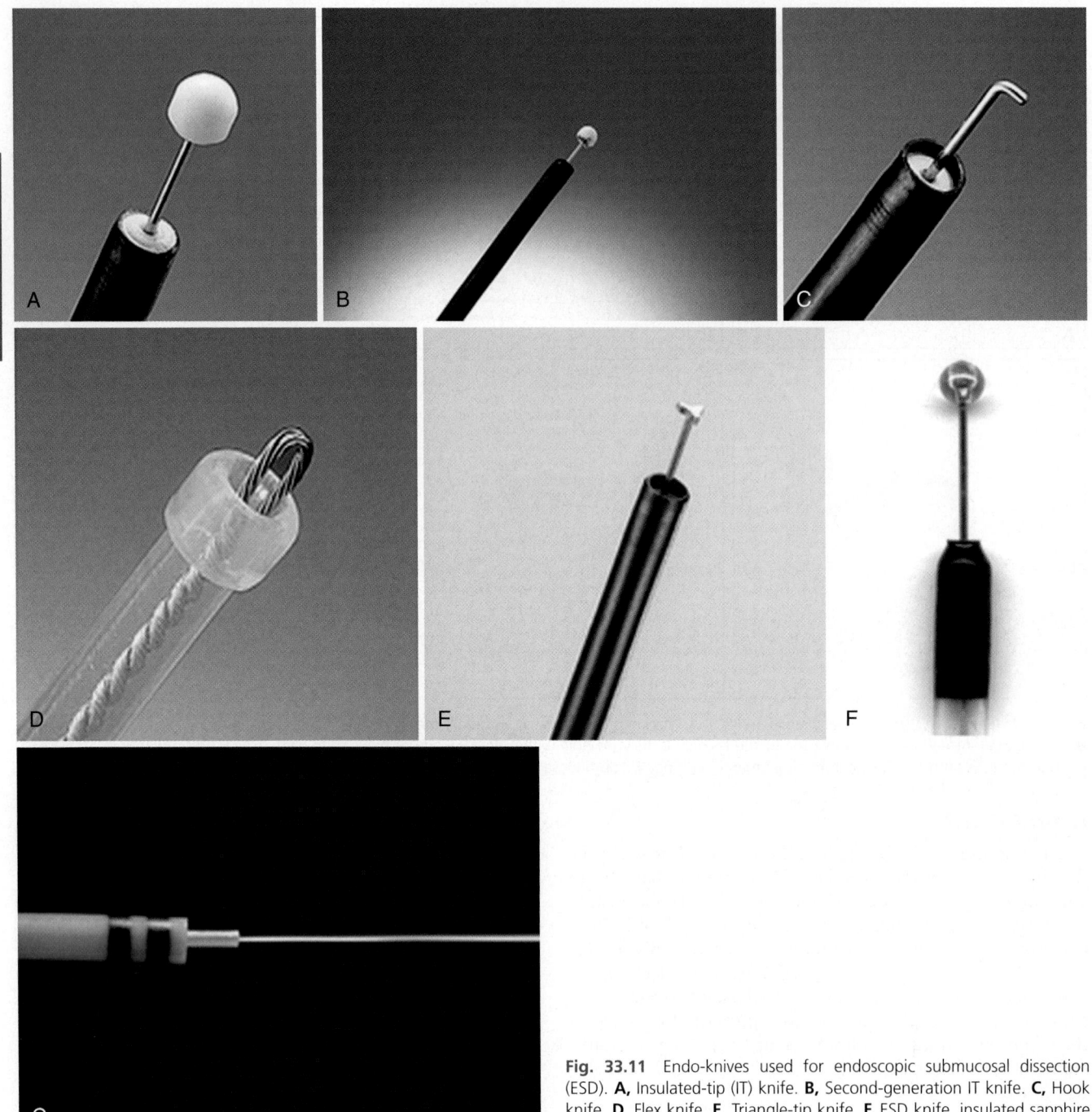

Fig. 33.11 Endo-knives used for endoscopic submucosal dissection (ESD). **A,** Insulated-tip (IT) knife. **B,** Second-generation IT knife. **C,** Hook knife. **D,** Flex knife. **E,** Triangle-tip knife. **F,** ESD knife, insulated sapphire ball tip. **G,** Hybrid knife.

7. Assessment of the results is based on the rates of complete removal or destruction, rates of en bloc resection, rates of recurrence, and survival.

The Japanese Research Society for Gastric Cancer has developed the following criteria for lesions that are suitable for endoscopic resection: (1) well differentiated, type I or IIa, limited to the mucosa, without histologic ulceration and less than 2 cm; (2) well differentiated, type IIc, limited to mucosa without ulceration and less than 1 cm. When these criteria are followed, the risk of lymph node involvement is only 1.7%. The use of morphologic staging is subjective, however, and its generalization has not been evaluated.

A retrospective evaluation of 210 cases of EGC treated with EMR and followed up for 14 years reported a 5-year survival of 86% and a 10-year survival of 56%; there were no cancer-related deaths.[119] EMR as a curative treatment has been evaluated in 102 patients.[108] No distant or local metastases were seen during 9 years of follow-up.

A total of 106 patients with EGC up to 2 cm in diameter were treated with complete resection of the lesion in a single procedure, either by en bloc resection for lesions less than 10 mm (64%), or by piecemeal resection for larger lesions (36%).[139] No recurrence after either technique was found in patients with tumor-negative margins. The overall recurrence

Depth	Mucosal cancer				Submucosal cancer	
	UL(−)		UL(+)		SM1	SM2
Histology	≤20	20<	≤30	30<	≤30	Any size
Differentiated						
Undifferentiated						

Fig. 33.12 Proposed extended criteria for endoscopic resection in the endoscopic submucosal dissection (ESD) era. SM, submucosal cancer; UL, ulcer.

☐ Guideline criteria for EMR ☐ Surgery
☐ Extended criteria for ESD ☐ Consider surgery

rate of cancer in this particular study was 2.8%. Tumors that recurred all were greater than 15 mm initially and treated with piecemeal resection. Because histologic reconstruction to confirm complete resection by piecemeal method is often difficult, patients should be followed very closely after piecemeal resection.

In a retrospective study, Amano and coworkers[140] evaluated endoscopic therapy in patients with EGC that does not meet the Japanese Research Society for Gastric Cancer morphologic criteria for lesions suitable for EMR. Endoscopic therapy consisted of EMR, thermal therapy, or both. The study included poorly differentiated and well-differentiated tumors 1 to 3 cm. Some patients with submucosal invasion limited to the most superficial layer (sm1) were included. Curative resection was achieved in 95%. The rate of cure in this group was statistically similar to the cure rate of cases that fulfilled the standard morphologic criteria for EMR resection (98%).[140]

Adequacy of EMR can be assessed by measuring the distance from the edge of the resected specimen to the margin of the cancer. In a prior study, no patient with a distance of more than 2 mm developed recurrence of the cancer, whereas 16% of patients with a distance of less than 2 mm developed recurrence.[141] Presence of cancer at the edge of the specimen was associated with a recurrence of 45.8%. No recurrence was observed if the distance from the edge of the specimen to the cancer was more than 7 mm, suggesting that adequate distance (preferably at least 2 mm) between the edge of the specimen and the cancer needs to be achieved to ensure a complete resection.[142] Margin-negative resections are more likely (81.2%) in cancers that are less than 1 cm in diameter than in cancers that are more than 2 cm in diameter.[142]

In a prospective analysis of 479 EGCs treated with EMR over an 11-year period at Tokyo National Cancer Center,[130] the following selection criteria were used: well-differentiated or moderately well-differentiated gastric cancer; morphologic types I, IIa, and IIc; no histologic evidence of ulceration; diameter of less than 3 cm with histologic confirmation of intramucosal carcinoma; no lymphovascular invasion; and clean margins. EMR was used to treat 405 patients, and complete resection was achieved in 69%. The recurrence rate was only 2%, and all recurrences were treated successfully with a modified combination therapy of EMR and laser. There was no subsequent recurrence in any of the 278 patients after a median follow-up period of 38 months (range 3 to 120 months). No cancer-related deaths were reported. More recently, EMR and ESD have become established alternatives to surgical therapy for EGC in Japan and Korea.[143–145]

The current criteria for endoscopic therapy are (1) elevated-type intramucosal cancer (0 to IIa) less than 20 mm; (2) depressed-type mucosal cancer without ulceration (0 to IIb, 0 to IIc) less than 10 mm; and (3) well-differentiated or moderately well-differentiated intestinal-type ADC. Depressed cancers were associated with lymph node metastases (86%) when there was submucosal infiltration, size of 20 mm or greater, or lymphatic vessel involvement.[146]

Extended indications for EMR in EGC have been proposed as follows[140]: (1) well-differentiated lesions up to 30 mm, without an ulcer or ulcer scar; (2) mucosal cancers less than 20 mm, with an ulcer or ulcer scar; (3) sm1 lesions less than 20 mm, without an ulcer or ulcer scar; and (4) poorly differentiated lesions less than 10 mm.

The risk for node metastasis is approximately 0.4% for differentiated cancers. Undifferentiated mucosal cancers should not be treated by EMR because the risk for node metastasis is approximately 4%. Poorly differentiated and signet-ring cell carcinomas less than 5 mm in size could be managed, however.[147] The proposed extended criteria for endoscopic resection in the ESD era are summarized in **Fig. 33.12**.

By expanding the criteria for EMR, the need for gastrectomy in EGC can be reduced. Because it is difficult to resect large and ulcerative lesions by conventional EMR, however, the technique of ESD was developed. Over the years, substantial experience in the use of this technique has been gained, and ESD with the IT knife has become a standard practice in Japan for the treatment of EGC.[148,149]

In Europe, ESD has been performed in 10 patients (9 EGCs and 1 adenoma, with a median diameter of 22 mm) using a new double-channel endoscope (the R-scope; Olympus Co, Tokyo, Japan). ESD was successful in six cases. Perforation occurred in two cases and were treated by surgery.[150] In another study, ESD was performed in 19 patients with gastric superficial lesions (15 to 30 mm), with high-grade (n = 15) or low-grade (n = 4) noninvasive epithelial neoplasia. ESD was performed in all cases, with 89% R0 resection and 79% en bloc resection rates observed. Major bleeding was reported in 1 case (5%); there were no cases of perforation. With a median follow-up of 10 months, a single recurrence (5%) was observed.[151]

Endoscopic resection has also been performed for undifferentiated-type intramucosal cancer.[152] In 38 patients with 42 undifferentiated intramucosal gastric cancers who declined surgical resection, ESD was performed with dedicated devices by experienced expert endoscopists. The en bloc resection rate was 83.3%; complete resection rate was 80.9%. Clinical remission was achieved in 92.8% with recurrence during follow-up seen in only 7.14%. In undifferentiated gastric cancer, grossly normal gastric mucosa surrounding the resected lesion could contain cancer cells beneath the epithelium[153]; this may explain why the complete resection rate of ESD for undifferentiated–type cancer is lower than that reported for well-differentiated cancer. The en bloc resection rate is better with ESD than with conventional EMR. The procedure time is longer in ESD, although this disadvantage might be improved with experience.[154]

POSTOPERATIVE CARE

Because of the extent of the resected area, a standard dose of proton pump inhibitor is administered for 8 weeks to prevent postoperative bleeding and to promote ulcer healing, and patients are typically placed on nothing per mouth (NPO) for 1 day, followed by clear liquids on the 2nd day and a soft diet for another 3 days.[155] A large ulcer after ESD was reported to heal within 8 weeks after resection with the patient receiving antacid treatment.[156,157]

COMPLICATIONS OF ENDOSCOPIC RESECTION

Complications of EMR and ESD include adverse events secondary to sedation and procedure-related complications that are specific but not exclusive to EMR and ESD.

Bleeding

Bleeding is the most common complication of EMR and ESD of gastric tumors. Immediate bleeding, which can be brisk, seems to be more common with resection of tumors located in the upper third of the stomach. The reported incidence of bleeding after EMR has ranged from 0.38% to 16.1%.[142] The discrepancy may be due to differences in definition of bleeding and to study methodology. Most institutions have reported the incidence of bleeding to be 10% to 16%, although studies based on surveys have reported a much lower incidence. In one large consecutive series, bleeding occurred in 7% of patients undergoing ESD.[158]

Most bleeding occurs during the procedure or within 24 hours after EMR. In the largest retrospective study dealing with predictors of bleeding after EMR of gastric tumors, the overall incidence of bleeding was 17.6%, with delayed bleeding occurring in 5.3%. In this study, the only statistically significant factor for predicting delayed bleeding was the occurrence of immediate bleeding during EMR.[159] Delayed bleeding is probably not due to inadequate initial hemostasis but rather to insufficient coagulation during resection because in this study the sites of delayed bleeding were not the same as the sites of immediate bleeding.[159] Size greater than 1 to 2 cm has been reported by some authors to be predictive of bleeding[160]; other studies have not found a positive correlation between size of lesion and risk of bleeding.[159,161] No significant association has been found between the risk of bleeding and different techniques used for EMR, morphology of the lesion (flat, raised, or depressed), type of electrocautery current used, amount of saline used, or location of the lesion.

Management of Bleeding after Endoscopic Resection

No maneuver has been shown to help prevent bleeding. Bleeding during endoscopic resection usually stops spontane-

ously. If significant bleeding occurs, the standard methods of endoscopic hemostasis should be attempted. A few caveats need to be remembered when treating this complication endoscopically. Cautery should be applied cautiously keeping in mind that the site has already received a significant amount of energy. Overvigorous delivery of additional coagulation current may result in a transmural burn or a perforation. Injection of diluted epinephrine (1 in 10,000 or 1 in 20,000) can also be used to control the bleeding, either as the only measure or to prepare the bleeding site for another maneuver, such as cauterization or placement of mucosal hemoclips.[159,160] One potential advantage of the latter maneuver is that hemoclips do not cause additional gastric wall injury to the resection bed. Application of clips during the procedure may preclude further endoscopic resection.

During ESD, immediate minor bleeding is common but can be successfully treated by grasping and coagulating the bleeding vessels with a hot biopsy forceps using 80-W soft mode coagulation (ICC200; ERBE).[162] Endoclips are also often deployed for brisk bleeding. Delayed bleeding, manifested by hematemesis or melena at 0 to 30 days after the procedure, is treated by emergent endoscopy, performed after fluid resuscitation, using similar techniques. Most bleeding (75%) occurs within 12 hours after the procedure and has been reported to be strongly related to tumor location and size.[159,163]

Patients who develop delayed bleeding should be managed as any patient who presents with upper GI hemorrhage. The initial objectives are to establish venous access and achieve hemodynamic stability. After the situation is under control, urgent endoscopic hemostasis can be attempted.

Perforation

Perforation typically occurs when part of the muscularis propria is inadvertently resected in the specimen. Transmural burns secondary to aggressive cauterization may also result in delayed perforation. The rates of EMR-induced perforation are highest for gastric lesions at 2.5% to 5% (vs. lesions in the colon at <1%). Reported rates of perforation are higher when performing EMR with an IT knife (5.6%) compared with the endoscopic aspiration technique (0.8%).[161] The overall risks of perforation during ESD is approximately 4%.[6]

Some caveats help to reduce the risk of perforation: (1) Avoid performing EMR in patients who have had prior attempts at endoscopic resection. Scarring secondary to prior cauterization may prevent proper lifting of the lesion from the underlying muscularis propria during submucosal injection. (2) Proper technique and an adequate volume of submucosal injection are important to provide a margin of safety. (3) Avoid repeat snaring of the resected tissue. (4) Abort the procedure if the patient experiences pain on closure of the snare because this may be an indication of full-thickness capture by the snare.

A randomized controlled study in a pig model with a new water-jet hybrid knife reported no ESD perforations (0 of 12) and may be a promising modality to reduce complications in gastric ESD.[137] The system is also convenient for the endoscopist to perform ESD without the need to exchange devices (knives and injection needles) during the procedure.

A surgical consultation should be obtained as soon as this complication is suspected. The earlier the diagnosis is established (within the first 6 hours), the better the prognosis. The standard of care for management of a recognized perforation is surgical; however, if the perforation is small and the patient is asymptomatic, endoclips could be used to close the defect, but this should be done early on.[161,164,165] Patients should be placed NPO and treated with broad-spectrum antibiotics.

Transmural Burn Syndrome

Transmural burn syndrome occurs when thermal injury to the muscularis propria and serosa is produced by excessive electrocoagulation during polypectomy or EMR and ESD. Transmural burn syndrome has been reported in 0.5% to 1% of colonic polypectomies, but the exact incidence in EMR and ESD is unknown.

Patients often present with symptoms and laboratory abnormalities that are indistinguishable from a perforation. It is crucial to exclude a perforation immediately before resorting to conservative management. A surgical consultation should be obtained. After a perforation has been excluded, patients should be placed on broad-spectrum antibiotics, intravenous hydration, and bowel rest. Serial abdominal x-rays should be ordered to monitor for the possibility of a late perforation. Most patients respond very well to conservative management.[166]

Luminal Stenosis

Luminal stenosis has been described as a delayed complication in patients who have had EMR mainly of an esophageal lesion,[167] but it could potentially occur after EMR and ESD of tumors located in the gastroesophageal junction and prepyloric area. This complication tends to occur after extensive resection when the mucosa of more than three-fourths of the luminal circumference has been excised. The mechanism of retraction seems to be related to the healing process. Temporary metal stent placement[168] and balloon dilations or a combination of both have been used effectively.[167] Incremental resections in multiple treatment sessions may help to minimize contraction of the lumen.

Ablation Techniques

NEODYMIUM:YTTRIUM-ALUMINUM-GARNET (ND:YAG) LASER

Lasers (*light amplification by stimulated emission of radiation*) are devices that produce a light energy that is focused into a unidirectional, single wavelength beam. The most common medical uses of lasers derive from the conversion of light to heat energy. The laser light beam can be used to cut, coagulate, or vaporize tissue depending on the wavelength of light, power density used to excite the lasing medium, and absorption and scattering. Neodymium:yttrium-aluminum-garnet (Nd:YAG), carbon dioxide (CO_2), Nd:holmium, and argon ion lasers are the most frequently used lasers in biomedical applications.

Laser energy can be delivered through flexible optic fibers at wavelengths of 1320 nm and 1064 nm. Because the emission is invisible, a helium-neon aiming beam is used in conjunction with Nd:YAG to visualize the focal target area.[169,170] To obtain photoablation, an optical fiber is passed through the operating channel of the endoscope, and the transmitted laser beam can be delivered in a contact or noncontact fashion. Tangential irradiation is impossible with this technique, so the location of some lesions may be more difficult to target.[171]

When performing laser therapy, safety eyewear is used to avoid ocular damage to endoscopy personnel. Adequate local exhaust ventilation and use of respiratory filter masks have been recommended to avoid respiratory exposure to aerosolized infectious pathogens resulting from vaporization of tissue.[172] Because of its limited portability, high cost, availability of less costly alternatives, and the need for specific training, laser therapy is not widely used today for endoscopic treatment of gastric neoplasms.

PHOTODYNAMIC THERAPY

Photodynamic therapy (PDT) also delivers energy via flexible optic fibers. The laser light activates a photosensitizing agent, releasing toxic singlet oxygen and causing tissue necrosis. The photosensitizer selectively accumulates in the target tissue. The only commercially available photosensitizer in the United States is porfimer sodium (Photofrin PDT).[173] Other photosensitizers include 5-aminolevulinic acid (5-ALA), zinc II phthalocyanine, aluminum sulfonated phthalocyanine, benzoporphyrin, meta-tetrahydroxyphenylchlorin (mTHPC), N-aspartyl chlorine e6 (NPe6), and motexafin lutetium. Among these different photosensitizers, mTHPC, porfimer sodium, and 5-ALA have been used extensively in gastroenterology. mTHPC is a potent, highly selective drug that has been used in the treatment of neoplasms, whereas 5-ALA, which induces very superficial necrosis, has been used to treat Barrett's esophagus.[174,175]

Porfimer sodium is administered at a recommended dose of 2 mg/kg intravenously and activated 48 hours later by a tunable dye laser at 630 nm.[173] 5-ALA is a heme pathway precursor that can be given orally or intravenously. 5-ALA is converted to the endogenous photosensitized protoporphyrin IX, which can be activated by red or green light.

LASER THERAPY FOR EARLY GASTRIC CANCER

Endoscopic laser therapy has been used to treat inoperable patients with EGC. In 13 patients with EGC, a complete response was achieved with Nd:YAG or PDT in 85% of the patients.[5] Sibille and colleagues[141] used Nd:YAG laser to treat 18 nonoperative patients with EUS T1 gastric cancer until a complete response (negative endoscopic biopsies) was achieved. The number of sessions varied from 1 to 15 sessions, performed every 2 weeks. Initial complete response was achieved in 16 (89%) patients after a mean of 1.7 sessions (range 1 to 4); two patients (11%) did not respond to therapy.

PDT was shown to achieve a complete response in eight EGC lesions diagnosed in seven nonoperative patients.[142] In another study, Takahira and associates[145] reported on the use of PDT with an excimer dye laser in 10 patients with 11 EGCs. A complete response was observed in 10 of 11 tumors (91%). Surgery was required in only one patient who had residual tumor after PDT. Nd:YAG laser therapy has also been used for photoablation of residual tumor after an incomplete EMR.[3,176]

LASER THERAPY FOR ADVANCED GASTRIC CANCER

Laser ablation therapy is more frequently used as a palliative modality in advanced gastric lesions. Successful palliation of bleeding or obstruction secondary to gastric cancer has been reported in 81% to 100%.[5,177,178] Relief of obstructing cancer in the gastric cardia using Nd:YAG laser has been reported.[179,180] Addition of external beam radiation and brachytherapy was found to increase the interval between laser treatments in advanced esophageal and gastric cardia adenocarcinoma.[181–183]

COMPLICATIONS OF ABLATION THERAPY

Bleeding is one of the most common complications of Nd:YAG laser therapy. A major bleeding rate of 12.5% after laser treatment of gastric tumors has been reported.[178] Perforations may occur in 1% to 9%, with a procedure-related mortality of up to 1%.[178] Stricture formation as a late complication of laser therapy (Nd:YAG and PDT) has been observed in 5% to 13%.[5] Pulmonary complications have been reported after PDT in up to 15%. Photosensitization, lasting up to 3 months, and severe sunburn have been reported in 5% to 7% of patients after PDT therapy.[173,184]

Argon Plasma Coagulation

APC uses a high-frequency current and an ionized argon gas for coagulating tissue. In the early 1990s, an APC delivery catheter that could be inserted through a flexible endoscope was invented by Farin and Grund.[151] Initially introduced as a hemostatic device, the technology subsequently was used for ablation of superficial neoplastic lesions. A noncontact coagulation device, APC can deliver a tangential current to coagulate a target lesion uniformly.[135]

The standard equipment consists of a high-frequency generator and an automatically regulated argon source. The APC current and argon gas are delivered via a flexible probe introduced through the operating channel of the endoscope. Straight fire and side fire probes are available. The recommended settings for ablation of gastric lesions using the APC 300/ICC 200 electrosurgical system (ERBE USA Incorporated Surgical Systems, Marietta, GA) are as follows: mode, auto coag; power setting, 60 to 80 W; coagulation type, forced; and argon plasma flow rate, less than 1.0 L/min. The VIO300D-APC2, a new second-generation APC system released by the same manufacturer, achieves similar results at power settings approximately half of the APC 300 unit.

ARGON PLASMA COAGULATION FOR EARLY GASTRIC CANCER

Compared with laser therapy, experience with APC for treatment of both early and advanced gastric cancer is limited with a shorter duration of follow-up.[185] APC as a curative treatment for EGC was used by Sagawa and colleagues[4] in 27 patients who were considered poor candidates for either surgical resection (17 patients) or EMR (10 patients) because of comorbidities including severe cardiac failure, marked thrombocytopenia, or anticoagulation therapy. No evidence of recurrence was observed in 26 treated patients (96%) at a median follow-up of 30 months. Only one patient had a tumor recurrence at 6 months, and this was successfully retreated with no evidence of recurrence after an additional follow-up of 39 months. Of the 27 patients, 12 (44%) had EGCs located in areas more difficult to access endoscopically, such as the posterior wall of the stomach or the cardia.[4] APC is also commonly used to ablate any residual tumor after EMR and ESD.[4,139]

ARGON PLASMA COAGULATION FOR ADVANCED GASTRIC CANCER

APC as part of a multimodality palliative approach for advanced gastric cancer has been reported.[186] Ten patients with gastric carcinoma in whom surgery would not have been curative were treated with APC for debulking of a partially obstructing tumor; a mean of 4.9 treatment sessions was required to achieve effective palliation and symptom relief.[186] In another study, 40 patients with superficial-type cancer were treated by APC only.[187] Intestinal-type intramucosal carcinoma disappeared in all patients after one or two sessions of APC. Residual tumor or recurrence was noted in four patients (10%)—three with submucosal invasion and one with an extensive, diffuse-type carcinoma. However, such lesions were locally controlled by follow-up APC.[187] APC has also been used to treat tumor ingrowth within self-expandable metal stents in patients with obstructing esophagogastric junction tumors.[188]

COMPLICATIONS OF ARGON PLASMA COAGULATION

APC therapy in 27 patients with EGC was not associated with any serious complications. Of 27 patients, 3 (11%) complained of abdominal fullness that was alleviated by intermittent suction or by continuous suction when a dual-channel upper endoscope was used.[4]

Enteral Stents

Enteral stents are indicated for malignant luminal obstruction of the GI tract. Patients who have gastric outlet obstruction secondary to gastric cancer can be treated with surgical palliative bypass (via laparoscopy in some centers).[189] Patients who are not good candidates for surgical palliation may benefit from percutaneous gastrostomy for decompression and enteral feeding.[190] Another alternative is the use of an enteral self-expandable metal stent (SEMS). SEMS have been used as palliative therapy for obstructing gastroesophageal junction tumors.[191] SEMS are made of various metal alloys in varying sizes and shapes. Covered and uncovered SEMS are available.[192] Many of the published series on placement of SEMS in the upper GI tract have used either modified or standard esophageal stents.[193,194]

A through the scope technique is used to place enteral SEMS, typically made of stainless steel or nitinol. Two important caveats for successful placement of SEMS are the ability to pass a guidewire across the stricture and the selection of a stent that is at least 3 to 4 cm longer than the obstruction, to allow an adequate margin on both sides of the obstruction.[195]

Other Gastric Neoplasms

Gastric Polyps

Gastric polyps are addressed in detail in Chapter 32.

Gastric Lymphoma
Epidemiology

GI lymphoma accounts for 4% to 20% of all NHL and 30% to 40% of all extranodal cases.[196] The incidence rate for NHL has been increasing with this trend being more prevalent for extranodal disease. Even though primary gastric lymphoma accounts for less than 5% of all gastric malignant neoplasms, an increase in incidence of primary gastric lymphoma has been observed in the United States.[197]

Time trend analysis based on a population-based registry has shown increased incidence rates for gastric (6.3%) and small bowel (5.9%) NHL; there is a concomitant decrease in GI NHL of unknown site, suggesting that the increased incidence at least partly may be a result of more accurate diagnosis. In this particular study, the most common site of GI NHL for all age groups was gastric (43.3%), followed by small bowel (27.4%) and large bowel (11.1%); NHL of unknown site accounted for the remaining 16.1%.[196]

Pathogenesis

An association between *H. pylori* infection and gastric NHL has been shown in several studies.[198,199] Acquired mucosa-associated lymphoid tissue (MALT) in the stomach provides the background for lymphoma to develop. *H. pylori* is the only well-established chronic antigenic stimulus that causes gastric MALT.[200] Parsonnet and colleagues[201] showed that prior *H. pylori* infection gives a statistically significant sixfold increased risk of developing gastric NHL, with the association being stronger for high-grade lymphoma. Complete regression of MALT after eradication of *H. pylori* infection has been described, with subsequent relapse of the lymphoma after reinfection with the organism.[200,202,203] The link between *H. pylori* gastritis and low-grade gastric lymphoma of the MALT type has also been supported by published data from case-control and epidemiologic studies.[202]

Although the rate of *H. pylori* infection in patients with gastric lymphoma has been found to be higher (91%) than in the general population (64%) in some areas throughout the world, the incidence of gastric lymphoma only partially parallels the incidence of *H. pylori* gastritis.[204] In some areas of Africa, the prevalence of *H. pylori* infection is very high, but the incidence of gastric lymphoma is very low. A study using population-based registries showed that the incidence of gastric lymphoma parallels the incidence of all NHL, indicating that *H. pylori* infection is not the only factor in the pathogenesis of MALT lymphoma.[204] A 22% rate of *H. pylori*–negative status based on histologic and serologic tests has been reported in patients with low-grade gastric lymphoma.[205] Rarely, low-grade lymphoma may develop in the background of *Helicobacter heilmannii*–associated gastritis.[206]

In some *H. pylori*–negative gastric MALT lymphomas, an association with autoimmune diseases such as Sjögren's syndrome has been described, but no association with viruses known to be present in other types of lymphomas has been detected.[207] Epstein-Barr virus infection, an early pathogen in the development of nodal lymphoma, is only very rarely found in gastric MALT lymphoma.[208] Occupational exposure to solvents and pesticides was suggested to play a pathogenic role in some gastric lymphomas in an Italian study.[198] The development of MALT that gives rise to gastric lymphoma is probably a multifactorial process involving both antigenic and host-related factors, but other mechanisms are unknown.

Clinical Features

Low-grade gastric lymphoma typically occurs in the fifth decade, whereas high-grade lymphoma occurs in the sixth decade, suggesting that the progression from low-grade to high-grade lymphoma takes about a decade.[209] Patients with gastric lymphoma generally present with nonspecific dyspepsia or with symptoms suggestive of peptic ulcer disease. Some patients may present with GI bleeding or anemia. The finding of an abdominal mass at presentation is rare.[209]

Endoscopic Diagnosis

Endoscopically, patients with low-grade lymphoma may display normal-appearing gastric mucosa, nonspecific macroscopic gastritis, thickened gastric folds, or ulcerative lesions. High-grade lymphoma generally displays large ulcers on more protruding tumors.[210] The diagnosis is based on gastric biopsies and enhanced by immunohistochemistry.[211]

Endoscopic Ultrasound Staging

EUS provides accurate staging of gastric lymphoma. Based on EUS criteria, gastric lymphoma can be divided into four types: superficially spreading (with thickening of the second or third layers or both), diffusely infiltrating (diffuse transmural irregular thickening of the gastric wall), mass-forming (localized hypoechoic mass with a clear margin located in the third layer or in the third and fourth layers), and mixed (combination of mass-forming and superficially spreading).[212] Superficially spreading and diffusely infiltrating lymphomas are seen only in patients with low-grade MALT lymphoma. Mass-forming lymphomas are of the same histologic type as intermediate-grade lymphomas, either diffuse large cell or mixed cell type.[212]

EUS is considered the most accurate technique for locoregional staging of MALT lymphoma.[212,213] EUS had a T staging accuracy of 91.5% when resected specimen histology was the "gold standard."[213] The accuracy of EUS for detection of lymph node metastasis was reported to be 83% compared with resected histology in the same study.[213]

A previous study evaluated the accuracy of a 12-MHz miniprobe for the staging of low-grade gastric MALT lymphoma compared with conventional EUS.[214] The study retrospectively reviewed 39 patients before treatment who had histologically confirmed low-grade MALT lymphoma. The accuracy of T and N staging using miniprobe and conventional EUS were similar in this study. The advantage of performing staging with the miniprobe is that this examination can be performed as a single-step procedure during diagnostic gastroscopy. We believe, however, that conventional EUS and EUS-guided FNA is the procedure of choice for staging MALT lymphoma because miniprobes cannot detect distant metastatic lymph node involvement (e.g., nodes in the celiac region) or provide a specimen for cytologic evaluation.[214,215]

Pathology

NHL are malignant neoplasms of the B and T lymphocytes and their precursor cells.[216] In Western countries, B-cell lymphoma is more common (>80%). In the Western world, B-cell lymphoma of the MALT type is the most common. Most of these lymphomas arise in the stomach.[202,217–219] In southern

Japan, T-cell lymphomas predominate, accounting for greater than 75% of GI cases.[202,217–219]

In the presence of *H. pylori* infection, B-lymphoid and T-lymphoid cells and neutrophils are brought to the gastric mucosa to form acquired MALT. In low-grade lymphoma, the autoreactive B-cell proliferation is secondary to a specific activation of reactive T cells by *H. pylori* and cytokines rather than to the bacteria per se.[220] The two main groups of gastric lymphomas are extranodal marginal zone B-cell lymphoma, MALT-type lymphoma, and diffuse large B-cell lymphoma.[221] Marginal zone B-cell lymphoma and MALT-type lymphoma are composed of a monotonous, diffuse infiltrate of small lymphoid cells, whereas diffuse large B-cell lymphoma is characterized by a diffuse infiltrate of large malignant lymphoid blasts resembling centroblasts, plasmablasts, and immunoblasts.[222]

Low-grade MALT lymphoma characteristically displays small cleaved cells or centrocytelike cells and is more frequently found in the stomach. As with nodal NHL, low-grade MALT lymphoma may progress to high-grade lymphoma. In the stomach, low-grade MALT lymphoma may extend over a large area or be multifocal.[223] A subset of patients with low-grade B-cell MALT lymphoma can have a focal high-grade component histologically. A lower survival rate has been found in this subset of patients.[224] Conventional biopsy specimens do not always yield a histologic diagnosis of low-grade B-cell MALT lymphoma.[211] EUS detection with EMR histologic confirmation has been reported in one patient.[225] Coexistence of gastric carcinoma and gastric lymphoma is uncommon but has been reported in the literature.[226–228]

Treatment

The strong association between *H. pylori* and B-cell lymphoma of MALT dictates that *H. pylori* eradication should be a routine treatment for superficial gastric lymphoma. A combination of two antibiotics (clarithromycin and metronidazole or amoxicillin) with a proton pump inhibitor results in more than 90% eradication of *H. pylori*.[229] When *H. pylori* eradication is achieved, more than 70% of low-grade MALT-type lymphomas regress at an early stage. Complete histologic remission of lymphoma can be achieved 2 to 18 months after *H. pylori* eradication.[203,205,230] In *H. pylori*–positive patients with localized gastric lymphoma who have no lymph node involvement assessed by EUS, a complete remission can be achieved in 79% of cases. A significant difference in response rate was found between lymphomas restricted to the mucosa and lymphomas involving the deeper layers.[205] Patients who have persistent tumor and fail antibiotic treatment and patients with *H. pylori*–negative status could benefit from radiotherapy or radical surgery with curative intent.[231] Elderly patients and patients in whom surgery is contraindicated should receive radiotherapy.[209]

ENDOSCOPIC THERAPY

Present experience using EMR to treat gastric lymphoma is very limited. Toyoda and associates[225] reported one patient with low-grade MALT lymphoma diagnosed by EUS and EMR to have a focal high-grade component. The ability of EMR to provide a histologic diagnosis and then confirm the depth of wall layer involvement allowed the appropriate therapy to be instituted (distal subtotal gastrectomy and extended lymph node [D2] dissection with Billroth I anastomosis). In a previous study, low-grade B-cell MALT lymphoma with a focal high-grade component was present in 27 of 233 (12%) patients. EUS and EMR may prove to be useful for identifying this subset of patients who have a worse postoperative 5-year survival rate than patients who have low-grade MALT lymphoma (80% vs. 96%).[224]

Carcinoid Tumor
Epidemiology

Epidemiologically, carcinoid tumor is a rare lesion, constituting only 0.5% of all malignancies. It is found in less than 1% of all cancer autopsy cases, and the approximate incidence is only 1 to 2 per 100,000 population.[197,232] The largest epidemiologic series to date indicates that the incidence of gastric carcinoid, as a percentage of all carcinoid tumors, has increased from 2.25% (1950–1971) to 5.58% (1992–1999).[233] The percentage of gastric carcinoid in relation to all gastric tumors also has increased from 0.4% in the early Surveillance, Epidemiology and End Results (SEER) data (1973–1999) to 1.77% in the late SEER data (1992–1999). It is unclear, however, if these findings represent a true increase in the incidence or are a result of increased awareness, more frequent use of endoscopy, or changes in reporting methods.[233]

Pathogenesis

Carcinoid tumors are slow-growing tumors that are derived from neuroendocrine cells known as enterochromaffinlike cells. The enterochromaffinlike cell is the main endocrine cell type of the corpus-fundus mucosa. Enterochromaffinlike cells are known to be highly sensitive to gastrin stimulus and able to trigger parietal cell acid secretion by releasing histamine.[234] Gastrin, fibroblast growth factor, and *H. pylori* all have been shown to have trophic effects on enterochromaffinlike cells. These factors potentially may be relevant in the development of carcinoids.[234,235]

Nearly 67% of carcinoid tumors arise from the GI tract, with the tracheobronchopulmonary system being the most frequent site for carcinoid formation outside the GI tract.[233] Most carcinoid tumors in the GI tract occur in the small intestines (41.8%), rectum (27.4%), or stomach (8.7%). A slight female predominance for this tumor has been found.[233]

The etiology of carcinoid tumor is unknown. Most tumors are considered to be due to sporadic somatic mutations, although there have been reports of a familial predisposition to the disease.[236] Carcinoid tumors have been classified into three types: tumors associated with chronic atrophic gastritis type A (type 1), tumors associated with multiple endocrine neoplasia type I and Zollinger-Ellison syndrome (type 2), and sporadic gastric carcinoid tumors unaccompanied by hypergastrinemia or any specific gastric pathology (type 3).[237]

Clinical Features

Clinical manifestations of carcinoid tumors are often absent or vague. In approximately 8% to 10% of patients, these tumors manifest with the carcinoid syndrome (flushing, watery diarrhea, abdominal pain, and wheezing). This syndrome is attributed to secretion of the bioactive mediator serotonin (5-hydroxytryptamine) into the systemic circulation from the primary tumor or, more commonly, from metastatic sites.[238]

An association between GI carcinoids and second primary malignancies has been reported with incidence ranging from 12% to 46%.[233,239] In the late SEER subset of data, carcinoid tumors in total were associated with other noncarcinoid tumors in 22.4%. Patients with gastric carcinoids had a decrease of 26% in the incidence of additional noncarcinoid neoplasms when the early SEER data (1973–1991) were compared with the late data (1992–1999). This findings prompted authors to speculate that the decrease might be related to higher identification and removal of these tumors endoscopically.[233] The most common site of second primary malignancy is the GI tract, which is involved in 32% to 62% of cases, followed by the genitourinary tract (9% to 22%) and the lung and bronchial system (9% to 13%). Adenocarcinoma of the colon has been reported as the most common second primary malignancy.[240]

It has been speculated that some bioactive substances secreted by carcinoids, such as epidermal growth factor, CCK, VIP, secretin, bombesin, and gastrin, can promote the growth of tumor cells. It is probable that, over time, prolonged exposure to such growth factors may promote phenotypic changes in susceptible cells and induce neoplastic transformation.[241] Metastases from carcinoid tumors have been reported to occur in approximately 29% of patients; most (61.2%) originate from the small intestine. After lymph node metastasis (89.9%), the liver is the most frequent site of metastasis (44.1%) followed by lung (13.6%), peritoneum (13.6%), and pancreas (6.8%).[242]

Endoscopic Diagnosis

Endoscopically, gastric carcinoid tumors may be present as polyplike lesions or, more frequently, as smooth, rounded submucosal lesions.[243] The presence of an irregular erythematous depression or ulceration on the lesion has been considered characteristic but not pathognomonic of gastric carcinoids.[244]

Pathology

Type 1 tumors associated with chronic atrophic gastritis type A are the most common type of gastric carcinoids, characterized by multiple tumors and hypergastrinemia.[237] The tumors are usually polypoid in appearance, are small (<1 cm), and are found in the body or fundus of the stomach. Type 1 tumors have a relatively benign course. Nodal involvement is reported in 16% of cases, and hepatic metastasis is reported in 4%.[245,246] Type 2 gastric carcinoids are typically also small lesions, but the adjacent mucosa is not atrophic. They have a low potential for malignancy. Type 3 carcinoids are usually solitary tumors greater than 2 cm in size; 40% are present in the antrum and prepyloric area. There is no hypergastrinemia or chronic gastritis. Type 3 tumors are characterized by deep invasion and high potential for metastasis, even when primary lesions are small.[237,247] Nodal metastasis is present in 55% of patients, and liver metastases are present in 25%. The 5-year survival is 50%. Histologically, tumors less than 1 cm or growth restricted to the mucosa are characterized as benign.[248]

Stromal Cell Tumor
Epidemiology

Gastrointestinal stromal tumors (GISTs) are rare; however, they are the most common mesenchymal tumors to arise in the GI tract. According to a population-based sample, the estimated incidence of GISTs is approximately 10 to 20 per 1 million per year.[249] The annual incidence in the United States has been estimated to be 5000 to 6000 cases per year.[250] The estimated incidence of malignant GISTs in southern Finland was 4 per 1 million.[251] GISTs rarely occur before age 40 and are slightly more common in men than in women. An association between GISTs and von Recklinghausen's disease has been suggested.[252] GISTs are most commonly located in the stomach (60%), with the remainder being found in the small intestine (20% to 25%), colon and rectum (5%), and esophagus (<5%).[250]

Pathogenesis

Morphologically, GISTs are a heterogeneous group of neoplasms that arise anywhere in the GI tract. They represent a family of tumors that probably originates from the intestinal pacemaker cell, also known as the interstitial cell of Cajal (ICC).[253] The ICC serves as a pacemaker system within the muscle layers of the gut and regulates GI motility.[254] In the normal gut, these cells express vimentin, CD34, and CD117. The observation that immunohistochemical staining for several of these markers is identical between the ICC and GISTs prompted Kindblom and colleagues[255] to propose that GISTs originate from the ICC or may originate from a pluripotential stem cell. The c-kit protein, or CD117, is now recognized as a very sensitive and specific marker for GI stromal cells.

Clinical Features

One-third of patients with GISTs are completely asymptomatic, and tumors are found incidentally during imaging, endoscopy, or surgical procedures being done for unrelated reasons.[249,251] Patients may present with vague symptoms, but the most common manifestations are intestinal bleeding (20% to 50%), abdominal pain (40% to 50%), or a palpable mass (25% to 40%).[251,256] Up to 30% of all GISTs are malignant. The most common site of extraintestinal metastasis is the liver, which is involved in 50% of malignant tumors, followed by lung (10%) and bone (<10%) involvement.[249]

Endoscopic Diagnosis

Most gastric stromal tumors appear as smooth, round, glistening masses covered with normal gastric mucosa. A defect in the overlying mucosa may occur when ulceration and resulting bleeding occur.[256] Endoscopic mucosal biopsy specimens are inadequate to establish the histologic diagnosis in most patients, reemphasizing need for EUS in evaluating suspected GISTs and other subepithelial lesions.

Endoscopic Ultrasound Diagnosis

On EUS, GISTs appear as hypoechoic masses arising from the muscularis propria layer (fourth layer); infrequently, lesions may originate from the muscularis mucosa layer (second layer).[257] When GISTs are occasionally found in the submucosal (third layer), they are thought to originate from the muscularis propria or the muscularis mucosa with subsequent extension into the submucosa.[258]

EUS features that may help to identify malignant tumors include size greater than 4 cm, irregular extraluminal borders, and presence of echogenic foci and cystic spaces. If at least two of these three features are present, the sensitivity of EUS for detecting malignancy is 80% to 100%.[259] Palazzo and colleagues[260] found that size less than 3 cm, homogeneous echo pattern, and regular margins were 100% specific for benign lesions. Whether EUS features alone can aid in the differentiation of high-risk versus low-risk tumors is less certain.[261]

EUS-guided FNA of suspected GISTs has been used widely to obtain a cytologic diagnosis. A single-center study by Ando and colleagues[262] compared EUS-guided FNA with subsequently resected specimens. Using the surgical specimens as the "gold standard" for malignancy or benignity, they found that EUS-guided FNA had an accuracy of 91.3% and specificity of 100%. Sensitivity was only 66.7%, however, with two malignant lesions missed at FNA. Hunt and coworkers[263] performed EUS-guided FNA in 40 patients for evaluation of spindle cell tumors. Of specimens, 17 stained positive for c-*kit*; tumors positive for c-*kit* were larger. Surgical resection was performed on 13 patients, 12 of whom had c-*kit*–positive tumors, and 3 of these 12 tumors had greater than 5 mitoses per 50 high-power fields. More recent data reinforce the idea that mutations in c-*kit*, high mitotic count, and larger tumor size are risk factors for poor prognosis in patients with localized GISTs and predict reduced relapse-free survival after curative resection.[261]

Pathology

The most common histologic variant among gastric GISTs is a cellular, spindle cell type of tumor consisting of uniform eosinophilic cells. Some of these tumors have a prominent nerve sheath tumorlike nuclear palisading pattern, whereas others show prominent perinuclear vacuolization with moderate to slight interstitial collagen.[250] Malignant GISTs may have a spindled, round cell, or epithelioid pattern, or a combination of these. Some malignant GISTs histologically resemble leiomyosarcomas, although they usually have a less eosinophilic cytoplasm.[250] Pathologic features that have been used to predict malignancy include mitotic activity, nuclear pleomorphism, degree of cellularity, nuclear-to-cytoplasmic ratio, tumor size (>5 cm have a high risk), mucosal invasion, ulceration, and tumor necrosis.[264]

Endoscopic Therapy of Submucosal Neoplasms

Submucosal tumors of the stomach are uncommon and are usually found incidentally during endoscopy. These tumors traditionally have been approached in one of two ways: (1) observation with or without an attempt to make the tissue diagnosis or (2) surgical resection. The advent of EUS has enabled the etiology of submucosal tumors to be determined noninvasively. Some tumors have EUS characteristics that are so pathognomonic that no additional diagnostic testing is needed. One example is a small lipoma that on EUS shows the classic hyperechoic texture of a lesion arising from the sub-

mucosa.[265,266] In other situations, the EUS features alone are inadequate to establish the correct diagnosis. Mesenchymal tumors as a group typically arise from the fourth layer of the muscularis propria as a hypoechoic lesion; however, the EUS features alone do not distinguish gastric stromal tumors from other types of mesenchymal tumors. In this situation, cytopathology and immunocytochemistry obtained by EUS-guided FNA are quite helpful to establish the diagnosis and guide therapy. Patients with symptomatic disease and any submucosal tumors of the stomach with EUS features suggestive of local invasion require surgical consideration regardless of FNA results.

A practical problem with EUS-guided FNA is the fact that small submucosal tumors of the stomach are often difficult to target. A small leiomyoma with tightly packed spindle cells may not permit adequate sampling using standard techniques. Newly introduced EUS-guided core biopsy needles theoretically provide a better tissue sample, but these needles are technically difficult to deploy, they often yield suboptimal results, and the technique is not feasible for small lesions. In some instances, surgical removal of a submucosal tumor may be the only practical way to provide a histologic diagnosis as well as being curative. Small (<1 cm) gastric submucosal tumors rarely involve the lymph nodes, and in the absence of suspicious EUS characteristics, simple observation and follow-up may be all that is required.

ENDOSCOPIC ULTRASOUND AND HIGH-FREQUENCY ULTRASOUND STAGING

Prior studies have shown the accuracy of EUS for the diagnosis of upper GI tract submucosal lesions.[265] More recently, the efficacy and safety of endoscopic resection of submucosal tumors based on EUS or HFUS probe findings also have been reported.[267] Prior reports and unpublished personal experience suggest that 20-MHz HFUS probes are useful for the evaluation of small submucosal lesions before EMR. Lesions larger than 2 cm may require the use of a lower frequency (12-MHz) probe or standard EUS-guided FNA for cytologic diagnosis and staging.[267]

ENDOSCOPIC MUCOSAL RESECTION

HFUS probe–assisted EMR has been performed in 26 of 28 submucosal tumors. A 20-MHz HFUS probe was used to evaluate the lesions and to confirm complete detachment of the lesion from the muscularis propria. All four gastric submucosal lesions (two carcinoids, one heterotopic pancreas, and one fibrovascular polyp) were successfully removed after saline solution injection into the submucosa. Two of the four (50%) benign gastric lesions involved the lower third of the submucosa (sm3), suggesting that deeply seated submucosal lesions are amendable to EMR therapy. Inability to separate the lesion completely from the muscularis propria by saline solution injection was noted in two rectal submucosal lesions, both of which were incompletely resected. Twenty-one of these lesions were removed by the lift-and-cut method, and six were removed using the cap technique. No complications occurred. There was no difference in complete resection rate with respect to location of the lesion in the submucosa (sm1, sm2, or sm3).[106] No recurrence was observed during a median follow-up of 21.5 months. These results suggest that even deeply seated *benign* submucosal lesions (sm3), as delineated by HFUS probe, are equally amendable to complete removal by EMR as mucosal lesions.

More recently, Ichikawa and colleagues[243] reported on the usefulness of EMR in the management of gastric carcinoid tumors. Five patients with type 1 gastric carcinoids underwent successful curative EMR. The depth of invasion was submucosal in three patients and mucosal in two patients by histologic evaluation of the EMR specimens. No evidence of recurrence was found during a mean follow-up of 32.6 months.[243]

Kojima and colleagues[267] also reported on their experience with EMR of submucosal tumors. Of 54 lesions studied, 23 (43%) were gastric (10 leiomyomas, 2 lipomas, 6 aberrant pancreas, 1 neurofibroma, 1 neurinoma, 1 leiomyoblastoma, 1 leiomyosarcoma, and 1 granular cell tumor). EMR was performed to remove 18 (78%) of the 23 gastric lesions. The other five (22%) patients had evidence of muscularis propria involvement by EUS, and EMR was used in these patients to resect the mucosa and expose the tumor for forceps biopsies. In this series, only one patient had bleeding after gastric EMR; this patient was managed successfully with endoscopic therapy.

Future Trends

In the past decade, there has been an explosion of technologic advances in the area of therapeutic endoscopy. The enhanced ability to stage GI neoplasms accurately by using noninvasive or minimally invasive endoscopic techniques has greatly benefited patients and allowed consideration of nonsurgical options for treating superficial gastric neoplasms. The interventional GI endoscopist is now poised to move beyond the traditional boundaries of endoscopic diagnosis and palliation to offer curative endoscopic resection for selected patients with gastric neoplasms.

EMR implies a limitation of the technique to treatment of mucosal disease. ESD is technically more difficult to perform, but the technique enables en bloc resection of lesions greater than 2 cm and is likely to improve the complete resection rate of EGC and to expand the indications of endoscopic resection to include undifferentiated mucosal cancers. More recently, investigators have been "pushing the envelope" to show the safety and efficacy of extending endoscopic resection to submucosal lesions, although the cumulative experience to date is still limited.[106,267] Concurrently, results in animal models indicate that full-thickness endoluminal resection and transluminal endoscopic surgery are technically feasible.[268,269] Successful translation of such innovative techniques into endoscopic practice in the near future will redefine the limits of endoscopic therapy for gastric neoplasms and blur the boundary between therapeutic endoscopy and surgery further.

References

The complete reference list is available online at www.expertconsult.com.

Chapter **34**

Endoscopic Management of Upper Gastrointestinal Familial Adenomatous Polyposis Syndrome and Ampullary Tumors

Roy D. Yen and Raj J. Shah

Video related to this chapter's topics can be found online at expertconsult.com.

Introduction

Classic familial adenomatous polyposis (FAP) is an autosomal dominant condition caused by mutation in the adenomatous polyposis coli (*APC*) gene that results in profuse adenomatous polyposis of the gastrointestinal (GI) tract, most marked in the colon. Attenuated FAP is associated with a smaller number of polyps in the colon and upper GI tract. The *MUTYH* mutation causes a recessively inherited polyposis condition, *MUTYH*-associated polyposis, which is characterized by a slightly increased risk of developing colon cancer and adenomas in both the upper and the lower GI tract. Patients with FAP and its variants generally undergo prophylactic colectomy during adolescence or early adult life. After colectomy, the proximal duodenum is the most common site of malignancy in FAP subjects.[1] The periampullary region is especially prone to adenomatous change, presumably related partly to the trophic effects of bile on the mucosa.[2–5] Duodenal adenomas develop in 40% to 100% of FAP patients. Less commonly, periampullary adenomas are sporadic (arising in non-FAP patients).

As with adenomatous polyps elsewhere within the GI tract, periampullary adenomas progress through the adenoma-carcinoma sequence and are premalignant. Although screening, surveillance, and removal of adenomas in the upper GI tract are required for FAP patients, the optimal intervals have not been determined. A consensus on the management of small (<1 cm) ampullary and periampullary adenomas in patients with either FAP or sporadic neoplasms has yet to be achieved.

Multiple reports have documented the outcomes of endoscopic surveillance and endoscopic approaches to treatment of periampullary lesions, including endoscopic snare resection and thermal ablation. Surgical options for advanced lesions include local transduodenal resection, pancreaticoduodenectomy, and pancreas-sparing duodenectomy. The appropriate management for each patient depends on many factors, including the size and number of lesions, degree of dysplasia, involvement of the pancreaticobiliary system, comorbidities, and local expertise.

Familial Adenomatous Polyposis Syndrome

FAP is an autosomal dominant condition with virtually complete penetrance, affecting approximately 1 in 8000 in the

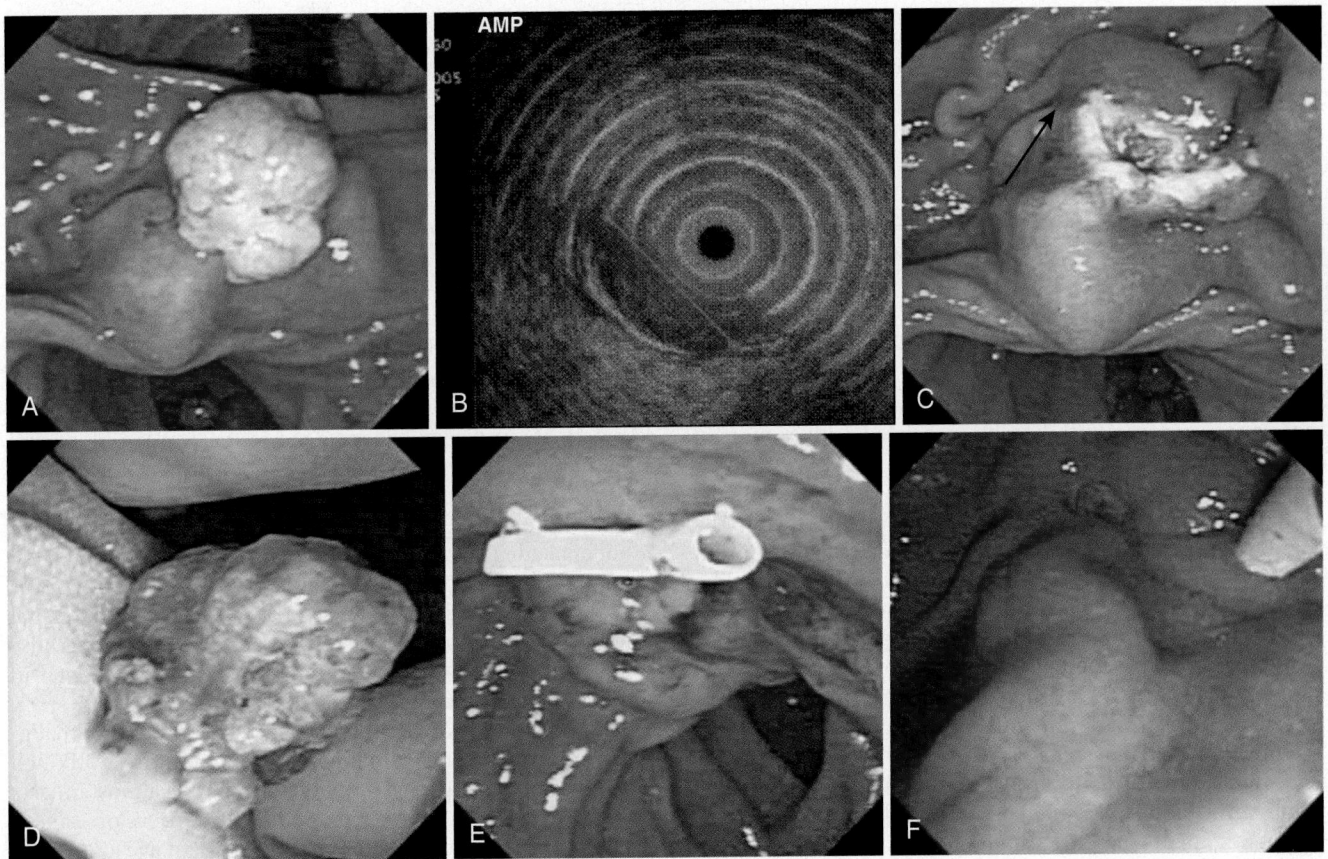

Fig. 34.1 En bloc resection of ampullary adenoma. **A,** Polypoid ampullary adenoma. **B,** Endoscopic ultrasound (EUS) image of ampullary adenoma with intact submucosal layer *(arrow)*. **C,** En bloc resection. **D,** Resected specimen. **E,** Prophylactic pancreatic stent placed. **F,** No adenoma found by surveillance biopsies at 1-month follow-up.

United States.[6] Mutation of the *APC* gene on the long arm of chromosome 5 is responsible for most cases of FAP.[7] The condition is classically characterized by the development of hundreds to thousands of adenomatous polyps in the colon with the inevitable progression of one or more of these adenomas to carcinoma. It is increasingly apparent, however, that an attenuated form of FAP exists. These patients generally present with fewer colorectal polyps developing later in life compared with classic FAP and often distributed more proximally in the colon. These patients develop upper GI disease, and the upper GI findings may be more marked in some patients than the findings in the colon.[8,9] Mutations in particular regions of the *APC* gene account for the attenuated forms of FAP.[8,10,11]

Extracolonic disease is common in classic FAP but varies in severity from family to family and between individuals within families. At one extreme is Gardner's syndrome, characterized by GI adenomatous polyps with other benign neoplasms, such as desmoid tumors, osteomas, and fibromas.[12] Gardner's syndrome also results from germline *APC* mutations and is best regarded as part of the spectrum of FAP. Turcot's syndrome is characterized by central nervous system tumors, often glioblastomas or medulloblastomas,[12] and colonic polyposis. The inheritance of this disorder has been difficult to determine[12] because the association of central nervous system tumors and polyposis may arise through germline mutation of more than one gene.[13] Germline *APC* mutations have been identified in some patients with Turcot's syndrome, particularly patients with cerebellar medulloblastomas and profuse colonic pol-

yposis.[13] For the purposes of this chapter, the term *FAP* incorporates Gardner's syndrome and cases of Turcot's syndrome attributable to *APC* mutations.

The colonic manifestations of FAP are cured by colectomy (although a risk of rectal cancer remains after ileorectal anastomosis or in any residual rectal mucosa after restorative proctocolectomy). After colectomy, extracolonic manifestations of FAP assume greater importance. The entire upper GI tract seems to be at risk of malignancy in FAP.[1] The duodenum is the most common site of malignancy in patients after colectomy. Duodenal cancer develops in 4.5% to 8.5% of these patients.[14,15] Adenomas and carcinomas have also been encountered in the distal ileal segment and within ileoanal pouches 5 to 10 years after proctocolectomy.[16]

Gastric polyps are a common finding in FAP. Multiple 3- to 5-mm fundic polypoid lesions are seen in at least 50% of patients (**Fig. 34.1**).[17] These *fundic gland* or *fundic cystic gland* polyps are hamartomatous lesions and were previously regarded as having no malignant potential. Histologic examination of fundic gland polyps reveals cystic dilation of fundic glands with generally no epithelial dysplasia.[18] However, Bianchi and colleagues[19] reported a series of 75 FAP patients undergoing upper endoscopic screening for adenomas. Fundic gland polyps, detected in 88% of patients and sampled by mucosal biopsy, showed dysplasia in 41% (3% with high-grade dysplasia). On multivariate analysis, the investigators found larger fundic gland polyps (>1 cm), higher Spigelman stage (**Table 34.1**), and antral gastritis were associated with

Table 34.1 **Spigelman Scoring System for Staging of Ampullary Adenoma**

No. Polyps	Polyp Size	Histology	Dysplasia	Points
1–4	1–4 mm	Tubular	Mild	1
5–20	5–10 mm	Tubulovillous	Moderate	2
>20	>10 mm	Villous	Severe	3

Stage 0, 0 points; stage 1, 1–4 points; stage 2, 5–6 points; stage 3, 7–8 points; stage 4, 9–12 points.

fundic gland dysplasia. Fundic gland polyps with size greater than 1 cm had almost 16 times greater odds for dysplasia compared with polyps 1 to 4 mm in size. Acid suppressive medication use was found to be associated with a marked decrease in dysplastic fundic gland polyps.

Similar findings were noted in a series of 24 pediatric patients undergoing screening endoscopy with 51% showing fundic gland polyps with dysplasia in 42%.[20] The investigators found that *APC* mutations between codons 1225 and 1694 may be associated with more aggressive gastroduodenal involvement in FAP. Several case reports also describe gastric adenocarcinoma arising from fundic gland polyps in patients with FAP and attenuated FAP.[21–24] Although a smaller series ($n = 29$)[21] revealed polyps (predominantly fundic gland) in 35% of patients in which all were hyperplastic without dysplasia, it is important to perform a thorough examination of the fundus to obtain a biopsy specimen or remove large fundic gland polyps (>1 cm or enlarging lesions on serial surveillance examinations) or polyps with atypical endoscopic appearances.

Gastric adenomatous polyps (predominantly in the gastric antrum) have been reported in 5% of patients with FAP in a British cohort[1] and 25% in a Japanese series.[25] The risk of gastric malignancy has been estimated to be 3.4 times that of controls.[26] However, this report was from Japan, where the epidemiology of gastric malignancy differs from that of Western societies. In a British study of 1255 subjects with FAP and mean follow-up of 22 years, only 7 developed gastric malignancy.[1] Nevertheless, just as adenomas are treated in other parts of the GI tract, if screening upper endoscopy is performed to assess for duodenal adenomas, inspection and biopsy or removal of suspected adenomas in the stomach should also be planned. Surveillance strategies of the upper GI tract for FAP patients are discussed subsequently.

Incidence of Sporadic and Familial Adenomatous Polyposis–Related Periampullary Adenomas

An understanding of the natural history of duodenal neoplasia in patients with FAP is essential to the development of surveillance strategies and decisions regarding management in this condition. Periampullary tumors represent 5% of GI tumors and 36% of resectable pancreaticoduodenal tumors.[27] A periampullary adenoma is an uncommon lesion in clinical practice, although not as rare as previously thought. An early review at the Mayo Clinic by Baggenstoss[28] found 25 of these lesions in 4000 consecutive autopsies (0.62%), suggesting that the lesion may be subclinical. A review of the case notes in this study suggested that only 6 (24%) of these 25 lesions might have been symptomatic.

Asymptomatic adenomatous change of the ampulla is extremely common in FAP patients, occurring in a high proportion of patients with one series showing adenoma in all of the patients studied.[29] The incidence of FAP-related duodenal and periampullary adenomas depends on the diligence of screening (see section on Diagnosis later). A review of the Johns Hopkins FAP registry indicated that the relative risk of duodenal adenocarcinoma in FAP compared with the general population was 330, and the relative risk of ampullary cancer was 123.[30] However, the combined absolute risk of duodenal cancer in FAP patients was only 1 per 1698 years. Because follow-up was incomplete and most cancers occurred later in life, the risk of malignancy may be underestimated. A study from the United Kingdom reported development of malignancy in 3 of 70 patients followed over 40 months.[31] Although adenomatous change in the duodenum may be almost universal in FAP, only a few patients apparently develop cancer. Several studies have indicated that the median age at onset of periampullary malignancy complicating FAP is in the 6th decade.[15,30,32] The literature on this subject often has inadequately differentiated sporadic from FAP-related periampullary adenomas.

Pathogenesis of Periampullary Adenoma

As an autosomal dominant condition, all nucleated cells in FAP patients contain one normal and one abnormal *APC* gene (a germline mutation). In the colon, a somatic mutation in the previously normal (wild-type) *APC* allele is generally an early event in carcinogenesis. Accumulation of other somatic mutations (in genes such as *TP53* and K-*ras*) drives the progression toward malignancy.[33] The situation with respect to periampullary malignancy seems to be similar except that somatic *APC* mutations may be relatively less frequent and K-*ras* mutations relatively more frequent.[34] Another study has shown *TP53* mutations associated with high-grade malignant change in periampullary tumors.[27] There may be other familial factors, possibly unidentified modifier genes, that influence the development of periampullary adenomas in FAP kindreds, partly explaining the familial segregation of periampullary disease observed within FAP families.[32] This segregation was independent of the specific *APC* mutation of the kindred.

Histology

Most periampullary lesions are tubular or tubulovillous adenomas that arise from the intestinal-type epithelium of the ampulla.[35] Foci of severe dysplasia or frank malignancy may be found within a lesion.[36] Other neoplasms of the ampulla are far less common; these include benign lesions (adenomyoma, leiomyoma, lipoma, lymphangioma, hemangioma, carcinoid, and paraganglioma) and primary and metastatic malignancies (lymphoma, melanoma, and metastatic small cell carcinoma).[37] A retrospective study by Bleau and Gostout[29] supported the temporal progression of periampullary adenomas to carcinoma, with diagnosis of adenoma at a mean age of 39, high-grade dysplasia at age 47, and malignancy at age 54.

Clinical Presentation

Lesions of the periampullary area may be asymptomatic or manifest relatively early with symptoms of pancreaticobiliary origin. Clinical presentation is usually a consequence of obstruction, resulting in abdominal pain, nausea, vomiting, cholangitis, or jaundice[37] or, less commonly, GI bleeding, iron deficiency anemia, or acute pancreatitis.[38] Courvoisier's sign is occasionally present, suggesting advanced disease.[39] Biochemical evidence of biliary obstruction is common in symptomatic patients.[40] The diagnosis is usually unsuspected before visualization of the ampulla, with most patients thought to have pancreatic malignancy, chronic pancreatitis, or choledocholithiasis.

Endoscopic Management of Periampullary Adenoma

Endoscopic management of periampullary adenomas can be separated into diagnosis, surveillance, and therapy. Colonic involvement in FAP can be asymptomatic, patients with FAP may have no family history (new mutations), and colonic manifestations of the disease may be delayed in attenuated forms of FAP.[33] For these reasons, all patients with apparently "sporadic" periampullary adenomas should undergo colonoscopy.

Diagnosis

In patients with FAP, diagnosis of upper GI and particularly periampullary adenomas requires proficiency in side-viewing duodenoscopy because forward-viewing endoscopy alone may miss 50% of gross lesions visible with the side-viewer.[29,41] Patients with FAP may have adenomas beyond the ampulla that are not seen with standard endoscopy. At least at index screening, it may be appropriate in FAP patients to include extended duodenoscopy with either a pediatric colonoscope or a push enteroscope. Biopsy specimens of the ampulla are necessary to detect early adenomatous change in light of the frondlike appearance of many normal papillae. Care should be taken to avoid the expected location of the pancreatic orifice (5 o'clock position) to reduce the risk of biopsy-related pancreatitis, and multiple biopsy specimens (at least six) are needed for adequate sampling. Nonetheless, ampullary biopsy carries a small risk of necrotizing pancreatitis and is not mandatory in an asymptomatic patient with an essentially normal-appearing ampulla. For larger lesions, mucosal biopsy alone may not sufficiently exclude invasive malignancy.[42] Additional cross-sectional imaging and endoscopic ultrasound (EUS) is often used to evaluate for invasive disease.

A small series of patients undergoing high-resolution endoscopy with chromoendoscopy suggested an improved yield of adenoma detection in periampullary and duodenal polyposis. Dekker and associates[43] evaluated 43 patients with

FAP who underwent screening endoscopy using high-resolution endoscopes. They found that the additional use of indigo carmine chromoendoscopy increased the detection of adenomas from a median of 16 adenomas per patient to 21 adenomas per patient ($P = .02$) and enhanced margin detection in 51%. The addition of chromoendoscopy resulted in upgrading of the Spigelman stage (see **Table 34.1**) in 12% of patients ($P = .03$). Itoi and colleagues[44] found that the use of either indigo carmine or narrow band imaging was superior to standard white light examination in 13 of 14 cases. In this study, visualization was categorized as difficult, fair, or excellent. Narrow band imaging had significantly higher proportion of "excellent" visualization of the tumor margin than indigo carmine chromoendoscopy ($P = .012$).

Because of the poor sensitivity of endoscopic biopsies in detecting malignant change, we routinely employ EUS to assess for depth of invasion and adjacent biliary or pancreatic involvement. Because we generally avoid diagnostic cholangiopancreatography, we pursue endoscopic retrograde cholangiopancreatography (ERCP) to assess for biliary or pancreatic ductal extension only when endoscopic ampullectomy is being considered during the same session. Although limitations of EUS include compression of the affected tissues and inability to "water-fill" the second portion of the duodenum adequately to assess for depth of invasion consistently, it has shown utility in the TNM (primary tumor, regional nodes, metastases) staging of periampullary malignancy with staging accuracy of 84%.[42,45-48]

Ito and coworkers[49] evaluated the role of EUS and intraductal ultrasound (IDUS) in preoperative or preendoscopic resection of ampullary neoplasms (adenomas and adenocarcinomas) and compared it with pathologic staging. The overall T staging accuracy of EUS was 63% (62% for pT1, 45% for pT2, and 88% for pT3-4) and of IDUS was 78% (86% for pT1 lesions, 64% for pT2 lesions, and 75% for pT3-4 lesions). Accuracy for determining intraductal biliary or pancreatic extension was similar between EUS and biliary IDUS (88% to 90%). We have also selectively employed cholangioscopy to assess for intraductal extension (**Fig. 34.2**).

For ampullary adenocarcinoma staging, comparative studies using EUS, computed tomography (CT), and magnetic resonance imaging (MRI) showed inconsistently higher accuracy of T staging by EUS but a surprising lack of difference in nodal staging.[50,51] In a study by Kahaleh and associates,[52] only EUS stage and a lack of a "lifting" sign were found to be predictive of malignancy (variables analyzed included gender, age, size of lesion, EUS T1 vs. T2 stage, and lifting) on univariate analysis, and only lifting was found to be a statistically significant predictor on multivariate analysis. Overall, these studies suggest that EUS and IDUS may be useful for assessing ampullary lesions by determining the extent of local invasion or intraductal involvement before consideration of endoscopic resection. However, the disadvantage of IDUS is the need for performing ERCP, which is unlikely necessary if invasive disease is identified by EUS or noninvasive imaging such as magnetic resonance cholangiopancreatography.

Surveillance

In 1950, Halsted and colleagues[53] advocated upper GI surveillance of FAP patients. Given the risk of progression to malignancy, concerns regarding residual adenomatous tissue after

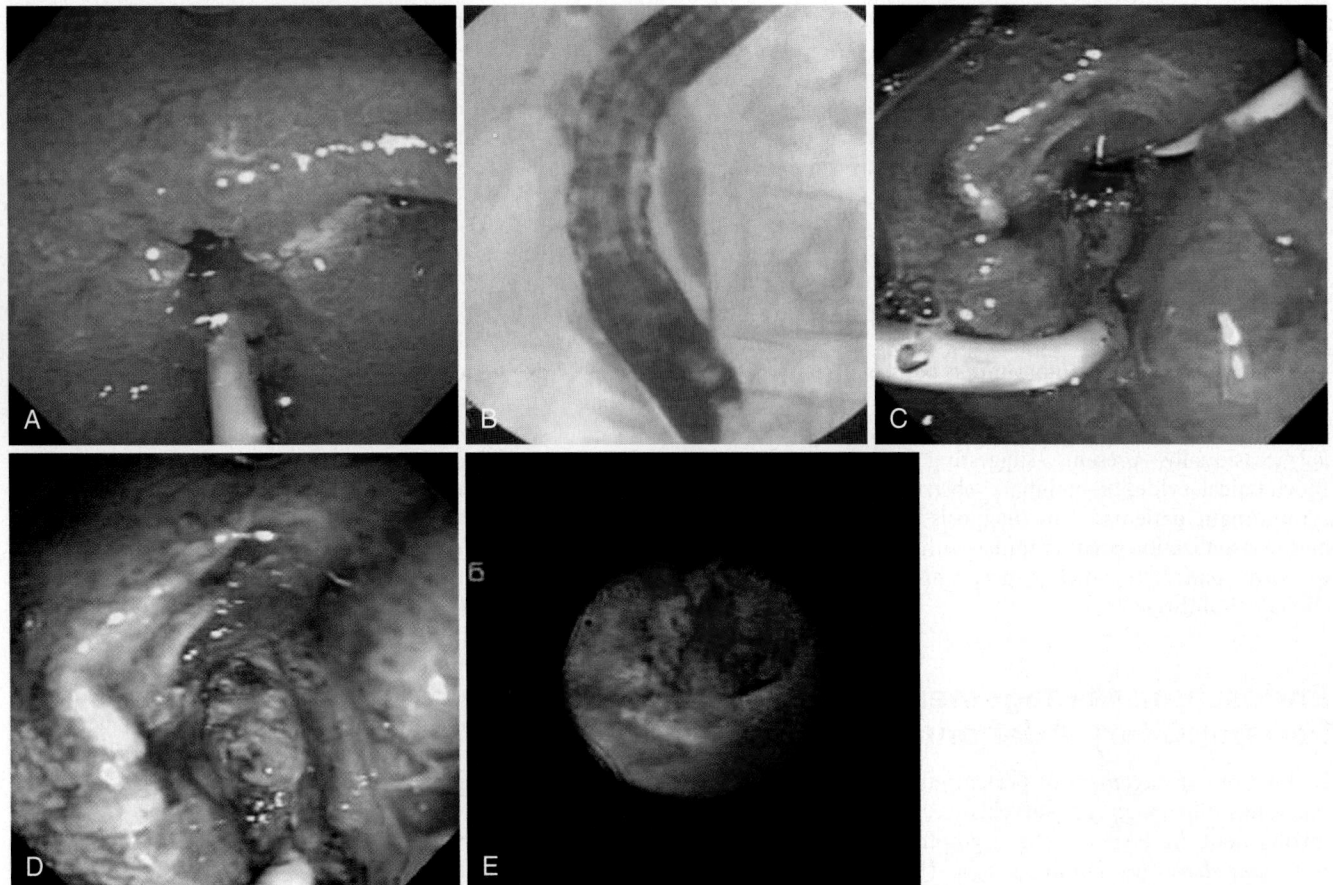

Fig. 34.2 Lateral spreading adenoma. **A,** Prophylactic stent placed after diagnostic pancreatogram. **B,** Suspected distal biliary stricture versus long intraduodenal bile duct segment. **C,** After biliary sphincterotomy to assess for intraductal extension. **D,** Methylene blue spray suggesting adenoma within biliary orifice. **E,** Cholangioscopy confirming intraductal extension of adenoma and distal biliary stricture.

ablation or resection, and the ongoing proliferative nature of these lesions, surveillance seems justified, although no studies have shown improved survival as a result. An ideal regimen for surveillance of these lesions is yet to be determined. As discussed previously, virtually all patients with FAP eventually have at least microscopic involvement of the ampulla, and most have multiple tiny adenomas spread over the proximal duodenum.

It may be impossible to remove all adenomatous tissue in FAP patients, and the aim of surveillance is to sample tissue to detect advancement to high-grade dysplasia. Larger lesions (>1 cm) are more likely to contain foci of high-grade dysplasia or malignancy. Depending on the degree of adenoma burden, we perform ablation of lesions larger than 5 mm and resection of ampullary adenomas greater than 1 cm. Sporadic adenomas occur as isolated lesions, and the aim of surveillance is to detect recurrence at a previous site of therapy.

The optimal time interval for surveillance in FAP patients remains to be determined. Spigelman and coworkers[54] retrospectively developed a scoring system to determine which patients are most likely to progress to malignancy and warrant more intense surveillance (see **Table 34.1**). Some authors have recommended surveillance intervals based on the Spigelman scoring system: 5 years for Spigelman stage 0–1, 3 years for stage 2, 1 to 2 years for stage 3, and consideration for surgery for stage 4.[55] In addition to the Spigelman stage, other authors

have modified this surveillance regimen based on the presence of any dysplasia.[19] Endoscopic surveillance should also include examination of the papilla with a side-viewing duodenoscope. Video capsule endoscopy for Spigelman stages 3 and 4 has also been suggested, but push enteroscopy during surveillance of the ampulla could be performed at the same endoscopic session.

Therapy

Endoscopic therapy for ampullary adenomas is a minimally invasive alternative to major abdominal surgery. The ideal technique for endoscopic therapy for periampullary adenomas has not been established. Excision has the advantage of submitting en bloc tissue for histologic examination followed by tissue ablation of residual adenoma at the conclusion of the initial endoscopic session and at follow-up examinations. Preliminary data from our series of 50 patients comprising FAP patients and patients with sporadic ampullary adenoma suggest that a positive resection margin or suspected residual adenoma treated predominantly with argon plasma coagulation at the index ampullectomy session does not preclude adenoma-free follow-up, owing mostly to vigilant surveillance and ablation techniques.[56]

The first step in endoscopic removal of the ampulla includes assessment of any intraductal extension of the adenoma, size, and endoscopic appearance that may suggest disease not amendable to resection (e.g., a firm, fixed lesion). If the lesion extends into the third layer of the duodenal wall or if it constitutes greater than 50% of the duodenal circumference, it is unlikely to be definitively treated with endoscopic treatment. The presence of these lesions can be determined by ERCP, EUS, and careful side-viewing duodenoscopy. Endoscopic removal of the ampulla may be performed either in a single piece (snare ampullectomy) or using a piecemeal resection technique.

Snare Excision

Snare excision removes the tumor en bloc (see **Fig. 34.1**). This technique has an advantage over piecemeal resection or preresection sphincterotomy by limiting cautery effect during histologic interpretation and potentially achieving a more accurate assessment of margin status. The procedure may be preceded by submucosal lift to raise the tumor. We add methylene blue to the solution, which enhances margin detection. Preresection cholangiopancreatography assists in assessing intraductal extension and provides a road map for pancreatic duct orifice identification and access after en bloc resection.

We prefer to perform postresection biliary and pancreatic sphincterotomies potentially to reduce subsequent orifice stenoses followed by prophylactic pancreatic and, when necessary, biliary stent placement. A concern with en bloc resection is the inability to identify the pancreatic orifice after ampullectomy. Methylene blue mixed in the contrast solution during pancreatography may assist in pancreatic orifice detection after resection. Other investigators have used indigo carmine staining to locate the pancreatic orifice.[57,58] Obtaining initial pancreatic duct access, advancement of a snare over an intraductal guidewire followed by en bloc resection has been described to permit prophylactic stent placement.[59] Whether this technique reduces pancreatitis complications compared with a conventional en bloc resection technique requires further study.

Piecemeal Resection

After cholangiopancreatography and dual biliary and pancreatic sphincterotomy (or pancreatic sphincterotomy alone), pancreatic stent insertion is performed. For smaller adenomas, extension of the sphincterotomies to the upper margin of the adenoma or to normal mucosa is attempted. Tissue is raised with a submucosal "lift," and the adenoma is snared piecemeal. A potential concern with this technique is residual adenoma. Caution is required when using cautery techniques, such as argon plasma coagulation, to ablate residual tissue around the pancreatic orifice. During endoscopic follow-up, a guidewire left within the pancreatic duct during side-by-side cautery ablation in this area may permit ablation and preserve access for prophylactic stent placement (personal observation). Given its relatively shallow depth of injury, argon plasma coagulation may be an attractive method for destroying residual tissue.[60]

Efficacy

We reviewed the medical literature on endoscopic snare resection of the ampulla. We searched PubMed for a combination

of key words: "ampullary adenoma," "ampullary tumor," "ampullary neoplasm," "ampullectomy," "endoscopic resection," and "papillectomy." Only published series with at least 10 subjects were included. Overall percentages are tabulated from the studies in which specific numbers are reported. In the last decade (2000–2009), 18 published series were found comprising 704 patients undergoing endoscopic snare resection of ampullary tumors.[52,57,58,61-75] **Table 34.2** summarizes these studies. The median number of patients in these studies was 23. Resected lesions ranged in size from 5 to 70 mm. When reported, patients with FAP or Gardner's syndrome constituted approximately 21% of study subjects. Adenocarcinoma found within resection specimens ranged from 0% to 47%[62] in these individual studies. This large variation largely depends on patient selection.

Thermal therapies (e.g., argon plasma coagulation, monopolar coagulation, snare tip cautery, or neodymium:yttrium-aluminum-garnet laser) have been reported as adjunctive therapy during the initial ampullectomy session. Thermal therapies were used in all but 1 of 14 evaluable studies.[57] Catalano and coworkers[69] reported a trend toward higher recurrence rates when index ampullectomy was performed without adjunctive ablative therapy. These methods are frequently used for retreatment of the ampullectomy site at follow-up.

Patient selection for endoscopic resection is necessary to optimize results. Generally, endoscopic snare resection was not attempted for distal biliary or pancreatic duct involvement; larger size (>3 cm); circumferential involvement of the duodenum; lateral extension; duodenal infiltration; endoscopic features of malignancy (spontaneous bleeding, friability, ulceration, depressed areas, erythema, or induration; **Fig. 34.3**); nonlifting after submucosal injection; histologic diagnosis of malignancy; coagulopathy; or significant comorbid conditions precluding a safe procedure. High-grade dysplasia without frank malignancy has not been considered a contraindication to endoscopic resection in most studies.

In one of the largest series to date, Irani and colleagues[63] evaluated 168 patients with ampullary lesions; 112 adenomas and 38 adenocarcinomas were found (18 nonadenomatous lesions were diagnosed and excluded from the analysis). Of patients, 41 (27.3%) were referred to surgery without ampullectomy. Of surgically treated patients, 20 patients had malignant mucosal biopsy specimens, 9 malignancies were identified at surgical resection, and 12 were large adenomas (of which two-thirds had high-grade dysplasia). Of the 150 patients with adenomatous lesions, 102 underwent endoscopic resection of the ampullary lesion. On univariate analysis, size smaller than 2 cm, younger age, absence of dilated ducts, and lack of lateral extension were factors affecting success of resection. On multivariate analysis, only size smaller than 2 cm and absence of dilated ducts were predictive of technically successful endoscopic resection.

With respect to resection technique, most studies have attempted en bloc removal of ampullary neoplasia for lesions smaller than 2 cm, whereas larger lesions often required piecemeal removal. In four studies that specifically described en bloc resection, success was achieved in 71.5% overall (range 54.5% to 94.4%).[58,61,70,75] In a study specifically describing piecemeal resection, Desilets and associates[72] described preampullectomy pancreatic sphincterotomy or stent placement and biliary sphincterotomy before resection in 13 patients (**Fig. 34.4**). After a mean of 2.7 procedures (mean follow-up

Table 34.2 Summary of Studies

First Author, Location, Year	No. Patients	Mean/ Median Size (mm)	FAP and Gardner's Syndrome	Resection Technique	Carcinoma	Pancreatitis	Complications			Technical Success	Mean/ Median Follow-up (mo)	Recurrence	Papillary Stenosis
							Bleeding	Perforation	Cholangitis				
Yamao, Japan, 2010[75]	36	14.3	11.0%	En bloc	22.2%	8.3%	8.3%	0.0%	0.0%	80.6%	17.9	3.4%	2.8%
Jung, Korea, 2009[61]	22	18	NA	En bloc	40.9%	18.2%	4.5%	4.5%	NA	77.3%	9.5	14.3%	NA
Boix, Spain, 2009[62]	21	10.0–50	9.5%	En bloc	47.6%	19.0%	4.8%	0.0%	NA	28.6%	15.9	16.7%	0.0%
Irani, U.S., 2009[63]	102	24	16.7%	En bloc (<2 cm)	7.8%	9.8%	4.9%	2.0%	1.0%	84.3%	34.7	7.8%	2.9%
Itoi, Japan, 2009[64]	14	14.1	25.0%	En bloc	7.1%	7.1%	14.3%	7.1%	NA	71.4%	NA	NA	NA
Eswaran, U.S., 2006[65]	37	10->50	32.3%	En bloc or piecemeal	5.9%	2.0%	7.8%	0.0%	NA	92.2%	NA	NA	NA
Katsinelos, Greece, 2006[57]	14	14.4	28.6%	Piecemeal for >2 cm	21.4%	7.1%	7.1%	0.0%	0.0%	78.6%	28.4	0.0%	NA
Bohnacker, Germany, 2005[66]	106	20	5.7%	Piecemeal for >2 cm	3.7%	12.3%	NA	NA	NA	73.0%	43	14.2%	NA
Han, Korea, 2005[67]	22	10.3	4.5%	Piecemeal for >2 cm	9.1%	0.0%	18.2%	4.5%	4.5%	72.7%	8.4	4.5%	4.5%
Harewood, U.S., 2005[68]	19	NA	NA	En bloc	NA	15.8%	NA	NA	NA	NA	NA	NA	NA
Catalano, U.S., 2004[69]	103	22.8	30.1%	Piecemeal for >2 cm	5.8%	4.9%	1.9%	NA	NA	80.6%	36	9.7%	2.9%
Cheng, U.S., 2004[70]	55	15	25.5%	En bloc or piecemeal	9.1%	9.1%	7.3%	1.8%	NA	100.0%	30	33.3%	3.6%
Kahaleh, U.S., 2004[52]	56	22.2	NA	En bloc or piecemeal	35.7%	7.1%	3.6%	NA	1.8%	85.7%	NA	NA	NA
Saurin, France, 2003[58]	24	16.5	0.0%	En bloc or piecemeal	0.0%	16.7%	12.5%	4.2%	NA	66.7%	81.7	6.3%	NA
Norton, U.S., 2002[71]	26	NA	57.7%	NA	3.6%	14.3%	7.1%	3.6%	NA	100.0%	13	9.5%	7.1%
Desilets, U.S., 2001[72]	13	21.5	53.8%	Piecemeal	0.0%	7.7%	0.0%	0.0%	0.0%	92.3%	19	0.0%	NA
Zadorova, Czech, 2001[73]	16	20–70	10.0%	En bloc	0.0%	12.5%	12.5%	0.0%	NA	100.0%	NA	18.8%	NA
Vogt, Germany, 2000[74]	18	15	NA	En bloc or piecemeal	0.0%	11.1%	11.1%	NA	NA	100.0%	75	44.4%	NA
Total	714		20.7%		11.9%	9.2%	6.8%	1.9%	1.2%	82.1%		12.1%	3.3%

FAP, familial adenomatous polyposis; NA, not available.

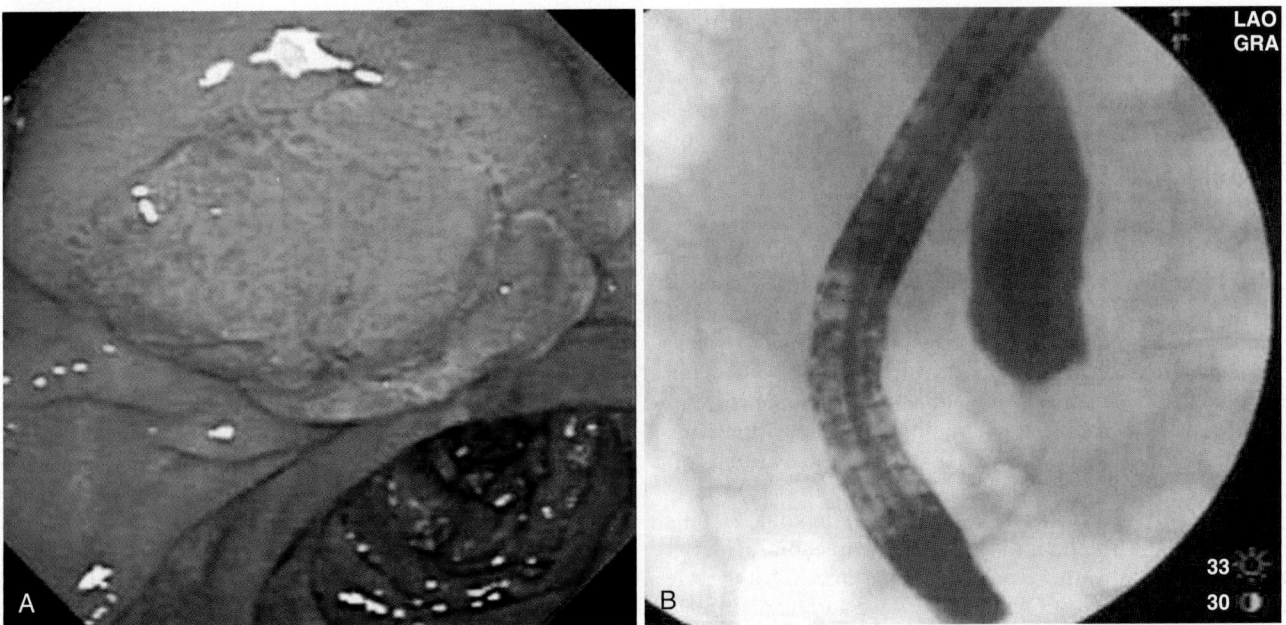

Fig. 34.3 Ampullary adenoma not amendable to resection. **A,** Firm and fixed texture. **B,** Endoscopic retrograde cholangiopancreatography (ERCP) showing distal biliary stricture.

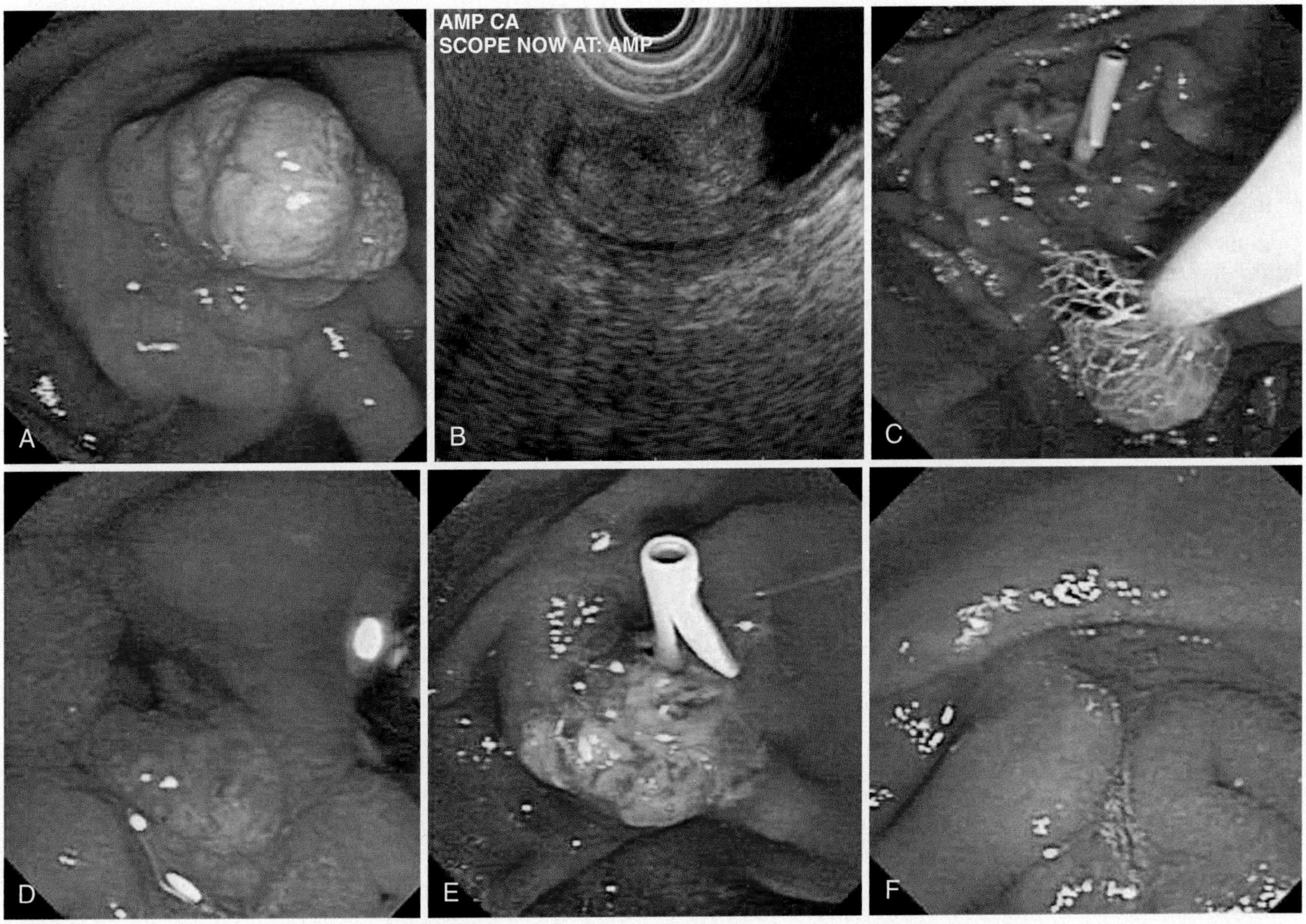

Fig. 34.4 Biductal sphincterotomies and pancreatic stent performed before ampullectomy. **A,** Polypoid ampullary adenoma. **B,** Endoscopic ultrasound (EUS) revealing adenoma limited to mucosa. **C,** Resection after biductal sphincterotomies and prophylactic pancreatic stent placement. **D** and **E,** Residual adenoma seen adjacent to pancreatic orifice on 1-month follow-up requiring argon plasma coagulation ablation and repeat prophylactic pancreatic stent placement. **F,** No residual adenoma found on surveillance biopsy specimens at 3-month follow-up.

19 months), 92% were disease-free. One patient developed mild pancreatitis.

Overall, of the studies reviewed, technical success of endoscopic resection of ampullary lesions was approximately 84% (range 28% to 100%) in individual studies depending on inclusion criteria and definitions of success. The inclusion criteria ranged from assessment following the index procedure alone to multiple treatments including adjunctive thermal ablative therapy to a negative resection margin alone. At follow-up (range 16 to 81 months), approximately 73% of patients were adenoma-free after endoscopic resection and adjunctive ablation. Patient selection was another key variable in the reported wide range for success among studies. Boix and associates[62] reported only 28.6% endoscopic success related mostly to inclusion of a high proportion of patients with carcinoma (10 of 21 [47.6%]) and intraductal extension (all of which failed endoscopic resection).

No definitive surveillance schedule after endoscopic ampullectomy has been established. After completion of serial endoscopic therapy to achieve adenoma-free histology, we suggest 6-month and subsequently annual to biennial intervals. Surveillance intervals in other series of endoscopic ampullectomies have varied. The median initial follow-up procedure for these studies was begun at 3 months. Subsequent surveillance procedures were most often scheduled every 3 months for at least 1 year. Of the studies reviewed, 12.1% (range 0% to 19%) of patients had recurrence treated mostly with repeat endoscopic resection or thermal ablation or both. The need for surgery after endoscopic ampullectomy was noted in approximately 16% (range 3% to 71%) of patients.

Endoscopic Complications

Complications of endoscopic snare resection of ampullary lesions have been classified as early or late. Early complications include bleeding, perforation, pancreatitis, and cholangitis. Late complications include papillary orifice stenoses. In the studies reviewed, bleeding has been reported in approximately 6% of patients, ranging from 0% to 18% requiring endoscopic hemostasis or transfusions. Perforation has been reported in approximately 2% (range 0% to 7%) of patients. Cholangitis has been reported in approximately 1% (range 0% to 4.5%) of patients. Only one mortality has been reported in the 18 studies.[52]

The most frequent complication with snare ampullectomy is acute pancreatitis. The studies reviewed reported pancreatitis in approximately 9% (range 0% to 19%) of patients. The only reported death from the reviewed ampullectomy series was due to complications of severe pancreatitis.[52] Although many series have reported routine pancreatic stent placement with ampullectomy, there is only one study to date that prospectively evaluated the effect of pancreatic stent placement on postresection pancreatitis. Harewood and colleagues[68] randomly assigned 19 consecutive patients undergoing en bloc resection of the ampulla to either pancreatic stent placement after ampullectomy or no pancreatic stent. Of 19 patients, 10 received a 5-Fr pancreatic stent after snare resection. Postresection pancreatitis occurred in three patients, all in the nonstent group ($P = .02$), with a median hospitalization of 2 days (range 1 to 6 days). Although our experience suggests that stent placement does not prevent pancreatitis, it is likely that it may help prevent severe pancreatitis. We prefer to place stents with an internal flange (one internal and two external or one internal with a full external pigtail) to reduce the risk of premature migration or dislodgment in the setting of a postprocedural bleeding event.

Surgical Therapy

Pancreaticoduodenectomy, pancreas-preserving duodenectomy, and surgical ampullectomy are surgical options for removal of ampullary and periampullary lesions and depend on depth and degree of adenoma burden or histology. These procedures are associated with significant morbidity and mortality.

Winter and associates[76] reported 450 patients who underwent surgical treatment. Of these patients, 77% had ampullary adenocarcinoma (41.1% of which had T2 disease). Almost 97% of the patients underwent pancreaticoduodenectomy (96.1% with R0 resection), and approximately 3% underwent surgical ampullectomy. Metastasis to regional lymph nodes (N1) was noted in 54.5%. Morbidity after surgery was reported in 52.2% for pancreaticoduodenectomy and 33.3% for ampullectomy ($P = .15$). The most common complications with pancreaticoduodenectomy included pancreatic leak (20.7%), delayed gastric emptying (16.0%), and wound infection (11.1%). Postoperative mortality was 2.1%.

Yoon and coworkers[77] reported their results for ampullectomy for early ampullary cancer. In their study, 98 patients underwent conventional Whipple's pancreaticoduodenectomy, 100 patients underwent pylorus-preserving pancreaticoduodenectomy, and 3 patients underwent pancreatic head resection with segmental duodenectomy. R0 resection was achieved in 95.5% of patients. Two deaths occurred (1%) from bleeding and sepsis. Postsurgical complications were experienced in 33.8%, including pancreatic fistula (9.5%), wound infection (6.5%), delayed gastric emptying (5.5%), bleeding (5.5%), intraabdominal abscess, biliary fistula, pneumonia, pleural effusion, and ileus. Lymph node metastasis in this select surgical series was high (33.3%).

Surgical ampullectomy is not a new technique, having been reported for ampullary lesions by Halsted in 1899 and used as a less invasive surgical alternative to pancreaticoduodenectomy.[40,42,78–80] Transduodenal resection may be inadequate therapy in many patients. Recurrence of benign adenomas has been reported in 25% to 33%.[40,42,80] FAP patients are a particularly difficult treatment group. Recurrent duodenal adenomas after transduodenal resection (mean recurrence in 13 months) led one group to conclude that this is inadequate therapy for these patients.[81] The potential for desmoid formation after surgery is another factor favoring the use of nonsurgical (i.e., endoscopic) techniques.

Grobmyer and colleagues[82] reported on their experience of surgical ampullectomy for 29 patients with preoperative adenoma ($n = 26$) and carcinoid ($n = 3$). However, 4 (13.7%) of the 29 patients were found to have carcinoma on surgical pathology and subsequently required pancreaticoduodenectomy. Morbidity was experienced by 45% and included wound infection, pneumonia, pancreatitis, pancreatic or biliary fistula, abdominal abscess, delayed gastric emptying, *Clostridium difficile* colitis, and deep vein thrombosis. There was one death (3.4%). Recurrence of adenoma was noted in 8%.

For patients with advanced ampullary disease who are inappropriate candidates for surgical or endoscopic therapy or have significant comorbidities precluding definitive resection, endoscopic palliation can be offered. Biliary or pancreatic obstruction from the mass lesion can lead to cholangitis, choledocholithiasis, pancreatitis, and small bowel obstruction with large mass lesions or infiltration of the duodenal wall by tumor. Stent placement across an obstructed lumen or for ductal decompression can be performed in the appropriate clinical setting.

Pharmacologic Treatment

A randomized controlled study showed that sulindac slows the progression of polyps in the colon of patients with FAP syndrome.[83] Similar findings have been reported with the use of the cyclooxygenase-2 (COX-2)–specific drug celecoxib.[84] A randomized placebo-controlled trial showed that celecoxib was an effective chemoprotective agent against sporadic colorectal adenomas[85]; however, it was associated with significant cardiovascular events. There is less compelling evidence for the use of nonsteroidal antiinflammatory drugs for progression of duodenal disease. The St. Mark's group randomly assigned 24 patients with advanced duodenal disease to sulindac, 200 mg twice daily, or placebo.[86] After 6 months of treatment, there was a reduction in epithelial proliferation in the sulindac group but no significant regression of large polyps. However, blinded review of videotapes showed significant regression of small polyps (<2 mm) compared with the placebo group.

This evidence supports the hypothesis that sulindac may also have an effect on polyp proliferation in the duodenum; however, it is unknown whether this would translate into a clinically significant benefit. The FAP Study Group randomly assigned 83 patients to one of two celecoxib groups (100 mg twice daily or 400 mg twice daily) or placebo.[87] Blinded, shuffled review of surveillance endoscopy by five panelists found a significant reduction in duodenal polyposis after 6 months of treatment with celecoxib, 400 mg twice daily. The cardiovascular toxicity of COX-2 inhibitors is well publicized, however, and use of these agents as chemopreventive agents must be cautiously considered.

Summary

Although randomized trials are lacking, there is an expanding body of literature supporting the use of endoscopic therapy to manage ampullary and periampullary adenoma as a minimally invasive option with lower morbidity compared with surgical therapy. Success and complications depend on careful patient selection, pretherapy assessment of disease extent, and endoscopist experience.

Acknowledgment

We would like to thank Drs. Ian Norton and David Koorey for their work on this chapter in the previous edition.

References

The complete reference list is available online at www.expertconsult.com.

Chapter **35**

Colorectal Cancer Screening and Surveillance

David Lieberman

Introduction

Colorectal cancer (CRC) is the second leading cause of cancer death in North America and Western Europe. Worldwide, there are more than 1 million new cases per year and more than 500,000 deaths. In the United States, 146,970 new cases and nearly 50,000 deaths were estimated to occur in 2009, representing about 14% of cancer deaths.[1] In their lifetime, 5% to 6% of adults develop CRC.

Survival is directly related to stage at diagnosis. Stage 1 (limited to mucosal and submucosa) has a 5-year survival of nearly 100%. Stage 2 (penetration to muscularis or serosa) has a 5-year survival of 80%. Stage 3 (lymph node involvement) has a 5-year survival of 30% to 70%. Finally, stage 4 (distant metastases) has very low 5-year survival. Early discovery improves survival. Because CRC is usually asymptomatic until late stage disease, the key to early discovery is the identification with screening of high-risk patients before symptoms develop.

Population-based screening can be costly and ineffective. Ideal screening employs relatively simple, inexpensive tests to risk-stratify patients followed by sensitive tests directed at individuals with highest risk. The criteria for population-based screening include factors summarized in **Table 35.1**. There is compelling evidence that population-based screening can reduce the incidence of and mortality from CRC.[2–5] Although there is considerable variation in screening recommendations in high-risk countries, some form of screening is recommended in Europe, Canada, Australia, and the United States.

Since 1985, there has been a slow but steady decline in CRC incidence in the United States. During this time period, screening rates have gradually increased to more than 50% of the U.S. population older than 50 years. From 2000–2005, the incidence of CRC declined by 6% in men and 9.4% in women. The annual percent reduction in mortality from 2002–2004 was 4.7%.[1]

Several different screening programs exist, each with advantages, limitations, and degrees of uncertainty. All CRC screening programs share a common final pathway for the evaluation of positive tests: colonoscopy. The role of endoscopy in colon

Table 35.1 Case for Screening

Criteria	Colorectal Cancer
Disease is common	5%-6% lifetime risk
Early detection can prevent mortality	5-yr survival
	Stage I: near 100%
	Stage II: 80%
	Stage III: 30%-70%
	Stage IV: 10%
Screening methods are shown to be effective	See text
	FOBT RCTs
	Sigmoidoscopy and colonoscopy case-control studies
Resources are available to provide screening in U.S.	FOBT: Yes; primary care setting
	Sigmoidoscopy: Yes; primary care or specialty clinic
	CT colonography: No; limited centers and fully trained radiologists
	Colonoscopy: Uncertain capacity (see text)
Resources are available to provide diagnostic tests for patients with positive screening	Colonoscopy resources are generally available if initial screening test positive
Screening is cost-effective	Models show cost-effectiveness
Screening methods are accepted by patients and providers	Yes: 50% adherence in U.S.

CT, computed tomography; FOBT, fecal occult blood test; RCT, randomized controlled trial.

Table 35.2 Probability of Invasive Colorectal Cancer by Age and Gender

	Male	Female
<40 yr	0.08 (1/1329)	0.07 (1/1394)
40–59 yr	0.92 (1/109)	0.72 (1/138)
60–69 yr	1.60 (1/63)	1.12 (1/89)
≥70 yr	4.78 (1/21)	4.30 (1/23)
Lifetime	5.65 (1/18)	5.23 (1/19)
Risk of death	2.45 (1/41)	2.45 (1/41)

Data from Jemal A, Siegel R, Ward E, et al: Cancer statistics 2009. CA Cancer J Clin 59:225–249, 2009.

Table 35.3 Incidence and Mortality of Colorectal Cancer by Race and Ethnicity

	Incidence*		Mortality*	
Race	Male	Female	Male	Female
White	58.9	43.2	22.1	15.3
Black	71.2	54.5	31.8	22.4
Asian	48.0	35.4	14.4	10.2
Native American	46.0	41.2	20.5	14.2
Hispanic	47.3	32.8	16.5	10.8
All	59.2	43.8	22.7	15.9

*Per 100,000 population.
Data from Jemal A, Siegel R, Ward E, et al: Cancer statistics 2009. CA Cancer J Clin 59:225–249, 2009.

cancer detection and prevention is paramount. Effective CRC screening depends on the availability of high-quality colonoscopy. This chapter discusses the epidemiology and pathogenesis of CRC and reviews the rationale for screening and surveillance in both high-risk groups and average-risk individuals.

Epidemiology of Colorectal Cancer

Age, Gender, and Race and Ethnicity

CRC represents the third most common form of cancer (excluding skin) among men and women and is the second leading cause of cancer death overall in the United States. There is a progressive increase in risk associated with age (**Table 35.2**). Age-adjusted incidence and mortality of CRC are higher in men. There is some evidence that natural premenopausal hormones or postmenopausal hormone replacement therapy may exert some protective effect in women.[6,7]

There is strong evidence that African American men and women are more likely to die from CRC than whites (**Table 35.3**).[1] African Americans are more likely to have advanced lesions at the time of diagnosis[8] and are more likely to have proximal CRC compared with other races.[9,10] The reasons for increased mortality in African Americans are unknown. Delays in diagnosis could be due to socioeconomic status or poor access to health care, although some compelling data suggest that there are biologic differences.[11,12] In a study of white and African American patients undergoing screening colonoscopy, African American men and women had higher age-adjusted prevalence of polyps larger than 9 mm.[8] These data support the hypothesis of biologic differences.

Variation by Country

Incidence rates vary around the world. The highest risk is in North America, Western Europe, Australia, New Zealand, Israel, and Japan (mortality 30 to 60 per 100,000). The lowest risk is found in India and most of Africa (mortality <10 per 100,000). Migrant studies have found rapid changes in incidence rates, suggesting that the disease is very sensitive to changes in environment. Incidence rates reach the levels of the host country within one or two generations.

Lifestyle and Medications

There is strong epidemiologic evidence that lifestyle factors have an impact on CRC risk. Diets that are high in fat and low in fiber and calcium may be associated with increased risk. Obesity, metabolic syndrome, low levels of physical activity, tobacco smoking, and heavy alcohol consumption have been associated with an increased risk of CRC. There is no evidence that modification of these factors reduces CRC risk; however, changes in most of these behaviors are generally good for overall health. There is strong evidence that individuals taking nonsteroidal antiinflammatory drugs and aspirin have a lower risk of developing colon adenomas and CRC.[13] However, these drugs have significant adverse effects, and are not recommended for routine CRC prevention.

Polyps and Colorectal Cancer Risk

Most CRC develops from adenoma precursors. Adenoma prevalence increases steadily with age and exceeds 35% in adults older than 75 years. There is a 5% to 6% lifetime risk of CRC, so most patients with adenomas apparently do not develop clinically detectable cancer during their lifetime. Polyp size and histology are directly associated with malignant risk. The risk of high-grade dysplasia in polyps smaller than 5 mm is 1.1%; for polyps 5 to 9 mm, the risk is 4.6%; and in polyps larger than 9 mm, the risk is 20%.[14] The risk of invasive cancer is less than 1% in polyps smaller than 1 cm and greater than 10% in larger polyps.[15] These data suggest that patients most likely to develop cancer are patients with advanced adenomas. Evidence from the National Polyp Study[16] supports the hypothesis that detection and removal of adenomas may prevent cancer incidence. All of these data have important implications for screening. Screening efforts directed at advanced adenomas would target patients with the greatest risk and potentially lead to significant reductions in cancer incidence.

Pathogenesis

Several genetic pathways may result in the development of adenomas and CRC. In 1990, a stepwise model of chromosomal instability was proposed by Fearon and Vogelstein.[17] More than 80% of sporadic CRC is associated with mutation of the adenomatous polyposis coli (*APC*) gene on chromosome 5. The mutation of this tumor suppressor gene most likely promotes the development of adenomas. In familial adenomatous polyposis (FAP), there is a germline mutation of this gene. Normally, this gene acts to phosphorylate beta-catenin, which leads to its destruction. Accumulation of beta-catenin leads to unregulated cell proliferation and suppression of apoptosis.[18,19] The progression of adenoma to cancer seems to require additional mutations (K-*ras*, chromosome 18, *TP53*). The observation that not all tumors acquire the same mutations strongly suggests that there are several genetic pathways to malignant invasion.

A second genetic pathway (15% to 20%) of sporadic cancer is due to mutation of mismatch repair genes.[20] These genes normally repair errors in DNA replication. Germline mutations are found in patients with hereditary nonpolyposis colorectal cancer syndrome (HNPCC). The key feature of this mutation in HNPCC is rapid development of polyps that progress to malignancy. In sporadic cancers, acquired mutation of these genes leads to microsatellite instability and malignant progression. Patients with large serrated adenomas

in the proximal colon may have *BRAF* mutations and hypermethylation, which may result in microsatellite instability and progression to malignancy.[21]

Another germline mutation in a base-excision repair gene, *MYH*, has been associated with recessive inheritance of multiple colorectal adenomas. The typical phenotype is a patient with 15 or more adenomas and no germline *APC* mutation.[22]

High-Risk Groups

Recognition of inherited syndromes and other high-risk diseases associated with CRC is key to appropriate screening and management (**Table 35.4**). It is important for primary care providers to recognize these syndromes and refer patients for appropriate screening and surveillance.

Perhaps the most important questions in the medical history are the following: (1) "Do you have a first-degree relative with CRC?" (2) "If yes, did any relative have cancer before age 50 years?" Patients with an index relative younger than 50 years old should be considered at risk for an inherited syndrome and warrant intensive screening at a young age. Recommendations for specific syndromes are summarized in **Table 35.4**.

Inherited Polyposis Syndromes

Patients with FAP have a germline mutation of *APC* on chromosome 5, predisposing them to adenoma formation. Most affected patients have more than 100 adenomas. All affected individuals (100%) develop CRC, and when the phenotype is recognized, colectomy should be considered. The average age of adenoma appearance is 16 years, and the age of CRC appearance is 39 years. In a variant of this syndrome, called *attenuated FAP*, mutations occur at either the 5′ or 3′ end of the gene. Phenotypically, patients have fewer polyps, with delayed onset of adenoma and cancer formation. Familial colon cancer in Ashkenazi Jews may be the result of a specific germline mutation of the *APC* gene (I1307K). This mutation seems to predispose to sporadic mutations at distant sites resulting in a high malignant risk.[19]

Family members should be advised to have genetic counseling and testing. Current tests detect 80% to 90% of FAP families. If the index patient has a retained rectum after subtotal colectomy, screening with sigmoidoscopy every 6 to 12 months is recommended. Index patients are at risk for other malignancies, the most common of which is duodenal or periampullary cancer (5% to 12% lifetime risk). Upper endoscopy with side-viewing instruments to visualize the ampulla is recommended beginning at age 20 to 25 years and should be repeated every 1 to 3 years. There is evidence that colon adenomas regress with cyclooxygenase-2 selective inhibition. Many experts recommend that patients use cyclooxygenase-2 inhibitors after colectomy, hoping to reduce the risk of upper gastrointestinal malignancy.

MYH-associated polyposis leads to development of multiple polyps that may be adenomatous or hyperplastic. Mutations of the *MutY human homolog (MYH)* gene, which encodes a member of the base excision repair system, occur. This system normally protects cells against the mutagenic effects of aerobic metabolism. Inheritance is autosomal recessive and

Table 35.4 Risk Stratification

Inherited Risk	Genetic Mutation	Lifetime Risk of CRC	Percentage of All CRC	Screening Recommendation
HIGH RISK				
FAP	*APC*	100%	1%	(1) Sigmoidoscopy in teenage years; (2) genetic screening can be considered; (3) colectomy if phenotype confirmed
HNPCC	Mismatch repair genes	80%	2%	(1) Colonoscopy beginning in 3rd decade at 2-yr intervals; (2) genetic screening can be considered; (3) awareness of extracolonic cancers
MYH-associated polyposis	*MYH*	Uncertain	Uncertain	Should be considered in polyposis syndrome if testing for FAP negative
Peutz-Jeghers syndrome	*STK11*	2%–13%	<1%	(1) Colonoscopy in teen years; (2) high risk for gastric and pancreatic malignancy
Juvenile polyposis	*SMAD4; DPC4*	Up to 50%	<1%	Colonoscopy in teen years
MODERATE RISK				
Chronic ulcerative colitis or Crohn's colitis	—	Up to 30%	<1%	Colonoscopy every 2 yr beginning 8–10 yr after onset of disease
Familial risk	—	≥10%	15%–20%	Begin screening 10 yr younger than age of index family member; colonoscopy preferred
Personal history of breast, uterine, ovarian cancer	—	Uncertain	<1%	No specific recommendation
AVERAGE RISK				
Age >50 yr with no family history of CRC	—	5%–6%	70%–75%	Begin screening at age 50 yr

CRC, colorectal cancer; FAP, familial adenomatous polyposis; HNPCC, hereditary nonpolyposis colorectal cancer.

should be considered in patients with 10 to 100 adenomas or hyperplastic polyps who have negative genetic testing for FAP.[22]

Hereditary Nonpolyposis Colorectal Cancer Syndrome

HNPCC accounts for about 2% of all colon cancers. Affected individuals inherit one of several mismatch repair gene mutations. There is evidence that regular screening of kindreds can substantially reduce the risk of CRC.[23] The clinical definitions have been modified over the years from the original Amsterdam criteria[24] to the Bethesda guidelines,[25] which provide a much less rigid clinical definition. Clinical suspicion should be high if there is a family member with CRC before age 50, multiple generations with CRC, and relatives with HNPCC-associated cancers (endometrium, small bowel, ureter, or renal pelvis). The findings of the Finnish Cancer Registry[26] reinforce the need to be aware of other cancers that may develop in these kindreds, including endometrial (60%); stomach (13%); ovary (12%); bladder, urethra, and ureter (4.0%); brain (3.7%); kidney (3.3%); and biliary tract and gallbladder (2.0%).

Patients who meet the Bethesda criteria should have genetic counseling. If the index family member has specific mismatch repair gene mutation, testing can be performed in other family members to determine who is at risk. Family members should have colonoscopy surveillance every 2 years beginning at age 20 to 25 years and then annually beginning at age 40 years. In addition, screening for upper gastrointestinal cancers with endoscopy and pelvic examinations with transvaginal ultrasound are recommended every 1 to 2 years.

Familial Risk

Epidemiologic data[27,28] show that individuals with a first-degree relative with CRC have an increased risk of CRC. Twin studies estimated that 35% of CRC arose from inherited factors and 65% arose from environmental factors.[29] A meta-analysis considered risk associated with familial risk.[30] The relative risk of CRC with an affected first-degree relative was 2.4. With more than one relative, the risk was 4.2. If CRC was diagnosed before age 45 years in the index family member, the relative risk was 3.8; diagnosis at age 45 to 59 years was associated with a relative risk of 2.2. If diagnosis was made after age 59 years, the relative risk was 1.8. The risk associated with second-degree relatives is less certain because this is difficult to study. An analysis from the Utah registry found a risk of 1.5 for patients with second-degree relatives with CRC.

Based on these data, family members should be screened with colonoscopy. If the index family member had cancer after age 60 years, screening should be initiated at age 50 years with colonoscopy and performed every 10 years if colonoscopy is negative. If the family member had cancer before age 60 years, screening should be initiated with colonoscopy at age 40 and then performed every 5 years. There is also evidence that family members of patients discovered to have adenomas before age 60 years may be at increased risk for CRC,[31] although this risk may be increased only if the index family member had advanced adenomas.[32]

Table 35.5 U.S. Colorectal Cancer Screening Recommendations for Average-Risk Individuals

Screening Test	ACS-MSTF-ACR	USPSTF	ACG	Recommended Interval
EARLY CANCER DETECTION TESTS				
gFOBT-SENSA	Yes	Yes	Yes	Annual
FIT—requires >50% sensitivity for CRC	Yes	Yes	Yes—preferred	Annual
Stool DNA—requires 50% sensitivity for CRC	Yes	No	Yes	ACS: uncertain ACG: 3 yr
CANCER PREVENTION TESTS				
	Cancer prevention tests preferred		Cancer prevention tests preferred	
Barium enema	Yes, but only if other tests unavailable	No	No	5 yr
CT colonography	Yes	No	Yes	5 yr
Flexible sigmoidoscopy	Yes—require insertion to 40 cm	Yes with FOBT every 3 yr	Yes	5 yr
Colonoscopy	Yes	Yes	Yes—preferred	10 yr

ACG, American College of Gastroenterology; ACS-MSTF-ACR, American Cancer Society–U.S. Multi-Society Task Force on Colorectal Cancer–American College of Radiology; CT, computed tomography; FIT, fecal immunochemical test; FOBT, fecal occult blood test; gFOBT, guaiac fecal occult blood test; USPSTF, U.S. Preventive Services Task Force.

Ulcerative Colitis and Crohn's Colitis

Although patients with inflammatory bowel disease represent less than 1% of all patients who develop CRC, patients with colitis represent a high-risk group. Risk is strongly associated with extent and duration of disease. The risk is very low in the first 8 years of disease. However, in patients with pancolitis, the risk increases by up to 0.5% to 1% per year so that after 35 years of disease, the cumulative risk of CRC may be 35%.[33] Patients with severe long-standing disease and primary sclerosing cholangitis may have a higher risk of developing CRC.[34]

Cancers that develop in patients with colitis are often flat and infiltrating, making endoscopic detection difficult. Current recommendations are to perform complete colonoscopy, beginning by year 8 of disease, and obtain four-quadrant biopsy specimens of otherwise flat mucosa at 10-cm intervals throughout the colon to detect dysplasia. Raised lesions require more intensive biopsy. There are data that patients with low-grade or high-grade dysplasia in flat mucosa have a high likelihood of having CRC, and colectomy is generally recommended. There is controversy regarding the approach to low-grade dysplasia. As patients age, they are likely to develop sporadic adenomas, which by definition are adenomas with low-grade dysplasia. Distinguishing a sporadic adenoma from a dysplasia-associated lesion or mass is often difficult. There is consensus that if a raised lesion is seen, a biopsy specimen of the lesion and surrounding flat mucosa should be obtained. If the surrounding mucosa is nondysplastic, it is assumed that the raised lesion is most likely a sporadic adenoma.

There are no randomized clinical trials to evaluate surveillance. There is some evidence that survival is better in patients enrolled in surveillance.[35] Recommendations to perform colonoscopy every 1 to 2 years for life are based on the steadily increasing cumulative risk of CRC with time. Patients with colitis limited to the rectum and left colon have a lower risk. Surveillance beginning at age 15 years is recommended.

Screening Strategies for Average-Risk Individuals

Screening recommendations for average-risk asymptomatic individuals vary around the world. In Asia, there are no specific guidelines. In Europe and Canada, most countries offer fecal occult blood test (FOBT), and some offer sigmoidoscopy (United Kingdom, Italy, Norway) or colonoscopy (Germany, Austria, Poland, Italy). In the United States, three guidelines[2–5] were published in 2008 and 2009 (**Table 35.5**).

Cancer screening is traditionally focused on early cancer detection (i.e., breast, prostate). However, because most CRC develops from adenoma precursors, there is an opportunity to prevent many cancers if precursor lesions are detected and removed.[16] More recent guidelines in the United States have preferred the use of tests that are likely to detect polyps and prevent cancer.[2,5]

Early Cancer Detection Tests

Fecal Occult Blood Test

Three randomized controlled trials showed that among patients who undergo FOBT compared with unscreened controls, cancers are discovered at an earlier stage, and mortality is reduced by 15% to 33%.[36–38] Standard guaiac fecal occult blood test (gFOBT) detects peroxidase activity of heme and is not specific for human blood. One-time testing with a standard guaiac test detects only 33% to 50% of patients with cancer (**Table 35.6**). A more sensitive guaiac test (SENSA) can detect more than 60% of patients with cancer (see **Table 35.6**).[2,4,39] Three separate stool samples per test have superior sensitivity compared with one or two samples. Patients with positive tests have a threefold to fourfold increased risk of cancer and should be referred for colonoscopy.

Table 35.6 Sensitivity (One-Time Test) of Colorectal Cancer Screening Tests

	Cancer	Advanced Adenomas*
STOOL-BASED TESTS		
Standard gFOBT[39,42,43]	33%–50%	11%
Sensitive gFOBT[2,4,39]	50%–75%	20%–25%
Fecal immunochemical test[3,5]	60%–85%	20%–50%
Stool DNA—old[42]	51%	18%
Stool DNA—new[43,44]	≥80%	40%
STRUCTURAL EXAMINATIONS OF COLON		
CT colonography[48]	Uncertain; likely >90%	90% if >10 mm
Sigmoidoscopy[55,57,58]	>95% distal colon	70%†
Colonoscopy[45–47]	>95%	88%–98%

CT, computed tomography; gFOBT, guaiac fecal occult blood test.
*Advanced adenoma defined as tubular adenoma ≥10 mm; adenoma with villous histology or high-grade dysplasia.
†Assumes that if an adenoma is detected in the distal colon, the patient would have complete colonoscopy, which would result in detection of some proximal advanced adenomas.
From Lieberman D: Screening for colorectal cancer. N Engl J Med 361:1179–1187, 2009.

Fecal immunochemical test uses antibodies specific to human hemoglobin, albumin, or other blood components and is more specific for human blood. There are many commercially available tests, most of which detect more than 50% of cancers with one-time testing. There are several uncertainties, including the number of stool samples, proper preservation of samples while awaiting testing, and the performance characteristics of the test in clinical practice.[39,40] It is unknown if fecal immunochemical test is superior to a less costly sensitive gFOBT.

Fecal blood testing has many important limitations. The detection rate for advanced adenomas is only 25% to 30%. One-time testing fails to identify most patients with important cancer precursor lesions. An effective program requires annual repeat testing for negative tests and referral for colonoscopy if tests are positive. Adherence in clinical practice is uncertain.[41] Although the initial cost of testing is low, efforts to ensure adherence to repeat testing, referral for colonoscopy, and the management of detected cancers contribute to the programmatic cost. Patients should understand the limitations of the test and the fact that many cancers and high-risk adenomas go undetected.

Stool DNA Test

Gene mutations associated with colonic neoplasia can be detected in stool samples. Proof of principle studies in a large screening cohort showed that more than 50% of cancers could be detected.[42] New versions of the test are promising but have not yet been evaluated in screening cohorts.[43,44] The stool DNA test fails to identify most patients with advanced neoplasia and should be viewed as an early cancer detection test.

Imaging Studies of the Colon

Barium enema accurately identifies late stage cancer but is a poor test for important cancer precursor lesions and is rarely used for colon cancer screening today. Imaging with *computed tomography (CT) colonography* has largely replaced barium enema. Helical CT scans render two-dimensional and three-dimensional images of the colon.[45–48] CT colonography can identify correctly 90% of patients with polyps 10 mm or larger with a false-positive rate of 14% when performed by properly trained radiologists.[48] Quality in other clinical practice settings is unknown.

CT colonography is a new technology with many uncertainties, as follows:

- *Who should be referred for colonoscopy?* There is consensus that all patients with polyps 6 mm or larger should be offered colonoscopy.[2] The management of patients with polyps 1 to 5 mm is controversial. CT colonography cannot accurately identify polyps of this size. Less than 2% of these patients have adenomas with advanced features, and cancer is rare.[49,50] No studies have shown the safety of following such patients with repeat CT colonography.
- *Detection of flat polyps with CT colonography is unknown, some of which may harbor malignancy.*[51]
- *Appropriate screening intervals after negative examinations or with possible polyps smaller than 6 mm are uncertain.*
- *Radiation exposure could increase the risk of developing cancers.*[52] Although low-dose regimens are used, there is concern about cumulative x-ray exposure, and some countries do not allow imaging for screening purposes.
- *The evaluation of extracolonic findings could be an important driver of cost.* Although 27% to 69% of persons screened with CT colonography have some other finding outside of the colon, most studies estimate that 5% to 16% of findings may be significant and require further evaluation.[2,4]
- *Cost-effectiveness is uncertain.* Several decision models find that screening with CT colonography would be costly. Key determinants of cost include the frequency of referral for colonoscopy and rate of evaluation for extracolonic findings.

Flexible Sigmoidoscopy

Case-control studies have found significant reduction in CRC mortality in patients who have undergone sigmoidoscopy—a benefit limited to the portion of the colon examined.[53] One small randomized trial showed a reduction in CRC incidence in patients exposed to sigmoidoscopy.[54] Screening colonoscopy studies show that sigmoidoscopy would fail to identify 30% or more of individuals with advanced neoplasia. There is evidence that sigmoidoscopy may be less effective with advancing age (>60 years old) because of higher prevalence of proximal neoplasia.[55] Large studies of sigmoidoscopy in the United States, United Kingdom, and Italy are not yet completed. Despite evidence of effectiveness, use of flexible sigmoidoscopy in the United States has declined over the past 10 years, coincident with the growth of screening colonoscopy.

Combined Flexible Sigmoidoscopy and Fecal Occult Blood Test

Although several cost-effectiveness analyses endorse the use of combined FOBT (annually) and sigmoidoscopy (every 5 years), there is little clinical experience with combined screening tests. The VA Cooperative Study[56] found that the combination of one-time sigmoidoscopy and FOBT would identify 76% of patients with advanced neoplasia, which represented only a small incremental improvement over sigmoidoscopy alone. There are no data regarding adherence to this complex screening program and no evidence that it is being used in clinical practice.

Colonoscopy

Colonoscopy is the most commonly used screening test in the United States. Worldwide experience has shown feasibility in different populations in North America, Asia, and Europe.[55,57–60] Among patients age 50 to 75 years being screened for the first time, 5% to 10% have advanced neoplasia, and 0.5% to 1.0% have cancer. Evidence from the National Polyp Study showed that detection and removal of adenomas could result in substantial reduction in incidence of CRC.[16] Case-control studies have shown that in patients exposed to colonoscopy, both CRC incidence and mortality are reduced.[61–63]

All of the current screening guidelines endorse the use of colonoscopy screening. Several important uncertainties remain, as follows:

- *Interval cancers may occur after colonoscopy*. In studies of patients with adenomas who had colonoscopy and polypectomy, 0.3% to 0.9% of patients developed cancer within 2 to 5 years of colonoscopy. There are several possible reasons. New fast-growing lesions with microsatellite instability may account for some interval lesions. Incomplete removal of neoplasia at baseline could lead to development of cancer at a prior polypectomy site. However, lesions missed at baseline colonoscopy represent the most common explanation in most interval cancers. Studies using CT colonography to evaluate optical colonoscopy showed that colonoscopy may miss 2% to 12% of polyps 10 mm or larger.[45–47] Flat lesions (see Chapter 36) may be difficult to detect at colonoscopy or incompletely visualized without chromoendoscopy.

- *The 10-year interval after a normal colonoscopy is based on expert opinion derived from indirect data*. Although case-control studies have suggested a 10-year benefit from endoscopic examinations of the colon, concerns about interval cancers noted previously have cast some doubt on whether a 10-year interval is appropriate for all patients. Studies of follow-up colonoscopy 5 years after a negative baseline screening examination reveal a low rate of advanced neoplasia.[64,65]

- *Quality in clinical practice is uncertain and may contribute to miss rates at colonoscopy*. Elements of quality[66] are summarized in **Box 35.1** and include both reporting indicators (does the element appear in the report, and is it reported in a reproducible manner) and performance indicators (examination completeness, polyp detection and removal, recommendations for follow-up, and adverse events). A study by the Clinical Outcomes Research Initiative[67] showed variability in reporting (despite use of a computerized report generator) and key outcomes such as completeness of examinations and polyp detection rates. Studies have shown that spending more time examining the colon during colonoscope withdrawal results in higher rates of polyp detection.[68] Further study is needed to validate key quality indicators.

New innovations in colonoscopy may make colonoscopy easier to perform (self-advancing instruments), able to view behind folds (3rd Eye, expanded wide vision angle), or detect polyps more accurately than white light alone (chromoendoscopy, narrow band imaging, autofluorescence). Further advances may enable "microscopic" endoscopy, which can characterize histologic features at the time of endoscopy. These innovations require further research.

Surveillance after Detection of Neoplasia

Surveillance after detection and removal of colon neoplasia (**Table 35.7**) should be viewed as part of a screening program. Recommendations for surveillance have an enormous impact on screening program cost and resource use.

Surveillance in Patients with Personal History of Colorectal Cancer

After the diagnosis and treatment of cancer, guidelines recommend surveillance colonoscopy within 1 year of curative resection, and every 3 to 5 years thereafter if the first colonoscopy is negative. This recommendation was based on a literature review of 24 studies, which found that 57 of 137 metachronous CRCs were found within 24 months of resection.[69] If a complete examination of the colon was impossible before treatment because of obstruction, a colonoscopy should be completed within 3 to 6 months of surgical treatment to rule out synchronous lesions.

Adenoma Surveillance

The rationale for surveillance after removal of adenomas is based on several lines of evidence, but connecting the dots of evidence is problematic. We know that patients with adenomas have an increased risk of developing CRC. Most CRC has

an adenoma precursor lesion. Numerous studies have shown that patients with adenomas who undergo colonoscopy and polypectomy have a high likelihood of having adenomas detected during follow-up examinations.[70] Some of these lesions may have been present at the baseline examination but may not have been detected or were incompletely removed, whereas others may represent new lesions. The rationale for adenoma surveillance is based on the premise that adenomas can develop into CRC and that after adenomas are removed at baseline colonoscopy, more adenomas are commonly found during follow-up examinations.

There are several flaws in this reasoning, however. In their lifetime, 30% to 50% of individuals develop adenomas and only 5% to 6% develop cancer. Most patients with adenomas do not develop cancer and would be unlikely to benefit from surveillance. How should patients who are likely to progress to malignancy (and benefit from surveillance) be identified? Risk stratification based on patient characteristics and the index polyp would be ideal. There is some preliminary evidence that patients who have only one or two small tubular adenomas are at low risk for development of new advanced adenomas during 5 to 6 years of follow-up.[55] Patients with multiple adenomas, large adenomas (≥10 mm), or adenomas with villous histology have a higher risk of having advanced adenomas during surveillance.[55,70,71] These data informed recommendations for adenoma surveillance, which are summarized in **Table 35.7**.[72]

Complications of Screening and Surveillance

Colon screening with fecal testing is not associated with direct adverse events. It may be argued, however, that failure to detect cancer if present results in delays in cancer diagnosis, which may adversely affect outcomes. Imaging studies with CT colonography or barium are rarely associated with adverse events in screening examinations. Perforations are uncommonly reported but have generally occurred in symptomatic patients. Sigmoidoscopy is also quite safe and rarely associated with perforation or bleeding. CT colonography and sigmoidoscopy are associated with some discomfort.

If the initial screening test is positive, all screening programs ultimately lead to colonoscopy. The safety of colonoscopy in diverse practice settings is uncertain. The overall rate of adverse events is 3 to 5 per 1000 colonoscopies.[73-83] The clinical studies summarized in **Table 35.8** have reported a limited set of adverse events, such as perforation (0.1 to 1 per 1000) and bleeding (0.5 to 6 per 1000). Most of these studies have included patients undergoing screening and diagnostic colonoscopy. Hospitalizations for other episodes such as cardiopulmonary events may occur in 1 in 1000 procedures and have been reported in a few studies. Few studies have fully evaluated events occurring within 30 days of colonoscopy.

Controversies in Screening and Surveillance

Age to Stop Screening

The 2008 U.S. Preventive Services Task Force guideline suggested that routine screening should stop at age 75 years and

Table 35.7 Surveillance Recommendations

Findings at Baseline Colonoscopy*	Recommended Interval for Colonoscopy
No polyps	10 yr
Hyperplastic polyps: rectum-sigmoid	10 yr
1–2 tubular adenomas <10 mm	5–10 yr
≥3 tubular adenomas	3 yr
Tubular adenoma ≥10 mm	3 yr
Adenoma with villous histology	3 yr
Adenoma with high-grade dysplasia*	3 yr
Invasive cancer†	1 yr
Incomplete removal of neoplastic lesion	3 mo

*Assumes complete examination to cecum, with preparation adequate to detect polyps >5 mm and complete removal of visible polyps.

†Assumes complete examination of the colon before resection of cancer. If complete examination was impossible, colonoscopy should be performed at 3 months to rule out synchronous lesions.

Data from Rex DK, Kahi CJ, Levin B, et al: Guidelines for colonoscopy surveillance after cancer resection: A consensus update by the American Cancer Society and the US Multi-Society Task Force on Colorectal Cancer. Gastroenterology 130:1865–1871, 2006; and Winawer SJ, Zauber AG, Fletcher RH, et al: Guidelines for colonoscopy surveillance after polypectomy: A consensus update by the US Multi-Society Task Force on Colorectal Cancer and the American Cancer Society. Gastroenterology 130:1872–1885, 2006.

Table 35.8 Serious Adverse Events of Colonoscopy: Studies from 2002–2009

Setting	Year	No.	Events per 1000 Colonoscopies		
			Bleeding	Perforation	Other Hospitalization*
VA Medical Centers, screening only, 30-day follow-up, U.S.[73]	2002	3196	1.9	0	1.0
Teaching hospital, Australia[74]	2003	23,508	2	1	—
Ambulatory surgical centers, U.S.[75]	2003	116,000	—	0.3	—
Medicare sample, age ≥65 yr, U.S.[76]	2003	39,286	—	2.0	—
Community, United Kingdom[77]	2004	9223	—	1.3	—
Community, Wisconsin, U.S.[78]	2006	12,407	2.0	0.16	—
HMO, California, U.S.[79]	2006	16,318	3.2	0.9	—
Community, screening only, Poland[60]	2006	50,148	0.26	0.1	0.7 hospitalizations
Outpatient, claims data, Ontario, Canada[80]	2008	97,091	1.6	0.85	—
Medicaid claims data, California[81]	2009	277,434	—	0.8	—
Claims data, 30-day follow-up, Manitoba, Canada[82]	2009	21,191	0.86	1.18	—
Medicare claims data, 30-day follow-up, U.S.[83]	2009	53,220; includes screening and diagnostic examinations	6.4	0.6	Cardiovascular events; increased only if polypectomy performed

*Other serious complications include cardiopulmonary and other events resulting in hospitalization.
Adapted from Lieberman D: Screening for colorectal cancer. N Engl J Med 361:1179–1187, 2009.

that no screening should be performed after age 85 years. This recommendation is based on a decision analysis that suggested benefit (prevention of colon cancer death) is reduced in elderly individuals, and potential for harm is increased. Nevertheless, CRC incidence and mortality continue to increase with advancing age. Many experts recommend that screening decisions be individualized based on patient comorbidity, likelihood of long-term survival, and a careful assessment of the risk of colonoscopy.

Customization of Screening

Women develop CRC and advanced neoplasia at a later age than men. The delay in onset of colon neoplasia may be related to natural hormonal protection before menopause or hormone replacement therapy after menopause. African Americans have a higher CRC incidence and mortality compared with whites[1] and have higher age-adjusted cancer precursor lesions compared with whites.[84] Current guidelines call for all men and women to be screened beginning at age 50 years, although one expert group advocated initiation of screening at age 45 for African Americans. There is a rational basis for considering customization of screening for women (delay initiation) and for African Americans (early initiation). However, there is also concern that current screening guidelines are complex and that adding another

layer of complexity with customization could paradoxically result in lower rates of screening.[2] The current guidelines place emphasis on ensuring that all individuals have access to screening.

Conclusion

CRC screening of asymptomatic individuals can reduce the incidence and mortality of CRC. High-risk patients with a family history of CRC need to be screened at an appropriate age with colonoscopy. For average-risk individuals, there are two types of screening tests: stool-based tests, which can detect early cancer, and structural examinations of the colon, which can detect early cancer and cancer precursor lesions. All programs ultimately lead to colonoscopy for positive tests. Effective programs depend on high-quality colonoscopy accurately performed by properly trained endoscopists with low rates of adverse events. In the future, the quality of screening will be defined by performance of key quality indicators with the goal of quality improvement.

References

The complete reference list is available online at www.expertconsult.com.

Chapter 36

II

Colonoscopic Polypectomy, Mucosal Resection, and Submucosal Dissection

Roy Soetikno, Tonya Kaltenbach, Shai Friedland, and Takahisa Matsuda

Video related to this chapter's topics can be found online at expertconsult.com.

"The work begins anew, the hope rises again, and the dream lives on."

Edward Moore Kennedy (1932–2009)

Introduction

A new wave of change in the field of colorectal neoplasms and colonoscopy is here, leading to the work in colonoscopic resection to begin anew. Nonpolypoid colorectal neoplasms (NP-CRN) are now widely recognized in Western countries (**Fig. 36.1**).[1] This finding requires numerous paradigm shifts in our clinical, educational, and research activities. The detection and diagnosis of NP-CRN necessitates the search for subtle nonprotruding findings during colonoscopy.[2] Treatment of NP-CRN requires mucosal resection technique, which is more complex than polypectomy. Because nonpolypoid neoplasms can be found throughout the gastrointestinal (GI) tract, all endoscopists must become familiar with endoscopic mucosal resection (EMR) techniques, and future generations must understand its theoretical basis, obtain the dexterity to perform it, and perfect it. Knowledge about the biology and outcomes of the management of nonpolypoid GI neoplasms

is to be acquired. Within the same period of time, new technology—high definition, high magnification, and image-enhanced endoscopy[3]—that is useful for the detection, diagnosis, and treatment of NP-CRN has become available and is increasingly employed. The technique of submucosal dissection, which has become a standard resection technique for early gastric cancer in Japan, is also being applied for the resection of certain types of colorectal neoplasms to achieve R0 resection—curative en bloc resection with all margins being free of neoplasms (**Fig. 36.2**)[4]—without surgery.

Advances in the ability to detect, diagnose, and treat all types of colorectal neoplasms are important. These advances provide hope that the benefit of colonoscopy screening to prevent colorectal cancer, one of the most common causes of cancer death worldwide, can be extended further. In the United States, it was estimated that there would be approximately 146,970 new cases of colorectal cancer in 2009 and 49,920 deaths caused by the disease. The lifetime risk of developing colorectal cancer in the U.S. population is about 6%, with 90% of cases occurring in individuals older than 50 years. The U.S. incidence of colorectal cancer is slightly higher in men than in women, but because women live longer than men, the total number of cases is higher in women. Colorectal

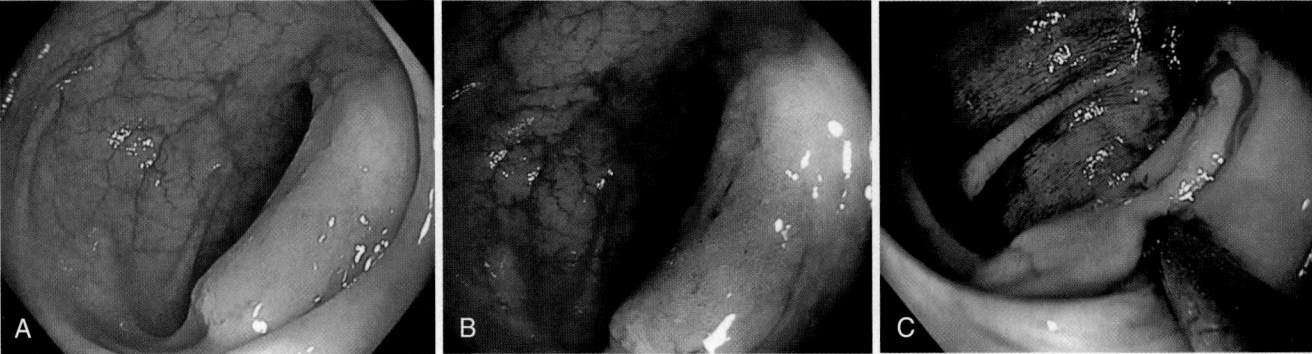

Fig. 36.1   **A,** Nonpolypoid colorectal neoplasm (NP-CRN) (slightly elevated) in the sigmoid colon. **B** and **C,** The border and surface pattern of the lesion were examined with image-enhanced endoscopy techniques using narrow band imaging (**B**) and diluted indigo carmine (**C**). The lesion was resected using mucosal resection technique; pathology showed adenoma.

	Method		
	Polypectomy	Mucosal resection	Submucosal dissection
Schematic (blue color denotes submucosal injectant)	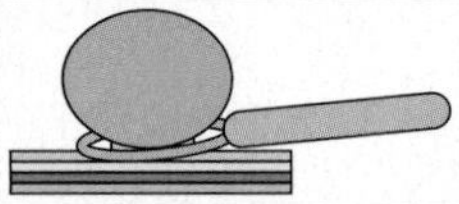	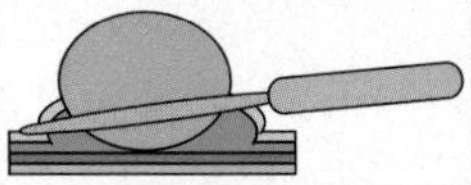	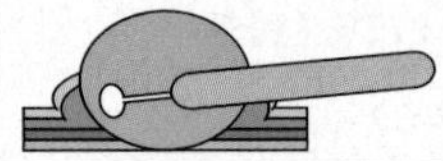
Instrument	Any type of snare	Injection needle Stiff snare	Injection needle ESD knife
Intended plane of resection	Mucosa	Submucosa	Submucosa
Cost, skills, time	+	++	+++

Fig. 36.2   General classification of methods of resection of colorectal lesions.

cancer incidence and mortality also vary by race and ethnicity, with the highest rate occurring in African Americans; an intermediate rate occurring in whites and Asian/Pacific Islanders; and the lowest rates occurring in American Indians, Alaska Natives, and Hispanics.[5] Most colorectal cancer deaths are believed to be preventable with screening colonoscopy and polypectomy.[6] The paradigm that a significant majority of colorectal cancers are thought to arise through the adenoma-to-carcinoma sequence[7] has been expanded with mismatch repair, serrated, and hybrid pathways.[8]

Neoplasms can be both polypoid and nonpolypoid, and NP-CRN has a higher risk to contain high-grade dysplasia or submucosal invasion at the time of colonoscopy compared with polypoid neoplasm.[1,9,10] It has been estimated that 25% to 40% of adults older than 50 years in the United States have at least one adenoma and that a small fraction of these adenomas progresses to cancer. Because it is impossible to predict which adenoma will become malignant, physicians attempt to remove all adenomas during colonoscopy. The National Polyp Study, which showed that removal of adenomas during screening colonoscopy can decrease the subsequent development of colorectal cancer by 90% compared with historical controls, provided a level of support to this current standard of practice.[6] It is our dream to be able to prevent the development of advanced cancer safely and efficaciously in every patient we treat.

Endoscopically, adenomas and early colorectal cancer can be classified as polypoid (protruded) and nonpolypoid (superficial) types (**Fig. 36.3**).[11] Colonoscopic polypectomy can be used to remove polypoid lesions. Colonoscopic mucosal resection, using the inject and cut technique, is a safe and efficacious technique used to remove nonpolypoid or sessile lesions. Colonoscopic submucosal dissection technique, which is used to remove diseased mucosa by dissecting through the middle to deeper layers of the submucosa, can refine our ability to remove lesions that are difficult, if not impossible, to remove using mucosal resection technique. In this chapter, we provide an in-depth survey of colonoscopic resection of polypoid and nonpolypoid colorectal lesions.

Differential Diagnosis

Colonic lesions are classified as either epithelial or nonepithelial. Epithelial lesions include neoplastic adenomas (serrated, tubular, tubulovillous, villous), carcinomas, and nonneoplastic polyps (hyperplastic, juvenile, hamartoma, inflammatory). Occasionally, numerous lesions are encountered during colonoscopy of patients who have polyposis syndromes, including familial adenomatous polyposis (adenomas), Peutz-Jeghers syndrome (hamartomas), juvenile polyposis (juvenile polyps), or Cowden's syndrome (hamartomas). In addition, patients with hereditary nonpolyposis colorectal cancer may harbor multiple advanced neoplastic lesions. Nonepithelial colonic lesions typically arise in the submucosal, muscularis propria, or serosal layers of the colonic wall and include lipomas, leiomyomas, carcinoids, lymphomas, and metastatic tumors. Indentations of the colonic wall by adjacent organs or endometrial implants on the serosa can also have the appearance of subepithelial lesions.

Careful endoscopic observation of the surface features of the lesion can often allow differentiation of epithelial from nonepithelial origin because nonepithelial lesions are usually covered by normal mucosa. With current videocolonoscopes, and especially with the addition of image enhancement and magnification endoscopy,[12] it is increasingly possible to distinguish reliably among hyperplastic polyps, adenomatous polyps, and superficial early adenocarcinomas. Colonoscopic resection may be viewed as a diagnostic procedure. Removal of the entire lesion, when possible, provides the most rigorous evidence that a malignancy was not missed, as it might be because of sampling error with standard biopsies. These procedures provide the definitive treatment when the lesions are removed completely. Subepithelial lesions sometimes can be removed safely when they are located above the muscularis propria, as evidenced by their endoscopic appearance, response to submucosal saline injection, and, if needed, endoscopic ultrasound (EUS). Generally, biopsy should be performed if possible in lesions that are not amendable to endoscopic resection to ascertain their histology, and the lesions should be endoscopically marked for surgical planning with submucosal tattoo and radiopaque clips.

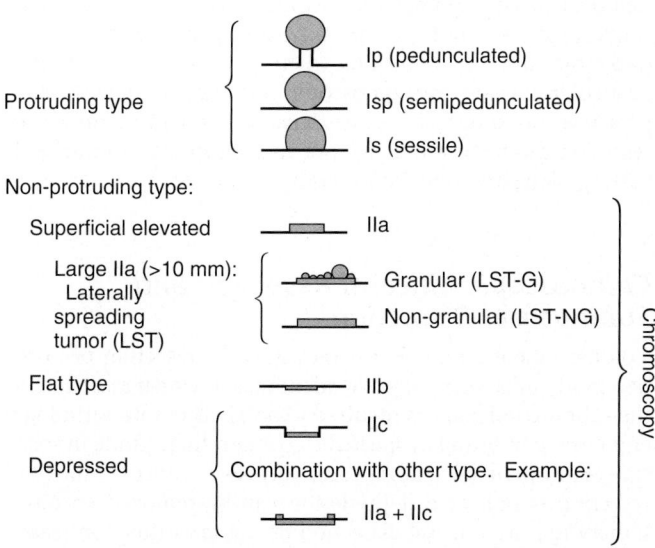

Fig. 36.3 Macroscopic classification of early neoplastic lesions of the colon and rectum. This classification provides a more precise schematic description of early neoplastic lesions. In addition to the commonly described pedunculated, semipedunculated, and sessile lesions, the classification provides the appropriate descriptors for flat and depressed lesions. The classification is particularly useful for the endoscopist in deciding treatment strategy of early colorectal carcinomas because the risk of submucosal invasion of these lesions corresponds to the endoscopic appearance and size. Image-enhanced endoscopy is useful to study the surface details and border of the nonprotruding type.

Clinical Features and Pathology

The macroscopic classification of adenomas and early colorectal neoplasms is crucial in the discussion of diagnosis and treatment of early colorectal cancer.[11,13] The classification by the Japanese Society for Cancer of the Colon and Rectum can provide a common descriptor of adenomas and early colorectal cancer (mucosal or submucosal cancer, regardless of lymph node status). The Paris classification has been promoted for worldwide use[14]—although a derivative from the Japanese categorization, its slight alterations in morphologic definitions make it difficult to infer directly the knowledge that has been meticulously collected by our Japanese colleagues. The application of a standard classification of colorectal lesions is the first step in stratifying which lesions are more likely to contain advanced pathology.

Based on their endoscopic appearance, we classify adenomas and early colorectal cancers as polypoid and nonpolypoid. The polypoid type consists of pedunculated, semipedunculated, and sessile polyps. The nonpolypoid type consists of superficially elevated, flat, and depressed lesions. Excavated superficial colorectal neoplasms are rarely observed. Superficially elevated nonpolypoid lesions are differentiated from sessile polypoid lesions both endoscopically (the height of the lesion is less than half the diameter) and histologically (the thickness of the lesion is less than twice that of the adjacent normal mucosa).[15] The term *flat* is often used to describe superficially elevated lesions. In the colon, however, *flat* generally connotes that the surface is flat, rather than that the lesion is at the same level as the surrounding mucosa (in the colon and rectum, in contrast to in the esophagus, early neoplastic lesions are rarely at the same level as the surrounding mucosa.)

In the Japanese literature and increasingly becoming common worldwide, flat lesions (IIa) larger than 10 mm are also called *laterally spreading tumors* (LST), although the term refers more to the growth pattern rather than the endoscopic appearance. In the United States, these large flat lesions are often called *carpet lesions*. LST with nodular or coarsely granular surfaces are called LST-granular. Other LST are called LST-nongranular. This distinction is important because LST-nongranular are more likely to contain invasive cancer, which is more difficult to assess endoscopically. LST-nongranular are also more difficult to resect and may require en bloc resection to ensure cure. In the Paris classification, semipedunculated lesions are lumped into the pedunculated category, and flat lesions are defined as lesions with height less than a closed biopsy forceps. Depressed nonpolypoid lesions, although rare, accounted for almost one-third of the invasive early cancers that were resected endoscopically by Kudo and colleagues,[16] who observed more than 14,000 colorectal lesions. Confirmatory reports have been published.[12,17] Epidemiology studies of flat and depressed lesions in Western countries have also shown that depressed lesions have a high likelihood of containing invasive cancer (**Table 36.1**).[18] More than 40% of small (6 to 10 mm) depressed lesions contain submucosal invasive cancer; virtually all large (>2 cm) depressed lesions have submucosal invasion (**Table 36.2**).[16] In comparison, submucosal invasive cancer is rare in flat lesions smaller than 10 mm. The risk increases to about 30% in LST larger than 2 cm. Protruding (polypoid) lesions have the lowest rate—slightly greater than 2%—of submucosally invasive cancer.[16]

Table 36.1 Series of Flat and Depressed (F&D) Neoplasms in Patients from Western Countries

Type of Study, Authors (Country)	No. Patients with F&D Neoplasms/All Patients (%)	No. F&D Neoplasms/All Neoplasms (%)	No. F&D Neoplasms with HGD/F&D Neoplasms (%)	No. F&D Neoplasms with Cancer/F&D Neoplasms (%)	No. F&D Cancers/All Cancers (%)
Prospective, Jaramillo et al[19] (Sweden)	55/232 (23.7)	109/261 (41.7)	12/109 (11)	3/109 (2.7)	3/17 (1.8)
Prospective, Fujii et al[20] (United Kingdom)	28 F&D lesions/210 patients	28/68 (38.2)	1/28 (3.5)	2/28 (7.1)	2/3 (66.7)
Prospective, Rembacken et al[21] (United Kingdom)	123 F&D lesions/1000 patients	123/327 (36.4)	16/123 (13.0)	4/123 (3.2)	4/6 (66.7)
Prospective, Suzuki et al[22] (United Kingdom)*	5 flat cancers/870 colonoscopies (0.57)	Not stated	Not stated	Not stated	5/45 (11.1)
Prospective, Saitoh et al[23] (U.S.)	48/211 (22.7)	57/139 (41)	Not stated	3/57 (5.2)	3/3 (100)
Prospective, Tsuda et al[24] (Sweden)	52/866 (6)	66/973 (6.8)	11/66 (16.67)	5/66 (7.5)	5/16 (31.3)
Prospective, Soetikno et al (U.S.)	170/1819 (9.4)	227/1535 (14.8)	11/227 (0.48)	4/227 (0.18)	4/12 (33)

Note: Only prospective studies with large numbers of patients are included.
*Study of colorectal cancer only.
HGD, high-grade dysplasia.
Modified from Kahng LS, Friedland S, Matsui S, et al: Flat and depressed colorectal neoplasms in the United States of America. Early Colorectal Cancer (Jpn) *2004.*

Table 36.2 Risk for Submucosal Invasions Correlated with Endoscopic Appearance and Size of Colorectal Lesions

Appearance	Size (mm)				
	<5	6–10	11–15	16–20	>20
Depressed	8.1%	40.7%	77.8%	84.6%	90%
Flat	0.04%	0.2%	1.8%	10.5%	21.4%
Protruding	0%	1.3%	8.5%	17.2%	31.2%

Modified from Kudo S, Kashida H, Tamura T, et al: Colonoscopic diagnosis and management of nonpolypoid early colorectal cancer. World J Surg *24:1081–1090, 2000.*

Indications and Contraindications

Indications

Endoscopists most commonly resect polypoid lesions using either a snare loop or a biopsy forceps. The malignant potential of an individual polyp is not fully known, and all polyps except diminutive hyperplastic-appearing polyps in the sigmoid and rectum are removed from otherwise healthy patients. However, the risks of polypectomy must also be considered. Treatment decisions must consider whether substantial risks exist and whether the patient's overall life expectancy is unlikely to be affected by the generally slow progression of colonic adenomas. The application of principles of statistics whereby the risks considered include the confidence interval must be used at the bedside (see later section). The natural history of progression through the adenoma to carcinoma sequence is estimated to be approximately 10 years,[26] so patients with advanced comorbid illnesses and limited life expectancy may not benefit from adenoma resection.

Colonoscopic Polypectomy

Generally, diminutive polyps measuring up to approximately 6 mm in diameter are easily removed with or without cautery, with use of a biopsy forceps or a snare. Intermediate sized and larger polyps are most commonly resected via a snare with monopolar cautery, although sessile polyps up to 1 cm can be removed by snare polypectomy with cautery (cold snare). Removal of large polyps may require piecemeal rather than single piece resection and prophylaxis against postpolypectomy bleeding. In addition, when polyps are sessile and particularly when the endoscopic appearance suggests the presence of superficial carcinoma, colonoscopic mucosal resection can be useful to achieve an appropriate submucosal cutting plane and resection margin.

Colonoscopic Mucosal Resection and Submucosal Dissection

Colonic mucosal resection is indicated for resection of non-polypoid and sessile polypoid adenomas in which resection at the submucosal plane is required to obtain accurate pathology and cure. For lesions suspected to contain high-grade dysplasia or superficial submucosal invasive cancer, mucosal resection is indicated if the lesion can be removed en bloc. Otherwise, submucosal dissection or surgery (after confirmatory biopsy) is indicated. The indications of colonoscopic mucosal resection and submucosal dissection are presented in **Box 36.1.** Nonpolypoid lesions can be difficult to capture with standard snare and polypectomy techniques. It may be impossible to perform en bloc resection of large flat lesions using standard polypectomy techniques. The application of electrocautery may lead to a burn into the muscularis propria. Resection of large sessile lesions carries similar risks. Mucosal resection technique using submucosal injection can ameliorate these technical difficulties and risks. Depressed lesions,

Box 36.1 Indications for Colonoscopic Mucosal Resection and Submucosal Dissection

I. A team to perform EMR or submucosal dissection safely and efficaciously is available.

II. The neoplasm does not have features of massive submucosal or advanced invasion.

III. EMR:
   A. Mucosal resection: Lesion (nonpolypoid or sessile) with adenomatous-appearing or villous adenomatous–appearing mucosa requiring resection at the submucosa to ensure cure. If the lesion is suspected to contain high-grade dysplasia or slight submucosal invasion, EMR is indicated, provided that the lesion is within the scope of EMR technique for en bloc removal.
   B. Submucosal dissection: Lesion requiring en bloc resection beyond the scope of EMR:
      1. Large, flat, nongranular lesion with slight depression
      2. Large, flat, granular or sessile lesion suspected to contain high-grade dysplasia or slight submucosal invasion
      3. Larger depressed lesions

IV. Pathologic evaluation provided proof of cure:
   A. Well-differentiated carcinoma (without poorly differentiated)
   B. Without lymphatic or vascular invasion
   C. Intramucosal cancer, regardless of size (limit of involvement in the United States)
   D. Minute submucosal invasion less than 1000 μm from the muscularis mucosa, or if the muscularis mucosa is absent, depth of measurement is performed from the surface of lesion (limit of involvement in Japan)
   E. Vertical and lateral margins are from carcinoma

EMR, endoscopic mucosal resection.

including small ones, are most likely to contain submucosally invasive cancer. Complete removal of small depressed lesions is the only way to determine accurately that invasive carcinoma is not present.

Because Western pathologists rely primarily on evidence of invasion to diagnose invasive carcinoma (as opposed to cellular and glandular morphology, as is common in Japan), mucosal resection technique is more appropriate to obtain a complete sample of small depressed lesions. The superficial submucosa is typically included in these resection specimens, allowing the pathologist to assess for submucosal invasion. Larger true depressed lesions often are invasive carcinoma. After a confirmatory biopsy and tattooing of the site, these lesions may be best managed with surgery. Mucosal resection is also used increasingly to remove submucosal lesions,[27] especially small (<1 cm) rectal carcinoids, where the risk of metastasis is low.[28,29]

Contraindications

Colonoscopy is usually inappropriate in patients who are pregnant[30] or have fulminant colitis, suspected intestinal perforation, fresh intestinal anastomosis, or recent myocardial infarction. Polypectomy and mucosal resection generally should not be performed in patients who have uncorrected bleeding disorders. Although polypectomy and mucosal resection were reported in one study to be relatively safe in lesions smaller than 1 cm, the technique used in that study involved submucosal injection before snaring and clipping to approximate the mucosal defect. Good bowel preparation is crucial for detection of subtle lesions and for resection of particularly large or difficult lesions when an elevated risk of perforation exists. Poor bowel preparation is also a contraindication for performance of complex polypectomy or mucosal resection.

Anticoagulation Therapy

Patients need individualized assessment, balancing the risks of interrupting anticoagulation for colonoscopic polypectomy or mucosal resection against the risks of significant bleeding during and after the procedure.[31,32] Patients at very high risk for thrombotic events, such as patients with recent coronary stent placements, should simply defer elective endoscopy until the thrombotic risk is lower. The American Society for Gastrointestinal Endoscopy (ASGE) has developed guidelines for management of anticoagulation.[33,34] Generally, patients at relatively low risk of thromboembolic complications can discontinue warfarin 5 days before the procedure and resume it shortly after standard polypectomy or 7 to 10 days after complex polypectomy or mucosal resection. The international normalized ratio should be 1.4 or less before polypectomy or mucosal resection of a large lesion. High-risk patients, such as patients with atrial fibrillation and concomitant valvular disease, should receive either standard intravenous heparin until approximately 6 hours before the procedure or low-molecular-weight heparin until approximately 24 hours before the procedure. Warfarin generally can be resumed on the night after the procedure with use of intravenous heparin resumed earlier at 2 to 6 hours after the procedure until the international normalized ratio is therapeutic.

Standard heparin has a short half-life compared with low-molecular-weight heparin, so it permits swift immediate reversal of anticoagulation should patients develop postpolypectomy bleeding. In our published experience of colonoscopic resection of small (<1 cm) colorectal lesions in anticoagulated patients, we withheld warfarin for approximately 36 hours only to avoid supratherapeutic anticoagulation resulting from dietary restriction and bowel purge. In this retrospective series, using various polypectomy techniques, including cold snare, standard snare with cautery, and inject and cut mucosectomy, followed by endoscopic clipping, the risk of major delayed bleeding in the resection of 5.1 ± 2.2 mm lesions was 0.8% (95% confidence interval 0.1% to 4.5%).[35]

Aspirin, Nonsteroidal Antiinflammatory Drugs, and Antiplatelet Medications

Limited data from the literature suggest that aspirin and other nonsteroidal antiinflammatory drugs (NSAIDs) in standard doses do not increase the risk of significant bleeding after colonoscopic polypectomy. ASGE recommends proceeding with standard polypectomy in patients taking these medications.[33,34] We are unaware, however, of any recommendations regarding polypectomy or mucosal resection of large or complex lesions. In our practice, patients with significant coronary disease continue to take aspirin, 81 mg/day, after large polypectomy or mucosal resection. The ASGE guidelines for management of platelet aggregation inhibitors, such as ticlopidine and clopidogrel, recommend discontinuation of these agents for 7 to 10 days. Patients receiving combination therapy (e.g., clopidogrel and aspirin) may be at an additional risk of bleeding. Reinstitution of antiplatelet agents should be individualized. Generally, when we believe that the risk of bleeding after endoscopic removal of a large or complex lesion is significant, we recommend that patients refrain from taking other NSAIDs and platelet inhibitors 7 days before the procedure and for 7 to 14 days after it.

Antibiotic Prophylaxis for Endocarditis

The ASGE and the American Heart Association guidelines state that antibiotic prophylaxis solely to prevent infective endocarditis is no longer recommended before endoscopic procedures, including diagnostic colonoscopy and colonoscopic polypectomy.[36]

Instruments

Snare Loop

Both the endoscopist and the endoscopy assistant must be familiar with the type of snare used. These individuals must understand and have tactile knowledge of the opening and closing of the snare, the closing pressure required to produce optimal coagulation, and the relationship between the size of the tissue being strangulated and the amount of snare being closed. Various snares, each with a slightly different feature, are used for polypectomy and mucosal resection. The choice is made based on personal preference, the size of the lesion, and the technique being used. The minisnare is often used for small polyps, and larger snares are used for larger polyps. Stiffer snares are used for colonoscopic mucosal resection so that flat or depressed lesions can be captured in the snare.[27,37]

Electrocautery

High-frequency electrical current is employed to facilitate cutting and to coagulate vessels at the resection margin.

Colonoscopic resection is typically performed with a monopolar snare. The metallic conducting snare serves as the active electrode, and the circuit is completed via a conducting grounding pad that is affixed to the patient's skin. In the case of polypectomy, when the snare grasps the polyp, electrical current is applied as the snare is closed to transect the stalk. Electrical current traveling through tissue heats it. The amount of heat transferred to each point in the tissue (per unit time) is given by the product of the square of the current density and the resistance. The current density is the amount of current passing through a unit area. Although the same total current passes through the stalk of the polyp and the grounding pad, the current density is much higher at the stalk because the cross-sectional area is smaller. As a result, the stalk is cauterized while the bowel wall and the rest of the patient's body generally are left untouched (**Fig. 36.4**).[38]

High-frequency electrical current greater than 300 kHz (300,000 cycles/sec) is used because lower frequencies can stimulate muscles, nerves, and the heart. The effect of the current on the tissue depends on the temperature achieved in the tissue, which depends on the shape of the electrode, the duration and waveform of the current, and the voltage. At temperatures between 50° C and 70° C, irreversible cell damage occurs. Between 70° C and 100° C, the tissue is coagulated; collagen is converted to glucose, and the glucose causes the coagulated tissue to become sticky. At temperatures greater than 100° C, the tissue is desiccated; intracellular and extracellular water is vaporized, and the tissue dries out, shrinks, and becomes sticky. During polypectomy, these effects are visualized as a shrinking and whitening of polyp stalks. If low peak voltage (<200 V) is used, the tissue is devitalized, coagulated, and desiccated. As the tissue is dehydrated, the resistance increases until current can no longer flow and no further heat ensues. In this mode, there is little or no cutting; in some clinical situations, the snare can become entrapped in the desiccated tissue.

For efficient electrosurgical cutting, temperatures greater than 500° C are required. At these high temperatures, intracellular and extracellular water is vaporized rapidly, and the cellular architecture is disrupted by steam pressure. Electrosurgery units generate vaporization by producing electrical arcs that jump between the active electrode (snare) and the tissue. The

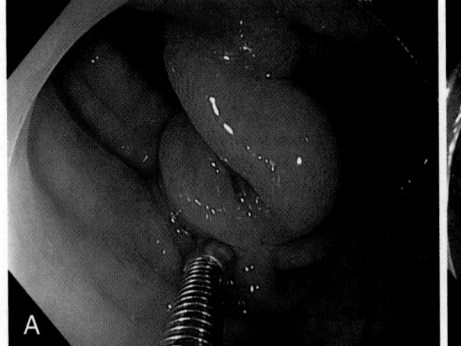 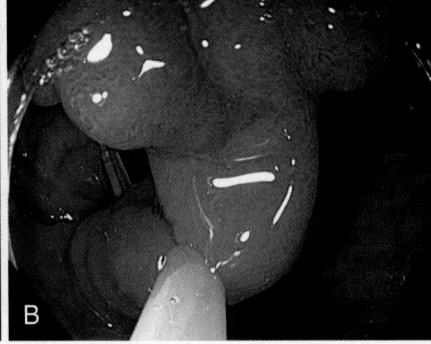 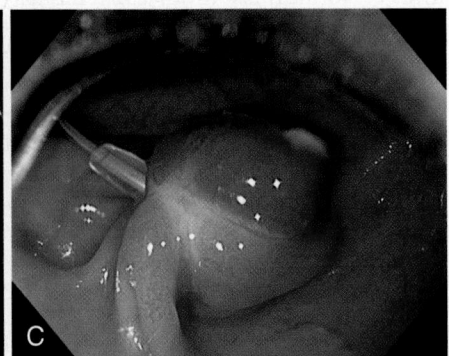

Fig. 36.4 The concept of electrocautery is important to master. In this case, application of understanding of the concept of current density—the amount of current per unit area—is shown. **A,** Current density is highest at the plane with the smallest area, in this case, cross-sectional area that has been strangulated by the loop *(arrow)*. The ideal way to snare a pedunculated polyp that has been looped is to tighten the snare as much as possible to make the snared plane smaller than the plane that has been looped. **B,** Care is given to snare with adequate distance from the deployed loop. **C,** In this case, the snare was not closed tighter than the loop, and cautery also occurred at looped area. This case also provides a reason to deploy the loop slightly away from the wall of the colon to prevent accidental coagulation necrosis.

electrical arcs focus the current on a small area on the tissue and result in a locally very high current density and temperature. At least 200 V are required to generate these electrical arcs; if the tissue is partially desiccated, the voltage required is substantially higher. Electrosurgical cutting is ideally performed without contact between the electrode and the tissue, leaving room for proper arcing to form; cutting occurs without mechanical pressure as tissue is vaporized.

During colonoscopy, the snare is typically in contact with the tissue. This contact can lead to lower resistance and high current, causing an inappropriate decrease in voltage that prevents electrical arcs from forming. The result is an unintended coagulation effect without cutting. Newer cautery units, such as the ERBE (Marietta, GA), automatically supervise the initial phase of cutting and provide the necessary current and voltage to ensure proper arcing. During electrosurgical cutting, there is also a coagulation effect, which depends on factors such as the electrode thickness and voltage. Thin electrodes (e.g., a needle-knife), low voltages, and rapid cutting result in little coagulation. Thicker electrodes (e.g., a thick snare loop) and higher voltages result in more intense coagulation. Uncontrolled rapid cutting with minimal coagulation can occur if mechanical pressure (e.g., by closing the snare rapidly) is applied; this phenomenon is also familiar to endoscopists from endoscopic retrograde cholangiopancreatography sphincterotomy, where it is called a "zipper" cut.

Most electrocautery units allow the endoscopist to choose between various cautery modes that are designed to produce predominantly cutting, predominantly coagulation, or a blend of both. However, factors such as the power level, tissue resistance, and speed of snare closure can alter the effect of the cautery. The "cutting" mode delivers a continuous sine-wave voltage pattern. When sufficient voltage is delivered to create electrical arcing, electrosurgical cutting ensues. "Coagulation" and "blended" modes actually deliver a higher voltage, but the delivery is intermittent: short pauses separating brief bursts of delivery. The duty cycle (the total proportion of time that current is delivered) is typically between 5% and 50% in coagulation modes and between 50% and 80% in blended modes. The higher voltages allow deeper coagulation during cutting, particularly in "coagulation" mode. An additional effect, fulguration (spray coagulation), can occur with very high voltages and low duty cycles when a series of random electrical arcs carbonize the tissue.

The use of submucosal injection during mucosal resection promotes a better distribution of current because the current can fan out from the resection site to the wide saline cushion. This fan out reduces thermal damage to the larger submucosal vessel and part of the colon wall immediately beneath the lesion.[39]

Argon Plasma Coagulation

Argon plasma coagulation (APC) is often used after EMR to cauterize the resection margins.[40] APC produces electrically conducting argon plasma by guiding argon gas through a delivery catheter that also contains an electrode for delivery of high-frequency current. APC generally creates uniformly deep zones of desiccation, coagulation, and devitalization that measure less than 3 mm deep in total. Because the argon plasma conducts the current, APC can be applied without tissue contact.[41–43] In a randomized, controlled study,

prophylactic APC to nonbleeding visible vessels at the en bloc polyp (5 to 20 mm) resection sites did not significantly decrease the rate of delayed postpolypectomy bleeding (4.3% in the control group vs. 2.5% in the APC group). The study excluded resections of pedunculated polyps, polyps smaller than 5 mm or larger than 20 mm, polyps that had immediate bleeding, and polyps with no vessels visible at the postresection site.[44]

Bipolar Instruments

Bipolar instruments, in which current flows between two electrodes in the instrument rather than from one electrode to a grounding pad, have the potential advantage of avoiding damage to deeper structures. Bipolar polypectomy snares are not currently widely used, although more recent studies have shown their potential utility in colonoscopic submucosal dissection. Bipolar coagulation devices are commonly used to treat bleeding vessels in peptic ulcer disease, and they can be employed to treat bleeding areas after polypectomy, although mechanical hemostasis using clipping or looping has been shown to be efficacious with perhaps less risk of perforation. Sufficient mechanical pressure should be applied to the vessel to compress it during cauterization, to prevent heat dissipation by flowing blood.

Other Instruments

Other instruments that are often used during polypectomy and mucosal resection include the standard sclerotherapy injection needle, endoclip,[44,45] endoloop,[46–48] Roth net,[49] and Tripod. Detailed examples of use of these instruments, which are important for colonoscopic resection, are described subsequently in the Techniques section.

Techniques

Adequate bowel preparation is important; split dosing of bowel preparation is very useful to clean the bowel adequately for the detection and diagnosis of NP-CRN and resection of all types of appropriate lesions. Techniques to prevent looping of the colonoscope during insertion are essential.[50] Familiarity with the patient, staff, equipment, and accessories is required. Various techniques are available to perform sophisticated colonoscopic polypectomy, mucosal resection, and submucosal dissection. These techniques, designed to increase the safety of resection, have allowed resections of lesions that in the past would have been accomplished through surgery. Interpretation of the pathology is vital, and preparation of the pathologic specimen requires the participation of the endoscopists at the completion of the procedure.

Estimation of Malignant Potential

Colonoscopic resection should be performed in patients whose lesions are most likely to benefit. Equally important, resection should be performed only when the endoscopist has the knowledge and expertise and supporting staff to complete the procedure. The assessment to determine the most likely pathologic findings and the depth of invasion is important in planning for colonoscopic resection. Lesions assessed to be noninvasive are most likely to benefit from endoscopic

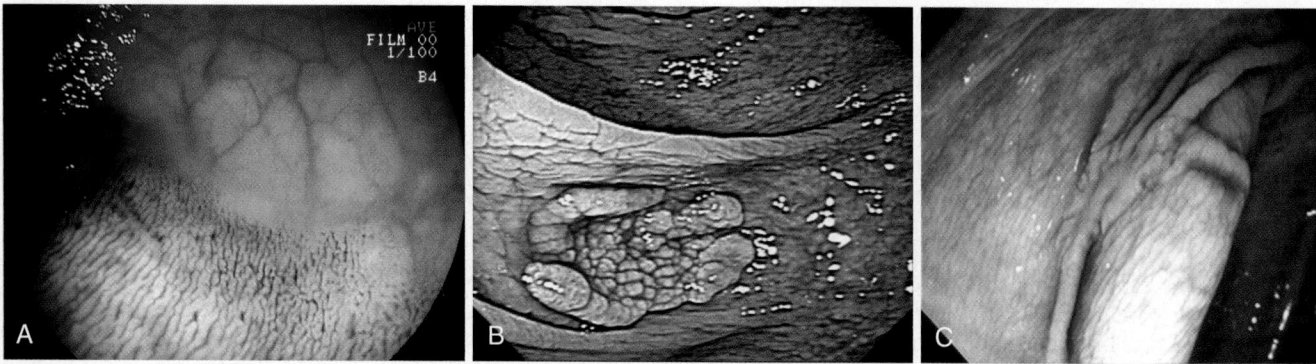

Fig. 36.5 Indigo carmine spray can be very useful for detecting and classifying flat and depressed lesions. **A,** Spraying a dilute solution of indigo carmine improves visualization of the grooves on the mucosal surface of the colon (innominate grooves). **B,** These grooves are also observed in hyperplastic lesions, as in this 15-mm lesion. **C,** Innominate grooves are not observed in neoplastic lesions. Indigo carmine also improves visualization of the border of this 5-mm depressed adenoma. *(From Palo Alto.)*

treatment. Lesions with minimal or moderate risk for submucosal invasion can be treated with endoscopy, provided that the endoscopist believes that the lesion can be safely removed in its entirety and that the potential benefits of endoscopic treatment outweigh the risks. Patients whose lesions are strongly suggestive of invasion should be referred to surgery after a confirmatory biopsy because endoscopic resection would expose them to unnecessary risks. Colonoscopic resection of neoplasms with massive submucosal invasive cancer is generally difficult; has a high risk of bleeding, perforation, recurrence, and metastasis; and should be avoided. Sometimes it is appropriate, after assessment of the lesion, to reschedule the patient for a dedicated resection procedure. Rescheduling allows appropriate discussion of the risks and benefits with the patient and ensures availability of the necessary equipment, endoscopy time, and personnel for the procedure.

Colonoscopy, in some cases with image enhancement, is generally adequate to assess cancer depth (**Fig. 36.5**). High magnification colonoscopy can be beneficial but generally is not available in Western countries. Colonoscopy with ultrasound is generally unnecessary because it does not provide a clear advantage in assessing depth of invasion over imaging with image enhancement. The assessment is based on several characteristics.

Appearance

The classification of a lesion helps in providing a general stratification of the risks for the lesion to contain high-grade dysplasia or submucosal invasive carcinoma. NP-CRN has up to 10 times higher risk of containing in situ or submucosal invasive carcinoma than a polypoid lesion of similar size. The larger the size, the more likely is submucosal invasion. The general appearance of the lesion can provide further clues regarding the likelihood for invasive cancer (**Figs. 36.6 and 36.7**). Firm consistency, adherence, ulceration, and friability are findings suggestive of invasion. In addition, the appearance of expansion of normal tissue immediately surrounding the lesion may indicate the presence of cancer creeping into the surrounding submucosa. Converging folds (two or more) toward the lesion can also predict submucosal invasion. Saitoh and colleagues[23] reported the diagnostic operating characteristics of endoscopic findings of depressed colorectal lesions. They observed that patients with one or more findings of

expansion appearance, deep depression surface, irregularity of depression surface, or converging folds toward the lesions are more likely to have deep submucosal invasion; the presence of one or more of these findings allowed endoscopists to determine deep submucosal invasion with a 91% accuracy. These investigators used indigo carmine to improve visualization of lesions, as described subsequently.

Image-Enhanced Endoscopy

Image-enhanced endoscopy is an integral part of colonoscopic resection of lesions.[3] It is part of standard practice in many progressive endoscopy units. Two types of image enhancement are available: equipment-based and dye-based. Equipment-based enhancement includes optical (Narrow Band Imaging; Olympus) or software (Fujinon Intelligent Chromo Endoscopy; Fujinon, and Tone Enhancement; Pentax) methods. Dye-based enhancement includes diluted indigo carmine and crystal violet; dyes are not used in most Western countries (**Fig. 36.8**). The equipment-based method is part of newer colonoscope systems, and dye-based image enhancement can be readily made available in any unit at low cost. Although equipment-based enhancement is sufficient in most cases, it cannot completely replace dye-based enhancement using diluted indigo carmine. The assessment of depth requires pooling of indigo carmine, and complex surface pattern analysis may require confirmatory dye spray.

Equipment-based and dye-based image enhancements are complementary to each other. First, image enhancement is useful to confirm the presence of a lesion. Second, it may be required to visualize and to define the border of NP-CRN. Third, image enhancement may be needed to visualize details of the surface pattern of the lesion because neoplasms cause abnormal growth patterns of glands, pits, and microvessels. Equipment-based enhancement allows endoscopists to visualize the microvessels that encircle the glands. Indigo carmine, by pooling in the pits, permits endoscopists to visualize the glands, which surround the pits. Image enhancement provides the opportunity to obtain endoscopic diagnosis: hyperplastic, adenoma or serrated adenoma, slightly invasive carcinoma, and advanced carcinoma. Indigo carmine chromoscopy is simple to use. A few milliliters of diluted solution of indigo carmine (0.1% to 0.4%) can be gently sprayed directly from a syringe through the accessory channel onto the tissue

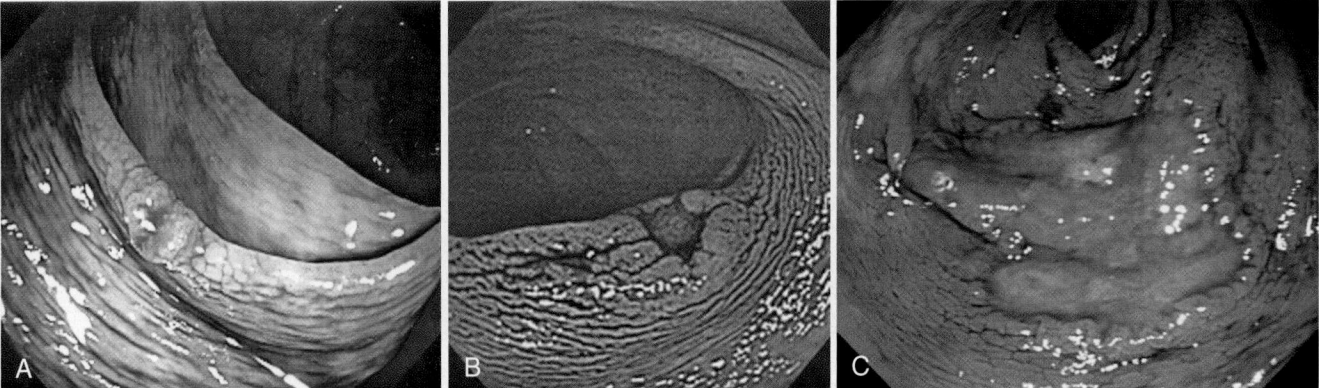

Fig. 36.6   Pseudodepression versus true depression. **A,** This adenomatous lesion has small depressions where indigo carmine solution pools. Small depressions without sharp borders, often referred to as *pseudodepressions,* are typically found in noncancerous adenomas. **B** and **C,** Extensive depressions with sharp borders are worrisome findings because they are often observed in cancerous lesions such as these two early adenocarcinomas. (*A* and *C, From Palo Alto; **B,** from Tokyo.*)

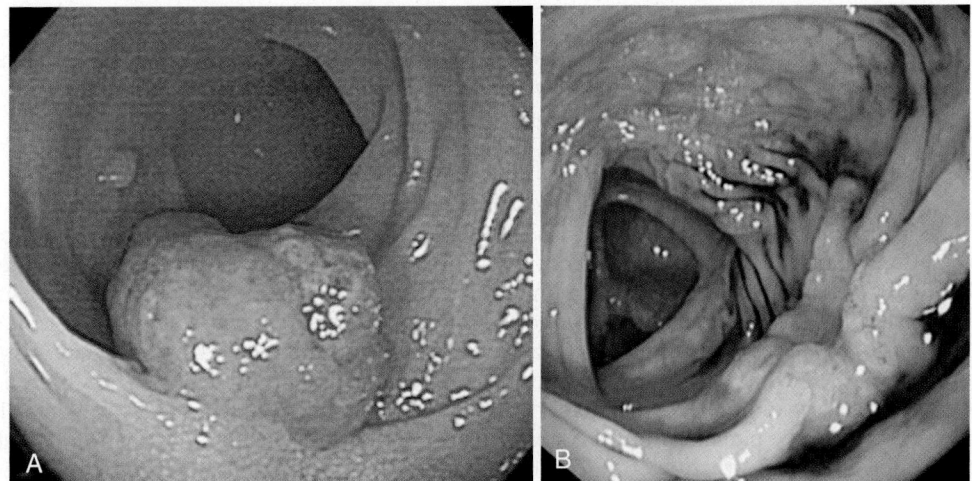

Fig. 36.7   Careful observation of the shape of a lesion is crucial to develop an appropriate treatment strategy. **A,** This sessile lesion has a *full* or *expansive* appearance and converging folds, suggesting the presence of invasive carcinoma in the deeper layers of the submucosa. **B,** Converging folds toward the lesion and central depression are present. The presence of converging folds is specific for invasion deep into the submucosa or beyond. Both of these lesions were treated surgically. (*From Tokyo.*)

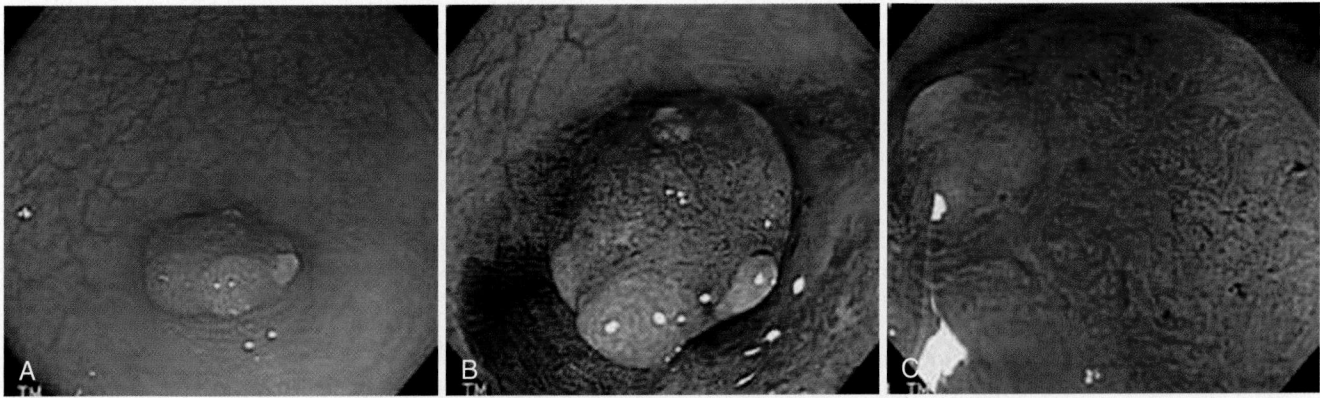

Fig. 36.8   Close-up observation of the surface of lesions using magnification endoscopy with crystal violet chromoscopy can improve endoscopic assessment. **A,** A 7-mm superficial elevated lesion with depression. **B,** Crystal violet has been applied. **C,** On close examination using magnification endoscopy (100×), the pit pattern was consistent with a deeply submucosal invasive pattern. The patient underwent surgical resection where a deep submucosal invasive adenocarcinoma metastatic to local lymph nodes (2/7) was removed. (*From Tokyo.*)

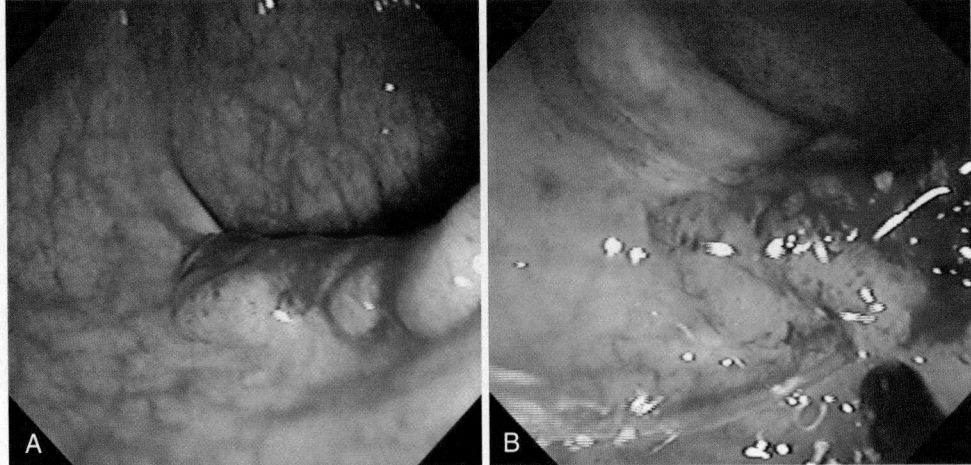

Fig. 36.9 **A,** Several previous attempts at endoscopic resection of this sessile rectal lesion were unsuccessful. The lesion has a full appearance that suggests invasive cancer, but prior pathology revealed only villous adenoma. **B,** Nonlifting sign. Injection of saline into the submucosa beneath this lesion does not result in lifting of the lesion; instead, a backflow of injected saline is seen jetting toward the endoscope. Analysis of the surgically resected specimen showed adenocarcinoma invading down to the muscularis propria. *(From Palo Alto.)*

surrounding the lesion; direct spraying may cause minor bleeding, which can obscure visualization of the pit pattern. Indigo carmine solution is not absorbed but rather pools in mucosal crevices and depressions.

Magnification Endoscopy

The ability to select lesions that warrant endoscopic removal is attractive (see **Fig. 36.5**). Hyperplastic lesions are left alone, adenomas and superficial early carcinomas are resected endoscopically, and invasive cancers are resected surgically. Closer examination of the surface mucosa using magnification endoscopy (100×) allows visualization of the pit pattern, which can provide insights as to the pathology of the lesion. Pit patterns may reflect the tangential structure of the glands of the lesion.[51] As the structural organization of the glands becomes disordered or even absent, as it does in invasive carcinoma, the lesion, as seen magnified from its surface, may have a disorderly pattern. Adenomas have sulci patterns. Hyperplastic lesions have a specific, orderly, enlarged round, oval, or stellar pit pattern.[52] The original classification of the pit pattern may be too complex to apply in routine clinical practice. A simpler classification that groups the patterns as nonneoplastic, noninvasive, and invasive has been reported but is yet to be used widely.

Nonlifting Sign

Observation of the lesion during and after submucosal saline injection during mucosal resection is a simple but important method to assess the potential for deeply invasive carcinoma (**Fig. 36.9**).[53–55] Lesions may not lift because of desmoplastic reaction, invasion from the lesion itself, or submucosal fibrosis from prior multiple biopsy, cautery, India ink injection, or ulceration. Several studies have reported the diagnostic operating characteristics of the nonlifting sign. The positive predictive value of the nonlifting sign is approximately 80%.[56] There is a correlate to the nonlifting sign when submucosal injection is not used; it is typically very difficult to capture in the snare deeply invasive lesions. Difficulties encountered

during attempted snare resection should alert the endoscopist to the possibility of deep invasion.

Endoscopic Ultrasound

Generally, endoscopic ultrasound (EUS) is not used in differentiating nonpolypoid mucosal lesions from submucosally invasive ones.[57–59] The information needed to decide whether or not to perform mucosal resection can usually be collected by observation during conventional colonoscopy, indigo carmine chromoscopy (with standard magnification), and tests for the nonlifting sign. EUS has been used to locate the blood vessels of large sessile or LST lesions. In this study, the information collected did not change the risks of postpolypectomy bleeding significantly.[60]

Techniques for Resection
Polypectomy
DIMINUTIVE (BABY) POLYPS

Diminutive polyps can be removed with various techniques, including single or repeated use of cold biopsy, hot biopsy (**Fig. 36.10**), cold snare,[61] hot snare (**Fig. 36.11**), or fulguration.[62] The optimal technique for complete eradication of all polyp tissue is unknown; the effect of routine removal during colonoscopy of diminutive (≤5 mm) polyps on colon cancer mortality is also unknown. However, documentation of adenomas is important for stratification of need for follow-up colonoscopy, which is based on assessment of risk of developing colorectal cancer.

PEDUNCULATED, SEMIPEDUNCULATED, AND SESSILE LESIONS

Pedunculated and semipedunculated lesions may be resected by snare-loop polypectomy at the middle or upper stalk. Sessile lesions can be resected by a similar technique at the base. Large polyps (>2 cm) or polyps with a thick stalk carry a higher risk of immediate or delayed bleeding. Prophylactic

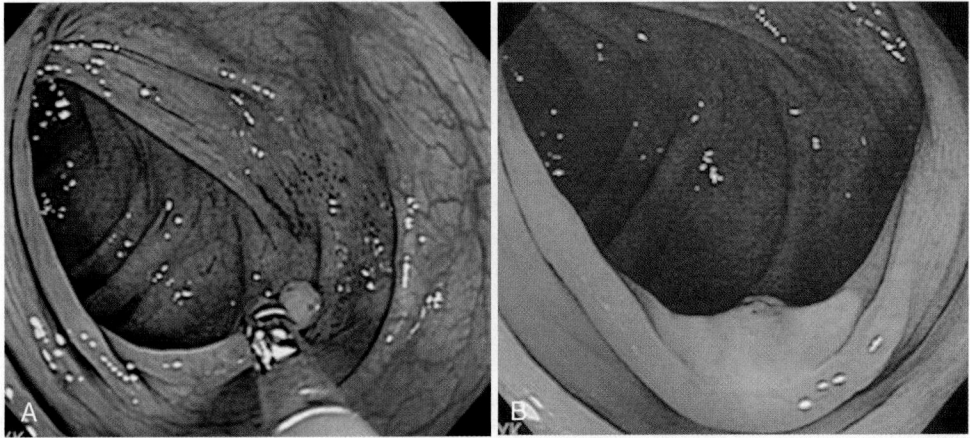

Fig. 36.10 Application of hot biopsy forceps to remove and cauterize a 5-mm adenoma. **A,** The lesion was captured using the forceps, and coagulation current was applied while the mucosa was tented up to form a pseudopedicle. Tenting causes the cautery effect to be concentrated at the pseudopedicle. **B,** The base of the lesion, which was previously the pseudopedicle, has been coagulated. *(From Tokyo.)*

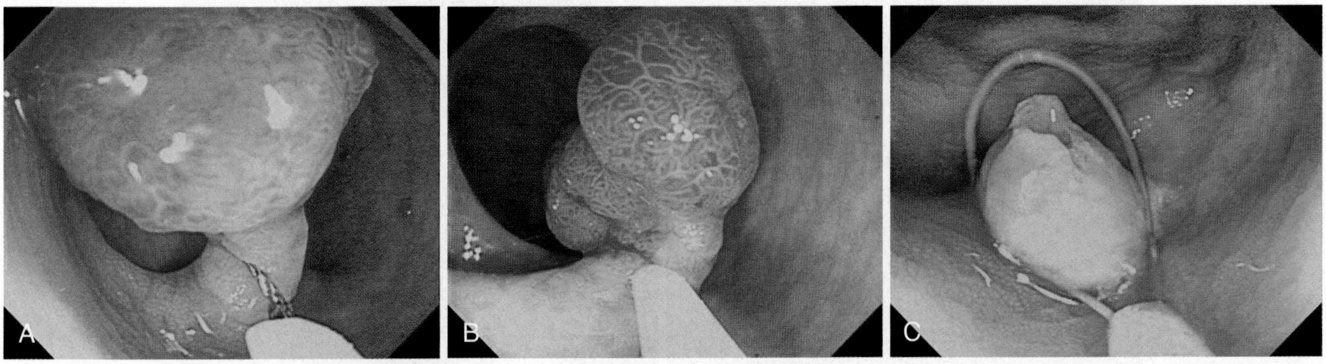

Fig. 36.11 Standard hot snare polypectomy of a thin-stalked pedunculated polyp. **A,** Snare loop has been positioned in the middle of the stalk of the polyp. **B,** As electrocautery was applied, the polyp was slightly tented, and care was taken to avoid having the head of the polyp touch the opposite wall. Touching the opposite wall could reduce the coagulation at the lower end of the stalk and might cause a contralateral burn. **C,** A stalk remnant with a well-coagulated surface is visible. Leaving some stalk remnant allows application of an endoloop for prevention of bleeding. Alternatively, had bleeding occurred immediately after snaring, the bleeding stalk remnant could have been cauterized further by grasping it with the snare. *(From Palo Alto.)*

treatment to strangulate the blood vessels before resection prevents immediate or delayed bleeding (**Fig. 36.12**).[46,47,63–66]

One prophylactic method is application of endoloops, which are detachable loops that are applied to the base of the polyp stalk to strangulate the vessels supplying the polyp. Iishi and colleagues[63] reported the use of endoloops in 47 patients and compared the rate of bleeding with 42 patients who did not have endoloops placed before polypectomy of pedunculated polyps with heads larger than 1 cm. No immediate or delayed bleeding was observed among patients who had endoloops; five (12%) patients in the control group had bleeding (one immediate, four delayed). Di Giorgio and colleagues[67] reported similar results (0% vs. 12% in patients who had and did not have endoloops placed) in a randomized trial with more patients. Another prospective, randomized study of large pedunculated colon polyps showed significantly lower and less severe delayed bleeding in the patients who underwent prophylactic detachable snare placement at the stalk base followed by conventional polypectomy and clip application in the residual stalk compared with the patients who underwent epinephrine injection alone followed by conventional polypectomy.[66] However, placement of the endoloop in pedunculated polyps

that have short stalks can be difficult (**Fig. 36.13**). Massive bleeding can occur if the endoloop slips right after snare polypectomy.[48,68] In addition, the endoloop is made of nylon, which can be too floppy for ensnaring the polyp.

Because massive colonic bleeding can easily cause immediate loss of visualization, other prophylactic techniques may be more appropriate (**Figs. 36.14 and 36.15**).[69] Seitz and colleagues[65] used diluted epinephrine to inject to the base of the stalk before polypectomy. Because the effect of epinephrine is transient, the site was then clipped. Other authors have reported safe use of single or multiple deployment of endoclips before polypectomy (**Fig. 36.16**).[63,70] The clips did not conduct current, perhaps because care was taken to avoid contact between the snare and the clips. En bloc resection is a key component to precise pathologic staging in cases of polyps containing invasive cancer. A case series of giant pedunculated polyps described a greater than 80% volume reduction after 4 to 8 mL of 1:10,000 epinephrine injections into both the polyp head and the stalk. The dramatic volume reduction decreased the need for piecemeal resection.[71] In addition to reducing bleeding, the prophylactic use of the endoloop or endoclip at the base of large pedunculated polyps to facilitate

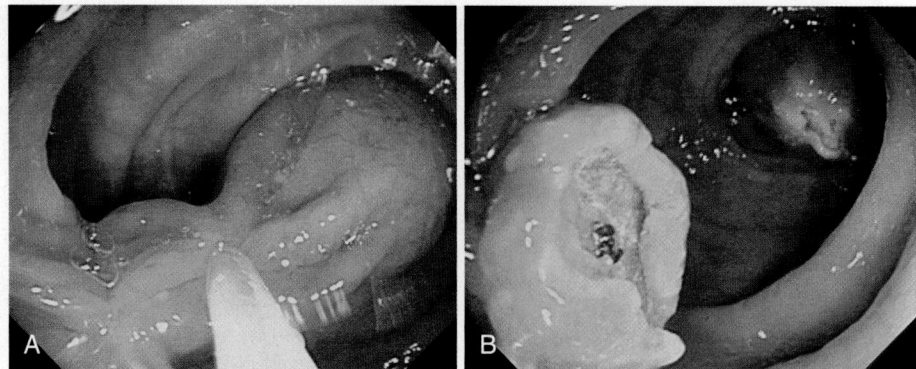

Fig. 36.12 Use of the endoloop to prevent postpolypectomy bleeding. The endoloop is used like a snare except it can be detached after its deployment at the base of the polyp. **A,** The endoloop has been applied at the base of a large pedunculated lesion. The electrocautery snare has been placed above the loop with sufficient room to prevent the endoloop from slipping off after transection. **B,** Resection site immediately after resection. A small blood vessel is visible. There was no bleeding after resection. The diagnosis was lipoma. *(From Palo Alto.)*

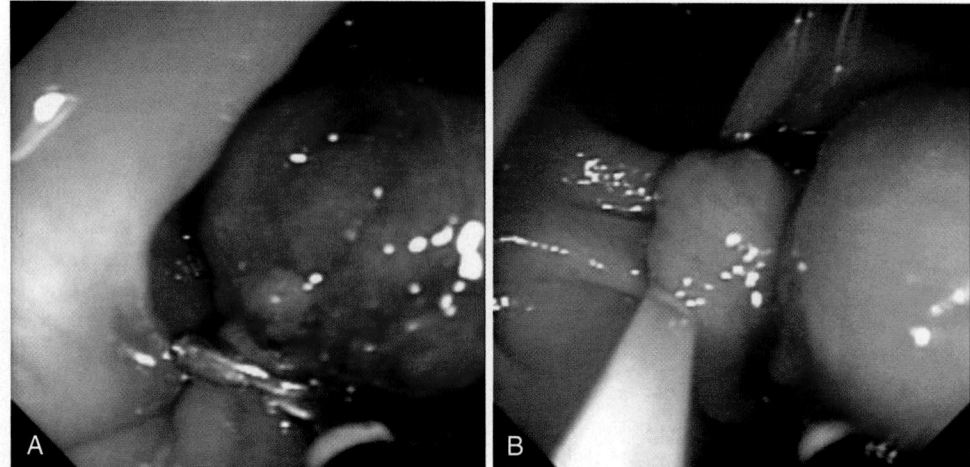

Fig. 36.13 Application of the endoloop can be difficult, especially with large pedunculated polyps in a narrow and tortuous sigmoid colon. The double-channel technique, also called *lift and ligate,* can be useful in these cases. **A,** The endoloop has been placed over the large polyp head, and a large grasper has been passed through the second accessory channel. **B,** The grasper was used to pull the polyp toward the endoscope and facilitate deployment of the endoloop. The polyp appeared dusky shortly after endoloop application, indicating that there was sufficient tension to cause ischemia of the polyp (not shown). Snare polypectomy was subsequently performed. The snare was placed well above the endoloop to prevent slippage of the loop. *(From Palo Alto.)*

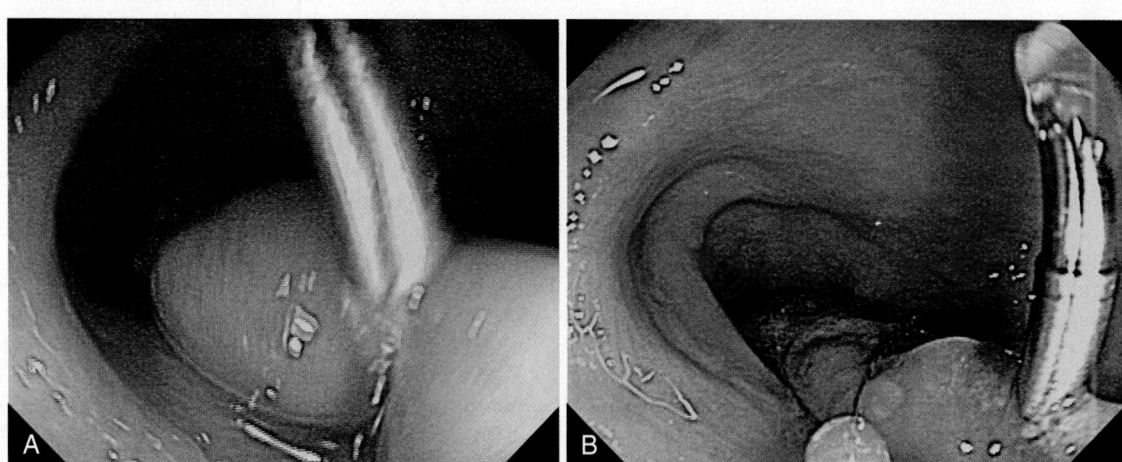

Fig. 36.14 An alternative to endoloops for preventing postpolypectomy bleeding is the endoclip. **A,** Single endoclip has been applied at the lower part of a long polyp stalk. **B,** The polyp appeared dusky after the endoclip placement, indicating effective strangulation of the stalk. The snare was subsequently positioned above the clip, and electrocautery was applied. It is important to avoid touching the clip with the snare during electrocautery application. *(From Palo Alto.)*

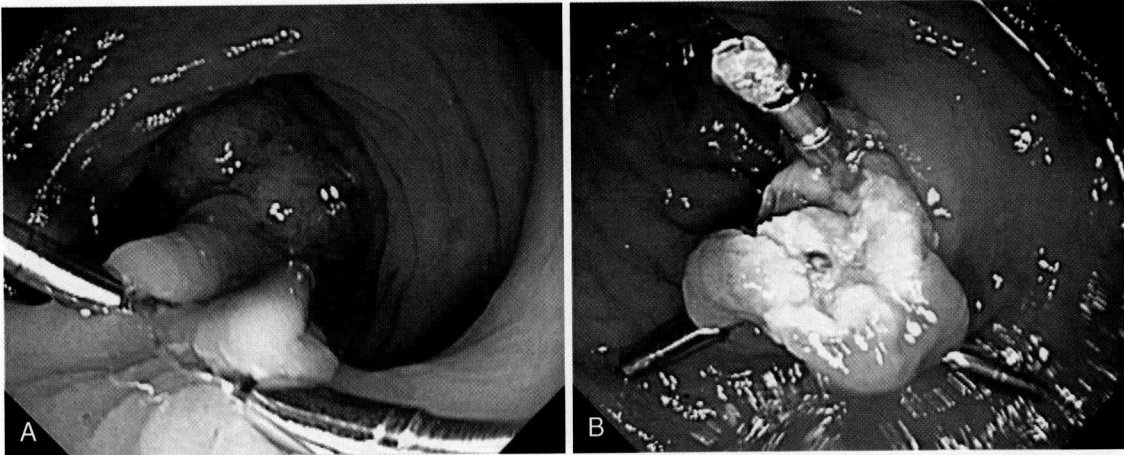

Fig. 36.15 Multiple endoclips can be used to prevent postpolypectomy bleeding from a thick-stalked polyp. **A,** Two endoclips were placed on opposite sides of the base of the stalk, causing the polyp to become dusky. **B,** A third endoclip was placed on the stalk remnant after transection to prevent bleeding. A sizable blood vessel was visible but was not bleeding. A fourth clip was subsequently placed on the vessel (not shown). *(From Palo Alto.)*

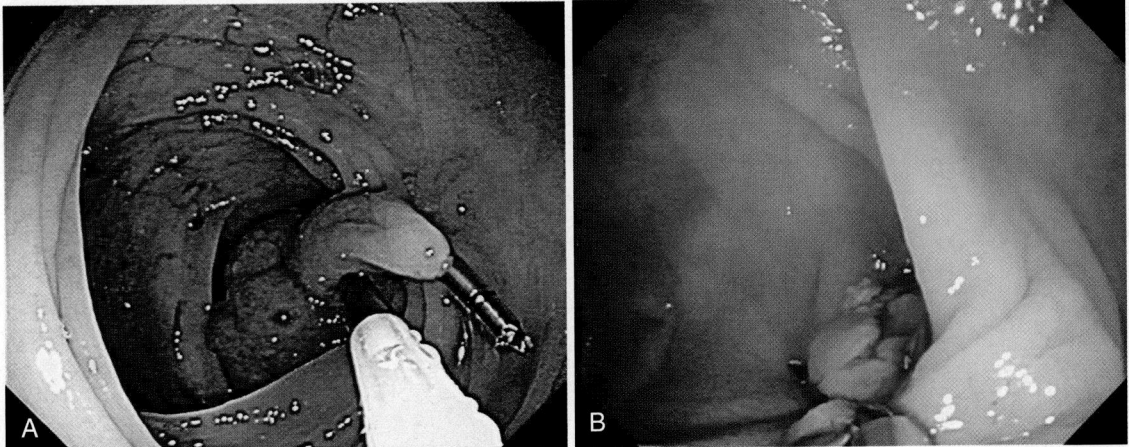

Fig. 36.16 Application of endoloops or endoclips may be difficult when the stalk is short. Diluted epinephrine can also be used to prevent immediate bleeding after polypectomy. **A,** Diluted epinephrine (1 : 10,000) was injected into the base of the stalk before resection. An endoclip had been previously applied to an area believed to contain a blood vessel. **B,** The effect of epinephrine was appreciated with the pale-appearing mucosa seen surrounding the resected site. Multiple endoclips were applied in a zipperlike sequence to clamp any possible large vessels. *(From Palo Alto.)*

en bloc rather than piecemeal resection has been described. The loop and let go technique may be useful for the treatment of large pedunculated lesions, especially colonic lipomas (**Fig. 36.17**).[72]

Mucosal Resection

Various resection techniques have been described.[27,37] The standard inject and cut technique, also known as saline-assisted polypectomy, is most common. The inject, lift, and cut technique is also popular in Japan. The simple suction technique has been used in many patients, some of whom had exceptionally large sessile or flat lesions. The mucosal resection technique using a ligation device is particularly useful for resection of submucosal lesions in the rectum.

INJECT AND CUT TECHNIQUE

The inject and cut technique requires submucosal injection to lift the diseased mucosa. The key aspects of submucosal

injection are to inject a sufficient amount and to recognize the presence of the on-lifting sign. The ideal solution, which would form a substantial bulge and would not dissipate quickly, has not been defined. Physicians in the United States routinely use saline (**Figs. 36.18 through 36.21**); physicians in Japan use Griseol, a mixture of saline and glycerol with a small amount of indigo carmine. Indigo carmine aids in the assessment of depth during and after resection. The remaining submucosa is blue-green in color, and deeper resections yield visualization of muscularis propria, fat, or other organs. Standard 25-gauge sclerotherapy needles are used. Tumor seeding has been reported in only one patient.[73] In our experience, performance of safe and effective mucosal resection demands that all necessary equipment and a trained assistant be present so that resection can be performed immediately after injection. We use a stiff standard snare. Whenever possible, we perform en bloc resections; if we must remove lesions piecemeal, we attempt to do so during a single session. We are able to resect most colorectal lesions using the inject and cut technique.

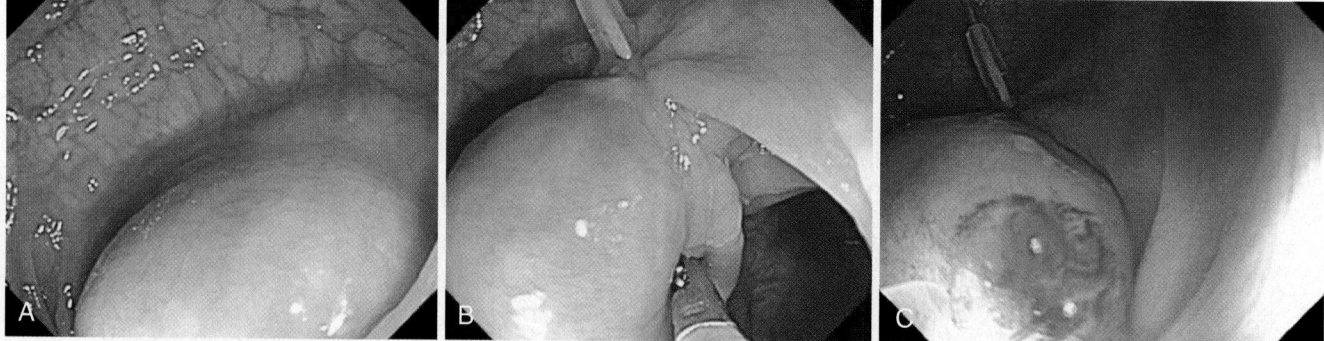

Fig. 36.17 Endoscopic polypectomy of colonic lipoma—well known to be benign—is known to carry a high risk of perforation. The ligate and let go technique is safe and efficacious to treat colonic lipoma.[72] **A,** Typical appearance of a colonic lipoma. Originally, the lesion was sessile (not shown), but by repositioning the patient to make it hanging, the lesion became pedunculated because its weight had pulled it from its point of attachment. **B,** Ligation of the point of attachment using an endoloop caused the lesion to become ischemic. **C,** Biopsy on biopsy showed the naked fat, confirming the diagnosis. There was no residual on follow-up colonoscopy a few months later.

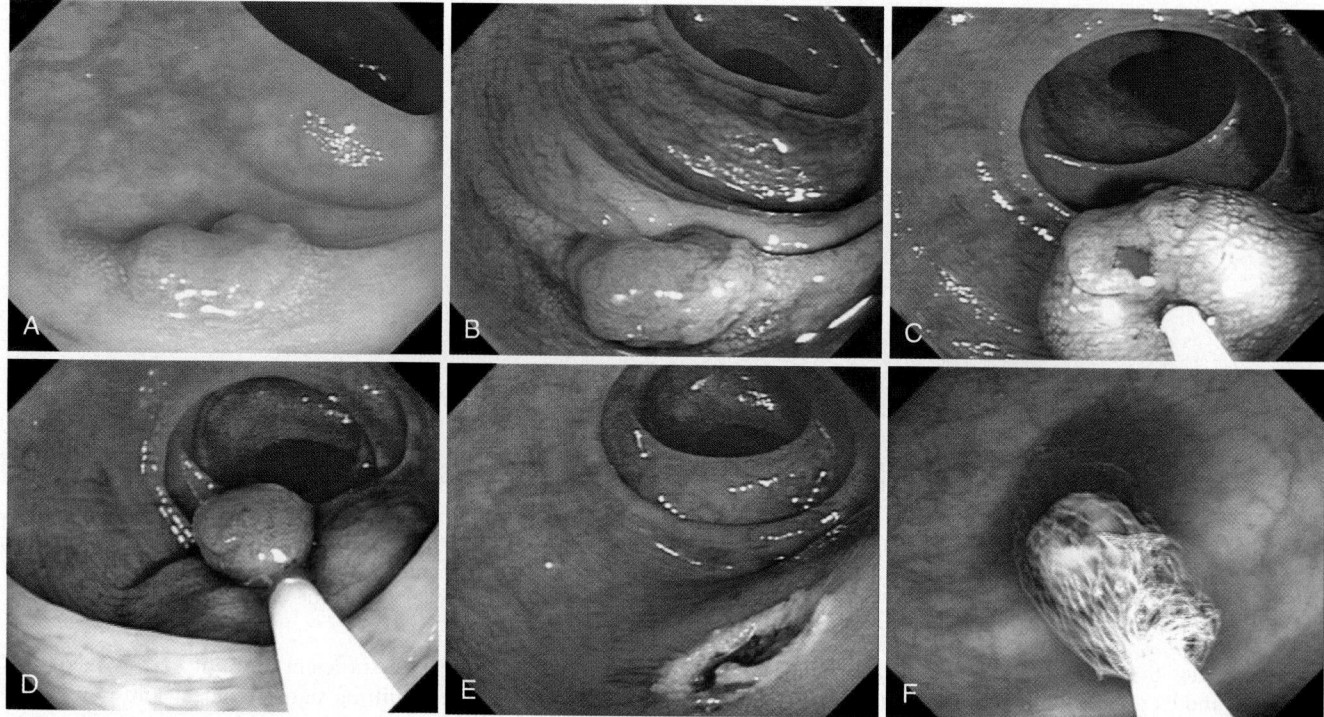

Fig. 36.18 The inject and cut endoscopic mucosal resection (EMR) technique. **A,** The lesion is carefully examined to assess for the potential of malignancy and depth of invasion. **B,** Indigo carmine was used to define the border of the lesion and to gain insight from the surface appearance. The lesion has a depressed surface, suggesting a high likelihood of malignancy. **C,** Saline solution (approximately 5 mL) was injected into the submucosa, lifting the lesion. **D,** A stiff snare was used to capture the entire lesion with a small rim of surrounding normal mucosa. **E,** The resection site was carefully examined by spraying additional diluted indigo carmine solution to examine for evidence of residual component. **F,** The lesion was carefully removed, without breaking it apart, using a Roth net. Maintaining the lesion as a single specimen is important to allow the pathologist to determine the resection margin if cancer is found. After the case had been completed, the specimen was pinned at its periphery onto a piece of wood with thin needles (not shown). EMR specimens are sectioned at 2-mm intervals to provide accurate staging. *(From Palo Alto.)*

SIMPLE SUCTION TECHNIQUE

The simple suction technique, developed by Soehendra and colleagues,[37,74,75] uses a special stiff 0.4-mm monofilament snare. The construction of this snare allows consistent placement of the snare parallel to the bowel wall and, with slight pressure, capture of the diseased mucosa. Piecemeal resections are performed without submucosal injections.

SUBMUCOSAL RESECTION WITH LIGATION

Submucosal resection with ligation[76] can be particularly useful for resection of submucosal lesions, such as carcinoid tumors in the rectum (**Fig. 36.22**).[28,77] After the endoscope is fitted with the ligation device, the target area is ligated, with or without prior deep submucosal injection. Standard polypectomy is performed below the rubber band. Small submucosal

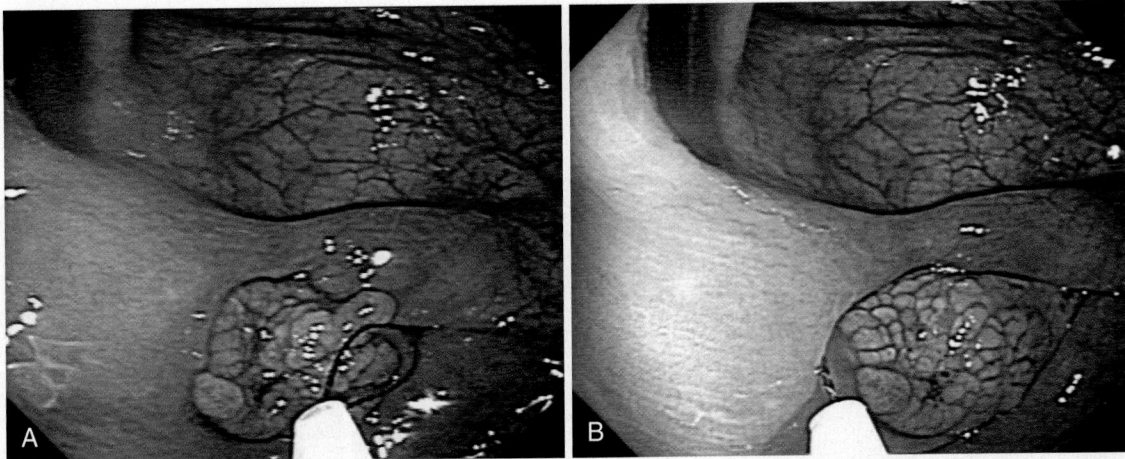

Fig. 36.19 The fulcrum technique was used in this case to ensure that the snare was placed in a plane parallel to the fold. Saline had previously been injected to lift the lesion. **A,** The tip of the snare was impacted slightly to the right of the lesion. The snare was slowly opened as the colonoscope was gently turned to the left. Close coordination between the endoscopist and the assistant is required to perform this maneuver. **B,** The snare was pushed toward the lesion, and air was suctioned slightly to draw the lesion into the snare. The snare was then slowly closed. Before cautery application, the snare was moved back and forth while examining the effect on the wall to ensure that muscularis propria was not entrapped in the snare. *(From Palo Alto.)*

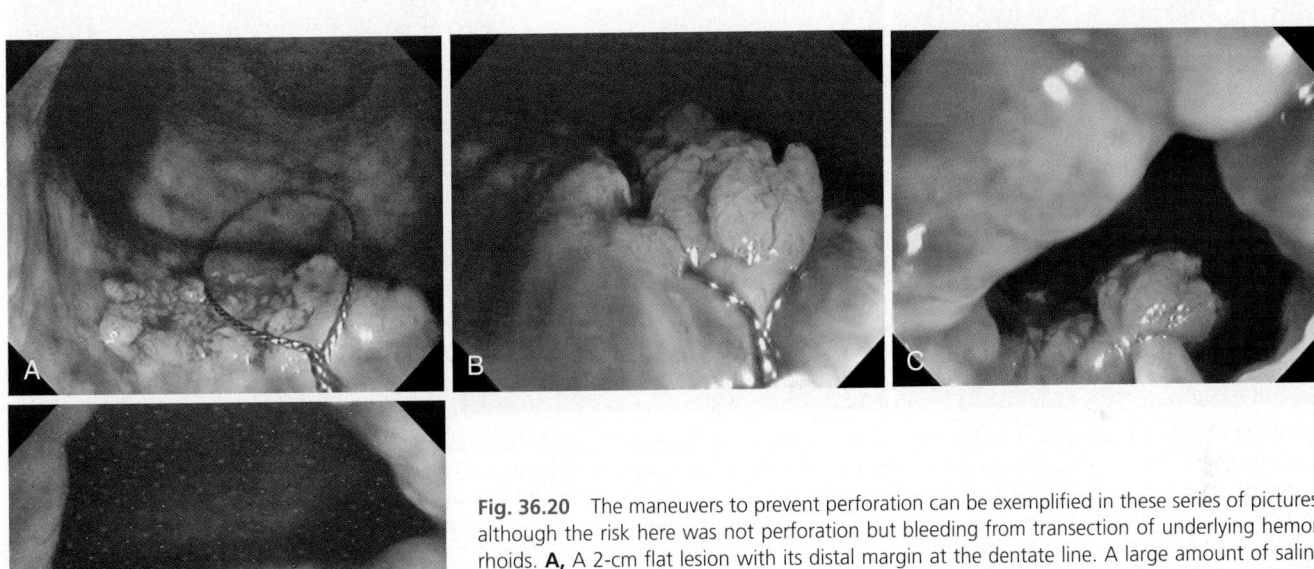

Fig. 36.20 The maneuvers to prevent perforation can be exemplified in these series of pictures, although the risk here was not perforation but bleeding from transection of underlying hemorrhoids. **A,** A 2-cm flat lesion with its distal margin at the dentate line. A large amount of saline had been injected to lift the lesion. **B,** The snare captured the lesion. **C,** The lesion was tented high into the lumen while the snare was loosened slightly. This maneuver was performed to release potentially entrapped structures deeper than the submucosa. **D,** Two separate resections were performed without bleeding. A small amount of residual tissue was found between the resection sites and was eliminated using the argon plasma coagulator (at 60 W). Histology showed a villous adenoma. On follow-up 1 and 2 years later, there was no evidence of recurrence (not shown). *(From Palo Alto.)*

lesions may require prior markings at their periphery, achieved by brief bursts of cautery using the tip of a snare, because such lesions may be difficult to find after the ligation device has been fitted to the endoscope.

OTHER TECHNIQUES

Other techniques that have been described but are not widely used include mucosal resection with cap[78-80]; inject, lift, and cut technique (double-channel EMR technique); and use of short endoclips to position the snare (**Fig. 36.23**).[81] Although

popular and efficacious for resection of superficial early cancer in the esophagus and stomach, EMR with cap or inject, lift, and cut can be risky to use in the colon.[78] The thin muscularis propria of the colon can easily be suctioned into the cap, potentially leading to perforation.

Submucosal Dissection

Endoscopic submucosal dissection (ESD) is the latest technique available for the resection of large nonpolypoid GI neoplasms.[82] The technique was initially developed for the

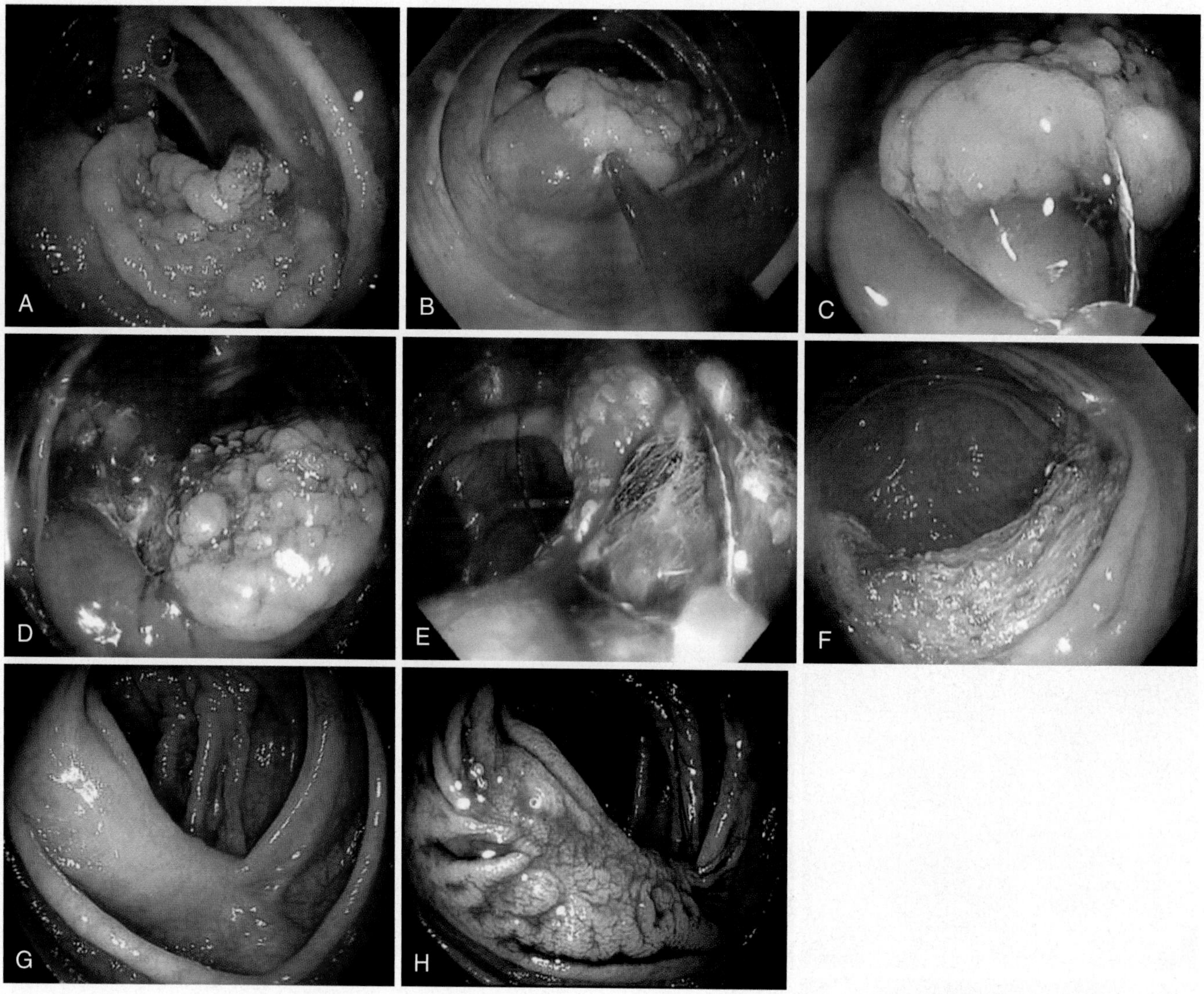

Fig. 36.21 Piecemeal resection of a large sessile lesion. A biopsy had been performed to document that the lesion was a large villous adenoma, as was suspected from its endoscopic appearance. **A,** The lesion was located adjacent to the ileocecal valve. **B,** A large amount (40 to 50 mL) of saline mixed with a few drops of 0.2% indigo carmine was injected into the submucosa to lift the lesion. Efforts were made to inject so that the lesion does not tilt away from the colonoscope. **C,** The first piece was resected using a stiff snare at the edge of the lesion. By resecting the lateral margin first, the endoscopist developed an understanding of the depth of the lesion and the location of the submucosal plane. **D,** A small piece of the lesion had been resected. The visible bluish layer was the submucosa. **E,** Subsequent resections were performed without proceeding deeper than the submucosa. The remaining large piece of the lesion was snared. Note the position of the snare: parallel with the bowel wall. **F,** Appearance after piecemeal resection, which was completed approximately 40 minutes later. Argon plasma was applied to ensure complete eradication of the villous adenoma. **G** and **H,** The area of prior resection on follow-up 3 months later. There was no residual adenoma.

resection of early gastric cancer that meets specified criteria in which the risks of lymph node metastasis approaches nil. However, in the colon and rectum, most neoplasms are benign and can be resected with minimal risks of recurrence. The indications for colorectal ESD are relatively uncommon (see **Box 36.1**).[4] Colorectal ESD is generally performed using various endoscopic knives, including the flex knife, bipolar knife, hook knife, and flush knife. The submucosal injectants used have also varied: saline with and without diluted epinephrine, glycerol, and hyaluronate. After generous submucosal injection, the procedure is begun with a circumferential cut to isolate the lesion with 3 or 4 mm of surrounding normal mucosa. After further submucosal injection, the submucosa under the lesion is dissected until the submucosa is divided

throughout. The lesion is removed en bloc. Numerous techniques have been described. By slow dissection of the submucosa under direct visualization, lesions that otherwise would be unable to be captured by a snare or lesions with submucosa fibrosis can also be removed.

The results of colorectal ESD performed by expert endoscopists are very encouraging. Saito and colleagues[83] reported the results of 200 colorectal ESDs measuring 38 mm on average, which took a median time of 90 minutes to resect. These investigators were able to obtain an en bloc resection rate of 84% with curative resection of 83%. They had a 5% perforation rate; except in one case (0.5%), the perforations were able to be treated by endoscopic clipping. Intraprocedure bleeding occurred in most patients and was treated

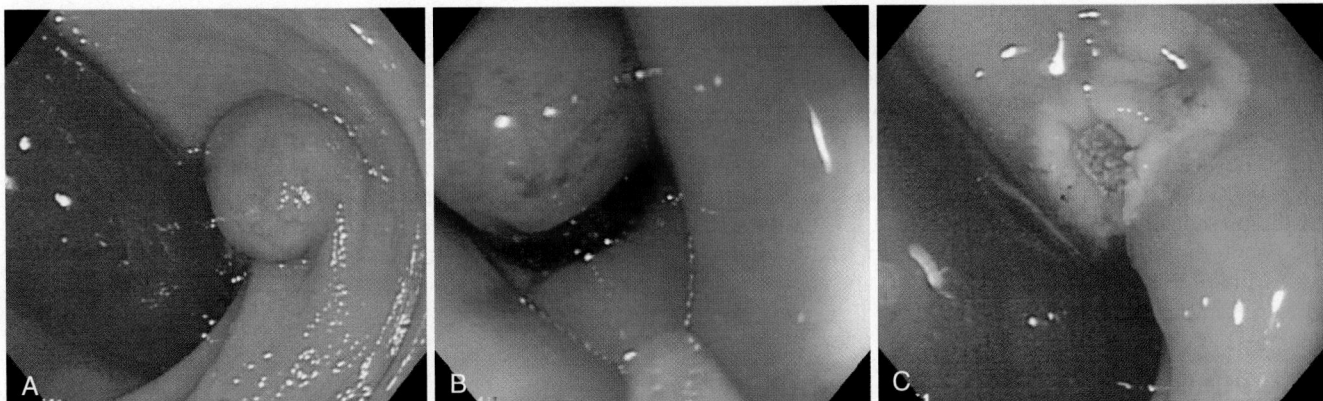

Fig. 36.22 Endoscopic submucosal resection of a small carcinoid tumor in the rectum using a band ligation device. **A,** Lesion. **B,** After deep submucosal injection of saline and placement of a band using the ligation device, a snare is seen transecting the lesion as cautery is applied. The lesion was contained within the resected specimen with a clear margin (not shown). By cutting immediately below the band, a deeper resection can be performed. *(From Tokyo.)*

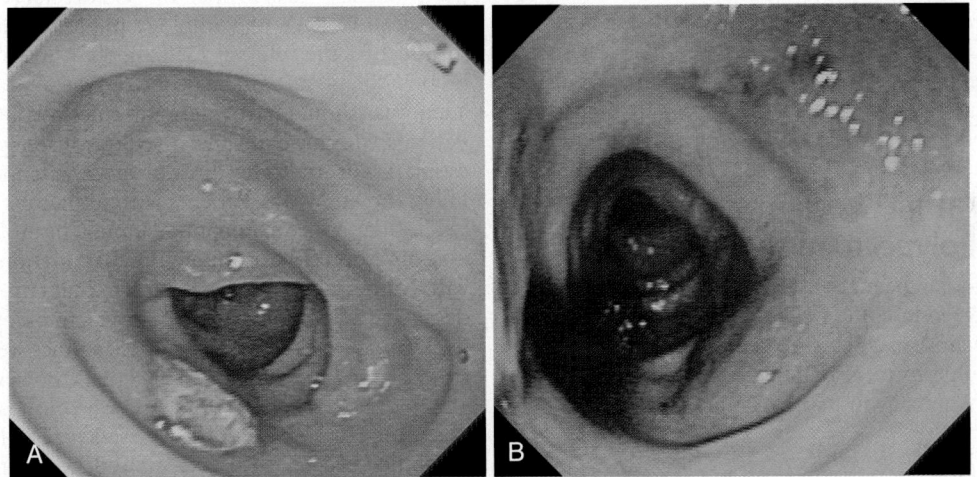

Fig. 36.23 India ink injection is used to mark an ulcerated depressed lesion *(inset)*. India ink solution was injected submucosally at three separate points. The depressed lesion was later shown to be an adenocarcinoma invading deep into the submucosa. Locations of the tattoos (distal, proximal, same level of the lesion) must be documented precisely, especially in cases of flat and depressed lesions. These lesions are often not palpable by the surgeon. Sometimes an endoclip is used in addition to India ink to mark the site on radiographs taken immediately after colonoscopy; this can assist in surgical planning, particularly when laparoscopic resection is contemplated in cases in the left colon. In these cases, the clip, as seen in the abdominal x-ray, can provide the precise location of the lesion. *(From Palo Alto.)*

endoscopically. Delayed bleeding occurred within the first 5 days after the procedure. Other authors have reported similar data showing high rates of en bloc resection and perforation, which can typically be treated with clipping, bowel rest, and antibiotics.[84]

The advantages of colorectal ESD include the ability to obtain a complete and accurate histologic assessment because the tissue is submitted with normal lateral margin and in one piece. In addition, the risk of recurrence in resection of benign lesions with clear margins is nil, and in lesions with minimal submucosal invasive adenocarcinoma, risk of recurrence can be estimated and stratified. Certain cases of well-differentiated adenocarcinoma that are slightly invasive into the submucosa without lymphatic or vascular invasion have minimal risks of invasion. Patients who have smaller risks of metastasis than surgery may be advised to undergo follow-up only. In Japan, ESD for the colon and rectum is indicated as long as the depth of invasion is less than 1000 μm from the muscularis mucosa.[85]

At the present time, the disadvantages of colorectal ESD are many, and they have become the barriers to its application in the Western countries. Colorectal ESD has a high risk of perforation (on average 5% to 6%, but up to 10%, in expert hands), although most perforations can be treated using endoscopic clipping, antibiotics, and bowel rest. Colorectal ESD requires additional training (25 to 40 gastric ESDs) and specialized devices and takes prolonged procedure time. In addition, patients are admitted to the hospital for approximately 5 days for supportive care and to ensure that complications occur in a monitored setting. Although the current technique and technology of colorectal ESD may pose some limitations, efforts are under way to simplify this modality. These efforts are aimed at eliminating the need for submucosal dissection, creating a modified technique of colorectal ESD that is less difficult and time-consuming.

ESD with snaring, described by Toyonaga and coworkers,[86] uses standard snaring technique after circumferential incision and trimming. The same authors have also described the results of EMR with a small incision. In this technique, after submucosal injection, a small mucosal incision was made using the tip of the snare. Snaring was then performed by pushing the snare lightly to the incision. These maneuvers, in effect, allowed the tip of the snare to be fixed and the opened snare to capture the surrounding normal mucosa of the lesion. At the present time, ESD with snaring and EMR with small incision techniques have been reported to lead to shorter procedure times, although data on bleeding and complication rate are still limited.

Techniques for Prevention and Treatment of Residual Lesions

Whenever possible, endoscopic resection should be completed in a single session. Mucosal resection of lesions that are highly suspicious for carcinoma should be resected en bloc. Such en bloc resection, if possible with surrounding normal mucosa, provides the ideal specimen for evaluation of involvement of the lateral and vertical margins. APC has been shown to be effective for treating small amounts of residual lesion.[40,87] More than one session may be needed to resect large sessile or flat lesions. Small recurrent lesions are often treated with repeat EMR, application of APC, or surgery.

Techniques for Identifying the Site of a Lesion or Polypectomy

The site of a lesion can be marked with India ink injected into the submucosa or endoscopic placement of a single or multiple radiopaque clips (see **Fig. 36.23**).[88,89] Both techniques are safe and simple to perform, although the endoclip may not be palpable and may not stay in place for a prolonged period.

Techniques for Retrieving the Specimen

The benefits of mucosal resection or polypectomy can be assessed only by a properly prepared pathologic examination. The Roth net is useful in recovering a specimen[90] from an en bloc resection of a flat or depressed lesion. Recovering such a specimen through the accessory channel may cause the mucosal resection specimen to be torn into smaller pieces. The Roth net can also aid in efficient recovery of a specimen from piecemeal resection of large sessile or pedunculated lesions. Smaller pieces can be collected through the accessory channel. The net, snare, basket, Tripod, and Pentapod are other accessories that can be useful for removal of large pedunculated polyps.

Techniques for Pathologic Staging

The benefits of polypectomy and mucosal resection can be realized only with first-rate pathologic assessment. Orientation of the specimen requires knowledge of the appearance of the lesion before resection. Orientation of the specimen by the endoscopist, especially in cases of mucosal resections of non-polypoid lesions, is required. To aid orientation, specimens from mucosal resections are flattened and fixed at their periphery with thin needles inserted into an underlying wood or Styrofoam block before immersion into formalin. The fixed lesion is sectioned serially at 2-mm intervals. Assessment of

a specimen containing carcinoma must include the depth of the lesion, neoplastic involvement of the lateral and vertical margins, histology, and involvement of the lymphatics or blood vessels or both. In the colon, involvement of the vertical margin is particularly important, more so than the involvement of the lateral margin, provided that there is no visible lesion remaining at the conclusion of the resection. The significant cautery effect at the lateral margin of the lesion during resection generally ablates any remnant cells. A repeat colonoscopy is needed to rule out evidence of residual or recurrent lesions.

Management and Surveillance after Polypectomy

Limited data are available to guide recommendations for surveillance after resection of adenomatous polyps.[91] The current joint guideline from the American Cancer Society, the U.S. Multi-Society Task Force on Colorectal Cancer, and the American College of Radiology published in 2008 is helpful in directing the interval for patients who have adenomatous lesions.[92] Patients who have one or two small (<1 cm) tubular adenomas should have follow-up colonoscopy at 5 to 10 years. Patients who have advanced (villous histology or high-grade dysplasia) or multiple (three or more) adenomas should have follow-up at 3 years. Patients with numerous adenomas, large sessile adenoma, malignant adenoma, or an incomplete colonoscopy should have follow-up examinations at short intervals. Numerous studies have shown that large sessile, flat, and depressed adenomas can be removed endoscopically with relatively good success.[16,65,75,93-95] These studies were conducted by expert endoscopists in referral centers, however.

After piecemeal resection, a repeat colonoscopy is typically performed in 3 to 6 months to assess for local recurrence. The postmucosectomy scar site should be examined carefully; image-enhanced endoscopy techniques may be useful to show the presence of the innominate grooves across the scar and normal pit or microvessel patterns. A resected specimen that was noted to contain adenoma at the index examination may contain advanced histology at a follow-up examination.[65,96] Khashab and colleagues[97] reported a high predictive value for long-term eradication in cases where the postmucosectomy scar site showed both normal macroscopic and microscopic (biopsy) findings. In cases with residual neoplasia, appropriate therapy with biopsy or repeat EMR is prudent, and another surveillance colonoscopy should be performed at 6 months. Subsequent examinations should be performed every 3 to 6 months until long-term eradication is confirmed, and then the patient should resume surveillance at the recommended guideline intervals. The rationale for such an intensive follow-up schedule is the relatively high rate of local recurrence described in the literature, particularly after piecemeal polypectomy.

A series of approximately 300 polyps larger than 3 cm that were resected endoscopically showed a recurrence rate of 17%, with most recurrent lesions successfully treated endoscopically.[65] In our efficacy study of standardized inject and cut EMR technique on 125 nonpolypoid lesions (117 flat and 8 depressed), we identified a 10% rate of local recurrence at the prior EMR site at the first surveillance colonoscopy, with ultimate eradication following one or two additional

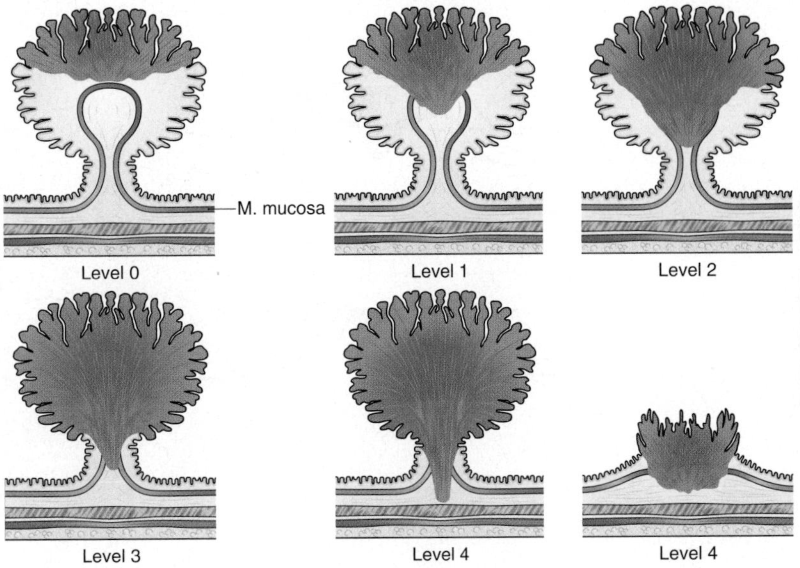

Fig. 36.24 Haggitt and colleagues[101] stratified the level of cancer submucosal invasion by the following criteria: *level 0,* carcinoma in situ (i.e., no extension below the muscularis mucosa); *level 1,* carcinoma invading through the muscularis mucosa but limited to the head of the polyp (i.e., above the junction between the adenoma and its stalk); *level 2,* carcinoma invading the level of the neck (i.e., the junction between adenoma and its stalk); *level 3,* carcinoma invading any part of the stalk; and *level 4,* carcinoma invading into the submucosa of the bowel wall below the stalk. In malignant sessile lesions, invasive carcinoma is considered as level 4.

colonoscopies. The recurrence is typically small. No lesion required surgery. Over a 4.5-year follow-up period, no patient developed or died of advanced colorectal cancer or distant metastasis.[2] The management of patients who have polypoid lesions containing invasive carcinoma is not straightforward. The risk of metastases of T1 lesions is approximately 10% to 15%.[98,99] Because most patients do not develop metastases, the decision of whether to perform surgery is complex. Immediate surgery performed shortly after initial local resection of T1 lesions confers a disease-free 5-year survival rate significantly higher than that of patients who had surgery only after local recurrence or lymph node metastasis from rectal cancer.[100]

Given the pathology findings, the endoscopist must assess whether the risk for lymph node metastasis is lower than that of partial colectomy. Various stratification methods have been reported; most distinguish patients at high risk and low risk to develop recurrence or metastasis. Published data often are collected from a few patients; even though they indicate that the absolute fraction of patients who developed metastases was low, great care must be exercised because the upper limit of the confidence interval of this fraction is often higher than the risk of surgery. Many studies grouped different types of lesions. The study by Haggitt and colleagues[101] that reported the level of invasion as the major prognostic factor is often cited to direct the management of polypoid lesions with submucosal invasion (**Fig. 36.24**). In this retrospective study, the authors concluded a low risk of metastasis or local recurrence when the level is less than 4. Generalizing their conclusions to endoscopic practice at large should be cautioned, however. The study involved a small number of patients—some had endoscopic treatment and others had surgery. The study lumped all patients who had sessile lesions that contained submucosal invasion into one group (level 4). Finally, Haggitt and colleagues[101] did not report the outer limit of the 95% confidence interval of their data (**Table 36.3**). When analyzed, patients with level 0 to 3 of invasion had up to 2.74% risk of developing metastasis, whereas patients with level 4 had up to 91% risk of favorable outcomes.

Because the risk of morbidity from surgery is less than 1% in patients with minimal comorbidity, the data by Haggitt and

Table 36.3 Statistical Limitations of the Haggitt* Study

Level of Invasion	Adverse Outcome (95% CI)	Favorable Outcome (95% CI)
0–3	0.9% (0–2.74)	99% (97.96–100)
4	25% (8.96–41.04)	75% (58.96–91.04)

*See reference 101.
CI, confidence interval.

colleagues[101] do not fully support that these patients should be uniformly advised to have watchful waiting. Similarly, a patient who has high risk for surgery with more than 10% risk of mortality may have a higher risk of dying from surgery than from developing metastasis (see **Table 36.3**). Detailed pathologic studies from Japan have found that the absolute depth of invasion should be considered because there is a gradual increase in the risk of lymph node metastasis with the depth of submucosal invasion.[16,102] Kitajima and colleagues[85] pooled the data from six institutions in Japan and classified the invasion according to **Fig. 36.25**. For pedunculated polyp, submucosal invasion was measured from an imaginary line drawn from the level 2 line of Haggitt's study to the deepest portion of the submucosa invasion. For NP-CRN, the muscularis mucosa was used as baseline, and the depth of invasion was the vertical distance from this line to deepest portion of invasion. When the muscularis mucosa could not be identified, the top of the lesion was used as baseline. For pedunculated lesions, they found that 0 of 53 patients (95% confidence interval 0% to 7%) with invasion limited to the head had lymph node metastasis. For the nonpedunculated lesions, 0 of 123 patients (95% confidence interval 0% to 3%) with depth of invasion less than 1000 μm had lymph node metastasis at the time of surgery. Similar to the data by Haggitt and colleagues,[101] this study was limited by the small sample size and length of follow-up.

Kikuchi and colleagues[102] stratified the risk of metastasis with the depth of carcinoma invasion from the muscularis

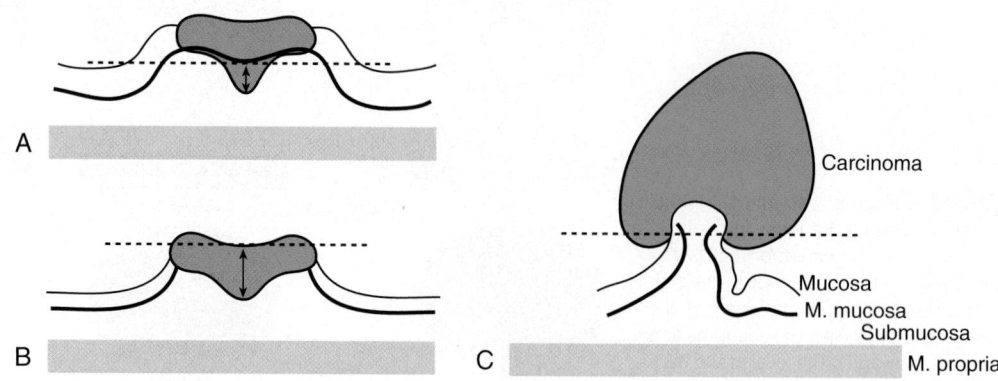

Fig. 36.25 Stratification of submucosal invasion of early colorectal cancer according to the General Rules for Clinical and Pathological Studies on Cancer of the Colon, Rectum and Anus. **A,** For nonpolypoid and sessile lesions, the vertical depth of the carcinoma is measured from the muscularis mucosa to the deepest point of invasion. **B,** If the muscularis mucosa has been destroyed by the carcinoma, the measurement is made from the surface of the lesion. Endoscopic therapy without surgery is accepted when the depth of the well-differentiated carcinoma without lymphatic or vascular involvement is less than 1000 μm and the lateral and vertical margins are negative. **C,** For pedunculated and semipedunculated lesions, the imaginary line is drawn according to level 2 invasion by Haggitt et al[101]: The lesion is considered to be head invasion only when the carcinoma did not infiltrate below the line. Endoscopic therapy is accepted without surgery in head invasion of well-differentiated carcinoma without lymphatic and vascular involvement.

mucosa and followed the patients for at least 5 years. Sm1 is slight mucosal invasion from the muscularis mucosa to a depth of 200 to 300 μm, sm2 is intermediate invasion, and sm3 is invasion near the inner surface of the muscularis propria. The investigators found that 64 patients with sm1 invasion (75% of whom had either semipedunculated or sessile lesions) had no evidence of metastasis during follow-up of at least 5 years. Other authors have developed stratification systems that combine depth and histology.[98,103] Favorable histology includes well-differentiated and moderately differentiated adenocarcinoma with carcinoma cells at least 2 mm from a clearly visualized margin. Unfavorable histology includes poorly differentiated adenocarcinoma, mucinous adenocarcinoma, and signet-ring cell carcinoma or one with adenocarcinoma cells within 2 mm from a clearly visualized margin. If the margins could not be assessed, the lesion was classified as unfavorable histology. No patients with favorable histology treated with endoscopic polypectomy had an adverse outcome. However, this study also involved only a few patients.

Additional factors have been suggested to be important in the patient risk stratification for local recurrence or metastasis. Tanaka and colleagues[104] reported that the absence of lymphatic or vascular involvement is highly predictive of a successful outcome. Masaki and Muto[105] showed that unfavorable histology (presence or absence of small nests of cancer cells with poorly differentiated or mucinous histology) at the invasive margin is predictive of adverse outcome. The management of small depressed lesions depends on the histology, lymphovascular invasion, and depth of invasion. Lesions larger than 1 cm often contain invasive cancer; patients who have such lesions are often referred directly to surgery.[16]

At the present time, the stratification of patients with lesions containing submucosal invasive cancer is not resolved.

Meticulous examination of the specimen by an experienced pathologist in close communication with the endoscopist helps to optimize the decision whether to recommend surgery. A patient with submucosal invasion must be well informed of the risks and benefits of endoscopic therapy and surgery, even in cases where the risk of metastasis is small.

Complications

Complications of polypectomy and mucosal resection include bleeding, transmural burn, and perforation. Familiarity with the endoscopic findings, symptoms, and signs of complications and treatment of complications is a prerequisite for performance of colonoscopic polypectomy and mucosal resection.

Postpolypectomy Bleeding

Postpolypectomy bleeding can occur during or after the procedure. The reported incidence varies according to the definition of *bleeding*, and the size and type of lesions resected. Significant bleeding was observed in 0.4% of hot biopsy specimens of diminutive polyps in one series. Other authors reported no complications in a series of more than 900 hot biopsy specimens of diminutive polyps. The overall risk is approximately 1% to 2% for snare polypectomy. Rosen and coworkers[106] reported a 0.4% risk of bleeding requiring hospital admission in a retrospective study involving 4721 patients who had polypectomies. Nivatvongs[107] reported 10 episodes of bleeding requiring blood transfusions among 1172 patients. Soehendra and coworkers[75] reported a 24% risk of bleeding in a series of 176 large (>3 cm) polypectomies. Most of these

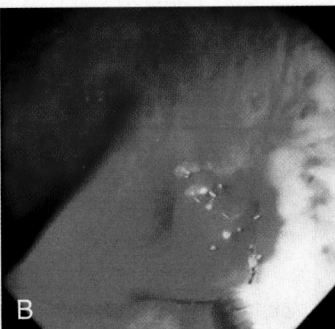
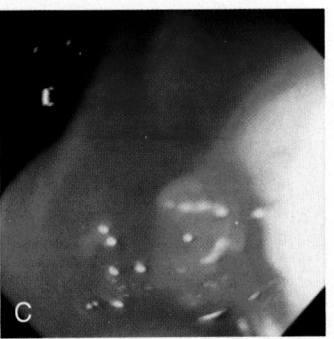
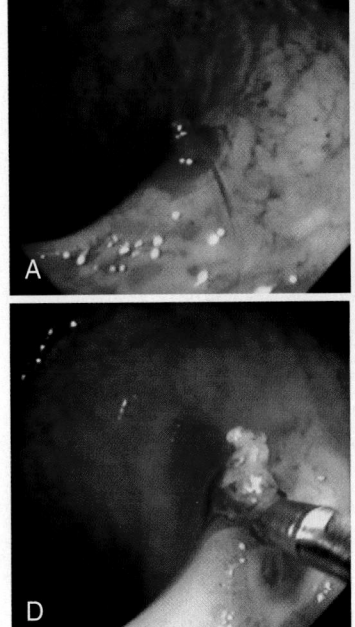

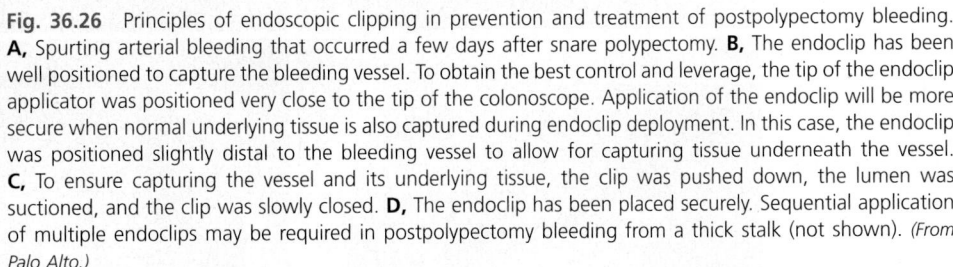

Fig. 36.26 Principles of endoscopic clipping in prevention and treatment of postpolypectomy bleeding. **A,** Spurting arterial bleeding that occurred a few days after snare polypectomy. **B,** The endoclip has been well positioned to capture the bleeding vessel. To obtain the best control and leverage, the tip of the endoclip applicator was positioned very close to the tip of the colonoscope. Application of the endoclip will be more secure when normal underlying tissue is also captured during endoclip deployment. In this case, the endoclip was positioned slightly distal to the bleeding vessel to allow for capturing tissue underneath the vessel. **C,** To ensure capturing the vessel and its underlying tissue, the clip was pushed down, the lumen was suctioned, and the clip was slowly closed. **D,** The endoclip has been placed securely. Sequential application of multiple endoclips may be required in postpolypectomy bleeding from a thick stalk (not shown). *(From Palo Alto.)*

hemorrhages occurred during the procedure, and all were successfully treated by endoscopic methods.

A variety of techniques are useful, including application of the endoclip or endoloop, use of APC, injection of diluted epinephrine, cauterization using monopolar or bipolar instruments, and repeat application of the snare or hot forceps biopsy to grasp the remnant stalk of pedunculated polyp. In cases in which endoscopic treatment fails, selective angiogram with the application of absorbable gelatin sponge (Gelfoam) emboli or surgery is employed. Our preferred technique for minor bleeding is APC; for significant bleeding, we use the endoclip or endoloop with or without prior injection of diluted epinephrine (**Fig. 36.26**). Parra-Blanco and colleagues[108] reported a case series showing the efficacy of endoclips to treat postpolypectomy bleeding. In cases with delayed bleeding, we typically would purge the bowel using 4 to 6 L of polyethylene glycol solution within 3 hours, immediately followed by a colonoscopy,[109] although Rex and colleagues[110] have reported successful colonoscopic treatment of delayed postpolypectomy bleeding without prior bowel purge.

Postpolypectomy Syndrome

Postpolypectomy syndrome, also called transmural burn syndrome, is thought to occur when cautery injury causes full-thickness necrosis of the bowel wall. Patients typically present with fever, localized abdominal tenderness (often with rebound tenderness), and leukocytosis. The onset of symptoms is commonly within a few hours of the polypectomy. The complication occurred in 6 (0.5%) of 1172 patients in one series[107] and in 9 (1%) of 777 patients in another.[111] Patients who are suspected to have postpolypectomy syndrome must be admitted for close observation by medical and surgical teams, bowel rest, and antibiotics. Most patients recover uneventfully. Abdominal radiographs and computed tomography (CT)

scans may show local changes such as air in the bowel wall but not within the peritoneum in the large amounts that would be seen with frank perforation. Localized perforation in the colon that is located in the retroperitoneum also may not be visualized using standard abdominal x-rays or manifested as diffuse free air or peritonitis.

Perforation

Perforation can occur when muscularis propria is included in the tissue grasped by a snare; this accident may happen, for example, when a large sessile polyp that is draped over a fold is grasped in its entirety. Techniques that may decrease the risk of capturing the muscularis propria have been summarized. Endoscopic clipping techniques have been shown to be useful in cases of fresh small perforation or, prophylactically, in cases where the resection appears too deep into the muscularis propria.[112] Most patients with colon perforation with diffuse peritonitis were reported to require surgery.[113,114] Patients who did not require surgery had smaller perforations owing to polypectomy, mucosal resection, or submucosal dissection rather than the large lacerations that are typically seen with diagnostic colonoscopy perforations. Delayed perforation can also occur as a result of tissue necrosis from cautery and requires surgery.

Future Trends

Advances in the technology and technique of colonoscopy have allowed us to manage increasingly complex colorectal lesions via endoscopy. Learning and using these new technologies and techniques may be demanding, but they enable us to perform endoscopic resections of lesions (**Fig. 36.27**) that previously would have required major abdominal surgery. The more sophisticated approaches can also improve recognition

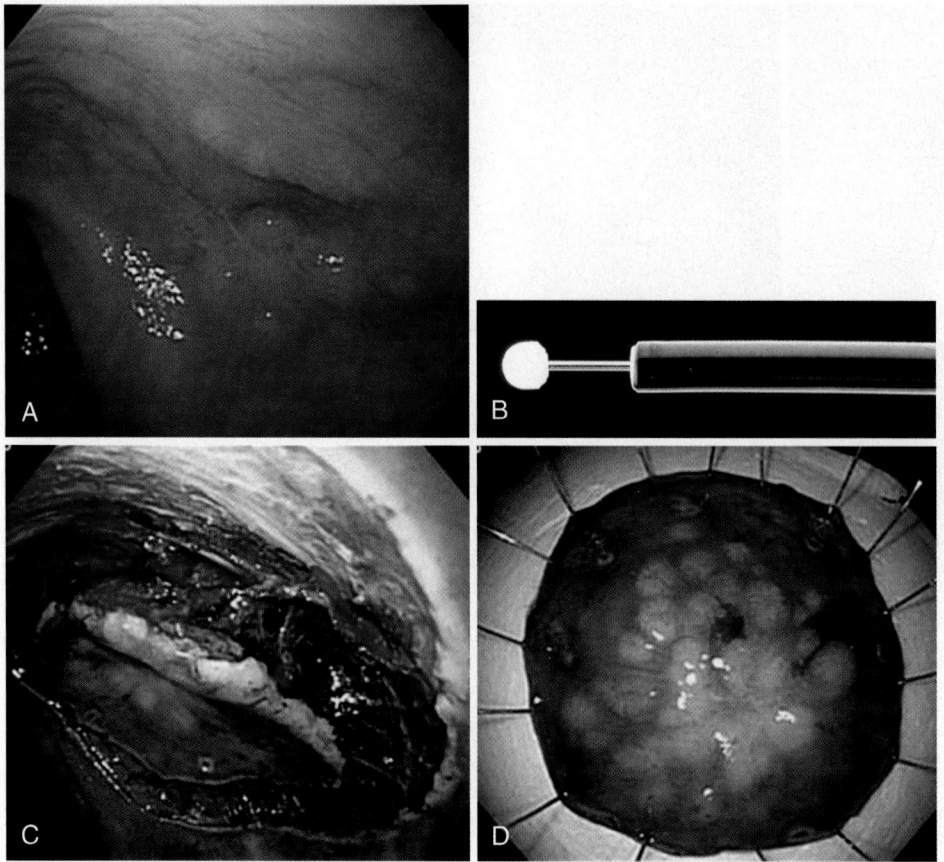

Fig. 36.27 En bloc resection of a large rectal localized lymphoma using the insulated-tip (IT) knife. **A,** The lesion seen after indigo carmine spray. **B,** IT knife is shown. **C,** Submucosal injection with diluted epinephrine and indigo carmine has been performed, and a circumferential incision has been made surrounding the lesion. **D,** After resection, the lesion is oriented, stretched, and pinned on a piece of Styrofoam by the endoscopist. The lesion was subsequently immersed in formalin. The pathologist sections the specimen at 2-mm intervals and notes their positions relative to each other. A precise determination of lateral and vertical depth of invasion can be reported. *(From Tokyo.)*

of the nonpolypoid lesions that were previously underappreciated in the Western countries and can assist in their treatment. Further developments will increase the potential of colonoscopic polypectomy, mucosal resection, and submucosal dissection. Extensive and long-term databases, using a common terminology for endoscopy and pathology,[115,116] are needed. Simplifications in the technology and techniques of the resections would allow them to be used more widely and ultimately benefit more patients.

References

The complete reference list is available online at www.expertconsult.com.

Section III

Pancreaticobiliary Disorders

Gregory G. Ginsberg

III

Chapter 37

Diagnostic Cholangiography

Evan L. Fogel, Lee McHenry, Jr., James L. Watkins, Stuart Sherman, Kyo-Sang Yoo, and Glen A. Lehman

Introduction

Endoscopic cannulation of the major papilla with imaging of the biliary tree and the pancreatic ductal system (endoscopic retrograde cholangiopancreatography [ERCP]) was first successfully accomplished with an end-viewing duodenoscope and reported in 1968.[1] Subsequent development of side-viewing endoscopes with a catheter-deflecting elevator greatly facilitated the technique. Diagnostic studies were supplemented by the first endoscopic sphincterotomies in the early 1970s.[2,3] These developments permitted less invasive diagnostic and therapeutic maneuvers in the bile duct previously limited to open surgical and percutaneous techniques. Although these procedures are more technically demanding than most other gastrointestinal (GI) endoscopic techniques, they are now being widely used and are the method of choice for many clinical problems involving the pancreatic ductal and hepatobiliary systems.

This chapter focuses on diagnostic endoscopic retrograde cholangiography (ERC). Radiographic visualization of the biliary tree is often key to establishing a clinical diagnosis and formulating a therapeutic plan.[4,5] With the aid of noninvasive imaging via transcutaneous ultrasound, computed tomography (CT), or magnetic resonance imaging (MRI),[6–13] thorough ductal filling at ERC is needed less frequently and is contraindicated in certain cases. Diagnostic ERC is just one portion of commonly combined ERCP and associated therapeutic maneuvers.

Endoscopic Retrograde Cholangiopancreatography

Indications and Contraindications

The role for diagnostic ERC alone has nearly disappeared as other, less invasive and noninvasive imaging techniques (e.g., CT scans, endoscopic ultrasound [EUS], magnetic resonance cholangiopancreatography [MRCP]) have become more widely used. Imaging of the biliary ductal system without anticipated therapy is clinically helpful in only a few clinical settings, such as cholestasis without dilated ducts. In certain settings, such as inflammatory bowel disease, patients with early sclerosing cholangitis may have ductal changes visible only via invasive cholangiography such as ERC (i.e., missed by noninvasive imaging). ERC is mainly indicated in clinical settings in which there is significant suspicion of obstructing, inflammatory, or neoplastic pancreatobiliary lesions that, if detected or ruled out, would alter clinical management. A general classification of indications is listed in **Box 37.1**.

Most contraindications of ERC are relative, and the degree of risk must be balanced against the potential benefit.[14–16] In certain settings, even very ill and unstable patients, such as with acute cholangitis with shock or sepsis from bile duct stones or biliary strictures, diagnostic (followed by therapeutic) ERCP may be lifesaving. ERC in patients with necrotizing acute pancreatitis and low clinical suspicion for ductal stones is considered relatively contraindicated because pancreatography may result in bacterial contamination of the pancreatic bed. Other relative contraindications include unstable cardiopulmonary disease or severe coagulopathy. Patients with comorbid life-threatening conditions can often have ERC performed in the intensive care unit (with or without fluoroscopy) if deemed medically necessary. ERC is generally not indicated in type III suspected sphincter of Oddi dysfunction (unless manometry is included).

Preparation for Endoscopic Retrograde Cholangiography

Preparation for ERC involves assembly of a skilled team that includes endoscopists, nurses, and radiology technical and physician support personnel. A quality fluoroscopic unit is needed. A variety of catheters, guidewires, and other therapeutic devices should be available.

Assembling the Team

We recommend that ERCP be done independently only by physicians with prior formal training in ERCP. An adequate number of examinations during training varies greatly with the trainee but should include at least 200 examinations.[17] This number includes at least 100 therapeutic examinations. Successful biliary cannulation rates should be at least 85% and preferably 90%. We recommend that nurses have experience with at least 1000 upper GI and colonoscopy examinations before "graduating up" to the ERCP suite. Nurses should train alongside experienced ERCP nurses for 100 to 200 examinations before independent guidewire and accessory management is undertaken. Two nurses are needed per examination: one for sedation and analgesia administration and one for

accessories management. Radiology technicians working in ERCP should maintain longevity and be team members rather than rotate frequently. In nearly all centers, a radiologist no longer assists in fluoroscopy or image acquisition except in the most difficult cases. Collaborative reading of final images may aid in the accuracy of final interpretation. Final reading by general radiologists with little pancreatobiliary training, experience, or interest may be counterproductive.

Patient Preparation

Patient preparation includes an updated medical history and physical examination; recent complete blood cell count, serum liver chemistries, serum amylase, and lipase; and at least one noninvasive imaging study of the upper abdomen with abdominal ultrasound, CT scan, or magnetic resonance cholangiography. Platelet count, prothrombin time, and partial thromboplastin time may be obtained if therapeutics are anticipated. However, a history of liver disease, renal disease, and bleeding are adequate to detect most patients with increased bleeding risk. Patients with a history of easy bruising, excessive bleeding after dental extraction, other postoperative bleeding, or family history of coagulopathy are best evaluated with the help of hematology consultation.

Risk factors such as anticoagulant therapy, prosthetic heart valves, and allergies must be addressed.[18] Patients with iodine allergy are at very low risk of allergic reaction[19]; nevertheless, some centers continue to use prednisone, 30 to 40 mg orally, 15 hours and 3 hours before the examination. Diphenhydramine (Benadryl), 25 mg intravenously, may be added if serious past reactions have occurred. Iodine allergy is not a reason to omit a needed examination, but limiting the volume of contrast medium used is logical. Air[20] can be successfully used for cholangiography if needed. If possible, aspirin and nonsteroidal antiinflammatory drugs should be avoided for 7 days before the procedure.

Fasting for 8 hours is generally recommended except for taking oral medications, such as blood pressure medication, the morning of the examination. Patients undergoing examination in the afternoon may have a clear liquid breakfast. Patients taking narcotics may need to fast for 12 to 16 hours or consume only clear liquids the evening before. Patients with constipation and patients who have had recent oral contrast agents may benefit from an oral laxative purge to clear the transverse colon of material, which may otherwise overlay and obscure viewing of the gallbladder, terminal bile duct, and pancreas. Broad-spectrum antibiotics are recommended (e.g., ciprofloxacin) for patients with obstructive jaundice, cholangitis, pseudocysts, fistulas, or immunosuppressed state. Quinolones are an attractive choice because they can be given orally. Oral simethicone solution is recommended 30 to 60 minutes before examination start time to decrease intraluminal foam, which may obscure visualization.

Informed Consent

Informed consent for ERCP must be obtained. It is both legally and ethically necessary to apprise the patient (and family members if applicable) of the risks, benefits, and alternatives of the anticipated procedure. **Table 37.1** lists potential complications of diagnostic and therapeutic ERCP and their relative frequency. Although legal standards continue to

Table 37.1 Approximate Frequencies of Complications from Endoscopic Retrograde Cholangiopancreatography (ERCP) and Sphincterotomy (%)

Complication	Average-Risk Patients		High-Risk Patients*	
	ERCP	Sphincterotomy	ERCP	Sphincterotomy
Pancreatitis	3	5	8	12
Bleeding	0.2	1.5	0.4	3.5
Perforation	0.1	0.8	0.3	1.5
Infection	0.1	0.5	2	2
Sedation reaction or cardiopulmonary	0.5	0.5	2	2
Total %†	3.9‡	8.3‡	12.7‡	21‡

*Certain patient characteristics and technical aspects of the procedure increase the risk of complications, including suspected sphincter of Oddi dysfunction, recurrent pancreatitis, difficult cannulation, precut sphincterotomy, coagulopathy, renal dialysis, cirrhosis, or advanced cardiopulmonary disease.
†Some patients have more than one complication.
‡Approximate severity of complications: mild, 70%; moderate, 20%; and severe, 10%.

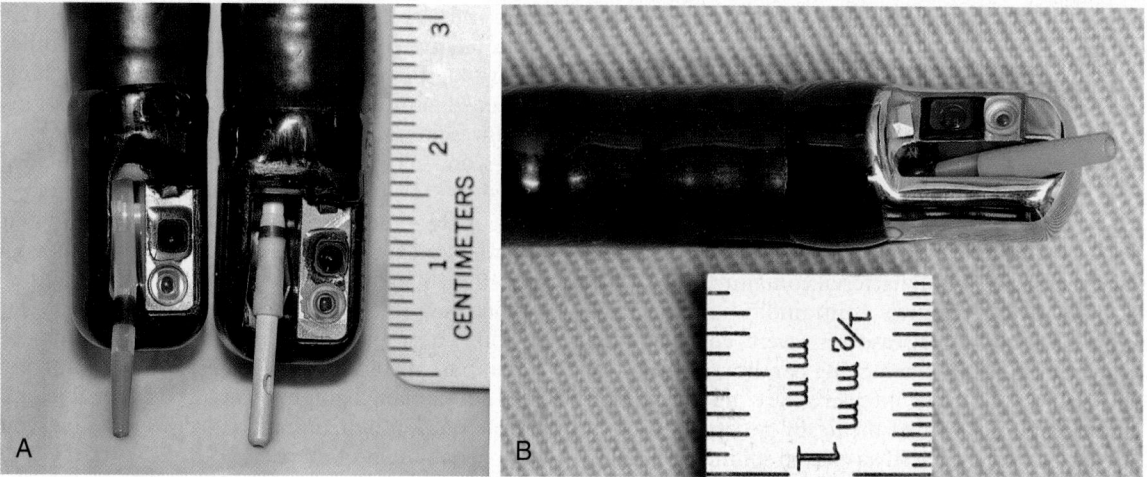

Fig. 37.1 A, Photograph of two side-viewing endoscopes used for standard endoscopic retrograde cholangiography (ERC). Biopsy channels range from 3.2 to 4.5 mm to accommodate a wide variety of accessories needed in diagnostic and therapeutic biliary studies. **B,** Newer generation Olympus pediatric videoduodenoscope for use in children weighing less than 10 kg.

evolve, we recommend that patients be informed of the potential complications and the relative frequencies of complications. In addition, we recommend that patients be told that a severe complication possibly may result in a prolonged hospital stay, intensive care unit monitoring, or open surgery and very rarely may result in permanent disability or death. Complication rates vary according to patient and procedure risk factors and the disease process being evaluated and treated. Patients with uncomplicated biliary stones, malignancy, or chronic pancreatitis have lower complication rates, whereas patients with acute recurrent pancreatitis and suspected sphincter of Oddi dysfunction have twofold to fourfold higher complication rates. Procedure techniques associated with higher complication rates include repeated cannulation attempts, repeated pancreatic duct injections, pancreatic parenchymal acinarization, and precut sphincterotomy (without associated protective pancreatic stent). Attention to details of the technique and patient selection can minimize, but not eliminate, complications. Morbidity can be limited by early recognition and treatment of complications.

Endoscopic Equipment

ERC can be performed with fiberoptic or video chip, side-viewing instruments. Endoscopes are 120-cm working length and generally categorized as diagnostic (approximately 10-mm diameter) or therapeutic (12- to 13-mm diameter). Video systems offer the advantage of television monitor viewing by all persons in the endoscopy suite; this offers better teaching capabilities and allows better coordination between the endoscopist and nursing assistants. Some newer generation endoscopes combine a large working channel diameter up to 4 mm with a standard 10- to 11-mm outer diameter (**Fig. 37.1**). A newer generation pediatric videoendoscope with outer diameter less than 7 mm is now available from Olympus America Inc. Most ERCP examinations are done with air insufflation. Limited data show that carbon dioxide inflation reduces postprocedure abdominal distention.[21] For patients undergoing Billroth II procedures, we generally start with a standard side-viewing duodenoscope, but an end-viewing endoscope is occasionally needed. In patients with a long Roux-en-Y gastroenterostomy or choledochojejunostomy, a 160-cm

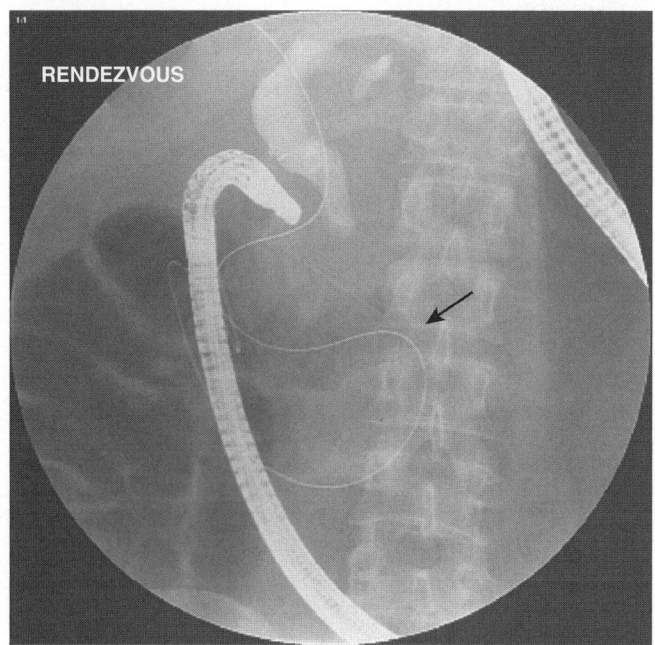

Fig. 37.2 A patient underwent gastric bypass surgery for obesity and developed biliary colic and suspected common duct stones. A pediatric colonoscope was passed by mouth but failed to pass retrograde back to the descending duodenum. A guidewire was passed percutaneous transhepatically into the duodenum, beyond the ligament of Treitz *(arrow)*, and on down into the jejunum. The wire was grasped, and the endoscope was pulled back to the papilla for stone therapy.

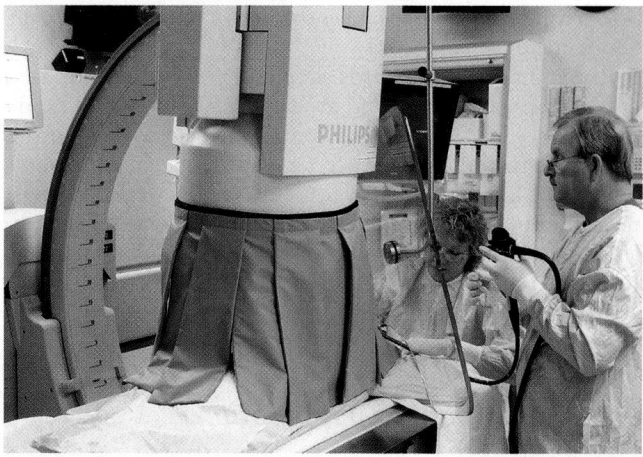

Fig. 37.3 Room set-up with C-arm x-ray unit. Table tilt and cradle, C-arm tilt, and rotation offer viewing in multiple angles. Note lead apron drape from image intensifier. Note see-through lead shield near the head of the patient.

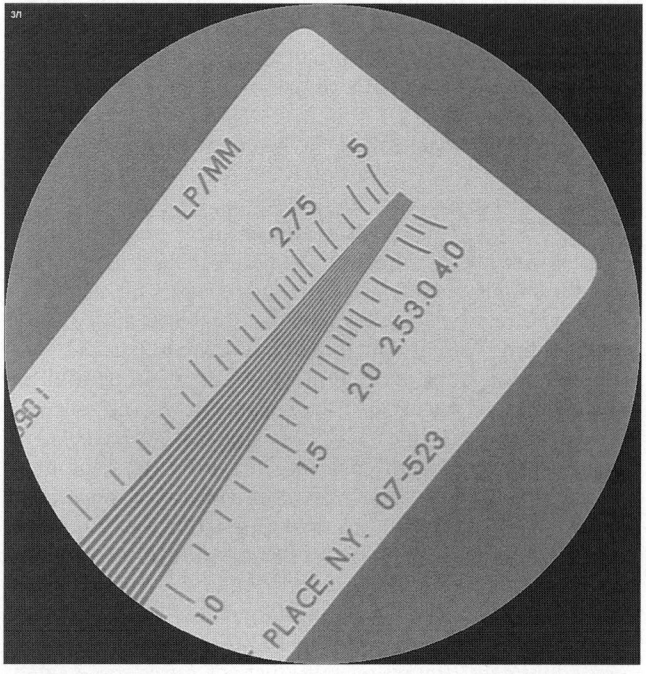

Fig. 37.4 Phantom used in determining line pair resolution during fluoroscopy or image acquisition. Greater than 2.5 line pair resolution is recommended for optimal endoscopic retrograde cholangiopancreatography (ERCP) resolution. (Courtesy of Joe Edmiston, Indiana University Medical Center.)

pediatric colonoscope or a 220-cm enteroscope can reach the bile duct in greater than half of patients.[22] Double-balloon enteroscopy has facilitated Roux-en-Y limb traversal.[23,24] The lack of a catheter-deflecting elevator and limited compatibility accessories make end-viewing endoscopy difficult in these settings. Rendezvous with transhepatic wire passage is occasionally helpful (**Fig. 37.2**).

Current-generation endoscopes are capable of undergoing submersion disinfection. After cleaning, endoscopes should be hung in vertical position to facilitate drying. In the past, *Pseudomonas* infections were directly linked to inadequate ERCP scope disinfection. Ideally, endoscopes should be cultured periodically. Patients developing infections after undergoing ERCP should be cultured for the presence of *Pseudomonas* species (see Chapter 4).

Radiology Suite

Few endoscopists have a dedicated suite for ERCP. We are aware of no manufacturer who markets a fluoroscopy unit specifically for ERCP. Most endoscopists schedule time in the radiology department and use general purpose or angiographic units. Film documentation is likely to disappear in the next decade, with digital formats viewed only on high-resolution monitors, which are becoming the new standard. Quality digital images now rival film quality. Flat tables with fixed overhead carriage have limited versatility. The preferred x-ray table includes the capability to tilt the patient's head up and down 30 degrees and has C-arm carriage, which allows axial, cranial, caudal, vertical, and horizontal movements, allowing viewing at multiple angles (**Fig. 37.3**). Because the

patient is usually positioned prone with the head at the "foot" of the table, ability to reverse the viewing image in both the vertical and the horizontal axes is helpful. In the past, endoscopists used older generation x-ray units, including portable C-arm units with limited image resolution. This practice is no longer acceptable because fluoroscopy and saved image quality are key to accurate diagnosis and management. High-quality ERCP imaging requires resolution equivalent to that for neuroradiology (brain blood vessels). Resolution of greater than 2.5 line pair per millimeter is strongly recommended for both fluoroscopy and final images (**Fig. 37.4**). This resolution is best accomplished with smaller diameter image intensifiers of 6 to 9 inches.

Radiation safety standards should be followed.[25] Monitoring of personal exposure and review of methods to limit exposure are needed. Attention to coning the field of view to the area of interest is good practice. Lead aprons or shields around the patient limit x-ray beam scatter. Use of newer generation pulse fluoroscopy gives intermittent viewing, which is slightly jerky but often adequate with one-tenth the radiation exposure. Appropriate lead aprons, lead glasses, and thyroid shields are recommended (**Fig. 37.5**).

Technique

Patient Positioning, Preparation, and Sedation

Most centers prefer to have the patient positioned in a prone or slightly left lateral decubitus position on a fluoroscopic table. Less often, supine position is preferred, such as in patients with recent abdominal incisions, patients with multiple abdominal drain tubes, and patients undergoing Billroth II procedures.[26] Intravenous access and monitoring equipment for blood pressure, pulse, and pulse oximetry are needed. Electrocardiogram (ECG) monitoring is desirable for patients with angina or a history of a cardiac arrhythmia and in other less stable patients.

Sedation and analgesia are achieved by slow intravenous administration of diazepam (10 to 40 mg), midazolam (2 to 10 mg), and meperidine (25 to 150 mg) or fentanyl (50 to 150 mg). The general ranges mentioned here are given over a 30- to 60-minute examination. Droperidol (2.5 to 10 mg) is a common supplement or alternative, particularly for alcoholics or persons regularly taking narcotics or benzodiazepines.[27] However, more recent concerns about arrhythmias and Q–T interval prolongation have limited the use of droperidol for endoscopy. Our policy is to use droperidol routinely for patients whose baseline ECG has a normal corrected Q–T interval.[28] More recently, propofol has been used for deep sedation and may offer better procedure tolerance and a much shorter recovery time than standard sedation. Propofol use, when administered by endoscopists and endoscopy nurses, is apparently safe for standard upper GI endoscopy and colonoscopy but has not been well studied for ERC.[29–31]

Visual monitoring in a darkened ERCP room with fluoroscopy equipment draped over the patient raises some safety concerns for ERC use. Topical pharyngeal anesthetic spray probably decreases gagging in patients. An antiperistaltic drug (e.g., glucagon or atropine) to inhibit duodenal motility is commonly needed. Drugs to treat bradycardia (e.g., atropine) and high blood pressure (e.g., labetalol) should be immediately available. Benzodiazepine and narcotic reversal agents should be immediately available in an "easy to administer" format. A fully equipped resuscitation cart must be close by. Pediatric cases can be done with success similar to adults. We prefer to use the pediatric endoscope with a diameter less than 8 mm for children weighing less than 12 kg, but we use the standard 10-mm diameter endoscope for all larger children.

Upper Gastrointestinal Endoscopy

Initially, a brief endoscopic examination of the esophagus, stomach, duodenum, and major duodenal papilla is done. The

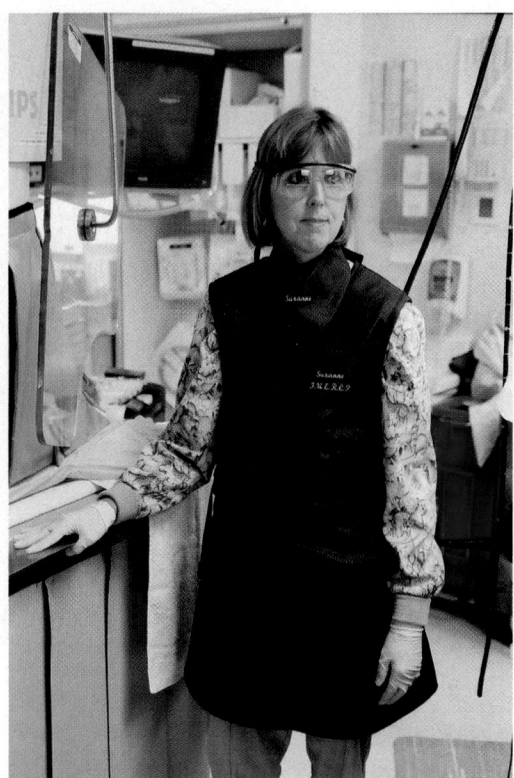

Fig. 37.5 Endoscopy assistant with lead apron, thyroid shield, and lead glasses for optimal radiation safety.

finding of a large ulcer or neoplasm may cancel the need for ERCP. One should attempt to exit the stomach with as little residual intragastric air as possible because a deflated stomach permits better en face papilla views. Other findings, such as tumor infiltrating the proximal descending duodenum, varices, a pseudocyst pressing on the gut wall, or edema of the medial wall of the duodenum, help to quantitate or localize disease processes. The major papilla is usually located on the medial aspect of the mid-descending duodenum but may reside anywhere from the duodenal bulb to the transverse duodenum. Care should be taken to observe for major papilla abnormalities (e.g., tumor, edema, enlarged orifice from stone or mucus passage). The location of orifices should be noted. A brief examination of the minor papilla may be helpful later in the examination if initial ERCP via the major papilla fails.

Before attempts at cannulation, fluoroscopic visualization (or still image acquisition) of the field of interest should be performed to look for stents, calcifications, masses, and residual contrast material (**Fig. 37.6**). The choice of initial cannulation tool is a personal preference (similar to choosing a tennis racket or golf club). One may begin with a simple single-lumen 5-Fr polyethylene catheter, without a guidewire, in many cases. The relative flexibility (not rigid), maneuverability, low cost, and simplicity are attractive features. A manometry catheter is initially used if ERCP findings are likely to be nonspecific or normal and if manometry is likely to be potentially helpful. If a sphincterotomy is almost certainly needed, a sphincterotome is a good starting tool. If the orifice appears small, a more tapered tip catheter or sphincterotome may be chosen. A few centers prefer various shaped metal tip catheters. Two-lumen or three-lumen catheters or sphincterotomes

Section III—Pancreaticobiliary Disorders 495

may be preferred because they have a separate lumen for a guidewire and contrast medium. A guidewire may be used at any point to aid cannulation or maintain intraductal stability. For biliary cannulation, 0.025-inch or 0.035-inch diameter wires are preferred. Soft-tipped wires have the advantage of less tissue trauma (e.g., fewer submucosal or other extraductal dissections). The specific devices used are much less important than the skill of the endoscopist (**Fig. 37.7**).

If the major papilla is not initially evident, gentle lifting of folds, greater air distention, and use of glucagon to inhibit peristalsis would likely expose the structure. If duodenal diverticula are present, the major papilla is most commonly on the diverticular rim, but the papilla is within the diverticulum per se in approximately 5% to 10% of cases (**Fig. 37.8**). The major papilla is then cannulated. Orientation of the

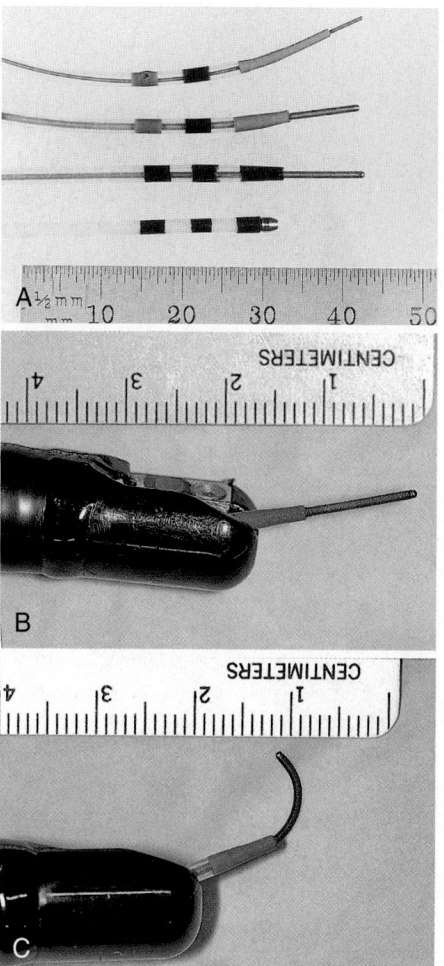

Fig. 37.7   **A,** A well-equipped biliary diagnostic unit contains a wide variety of guidewires with varying characteristics, different sizes (0.018-inch, 0.025-inch, and 0.035-inch diameter), variable hydrophilic tips, and some groomable wires whose tip shape can be changed. Also shown are 5-Fr catheters with variable tip taper or metal tip (bottom). **B,** Stainless steel wire of 0.035-inch diameter (with polytef [Teflon] coating) ungroomed (straight). **C,** Same wire as shown in **B** except tip has been manually groomed to curl cephalad for biliary cannulation assistance.

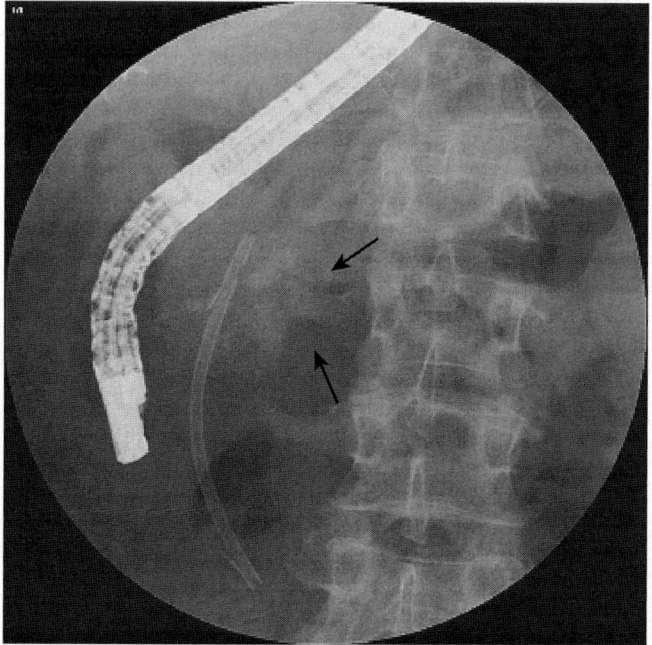

Fig. 37.6   Plain x-ray film of right upper quadrant showing post–shock wave lithotripsy pancreatic calcifications (arrows) and residual biliary stent. This film serves as a background view for all subsequent contrast agent injections.

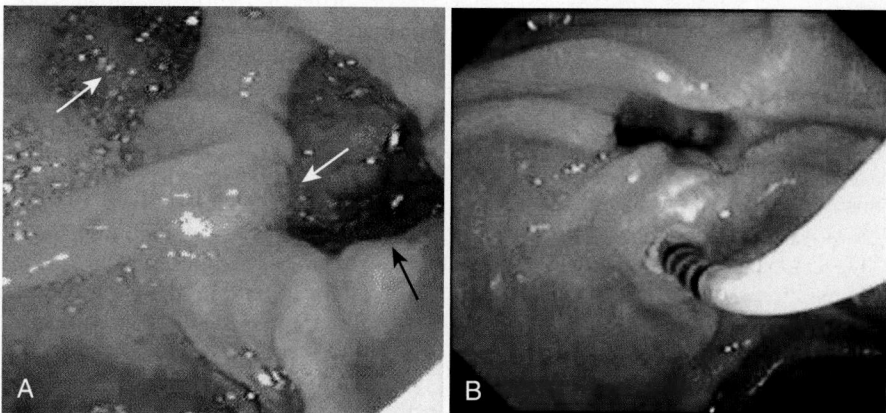

Fig. 37.8   **A** and **B,** Difficult biliary cannulation cases. Major papilla associated with duodenal diverticula. The papilla is most commonly on the rim of the diverticulum but may be located fully within the diverticulum and be much more problematic to cannulation. **A,** Bilobed diverticulum (white arrows) and major papilla orifice (black arrow). **B,** Papilla on 6 o'clock rim of diverticulum.

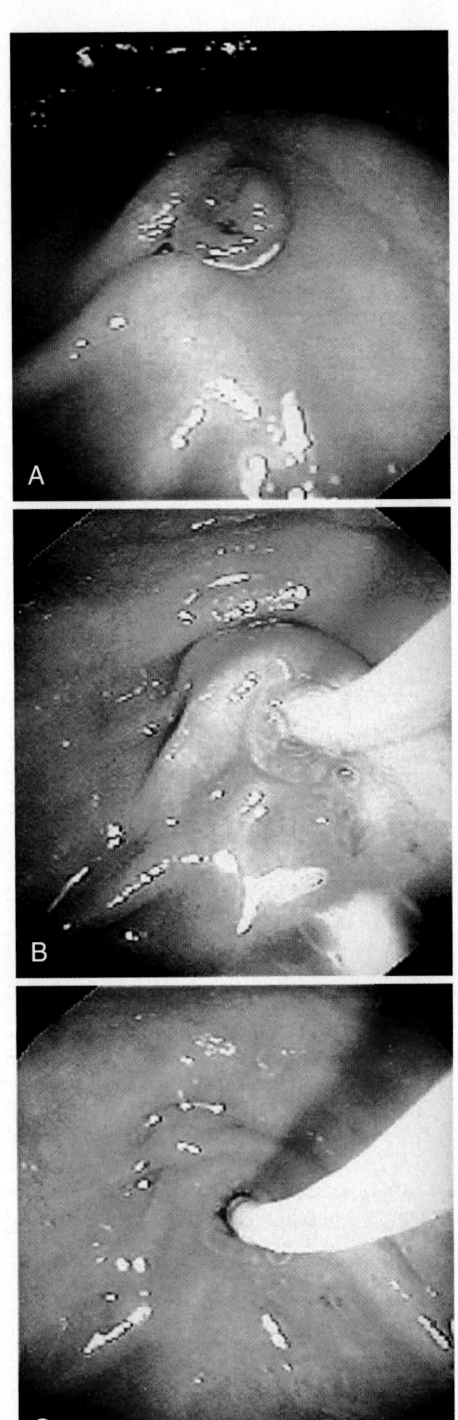

Fig. 37.9 A, Endoscopic view of 5-Fr catheter oriented toward the 11 o'clock position of the major papilla. **B,** The bile duct has been entered and bile aspiration confirmed by yellow color in the catheter lumen. **C,** The catheter was oriented more toward the 3 o'clock position to enter the pancreas.

catheter tip toward the 11 o'clock to 12 o'clock position (**Fig. 37.9**) would more likely enter the bile duct; orientation of the catheter toward the 3 o'clock to 5 o'clock position would more likely enter the pancreatic duct. Biliary orifice location may vary from 10 o'clock to 2 o'clock. Cannulation may be initially done by gentle impaction of the catheter tip in the papillary

orifice. Deep cannulation (>1 cm penetration of the catheter into the duct) more securely establishes an intraductal position, which allows contrast agent injection, fluid aspiration, patient position changes, and endoscope position changes without loss of access to the duct.

Selective Deep Biliary Cannulation

Pancreatic cannulation is easier than biliary cannulation. Selective biliary entry is mandatory in most cases of biliary pathology. We often start with a standard 5-Fr catheter and add a guidewire or a sphincterotome for assistance. If the cannulation angle fails to achieve adequate cephalad orientation, a sphincterotome or curved top guidewire generally helps to achieve that angle. There are increasing observations that initial use of a guidewire facilitates cannulation and decreases post-ERCP pancreatitis.[32] In patients with a prominent major papilla (protruding well into the duodenal lumen), the path of the biliary lumen is nearly always stair-stepped. Cannulation is initially cephalad, then more perpendicular into the wall, and then more cephalad again. The cannulation is partially accomplished by pulling the endoscope more cephalad, lowering the elevator, and moving the viewing lens very close to the papilla. A sharp guidewire may puncture the ampullary segment roof at the first cephalad-perpendicular junction. Gentle guidewire manipulations and more perpendicular catheter orientation are required.

Limited data indicate that cannulation may be facilitated in difficult cases with use of drugs (e.g., nitroglycerin) to relax the sphincter. If biliary entry is mandatory (obstructive jaundice) and initial attempts fail, precut entry is generally required (see Chapter 42). In this setting, the endoscopist must balance decisions regarding transfer to a more experienced facility[33,34] and consider percutaneous or surgical opinions versus proceeding with more aggressive endoscopic techniques.

Precut sphincterotomy[35–39] involves cutting the papilla to gain deep intraductal access to the biliary tree. This technique should be used by experienced endoscopists only and mostly applied in patients with a high clinical suspicion of obstructive pathology (e.g., impacted stone; **Fig. 37.10A**) or jaundiced patients with dilated bile ducts on noninvasive imaging after standard techniques fail. Precutting can be achieved by impaction of a short-nosed pull-type sphincterotome into the papillary orifice with sequential shallow cephalad cuts until the biliary orifice is identified. Similar sequential shallow cuts can be made with a needle-knife. We prefer to place a 3-Fr to 4-Fr, 6-cm long, no intraductal flange polyethylene stent into the pancreatic duct first, if possible, and use the stent to guide needle-knife cutting (**Fig. 37.10B**).

Contrast Medium and Image Acquisition

Standard ionic contrast medium (e.g., meglumine diatrizoate) at a 25% to 30% concentration is often called half-strength and is most commonly used for cholangiography. Half-strength contrast medium permits adequate visualization of small ducts of 2 to 6 mm diameter and allows filling defects (stones) to be seen in more dilated ducts. However, biliary stricture detail and peripheral intrahepatic ducts are better defined with full-strength contrast medium (50% to 60% concentration). Nonionic and lower osmolality contrast agents, which are more expensive, offer no safety advantage.[40] Many

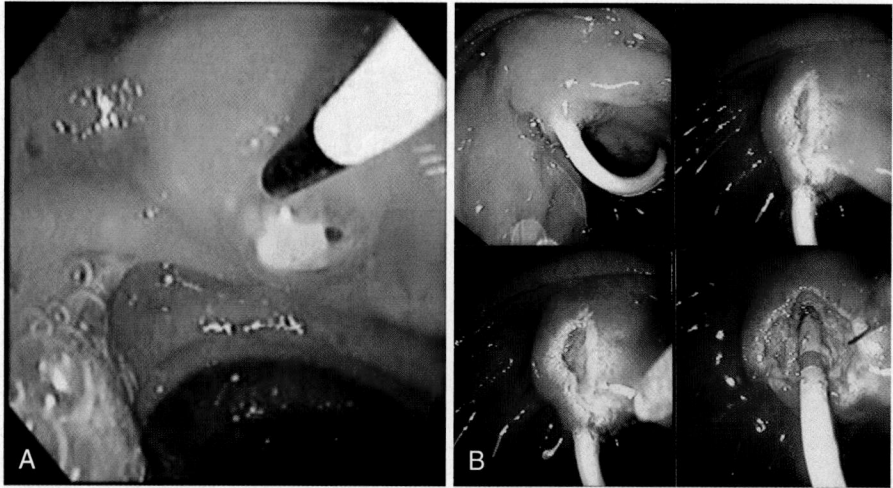

Fig. 37.10   A, Stone impacted in orifice. Needle-knife cut over stone being initiated. **B,** Endoscopic photos of technique of precut major papilla needle-knife sphincterotomy over indwelling pancreatic stent.

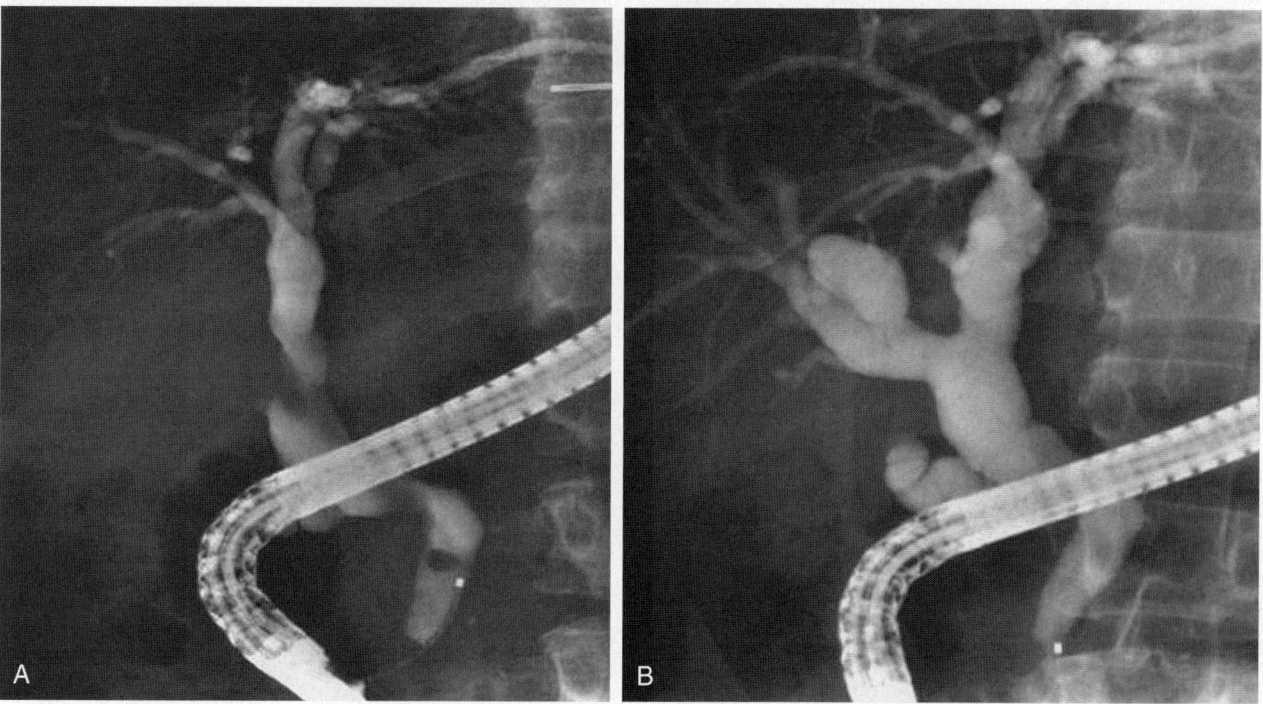

Fig. 37.11   A, Initial left lobe filling. This lobe fills preferentially because contrast medium is heavier than bile and flows down into the dependent left lobe with the patient prone. This could be mistaken for complete biliary filling. **B,** With the aid of tilting the patient head down 20 degrees and more volume, the right lobe is viewed.

manufacturers have abandoned marketing of inexpensive ionic agents making use of nonionic agents necessary.

We prefer 20-mL syringes because this avoids the need to exchange syringes as often (and potentially introduce air bubbles). With each syringe exchange, one should aspirate back to remove any air bubbles from the Luer connector and flush to ensure that the contrast medium extends to the catheter tip. Contrast agent injection is done with continuous fluoroscopic monitoring. Contrast medium is more dense than bile and flows along the most dependent route. The left lobe fills quickest (lowest) with the patient prone (**Fig. 37.11A**), the right lobe anterior segments fill next, and the right lobe posterior segments fill last (and may remain unfilled unless

adequate volume and injection force are applied) (**Fig. 37.11B**). The extent of ductal filling should be correlated with the clinical history and the need to know the ductal anatomy. High-resolution fluoroscopy is required to see fine detail of small ducts.

Multiple views of initial distal bile duct filling are recommended to see potential small filling defects (stones) that may be washed upstream (and no longer visible) or masked by more dense contrast concentration in a dilated duct (**Figs. 37.12 and 37.13**). Complete cholangiography requires filling of the peripheral intrahepatic radicles. The left lobe is more dependent in the prone position and fills preferentially. Right lobe filling may require tilting the patient's head down 15 to

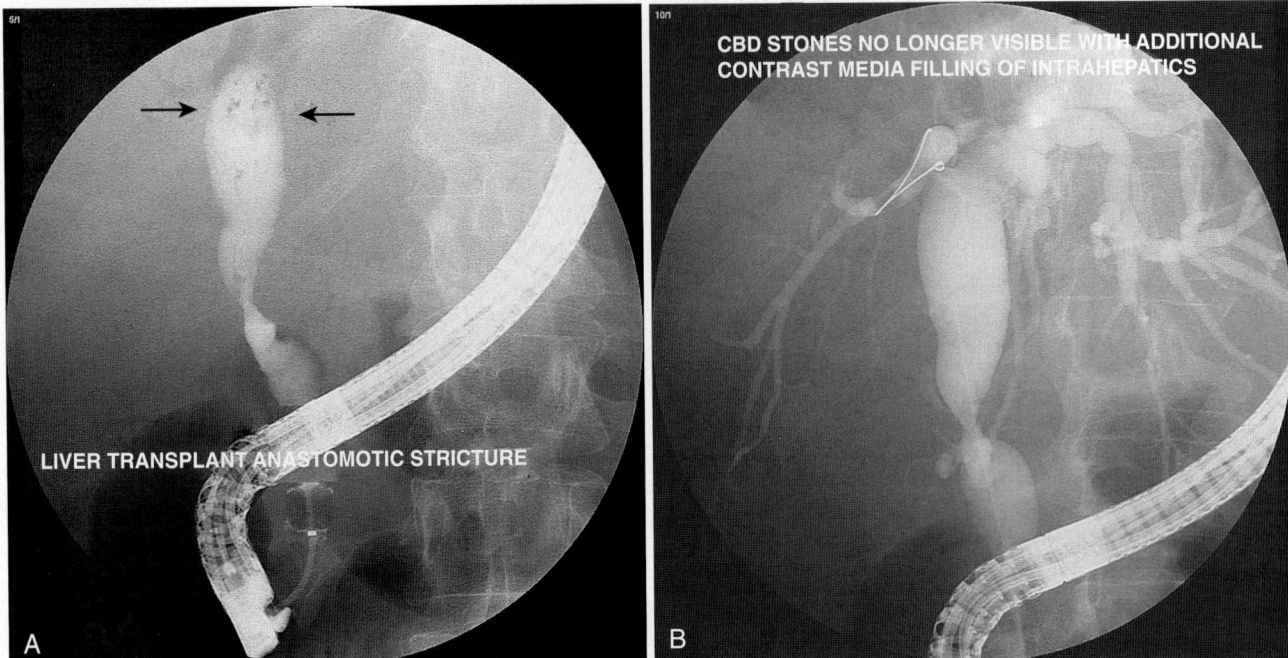

Fig. 37.12 Patients with suspected common duct stones (especially patients with dilated ducts) should have multiple early filling biliary films taken to observe stones (**A**) before the stones are potentially washed upstream or masked by dense contrast material (**B**). The patient has had a liver transplant with duct-to-duct anastomosis. There is stricture at the anastomosis.

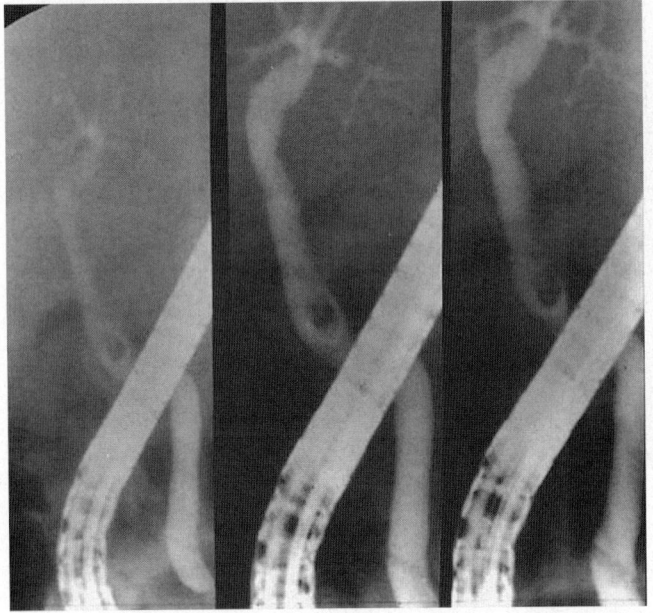

Fig. 37.13 Multiple early films with limited contrast agent injection provide the best opportunity to see small stones. The filling defect in this patient is a "pseudostone" representing the orifice of the cystic duct.

20 degrees on the fluoroscopy table, more forceful injection (a balloon occlusion catheter is helpful), selective right lobe cannulation, or turning the patient to the supine position. Contrast medium mixes slowly with gallbladder bile. Multiple films during early filling are recommended. Final films may be best taken in the supine position after withdrawal of the endoscope. Occasionally, delaying gallbladder films until 4 to 24 hours after completion of the procedure allows for passage

of intraluminal gas, giving better diagnostic film quality. In settings of tight biliary strictures, limited contrast medium filling upstream should be done until catheter access above the stricture is achieved (**Fig. 37.14**).[41-43]

Problem Solving

Table 37.2 reviews multiple general problems encountered with ERC and potential ways to solve them.[44-46] Biliary manometry usually is performed at the time of ERCP. All drugs that relax (e.g., anticholinergics, nitrates, calcium channel blockers, glucagon) or stimulate (e.g., certain narcotics, cholinergic agents) should be avoided for at least 8 to 12 hours before the study and during the manometry. Manometry is performed using a low-compliance infusion pump system and a 5-Fr catheter (see Chapter 49).

Normal Findings

A normal cholangiogram is shown in **Fig. 37.18**. Although there is controversy, the weight of evidence indicates that the biliary tree does not dilate after cholecystectomy in the absence of obstructing pathology. The common hepatic and common bile duct diameter on ERCP is commonly 2 to 3 mm greater than seen on CT or ultrasound. This difference is accounted for by filling (or overfilling) the ductal system with extra fluid (contrast medium) under greater pressure than physiologic secretory pressure.[47] Many centers accept the upper limits of normal diameter for the common bile duct as 10 mm in adults. The cystic duct commonly joins the common duct approximately halfway from the hilum to the papilla, but this junction may be quite variable. The intrahepatic radicles have a leafless tree–like branch pattern with marked variation in distribution. An aberrant, low insertion right hepatic duct,

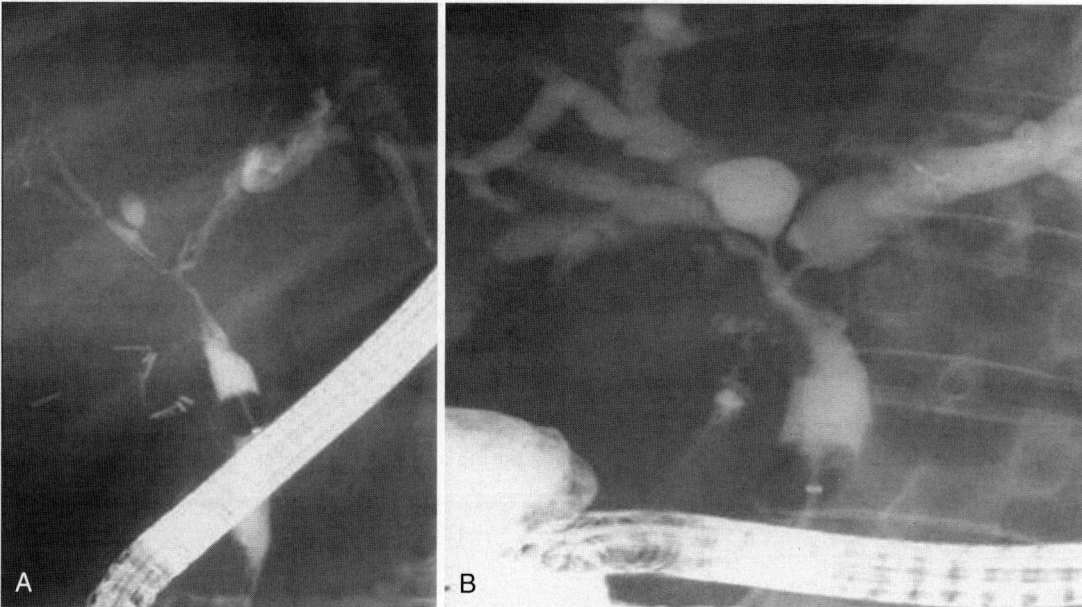

Fig. 37.14 **A,** Cholangiocarcinoma involving the hepatic hilum. Only a limited amount of contrast medium is injected above the strictures to avoid contamination. More contrast medium should be injected only after the guidewire is advanced above the stricture. If additional upstream information is needed, magnetic resonance cholangiopancreatography (MRCP) or computed tomography (CT) scan is recommended. **B,** Excessive intrahepatic filling above hilar stricture. Unless subsequent bilateral drainage is achieved, the patient is at higher risk of postprocedure cholangitis.

Table 37.2 Common General Problems and Challenges Encountered at Endoscopic Retrograde Cholangiography

Cholangiographic Challenge or Clinical Suspicion	Potential Steps to Solve Problem
Obese patient	Increase kilovoltage
	Take extra exposures (a few are likely to be adequate)
	Review still images before deciding on therapy (i.e., do not rely only on fluoroscopy view)
Patient moves frequently	Take multiple exposures (one is likely to be clear)
	Increase kilovoltage to shorten exposure time
Terminal (preampullary) CBD not well seen	If patient has cholangitis with risk of sepsis if greater filling done, pass stone retrieval balloon to mid-CBD, inflate balloon, and inject contrast agent downstream to balloon (need appropriate "below the balloon" injection port). Tilt head up 5–20 degrees (Fig. 37.15)
	If moderate amount of contrast agent already upstream in intrahepatic ducts, place catheter tip 1 cm above sphincter. Aspirate nonopacified bile until upstream contrast agent flows back into terminal CBD (Fig. 37.16)
Patient has typical postcholecystectomy pain, but ERCP (or MRCP) is normal	Perform manometry[37-39]
	Do not initiate ERCP if ducts are not dilated by noninvasive imaging and liver serum chemistries are normal, unless manometry is immediately available
Cannot find papilla	Check fluoroscopy to ensure endoscope tip is in descending duodenum. Be sure of surgical anatomy—Roux-en-Y gastrojejunostomy? Bile present—follow trail. Gently lift folds in candidate area. Find minor papilla, and search left and inferior. Give cholecystokinin or secretin to stimulate fluid flow
Left and right hepatic ductal systems overlap at hilum, not well defined	Fixed fluoroscopy table, roll patient to slight left posterior oblique position; use C-arm rotation to separate systems
Bile leak expected	Obtain multiple early images to locate leak site precisely before leak site contrast agent obscures view
	Limit injection to small amount of spilled contrast agent (Fig. 37.17A)
Air bubbles introduced	Observe where bubbles went and where collected; if distal CBD, tilt head down and aspirate bubbles, bile, and contrast agent from terminal duct
	Consider tilt head up and observe bubble passage into intrahepatic ducts

Continued

Table 37.2 Common General Problems and Challenges Encountered at Endoscopic Retrograde Cholangiography—cont'd

Cholangiographic Challenge or Clinical Suspicion	Potential Steps to Solve Problem
Contrast agent or air in duodenum or stomach detracts from image quality	Aspirate all contrast agent and air from duodenum before imaging; do this routinely when injecting contrast agent (Fig. 37.17B)
Endoscope repeatedly covers area of interest	Use C-arm (or patient positioning) to change angle
	Move endoscope from short (lesser curve) to long (greater curve) position
	Place catheter upstream to hilum, slowly back endoscope into stomach aspirating air and spilled contrast agent as if nasobiliary tube placement were being done
Pyloric or duodenal narrowing precludes endoscope passage	Pass guidewire and 5-Fr to 7-Fr catheter through the narrowing and ahead into transverse duodenum; an extra-stiff guidewire (Amplatz Super Stiff Guidewire; Boston Scientific, Billerica, MA) is especially helpful
	Pass endoscope over wire, paying attention to fluoroscopic alignment more than the endoscopic view

CBD, common bile duct; ERCP, endoscopic retrograde cholangiopancreatography; MRCP, magnetic resonance cholangiopancreatography.

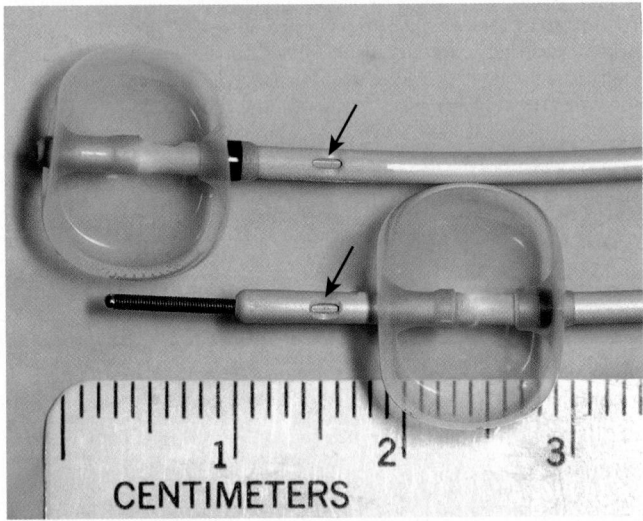

Fig. 37.15 Stone retrieval–type balloon catheters with injection port *(arrows)* above and below the balloon for selective filling of areas of interest above and below the balloon.

which connects to right posterior hepatic segments, is seen in 5% of patients (**Fig. 37.19**). These may be transected during laparoscopic cholecystectomy and give rise to problematic bile leaks from the disconnected segmental branch (**Fig. 37.20**). Because the transected duct does not fill on ERCP, MRCP may be more diagnostic.[48,49] Numerous other normal anatomic variants have been reported (**Fig. 37.21**)[49–51] and are beyond the scope of this chapter.

Biliary Stones

In white and African American patients, most stones are cholesterol or mixed type and occur in the gallbladder. These patients do not require ERC unless stones also occur in or migrate into the bile ducts.[52–57] **Fig. 37.22A** shows a 35-year-old female patient with multiple small stones in the gallbladder (transcutaneous ultrasound). **Fig. 37.22B** shows a single small ductal stone on ERC. Gallstone pancreatitis is one

common outcome of small stone (<5 mm diameter) passage. In this latter setting, more than 80% of patients spontaneously pass the stones from the bile duct into the duodenum. Selective use of ERC is recommended for patients who have persistent (≥12 hours) upper abdominal pain, persistent or worsening cholestasis, cholangitis, or dilated extrahepatic bile ducts.[58–66]

A meta-analysis of prospective randomized trials showed benefit of therapeutic ERCP in the setting of acute pancreatitis of suspected gallstone origin.[67] Additional noninvasive imaging is helpful but adds expense and should probably be reserved for higher risk patients (e.g., cardiopulmonary disease) and patients with relatively low probability (10% to 25%) of ductal stones. Patients with higher stone probability should have ERC without preceding MRCP or EUS (**Fig. 37.22C**).[68] A larger ductal stone is seen in **Fig. 37.23** in a patient after cholecystectomy. Intrahepatic stones[69–72] (with or without extrahepatic stones) are common in Asians. **Fig. 37.24** shows right segmental branches with large fusiform stones. A stone impacted in the cystic duct may compress the common hepatic or common bile duct and cause obstructive jaundice (Mirizzi's syndrome). **Table 37.3** reviews problems encountered in biliary stone cases and ways to solve them.

Biliary Strictures

Biliary strictures[73–84] are abnormal narrowings of the ductal system resulting from compression (e.g., chronic pancreatitis), scar formation (e.g., postoperative), or neoplasm (e.g., cholangiocarcinoma). These typically manifest clinically with cholestasis, obstructive jaundice, or cholangitis. The etiology of the stricture is usually evident from the history (e.g., recent biliary surgery, ethanol abuse, or elderly patient with weight loss). **Fig. 37.26** shows a smooth, tapered long narrowing within the head of the pancreas in a patient with calcific chronic pancreatitis. Laparoscopic cholecystectomy[85–87] is associated with thermal or mechanical injury, which results in stricture formation in 0.25% to 0.5% of patients. **Fig. 37.27** shows a typical postlaparoscopy stricture. Injuries at open cholecystectomy occur less frequently. Duct transections (**Fig. 37.28**) and duct resections are the most serious injuries.

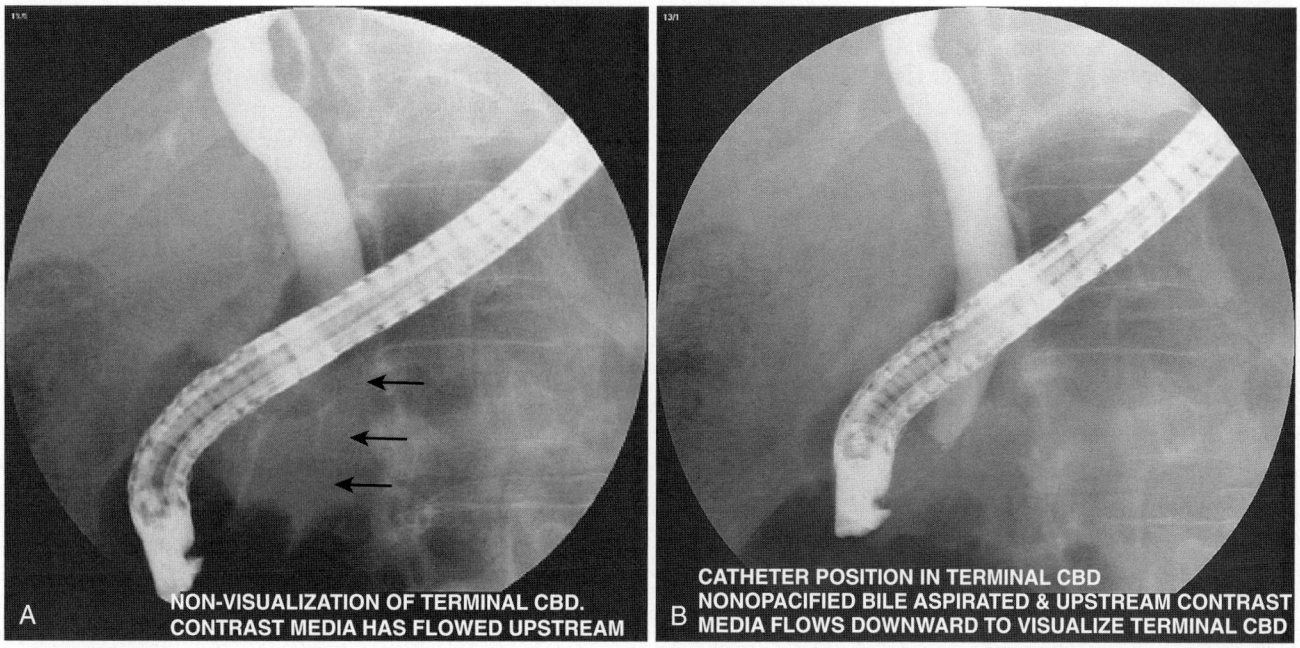

A NON-VISUALIZATION OF TERMINAL CBD. CONTRAST MEDIA HAS FLOWED UPSTREAM

B CATHETER POSITION IN TERMINAL CBD NONOPACIFIED BILE ASPIRATED & UPSTREAM CONTRAST MEDIA FLOWS DOWNWARD TO VISUALIZE TERMINAL CBD

Fig. 37.16 **A** and **B,** Terminal bile duct filling using aspiration technique to withdraw nonopacified bile from the terminal duct.

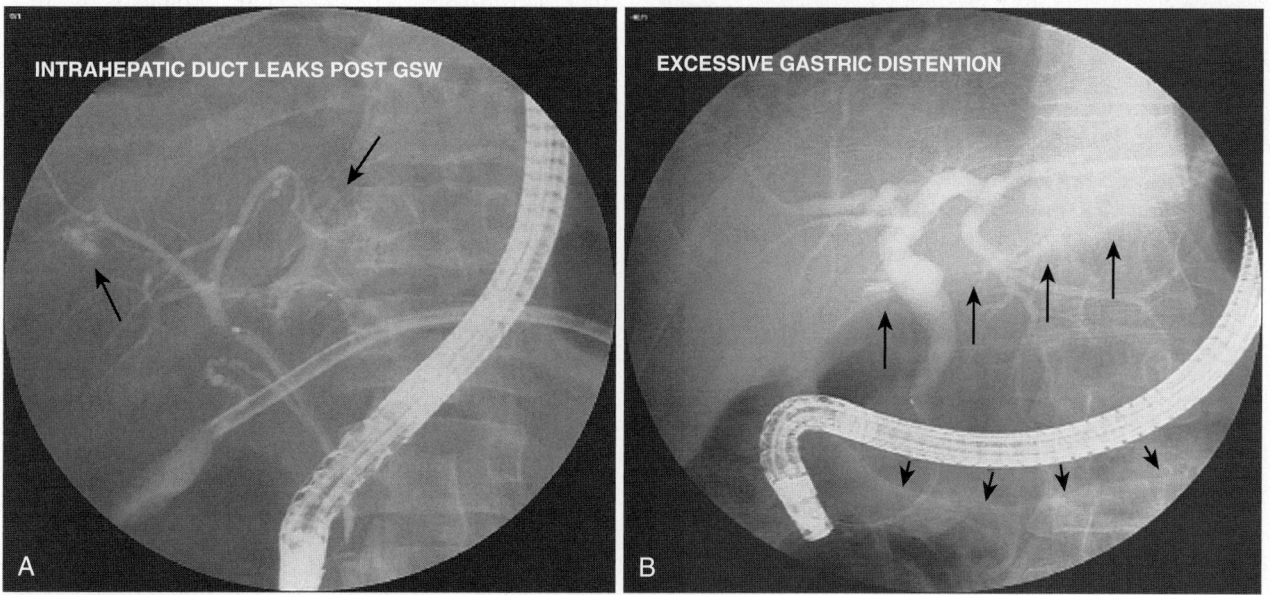

A INTRAHEPATIC DUCT LEAKS POST GSW

B EXCESSIVE GASTRIC DISTENTION

Fig. 37.17 **A,** Bile leaks. The patient had a gunshot injury to the liver with a small leak from the right lobe and a larger leak from the left lobe. **B,** Aspiration of duodenal and gastric air gives better ductal imaging. Excessive intragastric air partially obscures the terminal common duct.

Orthotopic liver transplant with duct-to-duct anastomosis results in pathologic narrowing at the anastomosis in 15% of patients (**Fig. 37.29**).[88,89] Primary sclerosing cholangitis[90–96] is characterized by multifocal extrahepatic or intrahepatic strictures, or both (**Fig. 37.30**). The gallbladder and cystic duct are spared.

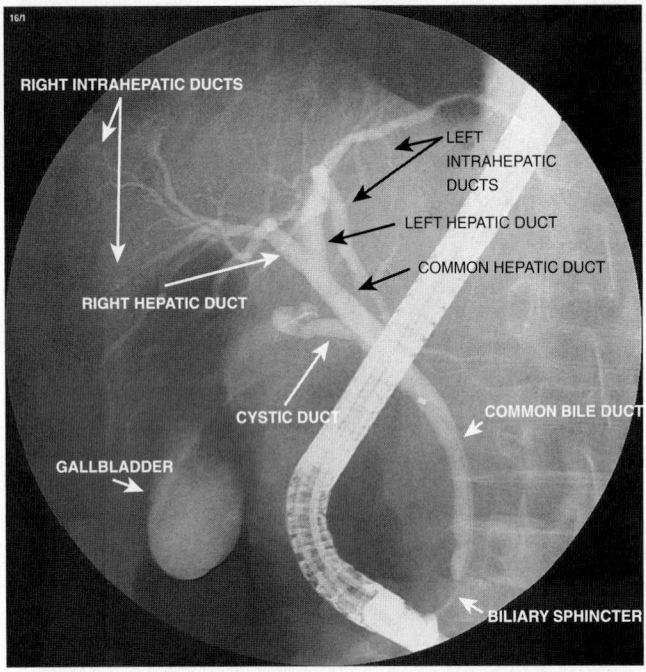

Fig. 37.18 Normal cholangiogram with ductal segments labeled. Colon gas overlaps the gallbladder making viewing suboptimal.

The goals of ERC in suspected primary sclerosing cholangitis are to (1) establish a diagnosis, (2) identify treatable dominant strictures, and (3) identify (or rule out) concomitant cholangiocarcinoma, which occurs in up to 40% of advanced cases going on to transplantation. Pancreatic ductal cell origin adenocarcinoma is the most common cancer encountered on ERC. Pancreatic cancer[97,98] of the head has the classic double-duct sign (**Fig. 37.31**). This sign may also be seen in patients with chronic pancreatitis. Tissue sampling[99–101] should be done on strictures that clinically have any suspicion of neoplasm. Brush cytology is easiest to obtain but detects cancer when present in only 30% to 50% of cases. Additional sampling with a second brush, forceps, or endoluminal needles each adds approximately 10% to the diagnostic sensitivity.

Biliary Leaks

Biliary leaks[102–108] result from surgery complications or trauma (penetrating or nonpenetrating). Laparoscopic cholecystectomy is most commonly associated with leaks from the cystic duct or duct of Luschka (**Fig. 37.32**). Bile leaks typically cause right upper quadrant pain, fever, mildly abnormal serum liver chemistries, and leukocytosis. A typical duct of Luschka leak is seen in **Fig. 37.33** with leak occurring from a small intrahepatic duct. A subhepatic contrast collection is seen in **Fig. 37.34** from a cystic duct leak occurring after laparoscopic cholecystectomy. **Table 37.4** reviews common problems encountered on ERC when dealing with strictures and leaks. Gallbladder disease is commonly found on ERC. **Fig. 37.35** shows stones of less than 2 mm diameter in a partially filled gallbladder. **Fig. 37.36** shows gallbladder stones and right colon filling via gallbladder fistula to the colon.

Text continued on p. 509

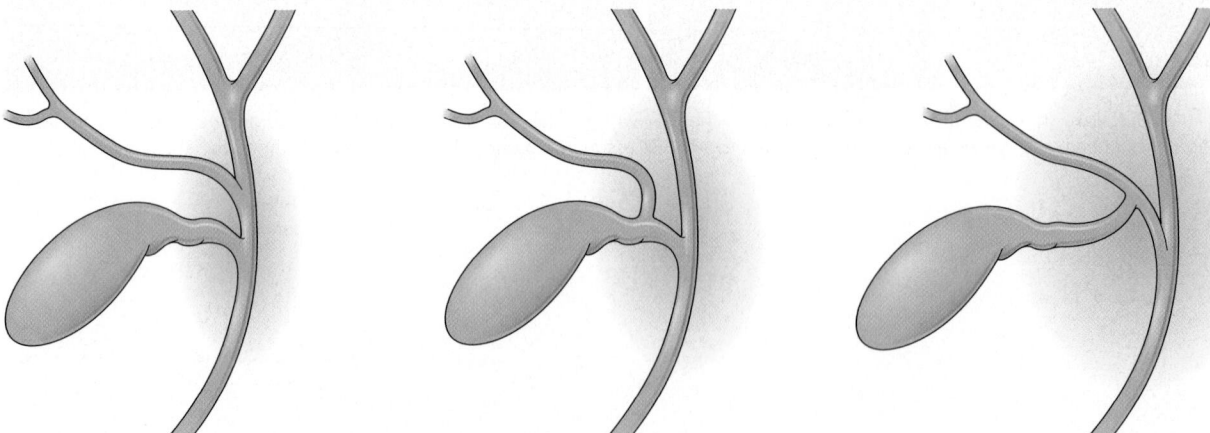

Fig. 37.19 Variations of the right posterior hepatic segment branch. *Left,* Cystic duct and aberrant right hepatic duct are adjacent to each other, but both are attached to main extrahepatic duct. *Center,* Aberrant right branch arises from cystic duct. *Right,* Cystic duct arises from aberrant right branch.

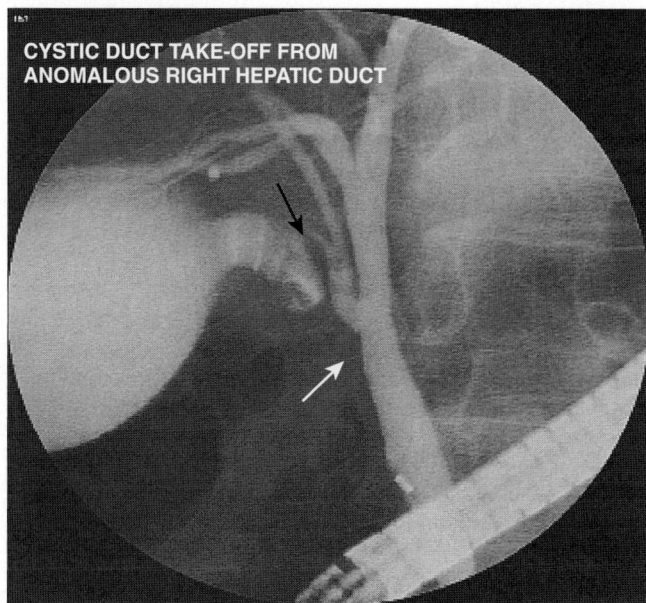

Fig. 37.20   Aberrant posterior segmental hepatic branch arising from mid-extrahepatic duct *(white arrow)*. The cystic duct take-off *(black arrow)* is from the aberrant right hepatic duct.

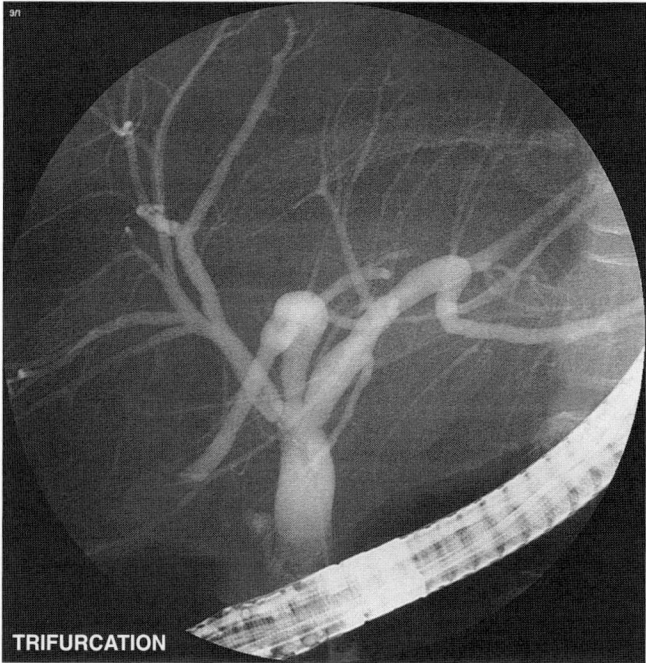

Fig. 37.21   Trifurcation of intrahepatic ducts at the hilum.

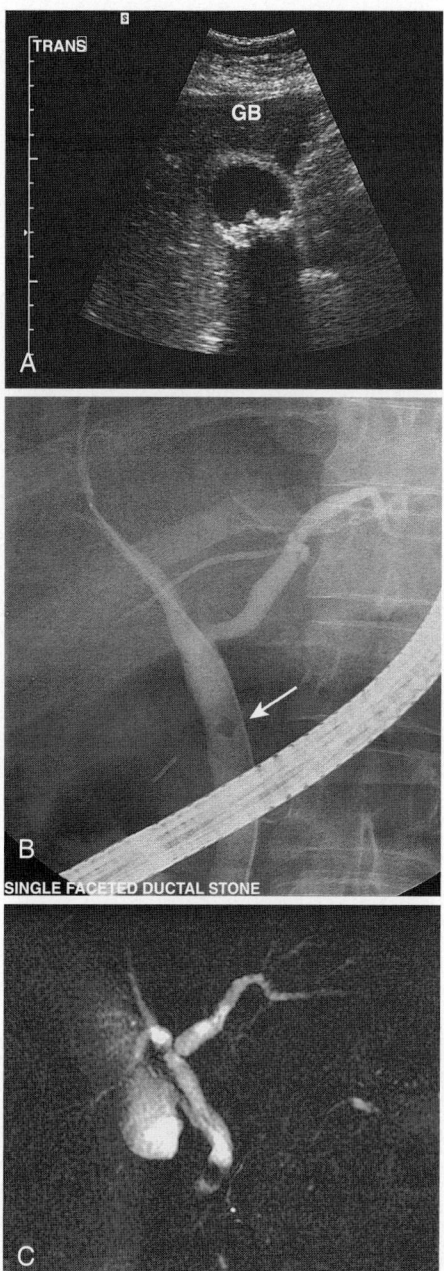

Fig. 37.22   **A,** Multiple small shadowing gallbladder stones seen by transcutaneous ultrasound. The gallbladder wall is thickened. **B,** Small common hepatic duct stone in a patient after cholecystectomy. **C,** Distal common bile duct stone detected by magnetic resonance cholangiopancreatography (MRCP).

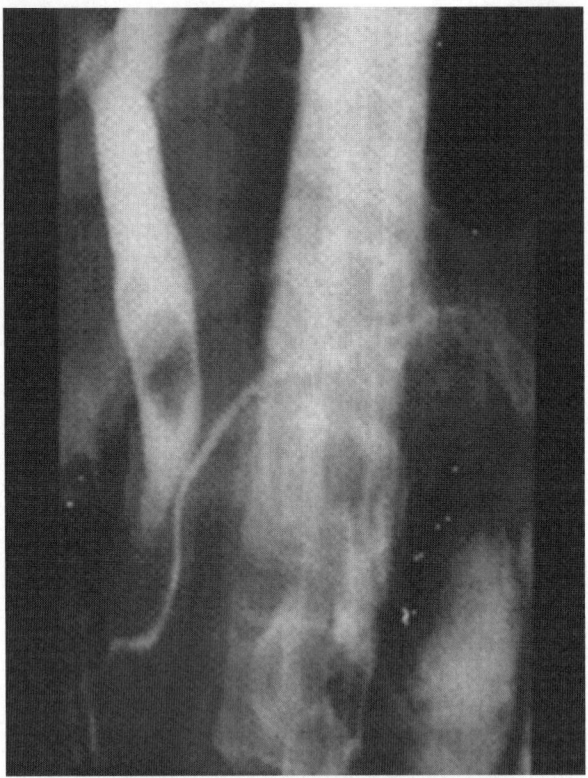

Fig. 37.23 Larger common duct stone in an elderly patient with long-standing biliary colic.

Table 37.3 Challenges for Optimal Viewing of Stones

Probable bile duct stones (most are in terminal CBD at beginning of examination)	Inject contrast agent with catheter tip in sphincter segment (not deeply cannulated)
	Inject contrast agent slowly
	Take film exposures early after only 1–2 cm of duct filled and again at each 1–2 cm further filling
	With patient prone, tilt table head up 5–20 degrees to keep contrast agent near papilla
Gallbladder stones	Take multiple early filling gallbladder films
	If overfilled, advance guidewire and catheter into gallbladder and aspirate excess contrast agent (Fig. 37.25)
	Take delayed films supine in 4–24 hr
Probable sludge seen in terminal CBD on early films	Stop contrast agent injection; aspirate bile through "see-through" (nonopaque) catheter and confirm granular material
Cholangitis manifesting with purulent bile (with or without sepsis)	Aspirate bile from CBD (send for culture) and replace aspirated bile (e.g., 30 mL with less than $\frac{1}{3}$ volume—10 mL of contrast media); limit intrahepatic filling; do definitive intrahepatic duct and stone evaluation later when cholangitis resolved

CBD, common bile duct.

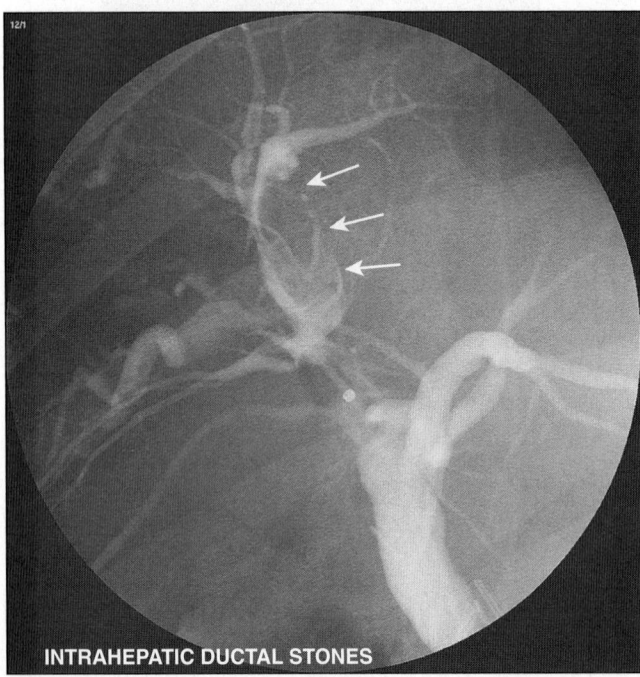

INTRAHEPATIC DUCTAL STONES

Fig. 37.24 Large intrahepatic stones in a white patient. Small common bile duct stones were also present. The gallbladder had been removed 5 years previously. These are much more common in Asian patients.

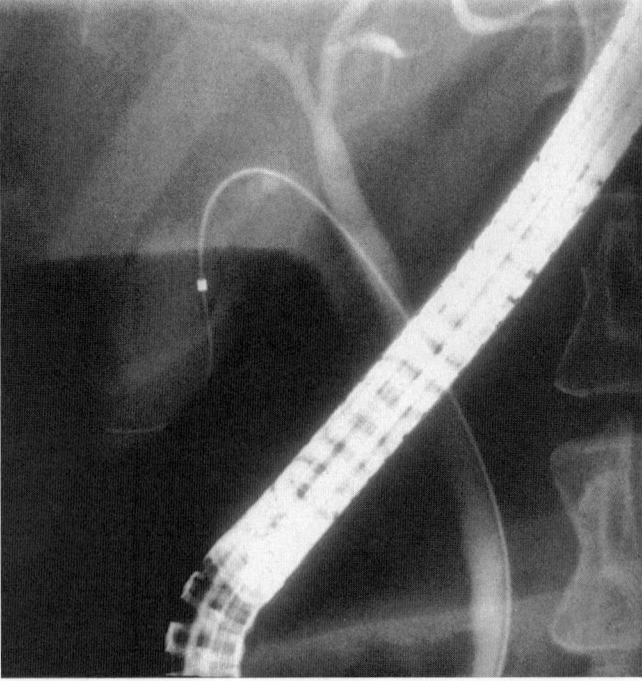

Fig. 37.25 Gallbladder aspiration done after passing a guidewire into gallbladder. This technique may be used to collect bile for crystals, inject contrast medium as needed, or aspirate excessive bile or contrast medium or pus.

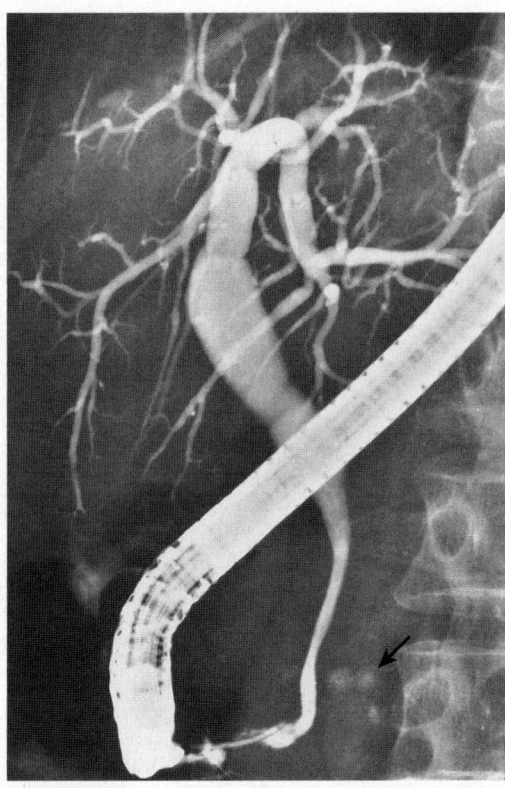

Fig. 37.26 Endoscopic retrograde cholangiography (ERC) showing long, smooth, tapered stricture within the pancreas with mild upstream dilation (the right lobe has not yet filled). Calcified stones *(arrow)* are seen in the head of the pancreas.

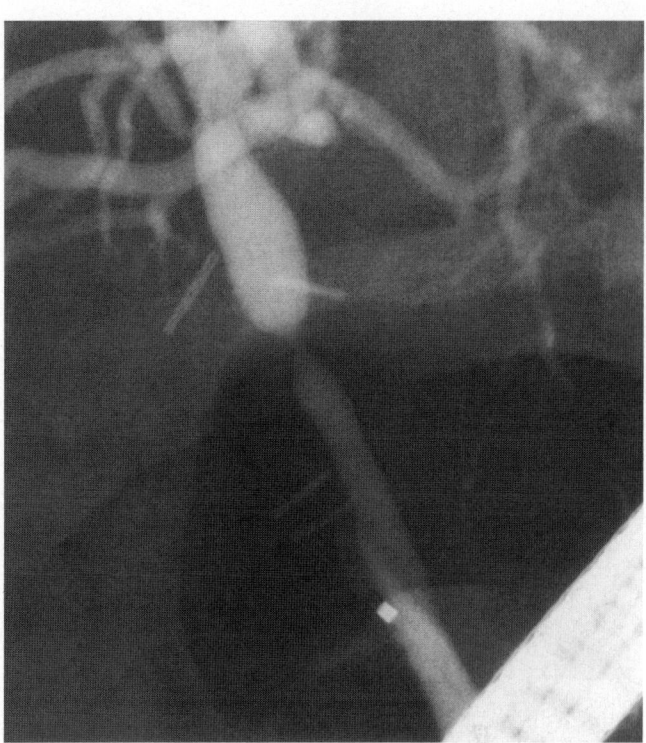

Fig. 37.27 Post–laparoscopic cholecystectomy. Short stricture of common hepatic duct seen with upstream dilation. The stricture occurred near clips and is probably due to a thermal injury.

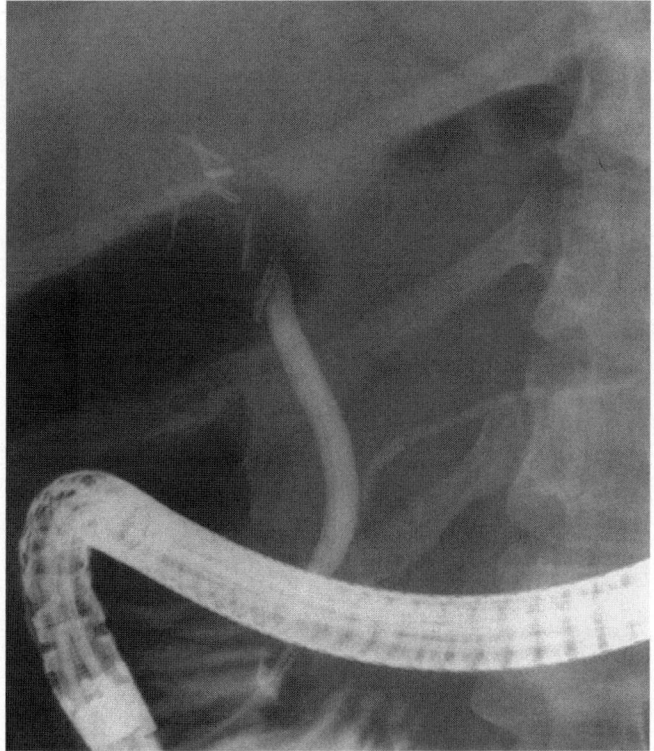

Fig. 37.28 Unintentional clip transection of the common bile duct at the cystic duct junction, which occurred at open cholecystectomy in a patient with prior upper abdominal radiation for lymphoma.

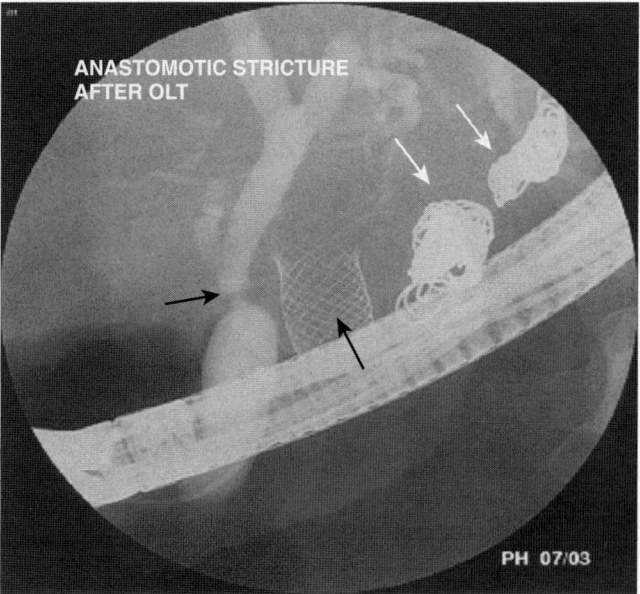

Fig. 37.29 Orthotopic liver transplant with duct-to-duct anastomosis. Narrowing of the anastomosis is seen just 10 days postoperatively *(long black arrow)*. Note endovascular metal stent (transjugular intrahepatic portosystemic shunt) used to treat prior variceal bleeding *(short black arrow)* and endovascular coils in the duodenal arcade from bleeding duodenal ulcers *(white arrows)*.

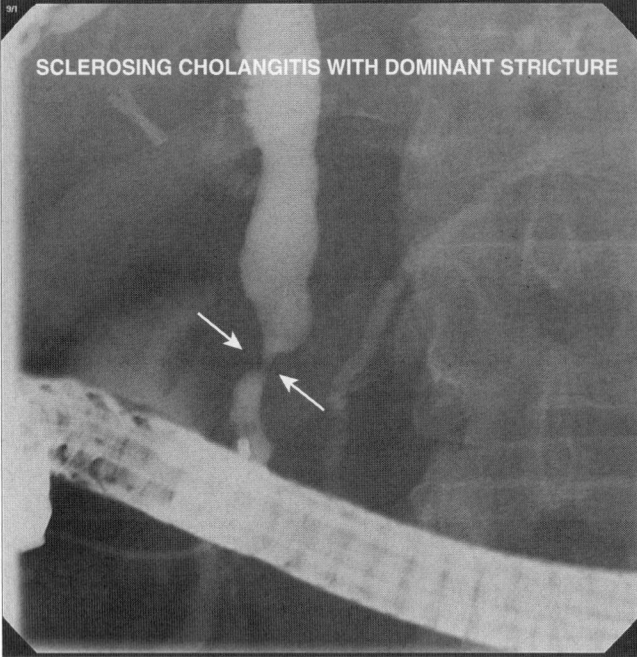

SCLEROSING CHOLANGITIS WITH DOMINANT STRICTURE

Fig. 37.30 Sclerosing cholangitis with dominant stricture. All diagnostic studies were benign.

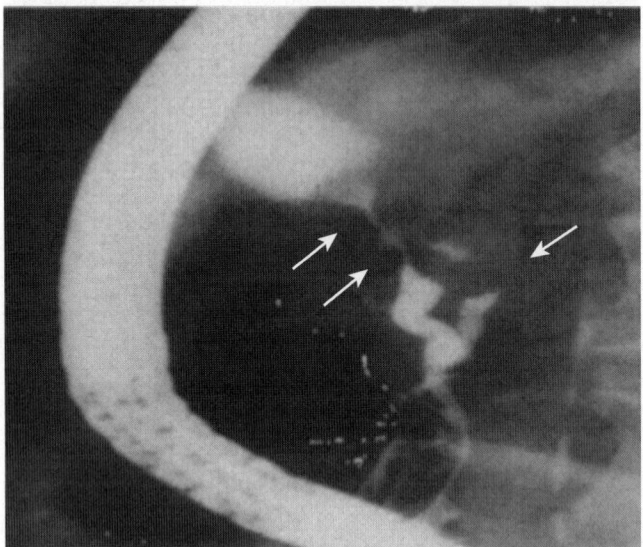

Fig. 37.31 Typical double-duct sign of pancreatic cancer. *Double arrows* indicate common bile duct narrowing. *Single arrow* indicates pancreatic duct narrowing. This sign may also be seen in chronic pancreatitis.

Table 37.4 Challenges in Detection and Optimal Viewing of Strictures

Hilar stricture	Take multiple early filling views with varying degrees of angulation; especially obtain Y confluens view with left and right main hepatic ducts separated
	Fill only a tiny amount of duct upstream initially, and get guidewire upstream before filling more; avoid thorough upstream filling (rely on MRCP or CT if that information clinically needed) unless guidewire and catheter already passed upstream and full stent drainage is certain
Common bile or common hepatic duct stricture with obviously dilated upstream ducts (per CT or MRI); need upper rim of stricture definition	Avoid thorough filling above stricture; advance large-diameter stone retrieval balloon above stricture, inflate, and fill downstream to balloon to see upper stricture definition better
Right lobe not filling—is obstruction present?	Inject more contrast agent with greater force (unless purulent bile)
	Advance catheter into right duct
	Consider aspirating bile from near hilum to "empty" right lobe to make space for contrast agent
	If prior sphincterotomy, use balloon occlusion
	Tilt head down 5–20 degrees
Probable sclerosing cholangitis setting or other intrahepatic stricturing; contrast agent preferentially enters gallbladder	Limit gallbladder filling in primary sclerosing cholangitis because post-ERCP cholecystitis may occur; inflate balloon catheter above cystic duct takeoff and inject upstream; after more aggressive intrahepatic filling, patient should remain on broad-spectrum antibiotics for 5–7 days
Sphincter segment appears narrow	This is usually a normal finding; dilated duct upstream or abnormal liver serum chemistries present suggests pathology
	Measure length of segment—>12 mm suggests scar or tumor narrowing; correlate with normal or abnormal appearance of papilla; brush cytology, manometry, sphincterotomy with viewing inside ampulla, or endoscopic ultrasound may be needed to clarify
Is postsphincterotomy biliary orifice adequate?	Do manometry, pull-through stone retrieval balloon; size with hydrostatic balloon (see Fig. 37.34)

CT, computed tomography; MRCP; magnetic resonance cholangiopancreatography; MRI, magnetic resonance imaging.

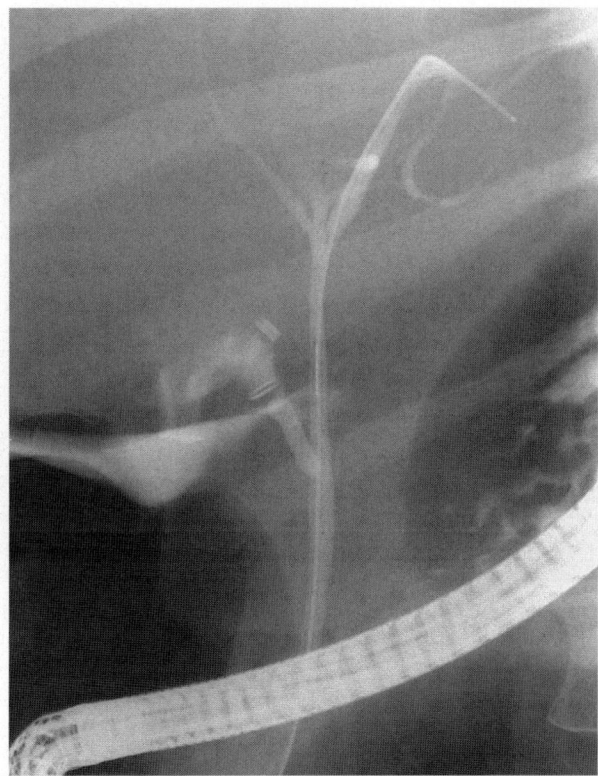

Fig. 37.32 Leak from cystic duct seen 2 days after laparoscopic cholecystectomy.

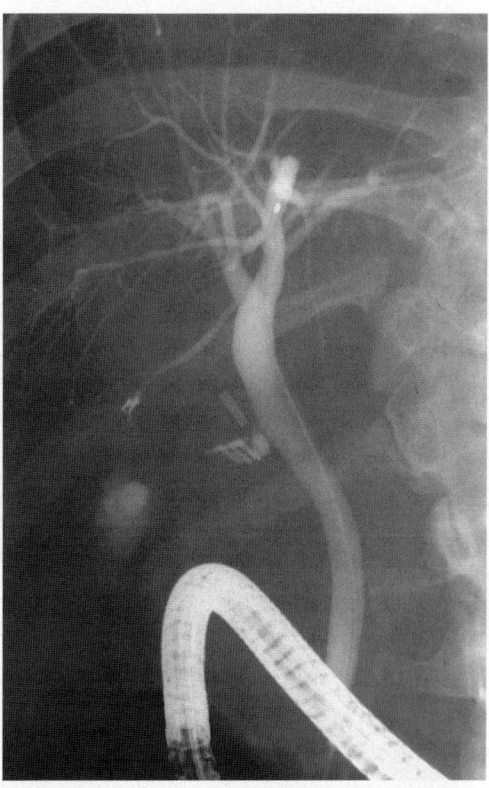

Fig. 37.33 Duct of Luschka leak seen 7 days after laparoscopic cholecystectomy. These ducts are in close proximity to the gallbladder bed and are exposed with free dissection of the gallbladder.

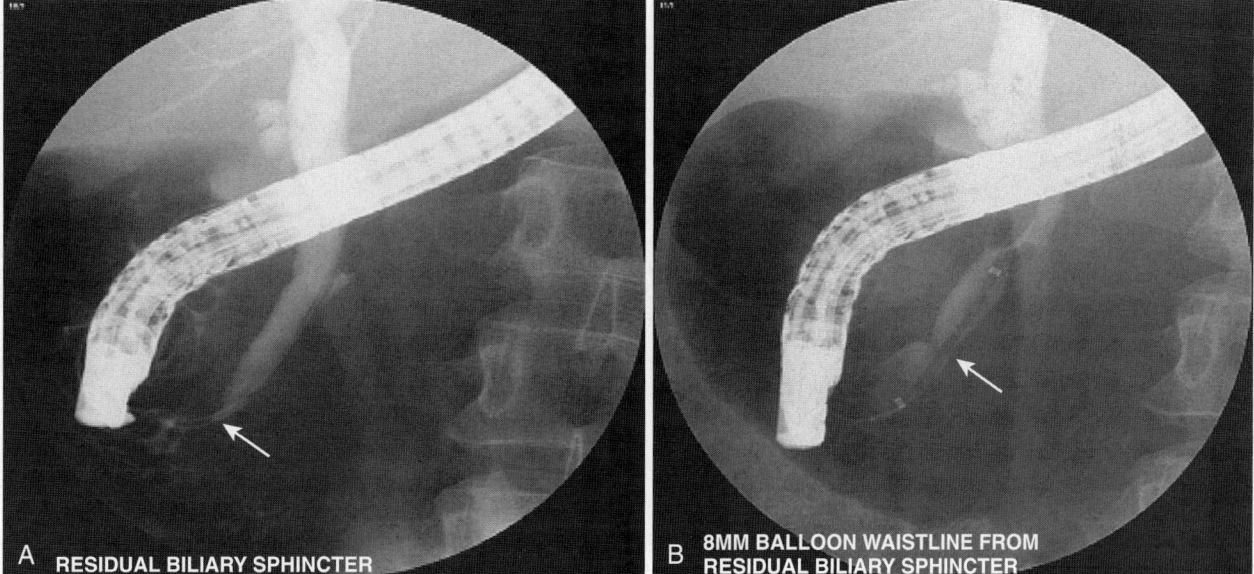

Fig. 37.34 After biliary sphincterotomy, the terminal bile duct may appear narrowed (**A**); however, true sphincter size is probably best determined by inflation of a hydrostatic balloon within the sphincter segment observing the residual waistline (**B**).

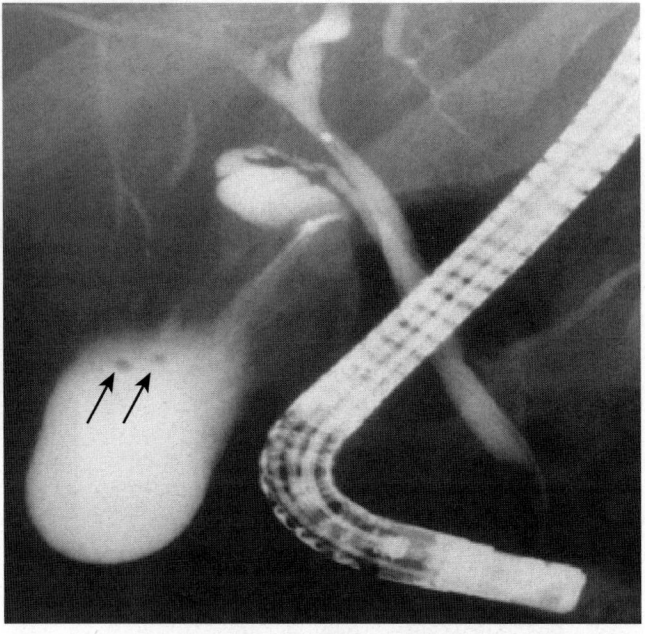

Fig. 37.35 Tiny gallbladder stones.

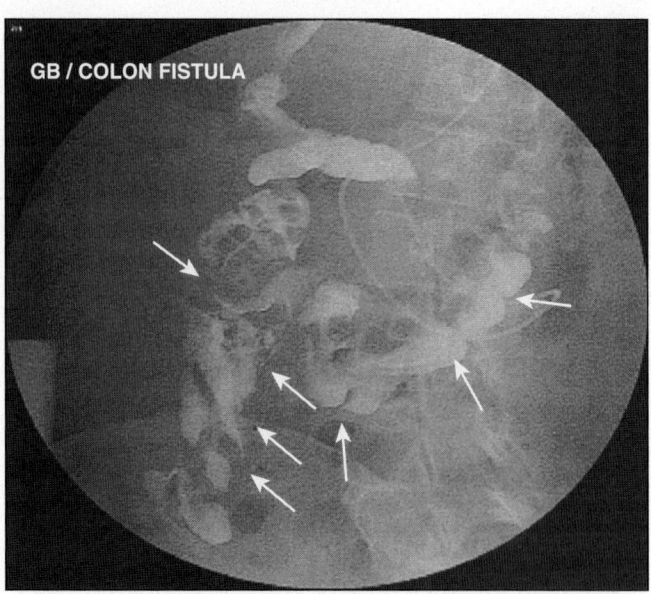

Fig. 37.36 Gallbladder colonic fistula *(top left arrow)* seen at endoscopic retrograde cholangiography (ERC). Colonic contrast medium is also seen *(multiple arrows)*.

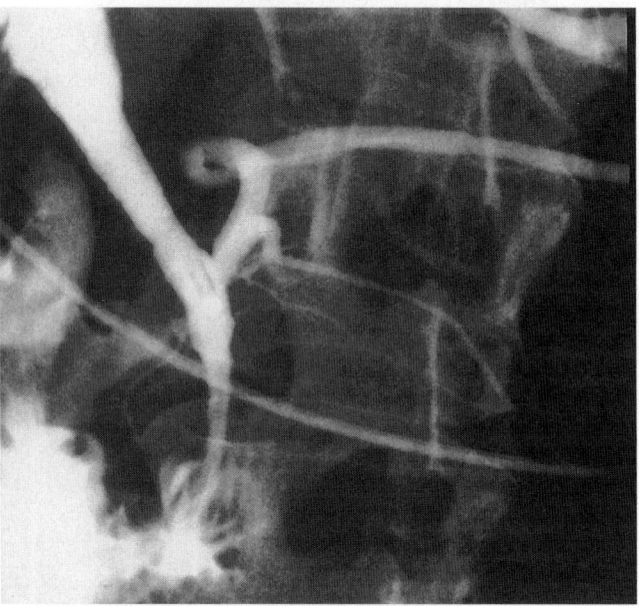

Fig. 37.37 Anomalous pancreatobiliary ductal junction with pancreatic duct joining the bile duct well outside the duodenal wall. Note the long common channel of at least 15 mm length.

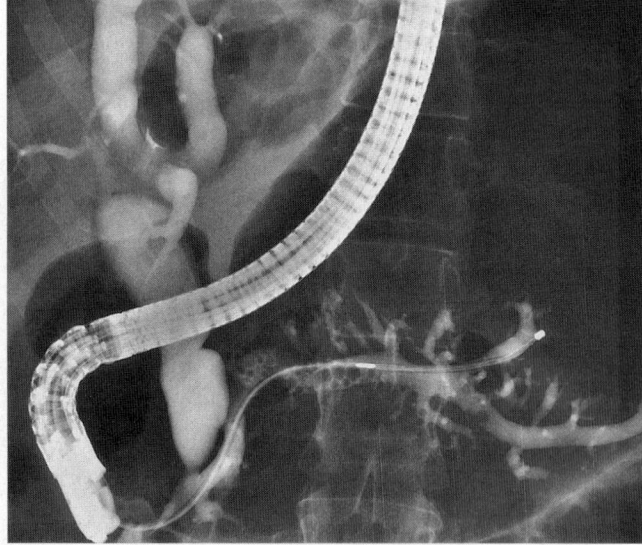

Fig. 37.38 Anomalous pancreatobiliary ductal union with (1) long common channel, (2) chronic pancreatitis, (3) bile duct entering apparent pancreatic duct, and (4) stricture at bile duct pancreatic duct junction with dilated bile duct upstream (choledochocyst is present at the hilum but is not pictured).

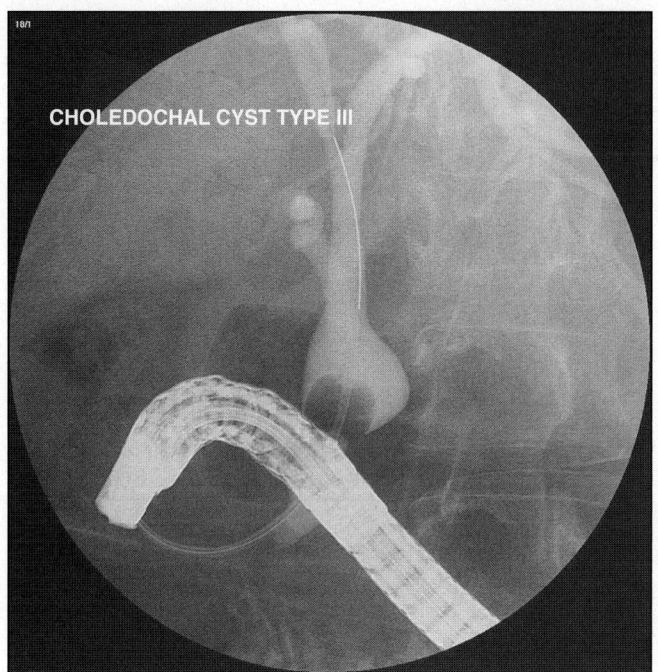

Fig. 37.39 Small type III choledochal cyst; 11-mm stone retrieval balloon is in cyst.

Anomalous Pancreatobiliary Ductal Union

Anomalous pancreatobiliary ductal union[109,110] occurs in approximately 2% of Asians but only 0.2% of whites. In this condition, the pancreatobiliary junction occurs outside the duodenal wall, and simultaneous biductal filling occurs from major papilla injection (**Figs. 37.37 and 37.38**). Approximately one-third of these patients have an associated choledochal cyst (**Fig. 37.39**). There is also an association with gallbladder cancer.

Summary

Obtaining a diagnostic cholangiogram at ERC is now less important in view of quality CT, EUS, and MRCP imaging. Nevertheless, the endoscopist should have the skills, knowledge, and equipment to obtain an excellent quality cholangiogram when clinically relevant. Attention to details, especially during initial ductal filling, and thorough filling aid in the effort. Appropriate clinical and endoscopic decision making is often possible only after a quality cholangiogram has been obtained.

References

The complete reference list is available online at www.expertconsult.com.

Diagnostic Pancreatography

Bret T. Petersen

Video related to this chapter's topics can be found online at expertconsult.com.

Diagnostic endoscopic retrograde pancreatography (ERP) evolved from a novel and cutting edge procedure in the 1970s to a widely used standard imaging tool in the latter 2 decades of the 20th century. The development of magnetic resonance imaging (MRI) and endoscopic ultrasound (EUS) contributed to the further evolution of ERP from a stand-alone diagnostic procedure to a highly therapeutic endeavor—the diagnostic uses being largely displaced by these alternative imaging modalities. Nevertheless, familiarity with the applications and findings of pancreatography is crucial to the skillful performance of endoscopic retrograde cholangiopancreatography (ERCP). This chapter reviews the indications for ERP, techniques involved in its performance, and normal and pathologic findings.

Indications

Despite the reduction in use of ERP and ERCP, indications have remained essentially unchanged over the past decade. As for all endoscopic procedures, ERP is indicated only when the potential findings would alter the management of the patient's condition in a meaningful way.[1,2] Appropriate indications have been published by national societies and interest groups[2] and revised for application in individual practice settings. Our standard indications for ERCP include investigation of symptoms strongly suspected to relate to the pancreas on the basis of associated abnormal laboratory or imaging tests, investigation of specific abnormalities on prior imaging or laboratory testing, and investigation of known pancreatic abnormalities

for which intervention is needed or anticipated (**Box 38.1**). Diagnostic ERCP alone is not indicated to confirm findings clearly shown on other testing if therapy would not be changed by its performance. ERCP alone also is not indicated for investigation of isolated abdominal pain when other tests are normal. A National Institutes of Health consensus conference addressing the clinical applications of ERCP emphasized that it is indicated for investigation of isolated abdominal pain only when equipment and skills are available for concurrent therapy and for manometric investigation for potential sphincter of Oddi dysfunction.[3]

Preparation

Pancreatography may be performed alone or in concert with diagnostic or therapeutic endoscopic cholangiography (ERCP). Patient preparation, sedation, and positioning for pancreatography are the same as for endoscopic cholangiography. Recommendations for fasting intervals before sedation and intubation vary among centers.[4] Most patients are asked to fast overnight; however, patients scheduled for afternoon procedures generally can be allowed a small clear liquid breakfast early in the day. Administration of antibiotics before the procedure is indicated in any patient with known or suspected parenchymal necrosis, duct obstruction, duct leak, or potential filling of poorly drained fluid collections or spaces such as peripancreatic fluid collections and pseudocysts.

Sedation for ERCP is usually accomplished by titrated parenteral administration of a narcotic and a benzodiazepine.

Box 38.1 Pancreatic Indications for Endoscopic Retrograde Cholangiopancreatography

Abdominal pain or laboratory or imaging studies suggesting pancreatic disease

History of acute pancreatitis of uncertain etiology

Current severe acute gallstone pancreatitis

Known pancreatic cancer—for palliation

Known or suspected pancreatic fistula or leak

Pancreatic insufficiency or malabsorption

Chronic pancreatitis, with pain, jaundice, or leak—for therapy or preoperative assessment

Pancreatic pseudocyst—for therapy or preoperative assessment

Recurrent abdominal pain—for manometry for suspected sphincter of Oddi dysfunction

Fentanyl is the narcotic of choice for most gastrointestinal (GI) endoscopy; however, compared with meperidine (Demerol), it has a shorter half-life and a greater stimulatory effect on the sphincter of Oddi.[5,6] Fentanyl is less advantageous for performance of ERCP, and meperidine tends to be the narcotic of choice. Midazolam (Versed) is the usual benzodiazepine for all GI endoscopy, including performance of ERCP. Midazolam has been shown to reduce sphincter of Oddi pressures[7,8] and is therefore not recommended during sphincter of Oddi manometry. Diazepam (Valium) does not influence the normotensive sphincter of Oddi, but little is known regarding its effects on the hypertensive sphincter. It is the preferred agent during manometric procedures.[9] Propofol has become a popular agent for use during endoscopy by virtue of its extremely rapid induction and reversal and the deep sedation it provides. For ERCP, propofol is typically administered by an anesthesia specialist. Propofol does not seem to influence sphincter pressures at commonly used doses and can be used for all aspects of ERCP practice.[10]

Optimal positioning for pancreatography is the same as for cholangiography. A fully anteroposterior view is usually optimal for fluoroscopic and radiographic imaging. When using fixed upright radiography-fluoroscopy tables, this view requires having the patient in a prone or supine position. Either the prone or the supine position can be used at times; however, endoscopes are adapted for approaching the papilla during prone intubation, and the risk for aspiration is least in this position as well. When circumstances prohibit the prone position and the supine position is used, endotracheal intubation may facilitate deep sedation and airway management. When using radiographic equipment with C-arm capabilities, the patient's position is less critical because anteroposterior views can be obtained from most angles. The lateral decubitus position may be better tolerated and potentially safer in many elderly or obese patients and patients with significant respiratory compromise.

Technique

Endoscope positioning within the duodenum is crucial for efficient performance of cholangiography or pancreatography. For cholangiography, the optimal lens position is below the papilla looking upward or backward toward the proximal second portion of the duodenum. The cannula follows an upward and slightly posterior trajectory to access the bile duct located in the 10 o'clock to 12 o'clock position relative to the papillary os. In contrast, for pancreatography via the major papilla, the optimal lens position is relatively en face to the papilla with a slightly anterior directed view. The cannula is directed in a slightly forward and upward trajectory to access the pancreatic duct, which lies roughly between 1 o'clock and 3 o'clock relative to the papillary os (**Fig. 38.1**) (see Videos).[11]

Cannulation of the major papilla is usually performed with the same equipment used in the biliary tree. Following apparent cannulation, fluoroscopically guided contrast agent injection should be more judicious and gradual than in the biliary tree. The normal pancreatic duct has a much smaller volume than the bile duct, and overfilling can occur after relatively small volumes of contrast agent have been injected; this may be recognized as acinarization, or filling of acini in a fluffy, more dense pattern throughout the distribution of the ducts (**Fig. 38.2**). Cannulation of normal side branches or of anomalous ductal systems can lead to overfilling of small segments almost immediately after injection is begun. Similarly, wire-guided cannulation must be more circumspect than in the bile duct because wire-induced perforation of a side branch can occur early, before contrast agent injection. When the appropriate position is confirmed within the desired system, more complete filling can proceed. Full-strength contrast agent is usually employed for pancreatography to optimize visualization of narrow ducts and fine detail.

In the setting of pancreatic fluid collections, for which formal drainage or surgery is not planned, caution should be employed to avoid excessive contamination of cysts that may not drain spontaneously. When difficult anatomy, pathology, or pancreas divisum prevents performance of pancreatography from the major papilla, it can be accomplished via the minor papilla approximately 90% of the time.[12] The minor papilla is usually located 2 to 3 cm proximal and slightly anterior to the major papilla. It is usually less apparent than the major papilla and may not have an obvious opening. If identification of either the papilla or the os is difficult, secretin can be administered (0.2 mcg/kg body weight by intravenous injection over one minute) to stimulate the flow of pancreatic juice into the duodenum, which occurs within minutes of administration.[13] Methylene blue can be sprayed on the duodenal wall to facilitate visualization of the focal source of drainage of clear pancreatic juice.[14] Once identified, the minor papilla can be approached with a nearly en face view using either a semi–long scope position or an extremely short scope position with slightly posterior orientation. Cannulation usually follows a slightly posterior and horizontal to mildly cephalad path.

Smaller caliber accessories are usually needed to image and access the pancreatic duct via the minor papilla. Accessories working with wires ranging from 0.018-inch to 0.025-inch caliber are generally used. A catheter with a short blunt needle tip (Cremer Catheter; Wilson Cook, Inc, Winston-Salem, NC) is often used to obtain a pancreatogram from an impacted position. However, this device does not accept a guidewire. A tapered tip sphincterotome-wire combination may be necessary to allow flexion toward an optimal axis for either impacted contrast agent injection or wire entry.

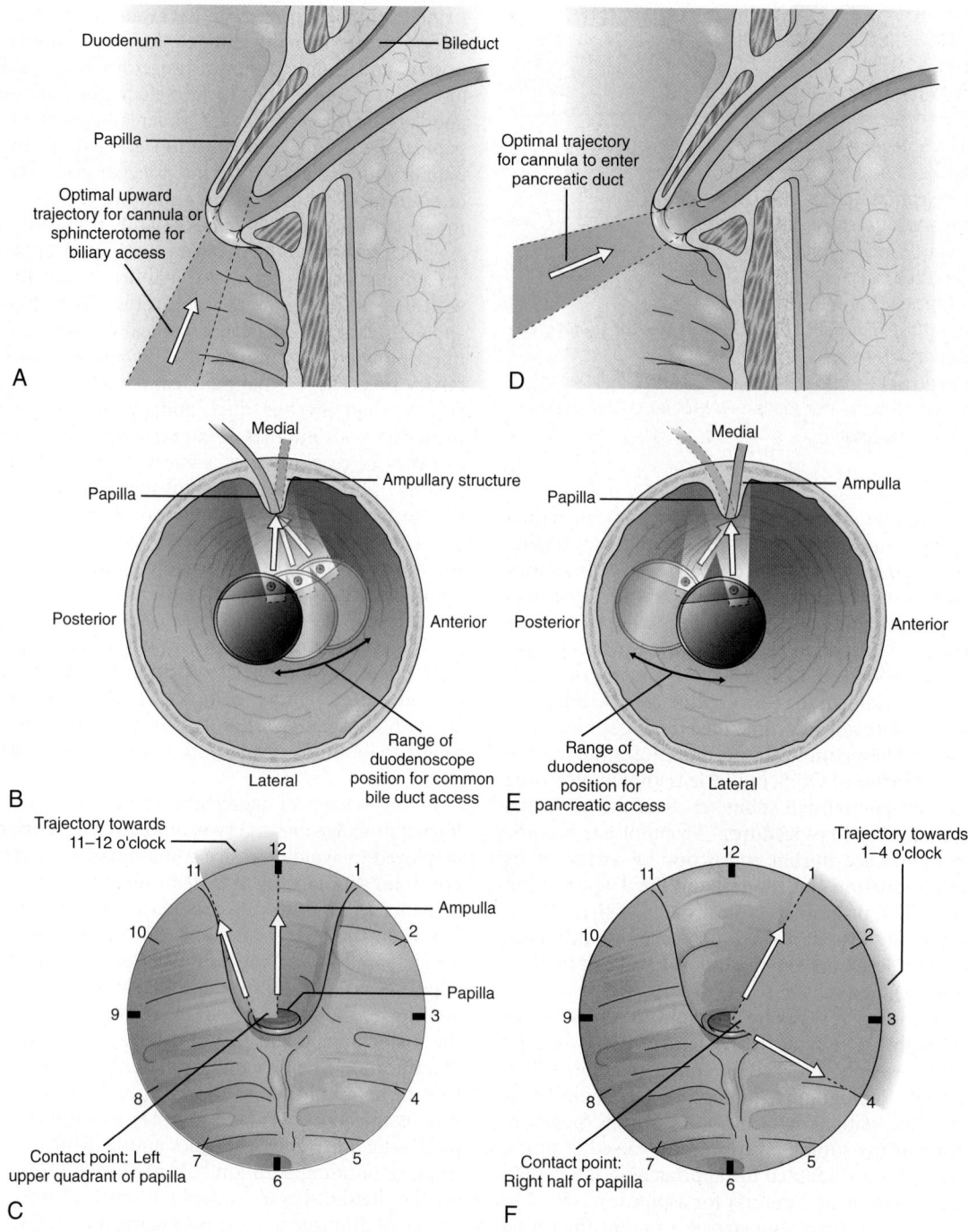

Fig. 38.1 **A–D,** Optimal trajectories for cannulation of the bile duct (**A**, **B**, and **C**) and the pancreatic duct (**D**, **E**, and **F**) as projected in transverse (**B** and **E**), coronal (**A** and **D**) and sagittal (**C** and **F**) sections.

Complications of Pancreatography

The complications of diagnostic pancreatography are similar to the complications seen with therapeutic pancreatography and ERCP in general; a major exception is the rarity of perforation and bleeding. Complications related to sedation and intubation are similar. Pancreatitis is the predominant concern. The performance of pancreatography during ERCP is one of the most consistently positive risk factors identified in studies of procedural pancreatitis.[15] Some studies note an even higher incidence with overfilling to the point of acinarization.

Investigation of patients with past episodes of pancreatitis, particularly procedure-related pancreatitis, and investigation of patients with suspected sphincter of Oddi dysfunction are also risk factors for post-ERCP pancreatitis.

Numerous studies have investigated medications and interventions intended to reduce the incidence of post-ERCP pancreatitis. The details are beyond the scope of this chapter; however, on rigorous study, most interventions have not proven useful.[15] Temporary prophylactic placement of a small-caliber pancreatic stent has been shown to reduce ERCP-related pancreatitis, or the severity of pancreatitis, in various

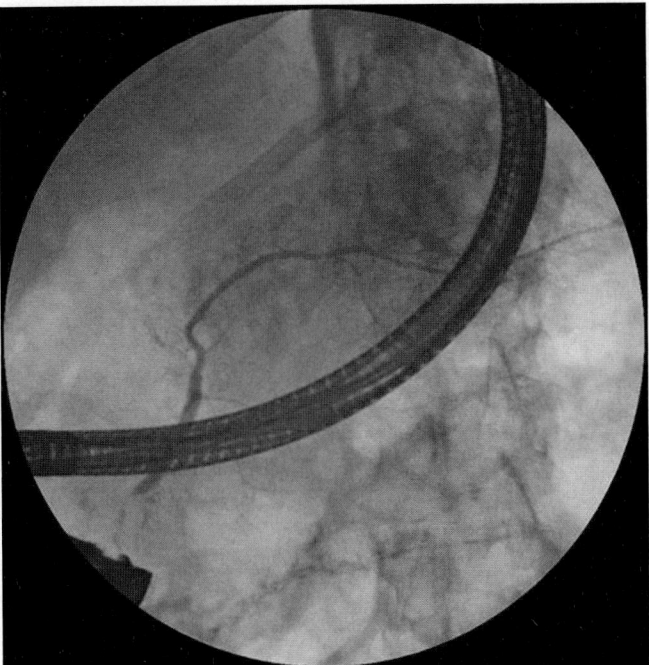

Fig. 38.2 Acinarization of the pancreatic body from overinjection of contrast material.

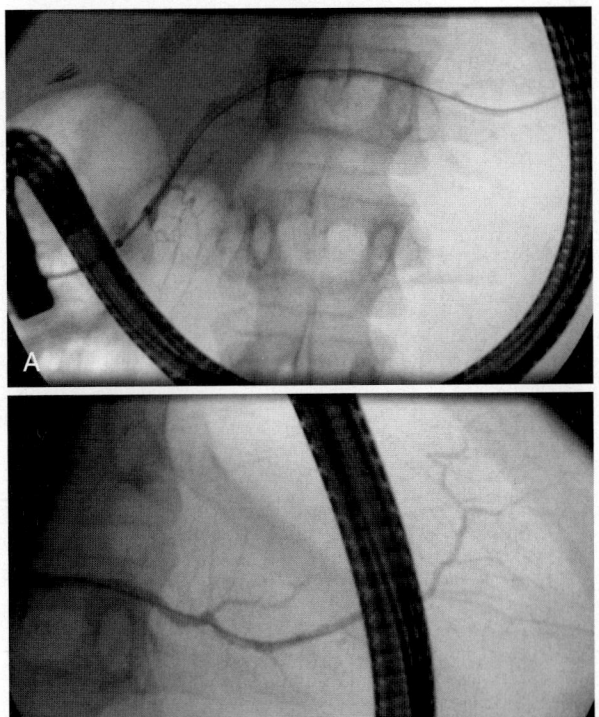

Fig. 38.3 **A** and **B,** Normal dorsal duct pancreatogram of head (**A**) and body and tail (**B**) regions.

patients,[16] including patients in whom needle-knife sphincter-otomy is used for access to the bile duct,[15] patients in whom sphincterotomy is performed for treatment of sphincter of Oddi dysfunction,[17] patients in whom sphincter dilation is performed for biliary stone removal,[18] and patients with other high-risk indicators including "difficult cannulation."[19]

Infection is a risk of pancreatography in predictable sub-groups of patients, particularly patients with necrosis, duct leaks, and communicating cystic spaces such as pseudocysts. Although minimal data exist to guide the use of antibiotics in these settings, risk-to-benefit considerations suggest potential benefit of prophylactic antibiotics in the peri-ERCP period. In the past, pancreatic pseudocysts were considered a relative contraindication to ERCP, unless surgical drainage was planned within 24 hours. Experience has not supported this concern, however.[20] Nonetheless, prudent practice might employ antibiotic prophylaxis and limited filling of chambers that would not effectively drain.

Normal Pancreatic Ductal Anatomy

Pancreatography provides a contrast-enhanced radiographic image of the shape, caliber, and distribution of the pancreatic ducts. It does not image the parenchyma of the gland. Occasionally, pancreatography grossly overestimates or under-estimates the size of the gland based on the degree of filling accomplished at the time of imaging and the actual length and distribution of the ducts. The ducts of interest usually include the main pancreatic duct of Wirsung, which drains from the tip of the tail through the pancreatic body and the ventral portion of the head to the major papilla; the accessory duct of Santorini, which extends from a major angle of the main duct, termed the *genu*, through the dorsal portion of the pan-creatic head to the minor papilla; an intermittently present

uncinate branch in the ventral portion of the head; and the many small side branches draining into the major and acces-sory ducts throughout the length of the gland.

Terminology for the linear extremes of the pancreatic duct is sometimes confusing because *proximal* and *distal* some-times correlate with direction of flow (distal bile ducts are at the major papilla), but in the pancreas, *proximal* and *distal* usually refer to relative distance from a point of reference at the duodenal wall (proximal pancreatic duct relative to or near the major papilla). In line with this classic use, surgical termi-nology uses *distal pancreatectomy* to refer to resections begin-ning with the tail. To avoid confusion, especially as may occur among three specialties providing procedural, radiographic, and surgical interpretations, it is clarifying to speak of *upstream* segments or locations as being toward the tail relative to another location and *downstream* segments or locations as being toward the duodenum.[21]

Globally, in the anteroposterior projection, the pancreato-gram extends in an oblique fashion from the tail, located left of the spine at the T12 level, to the major papilla located right of the spine at the L2 level (**Fig. 38.3**). There is significant variation, however, in both the overall extent and the course of individual portions of the main duct. Within the head, the duct runs cephalad about 15 degrees from parallel to the spine; in the body, it runs horizontally or perpendicular to the spine; and in the tail, it usually rises further at a gentle angle but may even descend.[22] The tail segment tends to be the most variable in course and shape. Occasionally, it is bifid, or split, left of the spine. In the anteroposterior projection, the retroperito-neal main pancreatic duct appears two-dimensional. However, oblique or lateral views show that it begins posteriorly in the

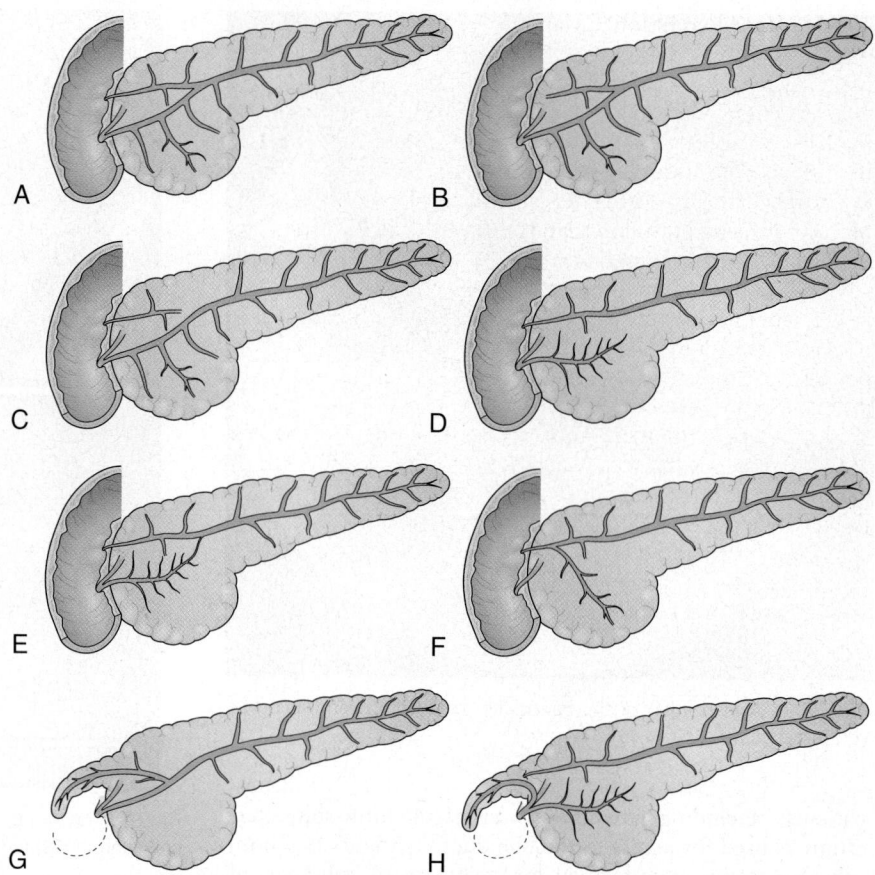

Fig. 38.4 Variations in dorsal and ventral duct migration and fusion. **A,** Normal. **B,** Normal with imperforate minor papilla. **C,** Normal with disjunction of the accessory duct. **D,** Pancreas divisum. **E,** Incomplete pancreas divisum. **F,** Pancreas divisum with no ventral duct. **G,** Annular pancreas with normal fusion of ventral and dorsal ducts. **H,** Annular pancreas with associated pancreas divisum.

tail, extends anteriorly around the spine, then extends back to a relatively posterior position at the genu and at the junction with the second portion of the duodenum. This excursion is highly variable and not useful for interpretation of displacement by adjacent space-occupying lesions.[23]

The main pancreatic duct is smooth with minor undulations and a general decline in caliber from the head to the tail. Focal nonpathologic indentations are sometimes noted at the genu, near the approximate junction with the accessory duct, and in the body, where it is in close proximity to the superior mesenteric vasculature.[24] The former is well described but uncommon, and the latter is infrequently reported. Numerous studies have reported the length and caliber of the pancreatic duct as obtained from postmortem and endoscopic studies.[25] Postmortem values tend to be slightly higher. With age, the duct caliber appears to increase slightly, while the length is stable. The length in normal glands averages about 16 to 17 cm, but it may range from 9 to 24 cm. When the main duct is less than 9 cm in length, obstruction should be suspected. The caliber of the pancreatic duct is most variable within the head of the gland, where the normal diameter is 3 to 4 mm but may range up to 6 mm, after correction for radiographic magnification. Accepted corrected diameters for the body and tail are 2 to 3 mm (up to 5 mm) and 1 to 2 mm (up to 3 mm).[26]

Visualization of side branches during pancreatography depends largely on technique and adequacy of contrast agent injection. Their visualization may be immaterial to the clinical question being addressed, or visualization may be crucial and of primary importance for resolution of clinical issues.

Depending on the indication, lack of side-branch filling may not be indicative of a suboptimal or inadequate study. Side branches are highly variable and asymmetric in the pancreatic head but quite regular and symmetric, with alternating junctions along the main duct throughout the body and tail. A postmortem study reported a mean of 56 first-order branch ducts (range 52 to 66).[27] Far fewer branch ducts are usually seen during even forceful pancreatography. A single large, inferiorly directed "uncinate" branch is seen in 55% to 62% of pancreatograms.[24,28] The accessory pancreatic duct is shown in only 14% to 62% of endoscopic pancreatograms, even though postmortem studies can show its presence in 100% of autopsy specimens.[25] It communicates with the main pancreatic duct in approximately 90% of specimens. Patency of the accessory duct and minor papilla together is highly variable. It is seen in more than 60% of general ERCP studies but in only 17% of studies in patients being evaluated for biliary pancreatitis, implying that when patent, the accessory duct serves to decompress the briefly obstructed main pancreatic duct.

Pancreatic Duct Variants

The pancreatic ducts are highly subject to abnormal formation during embryogenesis (**Fig. 38.4**). Most variants are of no clinical consequence, other than recognition when identified during diagnostic studies. Several risk the occurrence of pain or pancreatitis, however, on the basis of partial obstruction to flow of pancreatic juice after major stimulation. The most important and common variants occur as a result of either malrotation or malfusion of the ventral or dorsal embryonic pancreatic anlage. Normally, during the 6th to 8th week of embryogenesis, the smaller ventral pancreas rotates posteromedially as the duodenum rotates and migrates laterally. Once in a medial position neighboring the larger dorsal pancreas, the parenchyma and ducts fuse, yielding a main pancreatic duct comprising both dorsal and ventral segments. Failure of normal rotation and migration can yield an annular pancreas, in which some portion of the ventral pancreas remains behind in the path of migration (**Fig. 38.5**). The band of incompletely migrated duct and associated parenchyma typically form a partial to complete ring around the second portion of the duodenum, just proximal to the major papilla.

Many cases of annular pancreas remain asymptomatic, but more extreme variants can cause partial duodenal obstruction in infancy, childhood, or adulthood.[29] The preferred treatment for intestinal obstruction is duodenal bypass, rather than excision of the offending segment. Annular pancreas may also cause episodic pancreatitis, but its association with other abnormalities makes interpretation of the exact etiology

uncertain. Approximately one-third of cases are associated with pancreas divisum.

Pancreas divisum is the most common and important of the congenital variants (**Fig. 38.6**). It occurs as a result of incomplete fusion of the ventral and dorsal ducts after migration of the ventral anlage. Pancreas divisum occurs in approximately 7% (1% to 14%) of autopsy and pancreatography series. Approximately 20% of cases are incompletely divided, with persisting tiny communications via side branches of the dorsal and ventral systems. The technical approach to pancreatography via the minor papillae has been described previously. In pancreas divisum, the ventral duct may be generous, small, or nonexistent in up to 30% of cases. It should appear finely tapering with gradually smaller side branches, suggesting the appearance of a delicate Christmas tree. Abrupt termination of the main duct should prompt concern about a potential obstructing lesion. Dorsal ductography and EUS usually resolve this question.

The clinical importance of pancreas divisum relates to the fact that it precludes full evaluation of the dorsal ducts during pancreatography via the major papilla; it mimics and must be differentiated from small focal lesions obstructing the ducts near the junction of the ventral and dorsal systems; and when accompanied by relative stenosis of the minor papillae, it may contribute to partial outflow obstruction resulting in episodes of acute pancreatitis or solitary pain. Whether pancreas divisum causes important clinical problems is controversial. If so, the identification of the subset of patients in whom this relatively frequent anomaly produces clinical symptoms is a persistent challenge because only a few have a grossly abnormal dorsal pancreatogram. Delayed drainage during ductography and the use of secretin stimulation to identify prolonged duct dilation attributable to sphincter stenosis have not proven reliable.

The junction between the pancreatic duct and the bile duct at the major papilla is also highly variable (**Fig. 38.7**). Differences in junctional anatomy are primarily important for the challenges they present during selective cannulation of one or the other system during ERCP. A so-called anomalous pancreaticobiliary junction exists when the ducts unite proximal to the pancreatic sphincter and the duodenal wall. In this setting, there is no barrier for prevention of reflux of bile or pancreatic juice into the alternative system. This abnormality has been associated with the development of choledochal cystic dilation and acute idiopathic pancreatitis. Whether endoscopic sphincterotomy is adequately efficacious remains questionable because the junction is often above the boundary of safe incision. Duct

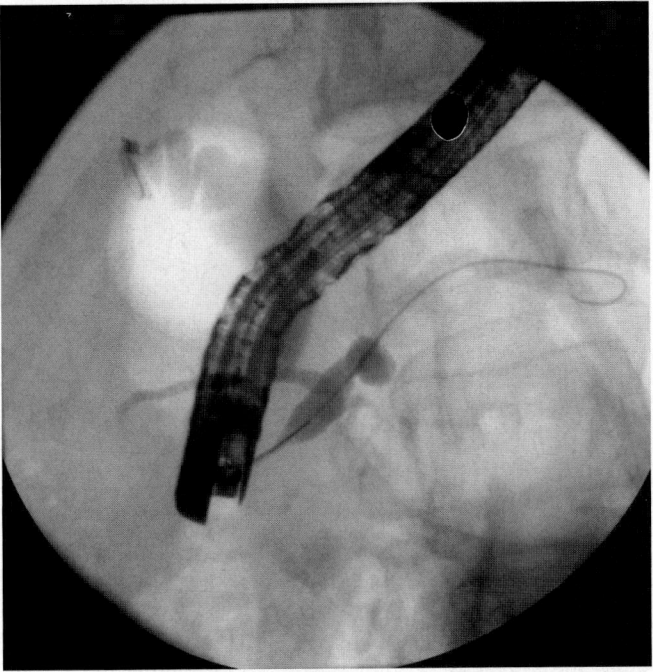

Fig. 38.5 Radiograph of a pancreatogram showing annular pancreas.

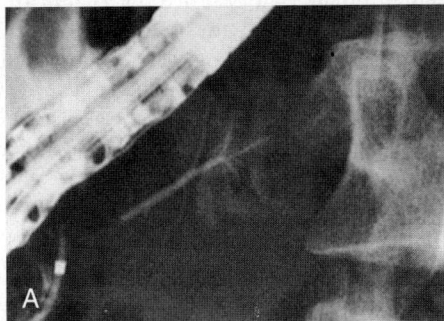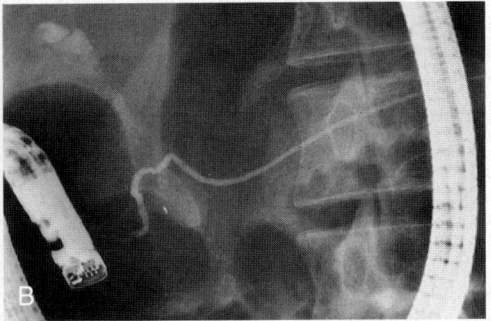

Fig. 38.6 Radiograph of a pancreatogram showing pancreas divisum. **A,** Ventral duct fills via injection into the duct of Wirsung at the major papilla. **B,** Dorsal duct fills via injection into the duct of Santorini at the minor papilla.

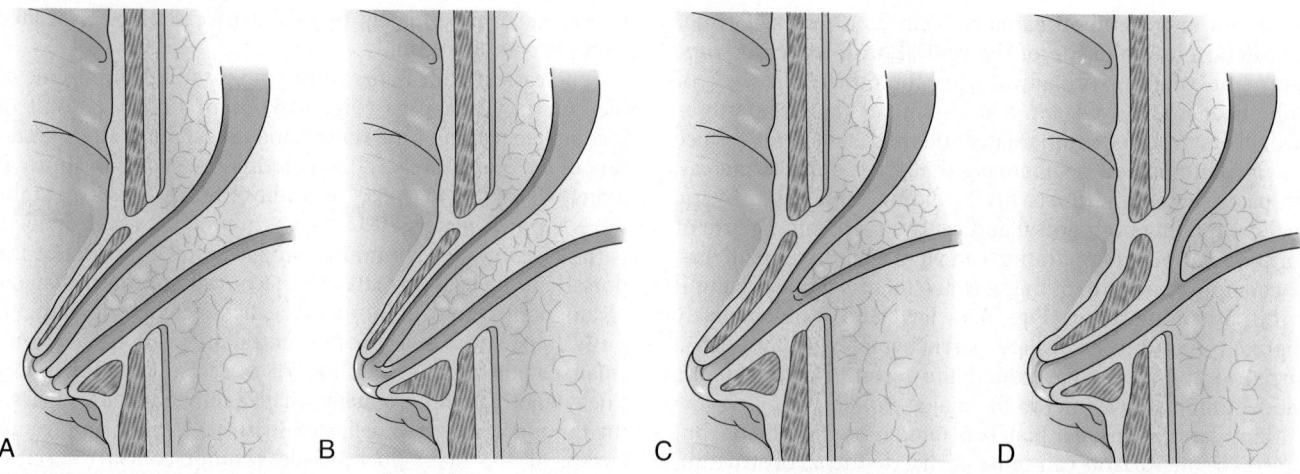

Fig. 38.7 Variations in the pancreaticobiliary junction. **A,** Separate openings on one papilla (infrequent). **B,** Fusion immediately at the duodenal surface of the papillary os (common). **C,** Fusion within a combined sphincter with a variable "common channel" length (usual). **D,** Fusion proximal to the ampullary sphincter yielding a common channel of greater than 15 mm (so-called anomalous pancreaticobiliary junction; this is rare).

duplications, with the resulting appearance of a bifid system, occur most commonly in the body and tail.[30] Duplications may be associated with unusual patterns of glandular parenchyma, but they are generally of no clinical consequence.

Periampullary Pathology Related to Pancreatic Disease

Pathologic appearances of the ampulla, the papilla of Vater, and the medial wall of the duodenum can be due to intrinsic conditions or can reflect underlying pathology within the neighboring pancreas or the pancreatic ducts. The most common extrinsic causes of an abnormal appearance are changes related to underlying malignancy or pancreatitis. Cancer within the head of the pancreas often encroaches on the periampullary region, causing mucosal and ampullary swelling, induration, and inflammation. In the absence of malignant ulceration, the changes are nonspecific and similar to changes seen with underlying severe acute or subacute pancreatitis. Severe pancreatitis often produces more prominent and widespread edema of the duodenal mucosa as well. Changes of the papillary os are uncommon and usually seen after stone passage from the bile duct. Transpapillary passage of white chalky pancreatic stones from the pancreatic duct is rarely seen endoscopically but has been noted during investigation of obstructive cholangitis in patients with chronic calcific pancreatitis and duct stones.[31] Observation of thick plugs of mucus extruding from a dilated papillary duct is pathognomonic of intraductal papillary mucin-producing neoplasm (IPMN) of either the bile duct or the pancreatic duct.[32] The latter is far more common (**Fig. 38.8**).

Pathologic Patterns Seen during Pancreatography

During pancreatography, recognition of pathology requires familiarity with normal findings and patterns of abnormalities that might be encountered. Various potential findings include (1) filling defects, (2) abnormalities in duct caliber or

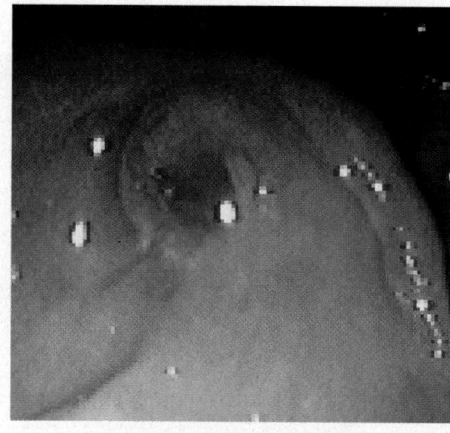

Fig. 38.8 Endoscopic image of mucus extruding from the major papilla in a patient with intraductal papillary mucin-producing neoplasm (IPMN) of the pancreas.

contour, (3) duct leaks, and (4) filling into cystic spaces. Each abnormality is associated with a differential diagnosis of possible causes, many of which overlap or contribute to multiple abnormalities (**Box 38.2**). Filling defects include stones, parasites, and mucus secreted by IPMN. Abnormalities in contour include partial or complete obstruction, duct dilation, and focal or diffuse irregularities secondary to malignancy or benign inflammatory processes. Leaks can be free, contained, or communicating with other organs as fistulas and occur as a result of trauma, surgery, endoscopy, and acute or chronic pancreatitis. Filling of cystic spaces can be within or extrinsic to the pancreas itself and may be associated with pseudocysts, central areas of necrosis within solid lesions, and communicating cystic neoplasms.

Pancreatic Neoplasia

Pancreatography is a key means of identifying neoplastic lesions of the pancreas. Pancreatic carcinoma produces characteristic duct abnormalities, most of which are nonspecific

Box 38.2 Pathologic Patterns Seen during Pancreatography and the Most Common Underlying Etiologies

Filling Defects

Stones (chronic pancreatitis)
Mucus (secreted by intraductal tumors)
Papillary tumors
Parasites

Abnormalities in Duct Caliber or Contour

Obstruction or stricture (tumor, stone, benign inflammatory lesions, extrinsic compression)
Dilation (downstream obstruction, intraductal mucus or stones)
Irregularity (acute or chronic pancreatitis)

Duct Leaks

Free leaks (trauma, surgery, endoscopy, acute or chronic pancreatitis)
Contained leaks (acute or chronic pancreatitis)
Fistulas (surgery, acute or chronic pancreatitis)

Filling into Cystic Spaces

Extrapancreatic spaces (pseudocysts)
Intrapancreatic spaces (pseudocysts, communicating cystic neoplasms, side-branch IPMN)

IPMN, intraductal papillary mucin-producing neoplasm.

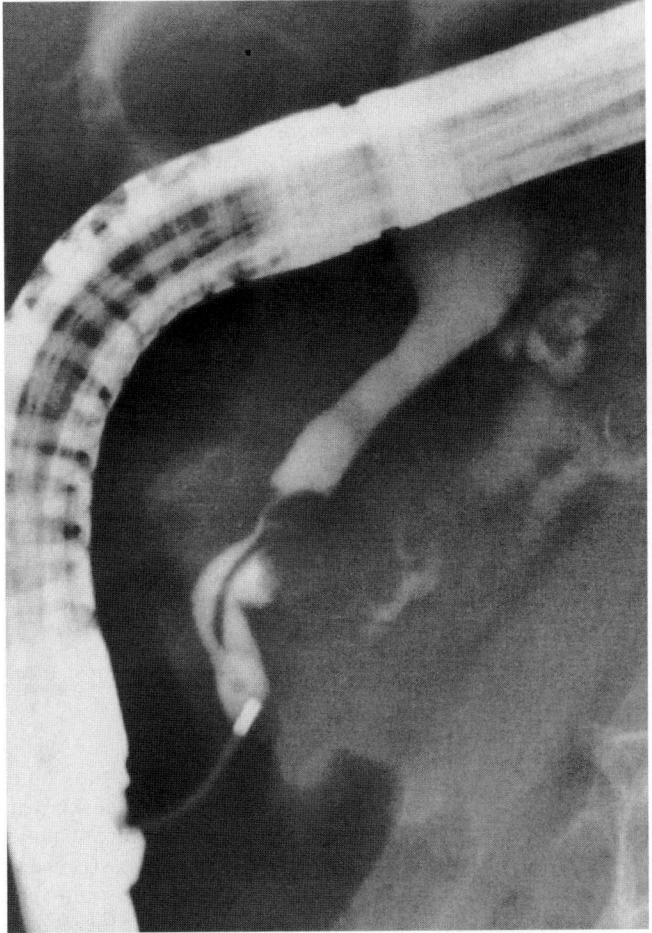

Fig. 38.9 The "double duct" sign of concurrent biliary and pancreatic duct obstruction, seen here with unusual deviation of both ducts produced by a small tumor of the periampullary region.

and must be differentiated from similar changes caused by chronic pancreatitis. Patterns include complete obstruction, focal stricturing or stenosis, irregular narrowing of moderate degree, distortion or obliteration of side branches, and stenosis with entry into necrotic cystic spaces.[33] The two dominant patterns are complete obstruction and focal strictures. Obstruction related to cancer may appear blunt, serrated, or abruptly pointed, whereas obstruction related to chronic pancreatitis may appear smoothly tapered, rounded, or concave from a meniscus sign related to intraductal stones. Malignant strictures tend to be more abrupt, with irregular contours, whereas strictures from chronic pancreatitis are either very short and suggestive of focal weblike scars or lengthy and smoothly tapered.[34]

In malignant obstruction or stenosis, the side branches are commonly absent near the lesion, dilated upstream from the obstruction, and normal downstream. In chronic pancreatitis, the side branches are intact but perhaps abnormal near the main duct lesion, and the main duct and side branches exhibit either dilation or chronic distortion upstream *and* changes of chronic pancreatitis *downstream* from the obstruction. Key findings for differentiating pancreatic carcinoma from autoimmune pancreatitis during pancreatography include the length of main pancreatic duct strictures (autoimmune pancreatitis > 3 mm, pancreatic carcinoma < 3 cm), presence (autoimmune pancreatitis) or absence (pancreatic carcinoma) of skip lesions, maximum caliber of upstream dilation (autoimmune pancreatitis < 3 to 5 mm, pancreatic carcinoma > 5 mm), and presence of demonstrable side branches in strictured segments of autoimmune pancreatitis but not in pancreatic carcinoma.[35] Successful interpretation varies among readers but can be learned and appropriately applied.[36]

The presence of concomitant neighboring abnormalities in both the pancreatic and the bile ducts is highly suggestive of malignancy. Findings may include dual obstruction or stenosis ("double duct" sign), displacement by tethering or compression, and effacement.[37] The double duct sign is highly suggestive and should be considered diagnostic of cancer until proven otherwise (**Fig. 38.9**). Lesions in the head are often first brought to attention by associated biliary obstruction and jaundice or pruritus. In this setting, ERCP often accesses the biliary obstruction for tissue sampling and palliative stent placement. If computed tomography (CT) or ultrasound findings are diagnostic of cancer, pancreatography is usually unnecessary. If no mass has been seen by cross-sectional imaging when ERCP shows a distal biliary stricture, it is very useful to obtain a pancreatogram at least within the pancreatic head, ideally including both uncinate and accessory branches. Cases of pancreatic carcinoma involving a nonfilling accessory duct with an otherwise "normal" pancreatogram have been reported.[38]

Of all the pancreatic neoplasms, findings with IPMN of the pancreatic ducts are among the most specific.[32] The characteristic production of mucus may occur silently, with eventual identification of dilated segments on cross-sectional imaging, or it may manifest clinically with episodes of pain or pancreatitis related to intermittent obstruction.[39] When IPMN involves the main pancreatic duct, pancreatography typically shows dilation and soft, bulky filling defects that can be stripped from the lumen with an occlusion balloon. When present only in side branches, the diagnosis is commonly suspected after cross-sectional imaging with CT or ultrasound. Contrast agent filling of segments harboring side-branch IPMN may require forceful injection above an occlusion balloon (see **Fig. 38.8**). This maneuver may not be justified, given the improving identification of this process by EUS. Gross papillary changes of the duct lining mucosa are infrequently evident radiographically but when present can be sampled with transpapillary biopsy and brushing to diagnose IPMN.

Transpapillary pancreatoscopy and intraductal ultrasound during ERCP have been described as useful in preoperative staging of the longitudinal spread of main duct IPMN.[40,41] Mucus markedly distorts the endoscopic view but wire-guided intraductal ultrasound identifies both the mucus and papillary changes if they are accessible. None of these endoscopic tools are highly sensitive for identifying the progression to invasive malignancy.[42]

Pancreatography in Acute Pancreatitis

Relative consensus now exists regarding the use of endoscopic cholangiography for acute pancreatitis. Despite the known risk of pancreatitis attributable to ERCP, performance of cholangiography in the setting of acute pancreatitis has been shown to be generally safe.[43] Cholangiography and sphincterotomy, as indicated by findings, are now accepted in the setting of severe acute pancreatitis with associated biliary obstruction or cholangitis.[44] These procedures may also be beneficial for severe biliary pancreatitis without biliary obstruction; however, data are mixed on this point,[45,46] and one study suggested detrimental effects in this setting.[47] Subsequent to resolution of one or more episodes of acute pancreatitis, pancreatography is useful for identification of potential etiologies, including biliary stone disease, anomalous anatomy (e.g., pancreas divisum, anomalous junction), occult neoplasia, and chronic pancreatitis.[48]

Venu and colleagues[48] reported use of ERCP and sphincter of Oddi manometry in 116 patients with recurrent idiopathic pancreatitis. A treatable cause of pancreatitis was identified in 37%, including a mixture of anatomic abnormalities, stones, and sphincter hypertension. As previously described, evolving guidelines propose that in this elective setting ERCP should be performed only if skills for therapy and performance of sphincter of Oddi manometry are also available. The use of pancreatography during episodes of severe acute pancreatitis is generally not indicated. However, smoldering pancreatitis that is not resolving and late morbidity related to strictures or leaks after improvement in the most severe inflammatory process are both settings in which pancreatography and associated therapies may be beneficial.[49–52]

Nonspecific findings that may be seen during acute pancreatitis, for which intervention is not indicated, include increased irregularity in contour of the main duct and side branches, perhaps less prompt filling of side branches, and occasional early parenchymal staining even before side-branch filling, suggestive of local necrosis. Duct leaks and strictures resulting from acute pancreatitis occur most frequently near the genu and likely result from focal necrosis at that site. Leaks identified within the first few weeks appear free within the retroperitoneum, whereas leaks identified after longer intervals enter more circumscribed spaces or mature pseudocysts. The timing of onset for duct leaks remains incompletely defined. Data from Neoptolemos and coworkers[53] suggested that most leaks occur after the 4th day. These investigators retrospectively stratified patients to modest versus extensive (>25%) glandular necrosis by CT scan then determined the incidence and timing of duct leaks based on pancreatography. No leaks were found among 89 patients with limited necrosis. In contrast, 7 of 16 patients in the extensive necrosis group exhibited leaks, including none of 4 patients studied before day 5 and 7 of 12 studied at day 5 or later.

In a prospective study of pancreatic duct integrity during acute pancreatitis, Uomo and colleagues[54] showed a 31% incidence of leaks by pancreatography performed during the 1st week (mean 4.2 days). Leaks did not correlate with need for surgical management. In both acute and chronic pancreatitis, it is useful to clarify whether leaks are being potentiated by downstream obstruction related to strictures or stones because this has implications for endoscopic and surgical management.

The details of therapeutic interventions are beyond the scope of this chapter. There is growing interest in the potential utility of early investigation and prophylactic intervention or early treatment for significant duct injury in severe necrotizing pancreatitis.[55] However, only limited data support this approach, and the potential for secondary infection of necrosis and peripancreatic tissues mandates that prospective studies be performed before this approach becomes common practice.

Pancreatography in Chronic Pancreatitis

The indications for pancreatography in chronic pancreatitis include (1) to establish a diagnosis, (2) to characterize the anatomy before surgical management, and (3) to characterize the anatomy as a component of endoscopic therapy. Pancreatography has been the "gold standard" for diagnosing chronic pancreatitis for several decades. Several classification systems for chronic pancreatitis have been proposed. Although none are perfect or all-encompassing, the Cambridge Classification of 1983 proposed a sequential gradation of ductal abnormalities[21] that remains perhaps the most straightforward and widely used. Pancreatograms are termed normal, equivocal, or indicative of mild, moderate, or marked pancreatitis on the basis of side-branch abnormalities; main duct abnormalities; or additional advanced irregularities including presence of cavities, complete obstruction, filling defects (stones), severe dilation (>1 cm), and segmentation ("chain of lakes") (**Figs. 38.10 and 38.11**).

The severity of pancreatographic findings correlates loosely with progression of disease and decline in pancreatic function. The main challenges in the interpretation of pancreatography for the diagnosis of chronic pancreatitis are the differentiation of normal from early disease with minimal changes and the differentiation of pancreatic carcinoma from chronic disease with focal stricturing. Comments on the latter have been made earlier. Mild changes on pancreatography—blunting, dilation, or shortening of the side branches—are the least specific and most subjective because they are highly dependent on technique and adequacy of filling and potentially a result of age-related changes or transient effects of acute injury. ERP is more sensitive for early changes of chronic

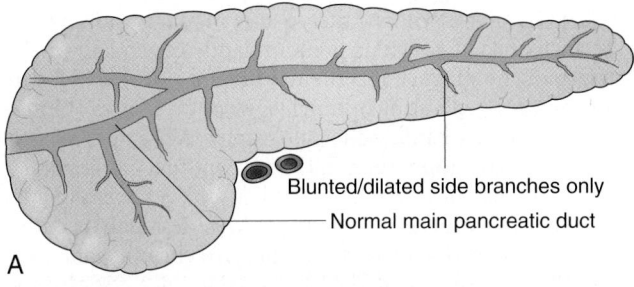

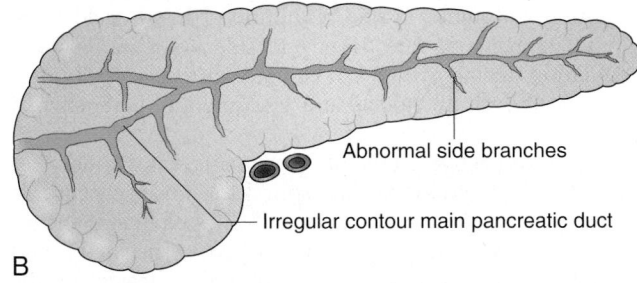

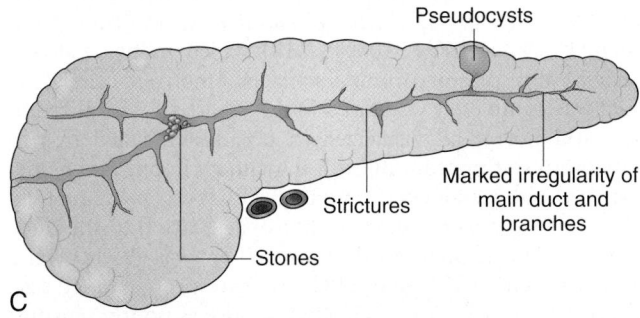

Fig. 38.10 Cambridge classification of chronic pancreatitis. **A,** Mild. **B,** Moderate. **C,** Marked.

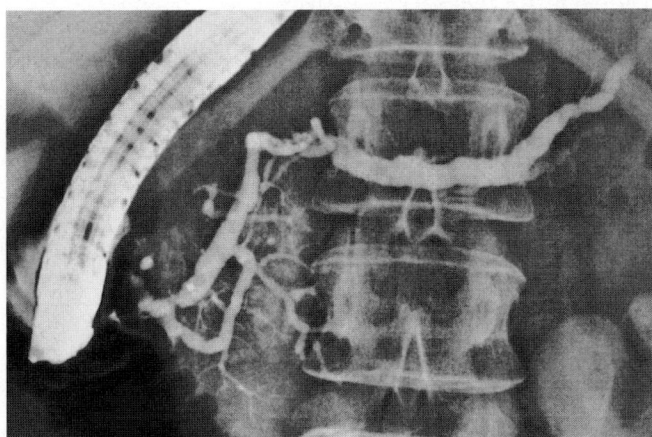

Fig. 38.11 Pancreatogram showing advanced grade of chronic pancreatitis.

pancreatitis than CT, transabdominal ultrasound, or magnetic resonance cholangiopancreatography (MRCP). EUS is both highly sensitive for early chronic pancreatitis and safe.[56] In centers with adequate EUS experience, it is becoming the procedure of choice for making this diagnosis when CT or MRCP are normal.

Pancreatic duct morphology is best characterized by pancreatography, and this remains the procedure of choice for anatomic characterization before surgery or in concert with other, less invasive therapies for pseudocysts, fistulas, leaks, and pancreatic ascites related to chronic or postnecrotic pancreatitis.[57,58] In a prospectively documented series of 41 patients with pseudocysts associated with chronic or resolving acute pancreatitis, Nealon and coworkers[59] showed that preoperative ERCP led to significant alterations in the surgical management in 24 patients (59%). In particular, ERCP led to pseudocyst drainage combined with concurrent drainage of the pancreatic duct in 19 patients and of the common bile duct in 11 patients with chronic pancreatitis. In the current era of transmural and transpapillary endoscopic drainage of pseudocysts, the role of endoscopic characterization of the pancreatic duct remains incompletely defined. Its utility is likely to be equivalent or greater than when used in concert with surgery.

Miscellaneous Settings

After pancreatic surgery, questions pertaining to anastomotic leaks and strictures are often best answered by pancreatography (**Fig. 38.12**). Duct decompression and drainage are feasible at the same procedure, similar to the procedure described for acute and chronic pancreatitis leaks. Resection procedures generally yield leaks at closure lines of main ducts, whereas surgical enucleation or excision procedures are more prone to

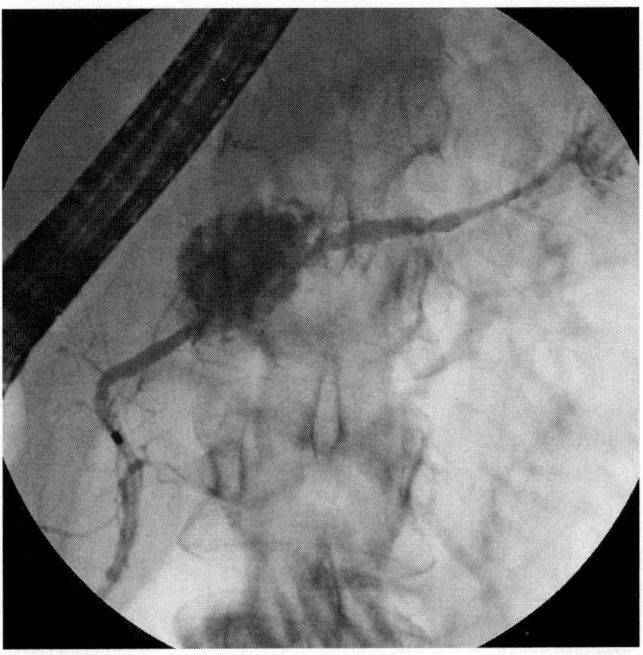

Fig. 38.12 Pancreatogram showing a postoperative leak from the region of the genu subsequent to enucleation of a neighboring small benign tumor.

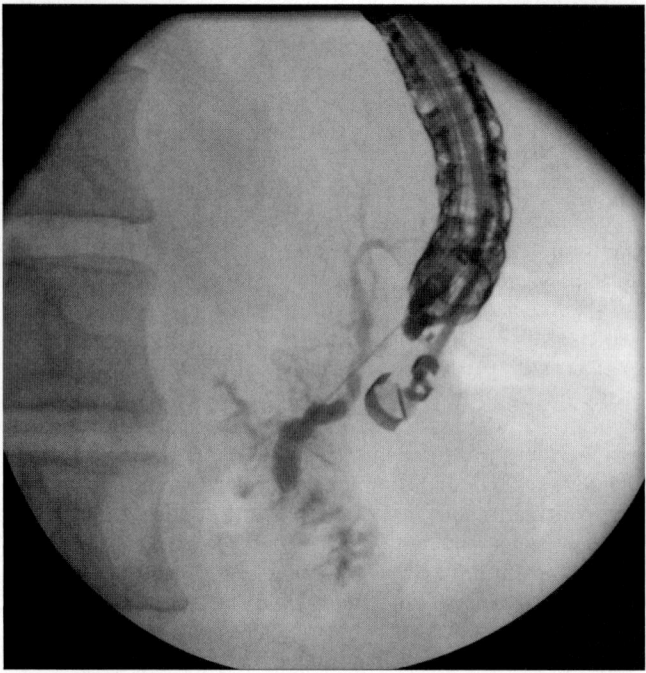

Fig. 38.13 Pancreatogram via direct endoscopic ultrasound (EUS)–guided transgastric puncture of the main pancreatic duct.

smaller side-branch or lateral main duct leaks. Pancreatography may also be useful for investigation and therapy of late postoperative anastomotic strictures. Pancreaticojejunal anastomoses fashioned in decompressive procedures, including the Peustow lateral pancreaticojejunostomy and the Frey procedure, can be studied via the pancreatic os at the major papilla. Pancreaticojejunal anastomosis employed in the Whipple procedure and the Beger procedure must be accessed via enteroscopy into an afferent limb or a Roux limb; this is significantly more difficult.

In our experience, ERP is successful in only 10% to 15% of patients after the Whipple procedure.[60] In most patients with post-Whipple anatomy, a pancreatogram can be obtained most easily via transgastric EUS-guided duct puncture (**Fig. 38.13**).[61] This maneuver is also used as a prelude to EUS-guided transgastric stent decompression of obstructed ducts resulting from cancer or chronic pancreatitis. These therapies may be accomplished in usual retrograde fashion after rendezvous passage of a guidewire or directly from stomach to pancreas.[61] Percutaneous duct access for pancreatography and associated therapies has also been described.[62]

Pancreatography is also very useful during investigation of blunt midabdominal trauma, from which mid–pancreatic duct leaks can occur owing to rupture of the gland over the spine. Identification and localization of traumatic leaks can guide surgical[63,64] or endoscopic management.

Magnetic Resonance Pancreatography

Each of the imaging modalities for the pancreas is associated with particular benefits and shortcomings. ERP is relatively invasive and is associated with moderate to significant risk, but it also provides the opportunity for efficient therapy of lesions

identified during the same study. EUS is relatively invasive but safer than ERCP. EUS offers opportunity for tissue and fluid sampling, therapeutic options for injection of anesthetic or ablative agents for neurolysis, and transgastric access for duct imaging and therapy. Both CT and MRCP provide optimal noninvasive imaging of the parenchyma and the neighboring organs. Based on differentiation of fluid density, MRCP more easily provides a diagnostic quality pancreatogram as well. Neither CT nor MRCP is a therapeutic modality, however.

Performance of MRCP is predominantly dependent on the strength of the magnet and the use of sophisticated software algorithms for generating optimal views of the region of interest. Magnetic resonance pancreatography (MRP) has slightly less spatial resolution than ERP, but optimal performance approaches that of endoscopic studies and is generally adequate for clinical decision making.[65] MRP is highly accurate for the diagnosis of pancreas divisum.[66] In chronic pancreatitis, MRP can show glandular and periglandular atrophy and inflammation, in addition to the status of the ducts. The duct distention and higher spatial resolution of ERCP yield more optimal imaging of fine detail and side branches. Secretin stimulation during MRCP can enhance distention and interpretation of both duct detail and assessment of parenchymal function.[67]

In a retrospective study of 32 patients who underwent ERCP, CT, and abdominal ultrasound for advanced chronic pancreatitis, Varghese and colleagues[68] assessed dual interpretations of MRP. They reported sensitivity, specificity, and diagnostic accuracy for detection of filling defects in the pancreatic duct (56% to 78%, 100%, 87% to 94%), ductal strictures (75% to 88%, 92% to 96%, 88% to 94%), and pseudocysts (100%, 100%, 100%). MRP failed in two patients because of respiratory motion artifacts. Among all others, the duct was completely visualized in 84%, partially visualized in 9%, and not at all visualized in 6%. ERCP failed in two patients, resulting from Billroth II anatomy in one and a duct stricture and pseudocyst in another. ERCP was inadequate in five (6%) patients because of poor opacification of the duct, which was insufficient for diagnosis. There was good correlation between MRCP and ERCP with respect to duct size. Varghese and colleagues[68] concluded MRP is poorly sensitive but specific for duct abnormalities and, when combined with CT or transabdominal ultrasound, can be sufficient for planning therapy in most patients with advanced chronic pancreatitis.

Helical CT and optimal MRCP yield equivalent results for detection of pancreatic neoplasms, vascular invasion, and neighboring lymphadenopathy.[65] Cystic tumors and the contents of tumors and fluid collections are more accurately characterized with MRCP than with CT. Most centers use MRCP (or CT) for diagnosis or characterization of advanced disease and for patients who are not good candidates for sedation and intubation or in whom the clinical suspicion is quite low. ERCP is reserved for patients in whom more subtle duct abnormalities are anticipated or endoscopic therapy is planned. Local preferences dictate which study is used for preoperative anatomic characterization.

References

The complete reference list is available online at www.expertconsult.com.

Difficult Cannulation and Sphincterotomy

Juergen Hochberger, Johannes Maubach, and Detlev Menke

Video related to this chapter's topics can be found online at expertconsult.com.

Introduction

In the era of magnetic resonance cholangiopancreatography and endoscopic ultrasound, endoscopic retrograde cholangiopancreatography (ERCP) has become a procedure with a primarily therapeutic focus (e.g., access to and through stenoses, removal of stones, or drainage of cysts).[1-4] If used as a diagnostic procedure, ERCP is more often performed to sample tissue by the introduction of cytology brushes or biopsy forceps or to facilitate direct cholangioscopy. Major papilla sphincterotomy is mandatory in most cases to achieve adequate access for the introduction of instruments and drainage catheters. General issues related to cannulation and sphincterotomy have already been discussed in Chapter 37. The present chapter focuses on variations of the standard technique that can be used by advanced endoscopists. The variations in technique have to be performed with caution and adapted to the individual case. Important general issues are discussed first.

Proper Endoscope

The standard endoscope for most indications is a therapeutic side-viewing duodenoscope with an instrumentation channel of 3.7 to 4.2 mm. There are only very rare situations in which a smaller diagnostic duodenoscope offers advantage, such as duodenal stenoses. For examination of a pediatric patient younger than 2 years and in a case in which the papillary orifice is localized on the inner side of a duodenal diverticulum, a standard 11.5-mm duodenoscope may be advantageous. A disadvantage of a smaller scope is a channel of only 2.8 to 3.2 mm, which makes the implantation of 10-Fr to 12-Fr stents impossible and the use of two guidewires difficult. A previous argument had been the better deflection of the elevator (Albarran's lever) using standard 6-Fr to 7-Fr catheters or tiny instruments. Changes in elevator design in the last decade have eliminated this problem with therapeutic duodenoscopes. However, grooming of standard catheters to facilitate cannulation of the common bile duct (CBD) can still be helpful in certain situations.

Access to and cannulation of the papilla in case of a Billroth II (BII) resection (**Figs. 39.1** and **39.2**) is generally possible with a comparable success rate using a prograde or a side-viewing endoscope; this is described later.[5-7] Gastroscopes work only in a few usually older BII patients without enteroenteric anastomosis, but gastroscopy may be helpful for initial inspection and orientation of the anastomoses. In patients with a very long afferent loop and in patients after gastrectomy with Roux-en-Y anastomosis, a pediatric colonoscope or enteroscope longer than 170 cm is needed in case of

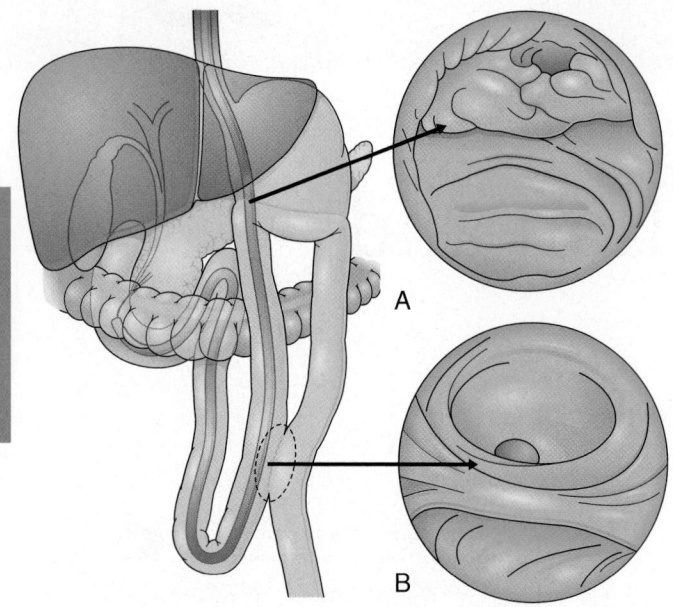

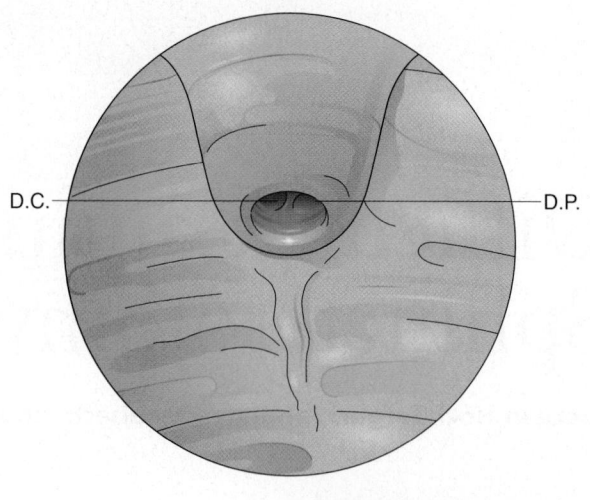

Fig. 39.1 Billroth II anatomy: endoscopic access. Endoscopic view at the gastrojejunal (**A**) and enteroenteral (Braun) anastomosis (**B**). The endoscopist should use an afferent loop and stay on the same side of the enteral wall when passing the enteroenteral anastomosis *(oval)*. *(Modified from Soehendra N, Binmoeller KF, Seifert H, et al:* Therapeutic endoscopy: color atlas of operative techniques for the gastrointestinal tract, *New York, 1997, Thieme Medical Publishers.)*

a forward-viewing endoscopic approach. Although the forward-viewing instrument facilitates intubation of the afferent loop at the gastroenteric anastomosis, it typically provides only a tangential view of the papilla.[8]

The duodenoscope offers the advantage of improved visual orientation to the ampulla. The elevator is helpful to manipulate and maintain accessories. A duodenoscope is preferred by many endoscopists if applicable.[5,8] In a difficult anatomic situation with a steep afferent loop, it can be helpful first to place a 0.035-inch, 450-cm guidewire (polytetrafluoroethylene-coated standard Seldinger wire; PNB Medical, Denmark) into the blind proximal end of the duodenal stump under radiographic control as a pathfinder for the side-viewing instrument.

Locating the Papilla

Although the natural position of the papilla is on the inner side of the duodenal C-loop in the midportion of the descending duodenum, it may be difficult to find in some instances. The papilla may be located toward the lower portion, which often requires a very "long" endoscope position. The papilla can be cloaked by duodenal folds, and often only the frenulum, as a caudal longitudinal extension, indicates that the papillary orifice may be close. In the search for the papilla, an atraumatic ERCP catheter or sphincterotome can be helpful to lift and separate folds. Duodenal diverticula have to be inspected carefully. One way to expose the inner side of the diverticulum is to push the mucosa gently from the outer rim of the diverticular ring caudally with an ERCP catheter. The papillary orifice often appears by being pulled from the inner side of the diverticulum toward the edge of the opening. Submucosal injection into the bottom of the diverticulum has

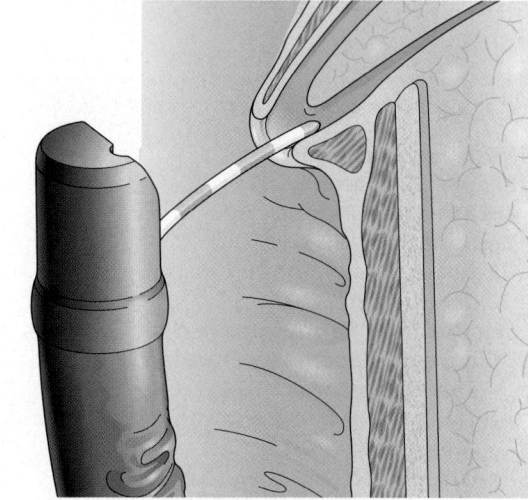

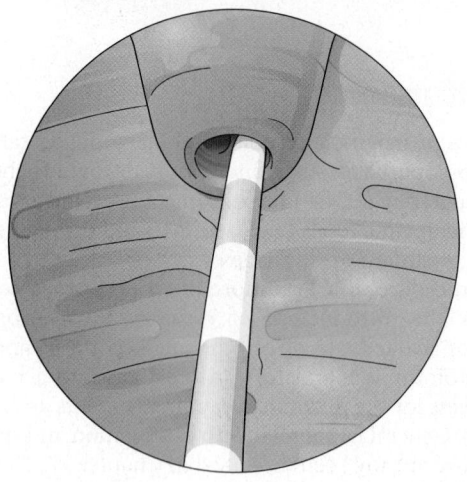

Fig. 39.2 Billroth II cannulation. View of the papilla from below with inverted anatomy. *(Modified from Soehendra N, Binmoeller KF, Seifert H, et al:* Therapeutic endoscopy: color atlas of operative techniques for the gastrointestinal tract, *New York, 1997, Thieme Medical Publishers.)*

been described to lift the papillary orifice. However, one should keep in mind the very thin wall of the diverticulum with the risk of potentially severe complications owing to needle perforation and retroperitoneal leak and a potential edematous compression of the papillary orifice.[9]

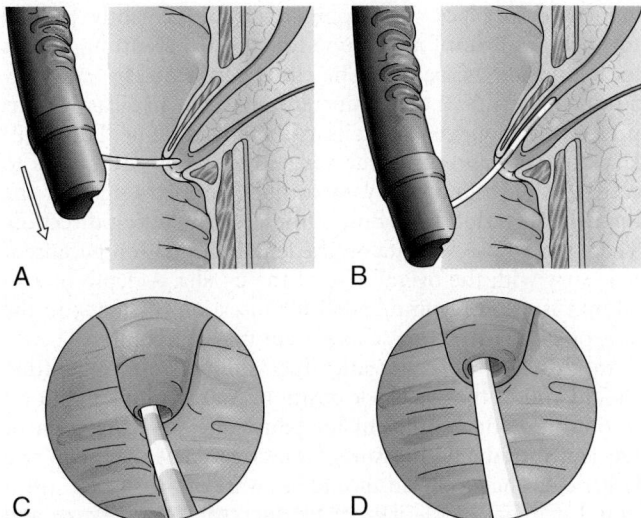

Fig. 39.3 For primary cannulation of the common bile duct using a standard catheter and a therapeutic duodenoscope, it often helps first to intubate the papillary orifice with the catheter (**A**) and then to change the angle of the catheter by gently advancing the endoscope (**B**). Alignment with the axis of the papilla is important in biliary cannulation (**C** and **D**). *(Modified from Soehendra N, Binmoeller KF, Seifert H, et al: Therapeutic endoscopy: color atlas of operative techniques for the gastrointestinal tract, New York, 1997, Thieme Medical Publishers.)*

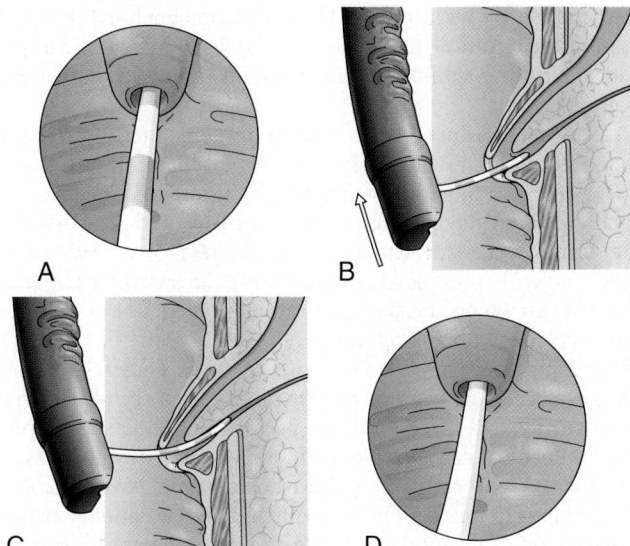

Fig. 39.4 **A–D,** Pancreatic cannulation. Flat position of the catheter facing the papilla at the same level (**A**). If common bile duct cannulation was performed first, pulling back the endoscope facilitates cannulation (**B** and **C**) and changes the direction of the catheter within the papilla (**D**). *(Modified from Soehendra N, Binmoeller KF, Seifert H, et al: Therapeutic endoscopy: color atlas of operative techniques for the gastrointestinal tract, New York, 1997, Thieme Medical Publishers.)*

In rare cases, it can take 20 minutes or longer to find the papilla. Sometimes, the papilla is located more proximally. This situation occurs after Billroth I resection. Very rarely, the papilla is located in the duodenal bulb. An edematous duodenum after an acute attack of chronic pancreatitis or advanced cancer of the head of the pancreas can make successful localization and cannulation of the papilla impossible. A radiologically guided percutaneous-transhepatic rendezvous procedure and endoscopic ultrasound–guided puncture into the biliary system are options in these cases.[10–14]

Park and coworkers[15] described using methylene blue to find the minor papilla orifice in patients with a complete pancreas divisum. After spraying dye onto the area of the papilla, pancreatic secretions wash away the dye from papillary orifice. Intravenous secretin (Secrelux, Sanochemia Diagnostics, D-41460 Neuss) can help in this case to stimulate pancreatic secretion and to identify the pancreatic orifice for minor papilla cannulation. Secretin is expensive, however, and should not be given in case of pancreatic obstruction or acute pancreatitis.

Cannulation

A well-sedated patient is the prerequisite for a smooth intervention. Before cannulation, the papilla should be observed carefully, and the endoscopist should imagine the natural course of the CBD. A long papillary roof delineating the distal bile duct above the horizontal fold (plica horizontalis) may be helpful in determining its axis and course (**Fig. 39.3**). For cannulation of the CBD, the papilla should be viewed from below, and the catheter direction should be steep and within the axis of the papilla. Curving the distal end of the catheter upward often facilitates achievement of this angle and eases biliary cannulation. The catheter tip is introduced into the papillary

orifice and gently pushed forward while the elevator is lifted and the bile duct is cannulated. For primary pancreatic duct cannulation (**Fig. 39.4**), the endoscope position remains at the level of the papilla, and the catheter direction is roughly horizontal. Although the course of the pancreatic duct leads toward the 5 o'clock position viewed from directly in front of the papilla, in our experience it can be helpful, in a native papilla, to turn the small wheel of the endoscope forward and cannulate the papillary orifice from the right to the left followed by only gentle injection of contrast material.

Catheter versus Sphincterotome Cannulation

The primary use of a catheter or a sphincterotome for biliary cannulation is controversial. The traditional first choice is a regular tapered 6-Fr catheter with a 4-Fr tip accepting a 0.035-inch wire that is used for biliary cannulation of the papilla and may serve for easier intrahepatic cannulation in biliary stenoses. The advantage of a prebent standard catheter over a 6-Fr sphincterotome is the higher flexibility and even less traumatic access owing to a high sensitivity even for narrow papillary channels. However, the use of a regular sphincterotome to initiate cannulation of the bile duct potentially allows variability and improvement of the vertical angle in which the bile duct is cannulated alongside the axial alignment.[16]

After correct adjustment is achieved, the catheter or sphincterotome is advanced toward the papilla. It is best to approach the papilla from a distance so that the natural curve of the sphincterotome is obvious on exiting the endoscope. The tip of the sphincterotome is gently introduced into the common channel. Bowing of the sphincterotome tip usually eases the tip into the mouth of the CBD; when this happens, a characteristic "give" often occurs. Relaxing the wire to straighten the tip and gently withdrawing the endoscope anchor the tip of the sphincterotome further within the distal bile duct. Simply advancing the sphincterotome now invariably leads to deep cannulation.

New devices are constantly being developed to improve the success rate of ERCP.[16,17] Two studies evaluated the use of a new steerable catheter (SwingTip; Olympus, Tokyo, Japan) to achieve bile duct cannulation. Igarashi and coworkers[18] reported successful cholangiography in 175 of 195 cases (90.5%) with a standard catheter; using the SwingTip catheter in cases in which the standard catheter failed, it was possible to carry out cholangiography in 11 of 17 patients (64.7%), increasing the overall success rate to 95%. Laasch and colleagues[17] conducted a prospective randomized controlled trial comparing the success rate in performing cholangiography and bile duct cannulation with three different catheters: a standard ERCP cannula, a short-nosed sphincterotome, and the SwingTip device. The study included 312 patients at two tertiary referral centers. Both steerable catheters were significantly better than the standard catheter for performing cholangiography ($P = 0.038$), but no differences were found between the SwingTip cannula and the sphincterotome. Steerable catheters were also more effective for deep cannulation of the bile duct, but the improvement did not reach statistical significance. Steerable catheters succeeded in 26% of the cases in which the standard cannula failed. The study also compared differences in the results obtained from an expert and a trainee endoscopist using the three catheters. Trainees experienced greater benefit from using steerable catheters, whereas experts were quicker in performing cholangiography and deep cannulation with the SwingTip device. The overall success rate was 97%, and pancreatitis occurred in 5.3% of cases.

Wire-Guided Cannulation

When routine maneuvers fail, the next step may be the use of a wire-guided sphincterotome.[16,19] The endoscopist positions the tip of the sphincterotome at the presumed mouth of the biliary orifice, and the assistant gently turns the wire. The J-tip of a 0.035-inch atraumatic hydrophilic guidewire (J-Terumo; Terumo Corp, Japan) is usually rotated in a clockwise direction. The tip of even the softest wire becomes stiff if forcefully pushed out of a catheter or if the sphincterotome lumen is pressed against tissue. One should gently press the sphincterotome or catheter toward the suspected CBD direction and leave enough room for the tip to flex slightly while the wire is rotated with a torquing device. When this technique fails, the options are to abort the procedure and review the indication or alternatives, such as proceed to access sphincterotomy or referral to another operator. A good reason for the endoscopist to stop at this point is limited experience and a low case volume.

Biliary and Pancreatic Standard Sphincterotomy

After deep cannulation of the CBD, the exact position of the catheter or sphincterotome is confirmed by injection of contrast medium. When sphincterotomy is confirmed, the instrument is withdrawn from the bile duct leaving a 0.035-inch

guidewire in place. The sphincterotome is gently pushed forward again until about one-fourth of the cutting wire is located inside the papilla. The cut is performed by smoothly advancing or lifting the sphincterotome. The papillary roof is preferentially opened along its axis and its midline. The papillary anatomy and axis may vary considerably from case to case. It may be necessary to torque the instrument in the opposite direction to maintain the desired cutting direction. There are no precise data on the length of incision because it may vary with the overall size of the papilla. A depth of 6 to 10 mm is often recommended for insertion of stents; in the case of stone extraction, a larger cut may be required.

In the case of pancreatic duct sphincterotomy, cutting should aim at the 1 o'clock position. An incision length of 3 to 6 mm is often sufficient for pancreatic stent insertion or relief of intraductal pressure. Stone treatment may require a larger cut. The physician should be aware of the shorter intramural segment of the pancreatic duct, smaller duct size, and increased risk of perforation. Similar to modern biliary sphincterotomy, the cutting wire should be introduced into the papillary orifice just deep enough to allow cut by diathermic current and gentle pressure.

Juxtapapillary and Periampullary Diverticula

Diverticula are the most common type of anomaly and are often found in elderly patients. Because of the distorted anatomy, it is often more difficult to cannulate the bile duct.

The papilla and the distal course of the bile duct may be located anywhere along the inferior rim or on the inner edge of the diverticulum. Aspiration of air may lead to a slight collapse of the diverticulum and may help delineate the location of the papillary orifice. We often take a standard catheter and push the duodenal mucosa close to the outer rim of the diverticulum caudally; this may lead to traction on the diverticulum itself and help expose the papilla at the opening of the diverticulum. The endoscopist needs to intubate the papilla quickly with the catheter, which stabilizes its position. The literature describes placing the patient in a prone position or pressing in the right upper abdominal quadrant as possible alternative steps. Injecting saline into the contralateral side of the diverticulum has been described and may lead to a protrusion and exposure of the papilla. However, the risk of retroperitoneal perforation needs to be considered.

Precut Sphincterotomy

Precut or "access" sphincterotomy employs techniques to gain access to the selected duct cannulation when other measures have failed. Specialized catheters and electrosurgical energy to cut papillary tissue are used to expose and gain access to the selective duct for cannulation.

The classic Erlangen-type precut sphincterotome is shaped like a standard sphincterotome, but its distal end is cut off to just below the cutting wire. Modifications include catheters with a 1- to 2-mm nose at the distal tip. The precut sphincterotome is placed in the papillary orifice and slightly lifted and gently pushed forward in the direction of the bile duct with diathermic current application. This technique can be

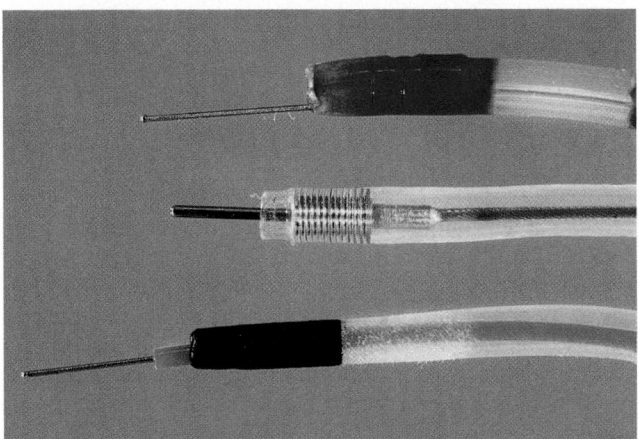

Fig. 39.5 Different types of needle-knives. Diameter and length of the cutting wire influence cutting properties: The thinner the wire knife, the faster and sharper the cut; the longer the wire, the potentially deeper the cut with relatively high risk of bleeding and perforation.

termed an "entry" cut to distinguish it from the following two freehand needle-knife techniques (**Fig. 39.5**).

Although needle-knife sphincterotomy has been considered a risk factor for ERCP-induced complications such as pancreatitis, bleeding, and perforation, series from centers with a high frequency of needle-knife precut sphincterotomies show that in experienced hands the needle-knife procedure does not have a higher complication rate.[19,20] The most common needle-knife technique is to place the needle tip into the papillary orifice, lift the upper lip of the papilla with slight tension on the needle-knife, and give short bursts of cutting current in the biliary direction. Another approach is sequential dissection of the roof of the papilla, starting at the papillary orifice with careful sweeping cuts of about 5 to 7 mm to dissect the papillary mound in a stepwise fashion. Subsequent dissections up to the plica horizontalis should allow separation of the cut edges of mucosa and submucosa with recognition of the red sphincter muscle. After careful opening of the papillary apparatus in the common sphincteric area, the circular structure of the biliary sphincter with an often dark central point indicates the desired orifice. It is now helpful to switch to a tapered cannula and probe the biliary sphincter atraumatically. A gush of bile to indicate successful bile duct access should not routinely be expected and usually occurs only in the case of an intrapapillary stone obstruction.

Billroth II Resection

ERCP in a patient with BII resection of the stomach may be challenging because of the more difficult endoscopic access in this altered anatomy. Advantages of the use of a prograde endoscope such as a pediatric colonoscope and a duodenoscope for cannulation and sphincterotomy were described earlier.

The endoscope is introduced alongside the minor curvature of the stomach, which often shows a longitudinal postoperative prominence. Routinely, visualization of the gastrojejunal anastomosis during introduction of the endoscope is useful to detect an early BII gastric stump cancer. The access to the bile duct in a BII patient is via the afferent loop.

Following the minor curvature of the stomach, the two orifices of the afferent and efferent loop appear in the form of an "8." The upper "o" of the "8" is usually the access to the afferent loop (see **Fig. 39.1**). Often, the angle of the fixation of the afferent loop to the stomach is very steep, and sometimes the opening of the afferent loop is seen only from below looking back in inversion to the stomach. One can easily slip from the afferent loop into the efferent loop—the endoscope takes on a U-shaped configuration. After only a brief loss of visualization, one may easily enter and follow the efferent limb for long distances without recognizing the error. When it seems impossible to intubate a steep afferent loop, one should exclude a terminal side-to-side gastrojejunostomy. This is the case in Whipple's resection of the head of the pancreas with a single jejunal loop attached to the stomach and Roux-en-Y anastomosis for biliary and pancreatic drainage. One or two 30-mL syringes filled with contrast material and injected (sequentially) directly through the instrumentation channel can help to find the course of a steep afferent loop. In the case of a terminal gastrojejunostomy such as in Whipple's resection, there is only a 1- to 2-cm blind end in the usual position of the afferent loop.

Advancing the scope toward the papilla, the afferent loop must be probed carefully and lifted with the tip of the endoscope. There is a significantly higher perforation rate of the small intestine, especially at the site of the anastomosis, leading to a higher overall complication rate for ERCP in cases of BII resection and Roux-en-Y anastomosis compared with ERCP in standard anatomy.[7,21] As described previously, the use of a forward-viewing instrument such as a gastroscope or pediatric colonoscope is preferable in the case of an unclear anatomic situation. Sometimes there is a corkscrewlike path of the first 5 cm entering the afferent limb at the gastroenteric anastomosis, which may be challenging for passage with a duodenoscope. Primary placement of a 4.5-m guidewire into the afferent limb via a prograde instrument is an option in these situations. The endoscope is withdrawn leaving the guidewire in place, which is followed endoscopically and radiographically side to side with the duodenoscope.

In the case of an enteroenteric (Braun) anastomosis, it is recommended to leave the stomach also via the afferent limb. When the enteroenteric anastomosis is reached, at least two lumens appear. Inverting the endoscope, a third lumen coming from the efferent limb and the endoscope coming from the afferent limb can be seen.

In the search for the correct route to the papilla, the trick is to follow the Kerckring folds of the afferent limb on the same side and not to cross the enteroenteric anastomosis. This recommendation holds true only in case the exit from the stomach was actually the afferent loop. Often the course of the afferent loop leaving the enteroenteric anastomosis on the way to the papilla is very steep, and this can lead to a U-shape of the endoscope with inability to propagate the endoscope further toward the papilla and risk of local trauma at the site of anastomosis at the maximum with perforation. Manual compression externally and a variable-stiffness pediatric colonoscope can help to intubate the afferent limb successfully at this point. On the way back, a clip marking the afferent limb of the enteroenteric anastomosis may help in localization for the next time ERCP has to be performed in the patient.

Concerning the ERCP procedure itself in a patient after BII resection or with a Roux-en Y anastomosis and intact duodenal anatomy (e.g., after tumor gastrectomy), the anatomy at the level of the papilla is reversed (see **Fig. 39.1A**). The papilla is approached from below instead of from above because usually the bile duct is now located at the 5 o'clock position. The pancreatic duct is reached via the 11 o'clock position. Using a side-viewing endoscope with the advantage of an elevator withdrawing the endoscope about 2 to 3 cm with a very flat tangential position toward the papilla often helps intubate the CBD. With regard to the reversed anatomy, the catheter tip should not be curved but should be straight.

There are different options for a sphincterotomy in a BII. The first option is to place a plastic stent into the desired bile duct and perform a needle-knife sphincterotomy onto the stent as a known possible technique from (minor) pancreatic sphincterotomy (see later). Careful dissection of the different tissue layers of the papilla as described previously is essential. The cutting direction is usually also opposite from the papillary roof toward the os in subsequent small cuts 3 to 5 mm long. The stent reduces the risk of cutting too deeply. However, care has to be taken not to slip to one or the other side of the stent with the needle-knife.

The classic option for BII sphincterotomy is a special Billroth II sphincterotome (Cook Medical, Winston-Salem, NC); the cutting wire is guided similar to in a standard sphincterotome for a path of 20 mm in the outside of the catheter. By advancing the handle apparatus, the cutting wire protrudes to form a "shark-fin" configuration. The cutting wire is advanced forward over a guidewire in the direction of the plica horizontalis in the middle of the papillary mound. However, this technique is not always as simple as it seems because the wire easily rotates and slips toward the duodenal side of the wall, and back rotation using a duodenoscope is not always that easy. Many endoscopists prefer the needle-knife technique on the stent. Variations of the latter technique include self-shaping a standard sphincterotome to allow a similar function as the commercial BII sphincterotome by overextending the cutting wire.[22]

Roux-en-Y Anastomosis and Double-Balloon or Single-Balloon Enteroscopy for Endoscopic Retrograde Cholangiopancreatography

The papilla can be reached using a pediatric colonoscope in only about 10% of all patients needing ERCP after gastrectomy.[5] For these cases, double-balloon enteroscopy and more recently single-balloon enteroscopy are good options.[23,24] Double-balloon enteroscopy can lead to successful ERCP in about 80% of cases with BII resections with long afferent limb and Roux-en-Y postsurgical anatomy.[25–28] For these cases, the therapeutic type of double-balloon enteroscope is preferred (Fujinon EN450T5; Fujinon Corp, Saytama, Japan).[29,30] However, special ERCP accessories with excess length have to be used. More recently, the prototype of a short 152-cm double-balloon enteroscope for ERCP (Fujinon EC450BI 5; Fujinon Corp) has been introduced. One advantage is the ability to use standard ERCP instruments, in particular, self-expandable metal stents and sphincterotomes.[28] Training in

double-balloon enteroscopy ERCP technique ex vivo has proved helpful for beginners.[31]

Cannulation and Sphincterotomy of the Minor Papilla

Minor papilla cannulation is indicated when complete pancreas divisum is suspected as a cause for acute recurrent or chronic pancreatitis. This congenital anomaly leads to drainage of the major dorsal part of the gland via the small minor papilla, whereas the major papilla exclusively drains the smaller ventral portion from the head region of the gland. Another indication for minor papilla cannulation can be an "incomplete" pancreas divisum (dominant dorsal duct) with only a very fine ductal connection of the ventral and dorsal pancreas and suspected increased intraductal pressure.

Because of its small size, cannulation of the minor papilla is more challenging. The minor papilla is sometimes hard to identify and often is only a 2-mm protrusion with a minute orifice (see the previous section on locating the papilla). The minor papilla is usually located 1 to 1.5 cm rostral to the major papilla and about 10 mm laterally to the right, often above the first or second horizontal fold in a groove. The major papilla should be identified first; then the endoscope has to be withdrawn slowly. The minor papilla should appear just below the superior angle of the duodenum. It is controversial whether a short or a long endoscope position is preferable. For cannulation, a 3-Fr Glo Tip or Bottle Neck catheter (Cook Medical) is helpful. Cannulation and contrast material injection should be carried out with caution so that interstitial edema is not created with the fine-tip catheter. Septotomy of the minor papilla may be performed with a wire-guided mini-sphincterotome (3.4-Fr Minitome; Cook Medical). The cut should not exceed 4 mm; some authors prefer a much shorter cut of 2 to 3 mm. The direction of the cut should aim at the 12 o'clock position (10 o'clock to 1 o'clock position). Because the minor papilla is usually very small and the orifice is difficult to cannulate, a two-step approach is often necessary: If primary cannulation fails, a 2-mm precut septotomy is performed toward the 12 o'clock position with no further attempt to cannulate or opacify the duct. After 2 to 3 days, cannulation is successful in most cases at repeat endoscopy.

A third approach is to first insert a 5-Fr (4-Fr to 7-Fr) stent. Septotomy is performed with a needle-knife using the stent as a guide rail. Because it is assumed that the stent reduces the risk of pancreatitis, it may be left in place for several days and can be removed in a second session.

Complications

Similar to success rates, complications associated with ERCP, and especially sphincterotomy, are volume-dependent. In sphincterotomy, bleeding, pancreatitis, and perforation are the most concerning complications. Bleeding may be attributed to an aberrant vessel in the roof of the papilla. The latter may occur as a variation of the normal anatomy in about 2.5% of cases.[32]

The reported incidence of pancreatitis occurring after ERCP and sphincterotomy ranges from 1.3% to 24.4% in nonselected series.[16,33,34] This varying incidence likely reflects differences in patient populations, indications, and endoscopic expertise and different definitions for pancreatitis and methods of data collection. Numerous patient-related factors are recognized as risks for post-ERCP pancreatitis in more recent large prospective studies, comprising 1966 cases, including the combination of female gender, normal serum bilirubin levels, and recurrent abdominal pain suggesting sphincter of Oddi dysfunction and previous post-ERCP pancreatitis.[32] Combinations of risk factors can substantially increase the odds ratio (e.g., to 16.2 for a difficult cannulation in a female patient with normal bilirubin). Among technique-related risk factors for post-ERCP pancreatitis, biliary sphincter balloon dilation, difficult cannulation, sphincter of Oddi manometry, and pancreatic sphincterotomy have also been recognized as significant risk factors.

Because the case mix in nonselected series does not significantly differ in the different studies, it is logical to assume that the different criteria adopted for defining post-ERCP pancreatitis play a key role in the reported wide variation of incidence reported for this complication. The occurrence and duration of pain and the amplitude of serum amylase after ERCP are critical points in the definition of post-ERCP pancreatitis. Although a consensus conference identified 24-hour persisting pain associated with hyperamylasemia greater than three times the upper reference limit as an indicator of pancreatitis, these two parameters are considered in a different manner in the studies available up to now. In a prospective study in which the incidence of post-ERCP pancreatitis was calculated by using the most widely used criteria, for both occurrence and duration of pancreatic pain and serum amylase amplitude, the incidence of postprocedure pancreatitis ranged from 1.9% to 11.7% depending on the criteria adopted.[32,35]

Pancreatic Stents for Prevention of Pancreatitis following Endoscopic Retrograde Cholangiopancreatography

As potential prophylaxis against post-ERCP pancreatitis, pancreatic drainage with stents or nasopancreatic tubes can reduce the risk or severity of post-ERCP pancreatitis in selected cases. In particular, patients with pancreatic sphincter hypertension benefit from a temporary endoprosthesis.[33,36] As a consequence, the implantation of a protective pancreatic stent (4-Fr to 7-Fr) has been postulated for prevention of pancreatitis after difficult cannulation or sphincterotomy or both.

Aizawa and Ueno[37] retrospectively analyzed the efficacy of temporary pancreatic duct stent placement for prevention of pancreatitis after endoscopic sphincter dilation for removal of bile duct stones. Endoscopic sphincter dilation was performed in 38 patients with a mean number of 2.2 ductal stones and a mean maximum stone size of 12 mm. Bile duct clearance was achieved in 37 patients after 52 sessions, using mechanical lithotripsy in 58% of the cases. Biliary drainage was augmented in 13 cases to prevent cholangitis. The success rate of insertion of pancreatic 5-Fr stents was 95%. Endoscopy was repeated after 3 days for removal of biliary and pancreatic prostheses, with the exception of a few cases in which there was spontaneous passage. In a historical control group of 92 patients, the success rates for endoscopic sphincter dilation without pancreatic stents were not provided. Medical treatment, such as oral administration of nifedipine 3 hours before treatment or subcutaneous low-molecular-weight heparin, showed no benefit compared with placebo.[35]

Cheon and associates[38] investigated the use of orally administered nonsteroidal antiinflammatory drugs (NSAIDs) in 207 evaluable patients randomly assigned to receive diclofenac, 50 mg, or placebo by mouth 30 to 90 minutes before and 4 to 6 hours after ERCP. The overall incidence of post-ERCP pancreatitis was 16.4%. It occurred in 17 of 102 patients in the control group (16.7%) and in 17 of 105 patients in diclofenac group (16.2%). There was no significant difference between the groups in the frequency or severity of post-ERCP pancreatitis in overall and high-risk patients; however, the power of the study was less than 45%.

Elmunzer and colleagues[39] performed a meta-analysis concerning the use of rectally administered diclofenac. They found four randomized controlled trials enrolling 912 patients. Meta-analysis of these studies showed a pooled relative risk for post-ERCP pancreatitis after prophylactic administration of NSAIDs of 0.36 (95% confidence interval 0.22 to 0.60); patients who received NSAIDs in the periprocedural period were 64% less likely to develop pancreatitis and 90% less likely to develop moderate to severe pancreatitis. The pooled number needed to treat with NSAIDs to prevent one episode of pancreatitis was 15 patients. No adverse events attributable to the use of NSAIDs were reported in any of the clinical trials. However, the investigators concluded that additional multi-center studies are needed for confirmation before widespread adoption of this strategy. At the present time, the best options for the clinician to reduce the risk of pancreatic complications after ERCP are awareness of specific patient-related and procedure-related risk factors before the procedure, referral of elective high-risk cases to an expert center, and, eventually, 4-Fr to 5-Fr nonpolyethylene protective pancreatic stent placement.

References

The complete reference list is available online at www.expertconsult.com.

Chapter 40

Endoscopic Retrograde Cholangiopancreatography Tissue Sampling Techniques

Douglas Howell

Video related to this chapter's topics can be found online at expertconsult.com.

Introduction

Tissue sampling at endoscopic retrograde cholangiopancreatography (ERCP) has been an area of controversy since the inception of therapeutic ERCP in 1973. Histologic diagnosis remains the most certain confirmation of the presence of malignancy; however, ERCP has been the only endoscopic procedure in which tissue biopsy and cytology are considered secondary, generally because the main goal of the intervention is to provide drainage for obstructive jaundice.

Nevertheless, ERCP may present a unique opportunity to establish a definite diagnosis of malignancy during a drainage procedure, which may save the patient subsequent unnecessary, painful, and expensive procedures.[1] Despite many years of study, imaging alone cannot make the diagnosis of malignancy.[2] This chapter covers this controversial topic including historical background, pathogenesis, techniques in tissue sampling, complications, and future trends and potential.

History

ERCP was developed in the late 1960s as a diagnostic technique to provide detailed radiography of the biliary tree and pancreatic ducts. ERCP remained primarily a diagnostic tool until 1973, when endoscopic sphincterotomy was performed in Japan and Germany. One of the first sphincterotomies performed in Germany by Demling and Classen was to introduce a biopsy forceps to sample a bifurcation stricture (Classen, personal communication, September 1992). Because of the

technical difficulties of introducing standard front-viewing endoscopic accessories over an elevator for retrograde cannulation, tissue sampling did not develop early in the history of therapeutic ERCP. Initial efforts were limited to simple aspiration of bile and occasionally pancreatic juice when deep cannulation was achieved. After placing a diagnostic catheter just below or into the stricture, aspiration of 10 to 50 mL of bile or 5 to 20 mL of pancreatic juice may be collected over 10 to 15 minutes. Shed cells within these biologic fluids occasionally yielded a definite diagnosis.

Specificity in early reports was uniformly 100%. Despite early enthusiasm, clinicians noted low yields when the technique was used in a clinical setting. Reports of sensitivity of only 6% to 32% in six published studies[3-8] have caused this technique to fall from practice in favor of the newer, higher yield approaches of brush cytology, fine needle aspiration (FNA) cytology, and endobiliary forceps biopsy.

Pathogenesis

Obstruction of the biliary tree by benign or malignant stricturing requiring temporary or palliative stent placement in the bile duct remains a major indication for ERCP, now that diagnostic ERCP has been largely replaced by lower risk imaging techniques of helical computed tomography (CT) and magnetic resonance cholangiopancreatography. As discussed elsewhere in this textbook, endoscopic ultrasound (EUS) has an important role in examining patients with pancreatic neoplasms in which the resectability remains uncertain after

Box 41.1 Staging of Extrahepatic Cholangiocarcinoma

Perhilar bile ducts (extrahepatic biliary tree proximal to the cystic duct origin)

TX	Primary tumor cannot be assessed		
T0	No evidence of primary tumor		
Tis	Carcinoma *in situ*		
T1	Tumor confined to bile duct, with extension up to the muscle layer or fibrous tissue		
T2a	Tumor invades beyond wall of bile duct to surrounding adipose tissue		
T2b	Tumor invades adjacent hepatic parenchyma		
T3	Tumor invades unilateral branches of portal vein or hepatic artery		
T4	Tumor invades main portal vein or its branches bilaterally; or the common hepatic artery; or the second-order biliary radicals bilaterally; or unilateral second-order biliary radicals with contralateral portal vein or hepatic artery involvement		
NX	Regional lymph nodes cannot be assessed		
N0	No regional lymph node metastases		
N1	Regional lymph node metastases (including nodes along the cystic duct, common bile duct, hepatic artery, and portal vein)		
N2	Metastasis to periaortic, pericaval, superior mesenteric artery, and/or celiac artery lymph nodes		
M0	No distant metastasis		
M1	Distant metastasis		
Stage 0	Tis	N0	M0
Stage I	T1	N0	M0
Stage II	T2a-b	N0	M0
Stage IIIA	T3	N0	M0
Stage IIIB	T1-3	N1	M0
Stage IVA	T4	N0-1	M0
Stage IVB	Any T	N2	M0
	Any T	Any N	M1

Distal bile duct (extrahepatic biliary tree distal to the cystic duct origin)

TX	Primary tumor cannot be assessed		
T0	No evidence of primary tumor		
Tis	Carcinoma *in situ*		
T1	Tumor confined to the bile duct histologically		
T2	Tumor invades beyond the wall of the bile duct		
T3	Tumor invades the gallbladder, pancreas, duodenum, or other adjacent organs without involvement of the celiac axis, or the superior mesenteric artery		
T4	Tumor involves the celiac axis, or the superior mesenteric artery		
NX	Regional lymph nodes cannot be assessed		
N0	No regional lymph node metastases		
N1	Regional lymph node metastases		
M0	No distant metastasis		
M1	Distant metastasis		
Stage 0	Tis	N0	M0
Stage IA	T1	N0	M0
Stage IB	T2	N0	M0
Stage IIA	T3	N0	M0
Stage IIB	T1-3	N1	M0
Stage III	T4	Any N	M0
Stage IV	Any T	Any N	M1

From American Joint Committee on Cancer (AJCC): AJCC cancer staging manual, ed 7, New York, 2010, Springer-Verlag (www.springer-ny.com).

Ampulla of Vater

EUS provides detailed images of the papilla of Vater. The papilla is best located during slow withdrawal of the echoendoscope from the third duodenum, using ultrasound rather than endoscopic landmarks. The ventral pancreas is visualized, and the bile duct or pancreatic duct lumens or both are identified. The ducts can be traced to the duodenal wall and papilla. Administration of intravenous glucagon and instillation of water into duodenum may improve visualization once the periampullary region has been located.

The submucosal apparatus of the papilla can be visualized as a round hypoechoic structure in duodenal submucosa composed of the sphincter of Oddi and the intramural ducts. The normal submucosal mound of the papilla is usually less than 6 mm in transverse cross-sectional diameter. The lumens of the bile duct and pancreatic duct are usually not visible within the papilla; they generally taper and disappear from view as they reach the duodenal wall. The finding of a visible ductal lumen in the papilla suggests obstruction of the papilla by a stone (see **Fig. 41.4**), stenosis, or tumor, but a ductal lumen can also be seen in choledochocele and intraductal papillary mucinous neoplasm (IPMN). IDUS has been used to study the ampulla and may aid in the local staging of some ampullary tumors. It identifies the sphincter mechanism and permits accurate measurement of its length. Ultrasound features do not distinguish normal from hypertensive sphincters.[40]

Ampullary Neoplasms

Adenomas of the papilla may occur on the duodenal surface of the papilla or within the papilla in the mucosa of the intraampullary ducts or in both places. They may spread into or arise from the periampullary bile duct or pancreatic duct. EUS findings include a mucosal mass on the duodenal surface of the papilla, enlargement of the submucosal ampullary apparatus secondary to intraampullary polyp, and thickening of the periampullary duct walls or an intraductal nonshadowing mass. These findings can be seen in ampullary adenoma and in T1 ampullary cancer, and the two entities are often difficult or impossible to distinguish with EUS.

The TNM staging of ampullary cancers is presented in **Box 41.2** and illustrated in **Fig. 41.7**. T1 carcinoma may be limited to the mucosal surfaces of the ampulla and intraampullary ducts but may also involve the sphincter mechanism of the ampulla. The presence of an irregular outer edge of the submucosal ampullary apparatus suggests a T2 lesion invading the duodenal submucosa or muscularis propria. T3 cancers invade the pancreas, extending either through the duodenal wall or directly from the periampullary ducts. A T4 tumor extends into peripancreatic soft tissue or other adjacent structures. Regional lymph nodes include not only nodes adjacent to pancreatic head but also porta hepatic and celiac nodes.

In one large series, EUS accuracy for T staging of ampullary malignancies was 78%.[41] Adenomas were considered T1 lesions, highlighting the difficulty in distinguishing adenoma from T1 cancer with EUS. Most errors in staging involved overstaging of T2 lesions or understaging of T3 lesions because of difficulty in assessing the presence of invasion into the pancreas. The presence of peritumoral pancreatitis and edema and shadowing and tissue thickening secondary to an indwelling biliary stent were the major factors limiting the accuracy of EUS. Tumor may be difficult to distinguish from the normally hypoechoic ventral pancreas, and invasion of the duodenal muscularis propria may be difficult to detect because in normal persons the muscularis propria is interrupted by the ducts as they cross into the papilla. Despite these limitations, EUS is more accurate than computed tomography (CT) or magnetic resonance imaging (MRI).[41-43]

Box 41.2 Staging of Ampullary Carcinoma

TX	Primary tumor cannot be assessed
T0	No evidence of primary tumor
Tis	Carcinoma in situ
T1	Tumor limited to ampulla of Vater or sphincter of Oddi
T2	Tumor invades duodenal wall
T3	Tumor invades pancreas
T4	Tumor invades peripancreatic soft tissues or other adjacent organs or structures other than pancreas
NX	Regional lymph nodes cannot be assessed
N0	No regional lymph node metastases
N1	Regional lymph node metastases
M0	No distant metastases
M1	Distant metastases

Stage 0	Tis	N0	M0
Stage IA	T1	N0	M0
Stage IB	T2	N0	M0
Stage IIA	T3	N0	M0
Stage IIB	T1-3	N1	M0
Stage III	T4	Any N	M0
Stage IV	Any T	Any N	M1

From American Joint Committee on Cancer (AJCC): AJCC cancer staging manual, ed 7, New York, 2010, Springer-Verlag (www.springer-ny.com).

IDUS is probably more accurate that transduodenal EUS for T staging of ampullary neoplasms. In one large series, IDUS had an overall accuracy of 89%.[42] IDUS visualized small tumors missed by EUS and was more accurate than endoscopic biopsies for diagnosis of ampullary neoplasm. IDUS was also accurate for differentiation of adenoma from T1 carcinoma. These results were achieved by experienced endosonographers, using IDUS at the patient's initial ERCP and before sphincterotomy, stent placement, or biopsy—an optimal algorithm for tumor imaging but difficult to replicate in most EUS referral centers.

Acute Pancreatitis

Diagnostic EUS has two roles in patients with acute pancreatitis: (1) timely diagnosis of common bile duct or ampullary stones in patients with acute gallstone pancreatitis and (2) differential diagnosis in patients with unexplained bouts of pancreatitis. In both cases, EUS can be used in place of diagnostic ERCP and may identify patients most likely to benefit from therapeutic ERCP. A prognostic role for EUS in acute pancreatitis has not been shown, although the use of intravenous ultrasound contrast agents may allow EUS diagnosis of pancreatic necrosis. The accuracy and cost-effectiveness of EUS for diagnosis of bile duct stones were discussed earlier in this chapter. When EUS is used to exclude ampullary stones, the ampulla must be examined from the second duodenum. A skilled examiner can perform a focused EUS of the extrahepatic bile duct in less than 10 minutes, and the patient can undergo therapeutic ERCP under the same sedation if a stone is shown. This strategy allows patients with suspected ductal stone to avoid the potential complications of ERCP if a stone is not present.

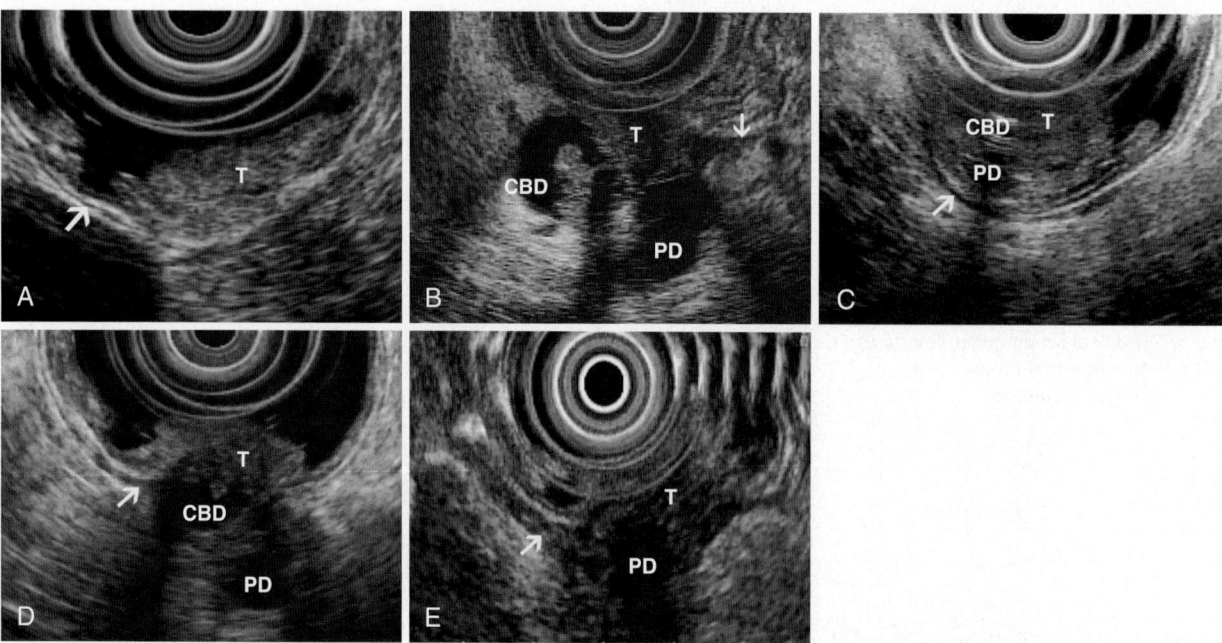

Fig. 41.7 Ampullary neoplasms. **A,** Adenoma on the surface of the ampulla. **B,** Ampullary tumor extending into the distal bile duct. **C,** T1 ampullary carcinoma involving the sphincter of Oddi. This lesion was mostly adenoma but contained foci of invasive carcinoma. **D,** T2 ampullary carcinoma invading the duodenal wall. **E,** T3 ampullary carcinoma invading the pancreas. *Arrow* indicates duodenal muscularis propria. *CBD,* common bile duct; *PD,* pancreatic duct; *T,* tumor.

One prospective trial investigating EUS in gallstone pancreatitis reported that it was accurate for diagnosis of gallbladder and ductal stones and predicted longer hospital stay in patients found to have peripancreatic fluid by EUS.[44] In another large series in which ERCP was used selectively, on the basis of EUS findings, patient outcomes were good, and recurrent biliary pancreatitis was uncommon.[45] EUS is also a useful tool in the evaluation of idiopathic pancreatitis, showing abnormalities in most patients.[3,46,47] Findings include missed biliary stones or sludge (see **Fig. 41.1**), chronic pancreatitis, pancreas divisum, pancreatic or ampullary malignancy, and pancreatic duct stones. EUS does not diagnose pancreatic sphincter dysfunction but may nevertheless supplant ERCP by diagnosing or excluding previously unsuspected gallbladder pathology, chronic pancreatitis, or pancreatic malignancy. EUS and MRCP seemed to have similar utility in one study.[48]

Chronic Pancreatitis

The traditional EUS features of chronic pancreatitis are listed in **Table 41.2** and illustrated in **Fig. 41.8**. This list of consensus criteria uses minimal standard terminology adopted by an international working group,[49] and good interobserver agreement has been shown for these criteria among experienced American endosonographers.[50] Investigators have also described other features not included in this list, including honeycombing (in which hyperechoic strands form a honeycomb pattern), heterogeneous echotexture, focal areas of hypoechogenicity, tortuous pancreatic duct, thickened pancreatic duct wall, and narrowing of the main pancreatic duct. The traditional EUS approach to diagnosis of chronic pancreatitis gives each feature equal weight and sums the number of features present.

The Rosemont criteria, proposed in 2009, offer an alternative approach to diagnosis based on major and minor criteria (**Table 41.3**).[51] In one study, the Rosemont criteria resulted in improved specificity and decreased sensitivity, although these changes were not statistically significant.[52] Definitions vary for some criteria. Hyperechoic foci have been defined as greater than 3 mm by some investigators[53] but as 1 to 2 mm by most others.[54,55] Main pancreatic duct dilation has been variably defined, often as a diameter of greater than 2 mm in the body or greater than 1 mm in the tail.[50] The Rosemont criteria offer semiquantitative definitions for many criteria (see **Table 41.3**). Criteria have been considered abnormal when visualized at either 12 MHz or 7.5 MHz by some investigators but at only 7.5 MHz by others. Findings must be interpreted with considerable caution when imaging the pancreatic head because some features (e.g., hyperechoic strands and visible side branches) are often seen in the normal pancreatic head, whereas others (e.g., cysts and stones) are not. Diagnosis is best made based on features seen in the pancreatic body and tail. Some investigators have seen visible duct side branches in the normal pancreatic body.[53]

Table 41.2 Traditional Endoscopic Ultrasound Features of Chronic Pancreatitis

Parenchymal Features	Ductal Features
Hyperechoic strands	Stones
Hyperechoic foci	Main duct irregularity
Lobularity	Hyperechoic main duct
Cysts	Visible side branches
	Main duct dilation

From The International Working Group for Minimal Standard Terminology in Gastrointestinal Endosonography: Minimal standard terminology in gastrointestinal endosonography. Dig Endosc 10:159–184, 1998.

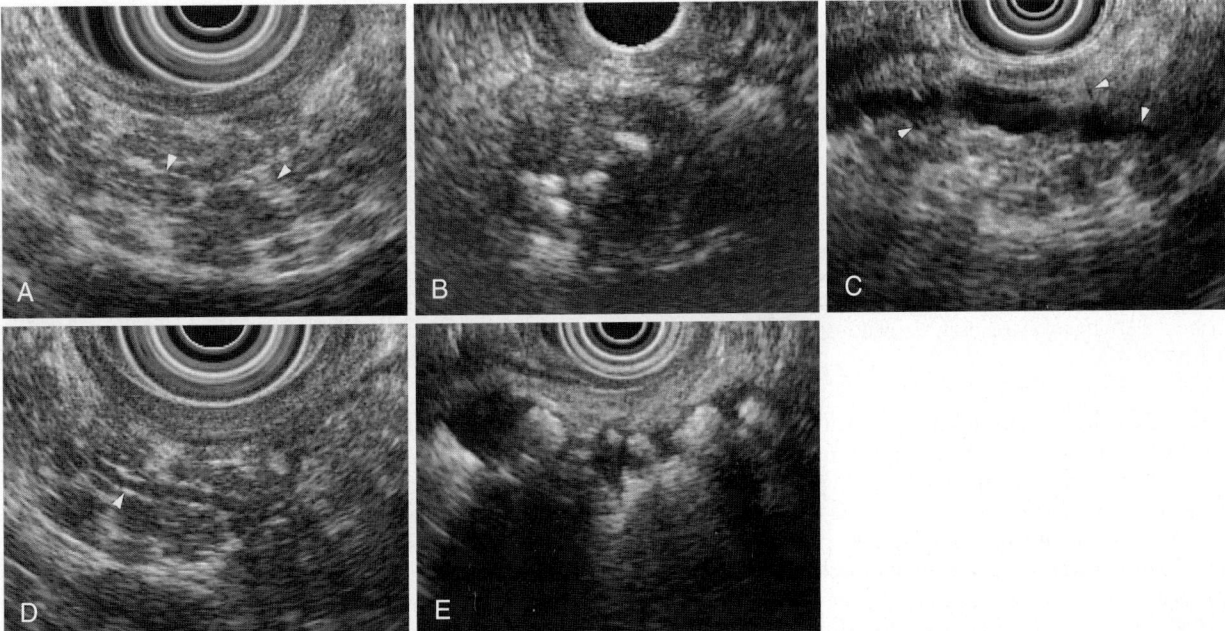

Fig. 41.8 Chronic pancreatitis. **A,** Hyperechoic strands *(arrowheads)* and contiguous lobulation. **B,** Hyperechoic foci in a hypoechoic pancreas. **C,** Dilated, irregular main pancreatic duct with visible side branches *(arrowheads)*. **D,** Hyperechoic, irregular main duct wall. **E,** Ductal stones.

Table 41.3 Rosemont Criteria for Diagnosis of Chronic Pancreatitis

Criterion		Definition	Criterion Weighting
Hyperechoic foci	with shadowing	Echogenic structures ≥2 mm in length and width that shadow	Major A
	without shadowing	Echogenic structures ≥2 mm in length and width with no shadowing	Minor
Lobularity	with honeycombing	Well-circumscribed, ≥5 mm structures with enhancing rim and relatively echo-poor center, ≥3 contiguous lobules	Major B
	without honeycombing	Well-circumscribed, ≥5 mm structures with enhancing rim and relatively echo-poor center, noncontiguous lobules	Minor
		Anechoic, round or elliptical structures with or without septations	Minor
Stranding		Hyperechoic lines ≥3 mm in length in at least 2 different directions with respect to the imaged plane	Minor
MPD calculi		Echogenic structures within main pancreatic duct with acoustic shadowing	Major A
Irregular MPD contour		Uneven or irregular outline and ectatic course	Minor
Dilated side branches		≥3 tubular anechoic structures each measuring ≥1 mm in width, budding from the main pancreatic duct	Minor
MPD dilation		≥3.5-mm body or 1.5-mm tail	Minor
Hyperechoic MPD margin		Echogenic, distinct structure >50% of entire main pancreatic duct in body and tail	Minor

Diagnostic Categories

Consistent with chronic pancreatitis	2 major A features, or 1 major A feature and major B, or 1 major A feature and ≥3 minor features
Suggestive of chronic pancreatitis	1 major A feature and <3 minor features, or major B and ≥3 minor features, or ≥5 minor features
Indeterminate for chronic pancreatitis	Major B and <3 minor features, or >2 and <5 minor features
Normal	<3 minor features, and no major features, dilated MPD and side branches, cysts

MPD, main pancreatic duct.

From Catalano M, Sahai A, Levy M, et al: EUS-based criteria for the diagnosis of chronic pancreatitis: The Rosemont classification. Gastrointest Endosc 69:1251–1261, 2009.

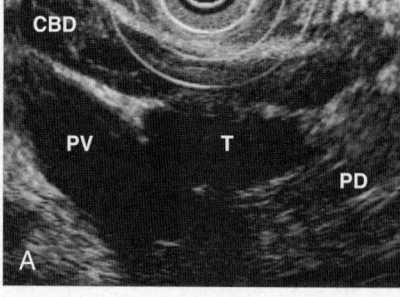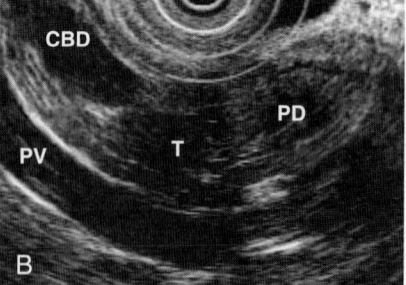

Fig. 41.9 Focal pancreatitis versus pancreatic cancer. Both lesions (T) caused biliary obstruction and were resected. **A,** Focal pancreatitis. **B,** T1 pancreatic adenocarcinoma. CBD, common bile duct; PD, pancreatic duct; PV, portal vein.

There are caveats regarding the specificity of EUS criteria for diagnosis of pancreatitis. EUS features of chronic pancreatitis have been reported in members of pancreatic cancer kindreds, in whom lobularity may correlate with the presence of pancreatic intraepithelial neoplasia in pancreatic branch ducts.[56–58] Focal areas of pancreatic hypoechogenicity can be due to focal inflammation but may also be due to neoplasm (**Fig. 41.9**). Acute pancreatitis may cause decreased parenchymal echogenicity (owing to edema), accentuating the echogenicity of the pancreatic duct wall and the interlobular septa

of the pancreas. For diagnosis of chronic pancreatitis, EUS should be performed after an acute episode of pancreatitis has resolved. Finally, ductal dilation and pancreatic fibrosis occur in older persons without clinical pancreatic disease.

Some EUS findings may be attributable to the effects of age, cigarette smoking, and alcohol on the pancreas rather than chronic pancreatitis. Although studies in normal volunteers have generally shown no parenchymal EUS abnormalities in young, asymptomatic individuals who do not use alcohol,[53,55,59] older patients with no history of pancreatic disease

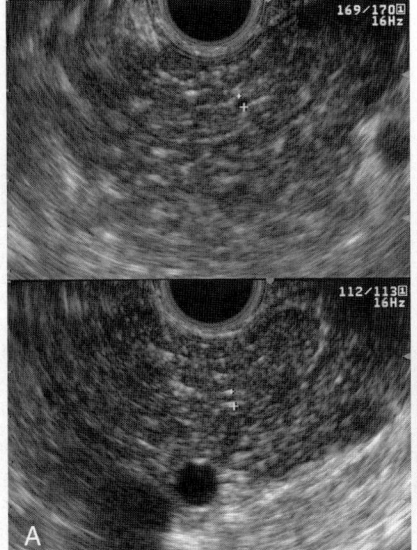

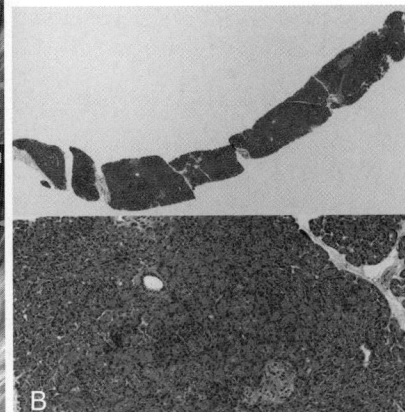

Fig. 41.10 Discrepancy between endoscopic ultrasound (EUS) and histology for diagnosis of chronic pancreatitis. **A,** Views of the pancreatic neck and body in a man with recurrent pancreatitis and chronic pain, showing hyperechoic strands and foci, contiguous lobulation, and a hyperechoic pancreatic duct wall. **B,** EUS-guided Tru-Cut needle biopsy of the pancreatic neck in the same patient shows normal histology.

undergoing EUS for other indications had on average two EUS features of chronic pancreatitis.[60] Autopsy data show that most alcoholic cirrhotics without a clinical history of pancreatic disease have pancreatic fibrosis.[61,62] EUS findings are strongly correlated with extent of ethanol ingestion; also, cigarette smoking correlates with increased number of EUS criteria.[63]

The accuracy of EUS for diagnosis of "early" or "minimal change" chronic pancreatitis is debated, and EUS has been compared with pancreatography, functional tests, and histology. Early studies comparing EUS with pancreatography concluded that the presence of three or more traditional criteria was the best threshold for EUS diagnosis of chronic pancreatitis.[53-55,64] These studies used pancreatography as a "gold standard"; however, the validity of pancreatography for diagnosis of early chronic pancreatitis is poorly validated: The commonly used Cambridge criteria for pancreatography interpretation are based on expert opinion, and autopsy studies have shown abnormalities on pancreatography in most people without a clinical history of pancreatic disease.[62,65]

Histologic comparisons have reached conflicting conclusions, with a retrospective study of surgical resection specimens concluding that the best threshold for diagnosis was the presence of three EUS criteria[66] and a prospective study of EUS-guided Tru-Cut needle biopsy concluding that histologic abnormalities were uncommon in individuals with three or four traditional EUS criteria (**Fig. 41.10**).[67] This discrepancy likely has several causes, including variations in EUS criteria, tissue sampling error, and differences in patient populations; the first study included patients with chronic pancreatitis of sufficient magnitude to require surgical resection, whereas the second study enrolled patients with chronic abdominal pain and a paucity of other objective findings. These studies are limited by the lack of consensus criteria for histologic diagnosis of chronic pancreatitis. There is histologic overlap between chronic pancreatitis and age-related pancreatic atrophy and fibrosis,[62] yet the presence of mild fibrosis was considered sufficient for histologic diagnosis of chronic pancreatitis in the first study.[66]

EUS has also been compared with pancreatic function testing (PFT) with conflicting results. In one early study, EUS and PFT correlated well in patients with advanced disease, but

PFT was often normal in patients with early chronic pancreatitis by pancreatography and EUS; it seemed that PFT was likely insensitive for diagnosis of early disease.[55] In a subsequent comparison from a large-volume PFT center, EUS fared poorly, appearing less sensitive than PFT for diagnosis of early disease.[68] More recently, endoscopic PFT has been compared with EUS; discordance between EUS and PFT was most likely in patients with two, three, or four traditional EUS criteria.[69] In some cases, EUS findings should be deemed indeterminate for chronic pancreatitis. This category, introduced by the Rosemont criteria (which rate the presence of three or four minor criteria as indeterminate), reflects clinical and histologic realities and the current state of knowledge. In such cases, PFT and repeat evaluation over time may be useful.

Solid Pancreatic Neoplasms

EUS is commonly used for diagnosis of pancreatic neoplasms. It images small tumors missed by other diagnostic modalities, provides local staging information, and permits immediate aspiration or biopsy of pancreatic masses and lymph nodes under real-time ultrasound guidance. This section reviews the role of EUS in patients with known or suspected pancreatic adenocarcinoma. Cystic neoplasms are discussed elsewhere in this chapter, and pancreatic neuroendocrine tumors are discussed in another chapter. To diagnose and stage pancreatic neoplasms accurately, the endosonographer must have a detailed understanding of pancreatic anatomy on ultrasound and the ability to identify important adjacent vessels reliably, including the portal vein, portal confluence, hepatic and gastroduodenal arteries, splenic vessels, and superior mesenteric vessels. Educational materials that teach this EUS anatomy are available.[70]

Adenocarcinoma

Pancreatic adenocarcinoma typically appears as a hypoechoic mass with poorly defined, irregular edges. The lesion often appears to obstruct the pancreatic duct. Large tumors may show poor echo penetration, making assessment for vascular

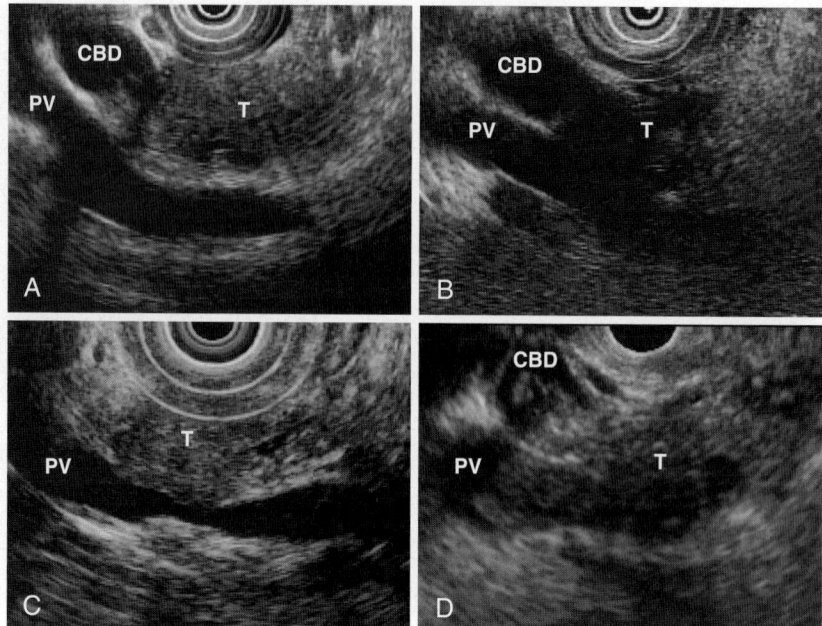

Fig. 41.11 Vascular involvement by pancreatic cancer. **A,** Normal tissue between tumor (T) and vessels of the portal confluence, with no evidence of invasion. **B,** Loss of echo plane between tumor and the portal vein (PV). **C,** Irregular vein wall and narrowed vein lumen. **D,** Tumor extending directly into the portal vein.

invasion difficult or impossible.[71] Infiltrating adenocarcinomas may cause a heterogeneous or hypoechoic parenchymal echotexture without a discrete mass. The finding of a hypoechoic pancreatic mass is not specific for adenocarcinoma and may be caused by focal pancreatitis. Acute or chronic pancreatitis can cause this appearance, and a focal mass is often seen in autoimmune pancreatitis. Benign pancreatic masses tend to have better defined edges than malignancies (see **Fig. 41.9**), and computerized image analysis has been used as an aid in differential diagnosis.[72] Analysis of blood flow in the mass using power Doppler and an echo-enhancing intravenous contrast agent has been reported to distinguish inflammatory masses from malignant masses accurately, but criteria vary,[73,74] and the technique seems unlikely to replace tissue acquisition for definitive diagnosis. EUS elastography of the pancreas does not seem to distinguish benign from malignant pancreatic masses reliably.[75]

EUS-guided aspiration of focal lesions is useful for preoperative differential diagnosis of a hypoechoic pancreatic mass, although a negative cytologic result does not fully exclude malignancy. EUS aspiration cytology has a sensitivity of about 80% for diagnosis of pancreatic cancer.[76,77] Analysis of cytologic aspirates for mutations and allele loss may improve the diagnostic yield further.[78,79] Early studies comparing CT and EUS showed that EUS was more sensitive for detection of pancreatic adenocarcinoma, particularly lesions less than 2 cm in diameter. Subsequent studies comparing contrast-enhanced helical CT with EUS, taken in aggregate, suggest that EUS remains superior.[80–82] Patients suspected to have pancreatic carcinoma but with no mass on CT should undergo EUS. In patients with an infiltrative rather than mass-forming malignancy, EUS may also fail to show a discrete lesion in the pancreas, although diffuse parenchymal changes are often seen. EUS-guided FNA of the pancreatic parenchyma may yield a diagnosis of malignancy in such cases, particularly if the aspirate is obtained near a ductal stricture.

EUS also permits assessment of the relationship between a pancreatic tumor and adjacent vascular structures. The finding

of normal tissue between a tumor and a vessel, or an intact echo-rich interface (echo plane) between the two, reliably excludes tumor invasion of the visualized vessel. Conversely, other findings suggest possible vascular involvement (**Fig. 41.11**), including loss of the echo plane between tumor and vessel, irregularity of the vessel wall, narrowing of the vessel lumen, echogenic material within the vessel lumen, and the presence of peripancreatic venous collaterals (**Fig. 41.12**). Although numerous studies have reported EUS accuracy of 75% to 100% for diagnosis of vascular invasion,[81] these studies relied on a reference standard of intraoperative assessment by dissection and palpation. The surgeon's intraoperative suspicion of vascular invasion may be incorrect, however, particularly if a tumor is densely adherent to a vessel without actual invasion.[83] Surgical resection of portal vein or superior mesenteric vein at the time of pancreatectomy has become an accepted technique, and patients undergoing venous resection have a survival comparable to patients not requiring venous resection.[84]

In a study comparing EUS with surgical histology of resected pancreatic masses, including masses undergoing venous resection, loss of echo plane was a poor predictor of vascular involvement (specificity <30%), and only half of resectable tumors with more advanced ultrasound features of vascular invasion required vascular resection.[85] A blinded review of EUS videotapes suggested that endosonographers were less accurate in their assessment of vascular invasion when they were denied access to other clinical information about the patient, including results of other imaging studies.[86] Taken together, these data suggest that EUS features of venous invasion are sensitive but not specific. EUS combined with a cross-sectional imaging study may provide more accurate local staging than either study alone.[87]

The 2002 revision of the TNM staging system for pancreatic carcinoma (**Box 41.3**) reflects current surgical philosophy and categorizes tumors as unresectable if there is local arterial invasion (stage III) or distant metastases (stage IV).[88] The classification distinguishes between tumors limited to

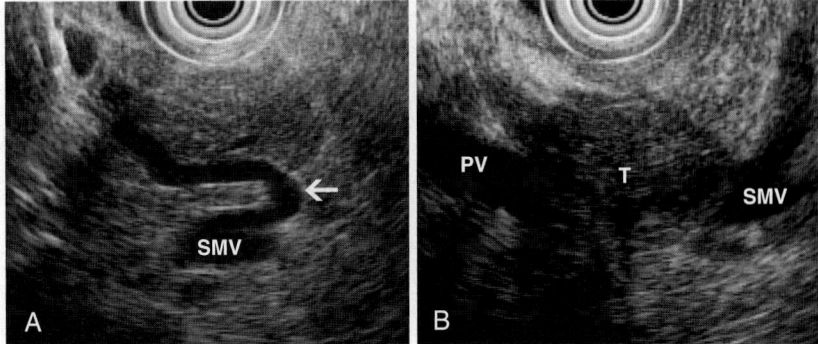

Fig. 41.12 Venous collaterals in pancreatic cancer. **A,** Large venous collateral *(arrow)* courses through the pancreatic head from the superior mesenteric vein (SMV), ultimately joining the proximal portal vein (PV). **B,** In a different image plane, a pancreatic adenocarcinoma (T) is seen obstructing the portal confluence.

Box 41.3 Staging of Pancreatic Adenocarcinoma

TX	Primary tumor cannot be assessed		
T0	No evidence of primary tumor		
Tis	Carcinoma in situ (includes PanIN III)		
T1	Tumor limited to pancreas, ≤2 cm in greatest dimension		
T2	Tumor limited to pancreas, >2 cm in greatest dimension		
T3	Tumor extends beyond pancreas but without involvement of celiac axis or superior mesenteric artery		
T4	Tumor involves celiac axis or superior mesenteric artery (unresectable)		
NX	Regional lymph nodes cannot be assessed		
N0	No regional lymph node metastases		
N1	Regional lymph node metastases		
M0	No distant metastasis		
M1	Distant metastasis		
Stage 0	M0	N0	M0
Stage IA	T1	N0	M0
Stage IB	T2	N0	M0
Stage IIA	T3	N0	M0
Stage IIB	T1-3	N1	M0
Stage III	T4	Any N	M0
Stage IV	Any T	Any N	M1

PanIN, pancreatic intraepithelial neoplasia.
From American Joint Committee on Cancer (AJCC): AJCC cancer staging manual, *ed 7, New York, 2010, Springer-Verlag (www.springer-ny.com).*

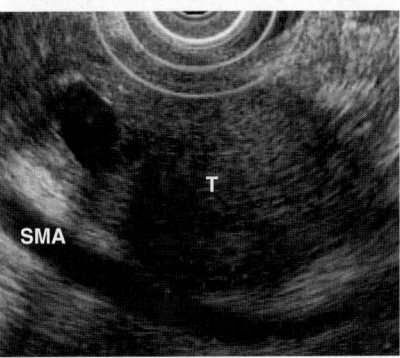

Fig. 41.13 Retroperitoneal margin in pancreatic cancer. A large pancreatic head cancer (T) extends close to the superior mesenteric artery (SMA). At surgery, the tumor was not adherent to the SMA and was resected, but the retroperitoneal margin was positive for malignancy.

the pancreas (T1 if ≤2 cm, T2 if >2 cm) and tumors that extend beyond the pancreas (T3 if not involving celiac axis or superior mesenteric artery, T4 if involving these arteries). Arterial but not venous invasion is considered when assigning T stage. T3 tumors, which extend beyond the pancreas, are considered resectable. Extension of tumor beyond the edge of the pancreas has become an important criterion for T staging of pancreatic cancer. Tumor extension is best seen during EUS when the pancreatic parenchyma has a different echotexture than surrounding fat. When the pancreatic parenchyma is isoechoic with surrounding fat, the endosonographer is able only to identify the edge of the pancreas where it abuts major peripancreatic veins or other organs. In such cases, it may be impossible to arrive at an accurate T stage on ultrasound, and CT or MRI may be more useful. When assessing the edge of the pancreas, particular attention should be given to the retroperitoneal margin of the

pancreatic head abutting the connective tissue between pancreas and superior mesenteric artery; this is the most likely site for a positive microscopic margin and subsequent local recurrence after resection of pancreatic head cancers (**Fig. 41.13**).[88]

EUS features of arterial invasion may suggest T4 disease, although the true specificity of these features for arterial invasion is unknown. EUS aids in the detection of nodal and liver metastases from pancreatic cancer. Compared with CT, EUS has equal or greater sensitivity for identification of abnormal lymph nodes and is usually the procedure of choice for sampling abnormal nodes. Regional lymph nodes (considered N1 when malignant) are the peripancreatic nodes, including nodes along the hepatic artery, celiac axis, pyloric region, and splenic region.[88] The presence of N1 disease is not considered a contraindication to resection in many referral centers because a "complete" resection seems to lengthen survival in such patients.[84,88] The finding of malignant nodes distant from the primary tumor is considered metastatic disease and generally excludes surgery. In this regard, EUS identifies mediastinal nodal metastases in up to 7% of patients with pancreatic adenocarcinoma.[89] A standard clinical approach to patients with suspected pancreatic cancer begins with a high-quality, contrast-enhanced CT or MRI examination. If liver lesions are shown, percutaneous or EUS-guided biopsy is the most direct approach to staging.

If a locally unresectable pancreatic mass is shown, EUS can provide confirmation of local staging and permits aspiration for tissue diagnosis. If an apparently resectable mass is shown, EUS may change staging by detecting liver or distant nodal

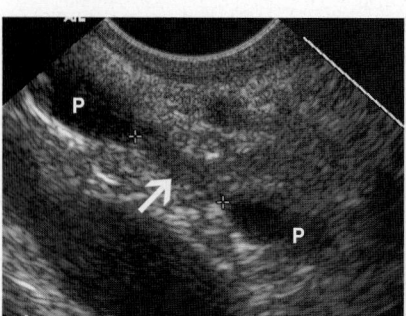 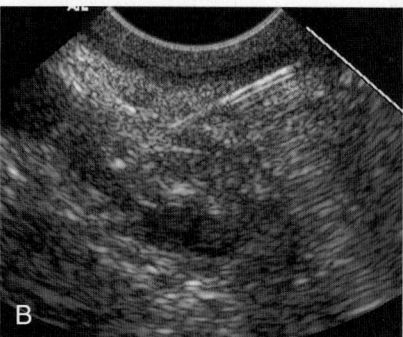 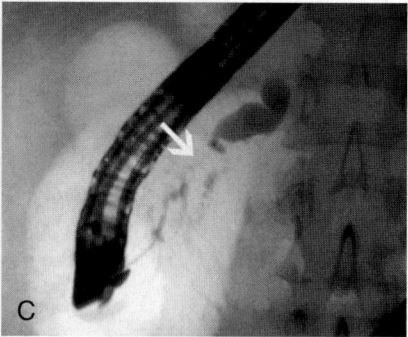

Fig. 41.14 Early pancreatic adenocarcinoma. **A,** Endoscopic ultrasound (EUS) shows a stricture *(arrow)* of the pancreatic duct (P), with thickening of the duct wall. **B,** EUS-guided fine needle aspiration (FNA) of the stricture was negative for malignancy. **C,** Intraductal biopsy specimens of the stricture *(arrow)* obtained during endoscopic retrograde cholangiopancreatography (ERCP) showed adenocarcinoma.

metastases in a few patients, and FNA of an apparently resectable mass shows a diagnosis other than adenocarcinoma in up to one-fourth of patients, potentially changing the management plan.[81,90] EUS-guided tissue acquisition is required to exclude cancer in some cases of autoimmune pancreatitis.[91] If pancreatic cancer is suspected, but no mass is shown on CT or MRI, EUS should be strongly considered for diagnosis of a small lesion missed by other modalities. Patients with small masses missed by other imaging techniques are probably the most likely patients to benefit from surgery.

Despite its overall excellent sensitivity for diagnosis of pancreatic cancer, EUS may fail to identify cancer arising in the setting of underlying chronic pancreatitis[90] or severe acute pancreatitis. Tumor may be difficult to differentiate from areas of inflammation. FNA is more useful than EUS imaging alone in this setting, although more needle passes may be required to make a diagnosis of malignancy.[92] Use of an intravenous ultrasound contrast agent may improve diagnosis in this setting; positron emission tomography also has been advocated. Infiltrating neoplasms that do not form a circumscribed mass can also be missed by EUS, as can early ductal malignancies (**Fig. 41.14**). FNA cytology is a reasonable diagnostic strategy in the absence of a mass, particularly when performed adjacent to an obstructed duct. When suspicion for malignancy remains high despite a negative EUS examination, other investigations (e.g., ERCP) may be warranted.

Other Solid Tumors

The most common variant of pancreatic adenocarcinoma is colloid carcinoma (or mucinous cyst adenocarcinoma), a solid tumor containing pools of mucus that may arise from a preexisting IPMN or mucinous cystadenoma. Colloid carcinoma may contain demonstrable cystic spaces on EUS (**Fig. 41.15**) and has a better prognosis after resection than typical adenocarcinoma. Metastatic cancer may manifest in the pancreas, including melanoma, breast, and renal cell carcinomas. Other uncommon solid tumors of the pancreas include lymphoma, acinar cell carcinoma, medullary carcinoma, osteogenic giant cell tumors, and pancreatoblastoma. The EUS features of these rarer tumors are not well described.

In contrast to adenocarcinoma, pancreatic neuroendocrine tumors typically appear as uniform, rounded, homogeneous masses with discrete edges. They may also appear cystic (**Fig.**

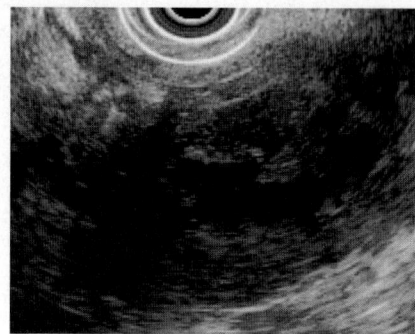

Fig. 41.15 Colloid carcinoma of the pancreas. The tumor contains cystic pools of mucus.

41.16). EUS is the most sensitive preoperative imaging test for diagnosis of pancreatic insulinomas and is an important modality in patients with multiple endocrine neoplasia type I who have numerous pancreatic gastrinomas, some of which are visualized only by EUS. EUS features suggestive of a malignant neuroendocrine tumor include an irregular central echogenic area and displacement or obstruction of the main pancreatic duct.[73] EUS-guided FNA is an accurate means of diagnosing functioning neuroendocrine tumors.[74] EUS of neuroendocrine tumors is discussed in more detail in Chapter 42.

Intraductal Papillary Mucinous Neoplasm

IPMN is a papillary growth of neoplastic epithelium in the main pancreatic duct or branch ducts. IPMN shares histologic and genetic features with pancreatic intraepithelial neoplasia, and both are precursor lesions for pancreatic adenocarcinoma, but IPMN is characterized by ductal dilation, mucin production, and more extensive ductal involvement.[93] IPMN occurs most commonly in the pancreatic head, but this neoplasm may be seen anywhere in the pancreas and may be multifocal. Histologically, IPMN ranges from hyperplasia of ductal mucosa (not a true neoplasia), to adenoma with low- or high-grade dysplasia, carcinoma in situ, and invasive carcinoma. Carcinoma is seen in more than 50% of cases of resected main duct IPMN but only about 15% of cases of resected

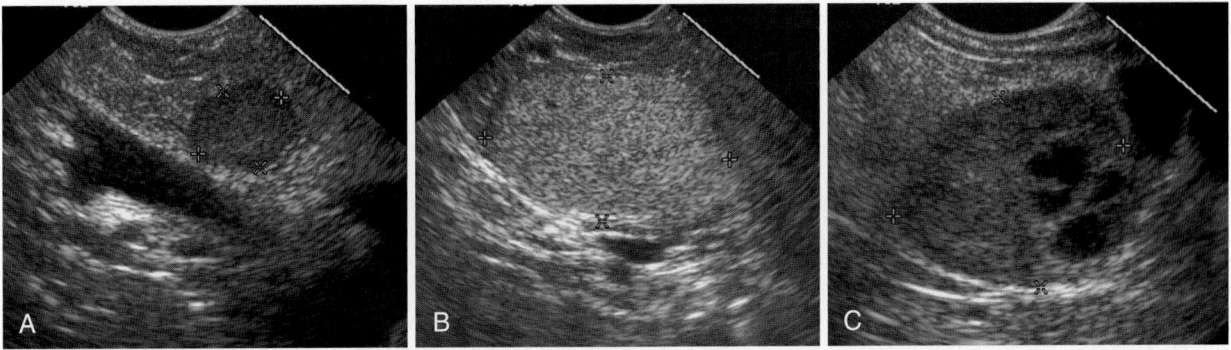

Fig. 41.16 Pancreatic neuroendocrine tumors (tumor margins indicated by measurement cursors). **A,** Gastrinoma. **B,** Insulinoma. **C,** Cystic islet cell tumor.

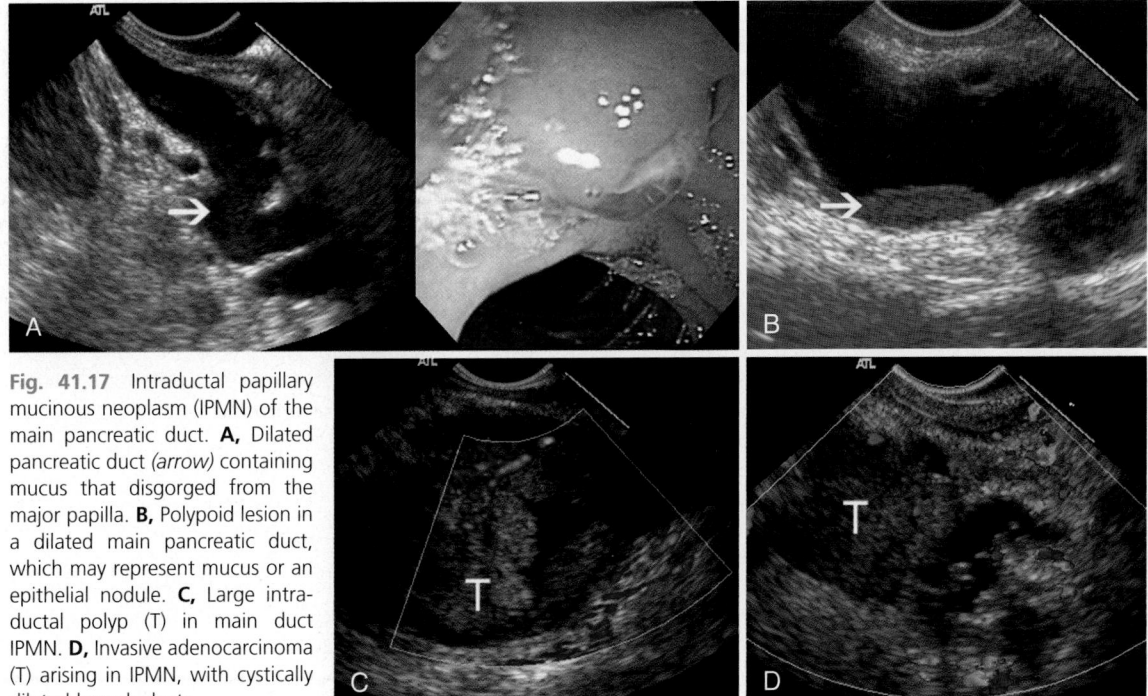

Fig. 41.17 Intraductal papillary mucinous neoplasm (IPMN) of the main pancreatic duct. **A,** Dilated pancreatic duct *(arrow)* containing mucus that disgorged from the major papilla. **B,** Polypoid lesion in a dilated main pancreatic duct, which may represent mucus or an epithelial nodule. **C,** Large intraductal polyp (T) in main duct IPMN. **D,** Invasive adenocarcinoma (T) arising in IPMN, with cystically dilated branch ducts.

branch duct IPMN,[94–97] and branch duct lesions appear less likely to progress over time.[95,98,99]

Diagnosis of main duct IPMN is clear-cut in a symptomatic patient with a markedly dilated main pancreatic duct containing polypoid filling defects, in which mucus is seen disgorging into the duodenum through a gaping ampullary orifice. Other, less classic presentations of main duct IPMN are increasingly recognized, including focal dilation or ectasia of the main pancreatic duct mimicking chronic pancreatitis or isolated polyps within the pancreatic duct. EUS shows the ductal dilation that is a hallmark of IPMN (**Fig. 41.17**). In main duct lesions, there is typically marked dilation of the duct without an obstructing mass, stricture, or stone. The main duct wall may be irregular or thickened, with visible side branches that are also involved. Faintly echogenic material may be seen in the duct lumen corresponding to mucin, and polypoid thickening of the duct mucosa may be evident, but these findings may be subtle or absent.

The differential diagnosis of main duct dilation includes chronic pancreatitis and downstream ductal obstruction by stone, stricture, or tumor, and the pancreatic duct should be traced during EUS looking for an obstructing lesion. Some branch duct IPMNs have a tubular branching structure that is clearly recognizable as a dilated ductal system, but others appear cystic rather than ductal (**Fig. 41.18**). EUS features that may suggest a diagnosis of branch duct IPMN include a connecting duct visible on ultrasound leading to the main pancreatic duct, pancreatic parenchyma rather than septa between the locules of a lesion, proximity to the pancreatic duct, or the presence of a branching architecture. In some cases, these features are absent, and the branch duct lesion appears to be a cyst without communication to the main pancreatic duct. IPMN should be considered in the differential diagnosis of any mucus-containing pancreatic cyst, particularly in men (in whom mucinous cystic neoplasm [MCN] is rare). Infiltrating parenchymal malignancy may be present in patients with

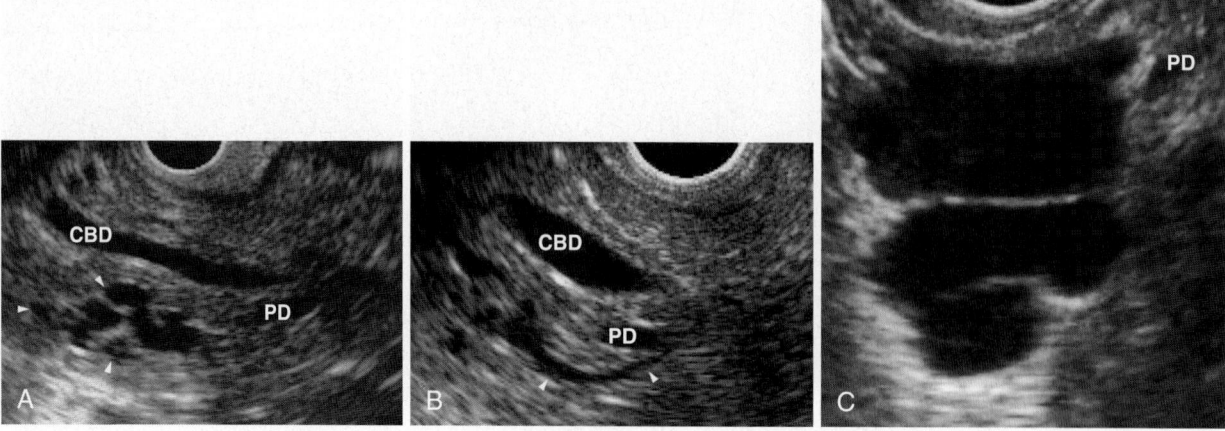

Fig. 41.18 Branch duct intraductal papillary mucinous neoplasm (IPMN). **A,** This oligocystic lesion *(arrowheads)* has a branching architecture, suggesting IPMN. **B,** In a different image plane, a connecting duct leading to the main pancreatic duct is seen *(arrowheads)*. **C,** Another branch duct IPMN but without distinguishing ultrasound features. CBD, common bile duct; PD, pancreatic duct.

Table 41.4 Differential Diagnosis of Pancreatic Cystic Lesions

Inflammatory	Cystic Neoplasms	Nonneoplastic Cysts	Vascular Lesions
Acute fluid collection	Serous cystic neoplasm	Cystic fibrosis	Splenic artery aneurysm
Walled-off necrosis	Mucinous cystic neoplasm	Polycystic kidney disease	Pseudoaneurysm
Pseudocyst	Intraductal papillary mucinous neoplasm	Lymphoepithelial cyst	
	Colloid carcinoma	Lymphangioma	
	Ductal adenocarcinoma with cystic degeneration	Epidermoid cyst (intrapancreatic accessory spleen)	
	Cystic neuroendocrine tumor	Endometrioma	
	Acinar cell cystadenocarcinoma	Hemorrhagic cyst	
	Papillary and cystic tumor	Congenital	
	Cystic teratoma	Tuberculosis	
	Leiomyosarcoma	Hydatid cyst	
	Pancreatoblastoma		

IPMN and should always be suspected when a patient with IPMN has obstructive jaundice. Hypoechoic pancreatic parenchyma associated with IPMN can be due to inflammation or malignancy, and EUS-guided FNA may clarify the diagnosis in such cases.

Pancreas Cysts and Fluid Collections

EUS is commonly used as an aid in the diagnosis of pancreatic cystic lesions. Although the differential diagnosis is extensive (**Table 41.4**), this discussion focuses on the most common cystic lesions of the pancreas. EUS features of pancreatic cystic lesions are listed in **Table 41.5**. On ultrasound, all cystic structures are characterized by increased through-transmission, with the appearance of enhanced echogenicity of the tissue beyond the cyst. The overall cyst architecture, the cyst wall, and the cyst lumen should be assessed during EUS. Unilocular cysts are usually round and have one cyst cavity, with or

Table 41.5 Ultrasound Features of Pancreatic Cysts

Architecture	Wall	Lumen
Shape	Presence of a wall	Echogenicity (anechoic, echogenic)
Unilocular, oligocystic, microcystic	Mural thickening (>1 mm)	Heterogeneity
Septa	Mural nodularity, mass	Sludge (layering, mobile)
Branching structure	Mural calcification	Intracystic mass
	Irregularity	Intracystic calcification

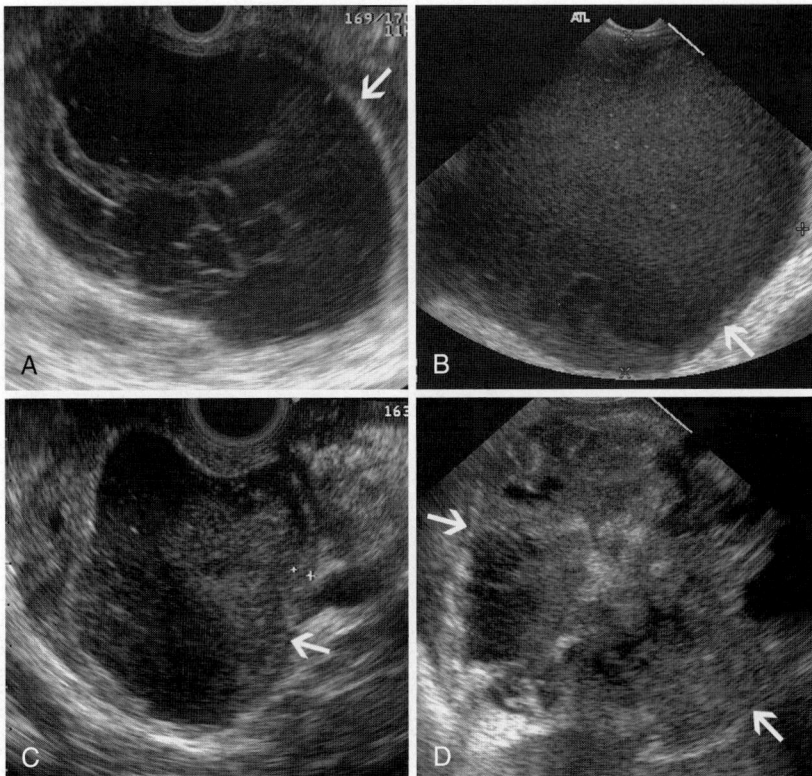

Fig. 41.19 Pancreatic fluid collections complicating pancreatitis. *Arrows* point to the collection wall. **A,** Acute fluid collection. This 12-day-old collection shows floating strands of retroperitoneal tissue and a thin wall. **B,** Pseudocyst with faintly echogenic contents. **C,** Pseudocyst with echogenic contents, which moved when the patient was turned. **D,** Organized pancreatic necrosis mimicking a solid lesion. This collection was subsequently drained and debrided endoscopically.

without incomplete septa. Oligocystic cysts contain more than one cystic space or locule separated by septa, but the individual locules are easily seen during EUS and can be counted. Microcystic cysts contain innumerable cystic spaces, some of which may be too small to be resolved by EUS.

Inflammatory Fluid Collections

Inflammatory fluid collections arise as complications of pancreatitis. Pathologically, they are distinguished from cysts by the absence of an epithelial lining. *Acute fluid collections* are less than 4 weeks old and do not replace pancreatic parenchyma; they commonly occur after acute pancreatitis and usually resolve spontaneously. *Pseudocysts* develop from an acute fluid collection or arise as complications of chronic pancreatitis; they are more than 4 weeks old and have a discrete wall. *Necrosis* is a nonperfused area of pancreatic parenchyma; when a wall develops around the necrotic region, it may be termed "organized" or "walled-off" pancreatic necrosis. Acute fluid collections often have a complex, heterogeneous appearance on EUS and may appear solid. They may have ill-defined borders, but a developing wall may be seen at the periphery of the collection as it matures. Pseudocysts are usually unilocular and have a well-defined wall; the pseudocyst lumen may be anechoic or may contain layering echogenic material (**Fig. 41.19**). Necrosis contains variable amounts of echogenic material, which sometimes fills the entire lesion, giving a solid appearance on EUS (see **Fig. 41.19**). The distinction between a cystic neoplasm and an inflammatory collection may be difficult to make with certainty by EUS appearance alone. Mural calcification can be seen in both chronic pseudocysts and cystic neoplasms. Echogenic material

in the cyst lumen may layer, suggesting sludge, but may also have the appearance of an intracystic mass.

The clinical history, findings on serial cross-sectional imaging studies, and results of EUS-guided FNA are often helpful in differential diagnosis. FNA of inflammatory collections may be complicated by infection of the collection, especially complex-appearing collections that cannot be aspirated completely. Fluid aspirated from an inflammatory collection may be clear or discolored and may contain gritty or particulate matter. A drop placed between two gloved fingers would typically not form a string. Fluid amylase is usually greater than 5000 U/L. Values for CA 19-9 vary widely in pseudocyst fluid and are usually not helpful for diagnosis, but values for carcinoembryonic antigen (CEA), CA 72-4, and CA 15-3 are typically low.

Serous Cystic Neoplasm

Serous cystic neoplasms are cystic growths that likely arise from centroacinar cells. Most serous cystic neoplasms are serous cystadenomas, although a few serous cystadenocarcinomas have been reported in the medical literature. In contrast to mucinous cystic lesions and IPMNs, these tumors lack k-*ras* mutations and have very low malignant potential.[93] Mutations of the von Hippel-Lindau *(VHL)* tumor suppressor gene have been implicated in their pathogenesis.[100] Most serous cystadenomas are microcystic, although they may also be oligocystic, unilocular, or (uncommonly) solid. A fibrous capsule or wall is usually not present.

Microcystic serous cystadenoma has a characteristic ultrasound appearance (**Fig. 41.20**). The lesion is rounded and contains innumerable small cystic spaces, with the largest

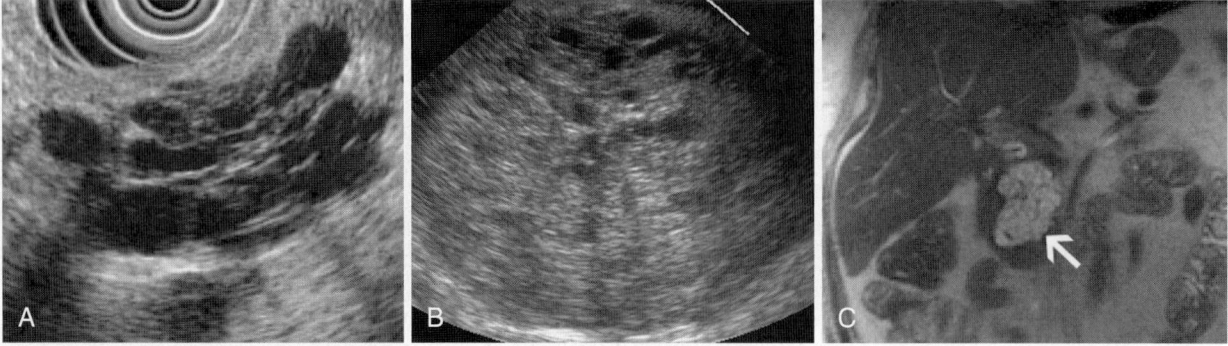

Fig. 41.20 Microcystic serous cystadenomas. **A,** Innumerable locules with intervening thin septa. The lesion has a discrete edge without a wall. **B,** Many portions of this microcystic lesion appear solid because of the microscopic size of some locules. **C,** Magnetic resonance imaging (MRI) of the lesion shown in **B** confirms the cystic nature of the entire lesion.

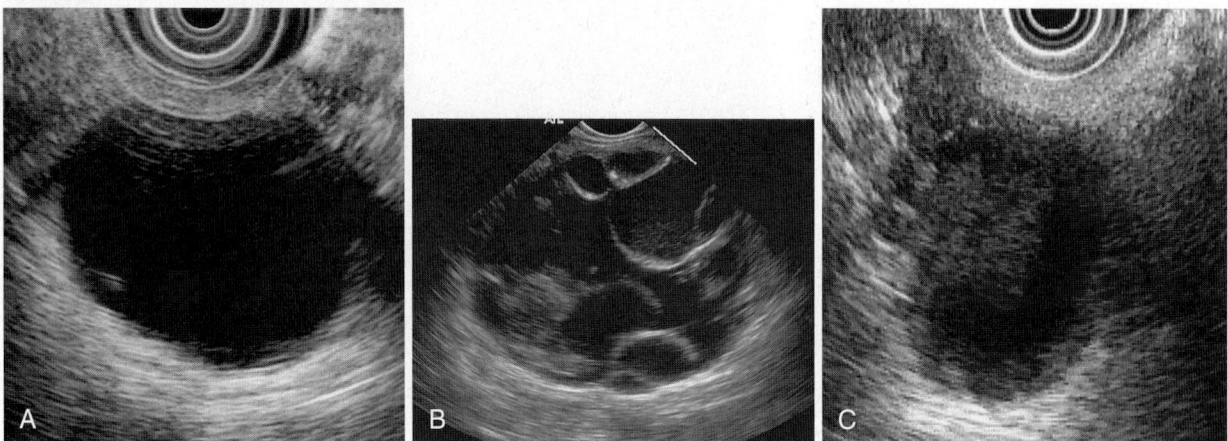

Fig. 41.21 Mucinous cystic neoplasms (MCNs). **A,** Unilocular mucinous cystadenoma. **B,** Oligocystic MCN with borderline features histologically. **C,** Mucinous cystadenocarcinoma, with a thickened wall, intracystic mass, and extension into adjacent pancreas parenchyma.

individual locule usually less than 2 cm in diameter. Central calcification may be seen in the lesion with a "sunburst" configuration. There is a discrete edge but typically without an identifiable wall. The absence of a wall is an important feature because cystic malignancies (e.g., colloid carcinoma and papillary and cystic neoplasm) may appear microcystic but often have a wall. In some portions of the lesion, the individual cysts are too small to resolve with EUS; in these areas, septa predominate, and the tissue has a relatively hypoechoic, solid appearance. Sometimes most of the lesion has this appearance, leading to misdiagnosis of a solid mass, but MRI can show the cystic nature of the lesion (see **Fig. 41.20**). Branch duct IPMNs may appear similar to oligocystic serous cystadenoma, and the two lesions can be confused with each other, especially when small. In contrast to the microcystic form, serous cystadenomas that are oligocystic or unilocular do not have ultrasound features that distinguish them from mucinous cystadenoma or inflammatory fluid collections.

Fluid aspirated from a serous cystadenoma is typically clear and watery and does not form a string. Little or no fluid may be obtained when the microcystic form is aspirated. Amylase level, CEA, and other tumor marker levels in the fluid are low, even in the macrocystic form.[101] CEA is low and is highly suggestive of serous cystadenoma or pseudocyst when less than

5 ng/mL.[102] Cytology may show glycogen-containing cells but is often nondiagnostic.[103]

Mucinous Cystic Neoplasm

MCNs are cystic growths with well-recognized malignant potential. Histologically, they are characterized by the presence of ovarian stroma. Ninety percent of MCNs occur in women. They are usually oligocystic, although a single large cyst may dominate. MCNs may be benign (mucinous cystadenoma) or malignant (mucinous cystadenocarcinoma) or have borderline features (MCN with moderate dysplasia).[93] Epidemiologic data suggest that these lesions begin as cystadenomas and grow slowly because patients with cystadenocarcinoma on average are 10 years older than patients with cystadenoma. In one large series, invasive carcinoma was present in only 18% of resected MCNs, and all such lesions were greater than 4 cm in diameter or had mural nodules.[104]

MCNs may appear oligocystic or unilocular on ultrasound (**Fig. 41.21**). When MCNs are oligocystic, some locules are generally greater than 2 cm in diameter. When the rim and septa of the lesion are thin and smooth, invasive malignancy is unlikely. Thickening, nodularity, or irregularity of these structures suggests the presence of mucinous cystadenocarcinoma (see **Fig. 41.21**), but these findings are nonspecific. Fluid aspirated from MCNs is often cloudy and tenacious, and a drop placed between two gloved fingers usually forms a string. Amylase level in the cystic fluid is usually low, and tumor marker levels in cystic fluid are elevated. CEA levels are generally elevated in fluid from MCNs.[102]

Occasionally, fluid aspirated from MCNs is not tenacious, perhaps because of digestion of mucins by pancreatic enzymes. A few MCNs communicate with the pancreatic duct, and fluid from the cyst in these cases may have high amylase levels without impressive elevations of tumor marker levels. The absence of typical findings on cystic fluid analysis does not exclude the diagnosis of MCN, particularly in a woman with no antecedent history of pancreatitis or imaging findings to suggest a pseudocyst.

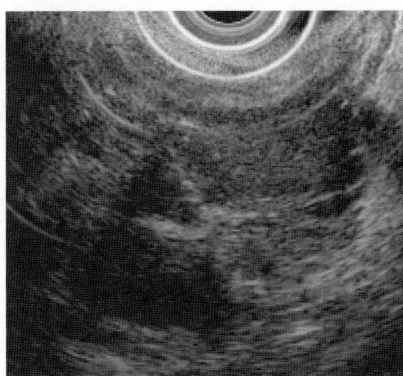

Fig. 41.22 Papillary and cystic neoplasm of the pancreatic head.

Intraductal Papillary Mucinous Neoplasm

Branch duct IPMNs may have the appearance of a cystic lesion on EUS. The lesion typically appears oligocystic and may be rounded. Clues to diagnosis include a branching architecture suggestive of a dilated ductal system and the presence of pancreatic tissue between the loculi of the lesion, rather than true septa. Careful examination may show the connecting duct leading from the lesion to the main pancreatic duct (see **Fig. 41.18**). These features are not always present, however. The Sendai criteria, which are consensus guidelines for resection of branch duct IPMNs, suggest that resection should be considered if one or more of the following criteria are present: cyst-related symptoms, main pancreatic duct diameter 10 mm or greater, cyst diameter 30 mm or greater, presence of intramural nodules, or cystic fluid cytology suspicious or positive for malignancy.[105,106] Patients with branch duct IPMNs may be at increased risk for development of typical pancreatic adenocarcinoma separate from the cystic lesion,[107] and the entire pancreas should be examined during follow-up examinations.

Fluid aspirated from IPMN has variable features. Generally, the fluid is either viscous with high tumor marker levels or thin and watery with low or midrange elevations of tumor marker levels. This variability is probably due to the communication between the lesion and the main pancreatic duct, resulting in a mixture of pancreatic juice and tumor secretions in the lumen of the lesion. Findings may vary from findings typically seen in pseudocysts to findings associated with MCNs.

Other Cystic Lesions

Solid pancreatic adenocarcinomas may undergo cystic degeneration, perhaps secondary to necrosis and liquefaction of portions of the tumor. About 15% of pancreatic adenocarcinomas are colloid carcinomas containing gelatinous pools of extracellular mucin[108]; these lesions often arise from MCNs or IPMNs and may appear heterogeneous or cystic on EUS. Uncommon cystic neoplasms of the pancreas include cystic neuroendocrine tumors (see **Fig. 41.16**), acinar cell cystadenocarcinomas, and papillary and cystic tumors (**Fig. 41.22**). These lesions typically have a discrete, thickened wall and a complex internal architecture, raising concern for an invasive neoplasm. The EUS appearance of these lesions is not specific for diagnosis. Acinar cell cystadenocarcinoma may be associated with elevated serum alpha fetoprotein levels. Little

information is available regarding the results of cystic fluid analysis in these less common cystic neoplasms. Among non-neoplastic cystic lesions, lymphangioma may be distinguished by the finding of milky white lymph fluid when the cyst is aspirated. The finding of squamous cells on cytology may suggest a lymphoepithelial cyst or teratoma.

von Hippel-Lindau Disease

von Hippel-Lindau disease is characterized by hemangioblastomas of the central nervous system and retina, renal cysts and carcinoma, pheochromocytoma, and multiple pancreatic lesions. The most common pancreatic findings in von Hippel-Lindau disease are serous cystadenoma and neuroendocrine tumor. Pancreatic lesions may be difficult to diagnose by ultrasound features alone because some microcystic serous neoplasms appear solid with a discrete edge, and conversely some neuroendocrine tumors may be cystic. EUS-guided aspiration and other imaging studies such as MRI and octreotide scanning may be useful.

Accuracy of Endoscopic Ultrasound for Differential Diagnosis

The ultrasound appearance of a pancreatic cystic lesion usually does not provide a specific diagnosis. Characteristic ultrasound features suggest a likely diagnosis when the classic features of microcystic serous cystadenoma or branch duct IPMN are seen. In oligocystic or unilocular lesions, however, ultrasound appearance alone is nonspecific for final diagnosis, and EUS appearance alone does not discriminate cysts of little or no malignant potential (pseudocysts and serous cystadenomas) from cysts with significant malignant potential over time (mucinous cystadenomas or branch duct IPMNs).[109] In one large surgical series, only 3% of asymptomatic cysts less than 2 cm in size were malignant, but half of the lesions were premalignant (MCNs or IPMN).[110] Follow-up is warranted in small, benign-appearing cystic lesions that are not resected.

Cystic fluid analysis may aid in the differential diagnosis of cystic lesions. Lesions containing thick mucinous fluid or numerous septa may be difficult to aspirate, with a plug of mucin or tissue filling the needle lumen. When sufficient fluid can be aspirated, multiple diagnostic studies should be obtained, including cytology, amylase, and CEA. Viscosity should also be assessed, either by measuring fluid viscosity or by placing a drop of fluid between two gloved fingers and

Table 41.6 Cystic Fluid Analysis for Diagnosis of Cystic Lesions*

	Pseudocyst	Serous Cystadenoma	Mucinous Cystadenoma	Mucinous Cystadenocarcinoma	IPMN
Amylase	High	Low	Low	Low	Variable
Viscosity	Low	Low	High	High	Variable
String sign	Negative	Negative	Positive	Positive	Variable
CEA	Low	Low	High	High	Variable
CA 72-4	Low	Low	High	High	Variable
CA 15-3	Low	Low	Low	High	—
CA 125	Low	Variable	Variable	High	—
CA 19-9	Variable	—	Variable	Variable	Variable

*Typical findings are shown[102,111]; results may vary in individual cases, as discussed in the text.
CA, Carbohydrate antigen; CEA, carcinoembryonic antigen; IPMN, intraductal papillary mucinous neoplasm.

determining if the fluid forms a string (the "string" sign). The typical results of fluid analysis for various cystic lesions are shown in **Table 41.6**. Routine cystic fluid analysis alone does not provide a confident diagnosis in many cases. Cytology is specific but insensitive for diagnosis of MCNs and IPMNs. A cystic fluid CEA value of greater than 800 mg/L is highly suggestive of a mucinous lesion, but only a few mucinous lesions show such high values[102]; an optimal cutoff of 192 ng/mL has an accuracy of 79% for diagnosis of a mucinous lesion, and extent of CEA elevation does not distinguish premalignant from malignant mucinous lesions.[111] Because IPMNs arise from the pancreatic ductal system, they show variable results of fluid analysis depending in part on the ratio of normal pancreatic juice to mucin in the aspirated specimen. The absence of typical findings on fluid analysis does not exclude a mucinous lesion.

A promising alternative approach to cystic fluid analysis involves analysis of cystic fluid DNA, including the optical density of cystic fluid (said to be a measure of DNA concentration), the presence of k-*ras* mutations, the amplitude of loss of selected alleles, and the presumed acquisition sequence of selected mutations.[112] In one more recent report, this approach distinguished mucinous from nonmucinous cysts and malignant from nonmalignant mucinous lesions with more accuracy than routine cytology and cystic fluid CEA concentration.[112] Most malignant lesions in this study had other indicators of malignancy, including presence of a solid component in 75% and positive EUS-guided FNA cytology in 75%. The investigators suggested that DNA analysis should be considered when cystic fluid cytology is negative, but the performance characteristics of DNA analysis were not reported in this subset of all study patients. Additional studies are needed before cystic fluid DNA analysis can be recommended as part of the clinical evaluation of pancreas cystic lesions.

Despite its shortcomings, EUS of pancreatic cystic lesions assists clinical decision making in many patients, particularly patients with small, incidentally detected cysts; patients with multiple cystic lesions; and patients with increased operative risk. The best EUS-guided diagnosis relies on a combination of the clinical history, the ultrasound appearance of a cyst, and results of diagnostic studies on cystic fluid. The decision to

proceed to cyst resection for definitive diagnosis hinges not only on EUS but also on the clinical presentation; the size of the lesion; and the age, symptoms, general health, and preferences of the patient.

Interventional Endoscopic Ultrasound of the Biliary Tree and Pancreas

Many EUS-guided therapeutic interventions for treatment of biliary and pancreatic disease have been described. CPB and pseudocyst drainage were the earliest and are now widely practiced modalities. More recent interventions include drainage of inaccessible biliary or pancreatic ducts, ablation of pancreatic cystic neoplasms, injection therapy of pancreatic malignancies, drainage of abscesses, placement of fiducial markers in pancreatic masses, retrieval of migrated pancreatic stents, thrombosis of pancreatic pseudoaneurysms, and transduodenal gallbladder drainage. Educational materials are available that show detailed EUS techniques for some of these procedures.[113] This section reviews selected interventions.

Celiac Plexus and Celiac Ganglion Block and Neurolysis

Treatment of pain by blockade or neurolysis of the celiac plexus has been performed for more than 100 years by percutaneous or surgical techniques. More recently, EUS-guided CPB or celiac plexus neurolysis (CPN) have been widely adopted. In both procedures, a local anesthetic is injected; for CPB, a steroid is usually added, and for CPN, ethanol is usually injected. Various injection methods and injectants may be used and are well summarized elsewhere.[114,115]

Traditional CPB and CPN procedures involve injections of the soft tissue surrounding the celiac axis, with diffusion of injected fluid into and around the celiac plexus; because celiac ganglia can be directly visualized by EUS in about 80% of persons,[116] direct ganglion injection has also been described.[117]

Few randomized, controlled trials of CPB or CPN have been done. In one prospective, randomized, double-blind trial, percutaneous CPN was more effective than sham injections.[118] Two randomized, prospective, nonblinded trials have compared EUS-guided CPB with percutaneous CPB, with both studies reporting better pain relief with the EUS approach.[119,120] A more recent prospective, randomized trial comparing two EUS techniques (central vs. bilateral injections) reported no difference in pain relief.[121]

Common side effects of CPB and CPN include orthostatic hypotension and diarrhea. Complications are uncommon and include retroperitoneal abscess and adrenal artery laceration.[122,123] Some experts administer prophylactic antibiotics before CPB. Spinal cord injury, with resultant paralysis and loss of bowel and bladder control, is a rare complication of CPB and CPN that probably occurs owing to spasm of a spinal artery. This complication has not been reported with EUS-guided approaches but probably rarely occurs with this modality as well. Direct injection of the celiac ganglia may theoretically decrease the risk of this complication.[117]

Drainage of Fluid Collections

Fluid collections are complications of pancreatitis and include acute fluid collections, pseudocysts, and walled-off necrosis. Endoscopic drainage is a preferred treatment modality for many of these collections, and a Seldinger technique for transgastric or transduodenal drainage is often preferred.[124] EUS may be used to guide endoscopic drainage of a pancreatic fluid collection, and the technique has been described in detail elsewhere.[113,125] Theoretical advantages of EUS guidance over standard endoscopic drainage include EUS examination of the lesion, possibly with FNA, to identify a cystic neoplasm mimicking a pseudocyst; avoidance of intervening vessels or varices that may lie in the path of planned transmural drainage; and better access to fluid collections that do not indent the lumen of the stomach or duodenum. In one large retrospective series, patients assigned to EUS-guided drainage because of a nonbulging collection or portal hypertension had similar outcomes to patients without these risk factors.[126] In two prospective, randomized trials, overall success of drainage was significantly higher with an EUS-guided approach compared with conventional endoscopic drainage, largely because nonbulging collections could be drained with EUS.[127,128]

Endoscopic drainage of pancreatic necrosis has traditionally had lower overall success rates than drainage of pseudocysts owing to the presence of solid necrotic material in the collection and the tendency for infection to occur when the collection has been inadequately drained. The emerging technique of endoscopic necrosectomy seems to improve the overall success of endoscopic treatment. Bleeding from vessels in the gut wall or retroperitoneum is the most common complication of endoscopic necrosectomy.[129] EUS miniprobes introduced into regions of pancreatic necrosis through a standard endoscope may identify vessels in the wall of the collection, theoretically decreasing the risk of vascular injury during endoscopic necrosectomy.

Ablation of Cystic Neoplasms

Cystic neoplasms of the pancreas are increasingly diagnosed, and some histologic types, including MCNs and branch duct IPMNs, have malignant potential. Standard therapy for these lesions is either observation or surgical resection. EUS-guided therapy of these lesions has been reported, including ethanol lavage of the cyst[130] and ethanol lavage followed by instillation of paclitaxel gel.[131] These therapies apparently result in decrease in the overall size of the cystic lesion; in one prospective study, ethanol lavage was superior to saline lavage.[132] It is unclear, however, whether these therapies ablate all neoplastic epithelium in the lesions or decrease the risk of pancreatic carcinoma. Most series have not used a standardized follow-up imaging protocol optimized to detect small remnant cysts. At the present time, EUS-guided ablation of pancreatic cysts remains investigational.

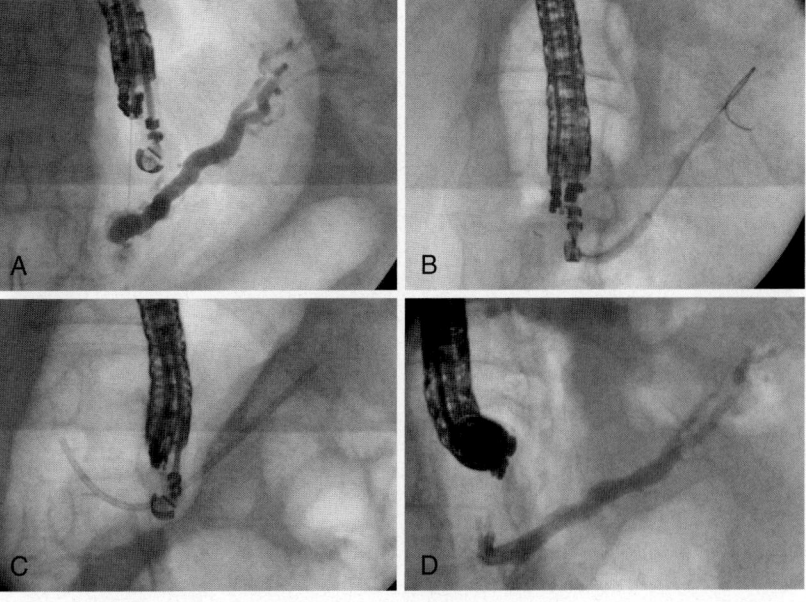

Fig. 41.23 Transgastric drainage of obstructed pancreatic duct. The patient presented with recurrent pancreatitis and chronic pain 6 years after a Whipple procedure for chronic pancreatitis. **A,** Transgastric puncture of the pancreatic duct under endoscopic ultrasound (EUS) guidance, with pancreatography. The pancreaticojejunal anastomosis is obstructed, and in this case a guidewire could not be manipulated across the stenosis. **B,** Transgastric balloon dilation of the tract from stomach to pancreatic duct. **C,** Placement of a 7-Fr plastic stent extending from the pancreatic duct to the stomach. **D,** At a subsequent stent exchange procedure, three stents are placed across the gastropancreatic fistula site.

Drainage of Biliary and Pancreatic Ducts

EUS can facilitate access to the biliary tree and pancreas and drainage of otherwise inaccessible ducts. EUS techniques may be used when ERCP fails or is unlikely to succeed (e.g., pancreatic duct access after a Whipple procedure). Techniques and instrumentation are evolving, and numerous procedural variations and technical subtleties are presented elsewhere.[113] It is possible to obtain an EUS-guided cholangiogram or pancreatogram in most patients requiring an EUS approach.[5,133,134] The goals of the procedure typically extend beyond ductal visualization, however, and injection of contrast material into an obstructed ductal system may be complicated by infection or leakage unless a drainage procedure is also performed. Passage of a guidewire through an EUS needle and across the site of ductal obstruction can be achieved in most patients.[5,133,134] A "rendezvous" procedure may be performed by leaving the guidewire in place, removing the echoendoscope, and passing another endoscope to grasp the end of the guidewire in the gut lumen and place a stent across the ductal obstruction over the guidewire.[5,133–135]

Alternatively, the drainage procedure may be performed through the echoendoscope, by dilation of the tract to the duct system over the guidewire and subsequent antegrade transgastric stent placement. If the site of ductal obstruction can be crossed with a guidewire, the stent may traverse the stomach wall, pancreas, and ductal obstruction, with the far end of the stent residing in the small bowel. If the site of ductal obstruction cannot be crossed with a guidewire, a stent may still be placed into the obstructed ductal system through the echoendoscope, accomplishing transgastric drainage (**Fig. 41.23**).[5] In patients with pancreatic duct obstruction after a Whipple procedure, placement of a transgastric stent that traverses the stomach wall and pancreas may facilitate future ductal access and stent exchange via the transgastric tract. Complications are frequent after EUS-guided ductal drainage procedures and include abdominal pain requiring hospitalization, infectious complications, and bleeding.[5,133,134] Urgent percutaneous or surgical procedures may be required if successful ductal drainage is not achieved. At the present time, these procedures are best reserved for patients whose clinical condition mandates ductal drainage, in whom other modalities (e.g., ERCP, percutaneous drainage, or surgery) are unfavorable.

References

The complete reference list is available online at www.expertconsult.com.

Endoscopic Ultrasound–Guided Fine Needle Aspiration of Pancreaticobiliary Lesions

V. Raman Muthusamy and Kenneth J. Chang

Video related to this chapter's topics can be found online at expertconsult.com.

Introduction

Many of the limitations of endoscopic ultrasound (EUS) as a pure imaging modality have been overcome by the development of EUS-guided fine needle aspiration (FNA). This chapter reviews the role of EUS-guided FNA in the diagnosis of pancreaticobiliary lesions such as pancreatic adenocarcinoma and cystic and neuroendocrine tumors of the pancreas and less appreciated applications, such as evaluation of biliary and ampullary cancers. The specific role of EUS-guided FNA in the staging of various pancreaticobiliary cancers is also discussed. Finally, this chapter addresses some of the exciting emerging applications of EUS-guided therapies such as fine needle injection (FNI). These new applications include celiac neurolysis, cyst gastrostomy, delivery of antitumor agents (via immune, viral, and gene therapies), accessing the pancreaticobiliary system when standard access is impossible, and assisting in radiation therapy via the placement of fiducial markers or directly performing EUS-guided brachytherapy. Technical considerations involving EUS-guided FNA and FNI are also addressed.

Endoscopic Ultrasound–Guided Fine Needle Aspiration in the Diagnosis of Pancreatic Tumors

Pancreatic Cancer

Adenocarcinoma of the pancreas is the fifth leading cause for cancer-related death in the United States. Despite improvements in medical and surgical therapy, the overall 5-year survival remains at 4%. The most favorable outcome is among surgical patients with small tumors without nodal, vascular, or systemic metastasis. These patients have 5-year survivals up to 25%. Optimally, earlier detection and precise preoperative staging would best stratify patients who would most likely

Table 42.1 Detection of Pancreatic Carcinoma by Body Imaging Tools

Size	EUS	US	CT	ERCP	AG
<20 mm (*n* = 10)	8/10	3/10	1/10	7/10	3/10
>20 mm (*n* = 136)	135/136	104/132	102/136	121/136	77/80
Total sensitivity	143/146 (98%)	107/142 (75%)	103/129 (80%)	128/146 (86%)	80/90 (89%)

AG, angiography; CT, computed tomography; ERCP, endoscopic retrograde cholangiopancreatography; EUS, endoscopic ultrasound; US, ultrasound.

benefit from surgery, while sparing the remaining patients from exploratory or palliative-only surgery.

EUS is considered one of the most useful diagnostic procedures among the body imaging tools for detecting pancreatic cancer. EUS was shown to be superior (sensitivity of 98%) to other imaging modalities, including computed tomography (CT), in 146 patients with pancreatic cancer (**Table 42.1**).[1] With the more recent introduction of spiral CT with dual-phase contrast, the detection rate for CT is improving. However, more recent comparisons between dual-phase spiral CT and EUS still favor EUS. The ability to obtain cytologic specimen by EUS-guided FNA has greatly aided in differentiating benign versus malignant lesions seen on EUS alone.

The application of EUS-guided FNA to the pancreas in particular has great clinical utility. CT-guided and ultrasound-guided percutaneous FNA have previously been the most commonly used methods for diagnosing pancreatic cancer. The sensitivity of percutaneous FNA ranges from 45% to 100%, with a specificity of up to 100%. However, obtaining a tissue diagnosis with CT or ultrasound guidance is limited by the ability to visualize the lesion. In our previous multicenter trial, 56% of patients with pancreatic carcinoma had CT scans that did not show a mass or revealed nonspecific enlargement of the pancreas.[2] Endoscopic retrograde cholangiopancreatography (ERCP) with cytologic brushing also has historically had a relatively low yield, with sensitivities between 30% and 56%. The overall sensitivity, specificity, diagnostic accuracy, negative predictive value, and positive predictive value of EUS-guided FNA for pancreatic cancer in this study were 83%, 90%, 85%, 80%, and 100%. These values were superior to CT alone (without FNA): 56%, 37%, 50%, 28%, and 65% (*P* < .05). There were four complications in 164 patients (2%), including two major (perforation, bleeding) and two minor (fever) complications. Comparison among the four centers showed that institutions in which a cytologist was present during the procedure had a significantly higher cytologic yield, sensitivity, and diagnostic accuracy.

Advantages of EUS-guided FNA include procuring a tissue diagnosis while obtaining additional tumor and nodal staging information, the avoidance of additional diagnostic testing or surgery, and the prognostic information gained from the staging information (**Figs. 42.1 through 42.4**). Another report from a large single-institution study of 144 pancreatic lesions undergoing EUS-guided FNA showed sensitivity, specificity, and diagnostic accuracy of 82%, 100%, and 85%.[3] More recently, helical or spiral CT has improved imaging of the pancreas. However, preliminary studies still show superiority of EUS compared with spiral CT.[4]

Despite these data, EUS and EUS-guided FNA still possess limitations. The most difficult diagnostic problem for any

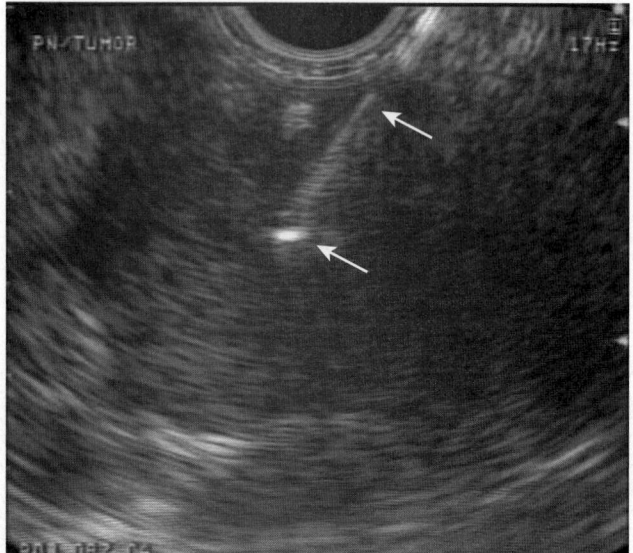

Fig. 42.1 Fine needle aspiration (FNA) (25-gauge) of neuroendocrine tumor of the pancreas.

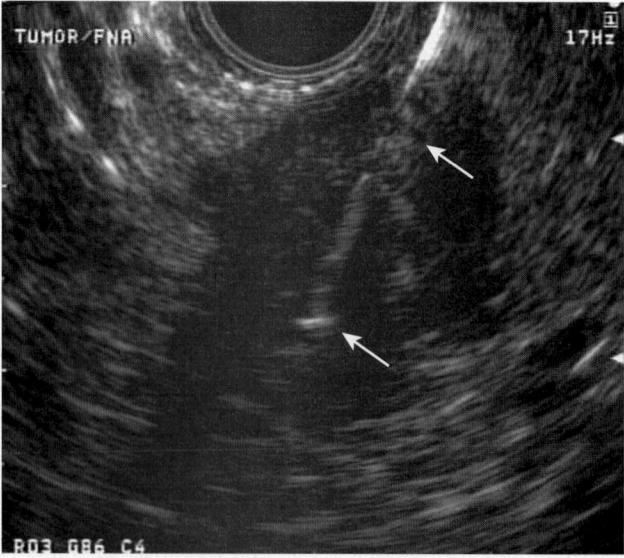

Fig. 42.2 Fine needle aspiration (FNA) (25-gauge) of solid pseudopapillary tumor of the pancreas.

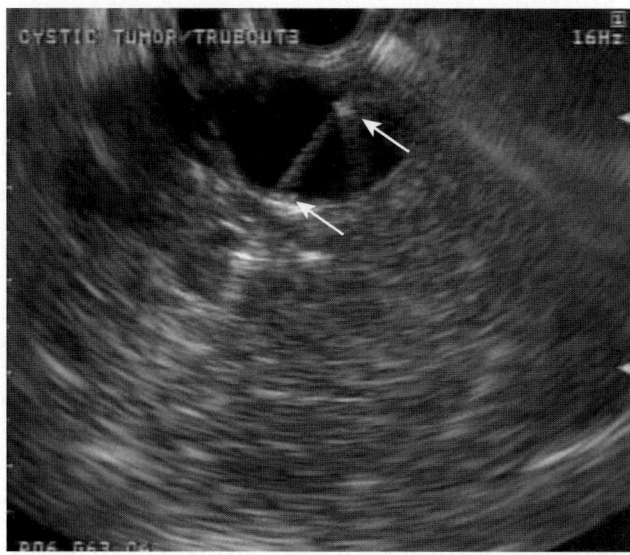

Fig. 42.3 Quick-Core (Cook Medical, Orange, CA) 19-gauge needle used to evaluate a pancreatic cyst. *(Courtesy of Cook Medical, Orange, CA.)*

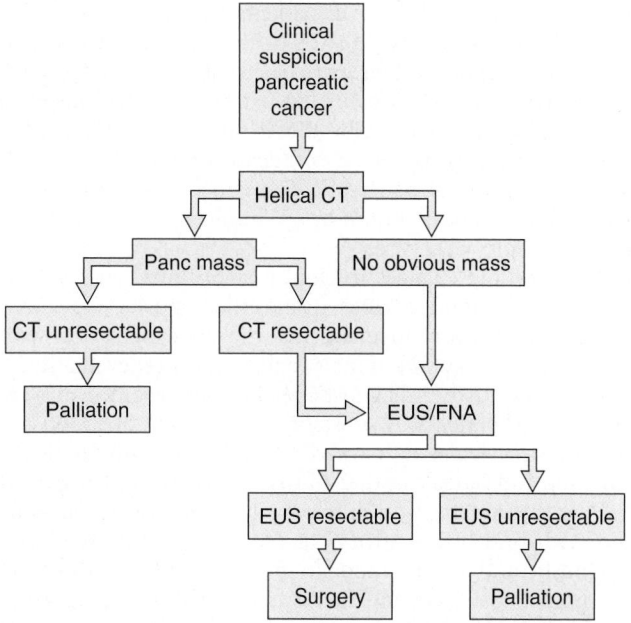

Fig. 42.5 Algorithm for diagnosis and staging of pancreatic cancer.

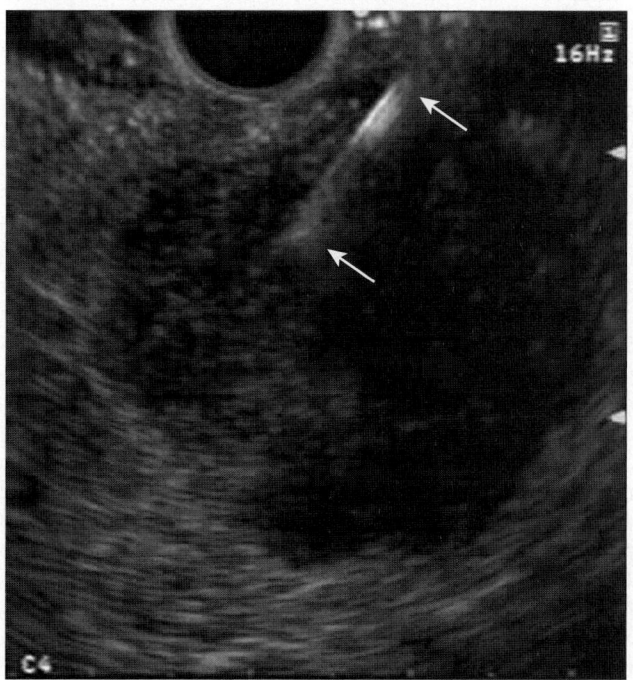

Fig. 42.4 Fine needle aspiration (FNA) (25-gauge) of metastatic liver lesion from pancreatic cancer.

acute pancreatitis (1 case).[5] A study of 116 pancreatic malignancies identified in patients with and without chronic pancreatitis found a sensitivity of EUS-guided FNA for malignancy of 89% in patients without chronic pancreatitis compared with 54% in patients with chronic pancreatitis.[6] An additional study of 282 patients with pancreatic mass lesions undergoing 300 EUS-guided FNA procedures also found reduced sensitivity in patients with chronic pancreatitis compared with patients without chronic pancreatitis (73.9% vs. 91.3%).[7] However, it was thought that this reduced sensitivity could be overcome with an increased number of FNA passes (median of five passes in patients with chronic pancreatitis patients vs. two passes in patients without chronic pancreatitis). An additional prospective study aiming to assess the number of passes to perform to maximize cytologic yield suggested that seven passes be made to optimize yield in pancreatic and miscellaneous (non–lymph node) lesions.[8]

These data have significantly affected the clinical algorithm of patients with known or suspected pancreatic malignancies. A clinical outcomes study was performed at a single center comparing the management and survival of 136 patients with pancreatic cancer between the pre-EUS and post-EUS eras.[9] EUS detected carcinomas that were either not seen or only possibly seen by CT in 34% of patients, and there were 75% fewer required operations for diagnosis. The median survival without liver metastases was also longer during the EUS period (102 days vs. 205 days; $P < .02$, log-rank test), probably secondary to lead-time bias.

We believe that all patients thought to have operable disease based on initial CT imaging should undergo EUS with or without FNA before surgical intervention (**Fig. 42.5**). Considering the possibility of a false-negative result (up to 20%, especially in the setting of chronic pancreatitis), we also believe that surgical intervention should not be precluded in a patient with a high suspicion of resectable pancreatic carcinoma and a negative FNA cytology. EUS-guided FNA of pancreatic

imaging test, including EUS-guided FNA, is the differentiation between pancreatic carcinoma and chronic pancreatitis. Although a positive FNA is almost 100% accurate, a negative FNA is only about 80% accurate. A multicenter, retrospective study of 20 cancers missed on EUS by nine experienced endosonographers found that although 60% (12 cases) of the cancers were missed because of underlying chronic pancreatitis, other factors associated with missed lesions included a diffusely infiltrating carcinoma (3 cases), a prominent ventral or dorsal split (2 cases), and a recent episode (<4 weeks) of lesions is also worthwhile in patients with a prior negative tissue diagnosis by ERCP or CT of the abdomen. Gress and colleagues[10] reported their experience with EUS-guided FNA of pancreatic mass lesions in 102 patients who had negative cytologic tissue diagnosis by ERCP sampling or CT-guided FNA. Among their patients, 57 of the 61 patients (93.4%) with a final diagnosis of pancreatic cancer had positive cytology results for adenocarcinoma by EUS-guided FNA. The false-positive results were zero.

The resulting changes in clinical algorithms can result in significant economic savings. In an earlier report, we reviewed a series of 44 consecutive patients who underwent EUS with or without FNA as part of their pancreatic cancer evaluation.[11] Surgery and further diagnostic testing were avoided in 41% and 57% of patients. A substantial cost saving of $3300 per patient was calculated. In a series of 216 consecutive patients, Erickson and Garza[12] studied the use of EUS with EUS-guided FNA as the initial approach to patients with obstructive jaundice. EUS and EUS-guided FNA not only proved useful as a diagnostic and staging modality but also served in directing the need for subsequent therapeutic ERCP, saving approximately $1007 to $1313 per patient. In addition, if EUS and EUS-guided FNA were not used at all, an extra $2200 would be spent per patient. In contrast to CT-guided FNA, EUS-guided FNA of the pancreas can be performed during the initial EUS procedure. The overall complication rate of EUS-guided FNA was reported to be 0.5% to 2.9%. An additional study comparing ERCP with brushing with EUS-guided FNA, laparoscopic biopsy, and CT-guided or ultrasound-guided FNA found that EUS-guided FNA is the best and most cost-effective initial method and the preferred secondary alternative method for the diagnosis of suspected pancreatic cancer.[13]

Several case reports have described malignant seeding of the needle tract after transcutaneous FNA. However, the true incidence has yet to be established. Theoretically, EUS-guided FNA of pancreatic cancers should have a lower chance of malignant seeding because of the short needle tract. A retrospective study comparing 46 patients diagnosed with pancreatic cancer via EUS-guided FNA with 43 patients diagnosed via CT-guided FNA seemed to confirm this hypothesis.[14] All patients underwent neoadjuvant therapy, followed by restaging CT and attempt at surgical resection if disease progression was absent. Despite no differences in tumor characteristics between the groups, the frequency of peritoneal metastases was 2.2% in the EUS group compared with 16.3% in the CT group ($P < .025$).

In pancreatic head lesions, EUS-guided FNA is usually performed from the second portion of the duodenum, a segment resected surgically along with the tumor during the Whipple procedure; this is another theoretical advantage of eliminating the needle tract and decreasing the risk of malignant seeding compared with the percutaneous approach. However, this advantage may not apply to pancreatic body and tail lesions, where the possibility of malignant seeding of the gastric wall (which is not resected in a distal pancreatectomy) could still exist. An additional advantage of FNA using EUS guidance is the ability to detect vascular structures around the targeted lesion by Doppler flow analysis immediately before FNA, minimizing the chance of bleeding complications. Bleeding that occurs during FNA is extremely rare, is self-limited, and usually resolves spontaneously. The safety of EUS-guided FNA is discussed further in the complications section.

Cystic Neoplasms

EUS can be helpful in distinguishing cystic neoplasms from pancreatic pseudocysts, although the specificity is not perfect.[15] The more problematic discernment is between serous and mucinous cysts, with the latter considered premalignant. The interobserver agreement for the interpretation of cystic lesions in the pancreas is quite low. The interobserver agreement on 31 pancreatic cyst cases among eight expert endosonographers was shown to be "fair" between endosonographers for diagnosis of neoplastic versus nonneoplastic lesions ($\kappa = 0.24$).[16] Agreement for individual types of lesions was moderately good for serous cystadenomas ($\kappa = 0.46$) but fair for the remainder. Accuracy rates of EUS for the diagnosis of neoplastic versus nonneoplastic lesions ranged from 40% to 93%.

EUS imaging alone is often inadequate for the clinical management of these patients. EUS-guided FNA of cystic contents can be analyzed for cytology, biochemistry, and tumor markers to aid in cyst classification. Because cytology is a relatively insensitive test, cyst fluid tumor markers such as carcinoembryonic antigen (CEA) have been employed to improve the sensitivity for the detection of malignancy. Cyst fluid CEA values are uniformly low in serous cystadenomas, higher in mucinous lesions, and markedly elevated in mucinous cystadenocarcinomas.[17] A multicenter European study reported a series of 67 patients who underwent EUS-guided FNA of pancreatic cysts and subsequently underwent surgery.[18] EUS alone (no FNA) correctly identified 49 cases (73%), whereas FNA correctly identified 65 cases (97%). Sensitivity, specificity, positive predictive value, and negative predictive value of EUS and EUS-guided FNA to indicate whether a lesion needed further surgery were 71% and 97%, 30% and 100%, 49% and 100%, and 40% and 95%. A value of the tumor marker for colorectal and pancreatic carcinomas (CA 19.9) greater than 50,000 U/mL had 15% sensitivity and 81% specificity to distinguish mucinous cysts from other cystic lesions and 86% sensitivity and 85% specificity to distinguish cystadenocarcinoma from other cystic lesions.

The most definitive data on cyst fluid analysis come from the Cooperative Pancreatic Cyst study, a multicenter U.S. trial that assessed 341 patients undergoing EUS-guided FNA of a pancreatic cystic lesion.[19] Surgical resection was performed in 112 patients, with a final histologic diagnosis of the cysts as follows: 68 mucinous, 7 serous, 27 inflammatory, 5 endocrine, and 5 other. The results of EUS, cyst fluid cytology, and cyst fluid tumor markers (CEA, marker for gastrointestinal (GI) and ovarian carcinomas [CA 72.4], marker for ovarian and endometrial carcinomas [CA 125], CA 19.9, and marker for breast carcinoma [CA 15.3]) were prospectively collected and compared. Receiver operator curve analysis of the tumor markers showed that cyst fluid CEA (optimal cutoff of 192 ng/mL) showed the greatest area under the curve (0.79) for differentiating mucinous versus nonmucinous cystic lesions and was the most useful cyst fluid tumor marker. The accuracy of CEA (88 of 111 [79%]) was significantly greater than the accuracy of EUS morphology (57 of 112 [51%]) or cytology (64 of 109 [59%]) ($P < .05$). No combination of tests provided greater accuracy than CEA alone ($P < .0001$). The study concluded that of the tested markers, cyst fluid CEA is the most accurate test available for the diagnosis of mucinous cystic lesions of the pancreas.

Table 42.2 Pancreatic Cyst Fluid Analysis

Diagnosis	Cytology	Amylase	CEA
Pseudocyst	Benign	↑↑↑↑	Low
Serous cystadenoma	Benign	Low	Low
Mucinous cystadenoma	Benign	Low	↑↑
Mucinous cystadenocarcinoma	Malignant	Low	↑↑↑↑

CEA, carcinoembryonic antigen.

Based on these data, we routinely send cyst fluid for cytology, amylase, and CEA (**Table 42.2**). Pseudocysts have very high amylase levels (often >50,000 IU/L) with normal CEA and benign cytology. Serous cystadenomas usually have benign cytology, normal CEA, and normal amylase. However, the specific detection of serous epithelial cells on cytology to make a definitive diagnosis in these lesions is rare (<20%) with EUS-guided FNA.[20] Mucinous cystadenomas usually differ from serous cystadenoma in having a high CEA. Mucinous cystadenocarcinoma classically has malignant cytology, a low amylase, and a very elevated CEA. Although there is still some overlap of the CEA levels in these three entities, we have found the recommended cutoff value of CEA greater than 192 U/mL to be very helpful in stratifying patients to surgical versus conservative management.

Several more recent studies have aimed to characterize pancreatic cysts via use of molecular markers within the cyst fluid. A small study of 27 patients comparing CEA with the presence of k-*ras*-2 or loss of heterozygosity mutations using surgical histology or cytopathology as a "gold standard" found CEA to be the most predictive of histology, with concordance among the three tests in only 35% of patients.[21] A larger study of 100 patients compared CEA with molecular criteria including DNA quantity, k-*ras*-2 point mutations, or two or more allelic imbalance mutations with pathology as the "gold standard." The study concluded there was poor agreement ($\kappa = 0.2$) between CEA levels and molecular analysis for diagnosis of mucinous cysts. The diagnostic sensitivity for CEA was 82% compared with 77% for molecular analysis but improved to 100% when results of CEA levels and molecular analysis were combined.[22]

A more recent large, prospective multicenter study of 113 patients presenting for EUS-guided FNA of a pancreatic cyst assessed cytology and CEA levels compared with a detailed FNA analysis that incorporated DNA quantification, k-*ras* mutation and multiple allelic loss analysis, mutational amplitude, and sequence determination.[23] Of 113 patients, 40 had malignant, 48 had premalignant, and 25 had benign cysts. Mucinous cysts were associated with a k-*ras* mutation (odds ratio 20.9) and with CEA levels greater than 148 ng/mL and allelic loss amplitudes of greater than 65%. Malignant cysts were associated with a DNA analysis that detected an allelic loss amplitude of greater than 82% and a high DNA amount (optical density ratio >10). The combination of a high-amplitude k-*ras* mutation followed by an allelic loss showed a specificity of 96% for malignancy, and all 10 of the malignant cysts with negative cytology were diagnosed as malignant by DNA analysis. The authors concluded that elevated amounts of pancreatic cyst fluid DNA, high-amplitude mutations, and specific mutation acquisition sequences are indicators of malignancy and that the presence of a k-*ras* mutation is also indicative of a mucinous cyst. They recommended DNA analysis should be considered when clinically suspicious cysts have a cytologic examination that is negative for malignancy.

The cytology from the fluid of malignant cysts is usually nondiagnostic. For analysis of the cyst fluid to be most useful, several methods have been developed to improve the cytologic yield obtained from EUS-guided FNA. We have found that targeting any solid component, including the cyst wall, may enhance the yield on FNA cytology. We examined 42 pancreatic cystic lesions on which EUS-guided FNA was performed.[24] The needle was advanced under EUS guidance into the cyst in the direction of the solid component and aspirated completely. Without withdrawal, the needle was advanced directly into the solid component. Fluid and solid cytologic samples were analyzed separately. All patients received prophylactic antibiotics. Of the 42 cysts, 12 were found to have a solid component (**Table 42.3**). Eight patients had both fluid and solid cytology showing benign cells. A single patient had malignant cells on both fluid and solid cytology. Three patients had benign fluid cytology but malignant (consistent with cystadenocarcinoma) solid cytology. The results of this study suggest an enhanced cytologic yield if the solid component is targeted.

In two small studies, the use of EUS-guided Tru-Cut needle biopsy (TCB) also seemed to enhance the diagnostic capability in cystic pancreatic tumors and lymphoepithelial cysts (see **Fig. 42.3**).[25,26] In addition, the use of a cytology brush was found to be superior to conventional FNA in 7 of 10 patients undergoing EUS-guided FNA of cystic neoplastic lesions of the pancreas in a single-center study.[27] Complications from this technique included one major and one minor intracystic bleed, with no infection or pancreatitis observed. Future techniques to enhance cytologic yield along with improved molecular methods of fluid analysis are needed to aid further our ability to characterize pancreatic cysts accurately.

Endocrine Tumors

EUS is very accurate in the detection of neuroendocrine tumors of the pancreas. Zimmer and associates[28] reported their results in localizing and staging neuroendocrine tumors of the foregut in 40 patients examined by EUS, somatostatin receptor scintigraphy (SRS), CT, magnetic resonance imaging (MRI), and transabdominal ultrasound. EUS showed the highest sensitivity in localizing insulinomas compared with SRS, ultrasound, CT, and MRI. The authors suggested that ultrasound and EUS should be the first-line diagnostic procedures if insulinoma has been proven by a fasting test. Further diagnostic procedures were unnecessary in most cases. Further

Table 42.3 Pancreatic Cyst Cytology (Fluid and Solid) in 12 Patients

Location	Size (cm)	Fluid Cytology	Solid Cytology
Head	3.1 × 2.5	Benign	Benign
Body	5.2 × 6.3	Adenocarcinoma	Adenocarcinoma
Body	1.9 × 2.6	Benign	Benign
Head	2.8 × 2.5	Benign	Benign
Body	3.2 × 1.9	Benign	Benign
Head	1.5 × 1.3	Benign	Adenocarcinoma
Body	5 × 3.5	Benign	Benign
Neck	4 × 4	Benign	Benign
Body	1.1 × 1.7	Benign	Benign
Body	8 × 8	Benign	Adenocarcinoma
Head	2.2 × 1.3	Benign	Benign
Neck	2.7 × 3.7	Benign	Adenocarcinoma

diagnostic procedures such as CT or MRI to search for distant metastases are necessary in large tumors or local invasive tumors. EUS shows the highest accuracy to detect or exclude pancreatic gastrinomas, but it fails to detect extrapancreatic gastrinomas in about 50%. The combination of EUS and SRS may give additional information. Zimmer and associates[28] recommended that the first-line diagnostic procedures in patients with gastrinoma should be SRS and CT or MRI. If no metastases are detected, EUS should be the next preoperative imaging procedure. In nonfunctional neuroendocrine tumors, EUS provides the best information on local tumor invasion and regional lymph node involvement.

EUS has also been shown to be cost-effective in the preoperative localization of pancreatic endocrine tumors. Bansal and colleagues[29] reported a case-control study of 36 patients who underwent preoperative EUS with a matched group of 36 patients who underwent surgical exploration immediately before the introduction of EUS. The EUS group had reduced charges for preoperative localization studies: $2620 versus $4846 per patient ($P < .05$). The lower cost was largely because of reductions in the number of diagnostic angiograms and venous sampling procedures performed. Surgical and total anesthesia times were decreased, as were the number of preoperative admissions for angiographic procedures. The cost-effectiveness ratio for the EUS group was $3144 per tumor localized compared with $5628 per tumor localized for the group treated before EUS became available ($P < .05$). The more specific utility of EUS-guided FNA in these patients was reported more recently (see **Fig. 42.1**).[30] EUS-guided FNA was performed in 10 patients with clinically suspected functioning neuroendocrine tumors (hormonal disturbances) to determine the location and to confirm the diagnosis cytologically. EUS identified 14 tumors in these 10 patients. In all but one patient, CT did not show the tumor or missed at least one of multiple lesions. Mean tumor size was 12 mm (range 4 to 25 mm). Tumor locations were pancreas ($n = 13$) and duodenal wall ($n = 1$). Of the 14 detected lesions, 11 were aspirated under EUS-guided FNA with accurate diagnosis in all cases. Surgical confirmation of EUS-guided FNA findings was available in seven patients. There were no complications related to EUS-guided FNA.

More recently, an additional study of 30 patients with 33 lesions identified intraoperatively found sensitivity, specificity, positive predictive value, negative predictive value, and accuracy rate of EUS in conjunction with FNA of 82.6%, 85.7%, 95%, 60%, and 83.3%.[31] EUS-guided FNA also seems to be highly effective and accurate in detecting the less common presentation of these lesions as cystic neuroendocrine tumors.[32] In addition to diagnosing neuroendocrine tumors via EUS-guided FNA, EUS may also be useful in marking these subtle lesions using EUS-guided fine needle "tattooing" before surgery to assist in intraoperative localization.[33] EUS-guided FNI may also be used in a therapeutic capacity for these lesions; a case of EUS-guided alcohol ablation of an insulinoma has been reported.[34]

Endoscopic Ultrasound–Guided Fine Needle Aspiration in the Staging of Pancreatic Cancer

In a prospective analysis, Mortensen and coworkers[35] found a 30% overall impact of EUS-guided FNA on clinical management in 99 consecutive patients with pancreatic cancer of whom 20 patients underwent EUS-guided FNA for staging purposes: 5 liver lesions, 1 malignant ascites, 13 lymph nodes, and 1 aspiration from retroperitoneal tumor infiltration. The remaining 25 patients had diagnostic FNA: 22 pancreatic and 3 duodenal. EUS-guided FNA was performed only if positive results would have a clinically relevant impact on the subsequent management of the patient. The clinical impact of EUS-guided FNA was 12% (12 of 99) for staging purposes and 86% (18 of 21) for diagnostic purposes.

The economic impact of EUS-guided FNA in the preoperative staging of patients with pancreatic head adenocarcinoma was shown in a decision analysis model.[36] The use of EUS-guided FNA prevented 16 surgeries per 100 patients compared with 8 surgeries per 100 patients if CT-guided FNA was performed for nonperitumoral lymph nodes. If the frequency of nonperitumoral lymph nodes was greater than 4%, EUS-guided FNA was the least costly procedure: $15,938 versus $16,378 for CT-guided FNA and $18,723 for surgery.

Lymph Node Assessment

According to a multivariate analysis, lymph node metastasis, intrapancreatic perineural invasion, and portal vein invasion are significant prognostic factors in patients with pancreatic cancer after curative resection.[37] A retrospective analysis of patients who underwent curative resection was conducted. Of 193 patients, 38 (20%) survived for more than 5 years; 5-year survival rates for stages I, II, III, and IV disease were 41%, 17%, 11%, and 6%. Subsequently, a subgroup analysis of nodal metastasis and intrapancreatic perineural invasion was performed in 126 patients with records of these histologic findings. In the group of patients without nodal metastasis, the 5-year survival rate for patients without perineural invasion was 75%, whereas the 5-year survival rate for patients with perineural invasion was 29%; the difference in survival of these subgroups was significant ($P < .02$). In the group of patients with nodal metastasis, the 5-year survival rate for patients without perineural invasion was 17%, whereas the 5-year survival rate for patients with perineural invasion was 10%.

EUS imaging alone cannot fully distinguish malignant from inflammatory nodes, limiting its specificity in lymph node staging. Various EUS criteria have been described to distinguish malignant from benign nodes. These parameters, including size, shape, borders, and echotexture have lacked specificity, however. We previously conducted a study correlating EUS features of lymph nodes with the respective EUS-guided FNA diagnosis (**Fig. 42.6**).[38] Computer analysis of EUS images of 48 lymph nodes in 47 patients using both linear array and radial scanning transducers was performed. Parameters included lymph node area, longest diameter, shape factor, and gray scale. There were 22 malignant and 26 benign nodes. When correlated with the FNA cytology results for each node, the only single criterion that was 100% specific for predicting malignancy was a longest diameter greater than 2.5 cm or an area greater than 2.5 cm^2. However, using this size cutoff, the sensitivity declined to only 18%. No single criterion has an acceptable sensitivity and specificity to circumvent the need for a tissue diagnosis by EUS-guided FNA.

A multicenter study of 171 patients undergoing EUS-guided FNA of 192 lymph nodes (46 benign, 146 malignant) has been performed.[39] The final diagnosis was ascertained by clinical follow-up (108 lymph nodes) or histopathology correlation (84 lymph nodes). The mean long axis dimension of benign lymph nodes was less than malignant lymph nodes (18 mm [5 to 37 mm] vs. 27 mm [5 to 80 mm]; $P < .001$). On average, two to three needle passes were made for each lymph node. The overall performance of EUS-guided FNA in lymph node assessment was sensitivity 92% (84% to 97% among four centers), specificity 93% (75% to 100%), and overall accuracy 92% (82% to 98%). If a long axis dimension of 15 mm was used for determining benign ($\leq$15 mm) versus malignant (>15 mm) lymphadenopathy, EUS alone had sensitivity (67%), specificity (50%), and accuracy (63%) all inferior to EUS-guided FNA ($P < .05$). In 89 patients, a total of 101 lymph nodes underwent EUS-guided FNA for the staging of lung cancer (14 patients) or primary GI or pancreatic malignancies (75 patients). When comparing EUS-guided FNA with EUS size criteria ($\leq$10 mm = benign), the sensitivity (90% vs. 91%; P = not significant) and accuracy (92% vs. 83%; P = not significant) for EUS-guided FNA were similar, whereas the specificity was superior to that of EUS size criteria alone (100% vs. 47%; $P < .001$).

Not only can EUS-guided FNA improve the specificity of lymph node metastasis with cytologic confirmation, but also more recently FNA has been used to detect genetic alterations in cytologic negative nodes. A prospective study was conducted to assess the clinical value of genetic staging of lymph node metastasis in patients with pancreatic adenocarcinoma who underwent curative surgery.[40] In the primary tumors in 18 of 25 patients with pancreatic adenocarcinoma, k-*ras* gene mutations were detected. Among these 18 patients, a mutated k-*ras* gene was also found in at least one lymph node in 13 patients. Of these 13 patients, 7 had no evidence of histologic nodal involvement, and 6 had histologic lymph node metastasis. Although there was no significant difference in overall survival rates between the pathologic node-negative and node-positive patients, overall survival of the five patients with nodes negative for the mutated k-*ras* gene was significantly better than overall survival of the 13 patients with genetically metastasis-positive nodes ($P < .001$). Overall survival of the six patients with genetically metastasis-positive nodes limited to the peripancreatic area was significantly better than overall survival of the seven patients with genetic metastasis in lymph nodes beyond the peripancreatic areas ($P = .018$). These findings suggest that detection of k-*ras* gene mutations in lymph nodes may be clinically useful to assess the accurate tumor staging and to stratify patients who may be at higher risk for recurrence after curative resection.

Finally, in addition to abdominal lymphadenopathy, a more recent study of 160 patients with pancreatic and periampullary cancers undergoing EUS staging found that 5% had malignant mediastinal adenopathy.[41] Only one of the eight patients with malignant adenopathy in the mediastinum had other sites of documented distal metastases by CT or positron emission tomography scan, although seven patients had a locally advanced cancer. These findings emphasize the importance of carefully examining the mediastinum for suspicious adenopathy routinely as a part of every EUS examination done to stage pancreatic cancer.

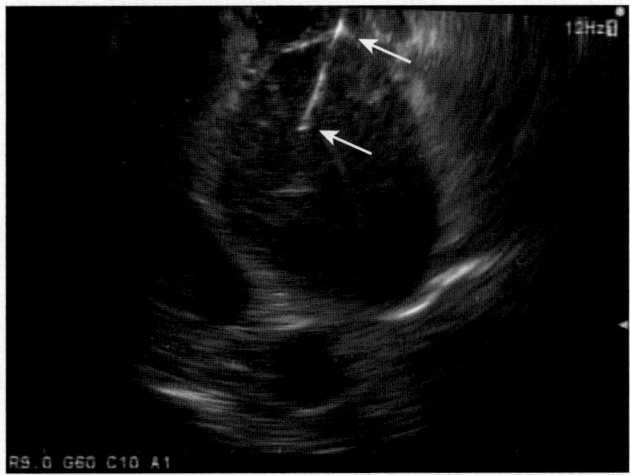

Fig. 42.6 Fine needle aspiration (FNA) (25-gauge) of a large subhepatic lymph node in a patient with cholangiocarcinoma.

Liver Metastasis

EUS is not traditionally thought to be clinically applicable in liver imaging. However, more recent data have suggested otherwise. A prospective study was conducted in which 574 consecutive patients with a history or suspicion of GI or pulmonary malignant tumor undergoing upper EUS examinations underwent EUS evaluation of the liver.[42] Focal liver lesions were found in 14 (2.4%) patients, and they underwent EUS-guided FNA (see **Fig. 42.4**). Before EUS, CT depicted liver lesions in only 3 of 14 (21%) patients. Seven of 14 patients had a known cancer diagnosis. For the other seven patients, the initial diagnosis of cancer was made by means of EUS-guided FNA of the liver. There were no immediate or late complications. This study showed that EUS can detect small focal liver lesions that are not detected at CT.

Findings of EUS-guided FNA can confirm a cytologic diagnosis of liver metastasis and establish a definitive M stage that may change clinical management. A retrospective questionnaire study regarding indications, complications, and findings of EUS-guided FNA of the liver was reported more recently, which included 21 EUS and FNA centers around the world.[43] There were 167 cases of EUS-guided FNA of the liver. A complication was reported in 6 (4%) of 167 cases, including death in 1 patient with an occluding biliary stent and biliary sepsis, bleeding in 1 patient, fever in 2 patients, and pain in 2 patients. EUS-guided FNA diagnosed malignancy in 23 of 26 (89%) patients who had a prior nondiagnostic FNA under transabdominal ultrasound guidance. EUS also localized an unrecognized primary tumor in 17 of 33 (52%) cases in which CT had shown only liver metastases. EUS imaging characteristics were not predictive of malignant versus benign lesions. The authors concluded that EUS-guided FNA of the liver apparently is a safe procedure with a major complication rate of approximately 1%. Additional studies have confirmed that EUS can detect previously undetected or additional lesions not visualized by other modalities[44-48] and correspondingly alter planned clinical management.[44,45] In addition, EUS-guided FNA achieves results comparable to or better than CT-guided FNA of hepatic lesions.[49]

Liver lesions typically have a much higher cytologic yield (requiring fewer needle passes owing to less inflammatory and fibrotic reaction compared with a primary pancreatic neoplasm) and give the highest staging information (see section on FNA technique). A study supporting these statements found a 94% diagnostic yield with EUS-guided FNA (31 of 33 lesions confirmed positive) of hepatic lesions with a mean of only 1.4 FNA passes taken.[50]

EUS-guided FNA of hepatic lesions is feasible and safe and should be considered when a liver lesion is poorly accessible to percutaneous FNA, when ultrasound-guided or CT-guided FNA has failed to make a diagnosis, or when a previously undetected lesion is seen at the time of EUS. If EUS detects a liver lesion de novo in the setting of staging pancreatic cancer, EUS-guided FNA should be attempted first, even before taking biopsy specimens of the primary pancreatic tumor, to provide the highest level of staging.

Ascites

The utility of EUS-guided FNA was evaluated for detection and aspiration of scant ascites among patients undergoing EUS for diagnosis and staging of GI malignancies.[51] EUS found ascites in 85 patients (15% of a series of 571 patients). CT performed before EUS identified ascites in only 18% of patients with ascites on EUS. Of the 85 patients, 31 underwent EUS-guided FNA paracentesis, and malignant ascites was diagnosed by EUS-guided FNA in 5 patients. The clinical impact was great in these patients because surgery was avoided.

Two additional studies have corroborated these findings. Kaushik and colleagues[52] identified ascites in 25 patients undergoing EUS for suspected or proven malignancy and diagnosed 16 cancers (64% of patients). Six of the nine patients with negative ascites on EUS-guided FNA had a diagnosed malignancy, but only one false-negative ascites cytology result occurred in these patients, yielding 94% sensitivity and 89% negative predictive value. DeWitt and colleagues[53] detected ascites on EUS in 60 patients being staged with known or suspected malignancy. Of these, MRI and CT detected ascites in only about 50% of patients who also had either of these examinations, and ascites was detected in only 27% of patients undergoing transabdominal ultrasound. Cancer was diagnosed in 16 (27%) patients. Of the eight patients who underwent subsequent surgery, three were found to have malignant ascites, illustrating the fact that a negative fluid cytology does not exclude the possibility of peritoneal carcinomatosis.

Two more recent articles have highlighted the fact that peritoneal implants may also be identified on EUS and that these can successfully undergo EUS-guided FNA with adequate specimen to confirm malignancy.[54,55] Some investigators have suggested that in patients with a small amount of ascites, a transrectal approach may be more sensitive in identifying and diagnosing malignant carcinomatosis.[56]

Endoscopic Ultrasound–Guided Fine Needle Aspiration in Biliary Lesions

Diagnosis and Staging of Cholangiocarcinoma

Cholangiocarcinoma is associated with a high mortality, and it is often difficult to obtain an accurate tissue diagnosis, with ERCP and brushings of the bile duct being the preferred modality for this purpose. The currently reported diagnostic yield from ERCP ranges from only 30% to 60%, and the diagnosis of malignant biliary stricture remains a challenge. EUS-guided FNA is now being used to diagnose and stage cholangiocarcinoma (see **Fig. 42.6**).[57,58] In the original case series describing the use of EUS in diagnosis of cholangiocarcinoma, 10 patients with bile duct strictures at the hepatic hilum, diagnosed by CT or ERCP or both, underwent EUS-guided FNA. Adequate material was obtained in nine patients. Cytology revealed cholangiocarcinoma in seven patients and hepatocellular carcinoma in one patient. One benign inflammatory lesion identified on cytology proved to be a false-negative finding by frozen section. Metastatic locoregional hilar lymph nodes were detected in two patients, and in one patient the celiac and paraaortic lymph nodes were aspirated to obtain tissue proof of distant metastasis.

In a second retrospective series of 238 patients with suspected or known biliary strictures, 35 patients with proximal bile duct strictures were identified. Of these, 27 were found to be malignant (23 cholangiocarcinomas, 3 gallbladder carcinomas, and 1 metastatic cancer), and 8 were benign. Of the 27 patients with malignancy, 17 underwent ERCP before EUS, and 10 underwent ERCP after EUS. A stricture was considered positive if a hypoechoic mass was seen on EUS around the common bile duct, or a positive tissue diagnosis was made by FNA. EUS-guided FNA was not done in one patient because ERCP had established the diagnosis. EUS-guided FNA obtained a tissue diagnosis of cholangiocarcinoma in 12 of 26 (46%) patients who had either negative brush cytology or an unsuccessful ERCP. EUS also correctly identified the eight benign strictures that had a clinical follow-up time of at least 8 months. There were no complications associated with EUS-guided FNA.

These studies suggest that EUS with FNA is safe and effective in evaluating proximal biliary strictures. Several additional studies, totaling 142 patients, have reported on the effect of EUS-guided FNA in evaluating biliary (including hilar) strictures, most of which had prior negative cytology with other tissue sampling modalities.[59-62] These studies have shown high sensitivities (80% to 90%) and overall accuracy rates (80% to 90%) with this technique. Even though the overall accuracy was high, this was due to the high percentage of malignancies in these series. One-quarter to one-third of patients with nonmalignant cytology on EUS-guided FNA were also ultimately diagnosed with malignancy. Given the low negative predictive values observed, a negative FNA result does not reliably exclude the possibility of malignancy. Nevertheless, this technique, when used in combination with ERCP, is extremely helpful in distinguishing benign from malignant strictures and in facilitating a definitive diagnosis by increasing tissue yield.

Another use of EUS-guided FNA is staging of cholangiocarcinoma via looking for perihepatic and distal lymphadenopathy. Assessing lymphadenopathy is not only important for staging patients before planned resection or chemotherapy, but it is also crucial in evaluating patients who are being considered for liver transplantation. A study comprising 44 patients with cholangiocarcinoma being evaluated with EUS before liver transplantation found 70 regional lymph nodes, with 9 of 70 nodes positive for malignancy[63]; this represented 8 of the 47 patients (18%). EUS detected 12 patients with lymph nodes not seen on standard imaging (CT or MRI). Of the 22 patients with negative lymph nodes by EUS and EUS-guided FNA, 20 (91%) had the EUS findings regarding their lymph node status confirmed. Two patients were found to have malignant perigastric lymph nodes at the time of surgery. An important additional finding of this study was that lymph node morphology and echo features did not predict malignant involvement and that EUS-guided FNA of all visualized lymph nodes in such patients is advised. Finally, in addition to cholangiocarcinoma, EUS-guided FNA has been found to be useful in diagnosing gallbladder masses, with sensitivity rates of 80% or greater for diagnosing malignancies.[62,64]

Diagnosis and Staging of Ampullary Cancer

Conventional abdominal imaging studies such as CT, MRI, and transabdominal ultrasound frequently fail to detect ampullary lesions. EUS is a sensitive modality for detecting and staging ampullary tumors. Accurate staging may be affected by biliary stent placement, which is frequently performed in these patients

with obstructive jaundice. Combined data from two centers reported the accuracy of ampullary tumor staging with multiple imaging modalities in patients with and patients without endobiliary stents.[65] Preoperative staging was performed in 50 consecutive patients with ampullary neoplasms by EUS plus CT (37 patients), MRI (13 patients), or angiography (10 patients) over a 3½-year period. Of the 50 patients, 25 had a transpapillary endobiliary stent present at the time of EUS examination. EUS was shown to be more accurate than CT and MRI in the overall assessment of the T stage of ampullary neoplasms (EUS 78%, CT 24%, MRI 46%). No significant difference in N stage accuracy was noted between the three imaging modalities (EUS 68%, CT 59%, MRI 77%). EUS T stage accuracy was reduced from 84% to 72% in the presence of a transpapillary endobiliary stent. This was most prominent in the understaging of T2 and T3 carcinomas.

A second retrospective study was published in which the role of EUS-guided FNA in the diagnosis and staging of ampullary lesions was reported.[66] EUS-guided FNA was performed in 20 of 27 (74%) patients with suspected ampullary tumors. EUS-guided FNA made the initial ampullary tissue diagnosis in seven patients (adenocarcinoma in five patients, adenoma in one patient, neuroendocrine tumor in one patient). In addition, EUS-guided FNA resulted in a change of the diagnosis from adenoma to adenocarcinoma in one patient. In one patient, EUS-guided FNA detected a liver metastasis not seen on CT. Overall, EUS-guided FNA provided new histologic information in 9 of 27 patients (33%).

Another study of 35 patients who underwent EUS-guided FNA of ampullary lesions, with follow-up available in 27 patients, revealed 13 patients with adenocarcinoma, 6 with atypical cells (4 suspicious for cancer and 2 consistent with reactive atypia), 2 with adenomas, 1 with carcinoid, and 13 with no evidence of malignancy.[67] Three false-negative studies were identified, yielding sensitivity 82.4%, specificity 100%, negative predictive value 76.9%, and overall accuracy 88.8% for EUS-guided FNA in diagnosing ampullary lesions.

A more recent study of 40 patients with adenoma and ampullary adenocarcinoma suggested that the use of intraductal ultrasound showed a trend toward improved T staging compared with standard EUS (78% vs. 63%), although this was nonsignificant ($P = .14$).[68] There was some concern that intraductal ultrasound may overstage lesions. Two recent studies comprising 68 patients found that EUS was comparable to CT or MRI in T and N staging of ampullary lesions.[69,70] Both studies showed about a 25% improvement in T staging accuracy with EUS, but this was not statistically significant because of the small number of subjects in each study.

Endoscopic Ultrasound–Guided Therapy for Pancreaticobiliary Lesions

Celiac Plexus Block and Celiac Plexus Neurolysis

Patients with significant abdominal pain who have unresectable pancreatic cancer may be candidates for EUS-guided celiac plexus neurolysis (CPN). Wiersema and Wiersema[71] described this novel technique and the impact on pain management of patients with pancreatic cancer. After visualizing the celiac trunk by the linear array echoendoscope and using a 22-gauge needle, injection of bupivacaine (0.25%) followed by ethyl alcohol (98%) can be performed on either side of the vessel. Of patients, 88% had persistent improvement in their pain score. Only minor complications were seen and consisted of transient diarrhea in four patients. This anterior transgastric approach for performing CPN is theoretically considered safer compared with the traditional CT-guided posterior method. Rare reported cases of paraplegia occurred with the posterior approach because of its proximity to the spinal column.

The effect of EUS-guided celiac plexus block (CPB) in controlling abdominal pain from chronic pancreatitis is less evident. Gress and colleagues[72] performed EUS-guided CPB in 80 patients with chronic pancreatitis. A mixture of bupivacaine 0.25% and 80 mg of triamcinolone (the substitution of steroid for alcohol distinguishes CPB from CPN) was injected using the above-described technique. Only 10% had benefit beyond 24 weeks. There were two major complications: peripancreatic abscess and bleeding from the celiac artery secondary to ethanol-induced arterial pseudoaneurysm. This technique was less effective in younger patients (<45 years old) and patients who had previous surgery for chronic pancreatitis. There was a slight economical advantage of EUS-guided CPB over the CT-guided approach ($1200 vs. $1400).

The findings of superior results with EUS-guided CPN in patients with cancer compared with EUS-guided CPB in patients with chronic pancreatitis were corroborated by a meta-analysis of eight studies of EUS-guided CPN comprising 283 patients and nine studies of EUS-guided CPB comprising 376 patients.[73] The results showed pain relief in 80.12% of patients with cancer and in only 59.45% of patients with chronic pancreatitis. A randomized trial of single versus bilateral injections of the same amount of medication during EUS-guided CPB in 51 patients with chronic pancreatitis was performed to determine if the suboptimal response rate in these patients could be improved. The results showed no difference between the injection techniques with regard to the overall response rates (56.5% for single injection, 53.6% for bilateral injection), the total duration of pain relief, or the onset of pain relief.[74]

Another study comparing single with bilateral injections that included patients with both chronic pancreatitis and pancreatic cancer and CPB and CPN in each group reached a different conclusion. This prospective, consecutive, nonrandomized study evaluated 89 patients receiving bilateral injections and compared them with 71 patients receiving a central injection. The group receiving bilateral injections had a mean pain reduction of 70.4%, which was significantly better than the 45.9% achieved by the group receiving a central injection.[75] Both groups had roughly equal numbers of patients with cancer and chronic pancreatitis and were similar in the percentages in each group undergoing CPB versus CPN. The only observed complication was in a single anticoagulated patient who developed self-limited bleeding secondary to a laceration of the left adrenal artery after a bilateral injection.

Routine bilateral injection may be preferred to routine central injection when performing a CPN or CPB in patients with abdominal pain secondary to pancreatic cancer or chronic pancreatitis. However, based on the available data, it is unclear whether this approach is beneficial in patients with benign pancreatic disease. The current technique of either bilateral or central EUS-guided CPN or CPB seems to be safe

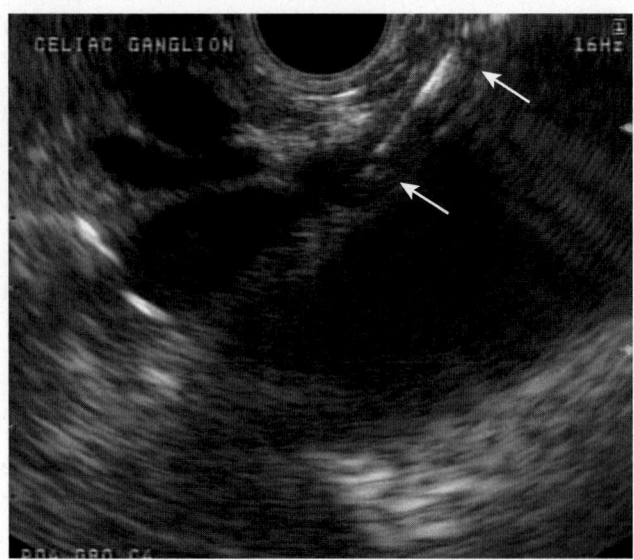

Fig. 42.7   Endoscopic ultrasound (EUS)–guided celiac ganglion neurolysis in a patient with chronic pancreatitis. The needle is seen within a celiac ganglion.

because others have more recently reported similarly low rates (1.8% [4 of 220]) of known complications including asymptomatic hypotension ($n = 1$), self-limited postprocedural pain ($n = 2$), or retroperitoneal abscess ($n = 1$).[76]

In 2006, two groups showed the ability of EUS to identify the celiac ganglia accurately.[77,78] This development potentially allows for a more focused delivery of medication to achieve neurolysis or nerve block (**Fig. 42.7**). In addition, it may allow for consideration of alcohol injection (CPN) for patients with pain from chronic pancreatitis. A subsequent prospective study of 200 patients undergoing EUS for various indications found that 81% had identifiable celiac ganglia at the time of EUS.[79] Female sex and no prior history of abdominal surgery were predictive of ganglion visualization. Among patients with visualized ganglia, linear echoendoscopes identified more ganglia per patient than radial echoendoscopes.

A retrospective study of 33 patients undergoing 36 ganglia injections (18 in patients with cancer, 18 in patients with chronic pancreatitis) found that 94% (16 of 17) of patients with cancer and 80% (4 of 5) of patients with chronic pancreatitis who received EUS-guided CPN into the ganglia reported pain relief compared with 0% (0 of 1) and 38% (5 of 13) when EUS-guided CPB was performed.[80] Patients with initial pain exacerbation secondary to injection of the ganglia seemed to have a significantly improved therapeutic response. These findings suggest that intraganglionic injections may improve response rates to EUS-guided CPN in patients with both benign and malignant disease. Prospective, randomized trials evaluating EUS-guided CPN and CPB into the ganglia are either under way or being planned. The results of these trials in patients with pain from benign and malignant pancreatic disease will serve to delineate better the efficacy and safety of this novel technique and to clarify its indications.

Cyst Gastrostomy

Endoscopic therapy for pseudocyst drainage is an established alternative for surgical and radiologic approaches. Since the initial report of EUS-assisted pseudocyst drainage,[81] the use of EUS as the sole tool for draining pseudocysts has been evolving. This approach became feasible with the development of larger accessory channel echoendoscopes. EUS-guided pseudocyst drainage technique overcomes many obstacles associated with the conventional endoscopic approach. In the absence of an apparent intraluminal bulge, common in cysts in the region of the pancreatic tail, cyst drainage can still be safely performed after an accurate measurement of the distance between the cyst and the GI wall, with a distance of less than 1 cm between the GI wall and cyst lumens recommended. EUS imaging with color flow and Doppler techniques can be used to define and avoid any intervening vessels.

These advantages theoretically can reduce the risk of hemorrhage and perforation. However, significant bleeding after EUS-guided cyst gastrostomy requiring angiographic embolization has been reported.[82] In cases where cystic neoplasms are a concern, cyst fluid aspiration should be performed before drainage. The level of tumor markers in the fluid, mainly CEA, and the concentration of amylase may assist in differentiating inflammatory from neoplastic cysts.[83,84] Careful assessment of the cyst is important and can exclude patients with cysts that may be malignant, patients with cysts that are unlikely to be technically feasible, or patients who are poor candidates for successful endoscopic therapy. Previous studies suggest that EUS may exclude 5% to 37% of patients referred for cyst gastrostomy for these reasons.[85,86]

We use a therapeutic linear echoendoscope and perform EUS-guided FNA with a 19-gauge needle of the cyst lumen, followed by, if needed, fluid aspiration for CEA and amylase analysis. The tract chosen should be less than 1 cm from lumen to lumen and be avascular. Subsequently, we place a 0.035-inch guidewire through the needle into the cyst and advance the wire under fluoroscopic guidance until multiple loops of wire are seen within the cyst. The FNA needle is backed out and replaced by an over-the-wire needle-knife, which is used to puncture the GI tract and enter the cyst. The needle-knife is exchanged over the wire for a 10-mm biliary dilating balloon, which is inflated for 3 to 5 minutes to provide an adequate opening to access and drain the cyst and to achieve tamponade of any bleeding that may occur. On balloon deflation, a large amount of fluid usually enters the gastric lumen and requires vigorous suctioning to maintain a luminal view. Once visualization can be maintained, the balloon is exchanged over the wire for a 10-Fr double-pigtail stent.

After the first stent is successfully deployed and confirmed in proper position via endoscopy and fluoroscopy, we reinsert the guidewire into the cyst alongside the first stent, and once it is properly coiled in the cyst on fluoroscopy, we place a second 10-Fr double-pigtail stent before completing the procedure. Nasocystic drainage is appropriate if evidence of infection or solid or thick debris is present within the cyst. Some authors have proposed placing fully covered self-expanding metal stents instead of one or two plastic stents and reported a 95% (17 of 18) technical success rate with 14 of 18 patients (78%) achieving complete resolution of pancreatic fluid collections with a mean time to final resolution of 77 days.[87]

Antibiotics should be administered during and after the procedure. Complications from this technique occur in less than 5% of patients undergoing the EUS technique, which appears reduced compared with direct endoscopic or surgical techniques.[86,88-90] Complications typically have included

hemorrhage, infection, perforation, or pneumoperitoneum. Stent migration into the cyst should occur rarely if pigtailed stents are used; however, should this occur, endoscopic stent retrieval and repositioning is feasible and has been reported.[91]

Several published studies have reported the efficacy of this technique. Giovannini and coworkers[92] drained 35 pancreatic cysts under EUS guidance, of whom 15 had pseudocysts and 20 had pancreatic abscesses. Of the 33 cysts drained via a transgastric approach, an extrinsic compression was seen in only one patient using a forward-viewing gastroscope. No major complications occurred except for a single case of a pneumoperitoneum, which was successfully managed medically. No bleeding was encountered. A 7-Fr nasocystic drain was placed in 18 of 20 cases of pancreatic abscess. Surgery was performed in the two other patients. In the pseudocyst group, placement of an 8.5-Fr stent was successful in 10 patients, and placement of a nasocystic drain was done in 5 patients. In one case, only cyst puncture and aspiration was performed. Over a mean follow-up of 27 months (range 6 to 48 months), one recurrence among the 15 pancreatic pseudocysts and two relapses of the 18 pancreatic abscesses were observed. The EUS-guided drainage success rate was 88.5% (31 of 35); only 4 patients with pancreatic abscesses underwent surgery.

In a related article, Seifert and associates[93] evaluated a new one-step device for stent placement using a large-channel echoendoscope (3.2 mm) for pseudocyst drainage in six patients. One of these patients had a pancreatic abscess. Transmural drainage was successfully done using modified 7-Fr diameter stents. No complications were encountered with the endoscopic interventions. One patient with necrotizing pancreatitis, who denied surgery, died secondary to sepsis. At follow-up of 3 to 13 months, the cysts had completely resolved in four patients. This study confirmed the feasibility and effectiveness of the EUS-guided one-step technique in draining various cystic lesions; however, larger studies are needed. In a subsequent study and using the one-step device through a 3.7-mm channel echoendoscope, the same group was able to place a 10-Fr stent in three patients and a 7-Fr stent in one patient, all with peripancreatic cystic lesions. One of the cysts had persisted for more than 3 months and was found to be a ganglioneuroma after surgical enucleation.[94]

Several comparative trials have been reported more recently evaluating endoscopic, EUS-guided, and surgical cyst gastrostomy. A retrospective study comparing 10 patients who had undergone a surgical approach with 20 patients who underwent EUS-guided cyst gastrostomy found no differences in clinical outcomes between the modalities but reported a reduction in postprocedure hospital stay (6.5 days for surgery vs. 2.65 days for the EUS approach), which resulted in a significant cost savings of $5738 per patient.[95]

A randomized controlled trial comparing two groups of 15 patients undergoing cyst gastrostomy has also been performed.[96] In the group undergoing pseudocyst drainage with conventional endoscopy, technical success was achieved in only 5 of 15 patients, with two bleeding complications and one death. All 10 patients with technical failures were crossed over to EUS-guided cyst gastrostomy, and technical success was achieved. The EUS-guided group had 14 of 14 patients achieve technical success (one cyst was correctly diagnosed as a biliary cystadenoma at EUS and excluded from drainage). No significant differences in clinical success rates or complications among the groups were noted, although the study appeared underpowered to make this determination.

A third study prospectively evaluated 99 consecutive patients presenting for endoscopic cyst gastrostomy. Patients without obvious portal hypertension and with a visible bulge on endoscopy underwent conventional endoscopic cyst gastrostomy ($n = 53$), and the remainder ($n = 46$) underwent the procedure with EUS guidance. Patients were followed prospectively, with cross-sectional imaging during clinic visits. Short-term (1-month) and long-term (6-month) results regarding effectiveness and complications were collected. No significant differences between the two groups regarding short-term success (93% vs. 94%) or long-term success (84% vs. 91%) were seen. Complications occurred in 19% of the EUS group and 18% of the conventional endoscopy group and consisted of bleeding ($n = 3$), infection ($n = 8$), stent migration ($n = 3$), and pneumoperitoneum ($n = 5$). All complications except one were managed conservatively.

Given these data, the EUS-guided approach seems to be more technically feasible overall, especially for pancreatic tail cysts, which often do not exhibit any intramural bulge and may be associated with reduced complication rates. Because the same stents are used for both endoscopic and EUS-guided approaches, it is not surprising that the clinical outcomes are similar when technical success is achieved. Although this technique is typically used for the drainage of uncomplicated pseudocysts, its use for the treatment of abscesses and pancreatic necrosis has also been reported.

Delivery of Antitumor Agents

We have examined the feasibility and safety of direct injection of allogeneic mixed lymphocyte culture (cytoimplant) in pancreatic adenocarcinoma under EUS guidance.[97] In a phase I clinical trial, eight patients with unresectable pancreatic adenocarcinoma underwent EUS-guided FNI of cytoimplants. Four patients were in stage II, three were in stage III, and one was in stage IV. Escalating doses of cytoimplants of 3 billion, 6 billion, or 9 billion cells were implanted using a novel EUS-guided FNI technique. The median survival was 13.2 months with two partial responders and one minor response. Major complications including bone marrow toxicity, hemorrhage, infections, renal toxicity, or cardiopulmonary toxicity were absent. Low-grade fever was encountered in seven of the eight patients and was symptomatically treated with acetaminophen.

Our study showed that local immunotherapy is feasible and safe. The technique of EUS-guided FNI was later applied to deliver antitumor viral therapy.[98] ONYX-015 (dl1520) is an E1B-55kD gene-deleted replication-selective adenovirus that preferentially replicates in and kills malignant cells. Over 8 weeks, 21 patients with locally advanced adenocarcinoma of the pancreas or with metastatic disease but minimal or absent liver metastases underwent eight sessions of ONYX-015 delivered by EUS injection into the primary pancreatic tumor. The final four treatments were given in combination with gemcitabine (1000 mg/m^2 intravenously). After combination therapy, 2 patients had partial regressions of the injected tumor, 2 had minor responses, 6 had stable disease, and 11 had progressive disease. No clinical pancreatitis occurred despite mild, transient elevations in lipase in a few patients. Two patients had sepsis before the institution of prophylactic

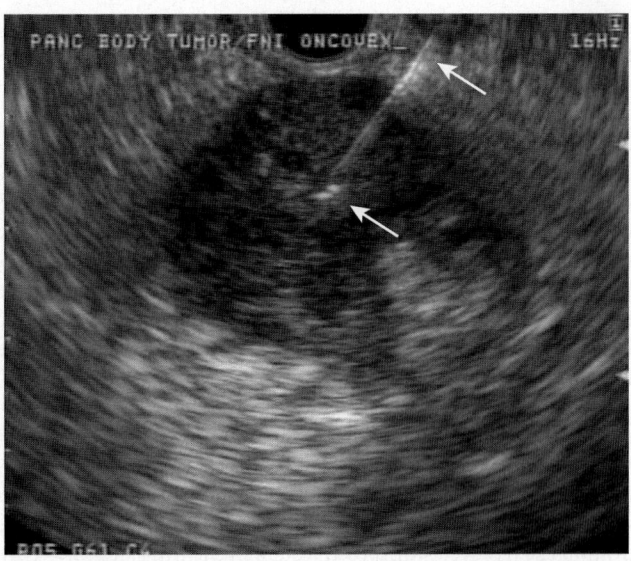

Fig. 42.8 Endoscopic ultrasound (EUS)–guided fine needle injection (FNI) using TNFerade in a patient with locally advanced pancreatic cancer.

oral antibiotics. Two patients had duodenal perforations from the rigid endoscope tip. No perforations occurred after the protocol was changed to transgastric injections only.

The most recent EUS-guided antitumor therapy involves novel gene therapies.[99] TNFerade, which involves a novel gene transfer approach, is the newest EUS-guided antitumor therapy (**Fig. 42.8**).[99-101] The attractiveness of this new approach is the potential to maximize local antitumor activity and minimize systemic toxicity. TNFerade was constructed as a second-generation (E1-deleted, partial E3-deleted, and E4-deleted) adenovector, expressing the cDNA encoding human tumor necrosis factor (TNF). To optimize local effectiveness further and minimize systemic toxicity, the radiation-inducible immediate response *Egr-1* (early growth response) promoter was placed upstream of the transcriptional start site of the human TNF cDNA. This vector was engineered to ensure that maximal gene expression and subsequent TNF secretion are constrained in space and time by radiation therapy. A synergistic "triple threat" is formulated: (1) 5-Fluorouracil chemotherapy is directly toxic to cancer cells and is a radiosensitizer, (2) external beam radiation destroys cancer cells and upregulates TNF production, and (3) TNFerade causes cancer cell death and is itself a radiosensitizer.

TNFerade in combination with radiation therapy has been studied in preclinical and early clinical (phase I) trials with encouraging results.[102,103] The study design consisted of a 5-week treatment of weekly intratumoral injections of TNFerade (4×10^9, 10^{10}, and 10^{11} particle units in 2 mL). EUS-guided FNI was compared with percutaneous approaches (CT or ultrasound). TNFerade was combined with continuous intravenous 5-fluorouracil (200 mg/m^2/day × 5 days/wk) and radiation (50.4 Gy). TNFerade was delivered with a single needle pass at a single site in the tumor for percutaneous approaches; up to four injections were given by EUS. The long-term results from a cohort of 50 patients showed that toxicities potentially related to TNFerade were mild and well tolerated.[100] Compared with two lower dose cohorts ($n = 30$), the higher dose group ($n = 11$) was associated with greater locoregional control of treated tumors, longer progression-free survival, a greater proportion of patients with stable or decreasing levels of CA 19.9, a greater percentage (45%) of patients undergoing resection, and improved median survival (6.6 months, 8.8 months, 11.2 months, and 10.9 months, in the 4×10^9, 4×10^{10}, 4×10^{11}, or 1×10^{12} particle units cohorts). At the 4×10^{11} dose, four of five patients whose tumors became surgically resectable achieved pathologically negative margins, and three survived more than 24 months.

Among patients receiving TNFerade who underwent resection, we achieved a complete pathologic response with no residual tumor at surgical resection.[101] However, this patient developed hepatic and bilateral pulmonary metastases slightly more than 1 year after resection and died 19 months after receiving the initial TNFerade injection.

We reported a survival analysis (from phase II and III clinical trials) of TNF treatment conducted at a single site. Between January 2003 and November 2008, 29 patients were treated: 20 patients with TNFerade plus standard of care (5-fluorouracil and radiation therapy) and 9 patients with standard of care only. TNFerade plus standard of care resulted in a median survival of 14.7 months versus 11.1 months for patients receiving only standard of care. These results are encouraging and are consistent with results across both multicenter trials that show a trend toward improvement in survival after the addition of TNFerade biologic to standard of care. A large, multicenter, randomized controlled trial evaluating the use of TNFerade in patients with locally advanced pancreatic cancer is ongoing.

Another oncolytic viral therapy for pancreatic cancer using a herpes simplex virus carrying the granulocyte-macrophage colony-stimulating factor gene (OncoVEXGM-CSF) has been developed (**Fig. 42.9**).[104] It remains to be seen which virus and encoded product combination will achieve the best results in this nascent field of viral oncolytic therapy.

Two additional therapies delivered by EUS-guided FNI have also been reported more recently. The first involves injecting immature dendritic cells into patients with pancreatic cancer to induce a T cell–dependent immune response.[105] Dendritic cells are powerful antigen-presenting cells that can initiate a strong tumor-specific immune response. Injections were done on days 1, 8, and 15 of each 28-day cycle. Seven patients with metastatic pancreatic cancer who were refractory to gemcitabine chemotherapy underwent EUS-guided FNI of immature dendritic cells; no complications were observed, and technical success was achieved in all cases. The median survival of 9.9 months in these patients was thought to be encouraging given their advanced disease at the time of the initiation of this therapy.

The second therapy involves treating cystic pancreatic tumors with ethanol lavage and paclitaxel injection.[106] This technique involves aspirating the cyst with a 22-gauge needle until it collapses while maintaining the needle tip within the cyst. The cyst is irrigated and lavaged with pure (99%) ethanol for 3 to 5 minutes, followed by reaspiration of all the injected ethanol and injection of the cyst cavity with a 3 mg/mL solution of paclitaxel diluted 1:1 with 0.9% saline. The amount of paclitaxel and saline solution reinjected was equal to the amount of fluid originally withdrawn from the cyst. A study of 14 patients with a median cyst size of 25.5 mm who were followed for a median of 9 months showed complete cyst resolution in 11 patients, partial resolution in 2 patients, and a persistent cyst in 1 patient. This technique holds promise for patients with indeterminate or mucinous cysts as an alternative to surgery or surveillance.

All of these new techniques and initial reports have established that EUS-guided FNI is an effective delivery system for antitumor agents. More definitive data regarding the clinical efficacy of these techniques are awaited.

Accessing the Pancreaticobiliary System

EUS-guided FNA and FNI can be used to access dilated pancreatic and biliary systems to perform cholangiography or pancreatography through contrast agent injection and provide decompression and drainage via the ampulla using rendezvous techniques or through the creation of transenteric fistulas. The initial EUS-guided injection of contrast agent through the duodenal wall into the common bile duct was first reported by Wiersema and colleagues[107] in 1996 as an alternative method for performing cholangiopancreatography in patients in whom ERCP had failed. This technique also has been used to provide ductal imaging and locate the minor papilla when it had not been identifiable at ERCP, using a combination of contrast agent and methylene blue.[108] Although technically feasible, direct injection of contrast agent into the bile duct or pancreatic duct for diagnostic purposes in the era of magnetic resonance cholangiopancreatography should be avoided unless subsequent therapy or drainage during the procedure is planned.

EUS-guided contrast agent injection followed by guidewire placement through either the duodenum or the stomach may also salvage difficult ERCP cannulations via EUS-guided rendezvous techniques, first reported by Mallery and colleagues in 2004.[109] In these techniques, a wire is passed across the major papilla to achieve biliary drainage or the major or minor papilla to achieve pancreatic duct drainage. Although the approach is usually transduodenal for biliary access and transgastric for pancreatic duct access, transhepatic cholangiography

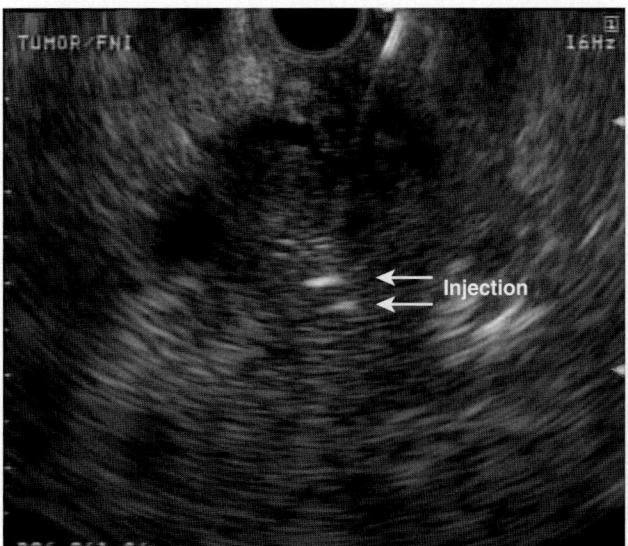

Fig. 42.9 Endoscopic ultrasound (EUS)–guided fine needle injection (FNI) of antitumor agent (OncoVEXGM-CSF) in a patient with pancreatic cancer.

performed from the stomach with subsequent rendezvous ERCP and stent placement has been reported.[110] Once the wire traverses the papilla, the EUS scope is replaced with a duodenoscope, and a second wire is passed adjacent to the EUS-placed wire into the desired duct, if possible. If this is not achievable, the EUS-placed wire is grabbed and brought through the biopsy channel of the scope, and the procedure is completed in the standard ERCP fashion.

A series of 23 patients undergoing EUS-guided cholangiography (13 via a transhepatic approach and 10 via a transcholedochal approach) with subsequent rendezvous ERCP found that drainage could be achieved in 21 patients, with transpapillary drainage being achieved in 18 and choledochoenteric fistula creation being required in 3. Complications included one bile leak, two cases of self-limited pneumoperitoneum, and one case of minor bleeding. The transhepatic approach was believed to be safer than the transcholedochal approach, possibly owing to reduced intraperitoneal spillage of bile.[111]

There are special situations after failed ERCP cannulation where EUS-guided passage of a wire into the pancreatic duct or biliary tree is needed to assist in transmural drainage as an alternative to percutaneous or surgical approaches. These cases usually occur when the major and minor papillae are inaccessible or not identifiable or when EUS-guided rendezvous attempts have failed, necessitating the need for alternative drainage techniques. Two reports showed the feasibility of therapeutic EUS-guided cholangiography or pancreatography with stent placement in patients with failed cannulation at ERCP. Burmester and coworkers[112] successfully performed EUS-guided cholangiography-assisted drainage in three of four patients with malignant biliary strictures in which ERCP was impossible. They used a modification of the one-step method for performing pancreatic pseudocyst drainage described by Seifert and colleagues.[93] The technique was performed by transgastric, transduodenal, and transjejunal approaches. Access and direct drainage via the proximal biliary tree has been described with EUS-guided hepaticogastrostomy.[111,112] These preliminary reports show that EUS-guided cholangiopancreatography with duct decompression can be successfully performed in patients in whom ERCP has failed.

Pancreatic duct decompression and drainage can also be achieved through the creation of enteropancreatic fistulas. Kahaleh and associates[113] performed EUS-guided pancreatography with subsequent gastropancreatic duct stent placement in two patients. These patients had complicated pancreatitis with pancreatic duct strictures where surgical reconstruction precluded access to the papilla. One patient developed upper GI bleeding 24 hours after the procedure, which was thought to be related to the needle tract. The bleeding was treated endoscopically. The second patient had no procedure-related complications. Both patients had improvement in symptoms 1 month after the procedure. Two larger series evaluating this technique in a combined 49 patients both achieved success rates of greater than 80%.[114,115] Four complications occurred (8% of patients): bleeding in two patients, pancreatitis in one patient, and a perforation in one patient.

We believe transmural pancreatic duct drainage procedures should be performed with great caution or avoided altogether in patients with a normal pancreas because of the increased risk of pancreatitis in these patients. Most experience with direct injection into the pancreatic duct and with pancreatic duct decompression has been in patients with established chronic pancreatitis in whom the risk of iatrogenic pancreatitis is less. Larger studies with long-term follow-up are needed to determine fully the safety and efficacy of these techniques.

Brachytherapy and Placement of Fiducial Markers

EUS-guided FNI has increasingly been used to facilitate or provide radiation therapy to malignant lesions. This technique has been used to place radiographic, or fiducial, markers within focal lesions in the mediastinum and abdomen to facilitate image-guided radiation therapy (**Fig. 42.10**). EUS-guided FNI is an attractive alternative to surgical or percutaneous placement of these markers because it has fewer risks and limitations. It particularly seems useful in accessing lesions in the posterior mediastinum and abdomen.

The fiducial markers used are typically 3 or 5 mm long cylindrical gold seeds with a 1.2 mm diameter that may be

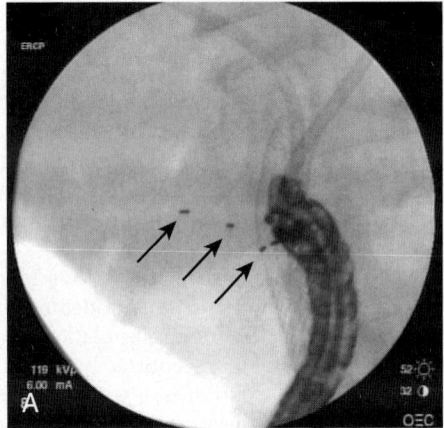
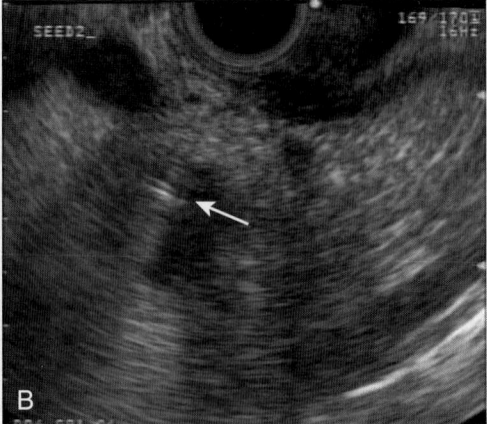

Fig. 42.10 **A,** Fiducial markers placed under endoscopic ultrasound (EUS) and fluoroscopy in a patient with locally advanced pancreatic cancer. Fluoroscopy image shows three markers in place. **B,** Fiducial markers placed under EUS and fluoroscopy in a patient with locally advanced pancreatic cancer. EUS image shows fiducial marker in place.

placed through a 19-gauge needle. Three to six seeds are placed preferably 2 cm apart in separate planes along the borders of the lesion to allow optimal lesion demarcation before focused radiotherapy. We typically place seeds one at a time, although multiple seeds can be placed during one needle injection if careful needle advancement is performed. Ideally, we prefer preloading the markers into the 19-gauge needle by retracting the stylet a few centimeters, inserting the seeds at the distal needle tip, and sealing the tip with bone wax. This approach avoids the air artifact that has been reported when the seeds are inserted into the needle handle and advanced into the lesion via the stylet after FNA of the target lesion has been performed.

EUS-guided fiducial marker placement was reported to have a high rate of success (85% [11 of 13]) in one more recent series of mediastinal and abdominal lesions for which fiducial marker placement was requested.[116] Fiducial markers could not be placed on two lesions because of the inability of the EUS needle to access the target lesion adequately or safely. In one lesion, an intervening blood vessel (the aorta) precluded needle advancement, and in the second lesion, a gastric outlet obstruction precluded accessing the lesion anatomically. The authors noted some difficulty passing a 5 mm long marker through the stiff 19-gauge needle when angulation of the tip of the scope was required, necessitating the placement of shorter 3-mm seeds in some cases.

A report of a prototype forward-viewing linear echoendoscope (XGIF-UCT 160 J-AL5; Olympus America Inc, Center Valley, PA) that was used to place fiducial markers in a perirectal lesion suggested this echoendoscope may facilitate advancement of the stiffer 19-gauge needle into targeted lesions, especially when the lesions are firm, allowing routine placement of the preferred 5 mm long seeds.[117] This facilitation with this echoendoscope may be due to the fact that the working channel is in line with the shaft of the echoendoscope, allowing for needle advancement and fiducial marker placement to be performed in a straight plane rather than tangentially.

EUS-guided FNI may also be used to place radioactive seeds within lesions to provide brachytherapy (**Fig. 42.11**). This technique also uses a 19-gauge needle in which the seeds are backloaded into the needle and sealed with bone wax before insertion into the echoendoscope. We initially reported on the successful placement of radioactive iodine (iodine 125) seeds via EUS-guided FNI in a patient with recurrent malignant lymphadenopathy after esophagectomy that was not visualized on CT imaging and required EUS for radioactive seed placement[118]; several more recent studies have focused on this technique for the treatment of advanced pancreatic cancer. EUS-guided brachytherapy was reported to have a 100% technical success rate in a series of 22 patients with locally advanced pancreatic cancer who received this treatment in conjunction with chemotherapy.[119] No complications occurred, and the authors noted a transient improvement in pain but no long-term survival benefit with this approach.

A second study of 15 patients with unresectable pancreatic cancer using EUS-guided FNI of iodine-125 seeds found 30% showed some clinical benefit, whereas 20% (3 of 15) had localized complications of pancreatitis and pseudocyst formation.[120] A more recent report in a porcine model suggests placement of iodine-125 seeds adjacent to the celiac ganglia via EUS-guided FNI may induce neuronal apoptosis and may provide palliation of pain in patients with advanced pancreatic cancer.[121] Future studies are needed to determine the utility and indications for this use of this novel technique.

Technical Considerations

The technique of EUS-guided FNA has been well described in the literature.[39,122–127] Specifically, the area of interest is visualized by EUS and placed within the center (or just slightly left of center on the monitor) of the imaging field. Doppler imaging is used as needed to identify vascularity of the lesion and to assess adjacent vascular structures. The needle, with the stylet slightly withdrawn to provide a sharp needle tip, is advanced through the endoscope biopsy channel and advanced into the lesion under direct ultrasound visualization, avoiding any possible intervening vascular structures. The central stylet is advanced to remove any tissue that may be present in the needle as a result of the transluminal puncture and subsequently completely removed. A 10-mL syringe is attached to

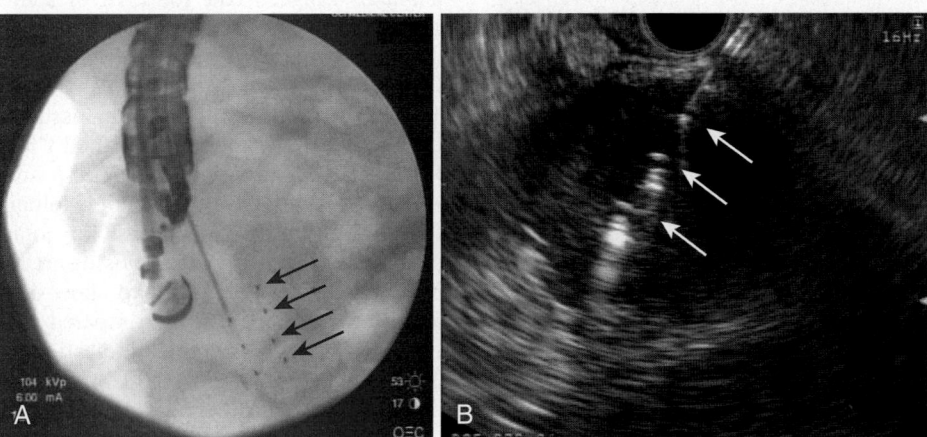

Fig. 42.11 **A,** Endoscopic ultrasound (EUS)–guided brachytherapy using a 19-gauge needle and radioactive iodine seeds *(small arrows)* in a patient with recurrent duodenal cancer. **B,** Corresponding EUS image shows placement of radioactive seeds.

the hub of the needle, and suction is applied as the needle is moved back and forth within the lesion (we typically perform 10 to-and-fro cycles). The suction is slowly released, the needle is retracted in the catheter, and the entire assembly is removed from the biopsy channel.

The aspirated material is sprayed onto glass slides (using an air-filled syringe); a set of two slides is processed immediately and reviewed by an attendant or nearby cytopathologist if available. If residual material is present within the needle, this is rinsed into a formalin container, which is collected and later processed into a cell block. More recently, we have adopted a slightly altered technique for solid pancreatic lesions that uses only the slow withdrawal of the stylet to provide negative pressure as the needle is moved back and forth within the lesion. We believe this technique may reduce the amount of blood in the specimen and improve the diagnostic yield.

Generally, placing the FNA needle directly into the center of the targeted lesion is appropriate. However, this may not be the optimal technique for large tumors, especially tumors arising from the pancreas. The center of large tumors may be necrotic, possibly from decreased oxygenation. If initial passes from the center show necrotic cells or acellular material, the endosonographer should realign the needle to target the periphery of the tumor. In addition, our experience suggests that targeting the precise site of obstruction of ductal structures seems to provide a particularly high-quality cellular specimen.

Studies regarding whether the choice of needle affects overall diagnostic yield or accuracy have yielded mixed results (**Fig. 42.12**). A study of 24 patients with solid pancreatic masses who underwent attempted tissue sampling with a 25-gauge, 22-gauge, and TCB (discussed subsequently) showed similar diagnostic accuracy rates of 91.7%, 95%, and 91.7% when technical success was achieved with each needle. However, technical success rates were significantly lower (50%) with the TCB, owing to its difficulty in accessing head and uncinate lesions, which lead to overall accuracy rates of 91.7%, 79.7%, and 54.1%. These findings suggested no statistically significant difference in overall diagnostic accuracy

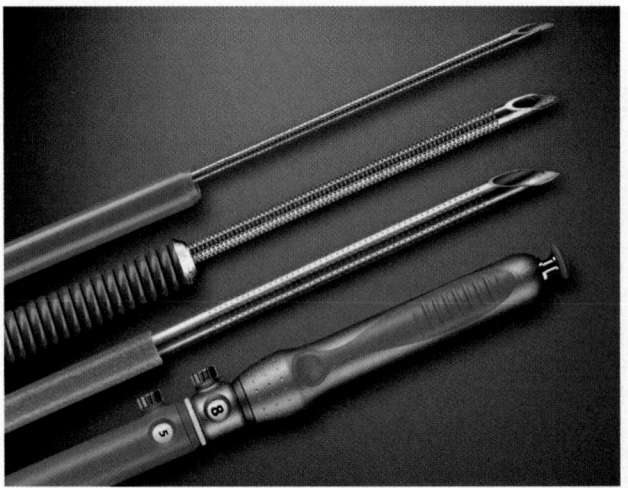

Fig. 42.12 EchoTip Ultra with HDFNA (Cook Medical, Orange, CA). *From top to bottom:* 25-gauge, 22-gauge, 19-gauge and handle. *(Courtesy of Cook Medical, Orange, CA.)*

between the 25-gauge and 22-gauge needles, although the authors commented that the 25-gauge needle was easier to use and was associated with significantly higher technical success rates compared with the 22-gauge needle for uncinate lesions.[128]

A similar study of 12 patients with pancreatic masses who underwent FNA with both 25-gauge and 22-gauge needles found no difference in cellularity with either needle, but three needle failures were seen in the 25-gauge group. A diagnosis was made in all cases.[129] A prospective, randomized controlled trial of 25-gauge ($n = 67$) versus 22-gauge ($n = 64$) needles for solid pancreatic masses found diagnostic accuracy rates of 95.5% versus 87.5% for the two needles. A similar number of passes was needed to achieve a diagnosis for each needle, and the findings were not statistically significant. The authors noted that the study may have been underpowered to detect small differences (up to 10%) in diagnostic accuracy.

In contrast to these data, two more recent larger studies have found significant improvement with the use of a 25-gauge needle in the diagnosis of solid pancreatic masses via EUS-guided FNA. The first study comprised 842 patients with pancreatic masses on EUS over a 6-year period who underwent EUS-guided FNA with a 22-gauge ($n = 540$) or 25-gauge ($n = 302$) needle. Sensitivity, specificity, positive predictive value, and negative predictive value were 84%, 100%, 100%, and 49% for the 22-gauge group and 92%, 97%, 98%, and 89% for the 25-gauge group. No complications were seen in the 25-gauge group; pancreatitis was reported in 2% of the 22-gauge group.[130] Our group reported on 100 patients with pancreatic masses undergoing EUS-guided FNA in each of two distinct time groups. The 22-gauge needle had sensitivity, specificity, positive predictive value, and negative predictive value of 88%, 100%, 100%, and 67% compared with 99%, 100%, 100%, and 93% for the 25-gauge needle. In patients ultimately diagnosed with a pancreatic malignancy, 95% achieved a diagnosis within two passes using a 25-gauge needle compared with only 88% achieving a diagnosis after six passes with a 22-gauge needle. No complications occurred in either group.[131]

Both of these latter studies and the randomized controlled trial suggest an 8% to 10% enhanced diagnostic yield with a 25-gauge needle. As a result, the specificity of the 25-gauge needle seems to be superior to the 22-gauge needle because of a reduction in the number of false-negative FNA results. We use a 25-gauge needle for FNA of solid pancreatic masses because of its apparent improved diagnostic accuracy, rapid diagnostic capability, and overall ease of use in traversing these firm lesions.

A more recent advance in our tissue sampling armamentarium was the introduction of the EUS-guided TCB in 2002 (**Fig. 42.13**). This needle containing an 18-mm tissue tray allows for histologic, rather than cytologic, analysis owing to the ability of EUS-guided TCB to obtain tissue cores that enable the assessment of both tissue architecture and cellularity. EUS-guided TCB seems to allow improved diagnosis of autoimmune pancreatitis compared with standard EUS-FNA.[132,133] Other suggested indications where EUS-guided TCB may be preferred over EUS-guided FNA include in the diagnosis of well-differentiated neoplasms, vascular lesions, and cystic or metastatic pancreatic tumors.[134]

Although EUS-guided TCB offers the theoretical advantage of diagnosing early chronic pancreatitis owing to its

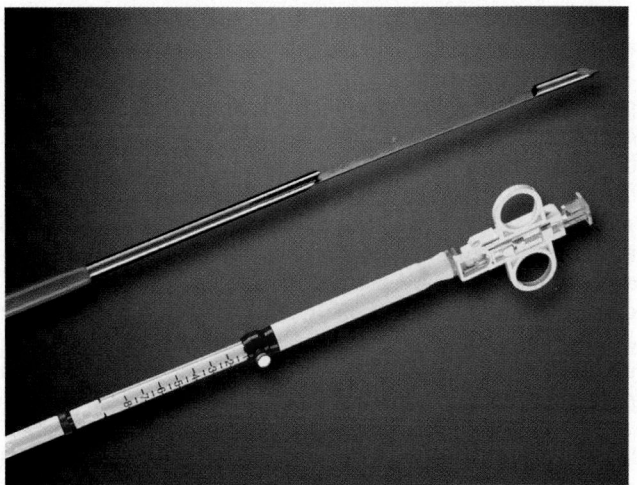

Fig. 42.13 Quick-Core (Cook Medical, Orange, CA) 19-gauge needle. *(Courtesy of Cook Medical, Orange, CA.)*

Table 42.4 Sequence Priority for Endoscopic Ultrasound–Guided Fine Needle Aspiration in a Patient with a Pancreatic Tumor

Target Site	Average No. Passes	Sequence Priority
Mediastinal lymph nodes	2 (range 1–5)	1
Ascites or pleural fluid	1	2
Liver	2 (range 1–5)	3
Distant (e.g., celiac) lymph node	2 (range 1–10)	4
Proximal lymph node	2 (range 1–10)	5
Pancreatic tumor	3–5 (range 1–19)	6

ability to obtain a core tissue specimen, the only study to date looking at this issue found that only 1 of 16 patients with suspected nonfocal chronic pancreatitis had tissue confirmation with EUS-TCB, leading the authors to discourage its use for this indication.[135] In addition, several studies have reported that although no significant difference was noted in diagnostic yields or accuracy between FNA and TCB,[136,137] the combination of the two modalities may be better than either alone.[138] As mentioned earlier, a comparative study of 25-gauge, 22-gauge, and TCB needles in 24 patients with solid pancreatic lesions showed EUS-guided TCB achieved the lowest accuracy rates, a result almost entirely due to the fact that EUS-guided TCB was deployed successfully in only 11 of 24 patients and in only 1 of 12 patients with head or uncinate lesions.[128]

The most recent and largest study of 113 patients undergoing EUS-guided TCB of pancreatic lesions also showed that EUS-guided TCB had a relatively poor sensitivity and overall diagnostic accuracy of 62% and 67.5%.[139] In contrast to prior reports, the size or location of the lesion within the pancreas in this study did not seem to affect the diagnostic yield. A multivariate analysis showed that only a transgastric approach for EUS-guided TCB and obtaining more than two passes improved diagnostic yield. No pancreatitis-associated complications were observed.

Although EUS-guided TCB offers the ability to obtain information about tissue structure, it seems to have a similar (and most likely reduced) diagnostic accuracy in assessing pancreatic lesions compared with standard FNA needles, likely owing to technical issues related to its deployment in the duodenum. It is best used for lesions greater than 2 cm in size that can be accessed via a transgastric approach. It seems relatively safe, especially with operator experience. Overall complication rates reported with EUS-guided TCB appear to be less than 2%, similar to complication rates reported for EUS-guided FNA.[140] We limit our use of this device to cases where information regarding the pancreatic tissue architecture is essential to the patient's clinical management or when a patient with a highly suspicious pancreatic lesion has a non-diagnostic EUS-guided FNA.

Prioritizing Lesions for Fine Needle Aspiration

There are situations when more than one lesion in a patient may be targeted for EUS-guided FNA. The priority and sequence for multiple lesions in a patient with a pancreatic primary are summarized in **Table 42.4**. The sequence priority is predicated on the principle of confirming the most advanced stage and economizing the number of passes.

If a patient has a pancreatic mass, a suspicious mediastinal lymph node, a celiac lymph node, and a lesion in the left lobe of the liver (no ascites), the endosonographer should approach the mediastinal lesion first. If this lesion is positive for cancer, this would give the most advanced staging information (although the liver lesion would also lead to M_1 stage), and biopsy of the other lesions would not be needed. However, if this lesion is negative, biopsy of the liver lesion, followed by the celiac node, and then the pancreatic mass itself would be needed to make the diagnosis and confirm the most advanced disease stage. This sequence also is the most efficient from a technical standpoint. The most difficult lesions to obtain adequate cytologic samples are pancreatic tumors and submucosal tumors. Lymph nodes and liver lesions are relatively easier because fewer passes are generally required to obtain an adequate sample.

Number of Passes

Pancreatic adenocarcinoma generally requires the greatest number of FNA passes to obtain an adequate specimen. Approximately three to five passes are required (range 1 to 19).[2] Pancreatic tumors may have extensive fibrosis (desmoplastic reaction) or necrosis, which decreases the cellularity of malignant cells. The number of passes required for pancreatic tumors may be related to the differentiation of the tumor. A study designed to assess prospectively whether any patient or EUS characteristics could predict the number of EUS-guided FNA passes needed for diagnosis of pancreatic malignancy has been performed.[141] Among 95 patients undergoing EUS-guided FNA of a pancreatic mass, the average number of needle passes into the mass (includes head, neck, body, and tail) was 3.44 ± 2.19 (range 1 to 10). Tumors that were well differentiated required an average of 5.5 passes to obtain an adequate specimen; this is significantly different from 2.7

passes for moderately differentiated tumors and 2.3 passes for poorly differentiated tumors ($P < .001$).

Based on this study, it was recommended that without a cytopathologist in attendance, five to six passes should be made for pancreatic masses. However, this approach would still be associated with a 10% to 15% reduction in definitive cytologic diagnoses, extra procedure time, increased risk, and additional needles compared with having "real-time" cytopathology interpretations. Lymph nodes and liver lesions generally require much fewer passes. In an earlier series of 171 patients, the median number of passes for lymph node was 2 (range 1 to 10).[39] Liver lesions in one series showed that the average number of passes was similarly 2 (range 1 to 5).[42] Lymph node and liver metastases generally do not exhibit the desmoplastic or necrotic reaction that is common for primary tumors of the pancreas.

Ascites and pleural fluid on average require only a single FNA pass to obtain a specimen for cytologic diagnosis.[51] The endosonographer should try to obtain as much fluid as possible (preferably >10 mL). The fluid is spun down to concentrate the cells on a slide. Making the diagnosis of peritoneal metastasis from ascitic fluid has a lower yield than solid lesions (approximately 50% false-negative rate, especially with small amounts of fluid). However, a positive cytology is still very helpful in staging the tumor as unresectable. Ascitic fluid, if present, should be aspirated first before any other abdominal lesions, especially given the possibility of contamination of the ascites from other lesions if they were to undergo FNA first. In the presence of ascites, FNA of the primary pancreas tumor, lymph node metastasis, or liver metastasis theoretically could contaminate the fluid. In addition, the process of preparing cytology slides from ascitic fluid requires an additional step of concentrating the cells by centrifugation. We often aspirate the fluid first, even before performing vascular staging, to allow sufficient time for cytologic interpretation before moving on to the second lesion. For the reasons of most relevant staging information and efficiency of FNA passes, the priority sequence for FNA is suspicious mediastinal adenopathy, ascites, liver metastases, distant and local lymph nodes, and primary pancreatic tumor.

The importance of dynamic "real-time" cytologic interpretation has been emphasized in numerous studies.[2,39,123,142] These studies have shown that centers with an attendant cytopathologist had higher cytologic yield and diagnostic accuracy compared with centers that performed passes on an empiric basis. Increasing the number of empiric passes may increase cytologic accuracy but at the expense of performing unnecessary passes with associated cost, time, and safety issues. A more recent abstract reported the experience of a single endosonographer practicing in two clinical sites, one with an attendant cytopathologist and one without.[143] In the site without an attendant cytopathologist, 17% of patients required repeat procedures compared with 2% of patients requiring repeat procedures in the site with a cytopathologist present ($P = .015$). This study further confirmed that on-site cytopathologic interpretation during EUS-guided FNA has a significant clinical impact by increasing the diagnostic yield of the FNA and suggests that EUS centers should allocate resources for on-site cytopathologic evaluation.

Needle Insertion and Suction

The technique of needle advancement can vary considerably from very fine motion of the needle handle, using only the fine motor pincher muscles of the thumb and index finger, to very large motions using a full hand grasp on the needle handle with gross motor elbow and shoulder movements similar to that of downward thrust with an ice pick. The optimal technique of advancing the needle varies according to three factors: (1) the consistency of the GI wall (wall parameter), (2) the size and consistency of the lesion targeted (lesion parameter), and (3) the proximity of surrounding vessels (vessel parameter). **Table 42.5** summarizes the needle advancement technique with respect to these parameters.

The amount of pressure to apply to the suction syringe also needs to be considered. For most lesions, 5 mL of continuous suction applied to a 10-mL syringe is optimal. One report assessing various syringe sizes and continuous versus intermittent suction of lymph nodes from an autopsy specimen showed that continuous rather than intermittent suction with

Table 42.5 Needle Advancement Technique for Endoscopic Ultrasound–Guided Fine Needle Aspiration

Wall Parameter	Lesion Parameter	Vessel Parameter	Needle Advancement Technique	Difficulty Level
Thin wall, taut (e.g., esophagus)	Small (e.g., lymph node)	Vessel immediately behind lesion	Very fine, slow pincer movements	Moderate
Thin wall, taut	Large (e.g., tumor)	No adjacent vessel	Slow, moderate movements	Easy
Thick wall, elastic (e.g., gastric fundus)	Small lesion or scant fluid	Vessel immediately behind lesion	Consider puncturing through stomach first (adjacent to lesion) with a very quick dartlike motion (or use spring-loaded device), then fine pincer movements to target lesion	Difficult
Thick wall, elastic	Large	No adjacent vessel	Very quick dartlike motion using wrist action directly into lesion	Moderate
Duodenum	Small	Adjacent vessel	Quick, pincer movement to avoid pushing scope tip away	Difficult
Duodenum	Large, firm tumor	No adjacent vessel	Very quick, hand grasp with elbow and shoulder "ice pick" motion	Difficult

smaller syringes (5- to 10-mL) provided optimal cellularity and that use of larger (20- to 30-mL) syringes did not improve the rate of obtaining a diagnostic specimen.[144] If a large amount of blood is present on the smear after the first pass, one should consider very little (2 to 3 mL) or no suction. Too much suction in a vascular lesion sometimes may result in an inadequate cytology specimen owing to the overwhelming amount of red blood cells.

Complications of Endoscopic Ultrasound–Guided Fine Needle Aspiration of Pancreaticobiliary Lesions

An important part of maximizing the yield of EUS-guided FNA is being aware of and avoiding potential complications. These complications include pancreatitis, bleeding, infection, seeding of malignant cells, and bile peritonitis. Initial data on the overall complication rates of EUS-guided FNA came from three large published series comprising more than 1000 patients.[3,39,145] One multicenter trial showed that complications associated with the procedure (457 patients) seem to arise predominantly from infectious or hemorrhagic events after puncturing pancreatic cystic lesions.[39] Five nonfatal complications occurred for a rate of 0.5% (95% confidence interval 0.1% to 0.8%) in solid lesions versus 14% (95% confidence interval 6% to 21%) in cystic lesions ($P < .001$). Another single-institution study among 333 patients who underwent EUS-guided FNA experienced only one complication (0.3%)—a streptococcal sepsis after puncture of a cystic pancreatic lesion.[3] A small risk (1 in 121 patients) of developing pancreatitis after EUS-guided FNA of the pancreas has been reported.[146] The overall risk of FNA is extremely low. Several more recent studies have reported on the specific risks of FNA of pancreaticobiliary lesions and are discussed subsequently.

The overall risk of pancreatitis from EUS-guided FNA appears to be less than 1%. A large retrospective series of 4909 patients undergoing EUS-guided FNA of solid pancreatic lesions from 19 centers over a 4-year period showed a 0.29% risk of pancreatitis.[147] This risk was 0.64% from the two centers that prospectively collected data and 0.26% from the 17 centers that retrospectively collected data, suggesting an underreporting of complications in the latter group. A subsequent prospective single-center study by the same lead author revealed a pancreatitis rate for solid pancreatic lesions of 0.85% (3 of 355).[148] The rates of pancreatitis are similarly low for cystic lesions; a large study of 603 patients with 651 pancreatic cysts undergoing EUS-guided FNA revealed only six cases of pancreatitis (0.92%) and an overall complication rate of only 2.2%.[149] Similarly, the complication rate from EUS-guided TCB is less than 2% and not significantly different from EUS-guided FNA.

Hemorrhage is a rare complication of EUS and EUS-guided FNA. Gress and colleagues[146] initially reported two cases of hemorrhage, resulting in one death, in 208 patients who underwent 705 FNA passes using both radial and linear echoendoscopes. In both cases, EUS was performed using a radial echoendoscope, which precluded visualization of the needle tip during FNA. In one case, bleeding extended into the gastric lumen, whereas bleeding occurred in the pancreatic head region in the other case.

A more recent study from Denmark reported on 3324 consecutive patients who underwent EUS procedures using curvilinear echoendoscopes over an 11-year period, of which 670 underwent EUS-guided FNA and 136 received EUS-guided interventions.[150] Only a single case of GI bleeding was reported in a patient with widespread pancreatic cancer who died 6 hours after EUS-guided FNA from massive GI bleeding. However, at autopsy, the FNA puncture site showed no signs of bleeding and no vessels in the puncture route, and the cause of bleeding could not be established.

A third study described self-limited, non–transfusion-requiring intraluminal bleeding occurring in 3 of 90 patients undergoing EUS-guided FNA of solid pancreatic masses.[151] These consisted of a small rim of blood after FNA, and one additional patient developed an intramural duodenal hematoma for an overall bleeding complication rate of 4.4%.

Limited data on extramural hemorrhage exist. One study reported 3 of 227 patients (1.3%) undergoing FNA had extraluminal hemorrhage at the site of aspiration.[152] The bleeding lesions included a large pancreatic islet cell tumor, a benign lymph node in a patient with esophageal cancer, and a recurrent benign pancreatic cyst in a patient with a history of a mucinous cystadenoma that had been surgically resected. The authors described the bleeding as an expanding echopoor region adjacent to the sampled lesions, although no clinically recognized sequelae of bleeding were noted. No predictive factors for bleeding were identified. The investigators applied 15 to 25 minutes of pressure at the puncture site via balloon inflation and echoendoscope tip deflection, although it is unclear if this had a tamponade effect on extraluminal bleeding.

A case of self-limited retroperitoneal bleeding after EUS-guided FNA of the pancreas has also been reported.[153] Self-limited intracystic hemorrhage after EUS-guided FNA of pancreatic cysts has been reported to occur in 6% (3 of 50) patients in one series,[154] and clinically evident hemosuccus pancreaticus has also been observed after EUS-guided FNA of a pancreatic cyst.[155] However, a more recent and larger series of 651 cysts undergoing EUS-guided FNA revealed only a single retroperitoneal bleed.[149] These data indicate that clinically significant bleeding after EUS-guided FNA of solid or cystic pancreaticobiliary lesions is extremely uncommon with current techniques.

As stated previously, EUS-guided FNA seems primarily to be associated with infectious complications when cystic lesions are aspirated. Initial studies reported infectious complications in 14% (3 of 22) of patients undergoing EUS-guided FNA of pancreatic cystic lesions.[39] As a result, routine preprocedure and postprocedure antibiotic prophylaxis was adopted for FNA of such lesions. A single case of streptococcal sepsis after EUS-guided FNA of a pancreatic cystadenoma was reported in a large single-center report of 317 patients undergoing FNA of 327 sites[3]; this infection occurred despite the use of prophylactic antibiotics and corresponded to an infectious complication rate of 0.3%. Fever, although infrequent, has also been reported in several studies after EUS-guided FNA. We reported 1 patient of 44 (2%) undergoing EUS-guided FNA for pancreatic lesions who developed fever after sampling of a pancreatic cystic lesion.[11] This patient did not receive antibiotics before FNA.

Another series showed that 2 patients developed fever and infection out of 355 patients with solid pancreatic masses undergoing EUS-guided FNA, yielding an infectious complication rate of 0.56%.[148] One of these patients had cystic spaces within a pancreatic adenocarcinoma and the other, who required surgical débridement, had acute pancreatitis with a focal lesion in the pancreatic tail. Bournet and colleagues[156] reported 1 patient of 224 undergoing EUS-guided FNA (0.45%) who developed fever and abdominal pain after aspiration of a mucinous cystadenoma, despite administration of antibiotics before the procedure. Similarly, Lee and colleagues[149] reported 1 of 603 patients undergoing aspiration of 651 pancreatic cysts who developed fever, pain, and leukocytosis, although it is unclear if this patient received antibiotics before the procedure. As a result of these data, current guidelines recommend the use of antibiotic prophylaxis for planned FNA of any cystic lesion but not for solid pancreaticobiliary lesions.

The risk of malignant seeding from EUS-guided FNA is also believed to be very low. However, a case of a focal gastric intramural recurrence at the site of an EUS-guided FNA of a pancreatic tail lesion that underwent distal pancreatectomy was reported 21 months after a surgical resection with negative margins.[157] Although seeding may occur with this technique, EUS-guided FNA seems to have a significantly lower potential for peritoneal seeding (2.2% vs. 16.3%) compared with CT-guided FNA, as mentioned earlier in the section on EUS-guided FNA of pancreatic lesions.[14]

EUS-guided FNA of the bile duct and gallbladder has been reported to cause bile peritonitis. A case of this complication requiring laparotomy was reported after FNA of a pancreatic head mass in which the obstructed bile duct was traversed with the FNA needle.[158] Another study evaluating EUS-guided FNA to diagnose gallbladder microlithiasis was halted after two of the first three patients developed bile peritonitis.[159] FNA of solid gallbladder masses in which the gallbladder lumen was avoided seems to be safe.[64] The specific complications associated with EUS-guided FNI and other therapeutic EUS interventions have been discussed earlier separately in the sections describing these techniques.

Conclusions

EUS-guided FNA is extremely useful in the diagnosis and staging of pancreaticobiliary lesions such as pancreatic cancers (with associated lymph nodes, liver metastasis, and ascites), cystic tumors, neuroendocrine neoplasms, ampullary cancers, and cholangiocarcinomas. In addition, this technique has been extended via techniques such as EUS-guided FNI into therapeutic modalities such as celiac plexus or ganglion block, cyst gastrostomy, achieving pancreaticobiliary access and drainage, assisting in or delivering radiation therapy, and delivering antitumor agents.

References

The complete reference list is available online at www.expertconsult.com.

Chapter 43 | III

Choledocholithiasis

James A. DiSario

Video related to this chapter's topics can be found online at expertconsult.com.

CHAPTER OUTLINE

Introduction 579
  Cholelithiasis 579
  Choledocholithiasis 579
Clinical Features and Diagnosis 580
  Biliary Sludge, Microlithiasis, and Crystals 581
  Gallstone Pancreatitis 582
  Suppurative Cholangitis 583
Treatment 583
  Surgery 583
  Endoscopic Therapy 583
Indications and Contraindications 585
Preoperative History and Considerations 585
Therapeutic Techniques 585
Unusual Situations 586

Pregnancy 586
Biliary Sludge, Microlithiasis, and Crystals 586
Gallstone Pancreatitis 587
Acute Cholangitis 588
Endoscopic Bile Duct Stone Extraction as Definitive Therapy with the Gallbladder In Situ 589
Endoscopic Balloon Dilation of the Sphincter of Oddi for Extraction of Bile Duct Stones 590
Balloon Dilation of the Intact Papilla 590
Difficult Stones 592
Postoperative Care 597
  Outpatient Endoscopic Retrograde Cholangiopancreatography 597
  Recurrent Stones 597
Complications 598

Introduction

Gallstone disease affects people of both genders from every society, race, and age group. It is estimated that 15% of Americans have gallstones. Approximately 700,000 cholecystectomies are performed each year in the United States, making it the most common reason for digestive disease admission to Western hospitals. More than 95% of biliary tract disorders are related to gallstones.[1] Most bile duct stones are gallstones that have passed into the bile duct.

Cholelithiasis refers to gallbladder stones, and choledocholithiasis refers to stones in the bile ducts. Noncrumbling concretions larger than 2 mm in diameter are considered stones, and biliary microlithiasis refers to particles 2 mm or less in diameter, although there is no universally accepted definition. Choledocholithiasis can be classified as primary stones, which develop in the bile ducts, or secondary stones, which pass from the gallbladder. Choledocholithiasis can be subdivided further by the location of the stones, which may be intrahepatic or extrahepatic. Of patients with symptomatic gallstone disease, 5% to 15% have bile duct stones, yet greater than 90% of patients with choledocholithiasis also have cholelithiasis. Sludge is a suspension of cholesterol monohydrate crystals, calcium bilirubinate granules, and other calcium salts with or without microlithiasis in gallbladder mucus. Sludge is a form of gallstone disease and may predispose to macroscopic stones or cause pancreatitis and other morbidity directly.[2]

Cholelithiasis

Most gallstones are composed primarily of cholesterol and are nodular and round with a golden color. A few gallstones contain mostly calcium bilirubinate and are round, hard, and black. Primary bile duct stones are composed of calcium salts of unconjugated bilirubin with variable amounts of cholesterol, protein, and bacteria. These stones are brown, are amorphous, and have an earthy texture. **Fig. 43.1** shows examples of stones extracted from the bile duct.

Choledocholithiasis

Epidemiologically, primary and secondary bile duct stones vary greatly. In Western societies, most bile duct stones are secondary, and the prevalence increases with age. Primary bile duct stones are more common in Asia. Primary stones are associated with bacterial contamination of the choledochus by biliary enteric anastomoses, sphincterotomy, stents, instrumentation, and portal bacteremia. Periampullary diverticula provide a site for bacterial proliferation with subsequent reflux into the bile duct (**Fig. 43.2**). Hemoglobinopathies may induce primary stones by providing a bilirubinate nidus for

579

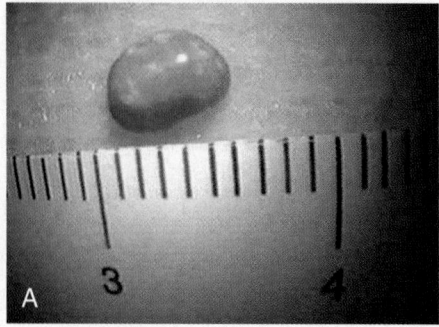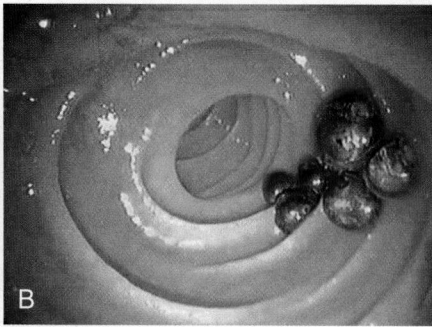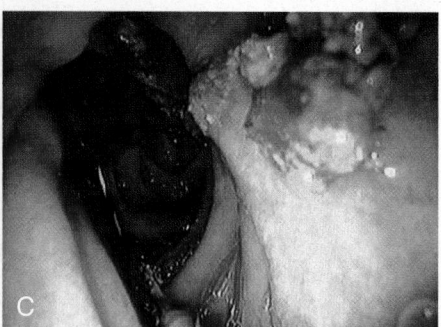

Fig. 43.1 A, Cholesterol and calcium stone ex vivo. **B,** Calcium bilirubinate stones in the duodenum. **C,** Brown, amorphous, earthy primary bile duct stone material in the duodenum.

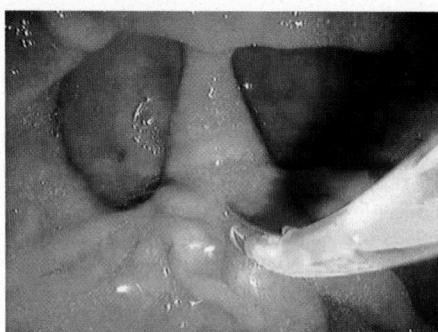

Fig. 43.2 A large periampullary diverticulum, which predisposes to choledocholithiasis. The bile duct is cannulated and can be seen traversing the diverticulum.

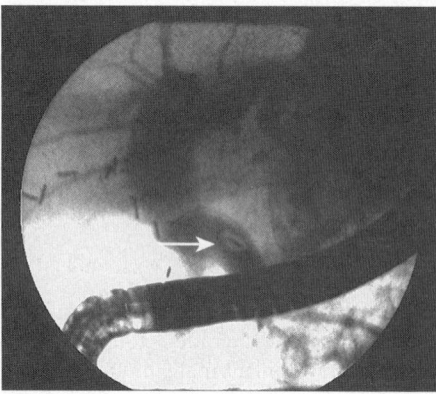

Fig. 43.3 Endoscopic cholangiography shows a radiolucent stone *(arrow)* in the common bile duct (CBD) that has a surgical clip from prior cholecystectomy as the nidus.

stone development. Foreign bodies including surgical clips and parasites may also introduce bacteria and serve as a nidus for stone formation, as shown in **Fig. 43.3**.[3]

Clinical Features and Diagnosis

The clinical presentation of biliary stones can be classified into three groups: (1) asymptomatic cholelithiasis or choledocholithiasis, (2) symptomatic gallstones (biliary colic), and (3) complications from gallstones (pancreatitis, cholecystitis, obstructive jaundice, cholangitis, gallbladder cancer, gallstone

ileus). No symptoms occur in 60% to 80% of persons with gallstones, and the risk of progression is small. However, once symptoms develop, 35% to 50% of patients have recurrence within 1 year, and nearly 2% per year have complications.[4]

Biliary colic precedes complications in 90% of cases. The natural history of choledocholithiasis is unpredictable and not well described. Many common bile duct (CBD) stones are asymptomatic and pass into the duodenum without incident, whereas others lead to biliary colic, jaundice, cholangitis, or pancreatitis.[5–7] Choledocholithiasis-associated biliary colic is similar to gallbladder-associated biliary colic. Untreated bile duct stone obstruction can cause secondary biliary cirrhosis, usually after about 5 years.[8]

The differential diagnosis is based on key clinical features, laboratory findings, and imaging studies. All foregut disorders may have similar symptoms, including esophageal, gastric, duodenal, hepatic, and pancreatic lesions. Additionally, colonic diseases, diaphragmatic and pleural diseases, and musculoskeletal disease may mimic biliary symptoms.

Bile duct stones typically cause elevations in serum transaminases, alkaline phosphatase, and total bilirubin and ductal dilation on transabdominal ultrasound studies. However, CBD stones can be present with normal laboratory values. Total bilirubin levels range from normal to very high, and duration of obstruction does not correlate with serum bilirubin. Complete obstruction may cause a steady increase in serum bilirubin. Alkaline phosphatase is usually elevated up to fivefold in symptomatic patients. Acute biliary obstruction usually causes an initial disproportionate increase in transaminases.[9]

Imaging studies are the standard for the diagnosis of biliary stone disease. Transcutaneous abdominal ultrasound is the initial imaging study obtained when gallstone disease is suspected; sensitivity and specificity are greater than 95% for cholelithiasis and about 50% and 98% for bile duct stones.[10] Spiral computed tomography (CT) is reported to be 82% sensitive and 97% specific for detecting bile duct stones, but many series have lower rates.[11,12] Meta-analysis data show magnetic resonance cholangiopancreatography (MRCP) to be 92% sensitive and 97% specific for stones, but sensitivity declines for concretions 5 mm or less in diameter **(Fig. 43.4)**.[12,13]

In a comparative study of 70 patients who underwent MRCP, transcutaneous ultrasound, or multislice CT, concordance was found between MRCP and ultrasound in 92% of cases for gallbladder lesions; however, statistically significant discordance occurred with ultrasound missing 16% of bile

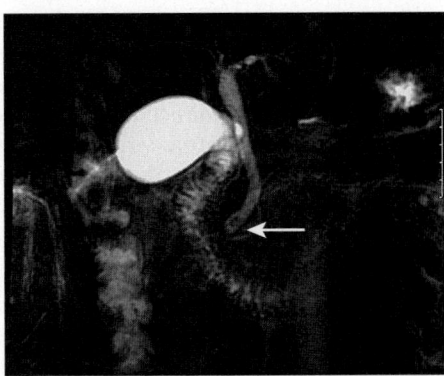

Fig. 43.4 Magnetic resonance cholangiopancreatography (MRCP) shows a 5-mm distal bile duct stone (arrow).

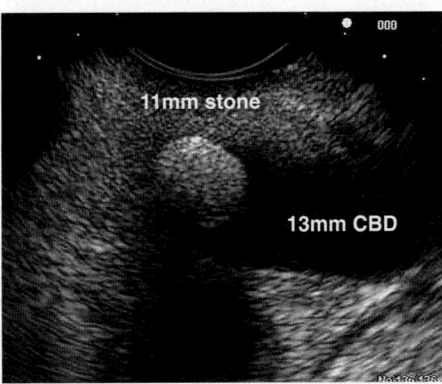

Fig. 43.5 Linear endoscopic ultrasound (EUS) image of a longitudinal section of the distal bile duct; a round bright echodense structure with shadowing represents a stone. (Courtesy of Iqbal Sandhu, MD.)

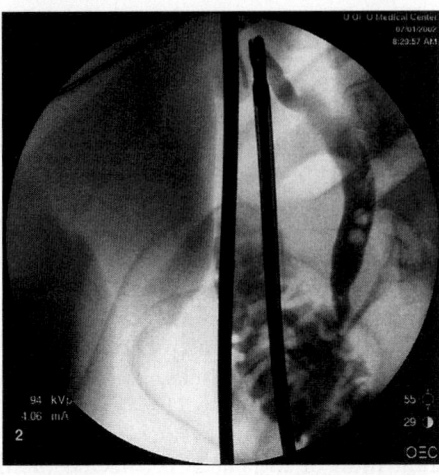

Fig. 43.6 Intraoperative cholangiogram with two radiolucent stones seen in the common bile duct (CBD). (Courtesy of Robert Glasgow, MD.)

duct stones. Although there was concordance between MRCP and CT gallbladder imaging in 87% of patients, statistically significant discordance for bile duct lesions occurred in 35% of patients.[14] Multiple studies show sensitivities and specificities for endoscopic retrograde cholangiopancreatography (ERCP) of 90% to 100% and 98% to 100%.[12] Endoscopic ultrasound (EUS) can be performed with a dedicated echoendoscope with either 360-degree radial imaging or linear imaging or with an intraductal probe. EUS is performed similar to a standard endoscopy with ultrasound imaging of the extrahepatic bile duct done through the duodenal bulb or descending duodenum as shown in **Fig. 43-5**. Reported sensitivities and specificities for EUS are 84% to 100% and 96% to 100%.[15]

Preoperative diagnosis of CBD stones is not always necessary. Many authors advocate intraoperative cholangiography (IOC) as the diagnostic modality of choice in the setting of cholecystectomy with suspected CBD calculi. Laparoscopic IOC is technically successful in more than 90% of cases and is about 80% to 90% sensitive and 76% to 97% specific (**Fig. 43.6**).[16,17] Fluoroscopic IOC has better diagnostic accuracy than static imaging. IOC is also used during cholecystectomy to verify biliary tree anatomy before dividing the cystic duct. IOC generally adds 5 to 25 minutes to the operation; however, it is usually faster, better tolerated, and less expensive than other invasive modalities.[17] Laparoscopic intraoperative ultrasound is less widely employed than IOC. Yet, it has no

radiation exposure, may be less time-consuming than IOC, and has sensitivity and specificity approaching 100%.[17,18]

Although 5% to 15% of persons who have cholecystectomy have bile duct stones, it is not cost-effective to perform universal IOC or ERCP, or both, for detection and treatment. Clinical, laboratory, and imaging studies are used to stratify for risk of harboring CBD stones. Numerous studies have identified risk factors and developed scoring formulas for risk. The most commonly detected factors are elevations in serum transaminases, alkaline phosphatase, and bilirubin, and bile duct dilation to 8 mm or larger on transabdominal ultrasound. However, only about 50% to 75% of persons predicted to be at high risk have choledocholithiasis.[1,19,20] MRCP or EUS may be useful to define the risk more precisely; however, these tests add cost, and EUS-guided stone extraction is experimental.[21] When stones are suspected preoperatively, the options for diagnosis and therapy are preoperative ERCP, IOC, and laparoscopic common duct exploration (LCDE). For stones detected by IOC and LCDE, intraoperative or postoperative ERCP can be done and obtain similar results. ERCP entails increased resource use, however.[22] Conversion to open common duct exploration is associated with significant morbidity and prolonged hospital and recovery times, and open common duct exploration should not be used routinely. Choledocholithiasis may be diagnosed after surgery with transabdominal ultrasound, CT, MRCP, EUS, or ERCP, depending on the index of suspicion, and subsequently treated with ERCP.[17]

Biliary Sludge, Microlithiasis, and Crystals

Biliary sludge, microlithiasis, and crystals are a form of gallstone disease and seem to have a natural history and clinical associations similar to macroscopic stone disease. Over the course of 3 years, 50% of persons with abdominal pain and sludge have spontaneous resolution of the sludge, 20% have sludge with no symptoms, 10% to 15% have symptoms develop or persist, and 5% to 15% acquire stones. Sludge, microlithiasis, and crystals account for about 75% of cases of acute recurrent pancreatitis in which the etiology is undiagnosed by history, physical examination, blood tests, and noninvasive imaging studies.[23–25] Cholesterol monohydrate crystals or calcium bilirubinate granules or both can be found in the gallbladder or bile duct after cholecystectomy in 67% to 89% of these patients.[25-27] These lesions are also associated with cholelithiasis not seen on noninvasive imaging studies, cholecystitis without macroscopic stones, and cholangitis.

The initial diagnosis of gallbladder sludge is often made by transabdominal ultrasound, which has been reported to be 86% sensitive at showing a dependent layer of nonshadowing, slowly mobile material.[28] MRCP is more sensitive than transabdominal ultrasound for the diagnosis of sludge and microlithiasis.[29] EUS is about 96% sensitive for detecting sludge and finds small gallbladder and bile duct stones missed on other studies.[28,30] Intraductal ultrasound probes are highly sensitive but may yield false-positive results. For lesions larger than 1.4 mm, intraductal ultrasound is 71% sensitive and 75% specific for microlithiasis validated by microscopy.[31] Direct microscopic examination of the bile is considered the diagnostic standard, is more sensitive than transcutaneous ultrasound or EUS, allows the determination of the type of particles in the sludge, and is required to diagnose microlithiasis in the absence of sludge. However, crystals may occur intermittently, and false-positive and false-negative results may occur.[2]

Duodenal aspiration after stimulation of gallbladder emptying is cumbersome and yields a contaminated specimen. ERCP with gallbladder cannulation and aspiration provides a relatively pure specimen and has the added advantage of allowing for imaging of the biliary tree and pancreas and sphincter of Oddi manometry when indicated.[32]

Gallbladder bile (B bile) is opaque dark green or black and is much more informative than lighter colored hepatic bile (A bile) for diagnosing microlithiasis and crystals (**Fig. 43.7**). Some authors have collected dark bile with cannulation of only the choledochus, but this may be time-consuming and unsuccessful.[33] Radiographic contrast material in the bile may cause false-positive microscopic examinations. I collect a pure bile specimen by gallbladder cannulation under fluoroscopic guidance before contrast injection into the gallbladder.

There is no consensus on the method of preparation, examination, and interpretation of bile specimens for microscopic crystal examination. Some authors have attempted to quantify the findings[33]; however, a qualitative examination is appropriate for clinical purposes.[2] One suggested protocol is to centrifuge a 10- to 15-mL specimen at 3000g for 15 minutes and make a slide from the sediment. The slide is examined by light and polarizing microscopy at 100× (two crystals or granules per field or four per slide is considered a positive test). Cholesterol monohydrate crystals are rhomboid plaques with a notch that are multicolored on polarized examination, and bilirubinate granules are amorphous and red-brown colored as shown in **Fig. 43.8**. Leukocytes may be indicative of acute or chronic cholecystitis. It is difficult and unnecessary to maintain the specimen temperature strictly at 37° C, so the specimen should be centrifuged as quickly as possible. The intact specimen should not be stored because bacterial contamination can occur in specimens at room temperature and refrigerated specimens, and cholesterol crystal precipitation develops in frozen bile. However, the sediment may be frozen for later examination if necessary.[2]

Gallstone Pancreatitis

Gallstones cause about 35% of cases of acute pancreatitis in the United States, and about 25% of these cases are severe with

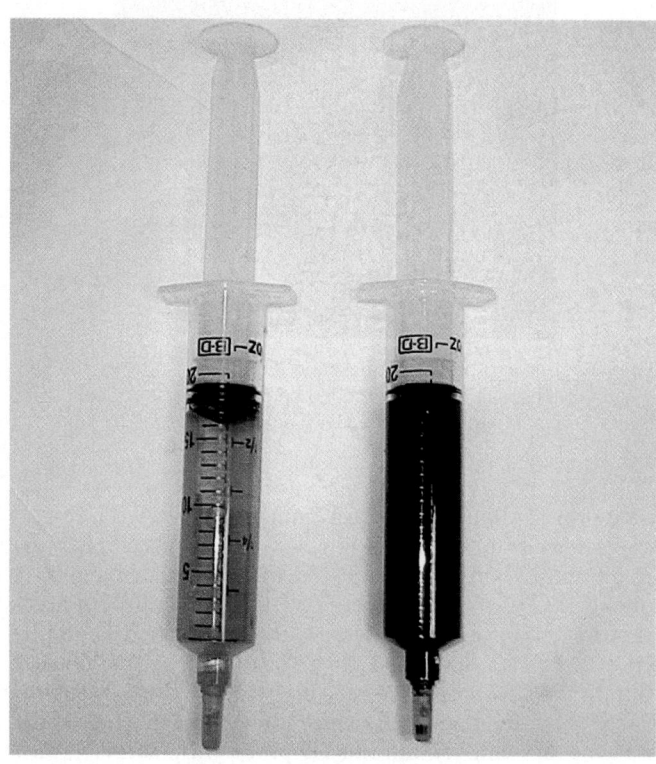

Fig. 43.7 Aspiration specimens of yellow hepatic bile (A bile) on the left and black gallbladder bile (B bile) on the right.

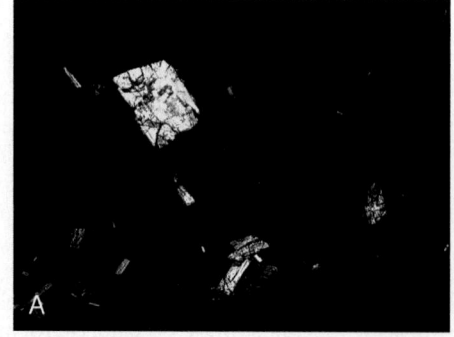
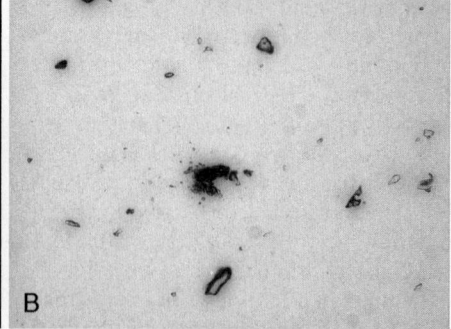

Fig. 43.8 **A,** Cholesterol monohydrate crystals seen with polarized microscopy. **B,** Amorphous bilirubinate aggregates seen with light microscopy.

mortality in 10%. Gallstones are recovered from the feces in 95% of patients with acute pancreatitis; however, only 7% of patients with gallstones develop pancreatitis.[34] Soon after the onset of pancreatitis, 78% of affected persons have bile duct stones found at surgery or ERCP.[35,36] However, delayed operations reveal CBD and impacted ampullary stones much less frequently.[37]

Small stones are thought to pass easily through the cystic duct and impact in the sphincter of Oddi; stones less than 5 mm in diameter are the most common.[38] The causal relationship between gallstones and pancreatitis is confirmed by the finding that cholecystectomy or endoscopic sphincterotomy with removal of bile duct stones prevents recurrences.[39] The pathophysiology may be due to obstruction of pancreatic juice outflow, reflux of offending substances into the pancreatic duct, or both.

The diagnosis of biliary pancreatitis is usually made by finding gallstones on transabdominal ultrasound in the absence of other known causes of pancreatitis, although EUS is more sensitive and specific and provides much better visualization of the bile duct.[35] Abnormal liver enzymes and bilirubin and bile duct dilation on transabdominal ultrasound are frequently found but are nonspecific.[40] It is important to stratify the severity of pancreatitis by various algorithms or failure of one or more organ systems because prognosis and therapy vary greatly between mild and severe cases. I use failure of one or more organ systems to categorize severe pancreatitis because algorithms are cumbersome and difficult to remember, include subjective criteria, and may require 48 hours of observation for a conclusion.[41]

Suppurative Cholangitis

Acute suppurative cholangitis develops in the setting of bacteria in the biliary system and bile duct obstruction. Bile duct stones are the cause of the obstruction in most cases. The bacteria enter the duct from the gut and proliferate resulting in increased intraductal pressure and forced translocation of bacteria and endotoxins into the hepatic sinusoids and bloodstream. In contrast to gallstone disease, women and men are affected equally with a median age of 50 to 60 years. Less frequently, benign and malignant strictures, obstructed stents, and side-to-side surgical anastomoses predispose to cholangitis. Mortality rates approach 100% in persons who fail conservative therapy and who do not have an adequate drainage procedure.[42]

The most common organisms are *Escherichia coli, Enterococcus, Klebsiella,* and *Enterobacter. Pseudomonas,* anaerobes, and skin and oral flora may be found after biliary instrumentation or surgery. Polymicrobial infection is more common in severe infections, and bile cultures are usually concordant.[42] The classic clinical presentation is Charcot's triad including fever, jaundice, and right upper quadrant abdominal pain; this occurs in 50% to 100% of patients. Reynold's pentad adds altered mental status and hypotension to Charcot's triad and occurs in less than 14% of patients. Typical laboratory abnormalities include leukocytosis, hyperbilirubinemia, elevated alkaline phosphatase, mildly increased transaminases, and occasionally elevated amylase.

Imaging findings on transabdominal ultrasound include stones or ductal dilation or both in 67% of patients. CT scans may show ductal dilation, the level of obstruction, and occasionally calcified CBD or gallstones or both. One study showed changes of papillitis to be 60% sensitive and 86% specific in homogeneous, hepatic contrast agent uptake to be 60% sensitive and 80% specific, and combined findings of papillitis and contrast agent uptake to be 97% specific for suppurative cholangitis.[43] MRCP is reported to show distinctive changes in 92% of patients; however, because MRCP is without therapeutic capabilities, the utility is unclear. EUS may be beneficial in a clinically stable patient when ERCP is unsuccessful or undesirable because of increased procedure risks or pregnancy. Percutaneous transhepatic cholangiography (PTC) is sensitive and specific in 90% or more of affected patients and allows for therapy. However, it should not be considered as a first-line procedure because of high complication rates. ERCP is the procedure of choice because it affords the opportunity to provide diagnosis and definitive therapy with acceptable morbidity and mortality rates.

Treatment

Surgery

The management of CBD stones varies widely around the world. Therapeutic determinants include individual patient presentation; operative risk; and available expertise for LCDE, open CBD exploration, and ERCP. Laparoscopic cholecystectomy is the preferred initial approach to cholelithiasis with the benefit of decreased pain, shorter length of hospital stay, more rapid return to full activity, and less cost than open surgery. LCDE seems to have similar advantages over open CBD exploration and is cost-effective compared with ERCP.[22] A transcystic duct approach is generally preferred to choledochotomy, resulting in shorter procedure duration and hospital stays and reduced need for T-tube placement. Some surgeons use a choledochotomy, however, depending on the stone. Stone extraction is generally achieved under fluoroscopic guidance with medical dilation of the sphincter of Oddi and flushing of small stones, by retrograde balloon or basket catheter techniques used to push stones through the native sphincter of Oddi, or after balloon dilation or antegrade sphincterotomy. Balloon dilation should be discouraged because of increased rates of pancreatitis. Choledochoscopic guidance may also be used with or without intracorporeal lithotripsy techniques.

LCDE results in stone clearance in 75% to 90% of cases, and T-tube placement or antegrade biliary stent placement is required for incomplete drainage. LCDE adds about 1 hour to the operation. Transcystic duct LCDE requires hospital stays of about 1.5 days, and transductal procedures generally result in stays of up to 7.5 days. Morbidity and mortality rates are 10% and 1%.[17] A treatment algorithm for preoperatively suspected bile duct stones managed by standard techniques is shown in **Fig. 43.9.** A treatment algorithm for bile duct stones requiring more specialized techniques is shown in **Fig. 43.10.** Stones detected after surgery are best managed by ERCP.

Endoscopic Therapy

ERCP with sphincterotomy is the most common method of treating bile duct stones in the United States, and more than 150,000 cases are performed each year. Overall, the procedure is ultimately successful in greater than 90% of patients with

Clinical suspicion
Gallbladder-in-situ
Postcholecystectomy
Laparoscopic cholecystectomy with intraoperative cholangiogram or ultrasound
ERCP with sphincterotomy
Success
No bile duct stones
Bile duct stones
Success
Open bile duct exploration
Fail
Laparoscopic bile duct exploration
Fail
ERCP w/sphincterotomy
Success
Success
Success

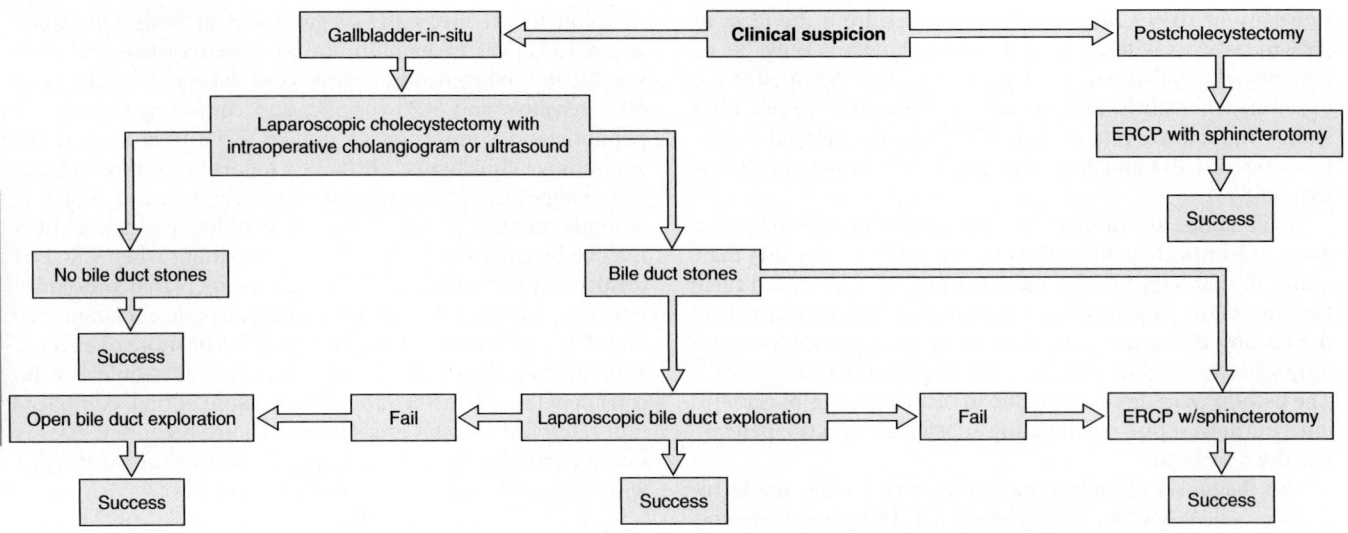

Fig. 43.9 Standard treatment for choledocholithiasis. ERCP, endoscopic retrograde cholangiopancreatography.

◆ERCP with sphincterotomy
Fail
Mechanical lithotripsy
Large balloon dilation
Fail
Fail
Endoscopic stents* temporary or palliative
Gallbladder-in-situ
Postcholecystectomy
Laparoscopic cholecystectomy with intraoperative cholangiogram or ultrasound
Extracorporeal shockwave lithotripsy
Fail
Peroral choledochoscopy with intracorporeal lithotripsy (laser, electrohydraulic)
Fail
Fail
◆ Open bile duct exploration
◆Laparoscopic bile duct exploration
Fail
Fail
Fail
Mechanical lithotripsy
Fail
T-Tube
Endoscopic stents*
Fail
Peroral choledochoscopy with intracorporeal lithotripsy (laser, electrohydraulic)
Fail
Extracorporeal shockwave lithotripsy
Fail
Trans T-Tube extraction, intracorporeal lithotripsy (laser, electrohydraulic)
Fail
Fail
Fail
Palliative stents (elderly, sick)
Fail
ERCP with sphincterotomy
Fail
Percutaneous transhepatic extraction, intracorporeal lithotripsy (laser, electrohydraulic)
◆ Entry point
* Stenting at any point can be either temporary or permanent (palliative)

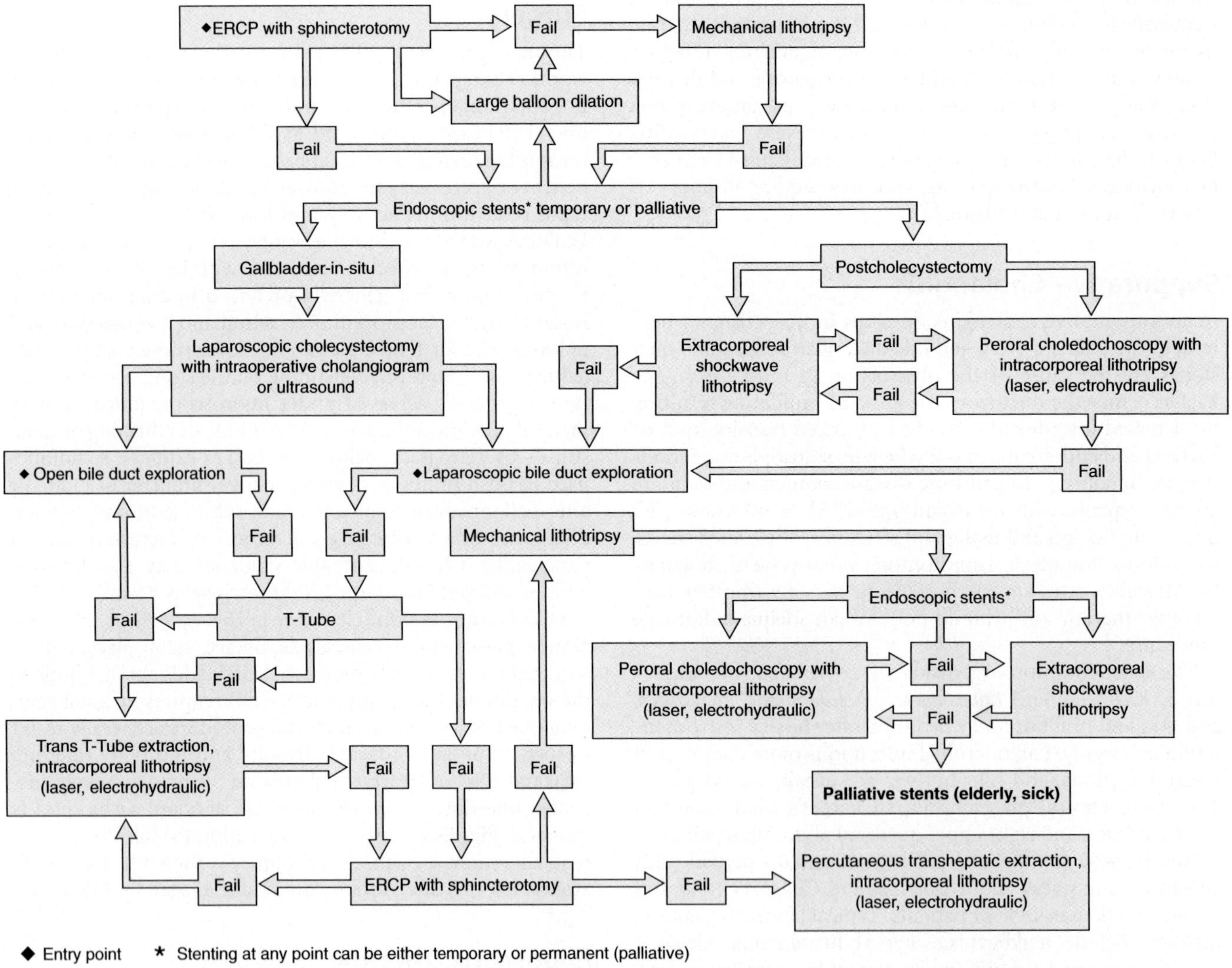

Fig. 43.10 Specialized treatment for difficult bile duct stones. ERCP, endoscopic retrograde cholangiopancreatography.

complications in about 10%.[44] Successful clearance of the biliary tree of all stones depends on the size and number of stones and experience of the endoscopists. Reported rates of successful bile duct clearance range from about 60% to greater than 90% at the initial procedure[45–48] to almost 100% with subsequent procedures at specialized centers.[49–57] Failed cases are usually due to the inability to access the major papilla owing to surgically altered anatomy. Morbidity occurs in only 3% to 5% of patients from initial ERCP with sphincterotomy performed for stones, especially when performed within 30 days of laparoscopic cholecystectomy.[48,58,59]

The underlying principle is to open the sphincter choledochus and remove the stones with balloon or basket catheters inserted into the bile duct under fluoroscopic and endoscopic visualization. Difficult and unusual circumstances may require the use of postsphincterotomy large-balloon dilation, mechanical lithotripsy, intracorporeal electrohydraulic or laser lithotripsy, or extracorporeal shock wave lithotripsy (ESWL). Long-term stent placement for palliation is appropriate for very high-risk patients.

Indications and Contraindications

ERCP is indicated as the standard of care for patients with known or suspected choledocholithiasis except for patients who have LCDE at the time of laparoscopic cholecystectomy. ERCP is also indicated urgently or emergently for patients with severe gallstone pancreatitis with biliary obstruction and patients with acute suppurative cholangitis. Absolute contraindications are the contraindications of endoscopy and ERCP in general, including bowel obstruction, perforated viscus, and patient refusal. Relative contraindications include coagulopathy, severe comorbidities, recent gastrointestinal anastomosis, and gastric outlet or proximal duodenal stenosis.

Preoperative History and Considerations

Bile duct stones are usually diagnosed by clinical history, serum hepatic and pancreatic enzymes, and imaging studies before ERCP is performed. However, there are circumstances where stones are suspected but not seen on imaging studies, in which case the ERCP is diagnostic and therapeutic if stones are found.

Considerations in the medical history include prior intestinal surgery with altered anatomy such as Billroth or Roux-en-Y anastomoses, which could require a different approach and special instruments. Stones are common in pregnancy, and pregnancy could alter the timing and technique of ERCP. Preprocedure coagulation studies are not generally recommended but are appropriate in patients receiving anticoagulants or with biliary obstruction, who may develop a coagulopathy secondary to vitamin K malabsorption, which is significantly exacerbated in patients receiving warfarin. It is wise to have the international normalized ratio corrected to 1.5 or less if sphincterotomy is anticipated.[60]

Indications for general anesthesia include sepsis with hypotension; severe acute pancreatitis; significant cardiopulmonary disease; macroglossia; dysmorphic facies; obstructive sleep apnea; morbid obesity; and narcotic, benzodiazepine, or alcohol tolerance. Other considerations include a bowel purge in patients who have recently had a CT scan or other barium contrast study because residual barium in the colon can compromise cholangiography. Prophylactic antibiotics are not recommended for routine bile duct stone removal. However, antibiotics that cover enteric gram-negative organisms, enterococci, and perhaps *Pseudomonas* are recommended for cases of bile duct obstruction when there is a possibility of incomplete drainage.[61]

Therapeutic Techniques

Stones are extracted after cannulation has been achieved; the stone is identified on cholangiography, and the sphincterotomy is performed. A balloon or basket catheter is advanced upstream to the stone. The balloon is inflated and retracted, bringing the stone with it into the duodenum as shown in **Fig. 43.11**. A basket is positioned so that it completely opens and deploys such that the stone is totally engaged. It is often helpful to move or jiggle the basket gently up and down the affected segment of the duct to entrap the stone. The basket is left in the fully opened position and retracted into the duodenum,

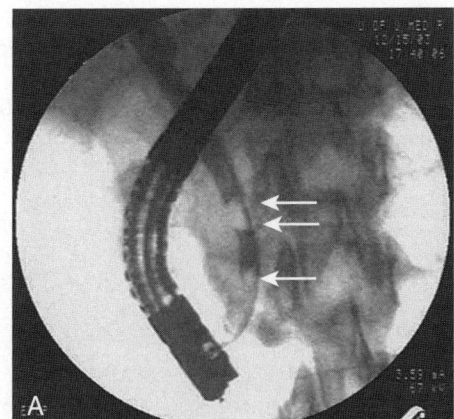
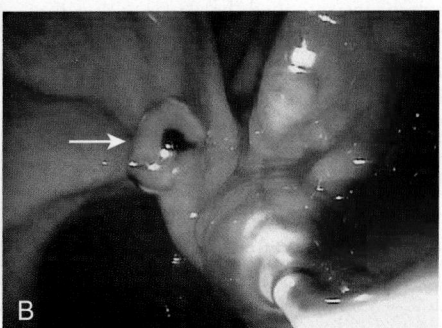

Fig. 43.11 A, Endoscopic retrograde cholangiogram with a balloon *(double arrows)* inflated in the common bile duct (CBD) above a stone *(single arrow)* in the distal bile duct. **B,** A mixed stone *(arrow)* extracted into the duodenum by the inflated balloon.

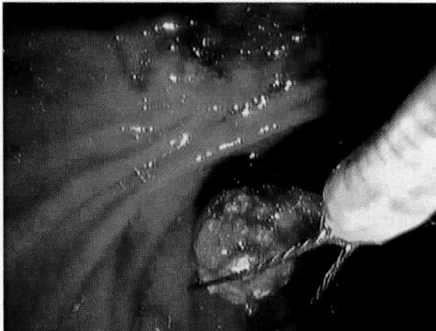

Fig. 43.12 A mixed stone is seen extracted within a basket in the duodenum.

bringing the stone with it (**Fig. 43.12**). If the stone continually slips out of the basket, the basket may be closed around the stone to get a better grip. If this maneuver is done, it is important that the stone be small enough to pass through the distal duct and sphincterotomy orifice or that the basket be compatible with mechanical lithotripsy, to prevent basket and stone impaction in the duct. If multiple stones are present, the most downstream stone should be removed first also to prevent this type of impaction.

It is important to keep the balloon or basket catheter in line with the axis of the bile duct during stone extraction. The viewing tip of the endoscope should be positioned directly below the papillary orifice abutting the opening. The catheter and stone are retracted to the most downstream portion of the duct. The catheter is held tightly against the endoscope with the third through fifth fingers of the left hand, and the endoscope is torqued clockwise and pushed inward, which directs the catheter and stone straight out of the duct. Alternatively, the endoscope may be pushed in slightly below the sphincterotomy orifice and the tip turned upward against the orifice in a slightly acute angle by turning the large up-and-down knob counterclockwise. The endoscope is retracted a little; the catheter is held tightly against the endoscope; and the up-and-down knob is firmly turned clockwise, which pulls the catheter and stone out along the axis of the duct.

If the balloon or basket catheter is simply pulled out with the endoscope in the standard position, the stone is likely to be forced against the superior aspect of the duct deep to the duodenal wall. The catheter then slips out inferiorly to the stone. The balloon can rupture against the bridge on the endoscope, or the basket may slip off of the stone and out. Primary bile duct stones have an earthy consistency and crumble with extraction. It is often necessary to sweep the duct repeatedly with a balloon and perhaps irrigate the biliary tree with saline. Brown stone debris extracted into the duodenum is shown in **Fig. 43.1C**.

When a stone is positioned loosely in the hepatic ducts, it may be possible to direct a guidewire upstream, pass a balloon catheter above the stone, and extract it in the usual manner. However, care should be taken to avoid further upstream force on the stone by hydrostatic pressure from contrast agent injection or from direct pressure from the instruments. If standard extraction is impossible, stones can often be retracted into the extrahepatic bile ducts by positioning a stone extraction balloon just downstream to the stone, inflating it to fit snugly into the duct, and then rapidly retracting it to create downstream suction to dislodge the stone.

Unusual Situations

Pregnancy

About 8% of pregnant women develop cholelithiasis and frequently have symptoms. Cholecystectomy can often be postponed until after delivery; however, choledocholithiasis poses significant risk of cholangitis and pancreatitis and generally requires therapy. Potential risks to the fetus include sedatives and analgesics; radiation exposure; and sequelae of procedural complications such as hypoxia, pancreatitis, and sepsis. There are several small series in the literature of ERCP during pregnancy including during the first trimester. Biliary sphincterotomy, stone extraction, and stent placement were frequently done. Most patients delivered healthy full-term infants. Therapeutic outcomes were generally successful with acceptable morbidity.[62]

A reasonable approach is to perform transabdominal ultrasound for pregnant women who develop right upper quadrant or epigastric pain, abnormal serum hepatic enzymes, unexplained acute pancreatitis, or biliary sepsis. If gallstones are found and there is no pancreatitis, cholecystectomy may be postponed until after delivery if the symptoms and biochemical tests resolve.[62] ERCP is indicated for choledocholithiasis or ductal dilation seen on ultrasound, persistent cholestasis, pancreatitis, or cholangitis. The patient should be considered for referral to a high-volume center with experience in these cases. Obstetric consultation should be obtained, and fetal monitoring should be considered during the procedure. The procedure may need to be performed in the supine or left lateral position. It may be wise to have an anesthesiologist administer the sedation or anesthesia and to consider endotracheal intubation if the patient is to be in the supine position.

Fetal radiation exposure should be minimized by lead shielding; using minimal fluoroscopy; and avoiding spot films, which give higher radiation exposure. Using these techniques, fetal radiation exposure can be contained to about 310 mrad, which is significantly below the accepted teratogenic dose.[63] Radiation exposure to the fetus may be monitored with a radiation dosimetry badge placed on the mother's abdomen over the uterine fundus.

Sphincterotomy and stent placement may be safely performed, and transpapillary gallbladder stent placement for cholecystitis has been suggested to postpone cholecystectomy until after delivery.[62,64] Some authorities advocate performing the procedure with no fluoroscopy. One technique is to use wire-guided cannulation with visualization of bile flow around the wire, through a small-caliber stent, or with aspiration through the sphincterotome. Sphincterotomy may be performed in the standard fashion or with a needle-knife over a stent. Stones can be removed with balloons, baskets, or mechanical lithotripsy.[65] Alternatively, a stent may be left in situ, and ERCP may be repeated after delivery.[66] Cholangioscopy has been used to confirm ductal clearance.[67] Ultrasound, rather than fluoroscopic, guidance has also been used.

Biliary Sludge, Microlithiasis, and Crystals

Traditional therapy for sludge, microlithiasis, and crystals is cholecystectomy, which generally cures relapsing pain and prevents recurrent pancreatitis. Ursodeoxycholic acid can dissolve cholesterol microlithiasis and crystals and prevents the recurrence of pancreatitis. However, the duration of effect is unknown.[2] Endoscopic sphincterotomy prevents or reduces episodes of recurrent pancreatitis caused by sludge, microlithiasis, and crystals.[33]

Gallstone Pancreatitis

The usual therapy for mild to moderate disease is supportive until pancreatitis resolves and then laparoscopic cholecystectomy with IOC generally during the same hospital stay. Severe disease is best treated with intensive care monitoring, prophylactic antibiotics for extensive necrosis, enteral nutritional support, and urgent biliary drainage for signs of bile duct obstruction (jaundice, persistently abnormal liver tests, and dilated bile duct) or cholangitis. Early biliary surgery is associated with high rates of morbidity and mortality in severe pancreatitis.[36] Cholecystectomy should be performed during the same hospital stay or as soon as possible afterward.

Urgent endoscopic retrograde cholangiography (ERC) with biliary sphincterotomy and stone extraction has been used to reduce morbidity and mortality.[68] There are six published peer-reviewed, randomized controlled trials of ERC compared with conservative management in patients with acute pancreatitis, and there are six meta-analyses of these studies with conflicting results. The conflicting results are due to heterogeneity of patients, inclusion criteria, severity of disease, and inability to confirm the presence of stones. There are also different methodologies and endpoints.[68-79] Extraction of obstructing stones is beneficial in relieving cholangitis and jaundice. There are several issues pertinent to interpreting this literature, as follows: (1) Does ERC prevent systemic or pancreatic morbidity? (2) Should ERC be done in all cases or only for cholangitis or biliary obstruction? (3) Is it beneficial to diagnose CBD stones with noninvasive imaging or EUS and then do ERC only if stones are seen? (4) Should sphincterotomy be done in all patients to provide drainage for unseen microlithiasis, sludge, or stones? (5) What is the optimal timing for ERCP?

Neoptolemos and colleagues[69] randomly assigned 121 patients from a single center with suspected biliary pancreatitis to have ERC with sphincterotomy for bile duct stones within 72 hours of admission compared with conservative therapy. Subgroup analysis of patients with severe pancreatitis showed a statistically significant decrease in morbidity and a numerical benefit in mortality. Fan and coworkers[70] randomly assigned 195 patients with pancreatitis of any etiology (including alcohol and hyperlipidemia) to receive ERC with sphincterotomy for choledocholithiasis within 24 hours of hospitalization or medical management. The overall outcomes were similar for the treatment and control groups; however, in patients with severe pancreatitis, morbidity was significantly less frequent at 13% versus 54% ($P = .003$). There was a trend toward improved mortality rates in the ERC group at 3% versus 18% ($P = .097$). Biliary sepsis occurred less commonly in patients with severe disease treated with ERC than conservative management at zero and 29% ($P < .001$). Issues with this study are inclusion of patients with pancreatitis of all causes and patients with cholangitis.

In a multicenter German study, 238 subjects were randomly assigned to ERC with sphincterotomy and stone extraction within 72 hours of symptom onset or conservative management. Patients with cholangitis or a total bilirubin of 5 mg/dL

or greater were excluded. Of 112 patients randomly assigned to conservative management, 20 went on to ERC, and 13 had stones extracted. The overall morbidity rates were similar between the ERC and control groups, but the data were not stratified by severity of pancreatitis. There were more serious complications in the treatment group, mostly because of respiratory failure ($P = .03$), but fewer episodes of cholangitis. Death occurred in 14 treatment and 7 control patients; most deaths were due to respiratory failure. Pancreatic morbidity rates were similar between the groups at 23% and 22%. The authors concluded that early ERC with sphincterotomy is not beneficial in patients with acute biliary pancreatitis and no obstructive jaundice or cholangitis. Problems with this study were that there were significantly fewer patients with stones and severe disease than in the other studies and that 19 of the 22 centers enrolled fewer than two subjects per year on average. The rate of respiratory failure in the ERC group was higher than in other studies. Considering the low volume at some centers and the undue rates of respiratory failure, questions have been raised about the degree of endoscopic expertise and potential for procedure-related aspiration.[71]

Zhou and colleagues[72] randomly assigned 45 patients with gallstone pancreatitis stratified by severity to have ERC within 24 hours or medical therapy. Sphincterotomy and extraction was done for small stones, and nasobiliary drainage was performed for large or no stones. Morbidity and length of hospitalization were significantly decreased in severe cases with ERC but not for mild disease. Issues with this study include the small sample size and that cholangitis was not explicitly excluded.

Another more recent randomized trial included 61 patients with gallstone pancreatitis and ampullary obstruction assigned to a control group of conservative therapy with selective ERC at 48 hours or a treatment group with ERC at 24 hours for persistent obstruction. In 9 of 31 control patients, obstruction did not spontaneously resolve, and 3 had ERC and sphincterotomy with no stones found. Among the treatment patients, obstruction resolved in 16, and 11 of 14 who had ERCP had stones removed. There was a statistically significant lower morbidity rate in the treatment group, and the authors concluded that these patients should have ERC within 48 hours. However, only 47% of the treatment patients had ERC.[73]

Oria and colleagues[74] randomly assigned 103 patients with acute gallstone pancreatitis with elevated bilirubin and dilated bile ducts but no cholangitis to ERC with sphincterotomy for stones or conservative management, and outcomes were stratified by severity. Bile duct stones were detected in 72% of the ERC group and 42% of the conservative group at subsequent surgery. There were no statistically significant differences between the groups in morbidity, CT index, local complications, or mortality. Limitations of the study are the small sample size and inclusion of patients with mild to moderate disease.

Van Santvoort and coworkers[80] performed a prospective multicenter, observational study of 153 patients with predicted severe biliary pancreatitis and no cholangitis. There were 81 patients who had ERC performed within 72 hours of admission for clinical indications. Morbidity occurred in fewer ERC patients with cholestasis than patients without cholestasis at 25% versus 54% ($P = .02$); this included fewer patients with greater than 30% of pancreatic necrosis at 8% and 31% ($P = .01$). ERC with or without papillotomy was also protective with statistical significance. For patients without cholestasis, morbidity rates were similar in the ERC and medically managed groups. Mortality rates were similar regardless of the treatment group. The authors opined that sphincterotomy may be beneficial in patients without choledocholithiasis seen at ERC by providing drainage for microlithiasis and sludge and stones that may have been missed.

There are six published meta-analyses of these randomized studies. ERC with or without sphincterotomy or conservative care was analyzed from four early trials including one published only in abstract. There were no exclusions for cholestasis or cholangitis. Morbidity and mortality rates were lower with ERC with statistical significance, and the number needed to treat to prevent complications and death was 7.6 and 25.5.[68-71] A Cochrane systematic review was performed on three trials with 511 patients. Treatment included ERC with or without sphincterotomy, and the analysis was controlled for cholangitis. The odds of having complications were reduced only in treated patients with predicted severe gallstone pancreatitis.[75] Petrov and colleagues[76] analyzed three trials with 450 participants and controlled for cholangitis. Early ERC, with or without sphincterotomy, in predicted mild and severe biliary pancreatitis did not lead to reductions in morbidity or mortality.

Another systematic review assessed local pancreatic morbidity. This review included five studies with 717 patients with mild or severe biliary pancreatitis. Early ERC did not significantly reduce the risk of local pancreatic complications.[77] Moretti and coworkers[78] reported a meta-analysis of five studies with 702 patients with predicted severe gallstone pancreatitis and determined that early ERC with or without sphincterotomy in patients with severe pancreatitis reduced complications with a number needed to treat of 3. Mortality was not significantly affected. There was no significant decrease in morbidity for mild disease. A meta-analysis by Uy and colleagues[79] involved two studies with 340 patients and was controlled for cholangitis; this showed no statistically significant benefit from early ERC.

Alternative approaches have been proposed. Liu and colleagues[81] randomly assigned 140 patients with suspected biliary pancreatitis to have EUS with ERC and sphincterotomy only for stones or ERC within 24 hours of admission. All patients in the EUS group had bile duct stones detected, but 14% were missed in the ERC group ($P = .001$). Additionally, standard transcutaneous ultrasound plus ERC missed cholelithiasis in six patients. The morbidity and mortality rates and lengths of hospital stay were similar between the groups. The authors concluded that EUS could safely replace diagnostic ERCP to select patients for therapeutic ERCP. Percutaneous transhepatic cholecystotomy was shown in a randomized trial to have similar outcomes to ERC in severe gallstone pancreatitis. The authors suggested percutaneous transhepatic cholecystotomy as second-line therapy if ERC fails.[82] The American Society for Gastrointestinal Endoscopy recommends the following for early ERC in acute biliary pancreatitis: (1) no early ERC in mild disease in the absence of clear evidence of a retained stone, (2) early ERC for concomitant cholangitis, (3) consideration of early ERC for evidence of obstruction, and (4) no recommendation for or against early ERC in patients with predicted severe acute biliary pancreatitis in the absence of overt biliary obstruction or cholangitis.[83] The American Gastroenterological Association

Institute and the American College of Gastroenterology have similar recommendations.[84,85]

From these data, ERC with sphincterotomy and stone extraction seems to improve outcomes in patients with severe biliary pancreatitis who have cholangitis or signs of biliary obstruction or both. The improved outcomes may be due to avoidance of and treatment for cholangitis or stone impaction or both; this may result in decreased systemic morbidity and progression to pancreatic necrosis. Some studies show a benefit to sphincterotomy even if no stones are present.[80]

Other series and expert recommendations favor reserving ERC and sphincterotomy for only patients who have stones seen on imaging studies including EUS. A rational therapeutic approach is to perform ERC within 24 to 72 hours in patients with severe pancreatitis and concomitant cholangitis or other signs of biliary obstruction. It is also reasonable to consider ERC in patients with mild to moderate biliary pancreatitis that appears to be associated with biliary obstruction and in patients with a persistent or deteriorating course. Sphincterotomy should be performed to prevent stone impaction in the absence of bile duct stones when cholecystectomy is not anticipated in the near future. This approach also applies during pregnancy to temporize until after delivery when cholecystectomy can be performed more safely.

One small study showed that about 90% of patients with gallstone pancreatitis do well for about 3 years after sphincterotomy and stone extraction without cholecystectomy.[39] Close follow-up is prudent in this circumstance. ERCP is not generally indicated for mild to moderate biliary pancreatitis without signs of obstruction. Laparoscopic cholecystectomy with IOC soon after the pancreatitis has resolved is optimal. Employing MRCP or EUS, or both, to diagnose stones in a less invasive fashion and then perform ERC on patients with positive results seems reasonable.[35,81,82]

Acute Cholangitis

Initial therapy is medical with supportive care, blood cultures, and parenteral vitamin K supplementation and empiric antibiotics. Up to 90% of patients respond to medical therapy within 12 to 24 hours and may then undergo semielective biliary drainage by ERC. Patients who do not respond require urgent or emergent drainage, preferably by ERC.[86-88] The choice of antibiotics should be based on local sensitivities and potential need for extended anaerobic coverage for elderly patients and patients with prior biliary instrumentation. Some appropriate regimens include monotherapy with fluoroquinolones (especially levofloxacin owing to expanded *Enterococcus* coverage), piperacillin/tazobactam, imipenem/cilastatin, or meropenem or therapy with extended-spectrum cephalosporins with or without metronidazole or clindamycin for enhanced anaerobic coverage. There are many other recommended regimens as well.[42]

Interventional radiographic drainage with PTC is successful in up to 90% of all patients with biliary obstruction, but morbidity, including bleeding, pseudoaneurysms, peritonitis, bile fistulas, infections, and strictures, occurs in 30% to 80%, and mortality occurs in 5% to 17% of patients with cholangitis.[89] ERC is more effective, has lower morbidity and mortality rates, and is preferred over PTC.[58,87] PTC may be indicated in unusual circumstances, however, such as intrahepatic stones, surgically altered duodenal anatomy, or failed ERC.

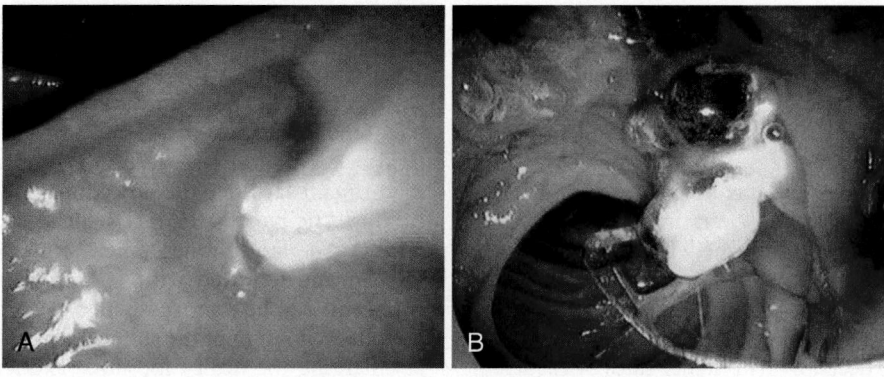

Fig. 43.13 A, Purulent drainage from the major papilla after cannulation indicative of suppurative cholangitis. **B,** Extracted stone with pus.

The traditional therapy for cholangitis is open surgery, but this is rarely performed as first-line therapy at the present time because of high rates of morbidity and mortality. In a randomized controlled trial in patients with cholangitis, Lai and colleagues[87] showed that ERC with sphincterotomy compared with open choledochotomy was associated with morbidity in 34% and 66% and in-hospital mortality in 10% and 32%. Operative mortality is associated with the severity of illness at the time of surgery with reported rates of 40% for emergent, 16% for urgent, and 3% for elective procedures.[86,90,91] Cholangitis may recur after open surgery with seemingly adequate drainage. In the setting of laparoscopic cholecystectomy, a systematic review showed that laparoscopic bile duct exploration is equivalent to ERC with sphincterotomy for bile duct stone clearance and morbidity and mortality but with shorter hospital stays.[22,90] However, the outcomes of laparoscopic bile duct exploration in patients with cholangitis are unknown because only a few patients with mild cholangitis are reported, and none had severe cholangitis. One-stage laparoscopic cholecystectomy with bile duct exploration seems appropriate for cholangitis patients with gallstones who respond to medical therapy and are clinically stable and good surgical candidates. Such surgery should not be performed in patients who are unstable or who have had prior cholecystectomy.[86,90,91]

ERC with sphincterotomy and stone extraction is the preferred procedure for patients with acute cholangitis who are critically ill or have had prior cholecystectomy. It is also appropriate for stable patients with cholelithiasis when expertise in laparoscopic bile duct exploration is unavailable. ERC may be performed in the standard fashion in stable patients with normal coagulation studies. However, patients with cholangitis frequently have septic shock with associated hypotension, multiorgan failure, disseminated intravascular coagulopathy, and coagulopathy from vitamin K malabsorption secondary to biliary obstruction. In these circumstances, it is generally best to provide temporizing biliary drainage rapidly with stent placement or a nasobiliary drain without sphincterotomy or stone extraction. I do these procedures under general anesthesia with endotracheal intubation. It is wise to aspirate and decompress the biliary system before injecting contrast material to avoid increasing the biliary pressure further with potential to exacerbate hematogenous seeding with bacteria and endotoxins. A stent may be placed in the normal fashion by passing a guidewire upstream to the obstructing stone and then inserting the endoprosthesis. Pus under pressure may be

seen to emanate around the cannulating catheter or through the stent (**Fig. 43.13**).

Nasobiliary drainage entails passing a guidewire above the obstructing stone and then advancing a 7-Fr drainage catheter over the wire and upstream to the stone. Pigtail catheters anchor above the stones and are more stable than straight catheters. The endoscope is removed over the drainage catheter while advancing the catheter to maintain position, without looping in the stomach, under fluoroscopic guidance. A 14-Fr tube is passed through a naris, grasped in the posterior pharynx, and pulled out through the mouth. The drainage catheter is digitally pinioned to the posterior pharynx to prevent dislodgment, and the proximal end is inserted into the oral end of the 14-Fr naso-oral catheter. The naso-oral catheter and the drainage catheter are pulled outward through the naris until it is straight in the pharynx while maintaining digital pressure for fixation of the drainage catheter in the posterior pharynx. The digital fixation pressure is released, the drainage catheter is aspirated and irrigated, and a cholangiogram is obtained to verify the position above the stone. The drainage catheter is fixed to the nose, face, and torso; connected to a bile bag; and set to gravity drainage. The catheter may be irrigated every 6 to 8 hours to maintain patency.

The outcomes of stent placement and nasobiliary drainage seem to be similar; I prefer stent placement because it is quicker, is easier, and has no external segment of the drain that could lead to accidental displacement.[88] Recovery is often rapid after drainage, and ERCP can be repeated with definitive sphincterotomy and stone extraction when the patient is stable and the coagulopathy has resolved.

Endoscopic Bile Duct Stone Extraction as Definitive Therapy with the Gallbladder In Situ

Patients with choledocholithiasis who are fit for surgery should have bile duct stone clearance and cholecystectomy. Endoscopic sphincterotomy with bile duct stone extraction cures the initiating episode related to choledocholithiasis. The need for subsequent cholecystectomy in patients with an intact gallbladder with gallstones has long been debated. After biliary sphincterotomy, there is a marked decrease in lithogenicity of gallbladder and hepatic bile, which has been proposed to decrease clinical events.[92] However, frequent symptoms and complications of leaving the gallbladder in situ include biliary colic, jaundice, cholecystitis, cholangitis, choledocholithiasis, pancreatitis bile leaks, and papillary stenosis. Predisposing factors include gallstones, complete opacification of the gallbladder at ERCP, bile duct dilation, and periampullary diverticula.[93–96]

McAlister and colleagues[97] performed a Cochrane systematic review to evaluate clinical observation with cholecystectomy only if symptoms occur versus scheduled cholecystectomy shortly after sphincterotomy in patients who had prior endoscopic biliary sphincterotomy. This analysis comprised 5 randomized clinical trials involving 662 participants. Patients who were managed expectantly had higher rates of recurrent biliary pain (relative risk [RR] 14.56, 95% confidence interval [CI] 4.95 to 42.78, $P < .0001$), jaundice or cholangitis (RR 2.53, 95% CI 1.09 to 5.87, $P = .03$), and subsequent ERCP or other cholangiography (RR 2.36, 95% CI 1.29 to 4.32, $P = .005$). Cholecystectomy was ultimately performed in 35% of the observational group. There were 26 (7.9%) deaths in the cholecystectomy group and 47 (14.1%) in the observational group representing a 78% increased risk of mortality (RR 1.78, 95% CI 1.15 to 2.75, $P = .01$). The survival benefit from scheduled cholecystectomy was independent of trial design, inclusion of high-risk patients, or inclusion of any one of the five trials.

Endoscopic Balloon Dilation of the Sphincter of Oddi for Extraction of Bile Duct Stones

Endoscopic balloon dilation of the sphincter of Oddi can be used to open the orifice to allow extraction of stones. This procedure may be done in the intact sphincter with a relatively small-caliber balloon for standard extraction of small stones and mechanical lithotripsy for large stones. Balloon dilation may also be done after sphincterotomy with large-caliber balloons for removal of large stones; this is discussed subsequently in the section on Large Stones.

Balloon Dilation of the Intact Papilla

Endoscopic sphincterotomy is the standard of care for opening the sphincter of Oddi and allows for removal of bile duct stones. Sphincterotomy is associated with short-term morbidity in about 5% of patients.[58] Medium-term (6 to 15 years) morbidity occurs in 6% to 24% of patients and can usually be managed with endoscopic techniques, but long-term outcomes remain largely unknown.[98–100] Endoscopic balloon dilation of the sphincter of Oddi has been proposed to prevent short-term and late occurring morbidity from sphincterotomy. Persons who may benefit most from this procedure are the young, healthy patients with laparoscopic cholecystectomy who have sphincterotomy for choledocholithiasis.

The technique of endoscopic balloon dilation involves passing a wire-guided balloon dilation catheter to bridge the biliary sphincter segment. The balloon is inflated with diluted radiographic contrast material to maximum pressure. Some experts advocate slow inflation to maximum pressure, which is maintained for 15 seconds before deflation to minimize pancreatitis risk. Although the benefits are unproven, this seems unlikely to increase morbidity.[101]

Fluoroscopy is generally used to document complete inflation with obliteration of the waist in the middle of the balloon. The diameter of the balloon is generally equal to the smallest diameter of either the stone or the duct; 6-mm and 8-mm balloons are the most common. Stones are removed with standard balloon and basket techniques (**Fig. 43.14**) Wire-guided instruments facilitate the procedure. Some authorities place a prophylactic pancreatic duct stent to reduce risks of pancreatitis.[102] For large stones, small-caliber dilation can be performed and followed with mechanical lithotripsy. Crushed fragments can be removed with extraction-balloon catheters.

Balloon dilation of the sphincter of Oddi is usually effective at enlarging the orifice for stone extraction. However, compared with sphincterotomy, it takes longer, has higher failure rates, requires increased use of mechanical lithotripsy, and is associated with higher morbidity rates owing to pancreatitis, including deaths.[46,48,103] Balloon dilation may induce edema or spasm, or both, with obstruction of the pancreatic duct or papillary edema and impaction of stones not extracted. Pancreatitis or cholangitis may result.[44,102,104] After sphincterotomy, most retained stones pass spontaneously. Some authors have proposed prophylactic placement of pancreatic duct stents to minimize balloon dilation–induced pancreatitis; but this has not been adequately studied.[102]

From four uncontrolled series of sphincter of Oddi balloon dilation involving 1296 patients, it appears that initial bile duct clearance was achieved in 72% of patients, with the remainder requiring two or more ERCPs and occasionally sphincterotomy, surgery, or other therapy. Mechanical lithotripsy was needed in 34%. Morbidity occurred in at least 7% to 19% and was mostly due to pancreatitis.[105–108] Problems with interpreting these studies include that three series seem retrospective with potential underestimation of complications.[105–107] All of these reports are from tertiary centers, the patients were relatively old, and standardized morbidity criteria were not consistently used.[44] Gabexate was given to decrease morbidity from pancreatitis in one series[108] and may have been used in others.[105–107]

Several randomized, controlled clinical trials from tertiary centers in Europe and Asia and a single multicenter study representing academic and community practices compared balloon dilation with sphincterotomy. The largest studies are summarized in **Table 43.1**.[45–48,109] The patients in the European and Asian studies were relatively old and sick, harbored large and numerous stones, often had periampullary diverticula, and did not always have cholecystectomy. Multiple procedures were frequently required, mechanical lithotripsy and precut sphincterotomy were often employed, procedures may have been terminated prematurely, and gabexate use was not always specified. The study methodologies were not always rigorous, lacking a predefined sample size, not verifying sequential enrollment or concealed allocation or both, and inconsistently using standardized criteria for overall and severe morbidity.[45,47,109] At least one dilation patient who experienced morbidity was excluded from analysis.[47] One study found no advantage to balloon dilation after 24 hours and after 12 months, and another study showed statistically significant increased rates of pancreatitis and overall morbidity with endoscopic balloon dilation.[45,109]

DiSario and colleagues[48] performed a randomized, controlled, multicenter, largely American study involving equal numbers of community and academic practices. The patients

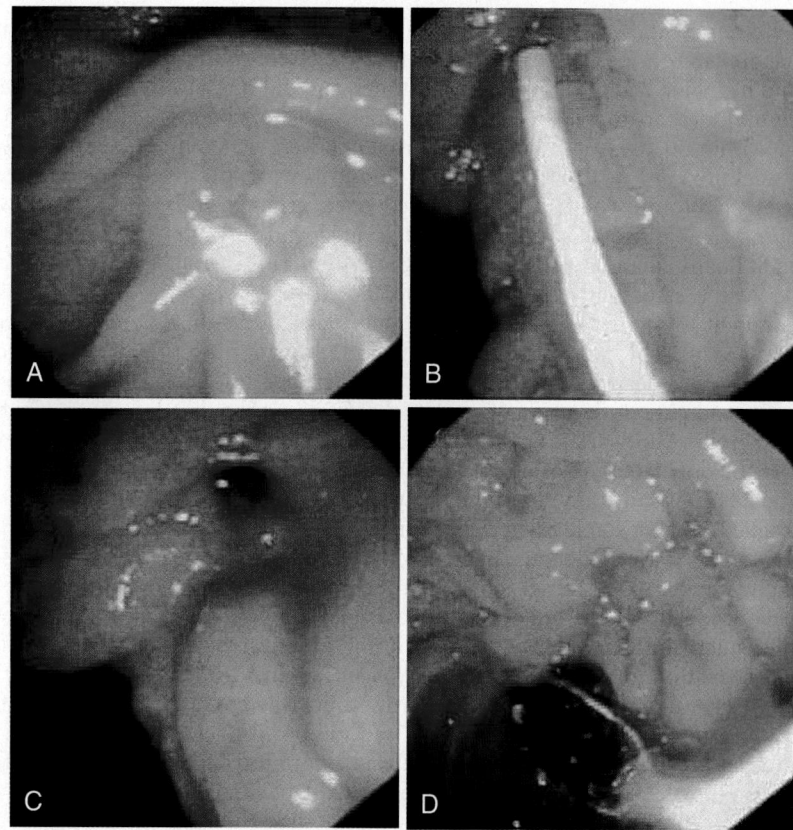

Fig. 43.14 A, Normal intact papilla. **B,** Inflated dilation balloon straightens the biliary sphincter. **C,** Opened papilla after dilation. **D,** Pigment stones are extracted with a basket.

Table 43.1 Randomized Studies of Balloon Dilation of the Sphincter of Oddi Compared with Sphincterotomy for Stone Removal

| | DiSario, et al[48] | | Bergman, et al[46] | | Fujita, et al[47] | | Vlavianos, et al[45] | |
	ED	*ES*	*ED*	*ES*	*ED*	*ES*	*ED*	*ES*
PATIENTS								
No.	117	120	101	101	117	120	117	120
Age, yr	47*	54*	72†	71†	47*	54*	47*	54*
Stones								
Size, mm	6*	5*	10†	9†	7*	7.3*	40% ≥10 mm	42% ≥10 mm
No.	1*	1*	2†	1†	2.5*	2.4*	39% ≥3	25% ≥3
Procedures								
Success‡	114 (97%)	111 (93%)	90 (89%)	92 (91%)	105 (76%)	113 (78%)	65 (63%)	63 (64%)
Crossover	11 (9%)	0	9 (9%)	0	0	3 (2%)	5 (1%)	1 (1%)
Morbidity								
Total	21 (18%)§	4 (3%)§	17 (17%)§	23 (23%)§	21 (15%)§	17 (12%)§	21 (15%)¶	17 (12%)¶
Severe	8 (7%)§	0§	4 (4%)§	3 (3%)§	‖	‖	≥1 (1%)¶	≥1 (1%)¶
Mortality	3 (2%)	0	1 (1%)	0	0	0	0	≥1 (1%)**

*Mean.
†Median.
‡Removal of all stones at the initial procedure.
§Consensus criteria.[44]
¶Partial consensus criteria.[44]
‖Incomplete data.
**Cardiopulmonary arrest.
ED, endoscopic balloon dilation; ES, endoscopic sphincterotomy.

were representative of patients having laparoscopic cholecystectomy in routine clinical practice in that they were younger and healthier, had fewer and smaller stones, and did not have complicated anatomy, and most had cholecystectomy before or within 30 days of ERCP. The procedures were generally straightforward without mechanical lithotripsy or precut sphincterotomy. The study had a predefined primary endpoint, sample size determination, and an independent Oversight Board. The study was stopped at the first interim analysis because a statistically significant difference in the primary endpoint was found with more overall morbidity in the dilation group. There were also significantly more severe complications, two deaths from pancreatitis, and greater resource usage and patient days away for normal activities in the dilation group. Multivariate analysis showed that balloon dilation was the only factor associated with complications.

The American study[48] and the study by Bergman and colleagues[46] from a single referral center in the Netherlands (see **Table 43.1**) have analogous methodology, and the results can be compared.[46,48] Overall and severe complications after balloon dilation occurred at similar rates of 18% and 4% in the Dutch study and 18% and 6.8% in the American study. However, the Dutch study showed overall and severe morbidity in 24% and 3% in the sphincterotomy group, whereas only 3.3% of American study participants had mild to moderate morbidity. These sphincterotomy-related morbidity rates reflect the older, sicker, and more complicated Dutch tertiary referral center patients and are much higher than the rates observed in younger and healthier patients treated in a broad spectrum of American practices.[48]

Two other large-scale multicenter studies showed less than 5% morbidity after sphincterotomy performed for stones.[58,59] Papillary balloon dilation was found to be the most significant risk factor for pancreatitis in well-designed, multicenter series of 1966 ERCPs with an adjusted odds ratio of 4.5 (95% CI 1.51 to 113.46, $P = .0027$).[110] A randomized, controlled clinical trial by Arnold and colleagues[104] also showed excessive overall and severe complication rates with dilation compared with sphincterotomy that compelled the authors to terminate the study prematurely. A Cochrane systematic review showed that balloon dilation compared with sphincterotomy for stone extraction imparts increased risks of pancreatitis and is slightly less successful.[103]

Complication rates for sphincterotomy are increased to 12% to 23% in the larger, referral center, randomized controlled studies owing to the complicated patients and procedures. These morbidity rates are similar to the morbidity rates of balloon dilation of 15% to 17% in these series, which is appropriate for that patient population.[45-47] However, these similarities reflect the selection bias of tertiary center patients and cannot be generalized to patients seen in routine practice. Morbidity rates for sphincterotomy from referral center patients are far greater than the 3% to 5% commonly seen in young and healthy patients undergoing laparoscopic cholecystectomy.[48,58,59]

The frequency and severity of morbidity of balloon dilation is unacceptable for routine clinical practice in the United States. Papillary balloon dilation has been proposed to avert the late-occurring complications of sphincterotomy, but it offers no clear benefit. There may be partial return of sphincter function 12 to 15 months after dilation. Chronic inflammation occurs 2 to 63 months after dilation with unknown

clinical significance.[111-114] Gallbladder motility seems normal 2 years after dilation but may be increased after sphincterotomy.[115] Bile duct flow assessed by quantitative cholescintigraphy 1 to 3 years after ERC is unaffected by dilation but is significantly increased after sphincterotomy.[116] Reflux of pancreatic enzymes into the bile duct as a measure of sphincter function was undetectable 1 year after either dilation or sphincterotomy.[117]

A multicenter Japanese study of 837 patients undergoing balloon dilation and followed for a mean of 4.4 years revealed biliary complications in 12.4% including recurrent stones in 8.8% and cholecystitis in 4.5%. Risk factors included lithotripsy at ERC and cholecystectomy either before or more than 30 days after ERC.[105] Another retrospective series of 686 patients revealed a statistically significant difference in late recurrence of stones after dilation in 8% and sphincterotomy in 17%.[114] A randomized study involving 104 patients followed for 16 months after ERC found similar rates of recurrent choledocholithiasis in 6.3% of dilation patients and 7.5% of sphincterotomy patients.[118] Another small randomized trial revealed stone recurrence in 25% and 6.3% of dilation and sphincterotomy patients at about 1 year; with about 5 years of follow-up, this changed to 6.3% and 26.7% for dilation and sphincterotomy patients.[119] Similar rates of morbidity of 29% for balloon dilation and 31% for sphincterotomy were reported at 10-year follow-up of the American multicenter, randomized study.[98]

Papillary balloon dilation may be appropriate for patients with severe coagulopathies and altered surgical anatomy that makes standard sphincterotomy more difficult and risky[120-122]; however, this approach may simply replace bleeding or perforation with pancreatitis. Pancreatic duct stent placement seems reasonable if papillary balloon dilation is used for these conditions. However, in routine clinical practice, balloon dilation of the sphincter of Oddi for extraction of bile duct stones is associated with high rates of morbidity and deaths from pancreatitis and should be avoided.

Difficult Stones

Standard techniques can be used to remove 85% to 90% of bile duct stones, the remaining 5% to 10% of stones are considered difficult. What constitutes a difficult stone is subjective but may include impacted stones, large stones, stones above strictures, intrahepatic stones, recurrent stones, and Mirrizi's syndrome. Various techniques are available for each of these circumstances.

Impacted stones at the ampulla first should be approached by attempting to pass a guidewire or catheter around the stone and upstream into the duct or by dislodging the stone slightly upstream by pushing with a catheter (**Fig. 43.15**). If a wire or instrument can be passed above the stone, a sphincterotomy can be performed, and the stone can be extracted in the usual fashion. If instruments cannot pass the impacted stone, an access or precut papillotomy may be required. Using a needle-knife or a sphincterotome with the cutting wire extending over the distal tip, the attenuated papillary tissue encasing the impacted stone is incised in the direction of the bile duct at the 11 o'clock position. The incision is freehand with repeated smooth and shallow cuts in the same incision line until access is gained. This procedure requires an experienced endoscopist with excellent control of the instruments. Once the incision

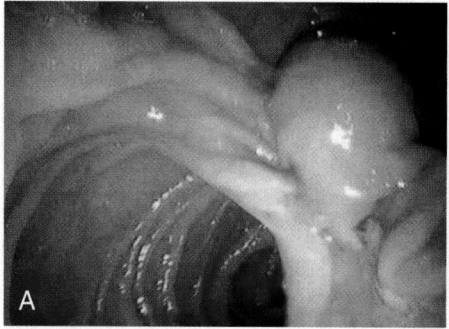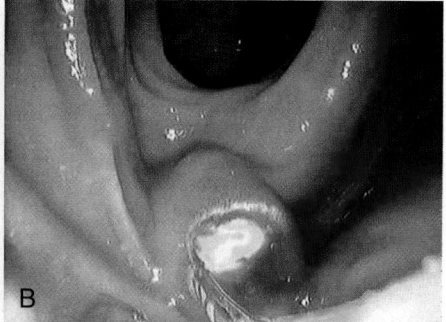

Fig. 43.15 A, Bulging major papilla resulting from an impacted stone. **B,** An impacted stone is seen at the orifice of the major papilla, and a sphincterotome is inserted below.

alleviates the impaction, the stone usually pops out spontaneously. However, it may be necessary to probe with the precut papillotome or an atraumatic guidewire until an instrument passes above the stone. Extension of the sphincterotomy can be performed with a standard sphincterotome.

Precut sphincterotomy is associated with increased rates of overall and severe complications compared with standard sphincterotomy. However, precutting is used to gain access to the duct in a complicated situation that requires therapy. The risks for precutting are less with a dilated bile duct and when the incision is made on an attenuated papilla, as is often the case with an impacted stone.[58,123]

Large Stones

Large stones are generally considered to be 10 mm or larger across the greatest span. They are often brown or mixed stones and are often impacted. Endoscopic extraction may be challenging because of the frequent presence of periampullary diverticula, the sheer volume of stone material, and the difficulty in entrapping very large stones in Dormia baskets. One series showed that only 12% of stones larger than 15 mm could be removed with standard sphincterotomy and techniques.[124] A large opening is required to remove large stones effectively. The first endoscopic maneuver is to create a large sphincterotomy or to extend a prior sphincterotomy. If a guidewire or catheter can be passed upstream to the stone, it can often be removed with standard techniques, mechanical lithotripsy, or stent placement to provide drainage and break the stone over time. A relatively new technique is to perform large balloon dilation after sphincterotomy and remove the stones in the usual fashion or with mechanical lithotripsy.[57] Alternatively, transendoscopic electrohydraulic lithotripsy (EHL), laser lithotripsy, or ESWL may be performed. One series of 108 patients with unsuccessful stone extraction by standard techniques showed success with mechanical lithotripsy in 33 patients, EHL in 65 patients, and ESWL in 7 of 10 patients with intrahepatic stones.[56]

LARGE-CALIBER BALLOON DILATION AFTER SPHINCTEROTOMY

The biliary orifice can be safely opened to 12 to 20 mm by performing large-caliber balloon dilation after sphincterotomy. The sphincterotomy separates the biliary and pancreatic components of the sphincter and prevents the inflated balloon

from compressing the pancreatic orifice. This approach does not seem to cause excessive rates of pancreatitis as with dilation of an intact papilla.[48] The technique is to incise the ampullary mound partially or completely. A complete incision is favored by many authorities to minimize balloon-induced trauma to the sphincter. Patients with prior sphincterotomy can have large dilation without extension.

A wire-guided large-caliber balloon dilator of the type used for esophageal and gastrointestinal dilation is inserted over a guidewire to bridge the orifice. The balloon should be about the same diameter as the stone but no larger than the diameter of the duct. These balloons often do not have a radiopaque tip, and care must be taken to avoid inadvertent ductal perforation unseen on fluoroscopy. The balloon is positioned along the axis of the duct by advancing the duodenoscope and applying rightward torque. The balloon is inflated with dilute radiographic contrast material while maintaining position with endoscopic and fluoroscopic visualization. Once inflation is complete and obliteration of the waist on the balloon is verified, it may be deflated and removed. There is no standard time of maintained inflation. The stones may be extracted with balloons, baskets, or mechanical lithotripsy.[57]

From a compilation of 12 series involving 842 patients with large stones who had sphincterotomy followed by balloon dilation to about 15 mm (range 12 to 20 mm), 92% had total stone clearance at the first procedure, and 12% required mechanical lithotripsy. Morbidity occurred in 7%, mostly owing to mild to moderate bleeding, pancreatitis, perforation, and pain.[125,126] Itoi and colleagues[125] showed that ERC with sphincterotomy with standard techniques and mechanical lithotripsy had a mean procedure duration of 40 minutes compared with sphincterotomy with large-balloon dilation, which took 32 minutes ($P < .05$). These procedures also required 22 minutes and 13 minutes of fluoroscopy ($P < .05$). In a randomized study of 27 patients with large stones assigned to sphincterotomy plus large-balloon dilation and 28 patients assigned to sphincterotomy and standard techniques, no statistically significant differences were detected in success at stone removal at the first procedure, use of mechanical lithotripsy, procedure duration, or morbidity. However, the small sample size limits the validity of this study.[127] Heo and colleagues[128] randomly assigned 200 patients with large stones to have small sphincterotomy and large-balloon (12 to 20 mm) dilation or sphincterotomy with traditional techniques. Similar results were found for ductal clearance (97% vs. 98%); large stone extraction (94% vs. 97%); mechanical lithotripsy

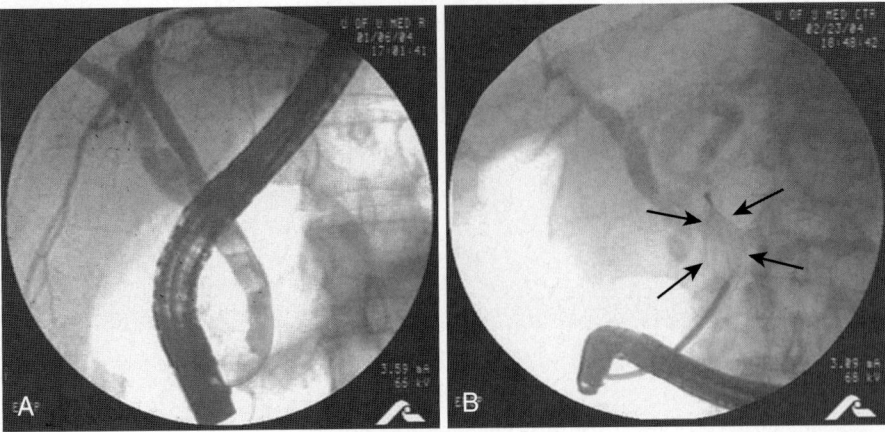

Fig. 43.16 A, Cholangiography showing medium to large stones. **B,** A stone (arrows) is entrapped in a mechanical lithotripsy basket. Note the metal sheath winched against the lower end of the basket.

use (8% vs. 9%); and overall morbidity (5% vs. 7%) including pancreatitis (4% vs. 4%), cholecystitis (1% vs. 1%), and delayed bleeding (0 vs. 2%).

INTRACORPOREAL LITHOTRIPSY

In mechanical lithotripsy, when the stone is too large to be pulled out of the sphincterotomy, it is entrapped in a basket with securely welded wires. The basket is winched down against a metal sheath until the stone abuts the sheath, and continued pressure from retraction of the basket shatters the stone or breaks the basket (**Fig. 43.16**). Devices that pass through the working channel of the duodenoscope are manufactured as a single unit or a sheath that can be inserted over the long wire shaft of a basket that has become impacted at the bile duct orifice and then attached to a winch. Mechanical lithotripsy results in complete bile duct clearance in about 80% to 90% of patients, but 20% to 30% require multiple procedures. This technique is less likely to be successful with larger or impacted stones.[129] Mechanical lithotripsy is a straightforward technology that should be present in all endoscopic units that perform stone extractions.

Intracorporeal lithotripsy can also be performed with EHL or laser probes under direct visualization via a cholangioscope passed through the duodenoscope. The probe can be aimed at the stone to prevent bile duct trauma. These techniques have traditionally required two endoscopists for the mother scope (duodenoscope) and the baby scope (4.5-mm or 3.0-mm cholangioscope). A light source and processing unit are required for each instrument as well as an irrigation system to maintain visualization and flush debris out of the bile duct. The endoscopist with the mother scope controls most of the motion of the baby scope, mainly with gentle torque on the duodenoscope insertion tube. The baby scope has tip deflection in only one axis. Single-user, partially disposable cholangioscopes are available that fasten to the duodenoscope. They have a reusable optical fiber, a working channel, and four-way tip deflection.[129,130] Another technique in development uses a small-caliber gastroscope directed into the bile duct with a fixation balloon in place of the duodenoscope and cholangioscope system.[131]

EHL produces shock waves by generating high-voltage sparks that vaporize fluid and transmit this energy through a small-caliber (3-Fr, 1-mm) probe. The probe is positioned about 1 mm from the stone. Shock wave energy is activated by a foot switch and is repeated until the stone is fragmented. Centering balloons and basket catheters are also available to aim the probe under fluoroscopic guidance without choledochoscopy.[132] However, aberrantly aimed shock waves can cause ductal trauma and perforation. EHL provides clearance of all stones and fragments in about 90% of patients with stones refractory to standard therapy. Morbidity is reported in about 9% of patients and is usually mild.[130,133,134]

Several laser lithotripsy systems have been used for bile duct stones. The most widely used are the holmium:yttrium aluminum garnet (YAG) and the frequency-doubled, double-pulse neodymium:YAG (FREDDY). High-power density laser light focused on a stone creates a plasma composed of a gaseous collection of ions and free electrons. An oscillating plasma bubble induces cavitation with tensile and compressive waves that shatter the stone surface.[129]

Holmium:YAG lasers are commercially available for treatment of bile duct stones. These lasers are commonly used for urinary tract stones. The laser delivers high-energy pulses of about 500 to 1000 mJ. Fibers come in several diameters ranging from 200 to 1000 μm and lengths of up to 4 m. Fibers are specifically designed for biliary use. The fibers must be used with a cholangioscope or centering balloon. Routine power settings are 0.6 to 1.0 J at 6 to 10 Hz for a total laser energy of 12 kJ. These are small, portable units that require no special plumbing. The FREDDY laser uses wavelengths of 532 to 1064 nm and generates up to 120 to 160 mJ (about 24 mJ at 532 nm). The pulse duration is 1.2 μsec at 160 mJ with single or dual pulse at adjustable rates of 1 Hz, 3 Hz, 5 Hz, or 10 Hz with standard 110 voltage AC. The recommended settings are 120 mJ single pulse and 3 to 5 Hz repetition rate, which can be increased to 160 mJ and 10 Hz. The fibers are 3.5 m long with a diameter of 420 μm and are reusable. The FREDDY laser causes minimal, if any, trauma to the duct and has been used with a cholangioscope and with centering balloons. These units are also mobile and do not require special plumbing.[129]

The holmium:YAG laser is reported to induce total clearance of intrahepatic and extrahepatic stones in 97% of patients from a compilation of several small studies.[129] There are reports of complications from the holmium:YAG laser, but it is reasonable to expect similar rates with EHL and other lasers. From two series involving 69 patients with large bile duct stones treated with the FREDDY laser under cholangioscopic (10%) or fluoroscopic (90%) guidance, complete clearance was achieved in 91% with a mean of 1.5 sessions. Mild morbidity occurred in 20% (nine cases of hemobilia, four cases of pancreatitis, and two cases of cholangitis).[129,134–136]

EXTRACORPOREAL SHOCK WAVE LITHOTRIPSY

ESWL focuses high-pressure shock wave energy at a desired point while minimizing the pressure in the adjacent tissue. There are different methods to generate the shock waves, but all systems require the shock waves to travel through water to minimize energy loss. The contact with the patient is with a water-filled compressible bag with a gel. When shock waves traverse the stone, the surface becomes cavitated, and changes in acoustic impedance release compressive and tensile forces resulting in fragmentation. The properties of the stone that determine fragmentation are the size, microcrystalline structure, and architecture and not the chemical makeup.[137]

The patient is positioned on the lithotripter, and the stone is identified by ultrasound or fluoroscopy. The shock waves are usually delivered from the back for the bile duct or over the liver for intrahepatic stones to avoid interposition of gas-filled intestinal loops. Prior placement of a nasobiliary drain for cholangiography or a biliary stent adjacent to the stone as a target is usually required. Prophylactic antibiotics and sedation and analgesia are given. The energy is delivered, and cholangiography is performed. If fragmentation has occurred, the debris is usually removed by endoscopic or percutaneous methods. If adequate fragmentation has not occurred, ESWL may be repeated at intervals of about 1 week.

ESWL can achieve complete removal of refractory bile duct stones in about 84% of patients and partial clearance in 12% of patients. Complete clearance is more difficult with larger stones but not with multiple stones.[138] About 13% of treated patients have stone recurrence within about 1 year; this may be due to retained fragments after ESWL. About 30% to 40% of treated patients have complications, including pain, hemobilia, cholangitis, sepsis, hematomas, pancreatitis, hematuria, ileus, and anesthesia effects. Mortality occurs in less than 1%; predisposing factors are advanced age, serious comorbidities, and concomitant cholangitis.[129] Randomized controlled studies show that intracorporeal laser lithotripsy is more effective at achieving complete ductal clearance than ESWL (about 92% vs. 66%). However, complete clearance was achieved in similar proportions of patients randomly assigned to ESWL (79%) and EHL (75%).[129] Crossing over to another lithotripsy modality improved the ductal clearance rates to 94% to 100%.[139–142]

PTC with antegrade instrumentation, choledochoscopy, or the modalities described previously is another option. PTC techniques achieve ductal clearance in 80% to 97% of cases but often require multiple procedures. Percutaneous tubes are usually left in place for several weeks. Minor complications are frequent and include pain, fever, and local infections. Serious morbidity from pancreatitis (10%), bleeding (2.5%), sepsis (2.5%), and pneumothoraces (0.5%) and deaths are reported. Other complications include subcapsular hepatic hematomas, hepatic artery aneurysms, cholangitis, peritonitis, bilomas, gallstone ileus, and premature tube displacement and may require surgery or other invasive procedures. Surgery for bile duct stones is generally reserved as a last resort.[129]

STENTS

Biliary drainage with nasobiliary drains or stents is required to prevent cholangitis when large stones cannot be removed at ERCP (**Fig. 43.17**). Nasobiliary drains are cumbersome to place and are uncomfortable and unsightly for the patient. Stents may be used to temporize until a definitive procedure is performed or as long-term therapy in patients with advanced age or serious comorbidities and a severely limited life span. Midterm to long-term morbidity and mortality rates are high, however, and careful patient selection is crucial. The stents may act as a wick allowing bile drainage through or alongside the stent when obstruction occurs. Friction from the stent may wear down or break stones. Sphincterotomy is performed, and one or two straight or pigtail 7-Fr or 10-Fr stents can be placed in virtually all cases. Stents placed for several months induce stone shrinkage and disappearance and facilitate removal at subsequent ERCP.[143] Ursodeoxycholic acid seems to facilitate this process.[144]

More recent cohort studies involving 196 elderly and sick patients treated with stent placement for refractory stones and followed for means of 2 to 39 months showed serious morbidity in 33%, usually resulting from cholangitis, and related mortality in 6%. Cholangitis developed at means ranging from 2 to 39 months.[145–148] In comparative studies, there were significantly higher late morbidity rates with stent placement than routine stone extraction (36% vs. 14%), EHL (63% vs. 8%), or surgery (36% vs. 8%) and elevated overall mortality rates with stent placement over EHL (74% vs. 41%).[49,146–148]

Hepatolithiasis

Primary intrahepatic stones are associated with ductal strictures, and secondary stones are gallstones or bile duct stones that have refluxed into the intrahepatic system. Primary stones occur mainly in residents of eastern Asia who are rural dwellers and of lower socioeconomic status. These stones are associated with parasitic infestations including *Clonorchis sinensis,* biliary infections, congenital factors, ductal abnormalities, and intrahepatic cholangiocarcinoma. In white patients, primary intrahepatic stones are associated with prior hepatobiliary surgery, strictures, cystic fibrosis, and Caroli's disease. The intrahepatic ducts are dilated and contain multiple stones, often of mixed composition. Patients have recurrent bouts of pain, fever, and jaundice that require repeated operations or other invasive therapies.[149]

Secondary intrahepatic stones may be treated with ERCP techniques with or without intracorporeal lithotripsy. However, primary stones are difficult to treat from a transpapillary approach because of duct angulation, multiple strictures, and peripheral stone impaction. Sphincterotomy should be avoided unless definitive therapy is ensured because of increased risks of recurrent cholangitis. However, clearance of intrahepatic stones was achieved in 64% of 36 patients treated with peroral cholangioscopic lithotripsy with morbidity in 1 (3%) and recurrences in 22% with almost 8 years of follow-up.[150]

PTC with intracorporeal lithotripsy results in complete stone clearance in 77% to 85% of patients with morbidity in

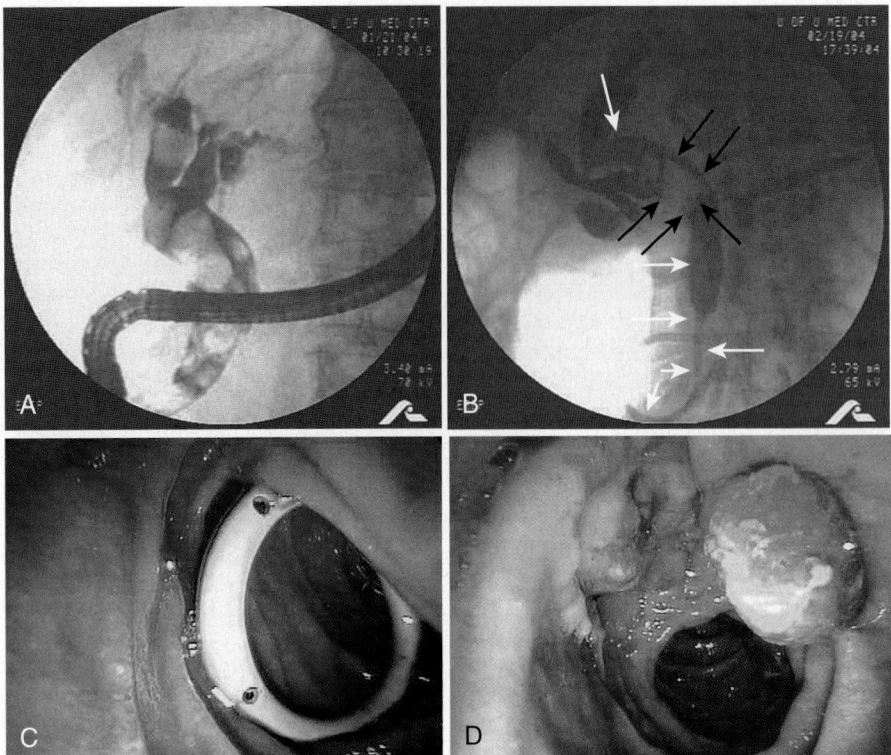

Fig. 43.17 A, Endoscopic cholangiography shows several large bile duct stones that could not be extracted with sphincterotomy and mechanical lithotripsy. **B,** A 10-Fr double-pigtailed stent has been placed *(white arrows)*. A large stone is shown *(black arrows)*. **C,** Duodenal end of pigtailed stent. **D,** A large, mostly cholesterol stone is successfully extracted with a basket 4 weeks later.

1.6% to 22%.[151,152] With 1 to 22 years of follow-up, recurrence of stones or cholangitis developed in about 63% and was directly proportional to duration of follow-up at a median of 11 to 18 years. Symptomatic recurrence was more frequent in patients with ductal dilation and strictures and occurred sooner in patients with strictures. Cholangitis and cholangiocarcinoma developed more often in patients with residual stones than patients without residual stones (44% and 16% vs. 6.6% and 0.7%).[151–152] ESWL has also been used successfully with lesser clearance rates.[50,51,139,141,142,153] In combination with intracorporeal lithotripsy, however, more than 90% of intrahepatic stones can be cleared.[44] Patients with stones associated with strictures do not respond as well.

Hepatic resection or hepaticojejunostomy, usually with intraoperative or postoperative choledochoscopy and lithotripsy, may be performed in selected patients with hepatolithiasis. Resection is generally indicated for segments with parenchymal atrophy, multiple abscesses, or intrahepatic cholangiocarcinomas. Patients with resection fare better than patients with biliary-enteric anastomoses, with operative morbidity in 20% and 16%, mortality in 2% and 6%, residual stones in 2% to 60% and 44% to 90%, recurrent stones in 16% and 33%, and cholangitis in 3% and 31%.[154,155]

Mirizzi's Syndrome

Mirizzi's syndrome is a rare disorder that occurs when a gallstone is entrapped in the gallbladder neck or cystic duct and causes obstruction or fistula of the bile duct. The appearance on direct cholangiography is an extrinsic obstruction with smooth tapering of the proximal and distal margins. Making the diagnosis requires an index of suspicion and careful interpretation of direct cholangiography and high-quality MRCP or intraductal ultrasound. Endoscopic therapy is challenging, and standard techniques usually fail. Bile duct stent placement and intracorporeal or extracorporeal lithotripsy can be successful, however.[156] Surgery is often complicated, and open conversion is often required. However, laparoscopic techniques are possible, and it is important to have a preoperative diagnosis to minimize the complications and conversion rates.[157]

Sump Syndrome

The sump syndrome is an unusual condition in which there is a choledochoduodenal fistula with downstream impaction of stones or food material, or both, in the bile duct remnant and sphincter segment. This condition may cause pain, pancreatitis, and cholangitis. Therapy is with endoscopic sphincterotomy, and excellent immediate and long-term results are obtained.[158]

Small Stones

Stones that are 3 mm or less in diameter are generally considered to be small (**Fig. 43.18**). The clinical significance of these lesions is uncertain and may be negligible. After ESWL, all stone fragments 3 mm or less in diameter and almost all stones 3.5 to 5 mm in diameter have been shown to pass into

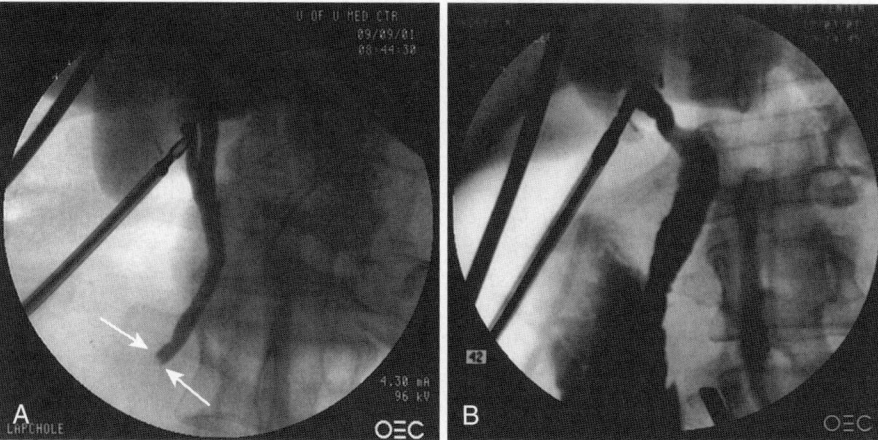

Fig. 43.18 A, Laparoscopic intraoperative cholangiography shows a 3-mm stone impacted in the ampullary segment *(arrows).* **B,** The stone has been flushed through after medical dilation of the sphincter of Oddi with glucagon, and the contrast material flows freely into the duodenum. *(Courtesy of Robert Glasgow, MD.)*

the duodenum with rare symptoms and no complications.[159] In a study of 539 cholecystectomy patients, 12% of the patients randomly assigned to have IOC had unsuspected bile duct stones detected with equivalent amounts expected in the control group. Similar symptomatic outcomes occurred in the IOC and control groups, and none of the control patients had clinically detected retained bile duct stones with 3 years of follow-up.[5] In another study of 163 preoperative patients with gallstones and abnormal liver test results and normal ERC, 49% had sphincterotomy with small bile duct stones found in 26%. With more than 3 years of postoperative follow-up, none of the sphincterotomy patients had biliary complications.[6] In another report, about 5% of 942 laparoscopic cholecystectomy patients who had routine IOC had filling defects indicative of stones, and a biliary catheter was left in place. A normal cholangiogram was seen at 48 hours in 26% and at 6 weeks in another 26%, but 48% had stones detected and removed by ERCP at 12 weeks.[7]

These data indicate that most small bile duct stones, particularly stones that are 3 mm or less in diameter, pass spontaneously without adverse sequela. However, if conservative management of these lesions is contemplated, clinical follow-up should be continued because small stones cause pancreatitis, and secondary biliary cirrhosis may develop in 1 to 3 years with intermittent ductal obstruction.[8,38]

Postoperative Care

Most patients undergoing ERCP are observed in a holding area or are hospitalized after the procedure. Postoperative management depends on the clinical situation and endoscopic maneuvers performed. Most patients who have had an uncomplicated ERCP with sphincterotomy for stones can be discharged on the same day with instructions to avoid anticoagulants, aspirin, nonsteroidal antiinflammatory drugs, and antiplatelet drugs to prevent hemorrhage. Patients at increased risk for pancreatitis because of younger age, female sex, small-caliber ducts, difficult cannulations, repeated pancreatic injections or instrumentation, or precut

sphincterotomy should be vigorously hydrated, given only sips of water, and provided with analgesics and antiemetics for 12 to 24 hours after the procedure. Patients with cholangitis who are adequately drained should receive antibiotics for 3 to 5 days after ERCP.[42]

Outpatient Endoscopic Retrograde Cholangiopancreatography

ERCP is regularly performed on an outpatient basis. Patients considered for same-day discharge must be stratified based on risk of complications. Good candidates are patients with few comorbidities and adequate support systems who reside in proximity to the hospital. Additional risk factors include suspected sphincter of Oddi dysfunction, cirrhosis, difficult cannulation, precut sphincterotomy, and combined PTC and endoscopic access. About 44% of complications in patients planned for same-day discharge develop within 2 hours, and 79% develop within 6 hours.[160] More recent studies show that up to 19% of planned outpatient procedures resulted in admission; most complications were detected in the endoscopy or recovery units, and few patients with complications returned from home.[161,162]

Recurrent Stones

Recurrent stones develop in about 10% to 20% of patients who have had sphincterotomy or papillary balloon dilation for stone extraction.[163–165] Recurrence is usually with brown stones, and the clinical presentation is often cholangitis. The problem may be due to bile stasis and repeated infections. Risk factors for recurrence include older age, periampullary diverticula, a largely dilated bile duct, biliary strictures, mechanical lithotripsy, and a gallbladder in situ. Clinical follow-up with serum enzyme levels and transabdominal ultrasound with ERCP for abnormal findings may improve stone extraction rates and decrease occurrences of cholangitis.[163,166,167] Surgery may be beneficial to remove stones that cannot be extracted by endoscopic means but has not been shown to decrease recurrence rates.[167]

Complications

ERCP with sphincterotomy for stones is successful in more than 90% of patients; morbidity is about 5%, and mortality is rare.[58] High-risk patients may safely and successfully undergo ERCP with sedation and analgesia for appropriate indications. Patients with significant comorbidities and morbid obesity who require ERCP benefit from general anesthesia with endotracheal intubation to minimize the risks of cardiopulmonary complications.[168] Patients with severe acute pancreatitis and suppurative cholangitis benefit from urgent ERCP and stone extraction or drainage but often require general anesthesia and maintenance of vital signs. Successful ERCP has been reported in five patients within 15 to 56 days after myocardial infarction for urgent indications without cardiovascular complications.[169] Patients with severe coagulopathies and thrombocytopenia with urgent indications for stone extraction should have attempts made to correct the problem with vitamin K, plasma, or platelet transfusions.[60] If the deficit cannot be corrected, stent placement or nasobiliary drainage may be performed without sphincterotomy, or papillary balloon dilation may be performed to minimize bleeding risks.[88,120]

References

The complete reference list is available online at www.expertconsult.com.

Benign Biliary Strictures and Leaks

Guido Costamagna

Video related to this chapter's topics can be found online at expertconsult.com.

Introduction

Accidental injuries of the bile ducts leading to biliary leaks and strictures may occur during any surgical procedure involving the biliary tract. However, the main cause of injury of the bile ducts at the present time is laparoscopic cholecystectomy (LC). Although LC has proved to be superior to open cholecystectomy in terms of shorter hospitalization, lower overall morbidity, faster recovery, and better cosmetic outcome, the risk of bile duct injury during LC is two to six times greater compared with open cholecystectomy.[1,2] Bergman and colleagues[3] described four types of postoperative bile duct injuries, as follows:

Type A: Cystic duct leaks or leakage from aberrant or peripheral hepatic radicles (minor lesions)
Type B: Major bile duct leaks with or without concomitant biliary strictures (major lesions)
Type C: Bile duct strictures without bile leakage (major lesions)
Type D: Complete transection of the duct with or without excision of some portion of the biliary tree (major lesions)

I refer to this classification in this chapter.

Epidemiology

LC was first performed by Mouret in France in 1987. The technique was standardized by two other French surgeons,

Dubois in Paris and Perissat in Bordeaux.[4,5] This new technique spread very rapidly around the world; in the United States, the percentage of cholecystectomies done laparoscopically grew from zero in 1987 to almost 80% in 1992.[6] The advent of LC also induced an estimated increase of at least 25% in the overall number of cholecystectomies performed,[7,8] so that the likely number of cholecystectomies performed at the present time in the United States is 800,000 per year.[9] The number of iatrogenic injuries to the bile duct has increased accordingly.[10]

Many reasons may explain the increased incidence of biliary complications at the beginning of the laparoscopic era, most related to the new technical skills required to perform laparoscopically what had been done by open surgery: bidimensional vision, loss of tactile sensations, different visual approach of the hepatic pedicle, difficult hemostatic maneuvers, abuse of electrocoagulation, and lack of confidence with the new instrumentation.[11] The rate of injuries seemed to be related to the surgeon's learning curve and his or her personal experience. An inversely proportional relationship between the number of cholecystectomies performed and the rate of injuries was suggested by earlier reported series.[1,12] In a review of 77,604 LCs performed in the United States, the incidence of biliary injuries decreased from 0.6% to 0.4% ($P < .001$) for surgical teams having an experience of more than 100 LCs.[1] A Belgian survey[11] suggested the number of 50 LCs as the threshold of a completed learning curve; however, the same authors emphasized that one-third of the biliary injuries in their

Table 44.1 Incidence of Major Biliary Lesions (Bergman's Type B, C, and D) during Laparoscopic Cholecystectomy (LC) (Multicenter Surveys)

Author	Country	Year	No. LC	Major Biliary Lesions (%)
MacFayden et al[2]	U.S.	1998	114,005	0.5
Nuzzo[13]	Italy	2002	56,591	0.31
Russell et al[6]	U.S.	1996	15,221	0.25
Z'graggen et al[16]	Switzerland	1998	10,174	0.31
Gigot et al[11]	Belgium	1997	9959	0.5
Wherry et al[17]	U.S.	1996	9130	0.41
Adamsen et al[18]	Denmark	1997	7654	0.74
Richardson et al[15]	Scotland	1996	5913	0.33

Table 44.2 Incidence of Minor Biliary Lesions (Bergman's Type A) during Laparoscopic Cholecystectomy (LC) (Multicenter Surveys)

Author	Country	Year	No. LC	Minor Biliary Lesions (%)
MacFayden et al[2]	U.S.	1998	114,005	0.38
Nuzzo[13]	Italy	2002	56,591	0.1
Z'graggen et al[16]	Switzerland	1998	10,174	0.93
Wherry et al[17]	U.S.	1996	9130	0.53
Adamsen et al[18]	Denmark	1997	7654	1.7
Richardson et al[15]	Scotland	1996	5913	0.28

country had occurred with surgeons with an experience of more than 100 LCs. When reviewing several multicenter series published before 1995, totaling 198,267 LCs, the incidence of biliary injuries was 0.55% in 13 European series and 0.49% in 17 series outside Europe.[13]

In the mid-1990s, the incidence of biliary injury seemed to be three times higher for LC than for open cholecystectomy. However, these figures most likely underestimated reality because there was a tendency not to declare all the lesions, as revealed by the low rate of reply to most surveys and by the increasing number of reported lesions in direct proportion with the collected replies.[14] At the present time, the incidence of biliary injuries has not substantially changed, even if a trend toward reduction has been reported by some authors.[6,15] The estimated overall incidence is 0.25% to 0.74% for major biliary lesions (**Table 44.1**) and 0.1% to 1.7% for minor biliary lesions (**Table 44.2**).[16–18] These figures are only partially explained by the still increasing number of LCs performed around the world and by the activity of young surgeons at the beginning of their learning curve. However, at least one-third of biliary injuries may be ascribed to technical mistakes during surgery.[19] The learning curve is not the only risk factor of LC.

Pathogenesis

An unintentional lesion of the bile duct also may occur during an "easy" cholecystectomy performed by an experienced surgeon. Intuitively, the likelihood of injuring the bile duct should increase when the cholecystectomy is difficult and the

surgeon is inexpert. Any cholecystectomy may become unexpectedly difficult during surgery; however, clinical and morphologic criteria exist that may be useful in predicting a cholecystectomy at higher risk of bile duct injury. Clinical criteria are obesity; previous abdominal surgery; cirrhosis; portal hypertension; age of the patient; and previous cholecystitis, cholangitis, or pancreatitis. Morphologic criteria revealed by preoperative abdominal ultrasound are related to the gallbladder status (scleroatrophic gallbladder, thickening of the gallbladder wall, gallbladder distention resulting from a stone in the infundibulum) and to the liver (hepatomegaly, atrophy or hypertrophy of the liver lobes). The presence of several criteria raises the chances of being confronted with a difficult cholecystectomy and the risk of concomitant common bile duct (CBD) stones.

Unrecognized CBD stones are one of the major risk factors of cystic duct leakage after LC. The mechanism and the cause of a biliary injury remain unexplainable in at least one-third of cases.[13] In more than 50% of cases, the injury occurs during the dissection of the cystic duct or during separation of the gallbladder neck from the CBD. Misinterpretation of the cystic duct and the CBD is the most common cause of injury.[12] Excessive traction on the gallbladder neck, especially if the tissues are not inflamed, may facilitate the injury of the CBD. Conversely, when the area is acutely or chronically inflamed or when a stone is trapped into the gallbladder infundibulum, the risk of CBD injury is higher during the dissection of the gallbladder neck from the hepatic pedicle. Other recurrent reasons for bile duct injury are related to incorrect hemostatic maneuvers in case of bleeding from the cystic artery;

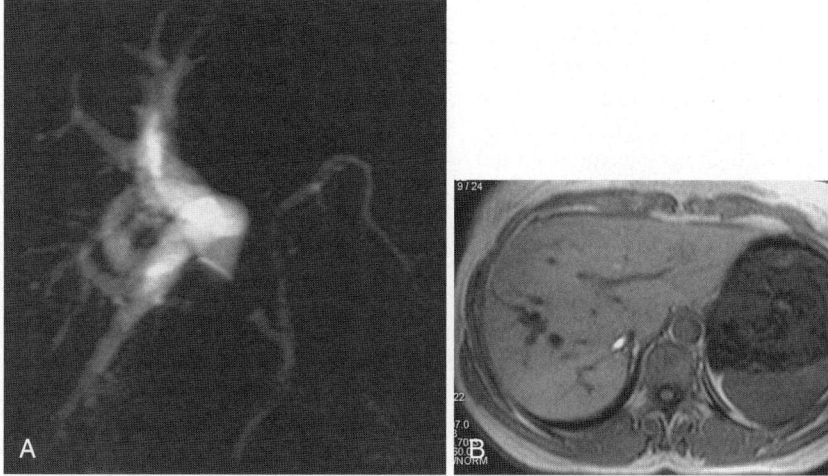

Fig. 44.1 This patient presented 2 years after laparoscopic cholecystectomy (LC) with only occasional minor right upper quadrant pain and slightly elevated liver function tests. **A,** Magnetic resonance cholangiography shows complete obstruction and dilation of the right biliary ductal system with normal common bile duct (CBD) and left biliary ductal system. **B,** Abdominal magnetic resonance imaging shows hypotrophy of the right liver and compensatory hypertrophy of the left liver.

inappropriate use of electrocautery; and other specific maneuvers, such as intraoperative cholangiography, cystic duct dilation, and transcystic CBD instrumental exploration.

An anatomic anomaly is often reported by the surgeon as having caused a biliary injury. Variations of the biliary anatomy, especially at the level of the main hepatic confluence, are present in 50% of patients (see the section on interpretation of intrahepatic cholangiography). Surgeons must be aware of such variations and must keep in mind the danger of injuring aberrant ducts originating in the right liver during dissection of the gallbladder pedicle. Aberrant ducts must not be interpreted as accessory ducts because the biliary distribution within the liver parenchyma is of a terminal type; this implies that there are no intrahepatic anastomoses between the ducts and that every injury of an aberrant duct would determine functional exclusion of the corresponding liver area. Injury to a small aberrant duct may still be considered a minor lesion; however, it would cause a bile leak into the peritoneal space with all the related consequences. Another cause of injury is clipping or ligation of an aberrant duct. This injury does not involve a bile leak but entails the functional exclusion of the corresponding liver area leading to its progressive atrophy and hypertrophy of the remaining liver parenchyma. This possible event may be clinically totally asymptomatic and noted only by an increase in biochemical parameters of cholestasis and cytolysis (**Fig. 44.1**). Although there is no indication of treatment in asymptomatic cases, if the obstructed ducts become infected, recurrent cholangitis is the typical clinical manifestation often requiring operative reestablishment of an adequate bile flow.

Clinical Features

Schematically, three main clinical pictures are characteristic of a bile duct injury: (1) external biliary fistula, (2) choleperitoneum, and (3) obstructive jaundice with or without the features of acute cholangitis. Various combinations of these clinical pictures may also be present. Most importantly,

although some of the clinical manifestations, such as uncomplicated jaundice or well-drained external bile leakage, do not require any emergency treatment, the presence of infection must be regarded as an important criterion that requires intensive care and rapid decisions to treat sepsis. Septic complications are the main reason for mortality in these patients in the postoperative period. External biliary fistula and choleperitoneum are both typical features of the immediate postoperative period, whereas obstructive jaundice may occur either immediately after surgery or later, within days to several years. When symptoms arise late after surgery because of a slow progression from injury to stricture, overt jaundice may be absent, and the clinical picture is typically that of anicteric cholestasis, with or without itching, and recurrent bouts of acute cholangitis.

The suspicion of bile duct injury is not always straightforward. When subtle symptoms such as abdominal dull pain, abdominal distention, low-grade fever, and nausea arise in the first days after LC, one should always suspect a possible complication. Intraperitoneal bile collections may initially produce very little or no specific symptoms, but they should be quickly suspected and eventually confirmed to identify the cause and to plan the best treatment for the individual patient. Hemobilia is a rare but alarming clinical presentation of a bile duct injury. The mechanism by which a biliary injury may be associated with hemobilia is often the perforation of a pseudoaneurysm of the right hepatic artery or one of its branches into the bile ducts. These pseudoaneurysms are the result of an inadvertent intraoperative injury of the artery produced by hemostatic maneuvers during a difficult cholecystectomy. In patients with an external biliary drainage or fistula, the bleeding may become suddenly and massively apparent through the drain and may occasionally require emergency treatment.

Differential Diagnosis

Strictures occurring long after surgery may need to be distinguished from malignant strictures and other benign conditions such as primary sclerosing cholangitis. The clinical history may be helpful only in cases in which the biliary injury had been recognized and eventually treated at the time of surgery. In this setting, the stricture is usually the result of progressive scarring at the site of surgical repair. In all other circumstances, the relationship with cholecystectomy should be questioned. However, clinical presentation may be helpful in discriminating postoperative and malignant stenoses; painless jaundice is in favor of a malignant disease, whereas development of overt jaundice in benign strictures is often heralded by a long period of anicteric cholestasis and relapsing attacks of mild to severe acute cholangitis. Stricture morphology may be very helpful in discriminating scars from neoplastic involvement of the bile duct. Postoperative strictures are usually short, with sharp, often asymmetric edges, and close to the cystic duct stump. Clips may be seen lying over the bile duct or located medially to it. Biopsy or brush cytology of the stricture may add information, but these procedures are seldom required because of their low sensitivity.

Treatment

In recent years, endoscopic retrograde cholangiopancreatography (ERCP) has acquired a pivotal role in the management of postsurgical biliary complications. Both of the major typical clinical presentations occurring in this setting may be addressed by ERCP: (1) biliary leak into the peritoneal cavity or external leak and (2) obstructive syndrome with cholestasis, cholangitis, or jaundice. ERCP is indicated to confirm the clinical suspicion of biliary injury and to obtain as much morphologic information as possible. ERCP is also increasingly used as a first-line therapeutic tool in complications that are amendable to endoscopic treatment.

Endoscopic Retrograde Cholangiopancreatography and Biliary Leak

The presence of a bile leak invariably indicates a break in the continuity of the biliary system. However, the severity of the injury (ranging from simple leakage of the cystic stump to complete transection of the bile duct) and the complexity of its repair are extremely variable. The magnitude of the bile output does not usually help in presuming the origin and the size of the leak. A direct cholangiogram is of utmost importance for accurate anatomic depiction and to classify the type of injury to plan therapy. The usefulness of magnetic resonance cholangiopancreatography (MRCP) in the delineation of postoperative biliary leaks[20] and of iatrogenic strictures[21] has been reported. However, in contrast to ERCP, MRCP has no therapeutic capability. MRCP may be recommended in anatomic situations in which the endoscopic approach is presumably difficult or occasionally impossible, such as in patients with a Billroth II anatomy and with Roux-en-Y hepaticojejunostomy.

ERCP provides a detailed morphologic picture of the biliary tree and, when indicated, offers immediate therapeutic options during the same procedure. In cases of biliary leaks, ERCP is usually required in the early postoperative period when the patient has fresh surgical scars (which are potentially painful,

especially if surgery has been converted to laparotomy) and has one or more external abdominal drains placed during surgery or in the postoperative period under ultrasound or computed tomography guidance; this is why the supine position is often preferred to the usual left lateral or prone position in performing ERCP. The supine position, although a little more demanding for the operator, is also preferable for interpretation purposes, especially in the case of complex hilar lesions. The anteroposterior radiologic projection, with the liver lying on the spine, substantially helps in identifying the anatomy of the main biliary confluence and of the segmental intrahepatic ducts. Use of the supine position also allows changing the patient position obliquely in case of superimposition of the biliary branches, which may create difficulties in interpretation.

In case of external biliary fistula through an abdominal drain, it is not advisable to start the procedure by injecting contrast medium through the drain (fistulography). In most instances, especially in minor lesions, the contrast medium freely flows into the peritoneal space without depicting the biliary tree. The presence of contrast medium overlapping the area involved by the lesion may hinder the correct interpretation of subsequent cholangiography and occasionally disguise the picture entirely. In contrast, fistulography is indicated whenever endoscopic cholangiography shows an incomplete filling of the biliary system resulting from a complete transection of the main bile duct or lack of visualization of a sectorial or segmental intrahepatic branch. As an alternative to contrast medium, which occasionally might not fill the missing branch, air may be used to obtain a pneumocholangiogram.[22]

The technique of ERCP in the setting of a suspected biliary injury does not substantially differ from the routine examination. Special attention should be paid to the injection of contrast medium, however, which should be slow and careful to allow precise delineation of the lesions. Massive injection of the biliary tree should be avoided. Minimal injection and early filling x-ray films are also important in detecting small residual CBD stones, which are present in 20% of patients with biliary leakage originating from the cystic duct stump. If the suspected lesion is located in an intrahepatic biliary branch, it is of paramount importance to obtain a complete intrahepatic cholangiogram; to achieve an adequate pressure of injection, especially if a sphincterotomy has been previously performed, the use of an occlusion balloon catheter is advisable. Intrahepatic biliary anatomy is better shown by multiple x-ray films taken in different projections. Percutaneous transhepatic cholangiography and MRCP should be reserved for patients in whom ERCP fails technically or fails to show the intrahepatic biliary anatomy because of proximal ductal disruption.[23]

Interpretation of Intrahepatic Cholangiography

The main biliary confluence is formed by the union of the right and left hepatic ducts that drain the bile originating in the right hemiliver and the left hemiliver. The main confluence is often incorrectly called *bifurcation* in the English literature; actually, although the portal vein and the hepatic artery carrying the blood to the liver have bifurcations, the fusion of ducts collecting the bile from the liver with a flow directed toward the CBD generates a *confluence*. According to the

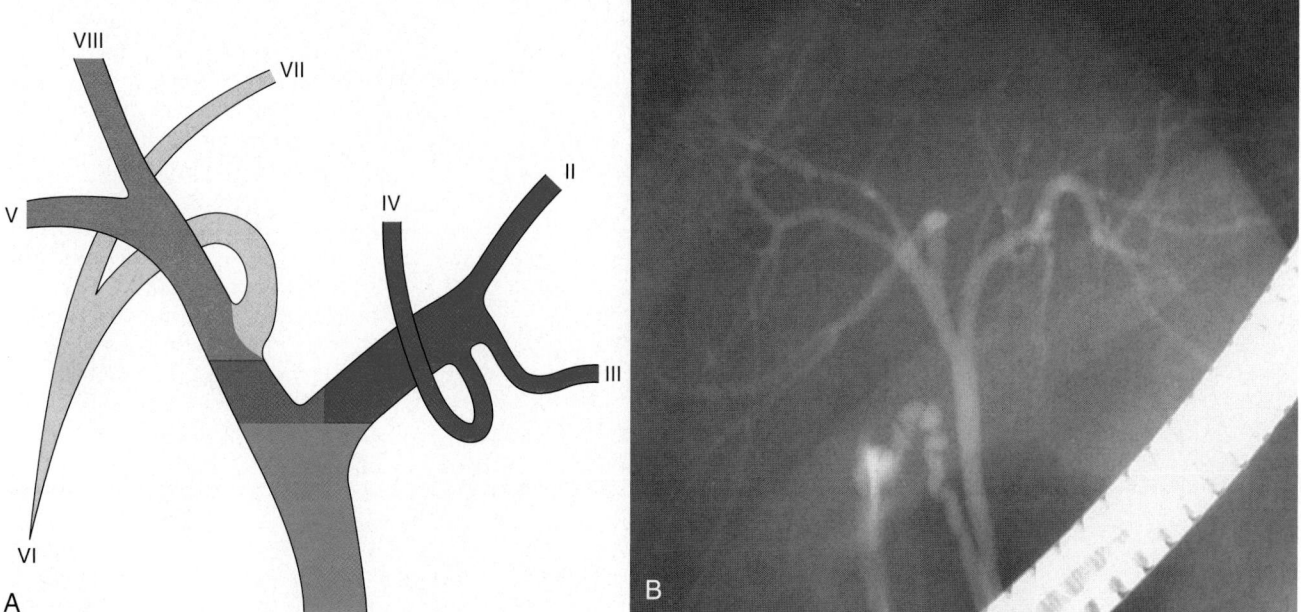

Fig. 44.2 **A** and **B,** Normal distribution of intrahepatic bile ducts: common hepatic duct *(light green)*, left hepatic ducts *(blue)*, right hepatic duct *(dark green)*, right anteromedial duct *(red)*, and right posterolateral duct *(yellow)*.

segmental liver anatomy described by Couinaud,[24] the left hepatic duct collects the bile originating from segments II and III (left anatomic liver lobe or left lateral sector) and from segment IV (quadrate lobe). One or more small ducts originating from segment I (caudate lobe) also join the left hepatic duct close to the main confluence. The anatomic variations occurring in the left hepatic system are rare and are irrelevant in this perspective. The right hepatic duct is shorter than the left hepatic duct and follows the same axis of the common hepatic duct. The right hepatic duct originates from the confluence of the right anteromedial sectorial duct (segments V and VIII) and of the right posterolateral sectorial duct (segments VI and VII). The right anteromedial duct is recognizable thanks to its orientation, which follows the same axis of the right hepatic duct, whereas the right posterolateral duct joins the right anteromedial duct on its medial aspect with a typical umbrella handle–like shape.

This normal anatomy (called "modal" by Couinaud) is present in approximately 60% of the population (**Fig. 44.2**). The main hepatic confluence is usually located high in the hilar region. A lower position at the level of the hepatic pedicle may also occur, causing a much closer proximity to the insertion of the cystic duct into the hepatic duct (**Fig. 44.3**). The main variations of the main hepatic confluence are the absence of the right hepatic duct with the anteromedial and posterolateral right ducts joining independently the left duct to form the confluence (**Fig. 44.4**) or with one of the two right sectorial ducts joining the CBD at a more distal level closer to the insertion of the cystic duct (**Fig. 44.5**). More rarely, an isolated segmental or subsegmental duct may join the CBD away from the main confluence, usually on the lateral aspect of the CBD close to the insertion of the cystic duct. Most aberrant ducts arise from the right liver and drain into the common hepatic duct or cystic duct within 30 mm of the hepatocystic angle.[25]

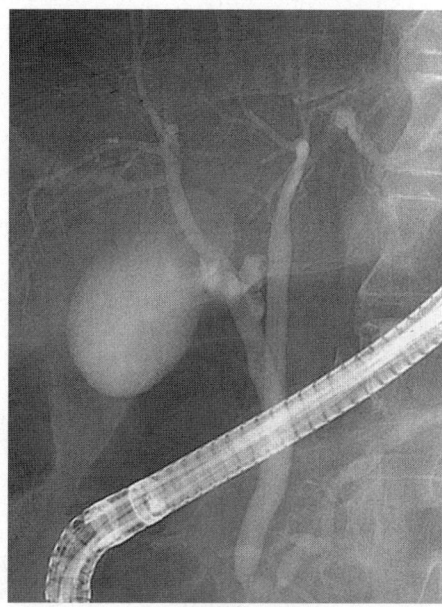

Fig. 44.3 Endoscopic retrograde cholangiopancreatography (ERCP) shows low main confluence with the cystic duct joining the right hepatic duct on its medial aspect.

These are the most dangerous anatomic variations for the surgeon during the dissection of the gallbladder pedicle. Apart from complete transection of the CBD (type D of the Bergman classification) (**Fig. 44.6**), which is typically an indication for open surgical repair, an attempt at endoscopic treatment may be envisaged in all other circumstances of biliary injury with concomitant bile leak. The basic principle of endoscopic treatment is abolition of the transpapillary pressure gradient, equalizing the bile duct and duodenal pressures and allowing flow of bile into the duodenum.[26]

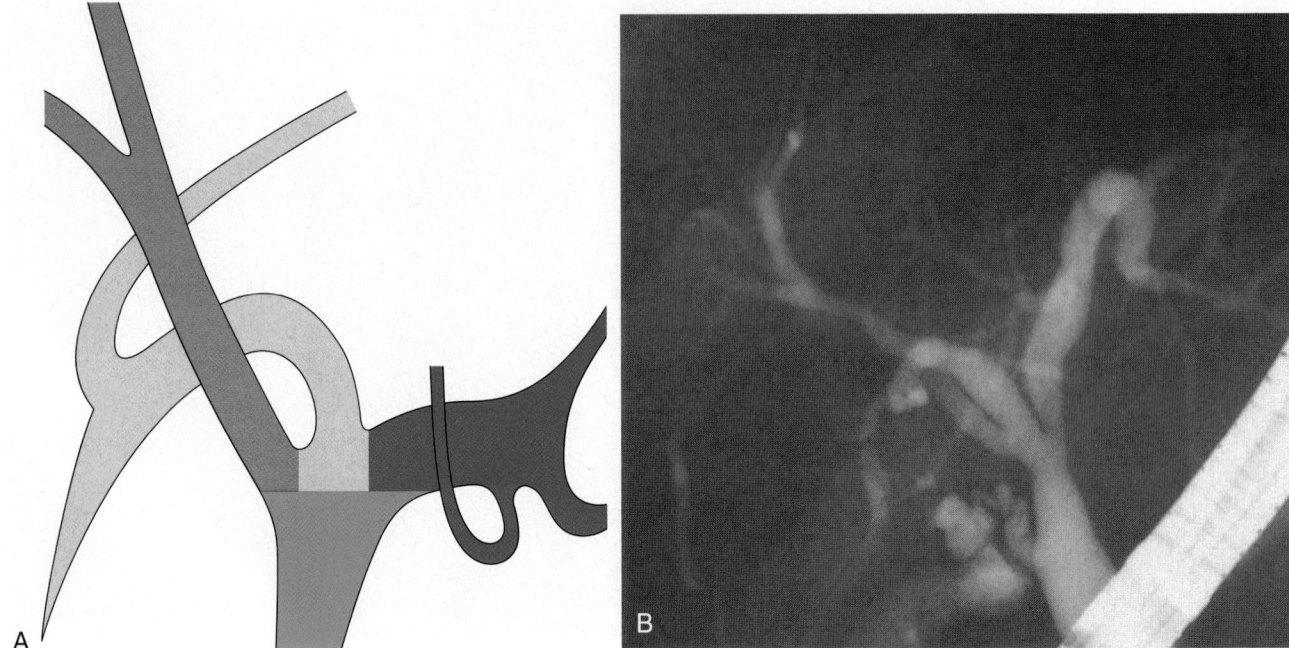

Fig. 44.4 **A** and **B,** Absence of the right hepatic duct. *Light green,* common hepatic duct; *blue,* left hepatic ducts; *red,* right anteromedial duct; *yellow,* right posterolateral duct.

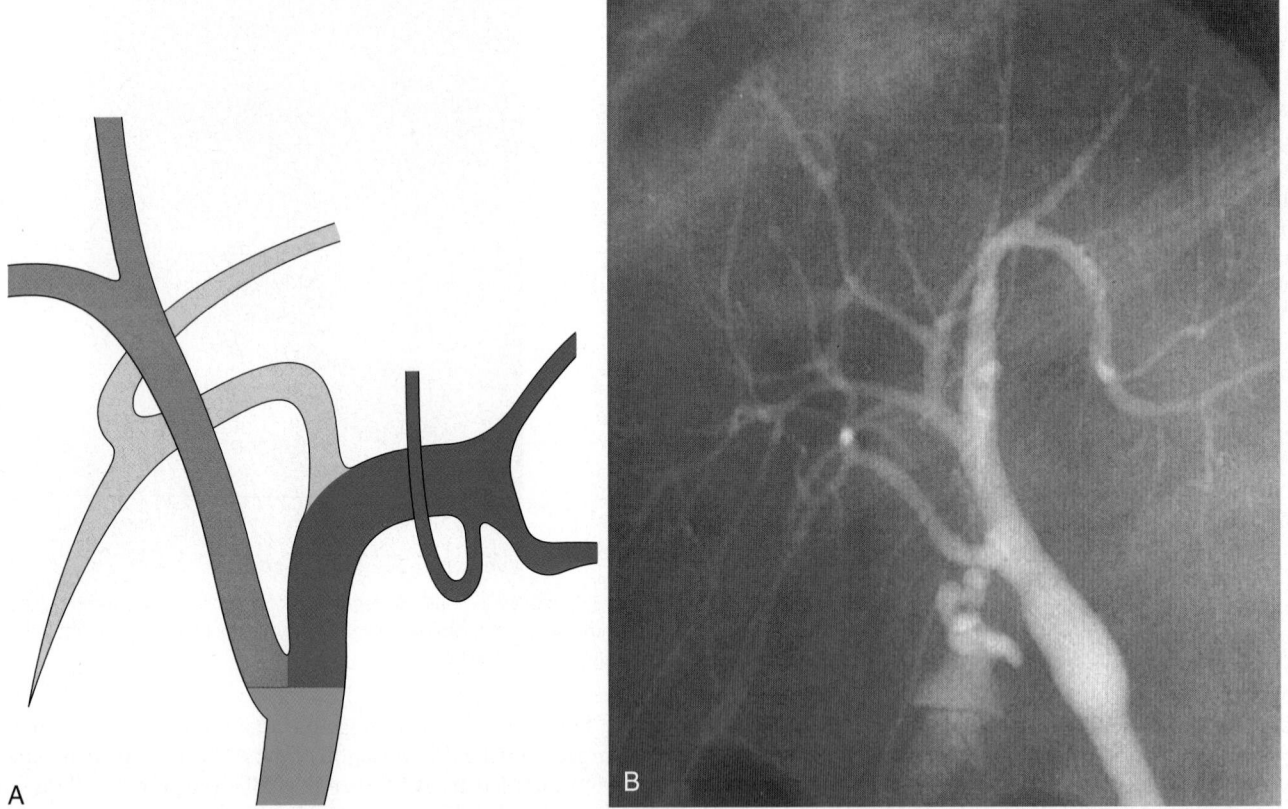

Fig. 44.5 **A** and **B,** Absence of the right hepatic duct. On endoscopic retrograde cholangiopancreatography (ERCP), the cystic duct joins the right anteromedial duct on its lateral aspect. *Light green,* common hepatic duct; *blue,* left hepatic ducts; *red,* right anteromedial duct; *yellow,* right posterolateral duct.

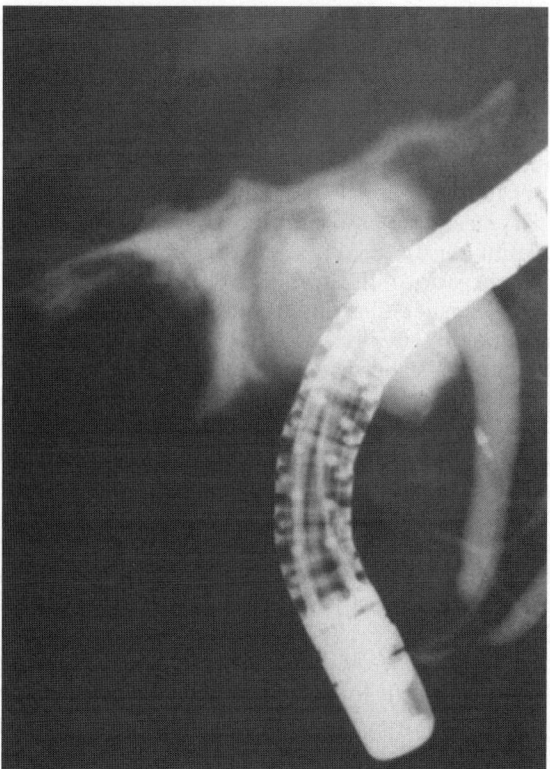

Fig. 44.6 Endoscopic retrograde cholangiopancreatography (ERCP) shows complete transection of the common bile duct (CBD) with contrast medium freely flowing into the subhepatic peritoneal space.

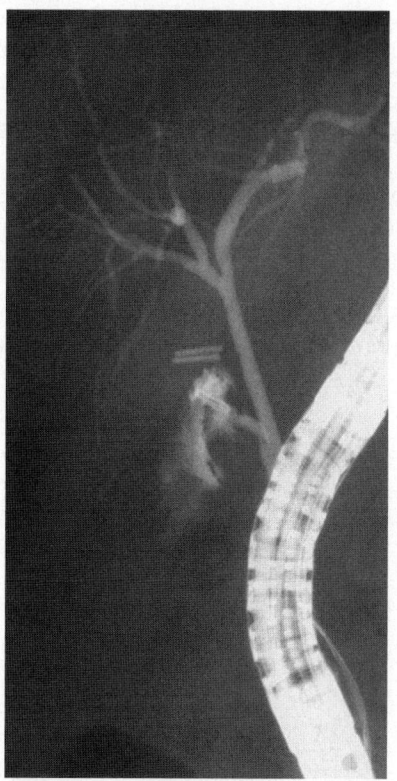

Fig. 44.7 Postoperative endoscopic retrograde cholangiopancreatography (ERCP) after laparoscopic cholecystectomy (LC), with leakage of contrast medium from the cystic duct stump.

Endoscopic Treatment of Minor Lesions

The largest part of biliary leaks from minor lesions originates from the cystic duct stump (**Fig. 44.7**). Bile leakage from the cystic duct stump may be due to stump dehiscence resulting from defective technique in clips positioning, inadvertent injury to the cystic wall below the closure, or partial disruption of the cystic duct implantation into the bile duct resulting from excessive traction. Biliary hypertension resulting from temporary impaction of a residual bile duct stone into the sphincter of Oddi in the early postoperative period is most likely the cause of cystic duct stump dehiscence in almost one-fifth of patients. Similarly, a simple spasm of the sphincter of Oddi theoretically may create enough pressure to induce dislodgment of clips placed on the cystic duct stump. Bile leaks can also originate from severed ducts of Luschka (small peripheral ducts connecting the intrahepatic system with the gallbladder lumen) (**Fig. 44.8**), small subsegmental ducts running in the gallbladder bed, and segmental or subsegmental aberrant branches joining the CBD in the proximity of the cystic duct.

Treatment of these leaks does not differ from treatment employed when the leak arises from the cystic duct stump (**Table 44.3**). The transpapillary pressure gradient can be equalized by endoscopic sphincterotomy (ES) alone,[27,28] ES and stent or nasobiliary drain (NBD) placement,[29] and stent[30,31] or NBD placement alone[31] without preliminary ES (**Fig. 44.9**). All methods seem to be equally effective in facilitating the closure of the biliary leak usually within 1 week of treatment.[3,26,30–33] The endoscopic approach of choice is

controversial. However, if stones are present in the CBD, ES and stone extraction with or without stent or NBD placement seems the most logical approach. However, each option has specific limitations. ES is associated with inherent immediate and potential long-term complications; stent placement requires a second procedure to remove the stent, which can also become clogged or can migrate; and NBD requires a prolonged hospital stay, is uncomfortable for the patient, and may be accidentally displaced. Advantages and disadvantages of the different options are summarized in **Table 44.4**.

To select the optimal endoscopic therapy, Sandha and colleagues[34] proposed classifying the bile leaks by ERCP into two categories: low-grade (identified only after intrahepatic opacification) and high-grade (observed before intrahepatic opacification). Of 104 low-grade leaks, 75 were treated by ES alone with a success rate of 91%. Of 100 high-grade leaks, 97 were treated by stent insertion with a final success rate (4 patients had to undergo retreatment) of 100%. The investigators concluded that this simple, practical endoscopic classification system might be clinically relevant in the choice of endoscopic therapy. Endoscopic local injection of botulinum toxin (Botox) to decrease the transpapillary bilioduodenal pressure gradient has also been reported.[35] Injection of 100 IU of botulinum toxin into the sphincter of Oddi was shown to lower CBD pressure significantly within 24 hours. This effect lasted for 2 weeks on average in the animal model.

Postoperative bile leaks from minor lesions (type A) are usually amendable to endoscopic management with a very high success rate. All methods seem to be equally effective in facilitating the closure of the leak within a few days.

Endoscopic Treatment of Major Lesions

Bile leakage in major lesions originates from a tear on the CBD or on one of the biliary branches that form the main hepatic confluence (type B). In both instances, ES alone may be inadequate to seal the leak. It is preferable to insert at least one large-bore plastic stent (10-Fr to 11.5-Fr) long enough to bypass the site of injury. The secondary intent of stent placement is to prevent the development of stricture at the site of

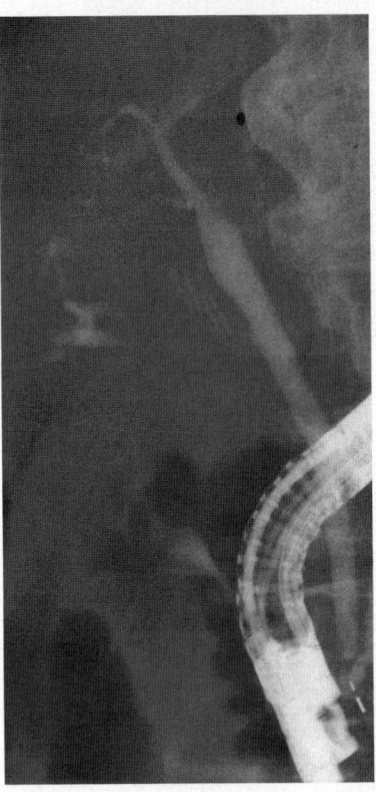

Fig. 44.8 Postoperative endoscopic retrograde cholangiopancreatography (ERCP) after laparoscopic cholecystectomy (LC) in a case of subhepatic bile collection. The common bile duct (CBD) is normal. Two clips are visible on the cystic artery and the cystic duct. A leak of contrast medium into the gallbladder bed originates from a duct of Luschka connecting a subsegmental branch that joins the CBD lower than the main confluence.

the injured bile duct wall.[23,26] For this purpose, the stent should be left in place for several months to allow the healing process to stabilize. In case of secondary stricture formation at the site of injury, the presence of a stent already in place facilitates successive endoscopic maneuvers to dilate the stricture. Therapeutic success may be obtained in 71% to 79% of cases (**Fig. 44.10**).[3,36,37]

Biliary stents have also been successfully used to reestablish the continuity of disrupted segmental branches at the level of the main hepatic confluence[22] and for leaks from aberrant bile ducts.[23,38] In major biliary injury with bile leakage, the primary therapeutic objective is to seal the leak to convert an acute problem into a stabilized condition. The high efficacy of the endoscopic approach in this setting justifies its use as a first-line treatment whenever possible. Treatment of postoperative bile duct strictures in the prelaparoscopic era was traditionally surgical. The role of ERCP was limited to the diagnostic phase and particularly to the definition of the level and extent of the lesion.[39]

Along with the increasing use of ERCP in the evaluation and treatment of acute complications of LC, therapeutic ERCP has been increasingly employed to manage postoperative strictures occurring both early and late postoperatively. The first nonoperative alternative in the management of bile duct strictures has been the percutaneous transhepatic approach. After establishment of percutaneous access to the intrahepatic bile ducts, the stricture is crossed with a guidewire, and pneumatic balloon dilation is performed. Although instantly very effective, this approach has a very limited value in the long-term because of the high rate of stricture recurrence.[40] Approximately one-third of patients undergoing this treatment modality experience complications, and stricture recurrence develops in at least 25% of cases during follow-up.[41,42] In another series published by the group at The Johns Hopkins University, the success rate of these procedures was only 55%, with 20% of patients having significant hemobilia.[43] The high recurrence rate after percutaneous pneumatic dilation is most likely due to the forceful disruption of the scar, which can add further traumatic damage to the tissue and consequential development of new local fibrogenic reaction.

The percutaneous approach has been progressively replaced by the endoscopic approach. The endoscopic approach avoids the need for liver puncture, which is the main cause of complications of the percutaneous approach; it is not more difficult when the intrahepatic bile ducts are not dilated or only slightly enlarged, which is often the case in postoperative strictures; and it is also feasible in case of liver cirrhosis, ascites, or

Table 44.3 Endoscopic Management of Biliary Leaks from Minor Lesions (Type A) after Cholecystectomy

Author, Year	n	LC (%)	Cystic (%)	Luschka (%)	Other (%)	CBDS (%)	ES (%)	ES + EP (%)	EP Only (%)	Success (%)
Bourke, 1995	85	62	79	6	15	18	33	67	0	95
Barkun, 1997	52	58	77	15	8	22	48	23	15	88
Ryan, 1998	50	78	72	8	20	22	12	26	62	100
Hourigan, 1999	53	85	68	17	15	11	15	15	70	96

CBDS, common bile duct stones; EP, endoprosthesis or nasobiliary drain; ES, endoscopic sphincterotomy; LC, laparoscopic cholecystectomy.

coagulopathy. The endoscopic approach avoids the need for long-standing percutaneous internal-external catheters, improving the patient's comfort and compliance. At the present time, the endoscopic approach is considered the first-line nonoperative alternative to surgical treatment; in addition, it never hinders the option of a surgical approach as a rescue therapy in case of failure. Which is the best therapeutic algorithm is still debated. Both surgery and endoscopic treatment may obtain good results. However, the two alternatives have never been systematically compared in a prospective randomized trial. It is also very unlikely that such a study will ever be conducted in the future because of the relatively low incidence of this pathology, its dispersion in several centers, and the heterogeneity of its clinical and morphologic presentation, which would make it very difficult to gather cases in homogeneous groups large enough for any comparison.

Description of Technique

Endoscopic treatment of postoperative biliary strictures is based on two technical steps: (1) getting over the stricture and (2) dilation of the stricture.

Getting over the Stricture

The morphologic requirement that allows getting over the stricture is the continuity of the CBD. In case of complete transection or obstruction of the bile duct, the endoscopic option alone is applicable in only a very few cases. A combined percutaneous and endoscopic approach with an aim at reconstructing the missing segment of the bile duct has been described.[44] A similar combined approach has also been described in the case of complete obstruction of the distal biliary stump; percutaneous puncture of the distal stump was performed under radiologic guidance with a device designed for nonbiliary use (a set marketed for placing transjugular intrahepatic portosystemic shunts).[45] However, because of the lack of standardization, these approaches cannot be recommended on a routine basis.

In most cases, and especially when symptoms develop a long time after surgery, the CBD is accessible by endoscopy, and the stricture is incomplete, getting over the stricture is the preliminary step to undertake dilation. This maneuver is often

Table 44.4 Endoscopic Options to Treat Postoperative Bile Leaks (Type A according to Bergman)

Procedure	Advantages	Disadvantages
ES	Treatment of associated CBD stones	Complications
Nasobiliary drain (days)	Avoids ES	Uncomfortable
	Allows check cholangiography	Prolongs hospitalization
Stent placement (wks)	Avoids ES	Repeat ERCP required
		Clogging, dislocation

CBD, common bile duct; ERCP, endoscopic retrograde cholangiopancreatography; ES, endoscopic sphincterotomy.

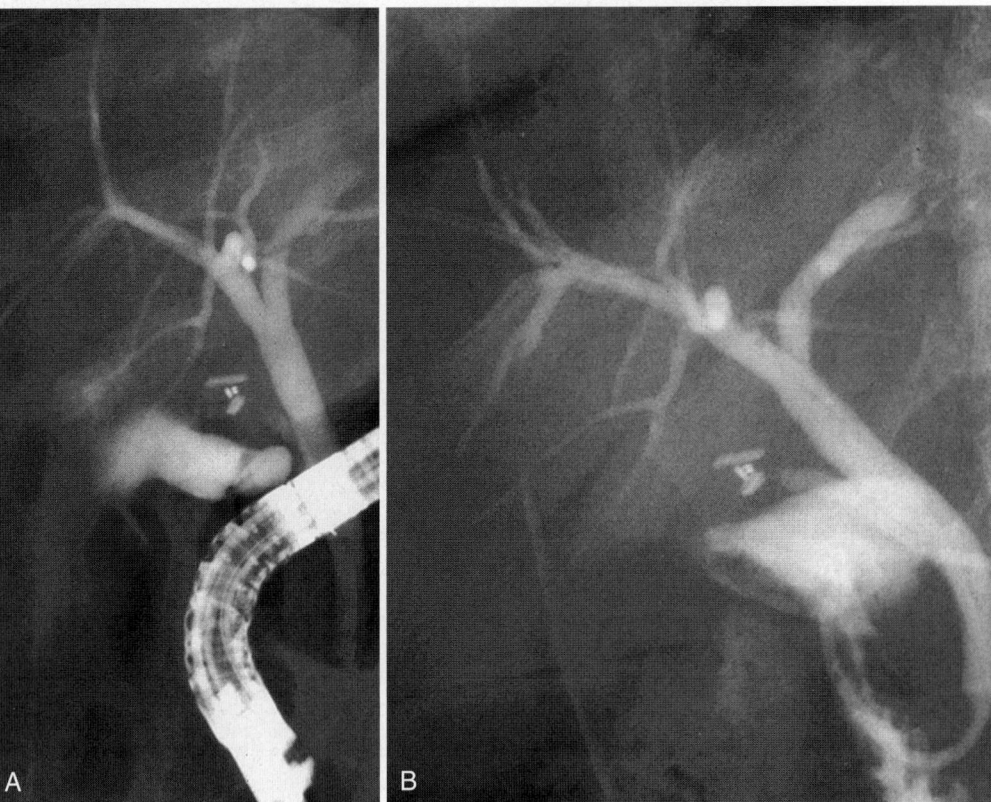

Fig. 44.9 Postoperative endoscopic retrograde cholangiopancreatography (ERCP) after laparoscopic cholecystectomy (LC) in a case of external biliary fistula through a subhepatic drain. **A,** Leak of contrast medium originating in the gallbladder bed (duct of Luschka) is seen. **B,** Check cholangiography performed 3 days after endoscopic sphincterotomy and nasobiliary drain placement. The leakage is no longer visible.

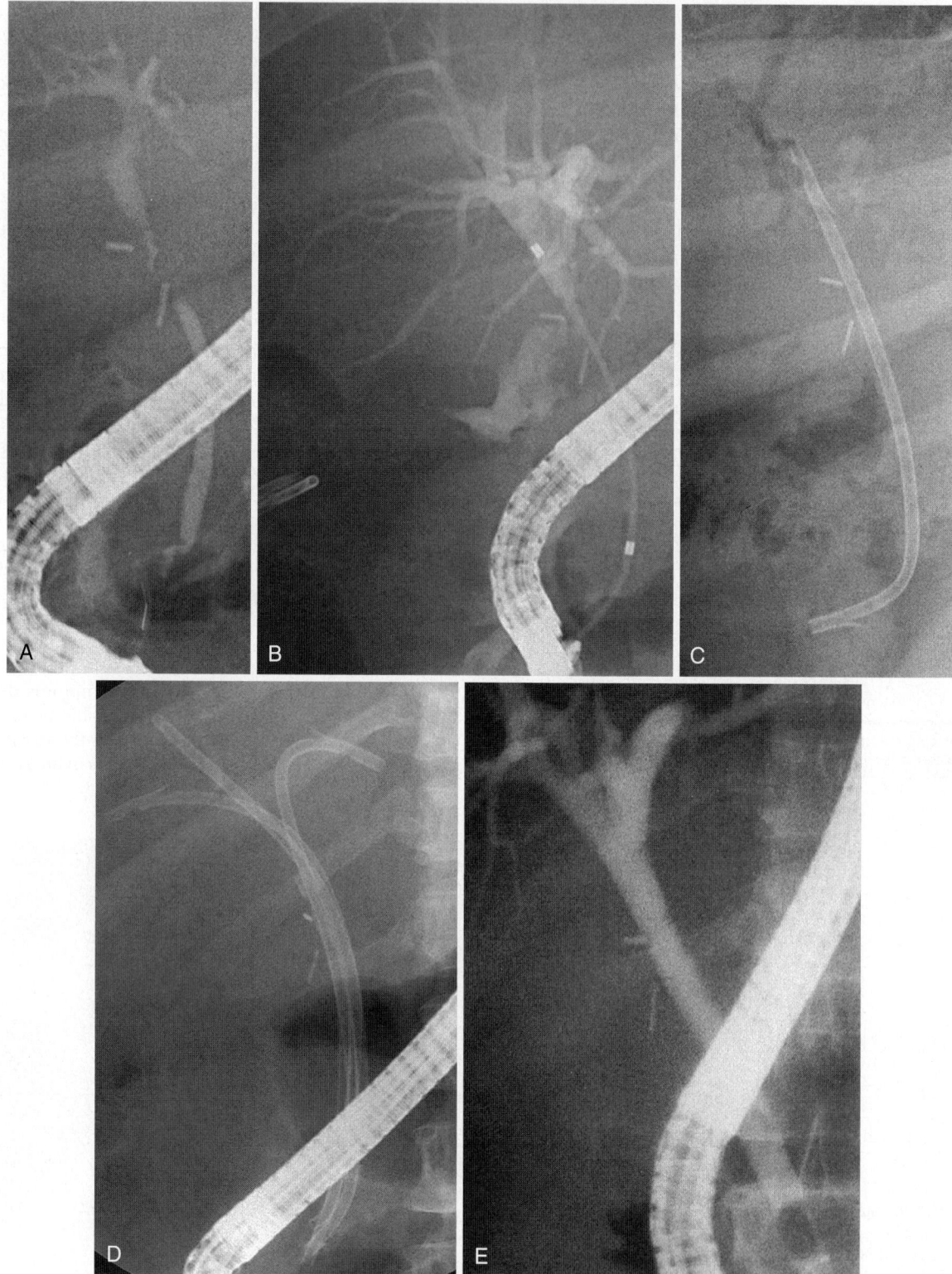

Fig. 44.10 Postoperative endoscopic retrograde cholangiopancreatography (ERCP) after laparoscopic cholecystectomy (LC) in a case of peritoneal bile collection and cholestasis. **A,** Stricture of the common bile duct (CBD) with clips overlapping. **B,** A catheter has been passed over the stricture using a guidewire; injection of contrast medium through the catheter clearly shows the site of biliary injury and the correspondent leak. **C,** A 10-Fr plastic stent has been placed. **D,** During the following months, three 10-Fr stents were inserted to dilate the stricture, one in each main biliary territory (anteromedial right, posterolateral right, and left biliary ducts). **E,** Balloon-occluded check cholangiography after removal of the three stents. The stricture has completely disappeared.

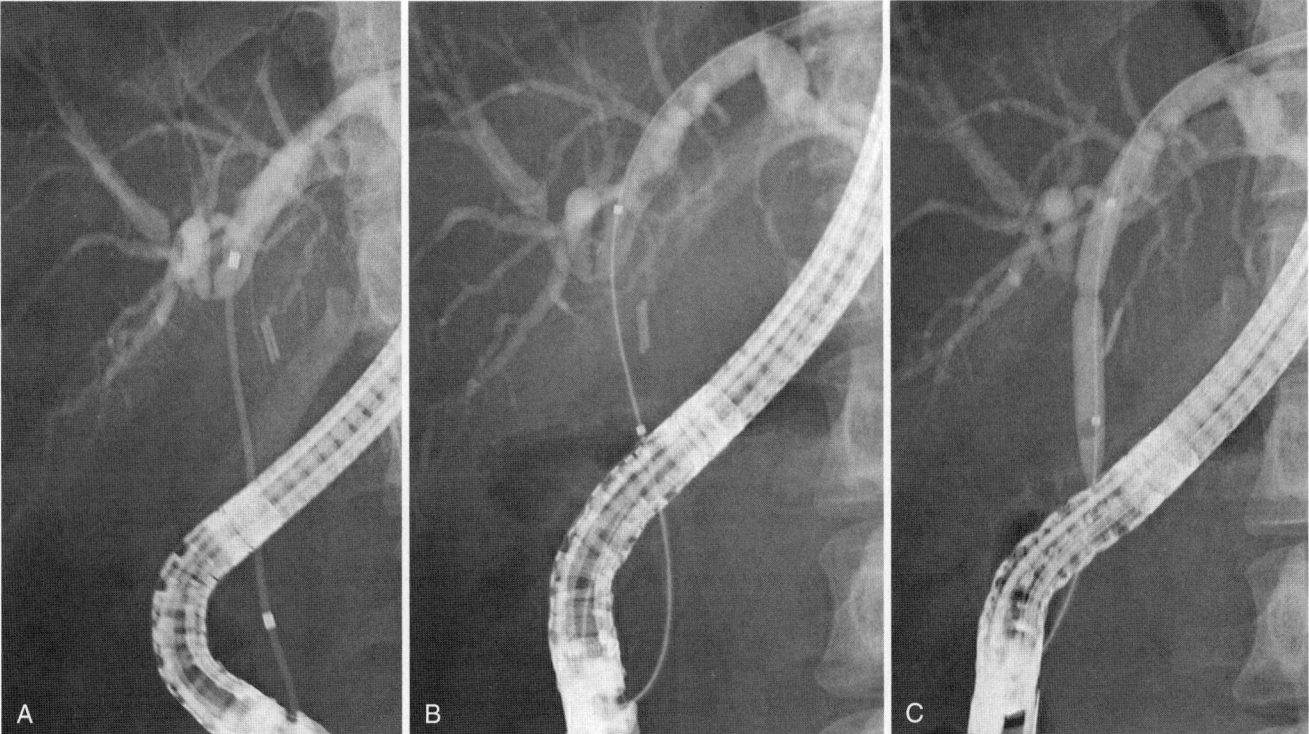

Fig. 44.11 Postoperative stricture after laparoscopic cholecystectomy (LC) converted to open cholecystectomy. **A,** At the level of the main confluence, a very tight stricture has been overcome by a catheter and guidewire. **B,** A balloon dilator has been passed through the stricture over the guidewire. **C,** Balloon dilation is performed. Notice the waist on the balloon indicating high stricture firmness.

much more difficult in postoperative strictures than in neoplastic strictures because the stenosis, even if commonly very short, may be asymmetric. The fibrosis makes it especially thin and tightened. It is often necessary to use thin hydrophilic guidewires (0.021 inch or 0.018 inch) with a straight or J-type extremity; their manipulation requires patience, skill, and optimal x-ray control.

The morphology of the stenosis has to be respected, and forceful maneuvers with stiff guidewires that may create false routes leading to the failure of the procedure should be strictly avoided. Changing the position of the patient may help in identifying radiologically the right pathway to follow with the guidewire. Pulling on a stone retrieval balloon inflated under the stricture may help in stretching the bile duct and in modifying the axis of the guidewire. Manipulation of bendable catheters or papillotomes may also be used to change the direction of the guidewire. When the stricture is passed, the hydrophilic guidewire is exchanged for a stiffer and more stable one to proceed to dilation.

Dilation of the Stricture

Dilation of the stricture has two objectives: (1) to reopen the bile duct to achieve a regular bile flow and (2) to secure the dilation to avoid restricture in the long-term. In the beginning of endoscopic treatment, only the first objective was pursued; in the percutaneous approach, the mainstay of treatment was pneumatic dilation alone.[46] However, it soon became clear that even if immediately very effective, pneumatic dilation alone was ineffective in granting good results in a long-term follow-up. At the present time, pneumatic dilation is mainly

used as a preliminary step before placement of one or more plastic stents (**Fig. 44.11**). The role of stent placement is to keep the stricture open for a long time (months to years according to different treatment strategies), while allowing scar modeling and its consolidation.[47]

Typically, two 10-Fr stents are placed, exchanged every 3 months to avoid cholangitis resulting from stent occlusion, and left in place for 1 year. In a retrospective study from the Amsterdam group reporting on the multidisciplinary experience obtained during a decade (1981–1990), the long-term results of endoscopic treatment were compared with the long-term results of surgery.[48] Surgery (Roux-en-Y hepaticojejunostomy) was performed in 35 patients, and endoscopic treatment was performed in 66 patients. Patient characteristics, type of initial injury, and level of obstruction were not significantly different in the two groups. At a mean follow-up of 50 months and 42 months for the surgical and the endoscopic groups, 83% of patients in both groups had an excellent (asymptomatic patient with normal or stable laboratory parameters) or good (single episode of cholangitis) result. Immediate complication rate was in favor of endoscopic treatment (8% vs. 26% for surgical treatment), whereas 21% of the patients had at least one episode of cholangitis resulting from stent malfunction during the stent period (two 10-Fr stents for 1 year with stent exchange every 3 months).

When analyzing the long-term results, it becomes immediately evident how the time interval between the end of treatment and the symptomatic recurrence of the stricture is much shorter in the group with endoscopic treatment compared with the surgical group (on average 3 ± 11 months vs. 40 ± 11 months), indicating possible undertreatment in the endoscopy group. However, this important study showed that endoscopic treatment may be considered at least as effective as surgical treatment in terms of long-term results, having the big advantage of not hindering any further surgery if necessary. Several other experiences of endoscopic treatment with plastic stents of postoperative biliary strictures have been published in recent years.[3,47–56] From the analysis of the available data, however, this treatment modality still seems far from standardized; the published experiences differ in terms of number of stents placed, their caliber, exchange intervals, and definition of treatment objectives and of outcomes. Examples of two different methodologic approaches follow:

- The treatment protocol used by the Amsterdam group (74 patients) is the classic one, entailing placement of two 10-Fr stents, exchanged every 3 months for 1 year (the period of stent placement).[53] Preliminary pneumatic dilation had been performed in approximately one-fourth of the patients before stent insertion. A combined percutaneous-endoscopic approach to bypass the stricture with a guidewire was required in only three cases. Stents were removed after 1 year.
- The protocol described by our group (55 patients)[52] involved the placement of the maximum possible number of stents (ideally 10-Fr) in relation to the tightness of the stricture and diameter of the CBD at every treatment session with a trimonthly interval. Treatment was continued until complete morphologic disappearance of the stricture at cholangiography (**Fig. 44.12**).

Preliminary balloon dilation was performed in 40% of the patients, almost always at the first treatment session. A combined percutaneous-endoscopic approach was required in three cases. The mean number of stents inserted was 1.7 (range 1 to 4) at the first session and 3.2 (range 1 to 6) at the end of the treatment. Disappearance of the stricture was checked 24 to 48 hours after removal of the stents by check cholangiography through NBD. Early complications developed in four

(9%) patients (three cholangitis, one pancreatitis), and stent occlusion that required early stent exchange occurred in eight (18%) patients. Mean duration of treatment was 12.1 ± 5.3 months (range 2 to 24 months). Follow-up included clinical evaluation, laboratory parameters, and liver ultrasound every 3 months during the 1st year and every 6 months in the following years.

- In the Amsterdam series, the technical success of stenting was 80%; however, only 44 patients (59% of the initial cohort and 75% of patients in whom an initial technical success had been obtained) concluded the 12-month stent period for different reasons. At a median follow-up of 9 years, 9 of 44 patients (20%) developed recurrent strictures. In eight of nine cases, recurrent strictures developed within the first 6 months of follow-up (median 2.6 months). On an intention-to-treat basis, this protocol was able to resolve definitively the bile duct stricture in 47% of the initial cohort. The results of this study suggest that endoscopic stent placement is not the best treatment option for patients with low compliance to repeated treatment sessions. Similar results, with 81% of patients symptom-free at a mean follow-up of 9.5 years, were reported in an abstract form by the Toronto group by using the same treatment protocol.[51]
- In our study, 42 of 55 patients initially considered were evaluable at a mean follow-up of 49 months after the end of treatment. Ten patients were excluded from the protocol because of complete CBD section ($n = 5$) or use of self-expandable metallic stents ($n = 5$). Another three patients were not evaluable for different reasons. Two patients died of unrelated causes during follow-up. Among the remaining 40 patients, there was no recurrence of symptoms caused by relapsing biliary stricture. One patient sustained two episodes of cholangitis but without stricture recurrence. By an intention-to-treat analysis, the success rate was 89% (40 of 45). Although the follow-up period in our

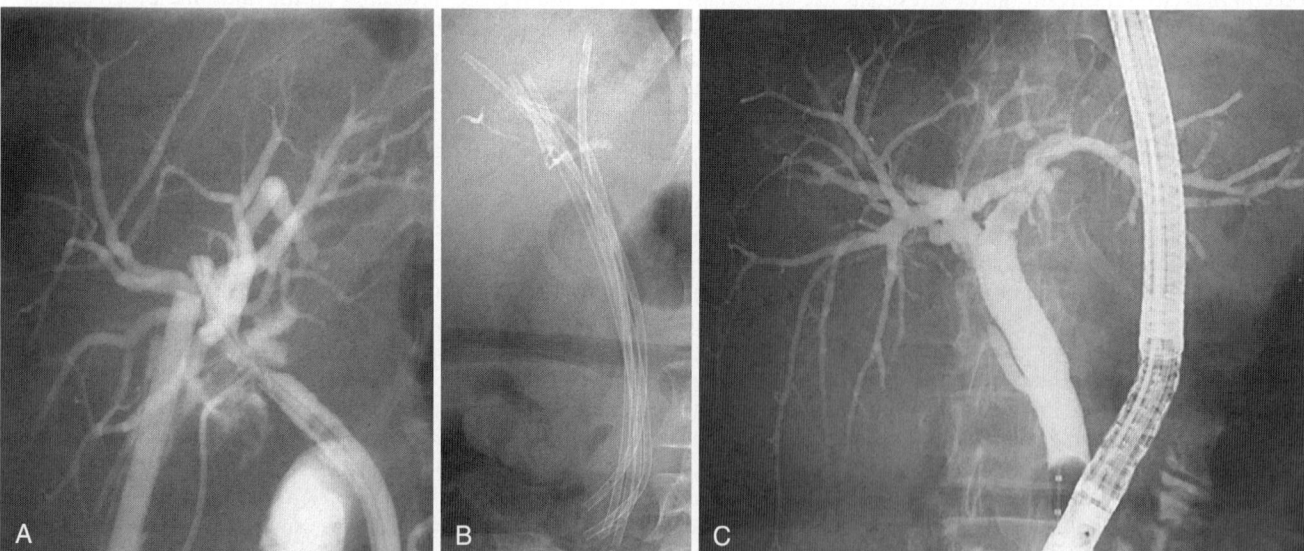

Fig. 44.12 Postoperative cholangiography through a T-tube drain placed at cholecystectomy to repair complete transection of the common bile duct (CBD) at the hilum. **A,** Stricture and leak of contrast medium around the CBD are visible. **B,** At the end of the fifth treatment, 10-Fr stents have been placed. **C,** Balloon-occluded cholangiography after stent removal. The stricture has disappeared completely.

series is shorter compared with the Amsterdam series, it is longer than the typical period during which all the recurrences after endoscopic treatment have been described (2 years). This more aggressive approach to endoscopic treatment with stents seems to improve long-term results for patients with postoperative biliary strictures. We reported more recently on the very long-term results of this aggressive approach in the same cohort of patients[57]; of 35 evaluable patients after a mean follow-up of 13.7 years, 7 (20%) had recurrent cholangitis owing to relapse of the stricture in 4 patients (all successfully retreated with stents) and newly formed bile duct stones in 3 patients. The remaining 28 patients remained completely asymptomatic with normal liver function tests and abdominal ultrasound.

Despite some controversies,[58] at the present time, multiple stent placement is a well-accepted strategy adopted worldwide for postoperative bile duct strictures.[59,60] According to the published data, endoscopic treatment with stents of major bile duct injuries and strictures is at least as effective as surgical treatment. The advantages of endoscopic treatment are its simplicity, reversibility, and minimal invasiveness. Endoscopic treatment should always be considered, whenever available, in the therapeutic algorithm of most patients with major bile duct injuries. For most patients, it may be the only treatment required. Endoscopy and surgery should be considered as complementary treatments. This complex and difficult pathology is best managed in centers in which a multidisciplinary approach is available.

Complications

Complications may occur during the first treatment session and are related to ES (acute pancreatitis, retroperitoneal perforation, and bleeding), which is usually performed to gain access to the bile ducts, or occur during the stent period. ES-related complications in this setting do not differ in frequency, severity, and management from complications encountered in other, more common situations, such as treatment of CBD stones. Complications arising during the stent period are mostly due to stent dysfunction—obstruction, migration, dislocation, and impaction. Acute cholangitis is the typical clinical manifestation of stent dysfunction. Cholangitis is usually mild and often self-limited in this setting but requires prompt endoscopic evaluation and reestablishment of correct bile drainage by stent repositioning.

A typical complication of long-term stent placement is the development of biliary sludge and stones above the stricture. This condition may cause cholangitis, but it may also be totally asymptomatic. In addition, liver function tests may be completely normal. The lack of symptoms and normal liver function tests may lead to unintentional prolongation of the planned stent period. Removal of all stones and sludge by basket or balloon extraction or both is mandatory before placement of a new stent or stents to avoid potential early reocclusion. To avoid stone formation, the trimonthly time schedule of stent replacement should not be prolonged. Patient compliance is crucial when dealing with postoperative bile duct stricture, and patients should always be fully informed of the inherent risks of not following the planned treatment program.

Future Trends

The main limitation of endoscopic treatment of postoperative bile strictures with the current method of multiple plastic stent placement is the need for repeat interventions over a long time (1 year on average). The ideal stent would allow progressive dilation of the stricture during weeks or months and would dissolve once the goal had been reached. Uncovered self-expanding metal stents (SEMS) have proved to be a bad alternative to plastic stents for several reasons.[54] First, SEMS invariably induce a hyperplastic response of the inflammatory tissue at the level of the stricture. This hyperplastic reaction ultimately leads to occlusion of SEMS, on average less than 1 year after their placement. Second, SEMS are usually not removable; treatment of secondary stricture resulting from hyperplastic reaction requires repeated balloon dilations and plastic stent placement. Third, biliary SEMS have been developed to produce abrupt recanalization of a stricture resulting from neoplastic invasion; the radial force exerted by the stent is much higher than the force desirable to induce progressive dilation of a scar, such as the scar of postoperative bile duct strictures.

Partially covered SEMS have the advantage of avoiding ingrowth of hyperplastic tissue at the level of the stricture and of being often removable[61]; however, no clinical experience is available. The advent of fully covered, removable SEMS has raised new interest concerning their potential use in benign conditions.[62] However, the experience in postoperative biliary strictures is still scanty and controversial.[63] Drug-eluting, self-expandable stents have been used in the vascular system to inhibit endothelial growth; it is conceivable that this technology might become available for use in the biliary system. Local release of antiinflammatory drugs able to control the fibrogenetic process that occurs during healing of a biliary injury may be valuable in this setting.

References

The complete reference list is available online at www.expertconsult.com.

Chapter **45**

Infections of the Biliary Tract

Jennifer J. Telford and David L. Carr-Locke

Video related to this chapter's topics can be found online at expertconsult.com.

Introduction

The histologic definition of cholangitis is inflammation of the bile duct. However, when used in practice, cholangitis refers to a characteristic clinical presentation associated with bile duct obstruction and bacterial infection. Other etiologies of bile duct inflammation have a preceding descriptor (e.g., parasitic cholangitis). All types of bile duct inflammation may be complicated by obstruction and secondary bacterial infection. The conditions predisposing to cholangitis are listed in **Box 45.1**.

Bacterial cholangitis accounts for most infections of the biliary tract. The underlying cause is usually extrahepatic bile duct obstruction from a stone or stricture and is readily managed by medical and endoscopic therapy. Less common forms of infectious cholangitis include recurrent pyogenic cholangitis, parasitic cholangitis, and acquired immunodeficiency syndrome (AIDS) cholangiopathy. Recurrent pyogenic cholangitis results from obstruction of the intrahepatic and extrahepatic biliary tract with repetitive episodes of bacterial cholangitis and is seen almost exclusively in Eastern Asia. Elsewhere in the world, patients with this condition present de novo or after emigration. Parasitic cholangitis affects individuals residing in areas endemic with pathogens that infest the biliary tract. AIDS cholangiopathy is characterized by

typical abnormalities on cholangiography combined with parasitic or viral infection of the biliary tract. Both parasitic cholangitis and AIDS cholangiopathy may be complicated by secondary bacterial cholangitis.

Cholecystitis usually results from obstruction of bile flow at the level of the cystic duct with subsequent mucosal inflammation of the gallbladder. Similar to cholangitis, migrated gallstones are the underlying etiology of most cases of cholecystitis. Acalculous cholecystitis is due to cystic duct obstruction from another cause or occurs in the absence of obstruction. Infection of the gallbladder is a common complication of cholecystitis but is rarely the underlying cause. Although the treatment of cholecystitis is usually surgical, there is emerging endoscopic experience in patients who are not surgical candidates.

Endoscopic Retrograde Cholangiopancreatography

Indications

The primary indication for endoscopic retrograde cholangiopancreatography (ERCP) in infectious cholangitis is to treat

Box 45.1 Conditions Associated with Cholangitis

Intraluminal Obstruction

Choledocholithiasis and hepatolithiasis
Biliary stent occlusion
Mirizzi's syndrome
Biliary parasites
Fungal ball
Hemobilia
Sump syndrome
Choledochal cyst

Nonneoplastic Stricture

Primary sclerosing cholangitis
Chronic pancreatitis
Pancreatic cyst or pseudocyst
Papillary stenosis
Recurrent pyogenic cholangitis
AIDS cholangiopathy
Ischemic stricture
Anastomotic stricture
    Liver transplant
    Bilioenteric anastomosis
Radiation
Postchemoinfusion
Tuberculosis

Neoplastic Stricture

Cholangiocarcinoma
Pancreatic carcinoma
Ampullary adenoma or carcinoma
Duodenal carcinoma
Carcinoid tumor
Small intestinal lymphoma
Kaposi's sarcoma
Metastatic disease

Iatrogenic

Post-ERCP
Postsphincterotomy
Posthepatojejunostomy
Post–transhepatic cholangiography
Post–T-tube cholangiography

AIDS, acquired immunodeficiency syndrome; ERCP, endoscopic retrograde cholangiopancreatography.

biliary obstruction through extraction of intraluminal material or stent placement across a biliary stricture.

Contraindications

Contraindications for ERCP in biliary tract infections are similar to other endoscopic procedures. Patients who are unable to tolerate conscious sedation because of cardiopulmonary disease require an anesthesia assessment. Patients with an allergy to contrast agents or iodine are at increased risk of a contrast allergy during ERCP. Premedication with steroids and use of a nonionic or low-osmolality contrast agent are recommended to reduce this risk.[1]

ERCP in pregnancy is apparently safe for both the mother and the fetus, whereas a delay in definitive treatment of cholangitis may be life-threatening. Radiation exposure to the fetus is limited by shielding the uterus with a lead apron, short periods of fluoroscopy, avoiding magnification, and avoiding hard copy radiographs.[2]

Equipment

To perform ERCP, a side-viewing endoscope, a duodenoscope, and fluoroscopy are required. Cannulation with a sphincterotome is recommended because most cases of biliary tract infection require a sphincterotomy. A guidewire is essential for selective cannulation of the intrahepatic ducts and the cystic duct and for accessing the biliary tree proximal to a stricture. To extract intraluminal debris, a biliary extraction basket and balloon and grasping forceps should be available. Mechanical lithotripsy may be necessary for crushing stones before extraction if the stone occurs proximal to a biliary stricture or the caliber of the distal bile duct is less than the stone diameter. Dilating catheters or a biliary dilation balloon, or both, and a selection of plastic and metal biliary stents are required to manage cholangitis secondary to a biliary stricture. A cytology brush and biopsy forceps are used to sample the stricture before stent insertion. Nasobiliary tubes are needed for biliary instillation therapy in certain forms of parasitic cholangitis. Duodenoscope-assisted cholangioscopy may be required to identify completely obstructed intrahepatic ducts, place a guidewire across a stricture, perform directed biopsies of a biliary stricture, and perform electrohydraulic lithotripsy (EHL).

Preparation

The patient should be given nothing per mouth (NPO) after midnight the day before ERCP. Coagulopathy should be corrected if possible. A decision to discontinue anticoagulants or antiplatelet agents should be individualized. There is insufficient evidence to support routine discontinuation of aspirin and nonsteroidal antiinflammatory drugs before therapeutic ERCP procedures. Patients with a history of a contrast allergy are given prednisone, 20 mg by mouth, 13 hours, 7 hours, and 1 hour before the procedure.[1] Conversely, the use of noniodinated contrast agents in place of premedication with steroids is favored by many clinicians. Antibiotics should be administered for prophylaxis of post-ERCP cholangitis if indicated.

Postprocedure Care

If complete endoscopic drainage is not achieved during the initial procedure, antibiotics should be continued until definitive therapy is performed by repeat endoscopic, percutaneous, or surgical biliary decompression. Biliary obstruction resulting from hilar strictures and intrahepatic duct strictures, particularly multiple strictures as seen in primary sclerosing cholangitis, often require antibiotics after the procedure.

The efficacy of antibiotics after successful endoscopic therapy of cholangitis is unknown. In a retrospective analysis of 80 patients with cholangitis who underwent endoscopic therapy, there was no difference in outcome between the group receiving antibiotics for 3 days or less and the group receiving antibiotics for more than 3 days after ERCP.[3] No placebo-controlled study addressing the use of antibiotics in cholangitis after endoscopic drainage has been done, and we generally do not continue antibiotics after successful endoscopic therapy.

Complications

Complications of ERCP include the complications inherent to any endoscopic procedure, including reactions to medications, cardiopulmonary complications, infection, perforation, and hemorrhage, and complications specific to ERCP, such as pancreatitis, postsphincterotomy hemorrhage, and biliary infection. Infectious complications of ERCP are post-ERCP cholangitis and long-term postsphincterotomy cholangitis. The rate of complications related to ERCP is 5% to 8%; risk of complications related to ERCP is 0.3%.[4,5]

Post–Endoscopic Retrograde Cholangiopancreatography Cholangitis

The risk of cholangitis immediately after ERCP is very low—0.7% in a large series from a single referral center where drainage of obstructed ducts is practiced aggressively.[6] The incidence of cholangitis increases 10-fold if diagnostic ERCP is undertaken without performing biliary drainage when an obstruction is found.[7] This increased incidence is due to contaminating sterile bile with enteric bacteria, which in the presence of obstruction results in cholangitis. Any obstructed segment of the biliary tract opacified during cholangiography should be drained. Improper disinfection of duodenoscopes or use of contaminated water also increases the risk of post-ERCP cholangitis and bacteremia, especially with *Pseudomonas aeruginosa*.[8,9]

Long-Term Postsphincterotomy Cholangitis

Surgical or endoscopic sphincterotomy is a risk factor for bacterial contamination of the biliary tract,[10] likely by facilitating transpapillary migration of enteric bacteria. *Escherichia coli* is the most common organism identified. Analysis of patients after cholecystectomy who underwent sphincterotomy revealed a predisposition for developing brown stones or sludge within the common bile duct (CBD) in association with bacteriobilia.[11] However, these data may be biased by predilection in choledocholithiasis prompting sphincterotomy in the first place.

Cholangitis

Bacterial cholangitis results from bile duct obstruction or previous biliary instrumentation. Enterobacteriaceae are the most common causative organisms, and blood cultures are positive in 50% of patients.[12] Isolation of enterococci or multiple organisms from bile is more common in patients with a biliary endoprosthesis[13] or bilioenteric anastomosis. Charcot's triad of right upper quadrant pain, fever, and jaundice is present in 70% of patients with acute bacterial cholangitis. The addition of hypotension and confusion constitutes Reynolds' pentad, which is present in less than 5% of patients with cholangitis but is significantly associated with mortality.[14] Right upper quadrant pain and fever may be absent in elderly

patients, diabetic patients, or patients treated with systemic corticosteroids.

Anatomy
Postoperative Cholangitis

Patients who have undergone bile duct reconstruction with creation of a hepatojejunostomy are at risk of postoperative cholangitis. This condition is especially prevalent in patients with biliary atresia.[15] Bacterial colonization of the hepatojejunostomy and stoma obstruction by food debris may be pathogenic factors.

Sump Syndrome

Sump syndrome occurs after creation of a choledochoduodenostomy to manage retained CBD stones in a dilated bile duct. The distal bile duct between the papilla and the anastomosis becomes a stagnant reservoir or sump into which sludge, calculi, and food can collect. The clinical presentation may include recurrent pain, cholangitis, hepatic abscess, or pancreatitis. Management with endoscopic sphincterotomy with extraction of debris from the bile duct is successful in most patients.[16] In case series, recurrence of symptoms has been noted in 0 to 19% and results from stenosis of the sphincter of Oddi.[17,18] A repeat sphincterotomy should be considered.[18]

Preparation

Prophylactic antibiotics are not recommended routinely in patients with biliary obstruction undergoing ERCP for prevention of endocarditis or post-ERCP cholangitis.[19,20] However, in patients with cholangitis, broad-spectrum antibiotics providing coverage of gram-negative bacilli and *Enterococcus* species are indicated until biliary drainage is successfully completed.

Procedure

ERCP is performed in the usual manner.

A scout film should be examined for pneumobilia, which may be present if a sphincterotomy had been performed previously, if gas-forming bacteria are present in the biliary tract, or if there is a biliary parasitic infestation with *Ascaris*.

After biliary cannulation has been accomplished, aspiration of bile and pus decompresses the biliary tract and reduces the risk of bacteremia from the pressure of contrast agent injection.

A specimen of aspirated bile can be placed in a sterile tube and submitted to microbiology for Gram stain and culture. Cholangiography usually shows the site and cause of biliary obstruction.

Intraluminal Obstruction

An adequate biliary sphincterotomy is required for removal of choledocholithiasis or other intraluminal debris.

Use of a balloon or basket for stone extraction is appropriate. Only the distalmost stone is removed on each sweep to prevent impaction.

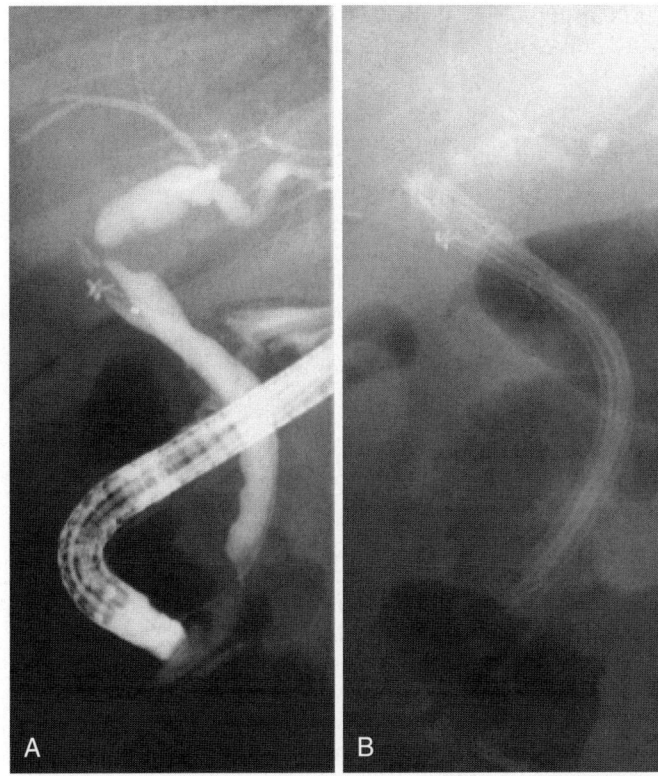

Fig. 45.1 A and **B,** Patient with cholangitis resulting from a benign postoperative bile duct stricture shown by endoscopic retrograde cholangiopancreatography (ERCP) (**A**) and after placement of three 10-Fr plastic stents (**B**).

Mechanical lithotripsy or DACP-assisted EHL is performed for stones larger than the distal bile duct. The stone fragments are removed as described previously.

Biliary Stricture

A guidewire is passed across the stricture.

The length of stent required is measured during withdrawal of the sphincterotome at the level of the biopsy channel.

The stricture is sampled by brushing or biopsy, either fluoroscopically guided or under direct vision during choledochoscopy.

Balloon or catheter dilation may be necessary to accommodate stent placement.

A stent is placed across the stricture to relieve obstruction (**Fig. 45.1**). Although a larger diameter stent is usually preferred, both stent size and type depend on the underlying etiology of the biliary stricture. For most benign strictures, the authors prefer a straight stent with internal and external flaps to prevent stent migration. For malignant strictures in palliative patients, a covered or uncovered self-expandable metal stent is another appropriate choice. Patients with strictures involving the biliary hilum should undergo stent placement into both the right and the left hepatic ducts when technically possible; this is accomplished by placing two guidewires, one into each ductal system, and sequential stent placement.

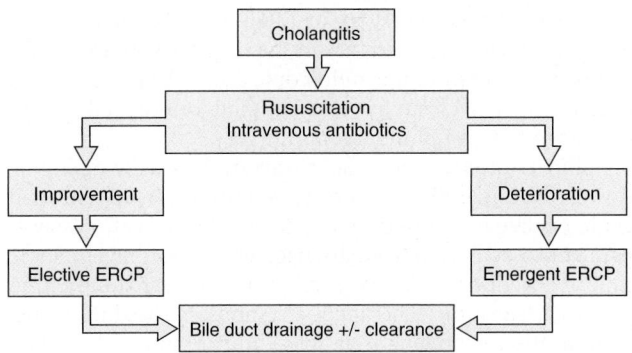

Fig. 45.2 Algorithm for management of cholangitis. ERCP, endoscopic retrograde cholangiopancreatography.

Drainage of bile and contrast agent through the stent should be noted endoscopically and fluoroscopically to ascertain successful decompression.

Stent Occlusion

An occluded plastic stent can be removed with a polypectomy snare through the biopsy channel of the duodenoscope.

An occluded metal stent should be trawled with a biliary extraction basket or balloon to remove any debris.

If metal stent occlusion is due to tumor ingrowth or overgrowth, deployment of another stent within the occluded stent may be performed.

Complications

Complications of cholangitis include hepatic abscess, distant metastatic abscess, bacteremia, systemic inflammatory response syndrome, and multiple organ dysfunction. There is a 10% risk of death.

Outcomes

Treatment of acute cholangitis includes resuscitation, antimicrobials, and biliary tract drainage (**Fig. 45.2**). Management of respiratory and circulatory insufficiency in a monitored setting and administration of broad-spectrum antibiotics should precede, but not delay, definitive biliary tract decompression in a severely ill or deteriorating patient.

Calculous Cholangitis

Biliary drainage can be accomplished endoscopically, percutaneously, or surgically. Endoscopic treatment, either sphincterotomy with stone extraction[21,22] or biliary stent or nasobiliary drain insertion, is superior to surgical treatment in patients with severe cholangitis. Endoscopic sphincterotomy with stone extraction resulted in increased survival compared with surgery in a retrospective cohort of patients with acute calculous cholangitis[21]; this was despite a higher number of concomitant medical problems and increased age in the patients managed endoscopically. Lai and colleagues[23] randomly assigned 82 patients with calculous cholangitis requiring emergent therapy to surgery or ERCP with nasobiliary catheter placement. The mortality in the surgical arm was significantly higher than in the endoscopic arm—32% and 10%. In addition, there were an increased number of nonfatal complications in the group undergoing surgery.

Sphincterotomy and stone extraction is usually attempted during the initial ERCP. However, in critically ill patients with acute cholangitis secondary to choledocholithiasis, it may be prudent to achieve biliary drainage endoscopically, by insertion of a stent or nasobiliary catheter, and defer stone extraction to a later time. Therapeutic response, procedure-related complications, and length of procedure are similar for biliary stents and nasobiliary catheters, but inadvertent catheter removal and patient discomfort are greater in patients who receive a nasobiliary catheter.[24] Approximately 10% of patients have cholangitis owing to stones that cannot be removed by standard means, including mechanical lithotripsy. These stones include large stones, stones located proximal to a stricture, or stones greater than the diameter of the distal bile duct. Options are endoscopic EHL, extracorporeal shock wave lithotripsy, endoscopic laser lithotripsy, and permanent biliary stent placement.[25–27] Increasingly, the use of adjunctive biliary balloon sphincteroplasty is being used to remove CBD stones safely and effectively. An occlusion cholangiogram at completion of ERCP may ensure clearance but carries a significant risk of bacteremia in this situation.

If all stones or stone fragments cannot be removed during the initial endoscopic session, a stent should be left in place to provide bile drainage and prevent further cholangitis (**Fig. 45.3**). Long-term stent therapy is no longer advisable because of the high incidence of cholangitis and related deaths.[28,29] Similar techniques can be employed in the cystic duct to treat Mirizzi's syndrome.[26,30,31] In a patient with cholangitis and gallstones but no evidence of choledocholithiasis on cholangiography, empiric endoscopic sphincterotomy does not appear to decrease the risk of subsequent episodes of cholangitis and results in a higher ERCP complication rate.[32]

Cholangitis Secondary to a Biliary Stricture

Biliary tract obstruction secondary to a malignant stricture rarely causes cholangitis, unless the bile has been contaminated with bacteria during a previous biliary intervention. Patients with strictures involving the biliary hilum should undergo stent placement into the right and the left hepatic ducts when technically possible because bilateral decompression would improve patient survival.[33] This is especially important if the biliary tract proximal to the stricture has filled with contrast material.

Cholangitis Secondary to Stent Occlusion

Plastic biliary stents develop a bacterial biofilm on their surface,[34] which leads to stent occlusion and risk of cholangitis. Uncovered self-expandable metal stents, by virtue of their larger diameter and composition, do not develop encrustation at the same rate and have a longer patency.[34] If metal stent obstruction does occur, it is usually the result of tumor ingrowth between the metal struts or tumor overgrowth at either end. Metal stents covered with a synthetic coating to prevent tumor ingrowth seem to have a similar or increased duration of patency (**Fig. 45.4**).[35]

Recurrent Pyogenic Cholangitis

Recurrent pyogenic cholangitis, also known as Oriental cholangiohepatitis, is a clinical syndrome comprising repetitive episodes of bacterial cholangitis resulting from intrahepatic biliary obstruction with calcium bilirubinate stones or strictures or both. The bile ducts in the left lateral segment of the liver are often the only ducts affected or the most severely affected. This segment may be anatomically predisposed to stasis because of duct angulations slowing bile drainage. Chronic obstruction eventually causes permanent dilation of the proximal biliary tract, often filled with intrahepatic stones. Bile stasis and bacterial contamination may result in the development of multiple hepatic abscesses. Enterobacteriaceae bacteria are the most frequent organisms cultured from bile. *P. aeruginosa* may be seen in patients who have previously undergone endoscopic or surgical biliary intervention. Anaerobes are less common. Growth of multiple organisms, although unusual in other causes of cholangitis, often occurs in recurrent pyogenic cholangitis.[36] Isolation of biliary parasites in patients with recurrent pyogenic cholangitis is common,[37,38] but it is unclear whether the parasite is an etiologic agent or an incidental finding.

Indications

ERCP is indicated to provide drainage to obstructed bile ducts when cholangitis is not responding adequately to supportive measures. Otherwise, ERCP in recurrent pyogenic cholangitis should be timed between episodes of acute cholangitis. The goal of endoscopic management is to treat biliary obstruction by stricture dilation and stone removal with the intent of decreasing the frequency of cholangitis.

Preparation

Prophylactic antibiotics have been recommended to decrease the risk of cholangitis during ERCP in patients with recurrent pyogenic cholangitis.[39] Magnetic resonance (MR) cholangiography before ERCP should be considered. The major advantage of MR cholangiography is complete visualization of the biliary tract including segments obstructed by calculi or strictures[40] that may not be apparent by ERCP. Detailed knowledge of intrahepatic segment anatomy is necessary to correlate MR imaging to the opacified ducts at ERCP and guide endoscopic management.

Procedure

Cholangiography during ERCP also accurately documents duct dilation, intraductal stones, and gallstones (**Fig. 45.5**). The intrahepatic ducts appear straightened and acutely angulated at branches, likely secondary to periductal fibrosis. There is often distinct tapering of the intrahepatic ducts proximally, described as the "arrowhead" sign, and decreased duct branching. Complete occlusion of an intrahepatic duct by a stone may be represented by segmental absence of contrast material and is better assessed by MR cholangiography.

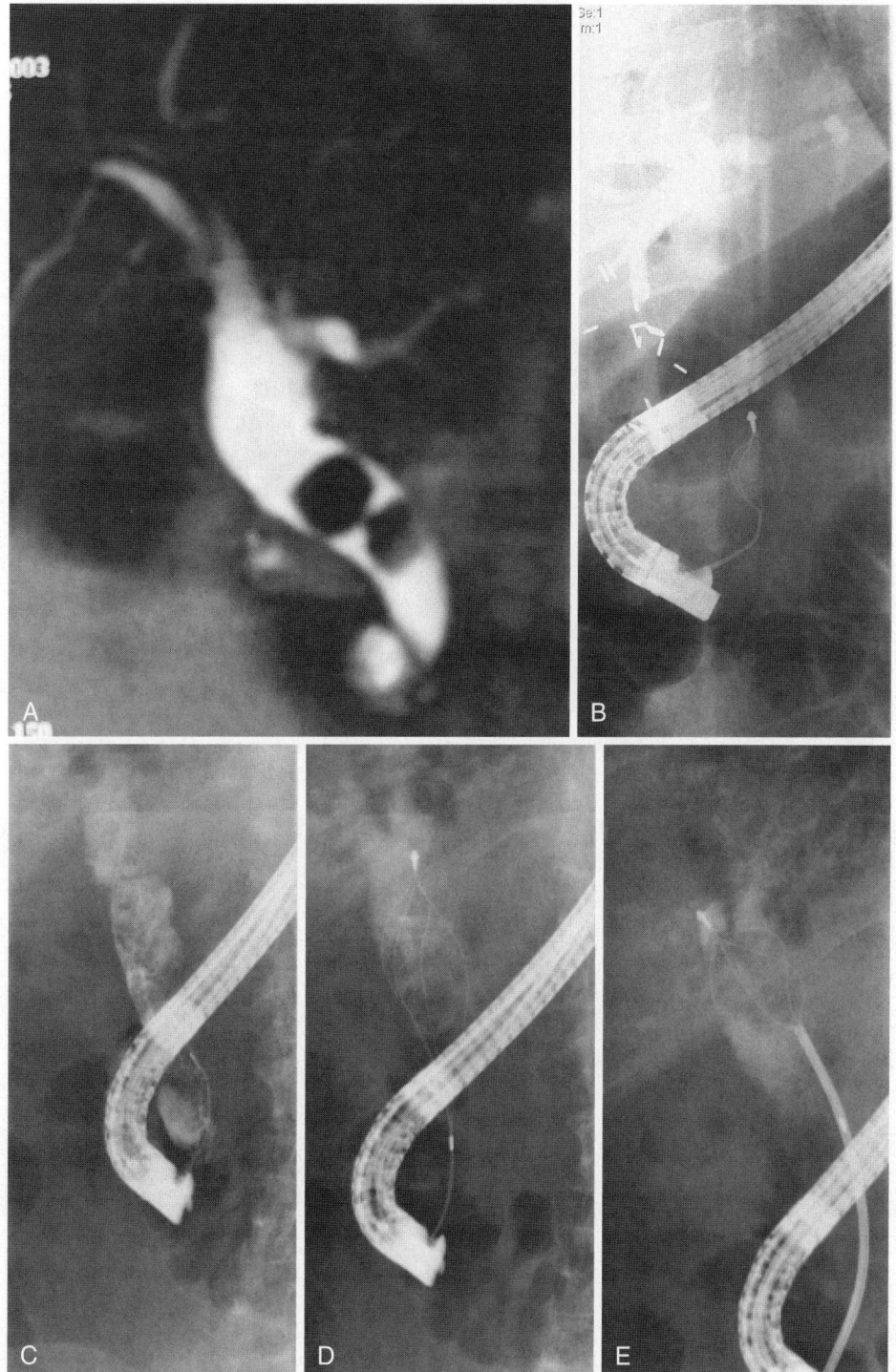

Fig. 45.3 A, Magnetic resonance cholangiopancreatography (MRCP) shows two large bile duct stones in a patient with cholangitis. **B,** Endoscopic retrograde cholangiopancreatography (ERCP) in the same patient with basket extraction of one of the stones. **C,** ERCP shows dilated bile duct packed with stones. **D,** Basket extraction. **E,** Mechanical lithotripsy.

ERCP is performed in the usual manner.

Obtaining a complete cholangiogram may be difficult because of intrahepatic duct obstruction by impacted stones or strictures or both. Occlusion cholangiography using a biliary balloon can be useful in this situation but carries a risk of cholangitis by contaminating obstructed ducts with contrast material and of bacteremia by increasing the intraluminal pressure. A complete cholangiogram should not be aggressively pursued if drainage of obstructed ducts is not intended.

An adequate endoscopic sphincterotomy is essential for definitive endoscopic management of recurrent pyogenic cholangitis.

Standard stone extraction techniques are attempted, but it is often necessary to place a guidewire into the desired hepatic or intrahepatic ducts.

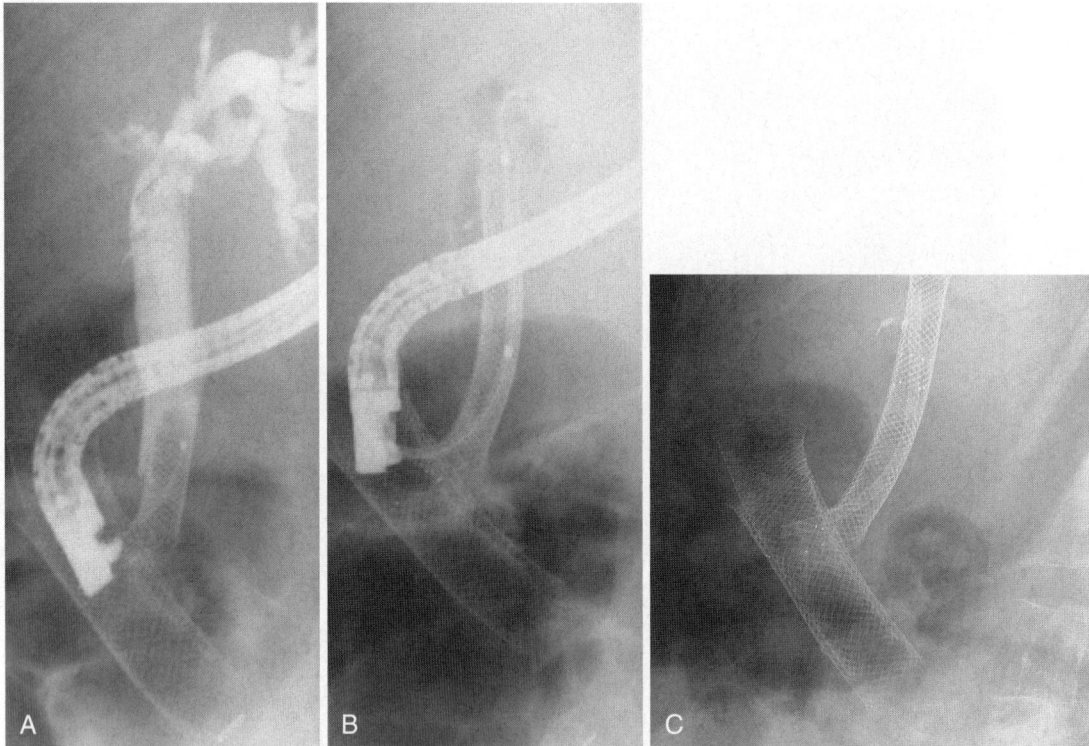

Fig. 45.4 Patient with cholangitis secondary to an occluded biliary metal stent (the patient also has three internal stents in the duodenum). **A,** Endoscopic retrograde cholangiopancreatography (ERCP.) **B,** Insertion of a 10-Fr plastic stent inside the metal stent. **C,** Final position of stent.

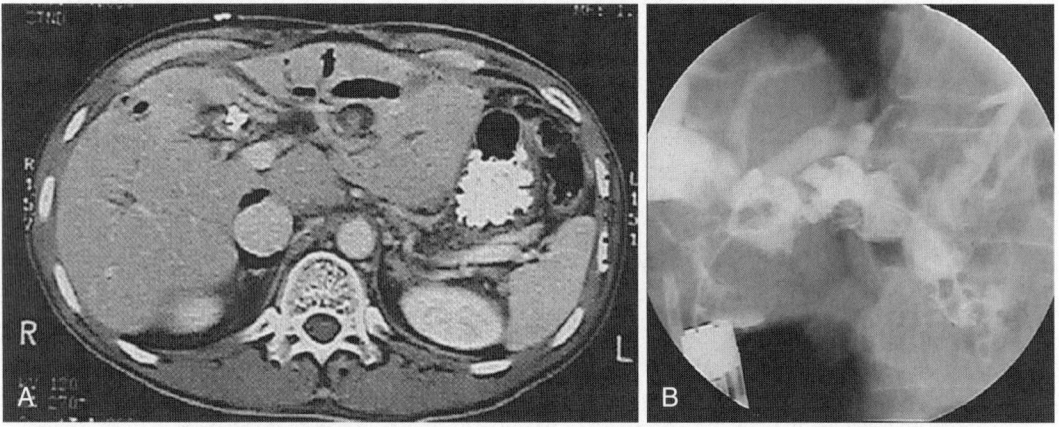

Fig. 45.5 Patient with recurrent pyogenic cholangitis. **A,** Computed tomography (CT) scan shows dilated air-filled left intrahepatic ductal system with stones and two stents. **B,** Endoscopic retrograde cholangiography (ERC) shows multiple lucent stones in the same system.

Removal of multiple stones is accomplished distal to proximal to reduce the risk of stone impaction. Given the propensity of pigment stones to fragment, extraction balloons or baskets may be used.

When extracting from smaller caliber intrahepatic ducts, it is necessary to have a variety of balloon diameters available or a multistep balloon that inflates in a stepwise fashion through a range of sizes. Baskets are more flexible and may reach deeply into difficult intrahepatic ducts, and when the size of a stone exceeds the caliber of the distal duct, basket lithotripsy can be used to fragment the stone before extraction.

If the aforementioned methods are unsuccessful, choledochoscopy should be considered.

The choledochoscope can assist in correct guidewire placement proximal to intrahepatic stones with subsequent exchange of the choledochoscope for an extraction device. Choledochoscopy also provides further therapeutic options for stones resistant to removal by conventional methods such as EHL. The stone debris is removed by balloon or basket extraction.

Strictures occur in the extrahepatic and intrahepatic ducts, often with proximal calculi. At or immediately distal to the hepatic duct confluence is a common site for strictures. It is essential to treat strictures before attempting proximal stone removal to prevent stone impaction at the stricture.

Either wire-guided balloon or catheter dilation is an acceptable method. The ideal posttherapy duct size should be equal to or larger than the proximal stones but is guided by the size of the duct distal to the stricture.

If the wire cannot be directed across an intrahepatic duct stricture, aligning the choledochoscope with the duct of interest and passing a guidewire through the accessory channel of the choledochoscope often provides access.

The choledochoscope can be exchanged for a biliary dilation balloon or catheter. Multiple endoscopic sessions may be required for adequate stricture dilation, and a stent should be inserted between procedures.

If a dominant stricture is evident on cholangiography, further evaluation to exclude cholangiocarcinoma should be undertaken; this includes biliary cytology brushing and biopsy under fluoroscopy or direct brushing or biopsy through the accessory channel of the choledochoscope. Another endoscopic finding that is suspicious for cholangiocarcinoma in recurrent pyogenic cholangitis is mucin within the bile duct.[41]

Parasitic biliary infestation may occur in recurrent pyogenic cholangitis. Endoscopic treatment of parasitic cholangitis is described subsequently.

Postprocedure Care

If complete drainage is not achieved, the patient is at risk of post-ERCP cholangitis, and prophylactic broad-spectrum antibiotics should be administered. Endoscopic therapy in recurrent pyogenic cholangitis is a temporizing measure and does not cure the underlying disease, and repeat interventions are required as stones and strictures recur.

Complications

The clinical course may be complicated by recurrent sepsis, hepatic abscess rupture with peritonitis,[37] portal pyelothrombophlebitis, and, rarely, hepatic failure.[42] Patients may present with acute pancreatitis, presumably secondary to obstruction of the pancreatic duct by a stone or parasite, but this is uncommon. In the long-term, patients are at risk of cirrhosis, atrophy of hepatic segments supplied by thrombosed portal branches, clinical manifestations of portal hypertension, and cholangiocarcinoma.[41,42]

Outcomes

ERCP has been successfully used in the treatment of recurrent pyogenic cholangitis for 25 years.[43] ERCP was traditionally used to provide a detailed "map" of the biliary tract, noting the location of stones and strictures, to guide definitive therapy. However, with the development of MR cholangiography, diagnostic ERCP should be reserved for situations in which MR imaging expertise is unavailable.[40] Endoscopic sphincterotomy with stricture dilation and stone extraction is uncomplicated for extrahepatic disease. The soft pigment stones readily deform and fragment, enabling delivery into the duodenum.

In contrast, management of hepatolithiasis is often technically challenging. Accessing intrahepatic branches obstructed by calculi or strictures to perform dilation or stone removal is frequently difficult. Obstructed intrahepatic ducts requiring treatment may not be apparent to the endoscopist. Intrahepatic ducts that have "vanished" proximal to a high-grade stricture or obstructing calculi are not always appreciated at

cholangiography. Duodenoscope-assisted choledochoscopy is very useful in this situation, not only to identify the presence of the obstructed intrahepatic branch but also to provide further therapy, such as EHL. These techniques of endoscopic therapy can also be applied percutaneously or through a surgically created biliary-enteric conduit as described subsequently. In the management of hepatolithiasis, multiple treatment sessions are usually necessary, conducted endoscopically or percutaneously, to perform sequential stricture dilation and to attempt complete stone removal. Percutaneous access to the biliary tree can be accomplished by formation of a transhepatic tract under ultrasound guidance. As the tract matures, biliary dilation catheters and stone extraction devices are passed into the biliary tree to provide therapy. Choledochoscopy and EHL are also possible by this route.

Complete clearance of hepatolithiasis is attained in 96% of patients after an average of six treatments.[44] However, one-third of patients have recurrent disease by 5 years. Cheung[45] reported 190 patients with residual hepatolithiasis after surgical choledocholithotomy and choledochoscopic lithotripsy who were treated via a T-tube tract. Treatment consisted of sequential biliary stricture dilation with stent placement between dilation sessions. After the strictures were adequately treated, choledochoscopy and EHL were performed to fragment intrahepatic calculi with basket retrieval of stone debris. Complete clearance was achieved in 88% of patients; 15% of these patients developed evidence of recurrent disease during a mean follow-up period of 4 years. Complications were mild and included hemobilia and fever. Biliary enteric bypass procedures for repeated access to the intrahepatic ducts involve creation of a Roux-en-Y hepatojejunostomy or choledochojejunostomy with one jejunal limb brought to the skin as a cutaneous stoma[46,47] or a jejunoduodenostomy.[48] Treatment of strictures and stones is possible using a duodenoscope, gastroscope, or choledochoscope (**Fig. 45.6**). When treatment is complete, the stoma can be buried subcutaneously, but it may be reaccessed by a simple surgical procedure in the event of disease recurrence.

Avoidance of hepatic resection and resolution of hepatic abscesses can be achieved; however, repeat therapy or hepatic resection are most likely to be required as stones and strictures recur.[47] Segmental hepatic resection is often used to treat localized disease, primarily involving the left lateral or right posterior segments. Initial stone clearance is 96% with a disease recurrence of 6% at 5 years.[44] The complications are greater compared with hepatic-preserving procedures and include hepatic insufficiency, postoperative hemorrhage, and bile leak. Liver transplantation is rarely performed in patients with recurrent pyogenic cholangitis.[49,50] Appropriate indications are advanced biliary cirrhosis or diffuse hepatic disease unresponsive to the aforementioned measures. The potential for disease recurrence in the transplanted liver is unknown. There is no evidence to support the use of long-term antibiotics or ursodeoxycholic acid in the management of recurrent pyogenic cholangitis.

Parasitic Cholangitis

Ascaris lumbricoides is a nematode or roundworm that matures within the small intestine and causes cholangitis by entering the bile duct across the major papilla. The

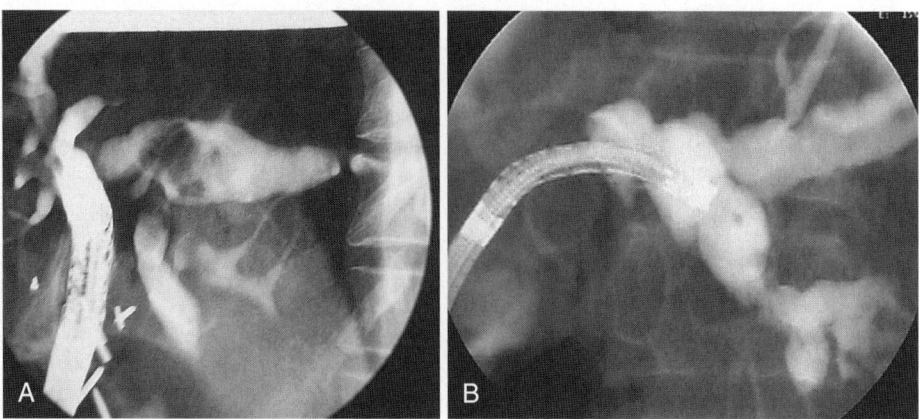

Fig. 45.6 Patient with recurrent pyogenic cholangitis, previously treated surgically with the creation of a cutaneous-jejunal-hepatic duct conduit. **A,** Gastroscope passed through the conduit shows a large left intrahepatic duct stone. **B,** After electrohydraulic lithotripsy and extraction of fragments.

trematodes *Opisthorchis sinensis, Opisthorchis viverrini, Opisthorchis felineus,* and *Fasciola hepatica* mature to adulthood within the human bile duct and are collectively known as liver flukes. *A. lumbricoides* and the liver flukes cause inflammation of the bile duct and secondary bacterial cholangitis by allowing ascending bacterial contamination of bile, obstructing the bile duct and stimulating choledocholithiasis. Hepatic infection by *Echinococcus* species frequently involves the biliary tract by hydatid cyst compression or rupture and direct extension of alveolar echinococcosis.

Ascaris Cholangitis

A. lumbricoides exists worldwide but is most prevalent in Asia, Africa, and South America as a result of crowded living conditions and poor sanitation. Ova are passed in the human feces and are ingested on contaminated fruit or vegetables. Previous endoscopic or surgical sphincterotomy,[51,52] bilioenteric bypass surgery,[51] and cholecystectomy[52] increase the likelihood of biliary involvement. *A. lumbricoides* causes inflammation of the bile duct and secondary bacterial cholangitis by allowing ascending bacterial contamination of bile, obstructing the bile duct and stimulating pigment stone formation. Migration into the gallbladder to cause acalculous or calculous cholecystitis seems to be facilitated by a low insertion of the cystic duct at the level of the ampulla and by pregnancy.[53]

Indications

ERCP is indicated in *Ascaris* cholangitis to remove worms from the biliary tract when anthelmintic therapy is unsuccessful or after medical therapy when the dying worm releases numerous eggs, and these, combined with the worm's own remnants, obstruct the biliary or pancreatic duct and act as a nidus for pigment stone formation (**Fig. 45.7**). The sequelae of *Ascaris* cholangitis, such as bile duct strictures and choledocholithiasis, may result in biliary obstruction necessitating endoscopic therapy.

Preparation

Parasite eradication should be attempted in all cases of documented infection, regardless of symptoms. Close contacts of

infected persons should submit stool specimens for analysis and be treated if positive.

Procedure

The goal of therapy is complete removal of the parasite and stones and treatment of strictures. If the diagnosis of parasitic cholangitis has not yet been established, aspiration of bile should be performed to evaluate for ova under microscopy.

ERCP is performed in the usual manner.

At duodenoscopy, the adult worm may be observed as a pale white or reddish yellow tubular structure up to 35 cm in length[12] either within the lumen of the duodenum or crossing the major papilla.

Pneumobilia may be evident on the scout film.

On cholangiography and pancreatography, *A. lumbricoides* appears as a tubular filling defect with tapered ends.

Real-time fluoroscopy may detect the erratic motility pattern typical of *A. lumbricoides,* particularly in the gallbladder.

Injection of contrast material may stimulate the worm to migrate distally into the duodenum.

Stones and strictures may also be present in the bile duct, and the pancreatic duct is usually dilated if involved.

In most instances, parasite extraction from the biliary tract necessitates an endoscopic sphincterotomy. However, because the enteric reinfection rate for *A. lumbricoides* after eradication is extremely high in endemic areas, sphincterotomy facilitates future biliary tract involvement and is relatively contraindicated. When the major papilla is patulous owing to worm migration, access and extraction is uncomplicated. With a papillary orifice of normal or decreased caliber from papillary stenosis, papillary balloon dilation is a useful compromise.

Worms that appear at the papilla, either spontaneously or in response to contrast agent injection, can be grasped with a biopsy forceps and pulled into the duodenum to the opening of the accessory channel on the duodenoscope. The endoscope and worm should be withdrawn, and the biopsy forceps should be opened to release the worm into a container for microscopy.

Worms located completely within the biliary tract can be removed with a biliary extraction balloon or basket. The

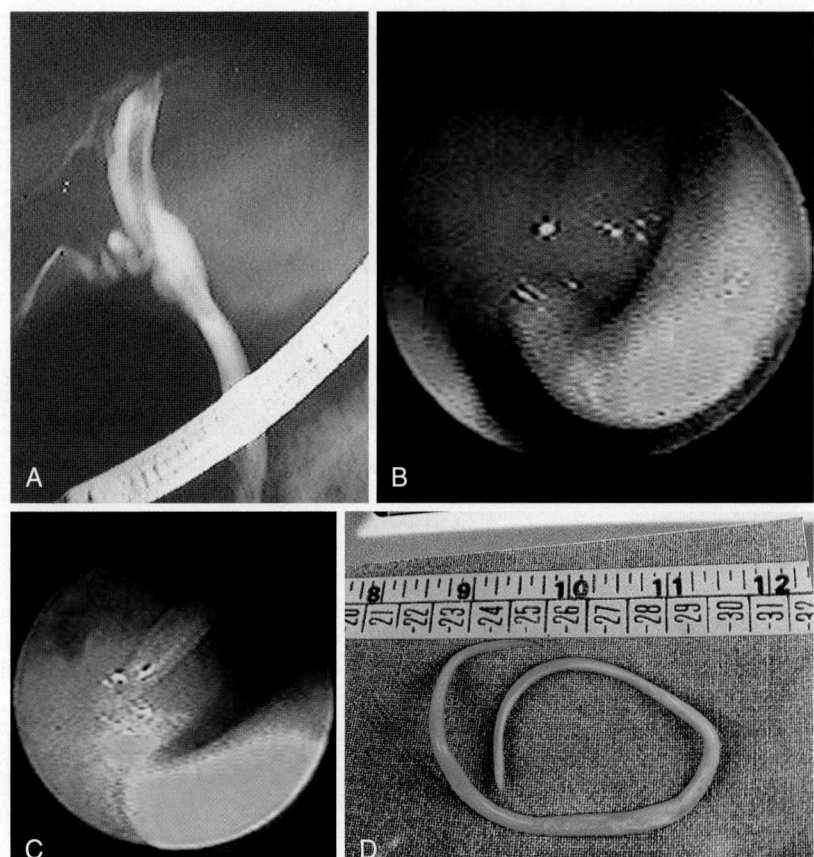

Fig. 45.7 A, Endoscopic retrograde cholangiopancrea-tography (ERCP) shows *Ascaris lumbricoides* within the proximal bile duct. **B,** Living *Ascaris* crossing the papilla. **C,** *Ascaris* crossing the papilla with the motile tip of the worm approaching the papilla. **D,** Extracted adult *Ascaris*. (**C,** *Courtesy of Dr. Angelo Ferrari, São Paulo, Brazil;* **D,** *courtesy of Dr. Alok Gupta, Kanpur, India.*)

ideal balloon diameter depends on the size of the bile duct. With either device, the worm should be brought to the papillary orifice and grasped using the biopsy forceps as described previously.

Polypectomy snares are liable to transect the worm and complicate extraction. If a worm is transected during extraction attempt or debris of dead worms is present in the bile duct, complete removal of all remnants is vital to prevent future episodes of cholangitis and stone formation.

Complications

In addition to infecting the biliary tree, *A. lumbricoides* para-sites also burrow through the bile duct wall into the liver parenchyma to form hepatic abscesses. Acute pancreatitis has been reported secondary to worms obstructing the pancreatic duct.[52]

Outcomes

ERCP is indicated for diagnosis and management of *Ascaris* cholangitis. ERCP enables sampling of bile to determine the presence of ova, which may be more sensitive than stool microscopy,[54] and to show the mature parasite within the biliary system (**Fig. 45.8**). Endoscopic extraction of biliary *A. lumbricoides* is successful and safe in 99% of patients.[52] Although endoscopic sphincterotomy increases the risk of reinfection, it is necessary for worm extraction in 95% of cases.[55] Surgical removal of *A. lumbricoides* from the biliary

tract was a common practice before the advent of therapeutic endoscopy. Present surgical indications include cholecystitis owing to worms or calculi and failure of endoscopic bile duct clearance.

Liver Fluke Cholangitis

Opisthorchis trematodes occur in Asia and Eastern Europe, whereas *Fasciola* flukes are prevalent worldwide. Human infection occurs from eating uncooked or undercooked fresh-water fish or plants such as watercress, alfalfa, and parsley. *Opisthorchis* enter the biliary tree through the major papilla, whereas *Fasciola* penetrate the intestinal wall into the peri-toneal cavity and enter the biliary tree transhepatically. Adult liver flukes most commonly reside in the intrahepatic branches but may be observed in the distal biliary tract. Infection of the gallbladder and pancreatic duct has also been reported.

Indications

ERCP is indicated for diagnosis of liver fluke cholangitis and endoscopic management including worm extraction and treatment of secondary bile duct strictures and choledocholithiasis.

Procedure

The goals and techniques of endoscopic treatment of liver fluke cholangitis are similar to *Ascaris* cholangitis. Because

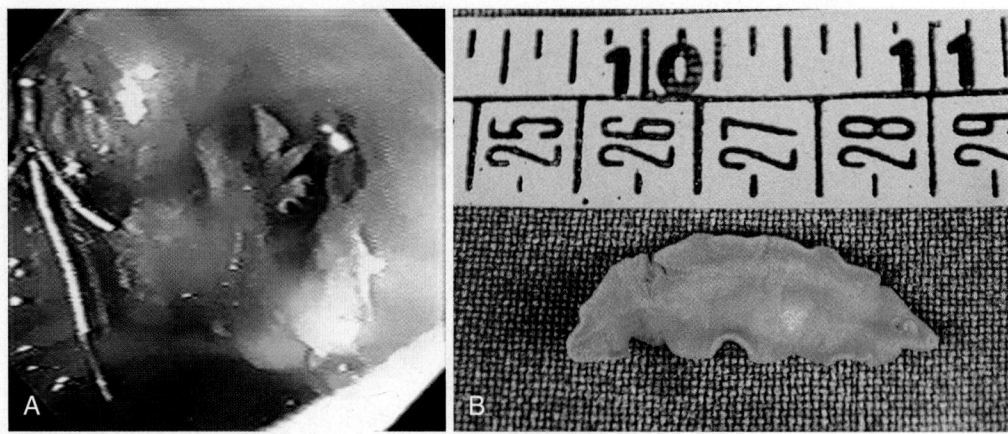

Fig. 45.8 A, *Fasciola hepatica* being extracted at endoscopic retrograde cholangiopancreatography (ERCP). **B,** Adult worm after extraction. *(**A,** Courtesy of Dr. Claudio Navarette, Santiago, Chile; **B,** courtesy of Dr. Alok Gupta, Kanpur, India.)*

liver flukes frequently inhabit the proximal biliary tree, their clearance can be challenging.

> ERCP is performed in the usual manner.
> Cholangiography may show saccular dilation of the intrahepatic ducts, often diffusely, with blunted terminal ends.[56] Filling defects represent the fluke, choledocholithiasis, or mucosal hyperplasia or dysplasia. The fluke has a filamentous curvilinear or elliptical shape and may be quickly obscured by contrast material.[54,56] The flukes are primarily in the secondary and tertiary branches of the intrahepatic ducts but may appear throughout the biliary tract and in the pancreatic duct.
> Contrast agent injection may wash adult flukes distally. They appear at duodenoscopy as brownish, flat, leaf-shaped organisms 1 to 2 cm long and usually less than 1 cm wide.[12]
> The flukes should be grasped with forceps and removed from the bile duct.[57]
> Endoscopic sphincterotomy is usually required for liver fluke extraction.
> Extraction of flukes should be undertaken with a biliary extraction basket or balloon. Wire guidance may be necessary to access the affected intrahepatic duct.
> Irregularities in the biliary wall should be sampled to evaluate for cholangiocarcinoma.
> Placement of a nasobiliary tube to perform biliary infusion of povidone-iodine has been described in the management of *F. hepatica* cholangitis.

Complications

Long-standing liver fluke cholangitis can lead to chronic liver disease with portal hypertension and, with *Opisthorchis* infection, cholangiocarcinoma.

Outcomes

Anthelmintic therapy is indicated in all infected individuals. Given the potentially severe complications and ongoing parasite transmission, even asymptomatic individuals should receive eradication treatment. ERCP enables sampling of bile to show the presence of ova, which may be more sensitive than

stool microscopy,[54] and demonstration of the mature parasite within the biliary system. Placement of a nasobiliary tube to perform biliary infusion of povidone-iodine has been described in the management of *F. hepatica* cholangitis.[58] Nine patients who had failed oral anthelmintic therapy became negative for stool ova after biliary administration of povidone-iodine. Surgical intervention is indicated for biliary or pancreatic obstruction after unsuccessful endoscopic therapy and for cholecystitis.

Echinococcal Cholangitis

Echinococcus granulosus accounts for up to 95% of all human echinococcal infections and is present throughout the world, particularly in regions where dogs are used to raise livestock. *E. granulosus, Echinococcus vogeli,* and *Echinococcus oligarthrus* form a unilocular cyst, the hydatid cyst, within the liver. The cyst is composed of three layers. The outermost layer is granulation and fibrous tissue produced by the host and may calcify over time. The middle layer is a laminated membrane. The innermost layer is the germinal layer of the parasite, which forms the daughter cysts and protoscolices. Biliary disease results from compression by the cyst or rupture of the cyst into the biliary tree. *Echinococcus multilocularis* cysts are not contained by an outer fibrous membrane and extend through the liver and into adjacent structures, such as the biliary tree, in a malignant fashion. Infection of the biliary tree occurs by invading into the bifurcation of the right and left hepatic ducts.

Indications

The indications for ERCP in biliary echinococcosis are listed in **Box 45.2**.

Procedure

The goals of ERCP are to document suspected *Echinococcus* cholangitis and treat biliary obstruction.

> ERCP is performed in the usual manner.
> Duodenoscopy may show glistening, white membranes within the duodenum.

The laminated membranes can be removed with biopsy forceps if protruding from the papilla.

On cholangiography, three patterns of filling defects have been reported (**Fig. 45.9**). The membranes appear filiform, the daughter cysts round, and hydatid sand as debris.[59] Endoscopic sphincterotomy should be performed if filling defects are shown.

The membranes, daughter cysts, and protoscolices should be removed with a biliary extraction balloon or basket.[60]

Saline irrigation through the sphincterotome facilitates removal of the protoscolices.

Placement of a nasobiliary tube allows instillation of hypertonic saline solution after ERCP. If technically possible, the nasobiliary tube should be advanced into the cyst cavity.

Biliary strictures resulting from hydatid cyst compression or alveolar echinococcosis invasion can be managed with stent insertion.

Endoscopic therapy may be required after surgical treatment or PAIR (puncture, aspiration of cyst contents, injection of scolicidal agent, reaspiration) to manage bile leaks, communication between the biliary tract and the surgical site with hydatid remnants causing biliary obstruction, or biliary strictures from scolicidal agents.[60]

Complications

E. multilocularis may invade into the portal venous system resulting in portal hypertension.[61]

Outcomes

Endoscopic management of biliary obstruction secondary to *E. granulosus* infection through extraction of hydatid debris

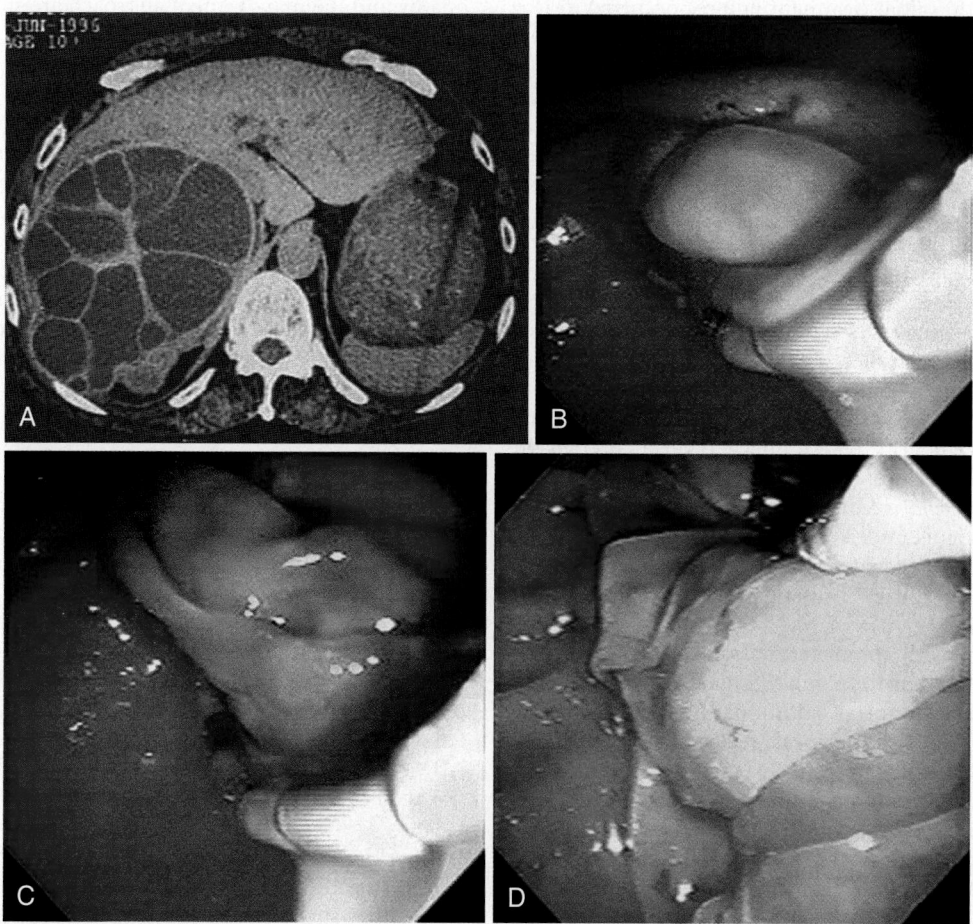

Fig. 45.9 A, *Echinococcus* (hydatidosis) infection shown in right lobe of the liver on computed tomography (CT) scan. **B–D,** Sequence of cyst wall extraction at endoscopic retrograde cholangiopancreatography (ERCP) after sphincterotomy. (*A, Courtesy of Dr. Nageshwar Reddy, Hyderabad, India; B-D, Courtesy of Dr. Claudio Navarette, Santiago, Chile.*)

or biliary endoprosthesis placement is successful at alleviating patient symptoms.[60] Case reports have documented resolution of a hydatid cyst communicating with the biliary tree after endoscopic extraction of cyst material followed by instillation of hypertonic saline solution via a nasobiliary tube placed in the cyst cavity and administration of albendazole orally.[62] In *E. granulosus* infection, approximately 30% of patients experience cure with medical therapy alone.[63,64] Successful therapy is more likely with small, simple cysts and treatment duration greater than 3 months.[63,65,66] Complete surgical excision by cystectomy, pericystectomy, or partial hepatic resection is usually curative in *E. granulosus* infection. Albendazole administered before surgery results in a higher number of nonviable cysts[66,67] and may decrease the risk of local recurrence or intraperitoneal seeding should spillage of cyst contents occur. Surgical mortality is 1% to 2%.[68] Complications include infection, bile leak, and leakage of cyst contents with hypersensitivity reaction and dissemination of disease.

Percutaneous evacuation with ultrasound-guided PAIR is widely used to treat unilocular *E. granulosus* cysts. Scolicidal agents employed for PAIR include 95% ethanol and hypertonic saline. Khuroo and associates[69] randomly assigned 50 patients to undergo cystectomy or PAIR and receive albendazole. At a mean follow-up of 17 months, the cyst diameter was similar in the two groups, but the surgical arm had significantly more complications and a longer length of hospital stay. After PAIR, initial treatment failures occurred in less than 1%, and probability of relapse ranged from 1% to 4.5%. Complications of PAIR include hypersensitivity reaction, infection, intraabdominal seeding, and fistula formation to adjacent organs. In a review of 765 abdominal hydatid cysts treated with PAIR, anaphylaxis occurred in four instances with one death, and minor complications occurred in 14%.[70]

ERCP should be performed before protoscolicide administration to ensure there is no communication between the cyst and biliary tree because contact with protoscolicidal agents produces sclerosing cholangitis and pancreatitis. Treatment with albendazole at least 4 hours before PAIR and up to 4 weeks following has been recommended.[70] The endoscopic management of *E. multilocularis* cholangitis consists of stent placement to relieve biliary obstruction. Sezgin and colleagues[61] have published the largest case series of hepatic *E. multilocularis* complicated by biliary strictures. Seven of nine patients underwent successful stent placement. The stent provided adequate biliary drainage but was ineffective in treating biliary fistula disease present in two patients.

Radical surgery with complete excision of larvae tissue is the only curative therapy for *E. multilocularis* infection. Treatment with albendazole for an additional 2 years postoperatively decreases the risk of local recurrence.[64,71] Patients deemed inoperable at diagnosis likely benefit from long-term albendazole therapy,[71] and a combination of palliative resection, aimed at lessening the mass of larvae tissue, and benzimidazole therapy is advocated.[72] Liver transplantation is a treatment option for unresectable alveolar echinococcosis. A retrospective study of European transplant centers reported 45 patients who underwent liver transplantation with an overall 5-year survival of 71% and disease-free 5-year survival of 58%.[73] Given the high probability of graft recurrence, long-term benzimidazole therapy should be considered in posttransplant patients.

Acquired Immunodeficiency Syndrome Cholangiopathy

AIDS cholangiopathy is a syndrome of right upper quadrant pain, elevated alkaline phosphatase, and typical cholangiography findings associated with human immunodeficiency virus (HIV) infection. Opportunistic infection of the biliary tract is likely a causative factor. *Cryptosporidium*, most commonly *Cryptosporidium parvum*, is isolated from the bile or stool in two-thirds of individuals with AIDS cholangiopathy,[74] but other organisms have also been associated, including *Microsporida*, cytomegalovirus, *Isospora*, *Cyclospora*, and *Mycobacterium avium intracellulare*.[75,76] Acalculous cholecystitis secondary to opportunistic infection of the gallbladder may occur alone or concomitant to cholangiopathy and is associated with similar underlying pathogens. Cholangiopathy is the AIDS-defining illness in a few patients, but most patients have had AIDS for at least 1 year.[77]

Indications

ERCP is the "gold standard" in diagnosing AIDS cholangiopathy (**Fig. 45.10**). The differential diagnosis of AIDS cholangiopathy and the management approach are shown in **Box 45.3** and **Fig. 45.11**, respectively.

Precautions

Protease inhibitors and benzodiazepines are both metabolized through the P-450 enzyme complex. Protease inhibitors decrease benzodiazepine metabolism, increasing their serum levels and potentiating their effects, including respiratory depression.[78] Because midazolam and diazepam are commonly used for sedation during endoscopic procedures, endoscopists should be cognizant of this drug interaction while administering benzodiazepines in patients receiving protease inhibitors.

Procedure

Cholangiography findings have been described as sclerosing cholangitis with segmental stricture formation to create a beaded appearance similar to primary sclerosing cholangitis. The patterns of biliary tract strictures are listed in **Table 45.1**. Papillary stenosis with intrahepatic strictures is the most common pattern observed.[75,77,79] Other reported cholangiography abnormalities include adherent polypoid filling defects; biopsy specimens of these defects show granulation tissue.[80] Pancreatography is abnormal in one-half of patients with AIDS cholangiopathy, revealing pancreatic duct strictures in the head of the pancreas.[75,81]

ERCP is performed in the usual manner.
The duodenum should be inspected for mucosal abnormalities such as erosions or ulcerations that may indicate enteric infection. Biopsy specimens of lesions or random mucosal biopsy specimens should be obtained and sent for microbiologic and cytologic analysis.

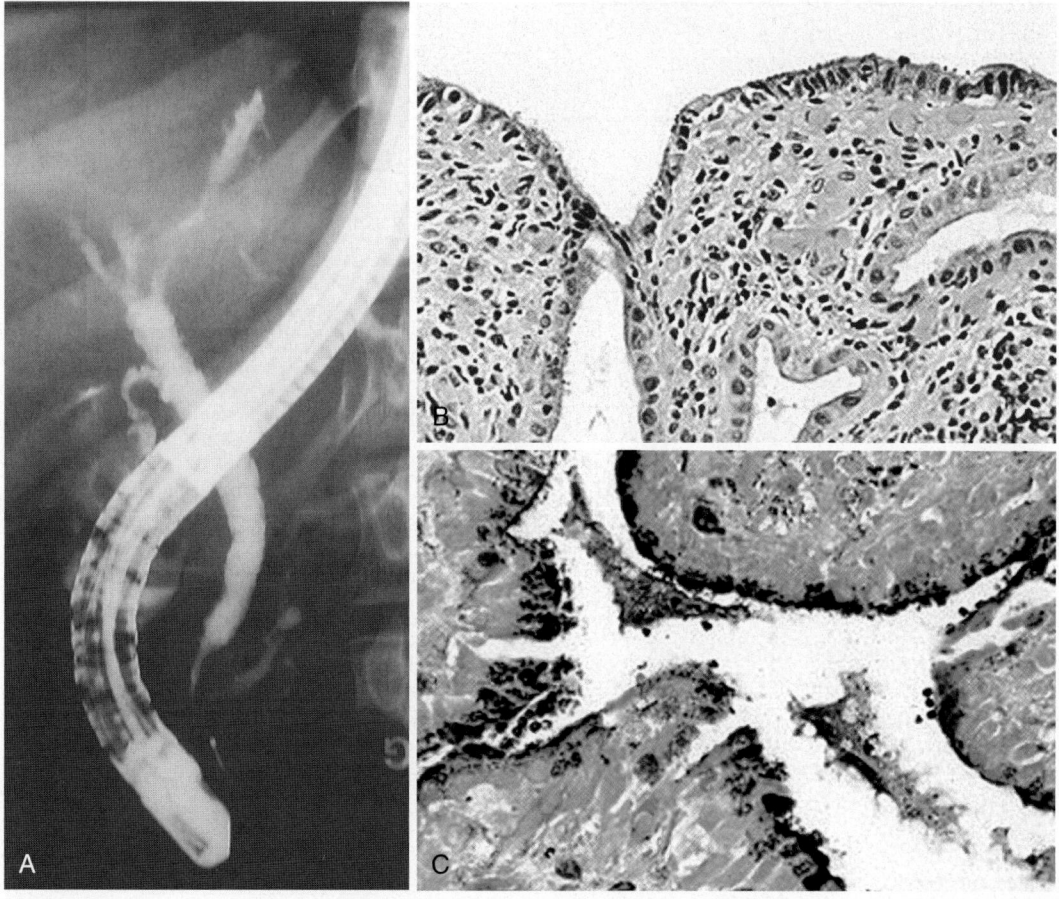

Fig. 45.10 A, Acquired immunodeficiency syndrome (AIDS) cholangiopathy shown by endoscopic retrograde cholangiopancreatography (ERCP) with narrowed distal bile duct and irregular bile duct walls. **B,** Relatively normal bile duct epithelium on biopsy and standard hematoxylin and eosin staining. **C,** Microsporidia shown on the surface as black with silver staining. *(Courtesy of Dr. Richard Tilson, Boston, MA.)*

Bile should be sampled after cannulation and submitted for analysis.

Evidence of papillary stenosis should be noted during cannulation and by observing bile drainage after cholangiography.

If papillary stenosis is present, an endoscopic sphincterotomy should be performed in a patient with abdominal pain, jaundice, or fever. Sphincterotomy is not beneficial in the absence of papillary stenosis.

Dominant strictures should be sampled for cytology with a cytology brush or biopsy forceps to exclude cholangiocarcinoma or another malignant process.

In a symptomatic patient, balloon or catheter dilation of the stricture may be performed, but long-term stent placement should be avoided to limit migration of enteric pathogens into the biliary tract.

When ERCP is completed, biopsy specimens of the major papilla may be obtained and sent for microbiologic and pathologic analysis.

Complications

Cholangitis with secondary fibrosis leads to bile duct stricture formation and papillary stenosis. Secondary biliary cirrhosis has not been described as a complication of AIDS cholangiopathy, perhaps because of the shortened life span of this patient population, but these patients may be at risk of cholangiocarcinoma.[82]

Outcomes

Aspiration of bile for culture and multiple biopsy specimens of the duodenum and papilla reveal an underlying pathogen in up to 92% of cases.[81] One study reported that isolation of *Cryptosporidium* or cytomegalovirus was more common when intrahepatic duct irregularities were present on cholangiography.[83] The medical management of AIDS cholangiopathy is divided into antimicrobial agents directed against the causative organism, highly active antiretroviral therapy (HAART) directed against the underlying HIV infection, and ursodeoxycholic acid.

Case series assessing the effect of treatment of cytomegalovirus, *C. parvum*, and *Microsporida* on patient symptoms, liver enzymes, and cholangiography findings have not been encouraging.[74,83,84] The use of HAART to restore the immune system has been effective in suppressing enteritis and possibly cholangiopathy associated with *C. parvum* and *Microsporida*, although eradication probably does not occur.[85] Castiella and associates[86] treated four patients with AIDS cholangiopathy with ursodeoxycholic acid (10 mg/kg body weight). At a mean

Box 45.3 Differential Diagnosis of Acquired Immunodeficiency Syndrome Cholangiopathy

Non–HIV-Related

Choledocholithiasis
Cholecystitis
Primary sclerosing cholangitis
Viral hepatitis
Chronic pancreatitis

HIV-Related

Medication hepatotoxicity

Opportunistic Infection

Acalculous cholecystitis
Peliosis hepatitis
Infectious pancreatitis
    Mycobacterial (MAI, tuberculosis)
    CMV

Opportunistic Neoplasm

Kaposi's sarcoma (papilla)
Lymphoma (papilla, pancreas, duodenum)
Adenoma/adenocarcinoma (papilla)

CMV, cytomegalovirus; HIV, human immunodeficiency virus; MAI, *Mycobacterium avium-intracellulare.*

Table 45.1 Cholangiography Findings in Acquired Immunodeficiency Syndrome Cholangiopathy

Finding	Frequency (%)
Papillary stenosis and intrahepatic duct strictures	33
Papillary stenosis alone	21
Papillary stenosis and intrahepatic and extrahepatic duct strictures	20
Intrahepatic duct strictures alone	12
Intrahepatic and extrahepatic duct strictures	8
Extrahepatic duct strictures alone	5
Papillary stenosis and extrahepatic duct strictures	1

Data from Benhamou Y, Caumes E, Gerosa Y, et al: AIDS-related cholangiopathy: Critical analysis of a prospective series of 26 patients. Dig Dis Sci 38:1113–1118, 1993; Bouche H, Housset C, Dumont JL, et al: AIDS-related cholangitis: Diagnostic features and course in 15 patients. J Hepatol 17:34–39, 1993; Cello JP: AIDS-related biliary tract disease. Gastrointest Endosc Clin N Am 8:963, 1998; Ducreux M, Buffet C, Lamy P, et al: Diagnosis and prognosis of AIDS-related cholangitis. AIDS 9:875–880, 1995; Farman J, Brunetti J, Baer JW, et al: AIDS-related cholangiopancreatographic changes. Abdom Imaging 19:417–422, 1994.

follow-up of 4.5 months, improvement in symptoms and alkaline phosphatase levels was observed in all patients.

Endoscopic therapy has been the most extensively studied treatment in AIDS cholangiopathy. Endoscopic sphincterotomy in patients with papillary stenosis results in improvement

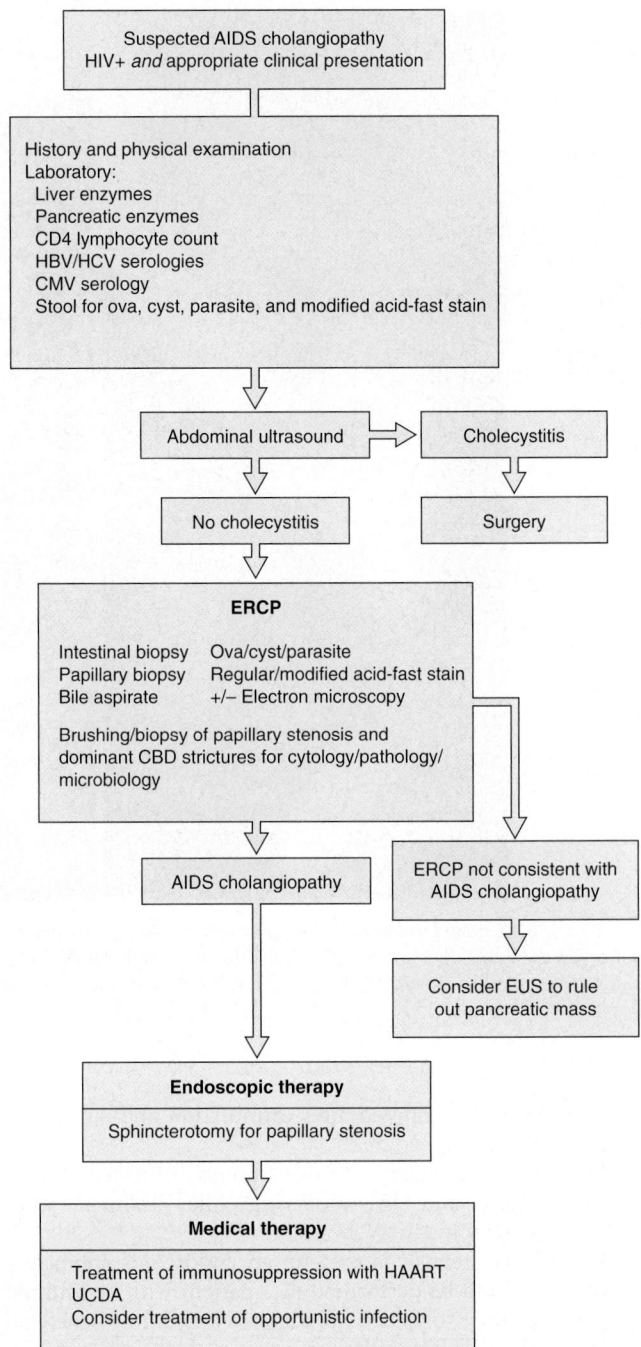

Fig. 45.11 Algorithm for management of suspected acquired immunodeficiency syndrome (AIDS) cholangiopathy. CBD, common bile duct; CMV, cytomegalovirus; ERCP, endoscopic retrograde cholangiopancreatography; EUS, endoscopic ultrasound; HAART, highly active antiretroviral therapy; HBV, hepatitis B virus; HCV, hepatitis C virus; HIV human immunodeficiency; UCDA, ursodeoxycholic acid.

of abdominal pain in 32% to 100% of patients.[81,83,87] Cello and Chan[88] reported improvement in pain scores at a mean of 9.4 months after sphincterotomy; this did not correspond to an improvement in liver enzymes or cholangiography abnormalities, both of which appeared to worsen. Patient survival after a diagnosis of AIDS cholangiopathy is not affected by the pattern of cholangiogram abnormalities or the presence of an endoscopic sphincterotomy but appears to be most strongly associated with the administration of HAART.[89]

Cholecystitis

Acute cholecystitis is an inflammatory injury to the gallbladder mucosa from bile stasis, ischemia, or infection. Bile stasis usually results from cystic duct obstruction by a gallstone or from decreased gallbladder motility. Less common causes of cystic duct obstruction are worms, hemobilia, and tumor. Decreased gallbladder motility and ischemia are implicated in the development of acalculous cholecystitis in critically ill patients. Infection of the gallbladder complicates cholecystitis in approximately 50% of cases but is not usually the causative factor, with the exception of parasitic and AIDS cholecystitis.

Indications

ERCP is indicated for gallbladder drainage in patients who are medically unfit for surgery and in whom percutaneous drainage is contraindicated or unsuccessful.

Preparation

Antibiotic coverage is directed against Enterobacteriaceae and *Enterococcus* species until directed therapy can be instituted against specific organisms identified in blood or bile cultures.

Procedure

ERCP is performed in the usual manner.
The cystic duct insertion is identified and entered. A guidewire may facilitate selective cystic duct cannulation.
Endoscopic cholecystography identifies calculi within the cystic duct and gallbladder.

Wire-guided balloon extraction of stones or placement of a biliary endoprosthesis through the cystic duct and into the gallbladder can be undertaken. Occasionally, an obstructing stone is dislodged into the gallbladder as instruments are advanced into the cystic duct.[90]

Irrigation of the gallbladder with 1% *N*-acetyl cysteine through a nasobiliary catheter has been described in acalculous cholecystitis.[91] The use of *N*-acetyl cysteine appeared to thin the gallbladder contents and enable gallbladder drainage and collapse around the catheter.

Complications

Complications of cholecystitis usually occur with secondary bacterial infection and include empyema, gallbladder wall necrosis resulting in a gangrenous gallbladder, perforation, and emphysematous cholecystitis. Gallbladder perforation may result in abscess formation, peritonitis, or fistula formation. Migration of a large gallstone through a cholecystoenteric fistula may lead to bowel obstruction, usually at the level of the ileocecal valve, referred to as gallstone ileus. Emphysematous cholecystitis refers to gas within the gallbladder wall owing to infection with gas-producing bacteria.

Outcomes

Cholecystectomy is the definitive therapy. Although patients may recover from an episode of acute cholecystitis, the risk of recurrent symptoms is 70% within the next 2 years.[92] Patients without serious concomitant medical problems should undergo cholecystectomy during the same hospital admission, usually 24 to 48 hours after admission. In particular, diabetics, given their increased risk of gallbladder necrosis and perforation, should be considered for cholecystectomy after their first attack of cholecystitis. Patients who are medically unfit for surgery and do not improve with supportive therapy require gallbladder drainage; this is generally achieved

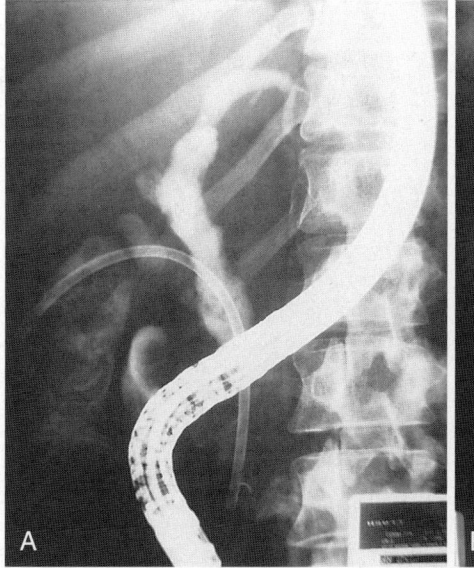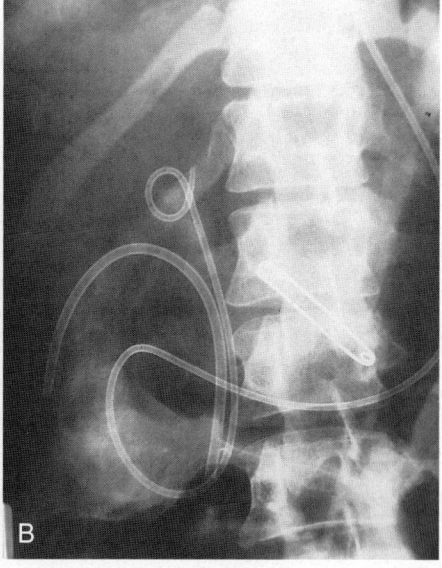

Fig. 45.12 Concomitant calculous cholangitis and cholecystitis. **A,** Endoscopic retrograde cholangiopancreatography (ERCP) shows a plastic stent draining the gallbladder. **B,** Radiograph obtained after ERCP shows addition of a nasobiliary tube draining the common bile duct (CBD).

by percutaneous cholecystostomy tube placement, although successful endoscopic drainage of the gallbladder has been described. Placement of a biliary endoprosthesis into the gallbladder during ERCP can alleviate symptoms resulting from recurrent biliary colic, calculous cholecystitis, acalculous cholecystitis, and gallbladder perforation (**Fig. 45-12**).[91-93] Endoscopic gallbladder drainage can be performed in the presence of coagulopathy and ascites when percutaneous cholecystostomy tube placement is contraindicated.

References

The complete reference list is available online at www.expertconsult.com.

Sphincter of Oddi Dysfunction

Stuart Sherman, Evan L. Fogel, James L. Watkins, Lee McHenry, Jr., and Glen A. Lehman

Video related to this chapter's topics can be found online at expertconsult.com.

Introduction

Since its original description by Oddi in 1887, the sphincter of Oddi has been the subject of much study and controversy. Its very existence as a distinct anatomic or physiologic entity has been disputed. Not surprisingly, the clinical syndrome of sphincter of Oddi dysfunction (SOD) and its therapy are controversial areas.[1,2] Nevertheless, SOD is commonly diagnosed and treated by physicians. This chapter reviews the epidemiology and clinical presentation of SOD and currently available diagnostic and therapeutic modalities.

Definitions

Postcholecystectomy pain resembling the patient's preoperative biliary colic occurs in at least 10% to 20% of patients.[3] These patients should have appropriate noninvasive and invasive (when clinically appropriate) evaluation to rule out common bile duct (CBD) stones, tumors, or strictures near the cholecystectomy site. Patients in whom these entities are ruled out have a high frequency of SOD. SOD refers to an abnormality of sphincter of Oddi contractility. It is a benign, noncalculous obstruction to flow of bile or pancreatic juice through the pancreaticobiliary junction (i.e., the sphincter of Oddi) resulting from a dyskinetic or stenotic sphincter of Oddi. SOD may be manifested clinically by

"pancreaticobiliary" pain, pancreatitis, abnormal liver function tests, or abnormal pancreatic enzymes. Sphincter of Oddi dyskinesia refers to a motor abnormality of the sphincter of Oddi, which may result in a hypotonic sphincter but, more commonly, causes a hypertonic sphincter. In contrast, sphincter of Oddi stenosis refers to a structural alteration of the sphincter, probably from an inflammatory process, with subsequent fibrosis.

Because it is often impossible to distinguish patients with sphincter of Oddi dyskinesia from patients with sphincter of Oddi stenosis, the term SOD has been used to incorporate both groups of patients. In an attempt to deal with this overlap in etiology and to determine the appropriate use of sphincter of Oddi manometry (SOM), a biliary clinical classification system has been developed for patients with suspected SOD (Hogan-Geenen SOD classification system; **Table 46.1**) based on clinical history, laboratory results, and endoscopic retrograde cholangiopancreatography (ERCP) findings.[4] A pancreatic classification has also been developed, but it is less commonly used (**Box 46.1**).[5] Both the biliary and the pancreatic classification systems have been modified,[6] making them more applicable for clinical use because biliary and pancreatic drainage times have been generally abandoned. Various less accurate terms—papillary stenosis, ampullary stenosis, biliary dyskinesia, and postcholecystectomy syndrome—are used in the medical literature to describe this entity. The last term,

Table 46.1 Hogan-Geenen Biliary Sphincter of Oddi Classification System (Postcholecystectomy) Related to the Frequency of Abnormal Sphincter of Oddi Manometry and Pain Relief by Biliary Sphincterotomy

Patient Group Classifications	Approximate Frequency of Abnormal Sphincter Manometry	Probability of Pain Relief by Sphincterotomy if Manometry:		Manometry before Sphincter Ablation
		Abnormal	*Normal*	
BILIARY TYPE I				
Patients with biliary-type pain, abnormal AST or alkaline phosphatase >2 times normal documented on two or more occasions, delayed drainage of ERCP contrast agent from the biliary tree >45 min, and dilated CBD >12 mm diameter	75%–95%	90%–95%	90%–95%	Unnecessary
BILIARY TYPE II				
Patients with biliary-type pain and only one or two of the previous criteria	55%–65%	85%	35%	Highly recommended
BILIARY TYPE III				
Patients with only biliary-type pain and none of the three previous criteria	25%–60%	55%–65%	<10%	Mandatory

AST, aspartate aminotransferase; CBD, common bile duct; ERCP, endoscopic retrograde cholangiopancreatography.

Box 46.1 Pancreatic Sphincter of Oddi Classification System: Patient Group Classification

Pancreatic Type I

Patients with pancreatic-type pain, abnormal amylase or lipase 1.5 times normal on any occasion, delayed drainage of ERCP contrast agent from the PD >9 minutes, and dilated PD >6 mm diameter in the head or 5 mm in the body

Pancreatic Type II

Patients with pancreatic-type pain but only one or two of criteria for type I

Pancreatic Type III

Patients with pancreatic-type pain only and no other abnormalities

ERCP, endoscopic retrograde cholangiopancreatography; PD, pancreatic duct.

Adapted from Sherman S, Troiano FP, Hawes RH, et al: Frequency of abnormal sphincter of Oddi manometry compared with the clinical suspicion of sphincter of Oddi dysfunction. Am J Gastroenterol 86:586–590, 1991.

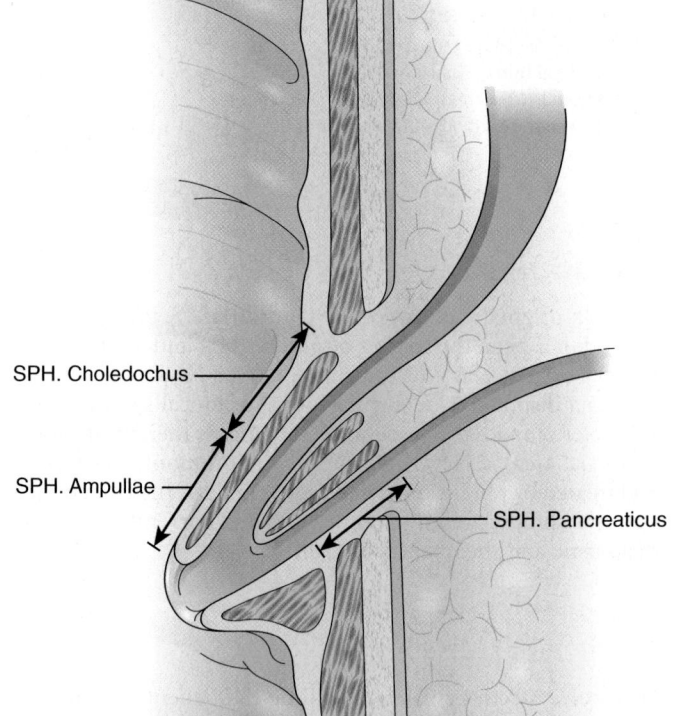

Fig. 46.1 Anatomy of sphincter of Oddi.

postcholecystectomy syndrome, is a misnomer because SOD may occur with an intact gallbladder.

Anatomy, Physiology, and Pathophysiology

The anatomy, physiology, and pharmacology of the sphincter of Oddi have been reviewed by Bosch and Pena.[7] The sphincter of Oddi is a small complex of smooth muscles surrounding the terminal CBD, main (ventral) pancreatic duct (of Wirsung), and common channel (ampulla of Vater), when present (**Fig. 46.1**). It has both circular and figure-eight components. The high-pressure zone generated by the sphincter is variably 4 to 10 mm in length. Its role is to regulate bile and pancreatic exocrine juice flow and to prevent duodenum-to-duct reflux (i.e., maintain a sterile intraductal environment). The sphincter of Oddi possesses both a variable basal pressure and phasic contractile activity. The former seems to be the predominant mechanism, regulating outflow of pancreaticobiliary secretion into the intestine. Although phasic sphincter of Oddi contractions may aid in regulating bile and pancreatic juice flow, their primary role seems to be maintaining a sterile intraductal milieu.

Sphincter regulation is under neural and hormonal control. Phasic wave activity of the sphincter is closely tied to the migrating motor complex of the duodenum. Innervation of the bile duct does not seem to be essential because sphincter function has been reported to be preserved after liver transplantation.[8] Although regulatory processes vary among species, cholecystokinin (CCK) and secretin seem to be most important in causing sphincter relaxation, whereas nonadrenergic, noncholinergic neurons, which at least partially transmit vasoactive intestinal peptide and nitric oxide, also relax the sphincter.[9] The role of cholecystectomy in altering these neural pathways needs further definition.

Luman and colleagues[10] reported that cholecystectomy, at least in the short-term, suppresses the normal inhibitory effect of pharmacologic doses of CCK on the sphincter of Oddi. The mechanism of this effect is unknown, however. Wedge specimens of the sphincter of Oddi obtained at surgical sphincteroplasty from patients with SOD show evidence of inflammation, muscular hypertrophy, fibrosis, or adenomyosis within the papillary zone in approximately 60% of patients.[11] In the remaining 40% with normal histology, a motor disorder is suggested. Less commonly, infections with cytomegalovirus or *Cryptosporidium,* as may occur in patients with acquired immunodeficiency syndrome (AIDS), or *Strongyloides* have caused SOD.

How does SOD cause pain? From a theoretical point of view, abnormalities of sphincter of Oddi pressure can give rise to pain by (1) impeding the flow of bile and pancreatic juice resulting in ductal hypertension, (2) inducing ischemia arising from spastic contractions, and (3) resulting in "hypersensitivity" of the papilla. Although unproved, these mechanisms may act alone or in concert to explain the genesis of pain. Patients with SOD have been shown to have lower perception thresholds in the referred pain area. Visceral and referred hyperalgesia may be important features in the pathogenesis of pain in patients with SOD.[12]

Epidemiology

SOD may occur in children or adults of any age; however, patients with SOD are typically middle-aged women.[13,14] Although SOD most commonly occurs after cholecystectomy, it may be present with the gallbladder in situ.[15] In a survey on functional gastrointestinal (GI) disorders, SOD seemed to have a significant impact on quality of life because it was highly associated with work absenteeism, disability, and health care use.[16] Using a brief symptom inventory and the 12-item short form health survey (SF-12), Winstead and Wilcox[17] found that patients with biliary SOD and unexplained recurrent pancreatitis had a significantly worse quality of life than nonpatients, high levels of somatic complaints, and a common history of sexual and physical abuse (20%).

Limited studies of the frequency of manometrically documented SOD in patients before cholecystectomy have been

done. Guelrud and colleagues[18] evaluated 121 patients with symptomatic gallstones and a normal CBD diameter (by transcutaneous ultrasound) by SOM before cholecystectomy. An elevated basal sphincter pressure was found in 14 (11.6%) patients. SOD was diagnosed in 4.1% (4 of 96) of patients with a normal serum alkaline phosphatase and in 40% (10 of 25) with an elevated serum alkaline phosphatase. Ruffolo and associates[19] evaluated 81 patients with symptoms suggestive of biliary disease but normal ERCP and no gallbladder stones on transcutaneous ultrasound by scintigraphic gallbladder ejection fraction and endoscopic SOM. Of patients, 53% had SOD, and 49% had an abnormal gallbladder ejection fraction. SOD occurred with a similar frequency in patients with an abnormal gallbladder ejection fraction (50%) and a normal ejection fraction (57%).

The frequency of diagnosing SOD varies considerably in reported series with the patient selection criteria, the definition of SOD, and the diagnostic tools used. In a British report, SOD was diagnosed in 41 (9%) of 451 consecutive patients being evaluated for postcholecystectomy pain.[20] Roberts-Thomson and Toouli[21] evaluated 431 similar patients and found SOD in 47 (11%). In a subpopulation of patients with normal ERCP (except dilated ducts in 28%) and recurrent pain of more than 3 months' duration, SOD was diagnosed in 68%. Sherman and colleagues[5] used SOM to evaluate 115 patients with pancreaticobiliary pain with and without liver function test abnormalities. Patients with bile duct stones and tumors were excluded from analysis. Of 115 patients, 59 (51%) showed abnormal basal sphincter of Oddi pressure greater than 40 mm Hg. These patients were categorized further by the Hogan-Geenen SOD classification system based on clinical presentation, laboratory results, imaging tests, and ERCP findings (see **Table 46.1**). The frequency of abnormal manometry of one or both sphincter segments was 86%, 55%, and 28% for biliary type I, II, and III patients. These abnormal manometric frequencies were very similar to the frequencies reported by others for type I and type II patients.[22,23] In biliary type III patients, the finding of an abnormal basal sphincter pressure has ranged from 12% to 59%.[6,24] Patient selection factors may be one explanation for this great variability.

SOD can involve abnormalities in the biliary sphincter, pancreatic sphincter, or both.[6,25] The true frequency of SOD depends on whether one or both sphincters are studied. Eversman and colleagues[6] performed manometry of the biliary and pancreatic sphincter segments in 360 patients with pancreatobiliary pain and intact sphincters. In this large series, 19% had abnormal pancreatic sphincter basal sphincter pressure alone, 11% had abnormal biliary basal sphincter pressure alone, and 31% had abnormal basal sphincter pressure in both segments (overall frequency of sphincter dysfunction was 61%). Among the 214 patients labeled type III by a modified Hogan-Geenen SOD classification system, 17%, 11%, and 31% had elevated basal sphincter pressure in the pancreatic sphincter alone, biliary sphincter alone, or both segments (overall frequency of SOD was 59%). In 123 type II patients, SOD was diagnosed in 65%; 22%, 11%, and 32% had elevated basal sphincter pressure in the pancreatic sphincter only, biliary sphincter only, or both sphincter segments. Similar findings were reported by Aymerich and colleagues.[26] In a series of 73 patients with suspected SOD, basal pressures were normal in both segments in 19%, abnormal in both segments in 40%, and abnormal in one segment but normal in the other segment in 41%. The negative predictive value of normal biliary basal sphincter pressure in excluding SOD was 0.42; when the pancreatic basal sphincter pressure was normal, the negative predictive value was 0.58. These two studies suggest that both the bile duct and the pancreatic duct should be evaluated when assessing the sphincter by SOM.

Although SOM has traditionally been thought to be reproducible,[27] two more recent studies have shown abnormal sphincter pressures in 42% and 60% in symptomatic patients restudied about 1 year after a normal study.[28,29] Dysfunction may occur in the pancreatic duct portion of the sphincter of Oddi and cause recurrent pancreatitis. As noted earlier, a pancreatic SOD classification system has been developed (see **Box 46.1**), but it has not been widely used.[5,6] Manometrically documented SOD has been reported in 15% to 72% of patients with recurrent pancreatitis, previously labeled as idiopathic[5,24,30]; this is discussed later in this chapter.

Clinical Presentation

Abdominal pain is the most common presenting symptom of patients with SOD. The pain is usually epigastric or right upper quadrant, may be disabling, and lasts for 30 minutes to hours. In some patients, the pain is continuous with episodic exacerbations. It may radiate to the back or shoulder and be accompanied by nausea and vomiting. Food or narcotics may precipitate the pain. The pain may begin several years after a cholecystectomy was performed for a gallbladder dysmotility or stone disease and is similar in character to the pain leading to the cholecystectomy. Alternatively, patients may have continued pain that was not relieved by a cholecystectomy. Jaundice, fever, and chills are rarely observed.

A symposium on functional disorders of the pancreas and biliary tree established the Rome III diagnostic criteria[31] for SOD. These criteria include episodes of severe abdominal pain located in the epigastrium or right upper quadrant or both and all of the following: (1) symptom episodes last 30 minutes or more with pain-free intervals, (2) recurrent symptoms occur at different intervals (not daily), (3) the pain builds up to a steady level, (4) the pain is moderate to severe enough to interrupt the patient's daily activities or lead to an emergency department visit, (5) the pain is not relieved by bowel movements, (6) the pain is not relieved by postural change, (7) the pain is not relieved by antacids, (8) other structural diseases that would explain the symptoms are excluded. The pain may manifest in one or more of the following ways: pain with nausea and vomiting, pain radiation to the back or right subscapular region or both, and pain awakens patient from sleep.

Physical examination is typically characterized only by mild epigastric or right upper quadrant tenderness. The pain is not relieved by trial medications for acid peptic disease or irritable bowel syndrome. Laboratory abnormalities consisting of transient elevation of liver function tests, typically during episodes of pain, are present in less than 50% of patients. Patients with SOD may present with typical pancreatic pain (epigastric or left upper quadrant radiating to the back) with or without pancreatic enzyme elevation and recurrent pancreatitis. The pain is often indistinguishable from biliary pain.[31] SOD may exist in the presence of an intact gallbladder.[18,19,32] Because the symptoms of SOD or gallbladder dysfunction cannot be reliably separated, the diagnosis of SOD is commonly made after cholecystectomy or less often after gallbladder abnormalities have been excluded.[31]

Clinical Evaluation

The diagnostic approach to suspected SOD may be influenced by the presence of key clinical features. However, the clinical manifestations of functional abnormalities of the sphincter of Oddi may not always be easily distinguishable from manifestations caused by organic ones (e.g., CBD stones) or other functional nonpancreaticobiliary disorders (e.g., irritable bowel syndrome).

General Initial Evaluation

Evaluation of patients with suspected SOD (i.e., patients with upper abdominal pain with characteristics suggestive of a pancreatobiliary origin) should be initiated with standard serum liver chemistries; serum amylase or lipase or both; and abdominal ultrasound, magnetic resonance (MR) imaging or magnetic resonance cholangiopancreatography (MRCP), or computed tomography (CT) scans. Serum enzyme studies should be drawn during bouts of pain, if possible. Mild elevations (<2 times upper limits of normal) are frequent in SOD, whereas greater abnormalities are more suggestive of stones, tumors, and liver parenchymal disease. Although the diagnostic sensitivity and specificity of abnormal serum liver chemistries are low,[33] evidence suggests that the presence of abnormal liver tests in type II biliary SOD patients may predict a favorable response to endoscopic sphincterotomy.[34]

CT scans and abdominal ultrasound are usually normal, but occasionally a dilated bile duct or pancreatic duct may be found (particularly in patients with type I SOD). With improvements in technology and more widespread availability, MRCP and endoscopic ultrasound (EUS) have been more commonly used to look for structural and parenchymal disease of the pancreas, pancreatic duct, and biliary tree. Standard evaluation and treatment of other, more common GI conditions, such as peptic ulcer disease, irritable bowel syndrome, and gastroesophageal reflux, should occur simultaneously. In the absence of mass lesions, stones, or response to medical therapy trials, the suspicion for sphincter disease is increased.

Diagnostic Methods (Noninvasive)

Because SOM (considered by most authorities to be the "gold standard" for diagnosing SOD) is difficult to perform, invasive, not widely available, and associated with a relatively high complication rate, several noninvasive and provocative tests have been designed to identify patients with SOD.

Morphine-Prostigmin Provocative Test (Nardi Test)

Morphine has been shown to cause sphincter of Oddi contraction, as assessed manometrically. Neostigmine (Prostigmin), 1 mg subcutaneously, is added as a vigorous cholinergic secretory stimulant to morphine, 10 mg subcutaneously, to make this challenge test. The morphine-Prostigmin test was used extensively in the past to diagnose SOD. Reproduction of the patient's typical pain associated with a fourfold increase in aspartate aminotransferase, alanine aminotransferase, alkaline phosphatase, amylase, or lipase levels constitutes a positive response. The usefulness of this test is limited by its low sensitivity and specificity in predicting the presence of SOD and its poor correlation with outcome after sphincter ablation.[35,36] This test has largely been replaced by tests thought to be more sensitive.

Radiographic Assessment of Extrahepatic Bile Duct and Main Pancreatic Duct Diameter after Secretory Stimulation

After a lipid-rich meal or CCK administration, the gallbladder contracts, bile flow from the hepatocytes increases, and the sphincter of Oddi relaxes, resulting in bile entry into the duodenum. Similarly, after a lipid-rich meal or secretin administration, pancreatic exocrine juice flow is stimulated, and the sphincter of Oddi relaxes. If the sphincter of Oddi is dysfunctional and causes obstruction to flow, the CBD or main pancreatic duct may dilate under secretory pressure; this can be monitored by transcutaneous ultrasound. Sphincter and terminal duct obstruction from other causes (stones, tumors, strictures) may similarly cause ductal dilation and need to be excluded. Pain provocation should also be noted if present. Limited studies comparing these noninvasive tests with SOM or outcome after sphincter ablation[37-42] show only modest correlation. Because of overlying intestinal gas, the pancreatic duct may not be visualized on standard transcutaneous ultrasound. Despite the superiority of EUS in visualizing the pancreas, Catalano and coworkers[43] reported the sensitivity of secretin-stimulated EUS in detecting SOD to be only 57%.

MRCP can also be performed to monitor the pancreatic duct noninvasively after secretin stimulation. It is also the best noninvasive test to obtain a cholangiogram and pancreatogram and evaluate for other structural causes for the patient's symptoms. Aisen and colleagues[44] showed that the pancreatic diameter increased significantly after secretin injection (monitored by MRCP), but the amount of increase and the duration of increase were similar for patients with normal and abnormal basal sphincter pressure. Pereira and colleagues[45] and Baillie and Kimberly[46] also found secretin-stimulated MRCP to be insensitive in predicting abnormal manometry. In contrast, in a pilot study of 15 patients with idiopathic pancreatitis, secretin-stimulated MRCP and SOM were concordant in 87%.[47] However, Testoni and colleagues[48] reported a disappointing negative predictive value for SOD and clinical success of sphincter ablation.

Quantitative Hepatobiliary Scintigraphy

Hepatobiliary scintigraphy (HBS) assesses bile flow through the biliary tract. Impairment to bile flow from sphincter disease, tumors, or stones (and parenchymal liver disease) results in impaired radionuclide flow. The precise criteria to define a positive (abnormal) study are controversial, but a prolonged duodenal arrival time, a prolonged hepatic hilum-to-duodenal transit time, and a high Johns Hopkins scintigraphic score are most widely used.[49-51] Four studies[49,52-54] showed a correlation between HBS and SOM. Taking these four studies as a whole, totaling 105 patients, the overall

sensitivity of HBS using SOM as the "gold standard" was 78% (range 44% to 100%), specificity was 90% (range 80% to 100%), positive predictive value was 92% (range 82% to 100%), and negative predictive value was 81% (range 62% to 100%). These promising results have not been reproduced by others, however.

Overall, patients with dilated bile ducts and high-grade obstruction seem likely to have a positive scintigraphic study. Esber and colleagues[55] found that patients with lower grade obstruction (Hogan-Geenen classification types II and III) generally have normal scintigraphy, even if done after CCK provocation. Pineau and coworkers[56] reported that 8 of 20 asymptomatic control subjects had an abnormal CCK-stimulated study. Using SOM as the "gold standard" in 29 patients with suspected SOD, two independent reviewers found the Johns Hopkins scintigraphic score to have a sensitivity of 25% to 38%, specificity of 85% to 90%, positive predictive value of 40% to 60%, and negative predictive value of 75% to 79% for diagnosing SOD.[57] The hepatic hilum-to-duodenal transit time had a sensitivity of 13%, specificity of 95%, positive predictive value of 50%, and negative predictive value of 74%. The duodenal arrival time mirrored the hepatic hilum-to-duodenal transit time findings. The value of adding morphine provocation to HBS was reported.[54] In 34 patients with a clinical diagnosis of type II and type III SOD, scintigraphy with and without morphine and subsequent biliary manometry were performed. The standard HBS scan did not distinguish between patients with normal and abnormal SOM. However, after provocation with morphine, there were significant differences in the time to maximal activity and the percentage of excretion at 45 minutes and 60 minutes. Using a cutoff value of 15% excretion at 60 minutes, the use of morphine during HBS increased the sensitivity and specificity for SOD detection to 83% and 81%.

The Milwaukee group reported their retrospective review of fatty meal sonography (FMS) and HBS as potential predictors of SOD.[58] In this study, 304 postcholecystectomy patients suspected to have SOD were evaluated by SOM, FMS, and HBS. A diagnosis of SOD was made in 73 patients (24%) by using SOM as the reference standard. The sensitivity of FMS was 21%, and the sensitivity of HBS was 49%, whereas specificities were 97% and 78%. FMS, HBS, or both were abnormal in 90%, 50%, and 44% of patients with Hogan-Geenen SOD types I, II, and III. Of 73 patients who underwent biliary sphincterotomy, 40 had a good long-term response. Among these patients with SOD, 11 (85%) of 13 patients with abnormal HBS and FMS had a good long-term response. This study suggested that although noninvasive tests are unable to predict an abnormal SOM with high sensitivity, they may be of assistance in predicting response to sphincter ablation in patients with SOD.

Cicala and colleagues[59] compared the reliability of HBS (hepatic hilum-to-duodenal transit time was measured) with SOM of the biliary sphincter in 30 postcholecystectomy patients (8 type I, 22 type II; 40% were men). HBS was abnormal in all 15 patients with abnormal maximal basal sphincter pressures and in 7 of 15 patients with normal maximal basal sphincter pressures. Of 14 patients with abnormal HBS who agreed to undergo biliary sphincterotomy, 13 were asymptomatic and had normal liver function tests, amylase levels, and lipase levels at 10 to 13 months of follow-up. All eight patients with abnormal HBS who refused to undergo sphincterotomy remained symptomatic. A favorable postsphincterotomy outcome was predicted by hepatic hilum-to-duodenal transit in 93% and by SOM in 57% of patients.

Although this study suggested that HBS is a useful and noninvasive test to diagnose SOD and is a reliable predictor of sphincterotomy outcome in postcholecystectomy biliary type I and type II patients, several concerns exist. Of enrolled patients, 40% were men, which is unusually high in the SOD population, and the frequency of abnormal maximal basal sphincter pressures in biliary type II patients was exceedingly low (36%). If the authors had used the mean basal sphincter pressure, which is the more commonly recommended manometric parameter for diagnosing SOD, the frequency of an abnormal SOM would likely have been even lower. This calls into question the authors' SOM technique and interpretation. In the absence of more definitive data, we and others conclude that use of HBS as a screening tool for SOD should not be recommended for general clinical use.[60] Abnormal results may be found in asymptomatic controls.[56] HBS does not address the pancreatic sphincter, which may be dysfunctional and a cause for patient symptoms. Use of HBS and other noninvasive methods should be reserved for situations in which more definitive testing (manometry) is unsuccessful or unavailable.

Diagnostic Methods (Invasive)
Endoscopic Retrograde Cholangiopancreatography

Because of their associated risks, invasive testing with ERCP and manometry should be reserved for patients with clinically significant or disabling symptoms. Invasive assessment of patients for SOD generally is not recommended unless definitive therapy (sphincter ablation) is planned if abnormal sphincter function is found. Cholangiography is essential to rule out stones, tumors, or other obstructing processes of the biliary tree that may cause symptoms identical to SOD. Once such lesions are ruled out by a good-quality cholangiographic study, ducts that are dilated or drain slowly suggest obstruction at the level of the sphincter. Various methods to obtain a cholangiogram are available. For noninvasive imaging, MR cholangiography is most promising, but quality varies greatly from center to center. Software development continues, and quality of images continues to evolve and improve. Direct cholangiography can be obtained by percutaneous methods, intraoperative methods, or more conventionally at ERCP.

Although some controversy exists, extrahepatic ducts that are greater than 12 mm in diameter (postcholecystectomy) when corrected for magnification are considered dilated. Drugs that affect the rate of bile flow and relaxation or contraction of the sphincter of Oddi influence drainage of contrast material and must be avoided to obtain accurate drainage times (if drainage time is desired). Because the extrahepatic bile duct angulates from anterior (the hilum) to posterior (the papilla), the patient must be supine to assess gravitational drainage through the sphincter. Although definitive normal supine drainage times have not been well defined,[61] a postcholecystectomy biliary tree that fails to empty all contrast material by 45 minutes is generally considered abnormal. Endoscopic evaluation of the papilla and peripapillary area can yield important information that can influence the

diagnosis and treatment of patients with suspected SOD. Occasionally, ampullary cancer may simulate SOD. The endoscopist should do tissue sampling of the papilla (preferably after sphincterotomy) in suspicious cases.[62]

Radiographic features of the pancreatic duct are also important to assess in a patient with suspected SOD. Dilation of the pancreatic duct (>6 mm in the pancreatic head and >5 mm in the body) and delayed contrast agent drainage time (9 minutes in the prone position) may give indirect evidence for the presence of SOD. ERCP alone is generally not indicated in the evaluation of abdominal pain of obscure origin in the absence of objective findings that suggest a biliary or pancreatic disease (i.e., type III patient).[63] Sherman and colleagues[64] found that only 10% of 197 patients with pancreaticobiliary pain, normal liver function tests, serum amylase, upper GI tract evaluation, and abdominal ultrasound or CT scan had an ERCP finding that might affect their therapy, including chronic pancreatitis (7%), gallbladder stones or sludge (2%), and a choledochal cyst (1%). Most of these findings could have been identified on noninvasive (MR imaging or MRCP) and less invasive (EUS) imaging tests. In view of the high procedure-related complication rate in these patients, the investigators concluded that ERCP alone could not be justified. In the National Institutes of Health State-of-the-Science Conference on ERCP, it was concluded that ERCP, if performed in type III patients, should be coupled with SOM.[65]

Intraductal Ultrasound

Intraductal ultrasound makes it possible to assess sphincter of Oddi morphology during endoscopy. The sphincter appears as a thin hypoechoic circular structure on intraductal ultrasound.[66] Limited studies so far reveal no correlation between the basal sphincter pressures (as detected at SOM) and the thickness of the hypoechoic layer.[67] Although intraductal ultrasound may provide additional information at the level of the sphincter, it cannot be used as a substitute for SOM.

Sphincter of Oddi Manometry

The most definitive development in understanding of the pressure dynamics of the sphincter of Oddi occurred with the advent of SOM. SOM is the only available method to measure sphincter of Oddi motor activity directly. Although SOM can be performed intraoperatively and percutaneously, it is most commonly done in the ERCP setting. SOM is considered by most authorities to be the "gold standard" for evaluating patients for SOD.[68,69] The use of manometry to detect motility disorders of the sphincter of Oddi is similar to its use in other parts of the GI tract. However, performance of SOM is more technically demanding and hazardous, with complication rates (in particular, pancreatitis) of 30% reported. Questions remain as to whether these short-term observations (2- to 10-minute recordings per pull-through) reflect the 24-hour pathophysiology of the sphincter. Despite some problems, SOM is gaining more widespread clinical application.

TECHNIQUE AND INDICATIONS FOR SPHINCTER OF ODDI MANOMETRY

SOM is usually performed at the time of ERCP. All drugs that relax (anticholinergics, nitrates, calcium channel blockers, glucagon) or stimulate (most narcotics, cholinergic agents) the sphincter should be avoided for at least 8 to 12 hours before manometry and during the manometric session. Current data indicate that benzodiazepines do not affect the sphincter pressure and are acceptable sedatives for SOM. Meperidine, at a dose of 1 mg/kg or less, does not affect the basal sphincter pressure but does alter phasic wave characteristics.[70] Because the basal sphincter pressure is generally the only manometric criterion used to diagnose SOD and determine therapy, it was suggested that meperidine could be used to facilitate conscious sedation for manometry. Droperidol[71] and propofol[72] are increasingly used for SOM, and it appears that these agents also do not affect the basal sphincter pressure. Similarly, ketamine, used in combination with meperidine and diazepam or midazolam, does not significantly alter the biliary and pancreatic basal sphincter pressure.[73] If glucagon must be used to achieve cannulation, an 8- to 15-minute waiting period is required to restore the sphincter to its basal condition.

Catheters sized 5-Fr should be used because virtually all standards have been established with catheters of this size. Triple-lumen catheters are state-of-the-art and are available from several manufacturers. Various catheter types can be used. Catheters with a long intraductal tip may help secure the catheter within the bile duct, but such a long nose is commonly a hindrance if pancreatic manometry is desired. Over-the-wire (monorail) catheters can be passed after first securing one's position within the duct with a guidewire. Whether this guidewire influences basal sphincter pressure is unknown. Some triple-lumen catheters accommodate a 0.018- to 0.021-inch diameter guidewire passed through the entire length of the catheter and can be used to facilitate cannulation or maintain position in the duct. A study in our unit found, however, that stiffer shafted nitinol core guidewires used for this purpose commonly increase basal sphincter pressure by 50% to 100%.[74] To avoid such artifacts, such wires need to be avoided, the wires need to be pulled back into the catheter during the recording period, or guidewires with a very soft core must be used.

Aspiration catheters, in which one recording port is sacrificed to permit both end and side-hole aspiration of intraductal juice, are highly recommended for pancreatic manometry (**Fig. 46.2**). Most centers prefer to perfuse the catheters at 0.25 mL/channel using a low-compliance pump. Lower perfusion rates give accurate basal sphincter pressures but do not give accurate phasic wave information. A new water perfused sleeve system, similar to that used in the lower esophageal sphincter, awaits further study in the sphincter of Oddi.[75] The perfusate is generally distilled water, although physiologic saline needs further evaluation. The latter may crystallize in the capillary tubing of perfusion pumps and must be flushed out often.

SOM requires selective cannulation of the bile duct or pancreatic duct (**Fig. 46.3**). The duct entered can be identified by gently aspirating on any port. The appearance of yellow fluid in the endoscopic view indicates entry into the bile duct. Clear aspirate indicates that the pancreatic duct was entered. It is preferable to obtain a cholangiogram or pancreatogram or both before performing SOM because certain findings (e.g., CBD stone) may obviate the need for SOM; this can be done simply by injecting contrast material through one of the perfusion ports. Blaut and colleagues[76] showed that injection of contrast material into the biliary tree before SOM does not significantly alter sphincter pressure characteristics. Similar evaluation of the pancreatic sphincter after contrast agent injection has not been reported. To ensure accurate pressure

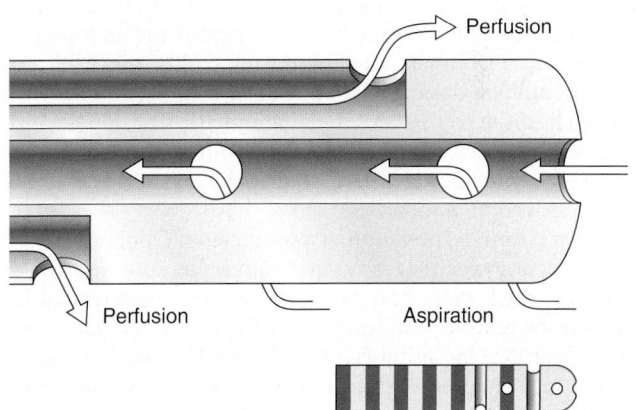

Fig. 46.2 Modified triple-lumen aspirating catheter.

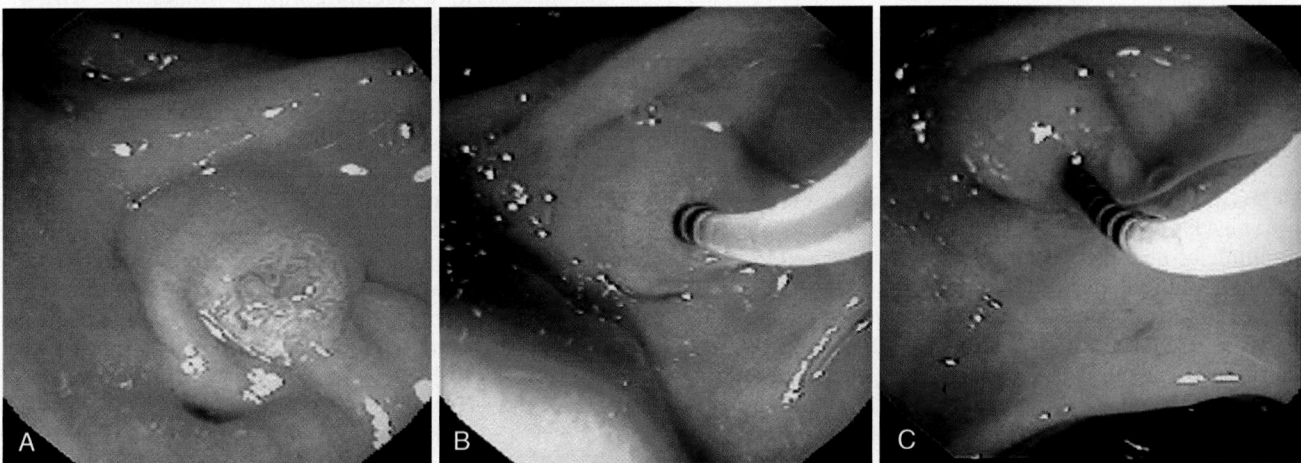

Fig. 46.3 Manometry. **A,** Normal major papilla. **B,** Biliary manometry. **C,** Pancreatic manometry.

measurements, one must ensure that the catheter is not impacted against the wall of the duct. When deep cannulation is achieved and the patient is adequately sedated, the catheter is withdrawn across the sphincter at 1- to 2-mm intervals by standard station pull-through technique.

Ideally, both the pancreatic and the bile ducts should be studied. Data indicate that an abnormal basal sphincter pressure may be confined to one side of the sphincter in 35% to 65% of patients with abnormal manometry.[6,26,77-80] One sphincter may be dysfunctional, whereas the other is normal. Raddawi and colleagues[77] reported that an abnormal basal sphincter was more likely to be confined to the pancreatic duct segment in patients with pancreatitis and to the bile duct segment in patients with biliary-type pain and elevated liver function tests. Abnormalities of the basal sphincter pressure ideally should be observed for at least 30 seconds in each lead and be seen on two or more separate pull-throughs. From a practical clinical standpoint, we settle for one pull-through (from each duct) if the readings are clearly normal or abnormal.

During standard station pull-through technique, it is necessary to establish good communication between the endoscopist and the manometrist who is reading the tracing as it rolls off the recorder or appears on the computer screen. Good communication permits optimal positioning of the catheter to achieve interpretable tracings. Alternatively, electronic manometry systems with a television screen can be mounted near the endoscopic image screen to permit the endoscopist to view the manometry tracing during endoscopy. After the baseline study is done, agents to relax or stimulate the sphincter can be given (e.g., CCK), and manometric or pain response can be monitored. The value of these provocative maneuvers for everyday use needs further study before widespread application is recommended.

Criteria for interpretation of a sphincter of Oddi tracing are standard; however, they may vary from center to center. Some areas in which there may be disagreement in interpretation include the required duration of basal sphincter of Oddi pressure elevation, the number of leads in which basal pressure elevation is required, and the role of averaging pressures from the three (or two in an aspirating catheter) recording ports.[4] Our recommended method for reading the manometry tracings is first to define the zero duodenal baseline before and after the pull-through. Alternatively, intraduodenal pressure can be continuously recorded from a separate intraduodenal catheter attached to the endoscope.

The highest basal pressure (defined as the pressure above the zero duodenal baseline; **Fig. 46.4**) that is sustained for at least 30 seconds is identified. The mean of the readings from the four lowest amplitude points in this zone is taken as the basal sphincter pressure for that lead for that pull-through. The basal sphincter pressure for all interpretable observations is averaged; this is the final basal sphincter pressure. The amplitude of phasic wave contractions is measured from the beginning of the slope of the pressure increase from the basal pressure to the peak of the contraction wave. Four representative waves are taken for each lead, and the mean pressure is determined. The number of phasic waves per minute and the duration of the phasic waves can also be determined.

Most authorities read only the basal sphincter pressure as an indicator of pathology of the sphincter of Oddi. However, data from Kalloo and coworkers[81] suggest that intraductal

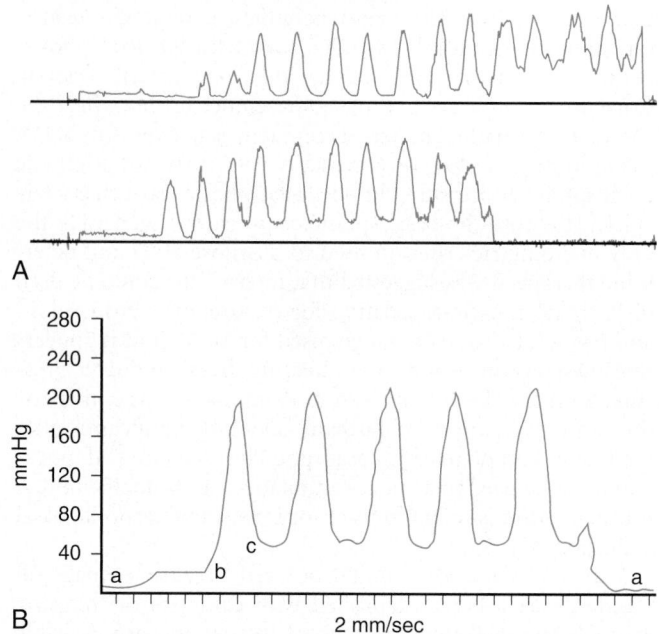

Fig. 46.4 **A,** Abnormal station pull-through at sphincter of Oddi manometry (SOM). The study has been abbreviated to fit onto one page. **B,** Schematic representation of one lead of the above tracing. Baseline duodenal 0 reference *(a)*. Intraductal (pancreatic) pressure of 20 mm Hg *(abnormal) (b)*. Basal pancreatic sphincter pressure is 45 mm Hg *(abnormal) (c)*. Phasic waves are 155 to 175 mm Hg in amplitude and 6 seconds in duration *(normal)*. *(Redrawn from Fogel EL, Sherman S: Performance of sphincter of Oddi manometry.* Clin Perspect Gastroenterol *4:165–173, 2001.)*

biliary pressure, which is easier to measure than sphincter of Oddi pressure, correlates with sphincter of Oddi basal pressure. In this study, intrabiliary pressure was significantly higher in patients with SOD than patients with normal sphincter of Oddi pressure (20 mm Hg vs. 10 mm Hg; $P < .01$). In a similar study, Fazel and colleagues[82] found that pancreatic duct pressure correlated with pancreatic sphincter pressure ($P < .01$). Pancreatic duct pressure was significantly higher in patients with SOD compared with patients with normal pressure (20 mm Hg vs. 11 mm Hg; $P < .001$). These studies must be confirmed, but they support the theory that increased intrabiliary or intrapancreatic pressure is a cause of pain in SOD.

The best study establishing normal values for SOM was reported by Guelrud and associates.[83] The study evaluated 50 asymptomatic control patients and repeated the evaluation on two occasions in 10 subjects. This study established normal values for intraductal pressure, basal sphincter pressure, and phasic wave parameters (**Table 46.2**). The reproducibility of SOM was confirmed. Various authorities interchangeably use 35 mm Hg or 40 mm Hg as the upper limits of normal for mean basal sphincter of Oddi pressure (this is 3 standard deviations above the mean). Although all authorities diagnose SOD when the basal sphincter pressure is 35 to 40 mm Hg or greater, some also make this diagnosis when there are greater than 50% retrograde contractions, tachyoddia (phasic wave frequency >7/min), or a paradoxical contraction response after an intravenous dose of CCK.[84]

Several studies have shown that pancreatitis is the most common major complication after SOM.[85-87] Using standard perfused catheters, pancreatitis rates of 31% have been

Table 46.2 Suggested Standard for Abnormal Values for Endoscopic Sphincter of Oddi Manometry Obtained from 50 Volunteers without Abdominal Symptoms

Basal sphincter pressure*	>35 mm Hg
Basal ductal pressure	>13 mm Hg
Phasic contractions	
Amplitude	>220 mm Hg
Duration	>8 sec
Frequency	>10/min

Note: Values were obtained by adding 3 standard deviations to the mean (means were obtained by averaging the results on two to three station pull-throughs). Data combine pancreatic and biliary studies.

*Basal pressures determined by (1) reading the peak basal pressure (i.e., the highest single lead as obtained using a three-lumen catheter) and (2) obtaining the mean of these peak pressures from multiple station pull-throughs.

Adapted from Guelrud M, Mendoza S, Rossiter G, et al: Sphincter of Oddi manometry in healthy volunteers. Dig Dis Sci 35:38–46, 1990.

reported. Such high complication rates have limited more widespread use of SOM. These data also emphasize that manometric evaluation of the pancreatic duct is associated with a particularly high complication rate. Rolny and associates[86] found that patients with chronic pancreatitis were at higher risk of postprocedure pancreatitis after pancreatic duct manometry. They reported an 11% incidence of pancreatitis after manometric evaluation of the pancreatic duct. Pancreatitis developed in 26% of patients with chronic pancreatitis undergoing SOM.

Methods that have been proposed to decrease the incidence of postmanometry pancreatitis include (1) use of an aspiration catheter; (2) gravity drainage of the pancreatic duct after manometry; (3) decrease in the perfusion rate to 0.05 to 0.1 mL/lumen/min; (4) limitation of pancreatic duct manometry time to less than 2 minutes (or avoid pancreatic manometry); (5) use of the microtransducer (nonperfused) or sleeve SOM system[75,88-91]; and (6) placement of a pancreatic stent after manometry, sphincterotomy, or both. In a prospective randomized study, Sherman and colleagues[85] found that an aspirating catheter (catheter that allows for aspiration of the perfused fluid from end and side holes while accurately recording pressure from the two remaining side ports) reduced the frequency of pancreatic duct manometry–induced pancreatitis from 31% to 4%. The reduction in pancreatitis rates with the use of this catheter in the pancreatic duct and the very low incidence of pancreatitis after bile duct manometry lend support to the notion that increased pancreatic duct hydrostatic pressure is a major cause of this complication.

When the pancreatic duct sphincter is studied by SOM, aspiration of pancreatic juice and the perfusate is strongly recommended. In a prospective randomized trial, Wehrmann and colleagues[88] found that microtransducer manometry was associated with a significantly lower incidence of postmanometry pancreatitis than standard (nonaspirating) perfusion manometry (13.8% vs. 3.1%; $P = .04$). A sleeve SOM catheter–based system was shown more recently to have similar accuracy as the standard triple-lumen SOM catheter with less artifact.[90] Because the sleeve assembly is reverse-perfused, no fluid enters the ducts potentially reducing the rate of postprocedure pancreatitis. In another prospective randomized trial,

Tarnasky and colleagues[92] showed that placement of a stent in the pancreatic duct decreased post-ERCP pancreatitis from 26% to 6% in a group of patients with pancreatic sphincter hypertension undergoing biliary sphincterotomy alone.

SOM is recommended in patients with idiopathic pancreatitis or unexplained disabling pancreaticobiliary pain with or without hepatic enzyme abnormalities. An attempt should be made to study both sphincters, but clinical decisions can be made when the first sphincter evaluated is abnormal. However, if the other sphincter is dysfunctional and not treated, the outcome of therapy may be suboptimal. Indications for the use of SOM have also been developed according to the Hogan-Geenen SOD classification system (see **Table 46.1**). In type I patients, there is a general consensus that a structural disorder of the sphincter (i.e., sphincter stenosis) exists. Although SOM may be useful in documenting SOD, it is not an essential diagnostic study before endoscopic or surgical sphincter ablation. Such patients uniformly benefit from sphincter ablation regardless of the SOM results (see the section on endoscopic therapy). Type II patients exhibit sphincter of Oddi motor dysfunction in 55% to 65% of cases. In these patients, SOM is highly recommended because the results of the study predict outcome from sphincter ablation. Type III patients have pancreaticobiliary pain without other objective evidence of sphincter outflow obstruction. SOM is mandatory to confirm the presence of SOD. Although this has not been well studied, the results of SOM may predict outcome from sphincter ablation in these patients.

Stent Trial as a Diagnostic Test

Placement of a pancreatic or biliary stent on a trial basis in hope of achieving pain relief and predicting the response to more definitive therapy (i.e., sphincter ablation) has received only limited application. Pancreatic stent trials, especially in patients with normal pancreatic ducts, are strongly discouraged because serious ductal and parenchymal injury may occur if stents are left in place for more than a few days.[93,94] Goff[95] reported a biliary stent trial in 21 patients with normal biliary manometry suspected to have type II and type III SOD. Stents (7-Fr) were left in place for at least 2 months if symptoms resolved and were removed sooner if they were judged ineffective. Relief of pain with the stent was predictive of long-term pain relief after biliary sphincterotomy. Pancreatitis developed in 38% of the patients (14% were graded severe) after stent placement. Because of this high complication rate, biliary stent trials are strongly discouraged. Rolny and colleagues[96] also reported a series of bile duct stent placement as a predictor of outcome after biliary sphincterotomy in 23 postcholecystectomy patients (7 type II and 16 type III). Similar to the study by Goff,[95] resolution of pain during at least 12 weeks of stent placement predicted a favorable outcome from sphincterotomy regardless of sphincter of Oddi pressure. In this series, there were no complications related to stent placement.

Therapy for Sphincter of Oddi Dysfunction

The therapeutic approach in patients with SOD is aimed at reducing the resistance to the flow of bile or pancreatic juice, or both, caused by the sphincter of Oddi.[13] Historically, emphasis has been placed on definitive intervention (i.e., surgical sphincteroplasty or endoscopic sphincterotomy). This approach seems appropriate for patients with high-grade obstruction (type I as per Hogan-Geenen criteria). In patients with lesser degrees of obstruction, the clinician must carefully weigh the risks and benefits before recommending invasive therapy. Most reports indicate that patients with SOD have a complication rate from ERCP, manometry, and endoscopic sphincterotomy of at least twice that of patients with ductal stones.[97,98]

Medical Therapy

Medical therapy for documented or suspected SOD has received only limited study. Because the sphincter of Oddi is a smooth muscle structure, it is reasonable to assume that drugs that relax smooth muscle might be an effective treatment for SOD. Vardenafil (Levitra), an inhibitor of phosphodiesterase type 5 and a smooth muscle relaxant used most commonly for male erectile dysfunction, was found to reduce basal sphincter pressure and phasic wave amplitude.[99,100] This drug has not been investigated in clinical trials, however. Sublingual nifedipine and nitrates have been shown to reduce basal sphincter pressures in asymptomatic volunteers and symptomatic patients with SOD.[1,101] Khuroo and colleagues[102] evaluated the clinical benefit of nifedipine in a placebo-controlled crossover trial. Of 28 patients with manometrically documented SOD, 21 (75%) had a reduction in pain scores, emergency department visits, and use of oral analgesics during short-term follow-up. In a similar study, Sand and associates[103] found that 9 (75%) of 12 patients with type II SOD (suspected; SOM was not done) improved with nifedipine. In a study of 59 patients with postcholecystectomy pain and suspected SOD treated with medical therapy for 1 year (nitrates or an antispasmodic or both),[30] 51% reported complete relief and 8 (14%) reported partial relief including 45%, 67%, and 71% type I, type II, and type III patients.[104]

Although medical therapy may be an attractive initial approach in patients with SOD, several drawbacks exist.[1] First, medication side effects may be seen in one-third of patients. Second, smooth muscle relaxants are unlikely to be of any benefit in patients with the structural form of SOD (i.e., sphincter of Oddi stenosis), and the response is incomplete in patients with a primary motor abnormality of the sphincter of Oddi (i.e., sphincter of Oddi dyskinesia). Finally, long-term outcome from medical therapy has not been reported. In a pilot randomized controlled trial, Craig and Toouli[105] found no benefit for extended-release nifedipine. Nevertheless, because of the relative safety of medical therapy and the benign (although painful) character of SOD, this approach should be considered in all patients with type III SOD and in patients with type II SOD and less severe symptoms before considering more aggressive sphincter ablation therapy.

Guelrud and colleagues[106] showed that transcutaneous electrical nerve stimulation reduces the basal sphincter pressure in patients with SOD by a mean of 38%, although generally not into the normal range. This stimulation was associated with an increase in serum vasoactive intestinal peptide levels. Electroacupuncture applied at acupoint GB 34 (a specific acupoint that affects the hepatobiliary system) was shown to relax the sphincter of Oddi in association with increased plasma CCK levels.[107] The role of electroacupuncture in the management of SOD has not been investigated.

Surgical Therapy

Historically, surgery was the traditional therapy of SOD. Most commonly, the surgical approach is a transduodenal biliary sphincteroplasty with a transampullary septoplasty (pancreatic septoplasty). During a 1- to 10-year follow-up, 60% to 70% of patients were reported to have benefited from this therapy.[108–111] Patients with an elevated basal sphincter pressure, determined by intraoperative SOM, were more likely to improve from surgical sphincter ablation than patients with a normal basal pressure.[109] Some reports have suggested that patients with biliary-type pain have a better outcome than patients with idiopathic pancreatitis, whereas others suggested no difference.[108,109] However, most studies found that symptom improvement after surgical sphincter ablation alone was uncommon in patients with established chronic pancreatitis.[109]

Morgan and associates[111] reported that chronic pancreatitis and younger age were independent predictors of poor outcome from surgical sphincter ablation. The surgical approach for SOD has largely been replaced by endoscopic therapy. Patient tolerance, cost of care, morbidity, mortality, and cosmetic results are some factors that favor an initial endoscopic approach. At the present time, surgical therapy is reserved for patients with restenosis after endoscopic sphincterotomy and when endoscopic evaluation or therapy is unavailable or not technically feasible (e.g., Roux-en-Y gastrojejunostomy). Among 68 surgical sphincteroplasties done at Medical University of South Carolina over a 5-year period, 51 had prior endoscopic sphincterotomy, and 17 had endoscopically inaccessible papillae because of prior gastric surgery. There was a trend toward improved outcome after surgical sphincteroplasty ($P = .06$) in patients who had previous gastric surgery and no prior ERCP compared with patients who had endoscopic sphincterotomy before surgery.[111] In many centers, however, operative therapy continues to be the standard treatment of pancreatic sphincter hypertension.[13,112]

Endoscopic Therapy
Endoscopic Sphincterotomy

Endoscopic sphincterotomy is the standard therapy for patients with SOD.[113] Most data on endoscopic sphincterotomy relate to biliary sphincter ablation alone. Clinical improvement after therapy has been reported to occur in 55% to 95% of patients (see **Table 46.1**). These variable outcomes are reflective of the different criteria used to document SOD, the degree of obstruction (type I biliary patients appear to have a better outcome than type II and type III patients), the methods of data collection (retrospective vs. prospective), and the techniques used to determine benefit. Rolny and colleagues[114] studied 17 type I postcholecystectomy biliary patients by SOM (**Table 46.3**). In this series, 65% had abnormal SOM (although not specifically stated, the biliary sphincter apparently was studied alone). Nevertheless, during a mean follow-up interval of 2.3 years, all patients benefited from biliary sphincterotomy. The results of this study suggested that because type I biliary patients invariably benefit from biliary sphincterotomy, SOM in this patient group not only is unnecessary but also may be misleading. However, the results of this study have never been validated at another center.

In contrast, results of several nonrandomized controlled trials[23,32,58,115,116] suggest that performance of SOM is highly recommended in biliary type II and type III patients because clinical benefit is less certain (**Table 46.4**). Several other case series have reported symptom improvement in 75% to 100% of type I patients undergoing biliary sphincterotomy.[59,117–120] Although most of the studies reporting efficacy of endoscopic therapy in SOD have been retrospective, three notable randomized trials have been reported. In a landmark study, Geenen and associates[121] randomly assigned 47 postcholecystectomy type II biliary patients to biliary sphincterotomy or sham sphincterotomy. SOM was performed in all patients but was not used as a criterion for randomization. During a 4-year follow-up, 95% of patients with an elevated basal sphincter benefited from sphincterotomy. In contrast, only 30% to 40% of patients with an elevated sphincter pressure treated by sham sphincterotomy or with a normal sphincter pressure treated by endoscopic sphincterotomy or sham sphincterotomy benefited from this therapy. The two important findings of this study were that SOM predicted the outcome from endoscopic sphincterotomy and that endoscopic sphincterotomy offered long-term benefit in type II biliary patients with SOD.

Confirming data were seen in a 2-year follow-up study by Toouli and coworkers.[122,123] In this study, postcholecystectomy patients with biliary-type pain (mostly type II) were prospectively randomly assigned to endoscopic sphincterotomy or sham after stratification according to SOM. At 2 years after endoscopic sphincterotomy, 85% (11 of 13) of patients with elevated basal pressure improved, whereas 38% (5 of 13) of patients improved after a sham procedure ($P = .041$). Patients with normal SOM were also randomly assigned to sphincterotomy or sham. The outcome was similar for the two groups (8 of 13 improved after sphincterotomy, and 8 of 19 improved after sham; $P = .47$). Sherman and associates[124] reported their preliminary results of a randomized study comparing endoscopic sphincterotomy and surgical biliary sphincteroplasty with pancreatic septoplasty (with or without cholecystectomy) with sham sphincterotomy for type II and type III biliary patients with manometrically documented SOD. The results are shown in **Tables 46.5 and 46.6**. During a 3-year follow-up period, 69% of patients undergoing endoscopic or surgical sphincter ablation improved compared with 24% in the sham sphincterotomy group ($P = .009$). There was a trend

---

Table 46.3 Biliary Sphincter Ablation in Type I Sphincter of Oddi Dysfunction (28-Month Follow-up)*

Basal Sphincter of Oddi Pressure	N	Asymptomatic or Improved after ES or SS
<40 mm Hg	6 (35%)	6 (100%)
>40 mm Hg	11 (65%)	11 (100%)

*15 ES, 2 SS.

ES, endoscopic sphincterotomy; SS, surgical sphincterotomy.

Adapted from Rolny P, Geenen JE, Hogan WJ: Post-cholecystectomy patients with 'objective signs' of partial bile outflow obstruction: Clinical characteristics, sphincter of Oddi manometry findings, and results of therapy. Gastrointest Endosc 39:778–781, 1993.

Table 46.4 Biliary Sphincterotomy for Type II and Type III Sphincter of Oddi Dysfunction Documented by Sphincter of Oddi Manometry: Results of Five Nonrandomized Trials

Author (Year)	Clinical Benefit	
	Type II	Type III
Choudhry et al (1993)[32]*	10/18 (56%)	9/16 (56%)
Botoman et al (1994)[23]	13/19 (68%)	9/16 (56%)
Bozkurt et al (1996)[115]	14/19 (78%)	5/5 (100%)
Wehrmann et al (1996)[116]	12/20 (60%)	1/13 (8%)
Rosenblatt et al (2001)[58]	22/30 (73%)	11/32 (34%)

*Six had cholecystectomy.

Table 46.5 Change in the Mean Pain Score*, Number of Hospital Days per Month Required for Pain, and the Percentage Improved in Patients with Manometrically Documented Sphincter of Oddi Dysfunction Randomly Assigned to Endoscopic Sphincterotomy, Sham Sphincterotomy, and Surgical Sphincteroplasty with or without Cholecystectomy

Therapy	Follow-up (yr)	Mean Pain Score		Hospital Days/Month		% Patients Improved
		Pretreatment	Posttreatment	Pretreatment	Posttreatment	
ES (n = 19)	3.3	9.2	3.9†	0.85	0.23‡	68%§
S-ES (n = 17)	2.2	9.4	7.2	0.87	0.89	24%
SSp ± CCx (n = 16)	3.4	9.4	3.3†	0.94	0.27‡	69%§

*Using a 0 = none to 10 = most severe linear pain scale.

†$P < .04$; ES and SSp ± CCx vs. S-ES.

‡$P = .002$; ES and SSp ± CCx vs. S-ES.

§$P = .009$; ES and SSp ± CCx vs. S-ES.

ES, endoscopic sphincterotomy; S-ES, sham sphincterotomy; SSp ± CCx, surgical sphincteroplasty with or without cholecystectomy.

Adapted from Sherman S, Lehman GA, Jamidar P, et al: Efficacy of endoscopic sphincterotomy and surgical sphincteroplasty for patients with sphincter of Oddi dysfunction (SOD): Randomized, controlled study. Gastrointest Endosc 40:A125, 1994.

for type II patients to benefit more often from sphincter ablation than type III patients (13 of 16 [81%] vs. 11 of 19 [58%]; $P = .14$).

Fig. 46.5 shows the recommended approach of the Rome III committee on functional disorders of the sphincter of Oddi[31] for the therapy of patients with types I, II, and II biliary SOD. Evidence is now accumulating that the addition of a pancreatic sphincterotomy to an endoscopic biliary sphincterotomy in patients with pancreatic sphincter disease may improve the outcome, as preliminarily reported by Guelrud and coworkers.[125] Soffer and Johlin[126] reported that 25 of 26 patients (mostly type II) who failed to respond to biliary sphincterotomy had elevated pancreatic sphincter pressure. Pancreatic sphincter therapy was performed with overall

symptomatic improvement in two-thirds of patients. Eversman and colleagues[127] found that 90% of patients with persistent pain or pancreatitis after biliary sphincterotomy had residual abnormal pancreatic basal pressure. Data from 5 years of follow-up revealed that patients with untreated pancreatic sphincter hypertension were much less likely to improve after biliary sphincterotomy than patients with isolated biliary sphincter hypertension. Elton and colleagues[128] performed pancreatic sphincterotomy on 43 type I and type II SOD patients who failed to benefit from biliary sphincterotomy alone. During the follow-up period, 72% were symptom-free, and 19% had partial or transient improvement.

Kaw and colleagues[129] presented preliminary data showing that response to sphincterotomy also depends on treating the diseased sphincter segment. Patients with pancreatic sphincter hypertension who fail to respond to biliary sphincterotomy can be "rescued" by undergoing pancreatic sphincterotomy (**Table 46.7**). More recent data from our unit[130] examined the outcome of endoscopic therapy in patients with SOD with initial pancreatic sphincter hypertension (with or without biliary sphincter hypertension). Patients were followed for a mean of 43.1 months (range 11 to 77 months); reintervention was offered for sustained or recurrent symptoms at a median of 8 months after initial therapy. Performance of an initial dual pancreatobiliary sphincterotomy was associated with a lower reintervention rate (70 of 285 [24.6%]) than biliary sphincterotomy alone (31 of 95 [33%]; $P < .05$). Confirmatory outcome studies, preferably in randomized trials, are awaited.

Many authorities argue that the current SOD classification systems might not be a good predictor of outcome.[84,131–133] In a study of 121 patients classified by the modified Milwaukee biliary classification system (18 type I, 53 type II, and 50 type III patients) and treated by biliary sphincterotomy with (49

Table 46.6 Clinical Benefit Correlated with Sphincter of Oddi Dysfunction Type

| SOD Type* | Patients Improved/Total Patients | | |
	ES	S-ES	SSp ± CCx
Type II	5/6 (83%)†	1/7 (14%)	8/10 (80%)†
Type III	8/13 (62%)	3/10 (30%)	3/6 (50%)

*SOD type based on Hogan-Geenen SOD classification system.
†P < .02; ES and SSp ± CCx vs. S-ES.
ES, endoscopic sphincterotomy; S-ES, sham sphincterotomy; SOD, sphincter of Oddi dysfunction; SSp ± CCx, surgical sphincteroplasty with or without cholecystectomy.
Adapted from Sherman S, Lehman GA, Jamidar P, et al: Efficacy of endoscopic sphincterotomy and surgical sphincteroplasty for patients with sphincter of Oddi dysfunction (SOD): Randomized, controlled study. Gastrointest Endosc 40:A125, 1994.

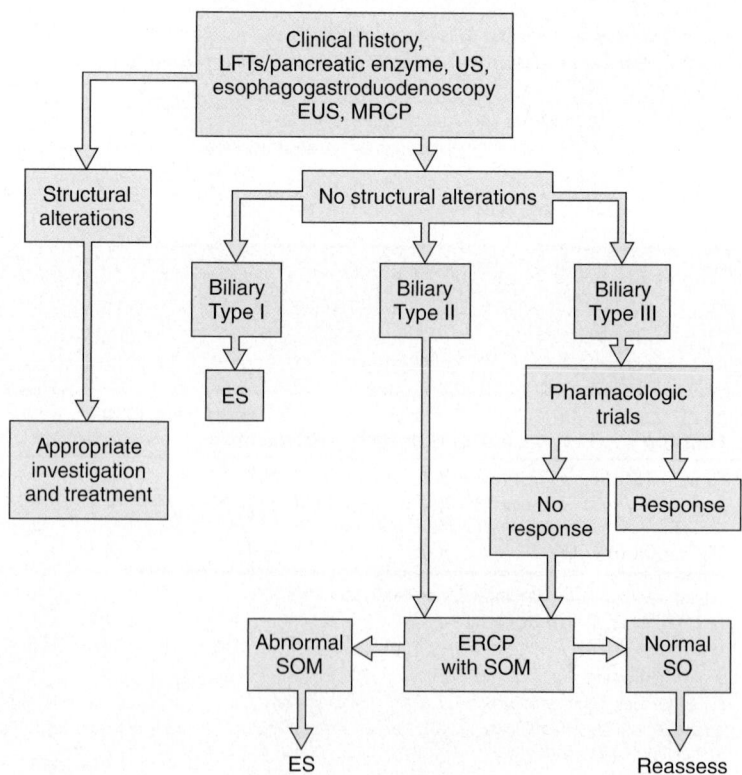

Fig. 46.5 Algorithm of the history, diagnostic work-up, and treatment of patients with types I, II, and III biliary sphincter of Oddi dysfunction (SOD). *(From Behar J, Corazziari E, Guelrud M, et al: Functional gallbladder and sphincter of Oddi disorders. Gastroenterology 130:1498–1509, 2006.)*

Table 46.7 Response to Sphincterotomy in Relation to Sphincter of Oddi Segment Treated (Follow-up 17 Months)

SOD	Biliary Sphincterotomy		Pancreatic Sphincterotomy	
	Total	Response	Total	Response
Biliary	10	8 (80%)	0	0 (0%)
Pancreatic	13	2 (15%)	11	8 (72%)
Combined	10	5 (50%)	5	3 (60%)
Total	*33*	*15 (45%)*	*16*	*11 (69%)*

Note: Overall benefit 26/33 (79%); patients with pancreatic or combined SOD who failed to improve after a biliary sphincterotomy underwent pancreatic sphincterotomy.

SOD, sphincter of Oddi dysfunction.

Adapted from Kaw M, Verma R, Brodmerkel GJ: Biliary and/or pancreatic sphincter of Oddi dysfunction (SOD): Response to endoscopic sphincterotomy (ES). Gastrointest Endosc 43:A384, 1996.

patients) or without (72 patients) pancreatic sphincterotomy, Freeman and colleagues[131] reported a good to excellent response in 69%. The response was not significantly different between biliary types I, II, and III. The authors found that significant predictors of a poor response to therapy were normal pancreatic manometry, delayed gastric emptying, daily opioid use, and age younger than 40 years. Abnormal liver function tests or dilated bile duct were not significant predictors of outcome. These results indicate that the response rate and enthusiasm for sphincter ablation must be correlated with patient presentation and results of manometry and balanced against the high complication rates reported for endoscopic therapy of SOD.

Most studies indicate that patients undergoing ERCP, manometry, and endoscopic sphincterotomy for SOD have complication rates two to five times higher than patients undergoing ERCP and endoscopic sphincterotomy for ductal stones.[97,98] Pancreatitis is the most common complication, occurring in up to 30% of patients in some series. Several prospective, multicenter studies examining risk factors for post-ERCP pancreatitis identified suspected SOD as an independent factor by multivariate analysis.[134] A suspicion of SOD tripled the risk of postprocedure pancreatitis to a frequency (23%) that was comparable to that found in other more recent prospective studies.[92,98,135–137] Placement of a prophylactic pancreatic duct stent has been shown to limit such complications.[92,138–140] These studies have also shown that the risk of pancreatitis is intrinsic to the patient group (patient-related factors) and events occurring during the procedure (procedure-related factors) rather than the SOM when the SOM is performed with an aspirating catheter. In multivariate analysis, SOM has not been shown to be a risk factor for pancreatitis.[141,142]

Balloon Dilation and Stent Placement

Balloon dilation of strictures in the GI tract has become a common procedure. In an attempt to be less invasive and possibly to preserve sphincter function, adaptation of this technique to treat SOD has been described. Because of the

unacceptably high complication rates, primarily pancreatitis, this technology has little role in the primary management of SOD.[143] Similarly, although biliary stent placement might offer short-term symptom benefit in patients with SOD and predict outcome from sphincter ablation, it too has unacceptably high complication rates and cannot be advocated in this setting.[95]

Botulinum Toxin Injection

Botulinum toxin (Botox), a potent inhibitor of acetylcholine release from nerve endings, has been successfully applied to smooth muscle disorders of the GI tract such as achalasia. In a preliminary clinical trial, botulinum toxin injection into the sphincter of Oddi resulted in a 50% reduction in the basal biliary sphincter pressure and improved bile flow.[144] This reduction in pressure may be accompanied by symptom improvement in some patients. Although further study is warranted, botulinum toxin may serve as a therapeutic trial for SOD with responders undergoing permanent sphincter ablation. In a small series,[145] 22 postcholecystectomy type III patients with manometric evidence of SOD underwent botulinum toxin injection into the intraduodenal sphincter segment. Of the 12 patients who responded to botulinum toxin injection, 11 later benefited from endoscopic sphincterotomy, whereas only 2 of 10 patients who did not benefit from botulinum toxin injection later responded to sphincter ablation. Such an approach requires two endoscopies to achieve symptom relief. Patients must have relatively frequent episodes of pain to assess the benefit from botulinum toxin. Further studies are needed before this technique can be recommended.

Failure to Achieve Symptomatic Improvement after Biliary Sphincterotomy

There are several potential explanations as to why patients may fail to experience symptom relief after biliary sphincterotomy is performed for well-documented SOD. First, biliary sphincterotomy may have been inadequate, or restenosis may have occurred. Although the biliary sphincter is commonly not totally ablated,[146] Manoukian and coworkers[147] indicated that clinically significant biliary restenosis occurs infrequently. If no "cutting space" remains in such a patient, balloon dilation to 8 to 10 mm may suffice, but long-term outcome from such therapy is unknown, and the risks may be considerable.[143] Prophylactic pancreatic stent placement may reduce the frequency of post–balloon dilation pancreatitis.[148] Second, as noted previously,[125–130] the importance of pancreatic sphincter ablation is being increasingly recognized. Third, patients may fail to respond to sphincterotomy because they have chronic pancreatitis. Tarnasky and colleagues[149] reported that patients with SOD were four times more likely to have evidence of chronic pancreatitis than patients without SOD ($P = .01$). Although SOD seems to be associated with chronic pancreatitis, a causal relationship has not been proven. These patients may or may not have abnormal pancreatograms. Intraductal pancreatic juice aspiration after secretin stimulation may help make this diagnosis.[150–152] EUS may show parenchymal and ductular changes of the pancreas in some of these patients suggesting chronic pancreatitis.[153] Fourth, some patients may be having pain from altered gut motility of the stomach, small bowel, or colon (irritable bowel or pseudo-obstruction variants). There is increasing evidence that upper GI motility disorders may masquerade as pancreatobiliary-type pain (i.e., discrete right upper quadrant pain). Multiple preliminary studies show disordered duodenal motility in such patients.[154–156] Soffer and Johlin[157] found that small bowel dysmotility occurred with greater frequency in type II and type III SOD patients who failed to benefit from sphincterotomy than in patients who did respond. This area needs much more study to determine the frequency, significance, and coexistence of these motor disorders along with SOD.

DeSautels and colleagues[158] suggested that type III patients have duodenal-specific visceral hyperalgesia with pain reproduction by duodenal distention. These patients were also shown to have high levels of somatization, depression, obsessive-compulsive behavior, and anxiety compared with control subjects.[159] Patients with SOD appear to have a higher than expected prevalence of irritable bowel syndrome,[160] and SOD may occur as part of a more generalized functional disorder of the gut. Patients with SOD not only have more somatization than controls, but also they may have an antecedent history of sexual or physical abuse similar to patients with irritable bowel syndrome.[161] Wald[15] suggested that selective treatment of the sphincter of Oddi cannot be expected to provide symptom resolution in such patients, and this may account for the high failure rate of sphincterotomy in many patients with type III SOD.

Sphincter of Oddi Dysfunction in Recurrent Pancreatitis

Disorders of the pancreatic sphincter may give rise to unexplained (idiopathic) pancreatitis or episodic pain suggestive of a pancreatic origin.[112] Although the pathogenesis of acute pancreatitis in SOD is uncertain, it is believed that the combination of pancreatic duct obstruction and increased exocrine juice flow are needed.[84] SOD is a frequent cause of recurrent pancreatitis previously labeled as idiopathic acute recurrent pancreatitis (IARP). It has been documented with manometry in 15% to 72% of such patients (**Table 46.8**).[6,24,30,162–171] Pancreatic sphincter manometry should be done in patients with IARP, particularly patients with normal biliary manometry and patients who have recurrent attacks after a biliary sphincterotomy. Isolated pancreatic sphincter hypertension is common among patients with IARP found to have SOD.[77,172] In addition, pancreatic sphincter hypertension may explain recurrent pancreatitis despite biliary sphincterotomy or surgical biliary sphincteroplasty.[172]

Biliary sphincterotomy alone has been reported to prevent further pancreatitis episodes in more than 50% of patients in some series. From a scientific, but not practical, viewpoint, care must be taken to separate out subtle biliary pancreatitis[173] that would similarly respond to biliary sphincterotomy. Because IARP is an episodic illness, long-term follow-up is necessary to conclude that a patient is "cured." Sphincter ablation is the recommended therapy for patients with IARP resulting from SOD. Historically, ablation has been accomplished surgically.[109] However, with increasing experience,

Table 46.8 Manometrically Documented Sphincter of Oddi Dysfunction Causing Idiopathic Acute Recurrent Pancreatitis

Author (Year)	Frequency
Toouli et al (1985)[165]	16/26 (57%)
Guelrud et al (1986)[166]	17/42 (40%)
Gregg (1989)[167]	38/125 (30%)
Venu et al (1989)[164]	17/116 (15%)
Sherman et al (1993)[168]	18/55 (33%)
Choudari et al (1998)[163]	79/225 (35%)
Kaw and Brodmerkel (2002)[169]	67/126 (53%)
Coyle et al (2002)[170]	28/90 (31%)
Total	781/2046 (38%)

Table 46.9 Pancreatic Sphincter Dysfunction and Recurrent Pancreatitis: Response to Sphincter Therapy

Treatment	Patients Improved/ Total Patients
Biliary sphincterotomy alone	5/18 (28%)
Biliary sphincterotomy followed by pancreatic sphincter balloon dilation	13/24 (54%)
Biliary sphincterotomy plus pancreatic sphincterotomy at later session	10/13 (77%)*
Biliary sphincterotomy and pancreatic sphincterotomy at same session	12/14 (86%)*

*$P < .005$ vs. biliary sphincterotomy alone.

Adapted from Guelrud M, Plaz J, Mendoza S, et al: Endoscopic treatment in type II pancreatic sphincter dysfunction. Gastrointest Endosc 41:A398, 1995.

endoscopic sphincterotomy has become the treatment of choice. Controversy continues to exist about the type of sphincterotomy that should be performed.[174]

The value of ERCP, SOM, and sphincter ablation therapy was studied in 51 patients with idiopathic pancreatitis.[69] An elevated basal sphincter pressure was present in 24 (47.1%) patients. There were 30 patients treated by biliary sphincterotomy ($n = 20$) or surgical sphincteroplasty with septoplasty ($n = 10$). Of 18 patients, 15 (83%) with an elevated basal sphincter pressure had long-term benefit (mean follow-up 38 months) from sphincter ablation therapy (including 10 of 11 treated by biliary sphincterotomy), in contrast to only 4 (33.3%; $P < .05$) of 12 patients with a normal basal sphincter pressure (including 4 of 9 patients treated by biliary sphincterotomy).

Guelrud and colleagues[125] found, however, that severance of the pancreatic sphincter was necessary to resolve pancreatitis (**Table 46.9**). In this series, 69 patients with idiopathic pancreatitis resulting from SOD underwent treatment by standard biliary sphincterotomy ($n = 18$), biliary sphincterotomy with pancreatic sphincter balloon dilation ($n = 24$), biliary sphincterotomy followed by pancreatic sphincterotomy in separate sessions ($n = 13$), or combined pancreatic and biliary sphincterotomy in the same session ($n = 14$). Of patients undergoing pancreatic and biliary sphincterotomy, 81% had resolution of pancreatitis compared with 28% of patients undergoing biliary sphincterotomy alone ($P < .005$). Sherman and colleagues[168] reported that only 44% of patients with SOD and IARP had no further attacks during a 5-year follow-up interval after biliary sphincterotomy alone. These data are consistent with the theory that many such patients who benefit from biliary sphincterotomy alone have subtle gallstone pancreatitis.

The results of Guelrud and colleagues[125] also support the anatomic findings of separate biliary and pancreatic sphincters and the manometry findings of residual pancreatic sphincter hypertension in more than 50% of persistently symptomatic patients who undergo biliary sphincterotomy alone. Kaw and Brodmerkel[169] reported that among patients with idiopathic pancreatitis secondary to SOD, 78% had persistent manometric evidence of pancreatic sphincter hypertension despite a biliary sphincterotomy. Toouli and coworkers[175] also showed the importance of pancreatic and biliary sphincter ablation in patients with idiopathic pancreatitis. In this series, 23 of 26 patients (88%) undergoing surgical ablation of both the biliary and the pancreatic sphincter were either asymptomatic or had minimal symptoms at a median follow-up of 24 months (range 9 to 105 months). Okolo and colleagues[176] retrospectively evaluated the long-term results of endoscopic pancreatic sphincterotomy in 55 patients with manometrically documented or presumed pancreatic sphincter hypertension (presumption based on recurrent pancreatitis with pancreatic duct dilation and contrast medium drainage time from the pancreatic duct >10 minutes). During a median follow-up of 16 months (range 3 to 52 months), 34 patients (62%) reported significant pain improvement. Patients with normal pancreatograms were more likely to respond to therapy than patients with pancreatographic evidence of chronic pancreatitis (73% vs. 58%).

Jacob and coworkers[177] postulated that SOD might cause recurrent episodes of pancreatitis, even though SOM was normal, and pancreatic stent placement might prevent further attacks. In a randomized study, 34 patients with unexplained recurrent pancreatitis; normal pancreatic duct SOM, ERCP, and secretin testing; and no biliary crystals were treated with pancreatic stents ($n = 19$; 5-Fr to 7-Fr, with stents exchanged three times over a 1-year period) or conservative therapy ($n = 15$). During a 3-year follow-up, pancreatitis recurred in 53% of the patients in the control group and only 11% of the patients with stent placement ($P < .02$). This study suggests that SOM may be an imperfect test because patients may have SOD, but it may not be detected at the time of SOM. Long-term studies are needed to evaluate the outcome after removal of stents, and concern remains regarding stent-induced ductal and parenchymal changes.[93,94] Because of the concern of stent-induced injury to the pancreas, trial pancreatic duct stent placement to predict outcome from pancreatic sphincterotomy is not recommended.[178]

Wehrmann and colleagues[179] evaluated the feasibility and effectiveness of botulinum toxin injection in patients with recurrent pancreatitis resulting from pancreatic sphincter hypertension. No side effects of the injection were noted in any of the 15 treated patients. At 3-month follow-up, 12 patients (80%) remained asymptomatic, but 11 developed a relapse at a follow-up period of 6 ± 2 months. These 11 patients underwent pancreatic or combined pancreatobiliary sphincterotomy with subsequent remission after a median follow-up of 15 months. This study showed that injection of botulinum toxin is safe, may be effective in the short-term, and may predict the outcome from pancreatic sphincter ablation in patients having frequent episodes of pancreatitis, but the need for definitive sphincter ablation in most patients limits its clinical use.

These data show that SOD is the most common cause of IARP when detailed endoscopic evaluation is performed. SOM should be considered the "gold standard" for diagnosing SOD. Complete sphincter evaluation requires manometric assessment of both the biliary and the pancreatic sphincters. Although the best endoscopic therapy of SOD in the setting of IARP warrants further investigation, there is mounting evidence that pancreatic sphincter ablation is necessary in most patients to achieve the best long-term results.

Conclusion

Knowledge of SOD and manometric techniques to assist in this diagnosis is evolving. Successful endoscopic SOM requires good general ERCP skills and careful attention to the main details summarized in this chapter. If SOD is suspected in a type III patient or a type II patient with mild to moderate pain level, medical therapy should generally be tried. If medical therapy fails or is bypassed, ERCP and manometric evaluation should be considered when expertise is available. Although the role of less invasive studies is uncertain, these are generally not advocated because of relatively low sensitivity and specificity. Sphincter ablation is generally warranted in symptomatic type I patients and type II and type III patients with abnormal manometry. Symptom relief ranges from 55% to 95%, depending on the patient presentation and selection. Initial nonresponders after biliary sphincterotomy alone has been performed may benefit from thorough pancreatic sphincter and pancreatic parenchymal evaluation. Data are accumulating to support pancreatic sphincter evaluation and therapy in expert centers, particularly in type III patients, to achieve optimal outcome. Patients with SOD have relatively high complication rates after invasive studies or therapy. A thorough review of the risk-to-benefit ratio with individual patients is mandatory.

References

The complete references list is available online at www.expertconsult.com.

III

Chapter 47

Acute Pancreatitis and Peripancreatic Fluid Collections

Todd H. Baron, Sr.

Video related to this chapter's topics can be found online at expertconsult.com.

Introduction

Acute pancreatitis may be clinically mild or severe. Clinically severe acute pancreatitis is usually a result of pancreatic glandular necrosis. The morbidity and mortality of acute pancreatitis are significantly higher when pancreatic necrosis is present, especially when infection of the necrosis occurs.[1] Patients with pancreatic necrosis must be identified so that appropriate management can be undertaken. The management of patients with necrotizing pancreatitis has shifted from early surgical débridement (necrosectomy) to aggressive intensive medical care. Specific criteria for operative or non-operative intervention have been developed.[2,3] Advances in radiologic imaging and aggressive medical management with emphasis on prevention of infection have allowed for prompt identification of complications and improvement in outcome for these patients.[4] Several types of pancreatic and peripancreatic fluid collections may arise as a result of acute pancreatitis,[5] including acute fluid collections, acute pancreatic pseudocysts, pancreatic abscesses, and organized pancreatic necrosis. This chapter reviews more recent advances in the diagnosis and treatment of acute pancreatitis and peripancreatic fluid collections.

Presentation and Classification of Acute Pancreatitis

Acute pancreatitis usually has a rapid onset manifested by upper abdominal pain, vomiting, fever, tachycardia, leukocytosis, and elevated serum levels of pancreatic enzymes. Gallstone and alcohol-induced pancreatitis are the most common causes in the United States. **Box 47.1** lists causes of pancreatitis. Several classifications of severity of illness for acute pancreatitis are used to identify patients at risk for developing complications (**Table 47.1**).[6,7]

Ranson's score consists of 11 clinical signs with prognostic significance; 5 signs are measured at the time of admission, and 6 signs are measured between admission and 48 hours later. There is good correlation between the number of Ranson signs and the incidence of systemic complications and the presence of pancreatic necrosis.[6] The Acute Physiology, Age, and Chronic Health Evaluation (APACHE) II score is a grading system based on 12 physiologic variables, patient age, and prior history of severe organ system insufficiency or immunocompromised state.[6] This score allows stratification of illness severity on admission and may be recalculated daily. Severe acute pancreatitis is present if there are three or more Ranson's criteria, if the APACHE II score is 8 or greater, or if clinical findings of one or more of the following are present: shock, renal insufficiency, or pulmonary insufficiency.[6] The Glasgow scoring system is another classification system.[7] In contrast to Ranson's criteria, the variables apply if they occur at any time within 48 hours. More recently, a bedside index for severity in acute pancreatitis (BISAP) score was developed.[8] The BISAP score has five variables: blood urea nitrogen greater than 25 mg/dL, impaired mental status, systemic inflammatory response syndrome, age older than 60 years, and pleural effusion detected on imaging. One point is assigned for each variable within 24 hours of presentation to yield a composite score of 0 to 5 (see **Table 47.1**).

Acute pancreatitis may be classified histologically as interstitial-edematous or necrotizing based on the inflammatory changes of the pancreatic parenchyma.[9] According to the International Symposium on Acute Pancreatitis in 1992, pancreatic necrosis is defined as one or more diffuse or focal areas of nonviable pancreatic parenchyma (**Fig. 47.1**).[9] Pancreatic glandular necrosis is usually associated with peripancreatic fat necrosis.[9-11] By definition, the presence of pancreatic necrosis represents a severe form of acute pancreatitis.[9] Approximately 20% to 30% of the 185,000 new cases of acute pancreatitis per year in the United States are necrotizing.[12,13]

Management of Mild Acute Pancreatitis (Interstitial-Edematous)

The management of patients with clinically mild or interstitial pancreatitis is almost entirely supportive. Patients with this form of pancreatitis generally have a self-limited course. There is no role for antibiotic therapy or nutritional support. The

Table 47.1 Severity Scores for Acute Pancreatitis

RANSON'S CRITERIA OF SEVERITY

At Admission	During Initial 48 Hours
Age >55 yr	Hematocrit decrease >10%
WBC >16,000/mm³	BUN increase >5 mg/dL
Blood glucose >200 mg/dL	Serum calcium <8 mg/dL
Serum LDH >350 IU/L	Pao₂ <60 mm Hg
Serum AST >250 IU/L	Base deficit >4 mEq/L
	Fluid sequestration >6 L

Score ≥3 is considered severe

APACHE II SCORE*

Score ≥8 is considered severe

GLASGOW CRITERIA

Within 48 hr of hospitalization
Age >55 yr
WBC >15,000/mm³
Glucose >180 mg/dL
BUN >45 mg/dL
LDH >600 U/L
Albumin <3.3 g/dL
Calcium <8 mg/dL
Pao₂ <60 mm Hg
Score ≥3 is considered severe

BISAP SCORE

BUN >25 mg/dL
Impaired mental status (Glasgow Coma Scale score <15)

SIRS—defined as ≥2 of the following
  Temperature of <36° C or >38° C
  Respiratory rate >20 breaths/min or Paco₂ <32 mm Hg
  Pulse >90 beats/min
  WBC <4000/mm³ or >12,000/mm³ or >10% immature bands

Age >60 yr
Pleural effusion detected on imaging

*Acute physiology score + age points + chronic health points.[5]
AST, aspartate aminotransferase; BISAP, bedside index for severity in acute pancreatitis; BUN, blood urea nitrogen; LDH, lactate dehydrogenase; Paco₂, arterial carbon dioxide tension; Pao, arterial oxygen tension; SIRS, systemic inflammatory response syndrome; WBC, white blood cell count.

Box 47.1 Causes of Acute Pancreatitis

Most Common

Choledocholithiasis
Ethanol
Idiopathic

Less Common

ERCP
Hyperlipidemia (types I, IV, and V)
Drugs
Pancreas divisum
Abdominal trauma
Hereditary (familial)
Sphincter of Oddi dysfunction

ERCP, endoscopic retrograde cholangiopancreatography.

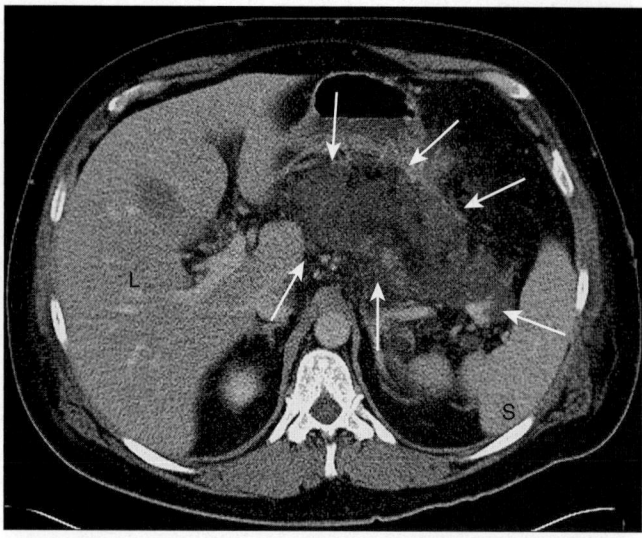

Fig. 47.1 Contrast-enhanced abdominal computed tomography (CT) scan of severe necrotizing pancreatitis. There is contrast enhancement of the liver *(L)* and spleen *(S)*; the normal enhancing pancreas has a similar density. In this case, there is little to no uptake into the pancreas *(arrows)*.

goal of management is to identify the etiology of the pancreatitis and to treat it appropriately. Identification of gallstones in the absence of other factors should be managed with cholecystectomy. Potentially offending drugs should be discontinued, and hyperlipidemia should be addressed. If there is alcohol abuse, a rehabilitation program should be offered to the patient. In some patients, an etiology for acute pancreatitis is not identified, and recurrent attacks occur. The management of these patients is controversial, specifically as it relates to sphincter of Oddi dysfunction and pancreas divisum. Data support pursuing endoscopic evaluation of these entities,[14] although there are no randomized trials proving effectiveness of endoscopic therapy.[15]

Identification and Clinical Importance of Pancreatic Necrosis

Pancreatic necrosis may be pathologically identified at surgery or autopsy. The radiographic diagnosis of pancreatic necrosis is determined by dynamic intravenous contrast–enhanced abdominal computed tomography (CT).[10] Because the normal pancreatic microcirculation is disrupted during acute necrotizing pancreatitis, contrast-enhanced abdominal CT shows a lack of normal contrast enhancement of affected portions of the pancreas (see **Fig. 47.1**)[16]; this may be better detected several days after initial clinical presentation. Contrast-enhanced abdominal CT is the "gold standard" for noninvasive diagnosis of pancreatic necrosis, with an accuracy of greater than 90% when more than 30% glandular necrosis is present.[10] The presence of radiographically detected pancreatic necrosis markedly increases the morbidity and mortality associated with acute pancreatitis.[17] As the percentage of glandular necrosis increases, the morbidity increases.

Theoretically, contrast medium may cause significant additional reductions of capillary flow, which has been shown to aggravate acute pancreatitis in experimental studies.

However, a more recent study in men with severe acute pancreatitis compared patients who did not receive contrast medium with patients who did. Patients in whom contrast medium was administered did not show deterioration of acute pancreatitis.[18] The overall mortality in severe acute pancreatitis is approximately 30%.[13] The mortality occurs in two phases. Early deaths (1 to 2 weeks after onset of pancreatitis) are due to multisystem organ failure from release of inflammatory mediators and cytokines.[1] Late deaths result from local or systemic infections.[19] As long as acute necrotizing pancreatitis remains sterile, the overall mortality is approximately 10%. The mortality rate at least triples if infected necrosis occurs.[12]

Patients with sterile necrosis and high severity of illness scores (Ranson's scores, APACHE II scores) accompanied by multisystem organ failure, shock, or renal insufficiency have a significantly higher mortality.[20] Myriad systemic and local complications of acute necrotizing pancreatitis may occur. Systemic complications have been detailed elsewhere[2] and include adult respiratory distress syndrome, acute renal failure, shock, coagulopathy, hyperglycemia, and hypocalcemia. Local complications include gastrointestinal bleeding, infected necrosis, and adjacent bowel necrosis. Late local complications that may require therapy include development of pancreatic abscess or pancreatic pseudocyst. Early therapy of acute necrotizing pancreatitis consists of the combination of aggressive supportive intensive medical care and prevention of infection using prophylactic antibiotics. Late management requires recognition of local infectious complications (pancreatic infection) and the initiation of aggressive débridement strategies. Infected necrosis develops in 30% to 70% of patients with acute necrotizing pancreatitis and accounts for more than 80% of deaths from acute pancreatitis.[1,3] The risk of infected necrosis increases with increasing amounts of pancreatic glandular necrosis and length of time from onset of acute pancreatitis, peaking at 3 weeks.[1,3]

Infection in Acute Necrotizing Pancreatitis

Because the development of infected necrosis significantly increases the mortality of acute necrotizing pancreatitis, prevention of infection is critical. In experimental acute necrotizing pancreatitis, pancreatic infection occurs primarily as a result of bacterial translocation from the colon.[21] Several animal studies have shown a decrease in pancreatic infection and mortality using orally administered antibiotics for "selective decontamination" of the gut or intravenous antibiotics with high pancreatic tissue penetration.[21–23] Similarly, human studies have shown benefits from orally administered antibiotics with or without rectally administered antibiotics for "selective decontamination" of the gut.[24,25] This regimen has not gained acceptance.

The use of systemic antibiotics for the prevention of pancreatic infection has been studied extensively. Numerous studies have been published in animals and humans regarding the use of prophylactic antibiotics. In addition, several meta-analyses have been performed showing conflicting results. The evidence does not show convincingly that the use of prophylactic antibiotics decreases mortality and need for surgery, although these do seem to decrease in

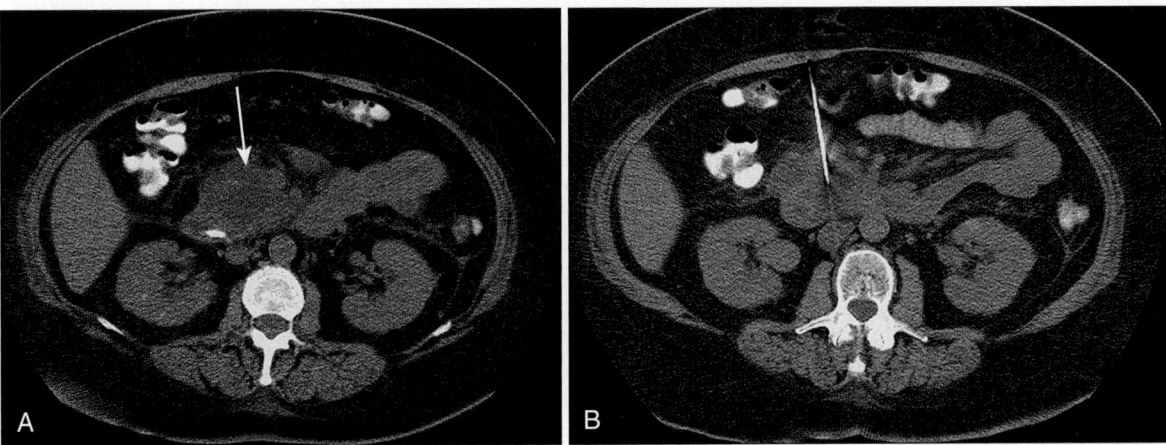

Fig. 47.2 Computed tomography (CT)–guided fine needle aspiration of suspected infected pancreatic necrosis. **A,** CT scan shows necrotic area *(arrow)* within the pancreatic head. **B,** Under CT guidance, an 18-gauge needle is passed into the necrotic area.

nonpancreatic infections.[26–30] At the present time, if administration of prophylactic antibiotics is chosen, intravenous antibiotics with excellent pancreatic tissue penetration (extended penicillins, carbapenems, or fluoroquinolones) is recommended. Duration of therapy of 2 weeks is advocated by some experts.

Sterile and infected acute necrotizing pancreatitis can be difficult to distinguish clinically because both may produce fever, leukocytosis, and severe abdominal pain. The distinction is important because the mortality in patients with infected acute necrotizing pancreatitis without intervention is nearly 100%.[12] The bacteriologic status of the pancreas may be determined by CT-guided fine needle aspiration of pancreatic and peripancreatic tissue or fluid (**Fig. 47.2**).[31,32] This aspiration method is safe and accurate with a sensitivity of 96% and specificity of 99%, and it is recommended in patients with acute necrotizing pancreatitis who experience clinical deterioration or who do not experience clinical improvement despite aggressive supportive care.[2] Ultrasound-guided aspiration may have a lower sensitivity and specificity[33] but can be performed at the bedside. Surveillance aspiration may be repeated on a weekly basis as clinically indicated.

Role of Endoscopic Retrograde Cholangiopancreatography in Severe Acute Gallstone Pancreatitis

Gallstone pancreatitis is caused by impaction of a stone within the common channel of the ampulla of Vater. In most cases, the stone passes without therapy. It is assumed that endoscopic retrograde cholangiopancreatography (ERCP) and biliary sphincterotomy would improve the outcome of gallstone pancreatitis because removal of an impacted stone would relieve obstruction to the flow of pancreatic secretions. Initial studies performing urgent (within 72 hours of admission) ERCP and biliary sphincterotomy (if a stone is identified) in patients with acute gallstone pancreatitis and choledocholithiasis showed an improved outcome in only the group of patients presenting with clinically severe acute

pancreatitis.[34] The improvement was attributed to relief of pancreatic ductal obstruction produced by an impacted gallstone in the common biliary-pancreatic channel of the ampulla of Vater. More recent studies suggest the improved outcome after ERCP and sphincterotomy in gallstone pancreatitis results from reduced biliary sepsis, rather than a true improvement in pancreatitis.[35,36]

In the presence of pancreatic ductal disruption, a frequent occurrence in acute necrotizing pancreatitis,[37] introduction of infection by incidental pancreatography during ERCP may theoretically occur, transforming acute necrotizing pancreatitis from sterile to infected. ERCP in patients with severe gallstone acute pancreatitis must be employed judiciously and reserved for patients with suspected biliary obstruction based on hyperbilirubinemia and clinical cholangitis because it is unlikely that the ampulla is obstructed in the presence of a normal serum bilirubin.[38,39] Other imaging modalities, such as endoscopic ultrasound (EUS) and magnetic resonance cholangiopancreatography, may be used in patients with severe biliary pancreatitis with the goal of selectively performing ERCP in patients with documented bile duct stones.[7,40] Whether empiric biliary sphincterotomy should be performed if bile duct stones are not identified is unknown, but this seems to be a reasonable approach.[41]

Nutritional Support for Acute Necrotizing Pancreatitis

To meet increased metabolic demands and to "rest" the pancreas, total parenteral nutrition (TPN) administered through a central venous catheter was used for nutritional support in patients with acute necrotizing pancreatitis. TPN does not hasten resolution of acute pancreatitis or preserve gut integrity, an important factor in preventing bacterial translocation. Randomized prospective studies of TPN and enteral feeding (through a nasoenteric feeding tube placed radiographically beyond the ligament of Treitz) instituted within 48 hours of onset of severe acute pancreatitis[42,43] showed that enteral feeding was well tolerated without adverse clinical effects and resulted in significantly fewer total and infectious complications. In a meta-analysis, enteral nutrition significantly reduced mortality, infectious complications, and pancreatic infections in patients with predicted severe pancreatitis compared with TPN.[44] The cost of nutritional support was threefold higher in the TPN group.[42] Acute phase response and disease severity scores were significantly improved after enteral nutrition.[43]

This form of enteral feeding seems to be preferable in patients with acute necrotizing pancreatitis in the absence of a significant ileus.[45] This approach has been extended to nasogastric feeding. In a review of four studies comprising 92 patients in which nasogastric feeding was compared with nasojejunal feeding, mortality and intolerance to feeding were similar.[46]

Enteral feeding is the preferred strategy with TPN reserved for patients when the gut has failed or administration of enteral nutrition is impossible for other reasons (e.g., prolonged ileus, complex pancreatic fistulas, abdominal compartment syndrome).[47] Various endoscopic techniques are available for placing nasojejunal feeding tubes in the setting of acute pancreatitis.[47] One method avoids the need to transfer the guidewire from the mouth to the nose. A small-caliber endoscope is passed transnasally into the duodenum.[48] A guidewire is advanced through the endoscope beyond the ligament of Treitz. The endoscope is withdrawn leaving the guidewire in place. The tube is passed over the guidewire with or without fluoroscopic guidance.

Interventions for Pancreatic Necrosis

The timing and type of pancreatic intervention for patients with acute necrotizing pancreatitis are controversial. Because the mortality from sterile acute necrotizing pancreatitis is approximately 10%, and surgical intervention has not been shown to reduce this figure, most investigators recommend supportive medical therapy in this group.[12] Conversely, infected acute necrotizing pancreatitis is traditionally considered uniformly fatal without intervention,[12] although small, retrospective studies found that antibiotic therapy alone was effective in a select group of patients.[49,50] Surgical pancreatic débridement (necrosectomy) remains the standard with which other drainage strategies are compared and may require multiple abdominal reexplorations.[45]

Necrosectomy should be undertaken soon after confirmation of infected necrosis. The role of surgery in patients with multisystem organ failure and sterile necrosis remains unproved, although this scenario is frequently cited as an indication for surgical débridement.[51] Additionally, the longer that surgical intervention can be delayed from the onset of acute necrotizing pancreatitis, the better the patient survival[52]; this is probably related to improved demarcation between viable and necrotic tissue at the time of operation. The role of delayed necrosectomy (after resolution of multisystem organ failure) in sterile acute necrotizing pancreatitis likewise is controversial. Some investigators advocate débridement in patients who remain systemically ill 4 to 6 weeks after onset of acute pancreatitis with fever, weight loss, intractable abdominal pain, inability to eat, and "failure to thrive."[2,53,54] Others believe that delayed necrosectomy is unnecessary as long as the process remains sterile.[54]

Surgical Débridement for Pancreatic Necrosis

Surgical methods for treatment of necrosis vary. There are three main types of surgical débridement: conventional drainage, open or semiopen procedures, or closed procedures.[45] Conventional drainage involves necrosectomy with placement of standard surgical drains and reoperation on demand (fever, leukocytosis, lack of improvement by imaging studies). Open or semiopen management employs necrosectomy and either scheduled repeat laparotomies or open packing that leaves the abdominal wound exposed for frequent dressing changes. Closed management involves necrosectomy with extensive intraoperative lavage of the pancreatic bed. The abdomen is closed over large-bore drains for continuous high-volume postoperative lavage of the lesser sac.

Most surgeons have abandoned the conventional surgical approach of débridement because inadequately removed necrotic tissue becomes or remains infected and results in a mortality of approximately 40%.[3] In all procedures except the closed technique, multiple operations are frequently required to remove the necrotic pancreatic and peripancreatic material.[3] Leaving the abdomen open avoids the need for formal laparotomies; packing may be changed in the intensive care unit. Repeated débridement and manipulation of the abdominal viscera using the open and semiopen techniques result in a high rate of postoperative local complications such as pancreatic fistulas, small and large bowel complications, and bleeding from the pancreatic bed. Pancreatic and gastrointestinal tract fistulas occur in 41% of patients after surgical necrosectomy and often require additional surgery for closure.[55,56] The mortality using open or closed techniques is approximately 20%.[3]

Alternative Débridement Methods

Alternative methods for débridement of pancreatic necrosis have been described. The precise role of these techniques in the management of patients with necrotizing pancreatitis still needs to be precisely defined, although they seem to be increasingly used as an alternative to surgery.

Percutaneous (Interventional Radiology) Therapy

Successful percutaneous therapy for infected acute necrotizing pancreatitis has been described using large-bore percutaneous catheters up to 28-Fr diameter in conjunction with aggressive irrigation.[57] At a mean of 9 days after hospital admission for necrotizing pancreatitis with medically uncontrolled sepsis, 34 patients had percutaneous drainage and irrigation catheters inserted into the pancreatic collection. An average of three separate catheter sites per patient and four catheter exchanges per patient was necessary for removal of necrotic material. Pancreatic surgery was completely avoided in 16 patients (47%). Control of sepsis with delayed elective surgery for repair of external pancreatic fistulas related to catheter placement was achieved in nine patients. Nine patients required immediate surgery for failure of percutaneous therapy. The mortality was 12% in these ill patients, many of whom had multisystem organ failure. In a similar fashion, Echenique and associates[58] described successful percutaneous drainage of

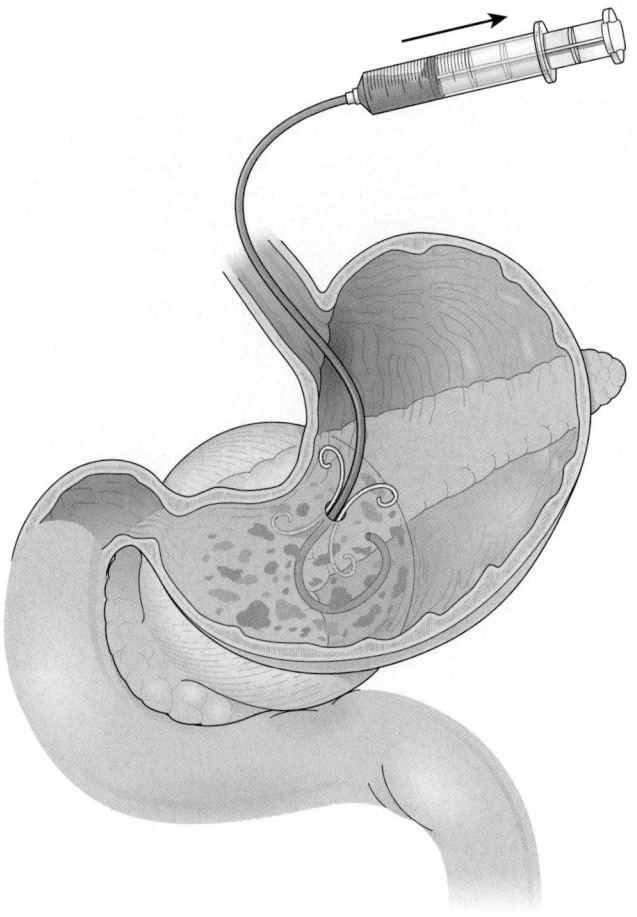

Fig. 47.3 Transmural drainage of organized pancreatic necrosis. Two stents are placed transgastrically alongside a nasobiliary irrigation tube. The transgastric tract is dilated to a large caliber (15 to 20 mm) to allow egress of solid material around the stents. *(Redrawn from Baron TH, Harewood GC, Morgan DE, et al: Outcome differences after endoscopic drainage of pancreatic necrosis, acute pancreatic pseudocysts, and chronic pancreatic pseudocysts. Gastrointest Endosc 56:7–17, 2002.)*

necrosis in 20 patients with documented necrosis. Solid debris was removed percutaneously using basket extraction techniques. Similar results have been obtained by other authors, although percutaneous therapy is most often used to improve immediate sepsis and delay necrosectomy.[59,60] Percutaneous access has also been used to allow subsequent passage of rigid endoscopes for débridement of necrosis.[61]

Flexible Endoscopic Therapy

Successful endoscopic drainage of symptomatic sterile or infected pancreatic necrosis several weeks after the onset of severe necrotizing pancreatitis has been described.[62] The initial descriptions used transmural placement (transgastric or transduodenal) of internal 10-Fr diameter drainage catheters plus a 7-Fr nasopancreatic irrigation tube into the retroperitoneum. The catheters are placed through a tract dilated up to 20 mm (**Fig. 47.3**). With this method, solid debris flows around the catheters through the transenteric tract. Complete nonsurgical resolution has been achieved in

84% of patients with this form of late, or "organized" pancreatic necrosis.[63,64]

Complications of endoscopic therapy (described in more detail in the section on peripancreatic fluid collections) include perforation, bleeding, and infection. Adjuvant percutaneous drains using this technique are often required to drain peripheral collections away from the body of the pancreas. Beginning in 2005, the flexible endoscopic approach evolved to incorporate direct endoscopic débridement.[65] Rather than relying on irrigation to débride necrotic material, the transmural entry site is dilated to a much larger diameter to allow passage of an upper endoscope directly inside the necrotic cavity to allow "direct" débridement (**Fig. 47.4**). Direct endoscopic necrosectomy has been shown to be superior to the initially described irrigation method with a higher success rate and less need for percutaneous catheters.[66] There are now many series on this approach with success rates of approximately 80%.[67–73]

Multiple procedures are nearly uniformly required before complete resolution is achieved. The drainage options for patients with pancreatic necrosis are expanding. The experience using newer, nonsurgical drainage procedures is limited, and no interdisciplinary comparative data exist. When deciding on the timing or treatment modality to be employed in these complex patients, the expertise of the local surgeon, interventional endoscopist, and interventional radiologist must be considered. Nonsurgical drainage of pancreatic necrosis, whether performed acutely in the first weeks or subacutely at 1 month or more after pancreatitis onset, should be undertaken only by expert interventional endoscopists or interventional radiologists familiar with the potential complications and time required for successful pancreatic drainage. Improperly drained sterile necrosis may lead to life-threatening infected necrosis. An upfront team approach in planning pancreatic interventions is useful because some patients may benefit from multimodality drainage. The decision to intervene should be based on infection of the necrosis or, in the setting of sterile necrosis, severe clinical symptoms such as gastric outlet obstruction, intractable abdominal pain, or failure to thrive.[74]

Long-Term Sequelae of Acute Necrotizing Pancreatitis

Despite the enormous cost of caring for patients with acute necrotizing pancreatitis, mean quality-of-life outcomes up to 2 years after treatment of pancreatic necrosis are similar to outcomes obtained with coronary artery bypass grafting.[75] The long-term clinical endocrine and exocrine consequences of acute necrotizing pancreatitis seem to depend on several factors including the severity of necrosis, etiology (alcoholic vs. nonalcoholic), continued use of alcohol, and the degree of surgical pancreatic débridement.[76] Exocrine function studies show persistent functional insufficiency in most patients up to 2 years after severe acute pancreatitis.[77] Use of pancreatic enzymes should be restricted to patients with symptoms of steatorrhea and weight loss secondary to fat malabsorption. Although subtle glucose intolerance is frequent, overt diabetes mellitus is uncommon.[78] Follow-up pancreatography frequently reveals obstructive pancreatic ductal abnormalities that may account for persistent symptoms of abdominal pain or acute recurrent pancreatitis (**Fig. 47.5**).[79]

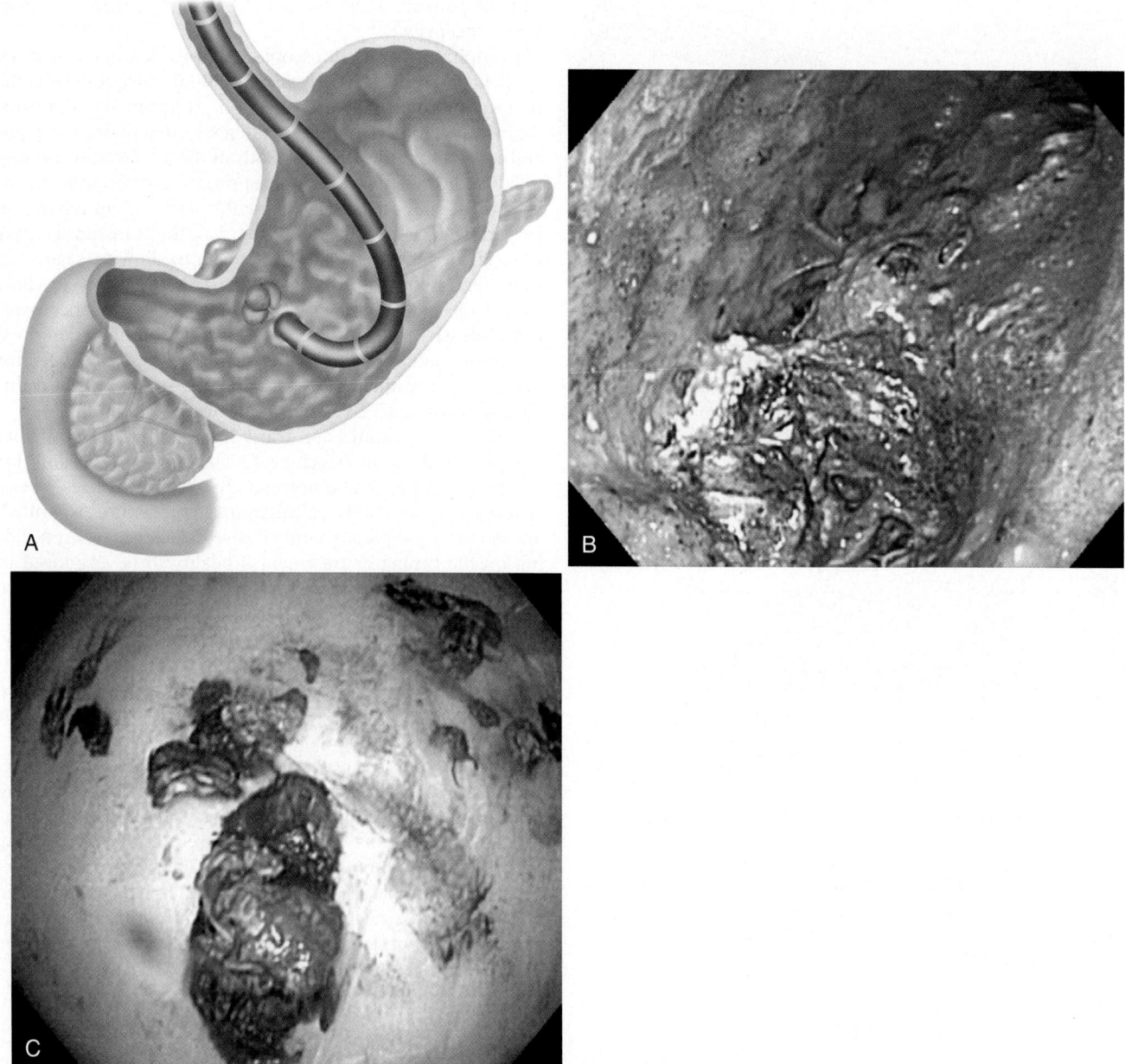

Fig. 47.4 Direct endoscopic necrosectomy. **A,** Direct endoscopic necrosectomy. A flexible endoscope is passed transorally then transmurally into the necrotic cavity. **B,** Endoscopic image taken within the necrotic cavity during direct endoscopic necrosectomy. **C,** Necrotic debris removed during direct endoscopic necrosectomy. *(From Baron TH, Kozarek R, Carr-Locke DL: ERCP. Philadelphia, 2007, Saunders, p 487.)*

Summary of Management of Clinically Severe Acute Pancreatitis

Box 47.2 summarizes the overall approach to the management of acute pancreatitis.

Pancreatic and Peripancreatic Fluid Collections

Pancreatic fluid collections (PFCs) arise as complication of acute and chronic pancreatitis or pancreatic trauma

(including postsurgical). PFCs that occur as a result of acute pancreatitis include acute fluid collections, pancreatic pseudocysts, pancreatic abscesses, and organized pancreatic necrosis (**Table 47.2**). These collections are amendable to endoscopic drainage. This section outlines the nomenclature, endoscopic drainage methods, and outcomes after endoscopic intervention of PFCs. Although there are other drainage options for these collections (percutaneous and surgical), these are not discussed in detail. Many gastroenterologists assume that any PFC arising as a consequence of acute pancreatitis represents a pancreatic pseudocyst. This assumption is incorrect, and it is important to recognize that several distinct entities fall

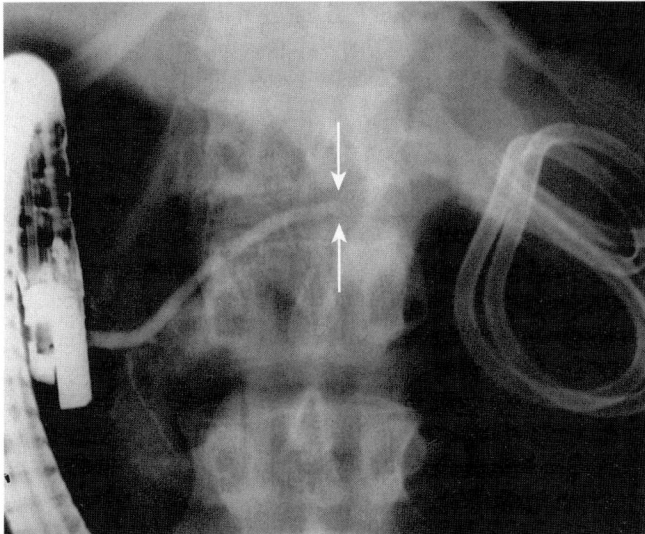

Fig. 47.5 Complete cutoff of main pancreatic duct (arrows) shown at endoscopic retrograde cholangiopancreatography (ERCP) at the time of removal of transgastric double pigtail stents (visible) after successful endoscopic drainage of organized pancreatic necrosis.

Table 47.2 **Types of Pancreatic Fluid Collections Complicating Acute Pancreatitis**

Term	Definition
Acute fluid collection	Collection of enzyme-rich pancreatic juice occurring early (within 48 hr) in the course of acute pancreatitis, located in or near the pancreas, and always lacks well-defined wall of granulation tissue or fibrous tissue
Acute pseudocyst	Collection of pancreatic juice enclosed by wall of nonepithelialized granulation tissue, arises as a consequence of acute pancreatitis, requires at least 4 wk to form, and is devoid of significant solid debris
Pancreatic necrosis (early)	Diffuse or focal area of nonviable pancreatic parenchyma >30% of the gland by contrast-enhanced CT, which is typically associated with peripancreatic fat necrosis
Organized or walled-off pancreatic necrosis (late)	Evolution of acute necrosis to partially encapsulated, well-defined collection of pancreatic juice and necrotic debris
Pancreatic abscess	Circumscribed intraabdominal collection of pus, usually in proximity to pancreas, containing little or no pancreatic necrosis, which arises as a consequence of acute pancreatitis or pancreatic trauma

CT, computed tomography.

Box 47.2 **Keys to Successful Management of Acute Necrotizing Pancreatitis**

Identify Necrosis

Clinically severe using severity of index scores
CT scan showing significant pancreatic necrosis—≥30% glandular necrosis by contrast-enhanced CT

Intensive Care Unit Management for Clinically Severe Acute Pancreatitis

Supportive care
Consider early use of antibiotics for radiographically documented pancreatic necrosis
Early endoscopic retrograde cholangiography for gallstone pancreatitis in the setting of jaundice or cholangitis
Nutritional support: Enteral feeding via nasoenteric tube beyond the ligament of Treitz (in the absence of significant ileus)

Identification of Infected Necrosis

CT-guided or EUS-guided fine needle aspiration

Débridement of Infected Necrosis

Operative management
Alternative débridement techniques (percutaneous or endoscopic) in selected centers with expertise

CT, computed tomography; EUS, endoscopic ultrasound.

Types of Pancreatic Fluid Collections

The types of PFCs occurring as a result of acute pancreatitis are acute fluid collections, pancreatic necrosis, pancreatic abscess, and pancreatic pseudocysts.

Acute Fluid Collections

Acute fluid collections arise early in the course of acute pancreatitis, are usually peripancreatic in location, and usually resolve without sequelae but may evolve into pancreatic pseudocysts (**Fig. 47.6**). Acute fluid collections rarely require drainage.[5,81]

Acute Pancreatic Pseudocyst

Acute pancreatic pseudocysts arise as a sequela of acute pancreatitis, require at least 4 weeks to form, and are devoid of significant solid debris (**Fig. 47.7A**). An acute pancreatic pseudocyst usually forms as a result of limited pancreatic necrosis that produces a pancreatic ductal leak (**Fig. 47.7B and C**). Alternatively, areas of pancreatic and peripancreatic fat necrosis may completely liquefy over time and become a

under the general terms of *peripancreatic* and *pancreatic fluid collections*. In 1985, Kozarek and colleagues[80] reported transmural (transgastric and transduodenal) placement of an endoprosthesis into pancreatic pseudocysts in four patients. Subsequently, a large body of literature describing endoscopic drainage of PFCs has emerged.

pseudocyst.[82] Despite the requirement of at least 4 weeks for a pseudocyst to form, this time period in and of itself does not define the collection as a pancreatic pseudocyst. In patients with significant pancreatic necrosis (≥30%), the early acute pancreatic necrosis and peripancreatic necrosis may evolve into a collection that resembles a pseudocyst radiographically but has been present for 4 or more weeks (see the next section on organized or walled-off pancreatic necrosis). By definition,

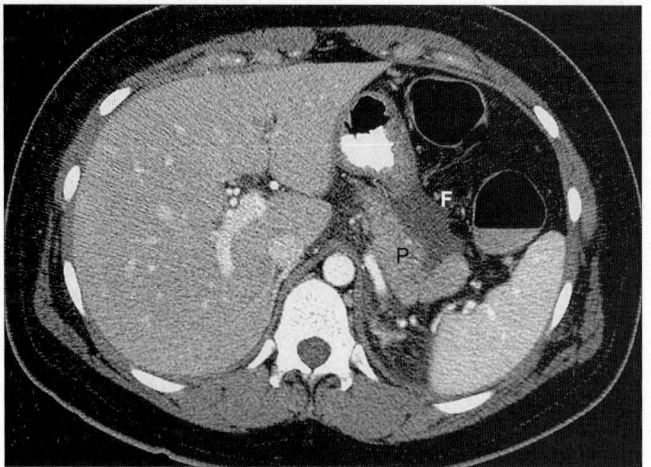

Fig. 47.6 Acute fluid collection. Fluid *(F)* is present adjacent to the pancreas and stomach. Normal enhancement of the pancreas *(P)* is seen.

if these collections contain significant solid debris, they are not pseudocysts, and endoscopic treatment of these collections by typical pseudocyst drainage methods may result in infectious complications because of inadequate removal of solid debris.[62,83]

Organized or Walled-off Pancreatic Necrosis

Pancreatic necrosis is defined as nonviable pancreatic parenchyma usually with associated peripancreatic fat necrosis.[9] In the earliest form, this entity is detected radiographically on contrast-enhanced CT by the presence of nonenhancing pancreatic parenchyma (see **Fig. 47.1**). Pancreatic necrosis is frequently accompanied by the development of major pancreatic ductal disruptions.[84] The collection may continue to evolve over several weeks and expand the initial area of necrosis and contain both liquid and solid debris (**Fig. 47.8**). The resulting collection has been referred to as organized or walled-off pancreatic necrosis to differentiate this process from the early (acute) phase of pancreatic necrosis.[62,63,85]

As mentioned previously, the radiographic appearance of organized pancreatic necrosis on CT may be similar to an acute pseudocyst. Because the underlying solid debris is frequently not discernible by CT,[86] its homogeneous appearance may lead one to embark on standard pseudocyst drainage methods, which do not remove the underlying solid material adequately. Serious infectious complications may result.[62,83,87] A more recent study showed that there are features on CT that can distinguish walled-off pancreatitis necrosis from

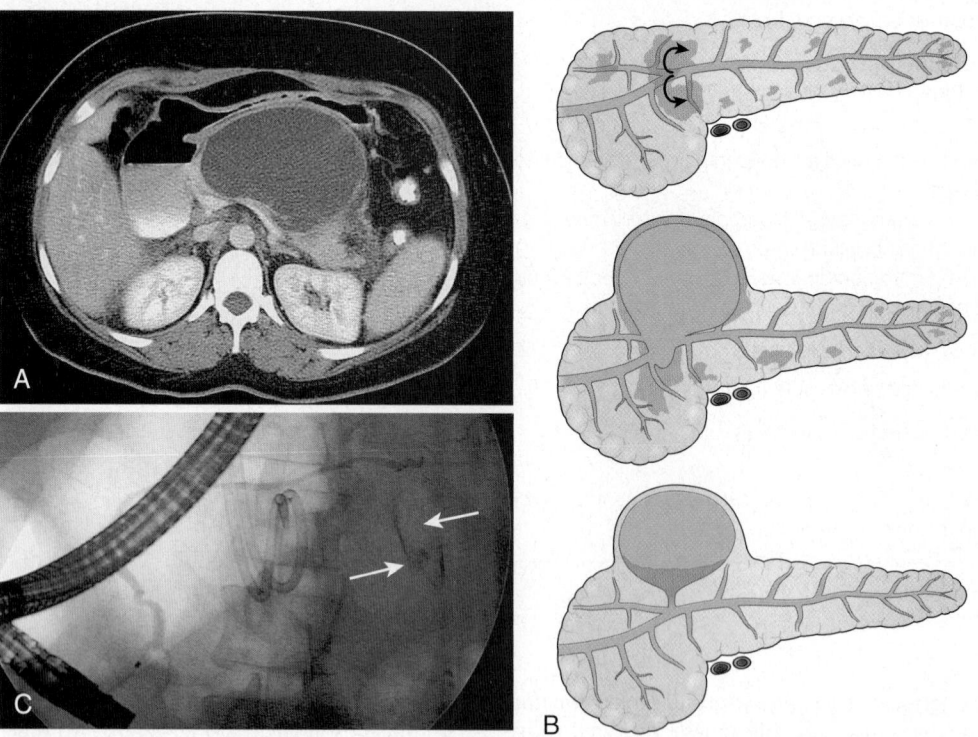

Fig. 47.7 Acute pseudocyst. **A,** Computed tomography (CT) scan shows homogeneous collection arising 4 weeks after clinically mild acute pancreatitis. **B,** Mechanism of formation of acute pancreatic pseudocyst. Limited necrosis of the main pancreatic duct produces a leak with accumulation of amylase-rich fluid. **C,** Pancreatogram in the same patient in **A** shows intact main duct with side branch leak *(arrows)*. *(B, Redrawn from Bradley EL 3rd, editor:* Acute pancreatitis: Diagnosis and therapy, *New York, 1994, Raven Press, p 73.)*

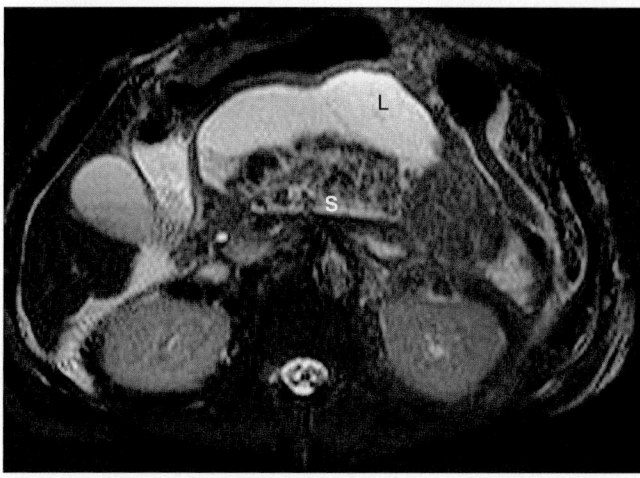

Fig. 47.9 Magnetic resonance (MR) imaging of pancreatic fluid collection (PFC) that appeared homogeneous by computed tomography (CT) scan. The patient had had severe necrotizing pancreatitis 6 weeks previously. The liquid component *(L)* has a whitish appearance, and the solid component *(S)* has a black appearance.

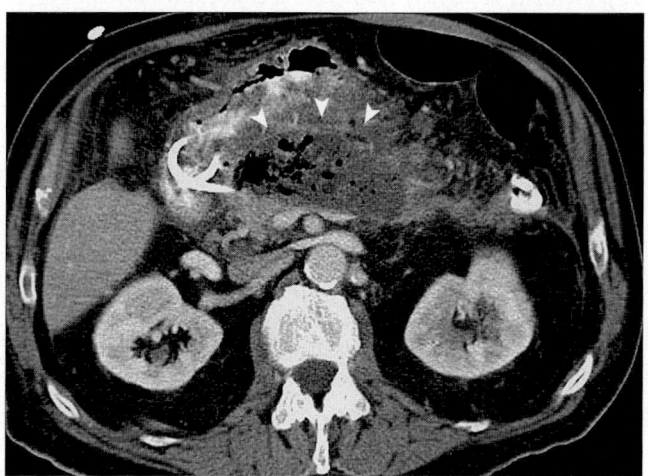

Fig. 47.10 Computed tomography (CT) scan obtained several days after endoscopic placement of transduodenal drainage catheter into pancreatic fluid collection (PFC). *Arrowheads* denote collection that contains nondependent air and debris.

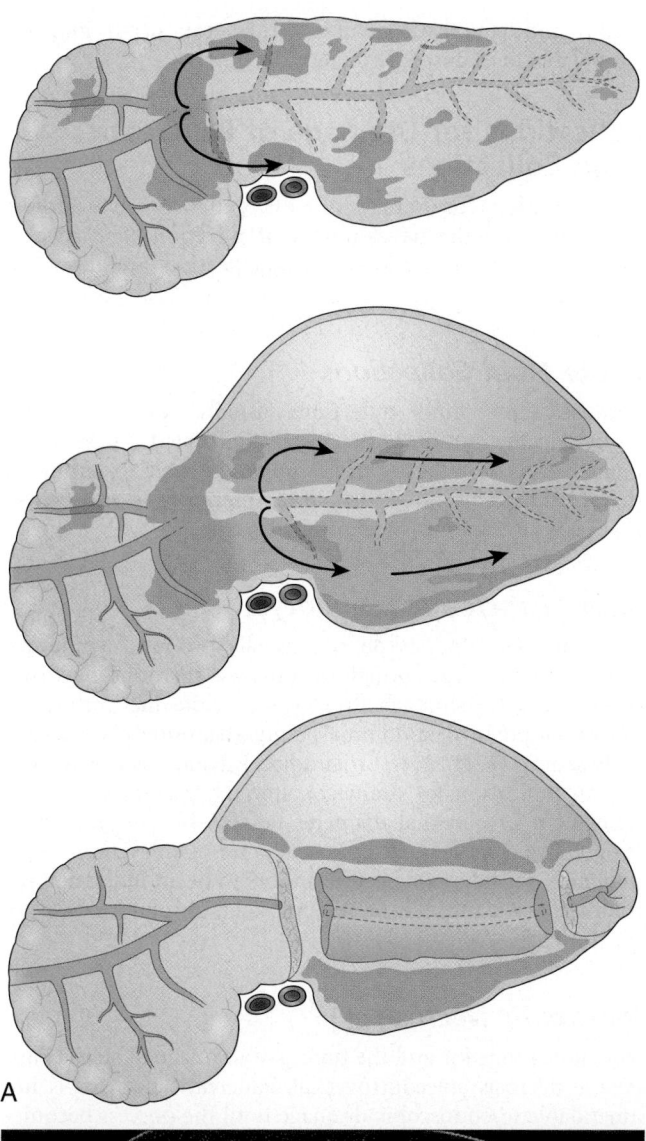

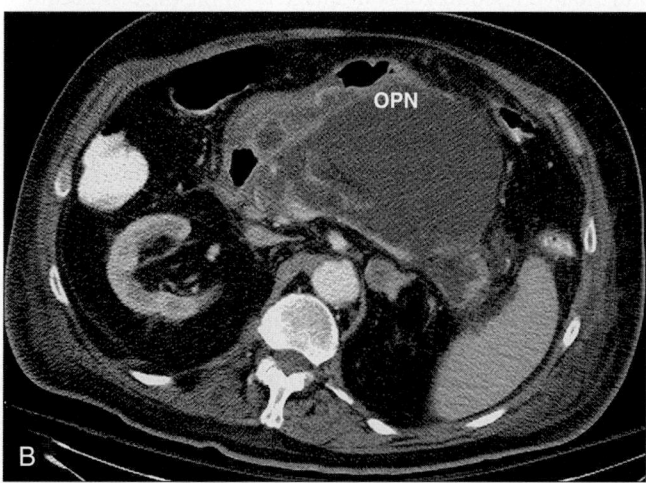

Fig. 47.8 Organized pancreatic necrosis. **A,** Formation of organized pancreatic necrosis. Mechanism of pancreatic duct disconnection is shown in bottom panel. **B,** Contrast-enhanced computed tomography (CT) scan shows large collection that has nearly replaced the pancreatic bed. This collection is consistent with organized pancreatic necrosis *(OPN).* (**A,** *Redrawn from Bradley EL 3rd, editor:* Acute pancreatitis: Diagnosis and therapy, *New York, 1994, Raven Press, p 73.)*

pancreatic pseudocysts.[88] The findings seen with walled-off pancreatitis necrosis include larger size, extension to the paracolic space, irregular wall definition, presence of fat attenuation debris within the collection, and pancreatic deformity or discontinuity. Other CT correlates that indicate the presence of walled-off pancreatitis necrosis include significant necrosis on an early contrast-enhanced CT scan obtained at the time of—or soon after—the initial bout of pancreatitis and evolution of changes on serial CT scans.

Magnetic resonance (MR) imaging before attempted drainage can also delineate the solid debris within the collection (**Fig. 47.9**).[88] Finally, a repeat abdominal CT scan after endoscopic drainage depicts solid material after some of the liquid component has been evacuated (**Fig. 47.10**).[87] Endoscopic findings at the time of drainage may alert the endoscopist to the presence of necrotic debris within the collection. If the collection is drained transmurally, solid material may be seen to flow from the collection; the presence of chocolate-brown or extremely turbid fluid (in the absence of clinical infection) also suggests underlying necrosis. During pancreatography, the finding of complete main pancreatic duct disruption suggests that pancreatic necrosis occurred during the initial course of pancreatitis and may be present in the collection. During contrast agent injection, either through the main pancreatic duct or transmurally, the finding of large filling defects within the collection denotes the presence of solid material.

If any or all of the aforementioned findings are recognized, appropriate steps must be taken to evacuate the underlying solid debris to prevent secondary infection (see section on endoscopic methods of drainage of PFCs later). Overall, one should consider the evolution of a pancreatic collection from the early phase of acute pancreatic necrosis toward a pseudocyst as a spectrum, with walled-off pancreatitis necrosis as an intermediate stage, but also realizing that some collections might not ever become completely liquefied.

Pancreatic Abscess

A pancreatic abscess is defined as a collection of pus in close proximity to the pancreas (**Fig. 47.11**). Some authors include infected pancreatic pseudocysts in the definitions of an abscess but not infected pancreatic necrosis. Pancreatic abscesses may arise from limited pancreatic or peripancreatic fat necrosis that subsequently liquefies and becomes infected.[5]

Chronic Pancreatic Pseudocyst

Chronic pseudocysts are a complication of chronic pancreatitis. Obstruction of the main pancreatic duct from strictures or stones results in upstream ductal blowout. Resultant symptoms requiring drainage are similar to the symptoms described for acute pseudocysts. In addition, symptomatic pancreatic

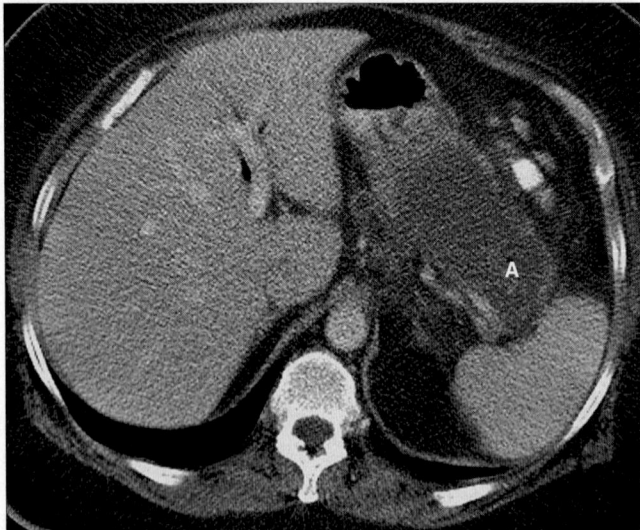

Fig. 47.11 Pancreatic abscess. This patient developed a septic episode 5 weeks after a bout of moderate acute pancreatitis. Cultures confirmed polymicrobial bacterial infection. The collection was successfully drained endoscopically via a transmural approach.

ascites and pancreaticopleural fistulas can occur and are amendable to endoscopic therapy.[89]

Indications for Drainage of Pancreatic Fluid Collections

The indications for drainage of a PFC generally are to address symptoms and the development of infection. The specific indications for drainage of each collection are discussed separately.

Acute Fluid Collections

Because acute fluid collections usually resolve without sequelae, intervention is not usually indicated unless documented infection occurs and is not responsive to antibiotic therapy. There are no reports in the literature of endoscopic drainage, although it is technically feasible.

Acute Pancreatic Pseudocyst

Pancreatic pseudocysts do not usually produce symptoms, unless they are large enough to compress surrounding structures such as the stomach, duodenum, or bile duct with resultant development of abdominal pain, gastric outlet obstruction, early satiety, weight loss, or jaundice. Pseudocyst size alone is not an indication for drainage, although pseudocysts larger than 6 cm in maximal diameter tend to be symptomatic.[90] Progressive enlargement of a pseudocyst in an asymptomatic patient is considered by some authors to be an indication for drainage.[91] An infected pseudocyst is an absolute indication for drainage.

Pancreatic Necrosis

The indications for and the timing of drainage of sterile pancreatic necrosis are controversial. Pancreatic necrosis is not amendable to endoscopic drainage until the process becomes organized, which usually occurs several weeks after onset of pancreatitis. If the process remains sterile, the general indications for drainage are refractory abdominal pain, gastric outlet obstruction, or failure to thrive (continued systemic illness, anorexia, and weight loss) 4 or more weeks after the onset of acute pancreatitis.[62] The severity of CT scan findings alone is not an indication for drainage. Because endoscopic drainage of these collections is more technically difficult, carries a higher rate of complications, and tends to involve more severely ill patients, the decision to intervene endoscopically in patients with sterile pancreatic necrosis must be carefully considered.

Alternative management options to endoscopic drainage include nutritional support with parenteral or enteral jejunal feeding and nonendoscopic drainage methods such as percutaneous or surgical drainage.[74] The final management option is usually based on local expertise and severity of comorbid medical illnesses. These patients ideally are best managed by a multidisciplinary approach.[87] Infected pancreatic necrosis is considered an indication for drainage. Infected necrosis may be indistinguishable clinically from sterile necrosis because of leukocytosis and fever. Percutaneous fine needle aspiration may be required to determine the bacteriologic status of the necrosis.

Pancreatic Abscess

By definition, a pancreatic abscess is infected and is an indication for drainage.

Evaluation before Drainage

Before embarking on endoscopic drainage of a PFC, the endoscopist must always ask the following questions:

1. Is the pancreatic collection an inflammatory collection? In other words, did the collection arise as a result of pancreatitis? There are many masqueraders of pancreatic pseudocysts, including cystic pancreatic neoplasms, duplication cysts, true pancreatic cysts, pseudoaneurysms, solid necrotic neoplasms (e.g., retroperitoneal sarcoma), and lymphoceles.[85,92,93] If the patient does not have a well-documented history of pancreatitis, the endoscopist should be wary that something other than a pseudocyst is present.[94]
2. Could the patient have an underlying pancreatic adenocarcinoma? An elderly patient who either presents with "idiopathic pancreatitis" complicated by pancreatic pseudocyst formation or develops a documented pancreatic pseudocyst in the absence of clinical pancreatitis should be carefully evaluated to exclude an underlying pancreatic neoplasm causing pancreatic ductal obstruction and upstream ductal leak.[95]

When the decision has been made to perform endoscopic drainage of a PFC, imaging and laboratory evaluation should be considered, including the following:

1. Oral and intravenous contrast abdominal CT scan allows assessment of the precise location of the collection in relation to the stomach and duodenum in anticipation of possible transmural drainage. Additionally, the relationship of the collection to potential intervening vascular structures can be assessed. Surrounding varices from splenic vein or portal vein thrombosis may also be visualized. The finding of inhomogeneity within the collection suggests the presence of underlying solid debris.[86]
2. EUS can be used before considering drainage of a PFC for two reasons. First, in a patient with a pancreatic collection following a documented episode of pancreatitis, EUS allows assessment of the collection for the presence of significant solid debris that may alter the management strategy. Second, if the endoscopist is uncertain as to whether the collection in question represents a true pseudocyst or other noninflammatory cystic lesion, EUS allows one to obtain a definitive diagnosis by using the ultrasound features and analyzing cyst contents aspirated during EUS.[96] When the endoscopist is certain that the lesion in question is a PFC and the decision has been made to proceed with endoscopic drainage, EUS may be used to guide transmural drainage as discussed in the next section.
3. MR imaging can determine the presence of solid debris to plan for irrigation methods or an alternative drainage strategy, depending on local expertise and necrosis drainage preferences.[88]

Coagulation parameters must also be considered.

Endoscopic Methods of Drainage of Pancreatic Fluid Collections

The following methods apply to endoscopic drainage of PFCs that do not have significant underlying solid debris (necrosis), such as acute pancreatic pseudocysts. The endoscopic management of organized or walled-off pancreatic necrosis is addressed separately. Endoscopic approaches to pseudocysts are transpapillary drainage,[97,98] transmural drainage,[99] and combined transpapillary and transmural drainage.[93,100] The decision to proceed with one approach over another is based on the anatomic relationship of the collection to the stomach or duodenum, the presence of ductal communication, and the size of the collection. If the stomach or duodenum is not in close apposition to the wall of the collection (within 1 cm by CT), it is not approachable transmurally. If the collection is very large, attempted transpapillary drainage alone in the presence of a ductal communication may result in infection because the transpapillary drainage process is relatively slow, and contrast agent injection introduces bacterial or fungal organisms or both into the collection. The endoscopic approach to patients with large pseudocysts (>6 cm) using combined transpapillary and transmural drainage is analogous to the treatment of large bilomas complicating laparoscopic cholecystectomy using percutaneous drainage for the biloma and endoscopic therapy to close the biliary ductal leak.

Transpapillary Approach

If the collection communicates with the main pancreatic duct, placement of a pancreatic endoprosthesis with or without pancreatic sphincterotomy is a useful approach, especially for collections measuring 5 to 6 cm or less that are not otherwise approachable transmurally.[101] The proximal end of the stent (toward the pancreatic tail) may enter the collection directly or bridge the area of leak into the pancreatic duct upstream from the leak (**Fig. 47.12**). Data suggest that complete bridging of the leak is the best approach.[102] The diameter of pancreatic stent used depends on the pancreatic ductal diameter but is usually 7-Fr. The advantage of the transpapillary approach over the transmural approach is the avoidance of bleeding or perforation that may occur with transmural drainage. The disadvantage of transpapillary drainage is that pancreatic stents may induce scarring of the main pancreatic duct in patients whose pancreatic duct is otherwise normal (i.e., patients with acute pseudocysts and small side-branch disruption).[103,104]

Transmural Approach

Transmural drainage of PFCs is achieved by placing one or more large-bore stents through the gastric or duodenal wall (**Fig. 47.13**). There is no standardized approach to this method of drainage, and some authorities believe that EUS evaluation is mandatory before performing endoscopic transmural drainage of PFCs.[107] EUS-guided and non–EUS-guided drainage is discussed.

Endoscopic Ultrasound–Guided Transmural Drainage

EUS may increase the success rate and reduce complications related to transmural entry of PFCs.[108] There are two ways

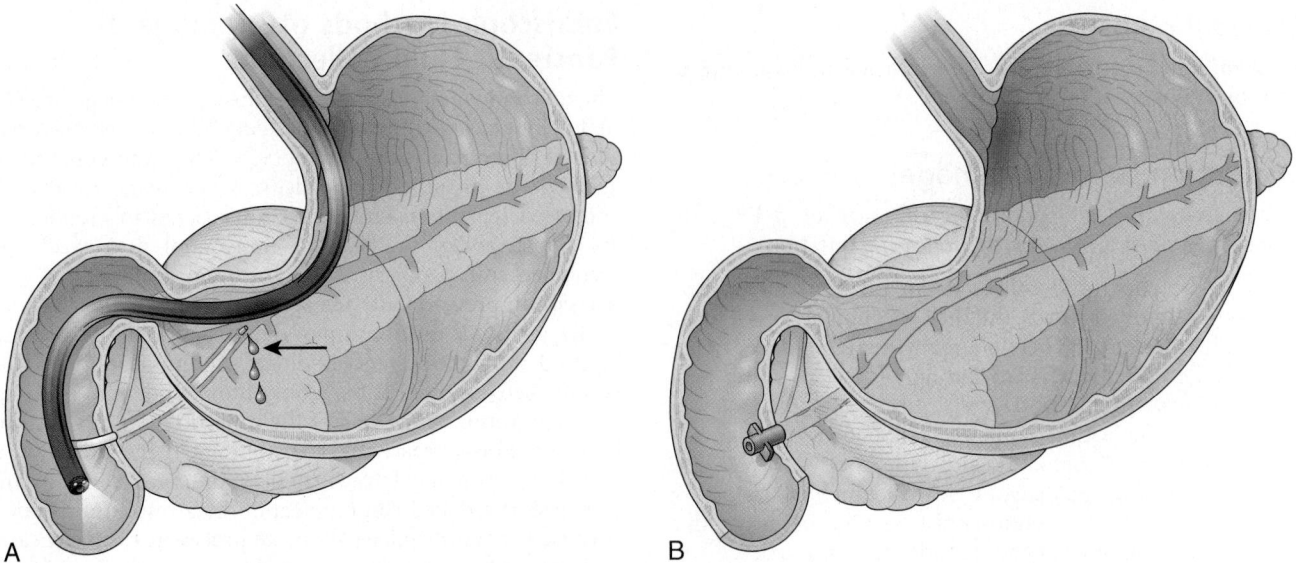

Fig. 47.12 Transpapillary drainage of pancreatic pseudocyst. **A,** Pancreatogram shows a leak off a side branch of the main pancreatic duct. **B,** Pancreatic duct stent is in place across the leak.

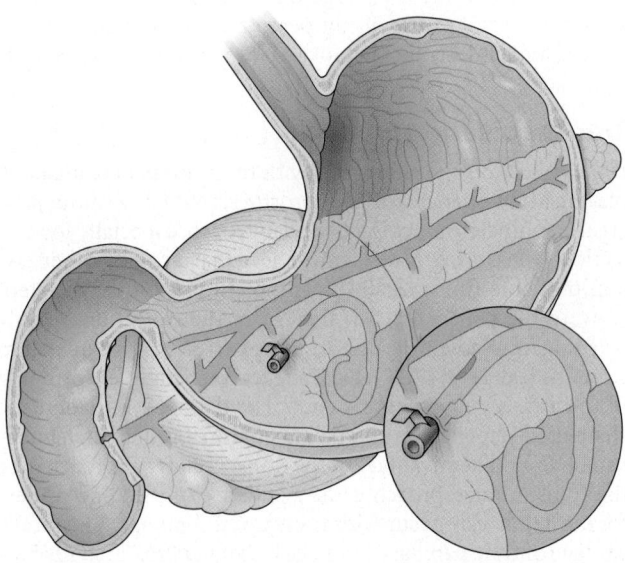

Fig. 47.13 Transmural stent in place through the posterior gastric wall into a pancreatic pseudocyst.

EUS can be used for transmural drainage of PFCs.[109] The first is to use the echoendoscope to localize the collection in relationship to surrounding structures and endoscopic landmarks; the echoendoscope is removed, and a therapeutic endoscope is used to perform transmural drainage by puncturing into the collection as described subsequently under non–EUS-guided drainage. The second is to perform the evaluation and entry into the collection using direct EUS guidance. Transmural drainage of PFCs can be performed entirely under EUS guidance using Doppler-equipped therapeutic channel echoendoscopes.[110] The lack of EUS availability does not preclude potential transmural drainage except in the following instances: small "window" of entry based on CT, especially in the absence of an endoscopically defined area of extrinsic compression or unusual location (**Fig. 47.14**); marginal, uncorrectable coagulopathy or thrombocytopenia; documented intervening varices; and failed transmural entry using non–EUS-guided techniques.[111]

Transmural Drainage without Endoscopic Ultrasound Guidance

Needle-knife electrocautery is used to enter the collection at the point of maximal endoscopically visible extrinsic compression with or without prelocalization using a needle.[112] Once entry into the collection has been achieved and a guidewire has been secured, the transmural tract is enlarged with a dilating balloon. The practice of enlarging the transmural tract with a sphincterotome has been abandoned because of the risk of bleeding.[113] Another method is localization and entry into the collection using a large-caliber needle without electrocautery employing the Seldinger technique (see Video).[101] This method seems to be safer because if the collection is not successfully entered with the needle (confirmed by aspiration of fluid or injection of radiopaque contrast agent), the needle is simply withdrawn without adverse sequelae. Similarly, if bleeding occurs on needle entry, if gross blood is aspirated, or if a visible hematoma develops, the needle is withdrawn to allow the vessel to tamponade. Another transmural entry site may be chosen during the same endoscopic session. Once the collection has been entered as confirmed by aspiration of fluid or injection of contrast agent, a guidewire is passed through the needle-knife or aspiration needle and coiled within the collection (**Fig. 47.15**). The transmural tract is dilated to 8 mm using standard biliary dilating balloons to allow placement of one or more double pigtail 10-Fr stents (see **Fig. 47.15**).

Follow-up

A short course of oral antibiotics is administered after uncomplicated attempted endoscopic drainage of noninfected pancreatic pseudocysts. Most outpatients do not require

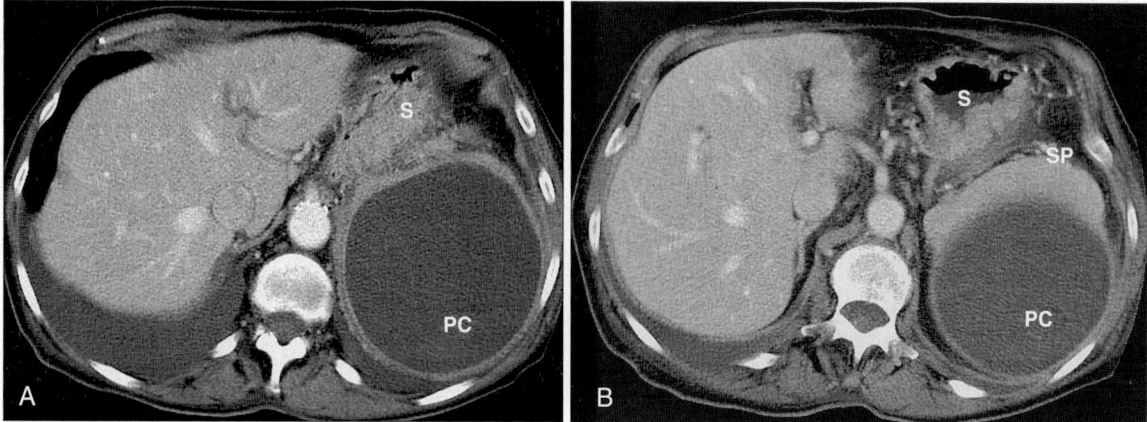

Fig. 47.14 Pancreatic pseudocyst best suited for endoscopic ultrasound (EUS)–guided drainage. **A,** Computed tomography (CT) scan shows pancreatic pseudocyst *(PC)* adjacent to collapsed stomach *(S)*. **B,** CT scan 1 cm below previous image. The spleen *(SP)* is visible. The narrow window would make attempted non–EUS-guided transmural drainage of this pseudocyst dangerous.

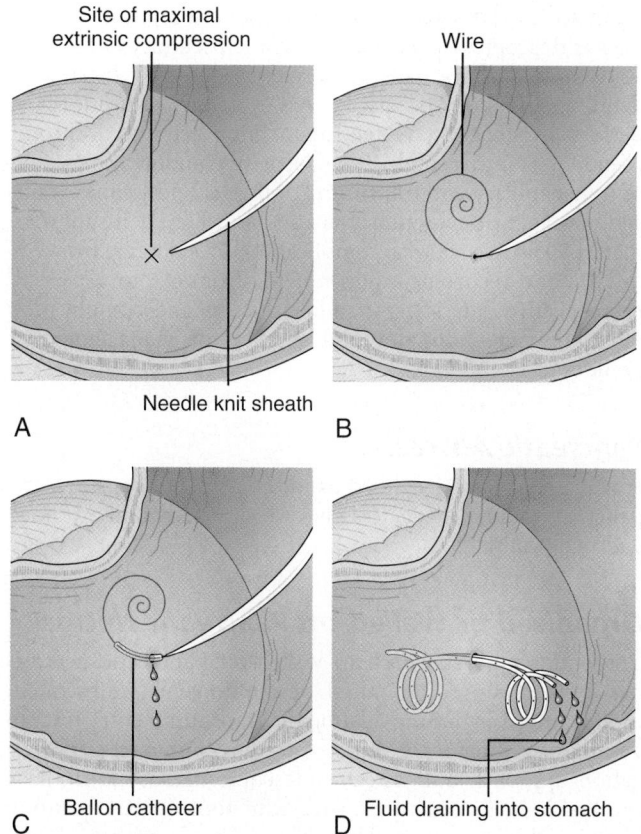

Fig. 47.15 Transmural drainage of pancreatic pseudocyst. **A,** Needle is placed through the posterior wall of the stomach or medial wall of the duodenum at the site of extrinsic compression. **B,** Guidewire is passed through the needle and coiled within the collection. **C,** Transmural tract has been balloon dilated. **D,** Two double pigtail stents have been placed through the wall into the pancreas. *(Redrawn from Baron TH, Morgan DE: Techniques in gastrointestinal endoscopy, Philadelphia, 1999, Saunders.)*

Endoscopic Drainage of Organized or Walled-off Pancreatic Necrosis

Because of the need to evacuate solid material, the endoscopic approach to drainage of organized or walled-off pancreatic necrosis differs from drainage of other PFCs. Generally, the transpapillary approach is inadequate to allow removal of solid debris. Transmural drainage is the preferred approach for these collections. After transmural entry into the collection as described previously, the gastric or duodenal wall is dilated to at least 15 mm on the initial endoscopy. Dilation allows a forward-viewing endoscope to be passed transmurally into the stomach for direct endoscopic necrosectomy as described earlier in the treatment of pancreatic necrosis (see **Fig. 47.4**). Two 10-Fr stents are placed to allow reaccess to the necrotic cavity for subsequent débridement. Although used much less often now, a 7-Fr irrigation tube can be placed into the collection (standard nasobiliary tube) for aggressive irrigation (see **Fig. 47.3**) allowing further débridement.

An alternative to nasocystic lavage is the placement of a percutaneous endoscopic gastrostomy tube with placement of a "jejunal" extension tube into the collection (**Fig. 47.16**).[115] The gastric port may be used for supplementing nutritional needs. Patients undergoing attempted endoscopic drainage of walled-off pancreatic necrosis should receive antibiotics before the procedure. It is recommended that outpatients be admitted to the hospital after the procedure for observation. Oral antibiotics are administered, and follow-up endoscopic débridement is performed until the collection has resolved as documented by follow-up CT. CT scans are obtained after the necrotic cavity appears to be completely débrided. The internal drains are endoscopically removed several weeks after complete resolution of the collection.

Complications of Endoscopic Therapy of Pancreatic Fluid Collections

Life-threatening complications that may arise after attempted endoscopic drainage of PFCs are listed in **Box 47.3**. It is recommended that endoscopic drainage of PFCs not be performed without the availability of surgical and interventional radiology support. The most feared complications of

hospitalization.[114] In the absence of suspected complications or worsening clinical course, a follow-up CT scan is obtained 4 to 6 weeks after the drainage procedure. The internal stents are endoscopically removed after documented radiographic resolution.

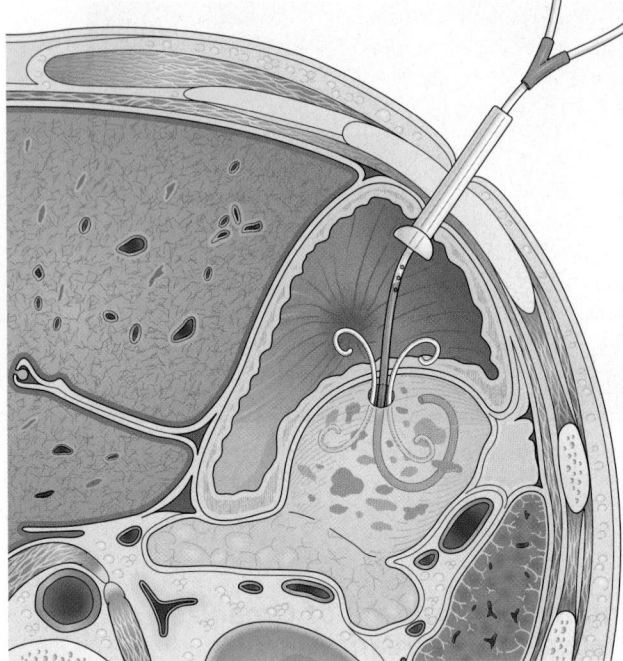

Fig. 47.16 Percutaneous endoscopic gastrostomy tube with jejunal extension tube placed through the posterior gastric wall into a necrotic pancreatic collection to provide irrigation. *(Redrawn from Baron TH, Morgan DE: Endoscopic transgastric irrigation tube placement via PEG for débridement of organized pancreatic necrosis. Gastrointest Endosc 50:574–577, 1999.)*

Box 47.3 Complications of Endoscopic Therapy of Pancreatic Fluid Collections

Bleeding
Perforation
Infection
Pancreatitis
Sedation complications
Aspiration
Stent migration or occlusion
Pancreatic ductal damage

---

transmural drainage are bleeding and perforation. Bleeding after transmural drainage may be managed supportively, endoscopically, surgically, or with angiographic embolization.[114] If perforation occurs during attempted transgastric drainage and is limited to the gastric wall (does not involve the collection), it may be successfully managed nonsurgically, provided that a stent has not been placed through the perforation; the gastric wall rapidly closes with conservative treatment consisting of nasogastric suction and antibiotics. Some authors believe that transduodenal perforation may be managed conservatively because the perforation is retroduodenal,[116] although this is not proven.

Infectious complications usually occur from inadequate drainage of fluid or solid debris. If endoscopic drainage was performed on a liquefied collection by the transpapillary route, stent exchange or upsizing of the stent or conversion to a transmural approach may resolve the infection. Similarly, if solid material was present and unrecognized during the initial procedure, placement of irrigation tubes or converting to a transmural drainage approach may resolve the infection. Occasionally, some patients require adjuvant placement of percutaneous drainage or irrigation catheters to manage infectious complications. Stent migration into the collection through the gastric or duodenal wall may occur during or after endoscopic stent placement. It is possible to retrieve the stent endoscopically if the collection has not completely collapsed and the transmural tract is still patent.

Results of Endoscopic Therapy of Pancreatic Fluid Collections

There are no prospective studies comparing endoscopic drainage with conservative (medical) therapy, percutaneous drainage, or surgical drainage.

Pancreatic Pseudocysts

The success rates, recurrence rates, and complication rates after endoscopic drainage of pancreatic pseudocysts are variable. Most authors have not used standardized criteria for defining pseudocysts, have used variable indications to perform drainage, have tended to lump acute and chronic pseudocysts into a single group, or have combined the results of transpapillary and transmural drainage. Endoscopic drainage of pancreatic pseudocysts can be achieved in approximately 90% of cases with complication rates ranging from 5% to 10% and recurrence rates ranging from 6% to 18%.[117,118] Retrospective data suggest similar success and complication rates between endoscopy and surgery for management of pseudocysts.[119–121]

Pancreatic Abscesses

Pancreatic abscesses defined as infected pseudocysts or peripancreatic liquefied necrosis have been successfully drained endoscopically.[65,122–124]

Organized or Walled-off Pancreatic Necrosis

The endoscopic approach to walled-off pancreatic necrosis has evolved since the initial descriptions.[62,114] Subsequent modifications including dilating the transmural entry tract to 15 mm or greater at the initial procedure with a primary irrigation approach and direct endoscopic necrosectomy have resulted in better outcomes. Successful nonsurgical resolution is achieved in approximately 80% to 85% of patients.[66–68,70]

Outcome Differences after Endoscopic Drainage of Pancreatic Fluid Collections

There are differences in success rates, complication rates, recurrences, and hospital stay for drainage of acute pseudocysts, chronic pseudocysts, and walled-off necrosis.[114] These differences are due to differences in pathology, pathophysiology, and severity of illness between the groups. Patients with pancreatic necrosis tend to be more severely ill, and endoscopic evacuation of solid debris is less efficient than evacuation of liquid. In terms of recurrence rates, acute pancreatic ductal disruptions occurring in patients with necrosis frequently lead to a disconnected duct syndrome whereby the head and tail of the pancreas are not in communication.[62,87] This situation leads to recurrent collections from the undrained viable pancreatic tail. Patients with acute pseudocysts tend to have less severe ductal abnormalities and lower recurrence rates. In addition to the type of pancreatic collection, the experience of the endoscopist seems to play a role in the success rate of drainage.[125] Future prospective studies assessing skill acquisition are required to define the minimum number of collection drainage procedures at which competence can be achieved.

Conclusion

Pancreatic necrosis is being increasingly recognized because of physician awareness and improved radiologic imaging. The identification of pancreatic necrosis is important because the morbidity and mortality from acute pancreatitis are markedly increased when necrosis is present. Aggressive medical care with use of antibiotics and limitation of surgery or other types of pancreatic débridement to patients with infected necrosis are the mainstays of management (see **Table 47.1**). PFCs are heterogeneous, with different underlying pathologies and pathophysiologies. Each type of PFC is amendable to drainage, although not in every patient. Collections with only a fluid component that are distinguished by either apposition to the gastric or duodenal wall by CT or communication with the main pancreatic duct by pancreatography can be drained endoscopically using transmural or transpapillary approaches. Collections containing significant amounts of solid debris that are treated endoscopically require débridement techniques to evacuate solid debris. Endoscopists considering endoscopic therapy of a pancreatic collection must identify the type of collection being drained and exclude masqueraders of PFCs, such as cystic neoplasms. EUS-guided drainage may decrease the complications of bleeding and perforation during transmural entry of PFCs. Refinement in endoscopic techniques to improve the safety and efficacy of endoscopic therapy and comparative studies with other drainage methods are needed.

References

The complete reference list is available online at www.expertconsult.com.

Acute Relapsing Pancreatitis

Michael K. Sanders and Adam Slivka

Video related to this chapter's topics can be found online at expertconsult.com.

Introduction

Acute pancreatitis is caused by acute or chronic alcohol intake or cholelithiasis in 80% of cases.[1,2] In the absence of alcohol or gallstones, numerous established and putative etiologies must be considered, any one of which can cause recurrent attacks of acute pancreatitis.[3] In instances in which the underlying etiology eludes detection and leads to a second attack, the term *acute relapsing pancreatitis* (ARP) is applied. **Table 48.1** lists the etiologies of ARP categorized by entities typically managed medically versus entities that respond to endoscopic therapy to prevent recurrences. This chapter focuses on the etiologies of ARP responding to endoscopic therapy. We also provide a brief update on the newly discovered and expanding body of knowledge of genetic causes of ARP, autoimmune ARP, and celiac-associated ARP. Endoscopic management for the genetic conditions is usually reserved for complications that develop from chronic pancreatitis (CP) and is discussed in Chapter 49. For a summary of all etiologies of ARP, readers are directed to the comprehensive review of Somogyi and coworkers.[4]

The initial work-up of a first attack of pancreatitis depends on the severity of the attack, special circumstances relating to the presentation, and the demographics of the patient. This work-up includes a core, common for all patients, and variations based on the individual case; the work-up must reflect a balance between rigor and reason. A detailed history is the most important part of the initial evaluation and should include alcohol intake, a detailed review of medications, postprandial onset of symptoms suggestive of a biliary source, review of epiphenomena suggestive of malignancy, a family history, an associated autoimmune or metabolic disorder, and a history of trauma. Physical examination may detect xanthoma or xanthelasma suggestive of hyperlipidemia, signs of alcohol-related liver disease, or a neck mass of parathyroid origin. Laboratory work and selective imaging should be used to confirm or exclude the differential diagnosis generated by the history and physical examination and to direct therapy.

An initial complete history and physical examination, routine blood work including liver function tests and corrected or ionized calcium and triglyceride levels, and transabdominal ultrasound or computed tomography (CT) scan reveal an etiology in 70% to 90% of cases of pancreatitis.[2,5–8] In younger patients (<40 years old), transabdominal ultrasound may suffice, but in older patients, a CT scan of the abdomen is advised because a pancreatic or ampullary neoplasm may manifest with ARP.[9,10] Without an adequate initial work-up and directed therapy, more than half of patients with an initial attack of acute pancreatitis experience recurrent attacks or develop CP.[5,11] In patients with gallstone pancreatitis, treatment of the index attack and prevention of further attacks may involve endoscopic sphincterotomy (ES) with bile duct stone extraction and laparoscopic cholecystectomy to remove the stone reservoir.[6,7] Patients who remain untreated have a 33% to 66% chance of a recurrent attack.[8,11–13]

Table 48.1 Putative Etiology of Acute Relapsing Pancreatitis

Medical Management	Endoscopic or Surgical Management
Alcohol	Annular pancreas
Autoimmune	Biliary stones or microlithiasis
Celiac disease	Choledochocyst and choledochocele
Drug-induced	Pancreas divisum
	Pancreatic and ampullary neoplasms

Genetic
  Hereditary pancreatitis
  CFTR mutations
	Periampullary diverticulum

SPINK mutations Tropical pancreatitis	Sphincter of Oddi dysfunction
Hypercalcemia	
Hyperlipidemia	
Infectious	
Vascular	

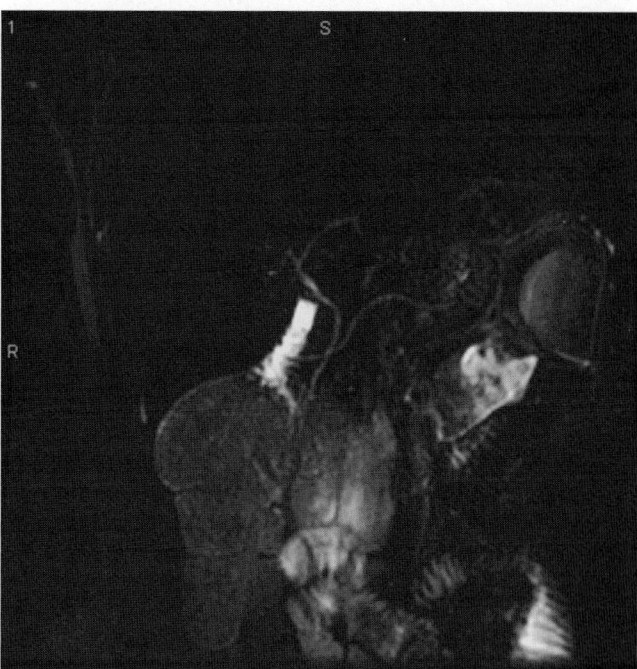

Fig. 48.1 Magnetic resonance cholangiopancreatography (MRCP) in a patient with acute recurrent pancreatitis shows pancreas divisum. The dorsal pancreatic duct is clearly seen crossing over the bile duct and entering the region of the minor papilla. The ventral duct is not seen, and the common bile duct appears normal.

Work-up of Acute Relapsing Pancreatitis

If the initial work-up after an index attack of pancreatitis is negative and successive attacks occur, a more extensive evaluation reveals a diagnosis in about two-thirds of patients. This evaluation may start with various blood tests depending on the individual scenario, followed by magnetic resonance (MR) imaging, magnetic resonance cholangiopancreatography (MRCP), or endoscopic ultrasound (EUS), and culminate in endoscopic retrograde cholangiopancreatography (ERCP). At each step of escalating invasiveness, the balance between the yield and the potential complications of the intended investigation should be carefully considered in discussions with the patient.

After an initial unrevealing evaluation for acute pancreatitis, ERCP reveals an etiology in approximately 70% of patients.[5,14] Although some experts advocate performing ERCP in all patients after a single attack of pancreatitis, most agree that ERCP is warranted only after a severe attack in which the etiology is not obvious or after recurrent attacks.[15,16] The utility of this test lies in its unique ability to diagnose and treat biliary microlithiasis, sphincter of Oddi dysfunction (SOD), and pancreas divisum, the most commonly encountered diagnoses in the work-up of ARP. Less often, pancreatic and ampullary cancers; duodenal diverticulum; pancreatic duct strictures or stones; and congenital malformations such as choledochocele, annular pancreas, and anomalous pancreaticobiliary junction may be encountered. ERCP is risky because it causes acute pancreatitis in 3% to 20% of patients[17,18] depending on the indication and maneuver performed. Acute pancreatitis is more frequent when ERCP is performed for diagnostic purposes, particularly when coupled with treatment of SOD, compared with other indications, most notably bile duct stones.[19] Other risk factors include multiple or high-pressure injections of contrast agent into the pancreatic duct, therapeutic intervention, a past history of pancreatitis, and

operator inexperience.[20] In a referral center treating 279 patients with acute pancreatitis over a 5-year period, ERCP was the causal factor in 4% of cases.[21] However, 3 of 11 patients in the subgroup with ERCP-related pancreatitis died.

MRCP is replacing diagnostic ERCP in many centers because of ERCP-related complications.[22] With heavily T2-weighted images, fluid within the bile and pancreatic ducts produces an image akin to an endoscopically generated cholangiopancreatogram. MRCP is accurate in detecting common bile duct stones[23,24]; its role in the evaluation of ARP includes the identification of anatomic abnormalities such as pancreas divisum (**Fig. 48.1**), choledochocysts, annular pancreas, and anomalous pancreaticobiliary junction.[24–27] However, ERCP continues to be used in the diagnostic evaluation of ARP because of the ability to visualize the ampulla, to sample tissue and bile, and to perform sphincter of Oddi manometry.

EUS uses higher frequencies than conventional abdominal ultrasound, and the image quality is not compromised by intestinal gas, providing a higher sensitivity and specificity for detecting cholelithiasis than conventional ultrasound.[28–30] It has been shown to be as accurate as ERCP in the diagnosis of choledocholithiasis,[31] and the positive predictive value for biliary tract disease including microlithiasis in the gallbladder and biliary sludge (**Fig. 48.2**)[32,33] is about 98%.[14] It remains the endoscopic procedure of choice for visualizing the pancreas,[34–38] and it is the most accurate technique for the detection and local staging of pancreatic carcinoma.[39,40] EUS is also useful in detecting changes in the pancreatic parenchyma and ducts.[38,39]

In patients with ARP, EUS correctly identified a cause of acute pancreatitis in 155 of 168 patients in whom a cause was found by a multidisciplinary diagnostic approach, involving

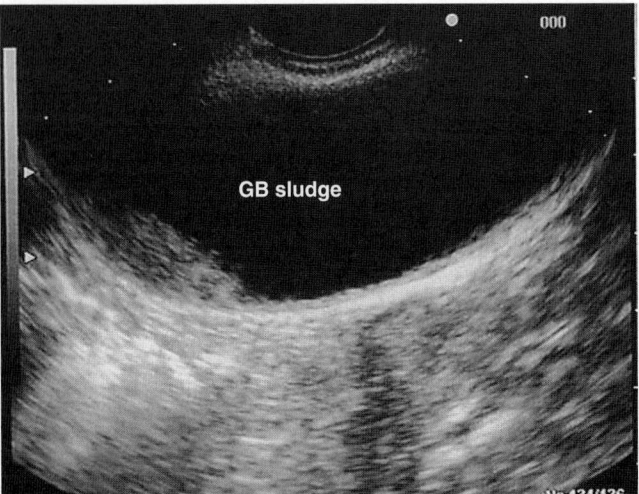

Fig. 48.2 Gallbladder sludge was found at endoscopic ultrasound (EUS) using a convex linear array echoendoscope in a patient with acute recurrent pancreatitis and normal transabdominal ultrasound. *(Courtesy of Dr. Kevin McGrath, University of Pittsburgh Medical Center.)*

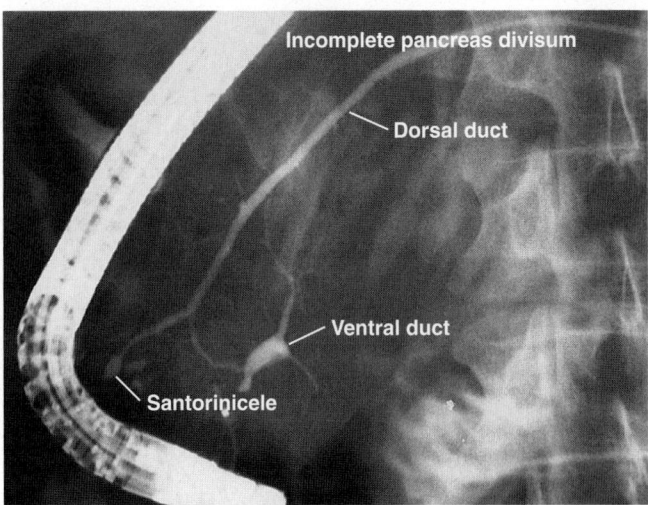

Fig. 48.3 Endoscopic retrograde cholangiopancreatography (ERCP) performed on a patient with acute recurrent pancreatitis shows incomplete pancreas divisum. The ventral duct and dorsal duct are connected by a small branch duct. At the distalmost portion of the dorsal duct, a cysticlike outpouching, called a santorinicele, is also seen. This patient responded to endoscopic minor papillotomy.

ERCP, bile crystal analysis, surgery, and medical follow-up. EUS may also be useful in the detection of pancreas divisum,[41] SOD,[42] and anomalous pancreaticobiliary junction,[43] but more data are required before the performance characteristics of EUS for these diagnoses is known. Given the high yield and lower complication rate compared with ERCP, EUS is being used earlier in the work-up of ARP. However, a consensus has not been reached so far regarding the exact place for EUS in the diagnostic algorithm for ARP. Increasingly, EUS evaluation of the pancreas, ampulla, and biliary system is being used to detect potentially diagnosable and treatable causes of ARP before use of ERCP.

Additional laboratory work-up after negative routine testing may include genetic testing for hereditary pancreatitis (HP) and cystic fibrosis (CF) and autoimmune markers. The mainstay of management for patients with ARP is to discover the etiology and perform an intervention that prevents recurrence because there is no specific therapy to treat an acute attack of pancreatitis.

Pancreas Divisum

Introduction

The term *pancreas divisum* refers to two pancreatic ductal systems that do not unite during embryologic organogenesis and drain separately via the two duodenal papillae—the dominant dorsal system through the minor papilla and the smaller ventral system through the major papilla (see **Fig. 48.1**). Incomplete pancreas divisum is a threadlike communication between dorsal and ventral pancreatic ducts and, when symptomatic, is treated similar to complete pancreas divisum (**Fig. 48.3**).

Epidemiology

Pancreas divisum is the most common congenital anomaly of the pancreas and may be found in 7% to 14% of autopsy

Table 48.2 Reported Incidence of Pancreas Divisum and Associated Acute Relapsing Pancreatitis

Author (Year)	No. ERCP Procedures	Incidence of Pancreas Divisum (%)	Idiopathic Pancreatitis as Indicated for ERCP (%)
Cotton (1980)[48]	810	5.8	25.6
Sugawa et al (1987)[77]	1529	2.7	2.4
Delhaye et al (1985)[221]	5333	5.7	5.3
Bernard et al (1990)[47]	1825	7.5	50
Burtin et al (1991)[222]	1049	5.9	12

ERCP, endoscopic retrograde cholangiopancreatography.

series.[44-46] The frequency of pancreas divisum among ERCP series varies greatly (2.7% to 7.5%) and depends on the population studied and the diligence with which complete pancreatography is pursued. Pancreas divisum is reported to occur less often in Asians (1% to 2%)[47] and blacks (2%).[48] The clinical significance of pancreas divisum is controversial. Although estimates reveal that less than 5% of the population with pancreas divisum ever develops pancreatic symptoms, authorities recognize its association with ARP, CP, and abdominal pain.[49-51] Patients undergoing pancreatography for documented pancreatitis are substantially more likely to have pancreas divisum than patients who have incidental pancreatograms during ERCP or for unexplained chronic abdominal pain.[52] **Table 48.2** summarizes the larger ERCP series of patients with pancreas divisum and pancreatitis. Caution should be exercised when assigning causation to pancreas divisum in patients with ARP given its prevalence in the population, and other known causes of pancreatitis should be sought for and excluded.

Pathogenesis

Because most exocrine flow is routed through the minor papilla in this ductal anomaly, it is hypothesized that in some patients an increased resistance to flow across this small orifice results in dorsal duct hypertension and clinical symptoms.[53–56] The resulting increased dorsal duct pressure may also make the pancreas more prone to injury from alcohol and drugs.[57,58] Surgical and endoscopic procedures aimed at decreasing resistance to flow across the minor papilla have been reported with varying success. Another mechanism by which pancreas divisum may lead to ARP is a decrease in the cystic fibrosis transmembrane conductance regulator protein (CFTR) function.[59] The association between loss of CFTR function and ARP is discussed later in the section on genetic causes.

Diagnosis

ERCP remains the "gold standard" for diagnosing pancreas divisum. A characteristic ventral pancreatogram with an attenuated duct that arborizes strongly suggests pancreas divisum. Caution must be exercised in patients with an obstructed pancreatic duct that may look like pancreas divisum. Pancreas divisum is confirmed by locating the minor papilla and injecting contrast agent into the dorsal duct (see Video). The minor papilla is usually located 2 cm proximal and 2 cm medial to the major papilla. It is best seen with the duodenoscope passed in a long position, without reducing the loop along the greater curve of the stomach. Occasionally, the minor papilla cannot be identified. The use of intravenous secretin (0.2 mcg/kg) during ERCP may stimulate the exocrine pancreas and help identify the minor papilla as a point origin of clear liquid "squirting" into the duodenum.[60] The prior application of methylene blue to the periampullary mucosa before intravenous secretin has been suggested to assist in the identification of the minor papilla.[61] Cannulation of the papilla may be difficult, and various tapered or metal-tipped catheters and papillotomes have been developed (**Fig. 48.4**). The success of minor papilla cannulation is optimized when the diagnosis is predetermined; this calls for noninvasive diagnostic modalities to avoid repeat ERCP. MRCP is best suited for this purpose. The use of intravenous secretin improves pancreatic duct visualization during MRCP.[62,63] The diagnosis of pancreas divisum may be made by CT (**Fig. 48.5**) or EUS, but the accuracy of diagnosis of these modalities is unknown.

Clinical Presentation and Treatment

The earliest attempts at treatment for patients with presumed symptomatic pancreas divisum were surgical. The surgical procedures first performed to reduce resistance to exocrine flow consisted of a transduodenal minor and major sphincteroplasty with cholecystectomy. More recently, a transduodenal minor sphincterotomy or sphincteroplasty alone[64] has evolved as the surgical treatment of choice. The clinical presentation of ARP, the presence of minor papilla stenosis either

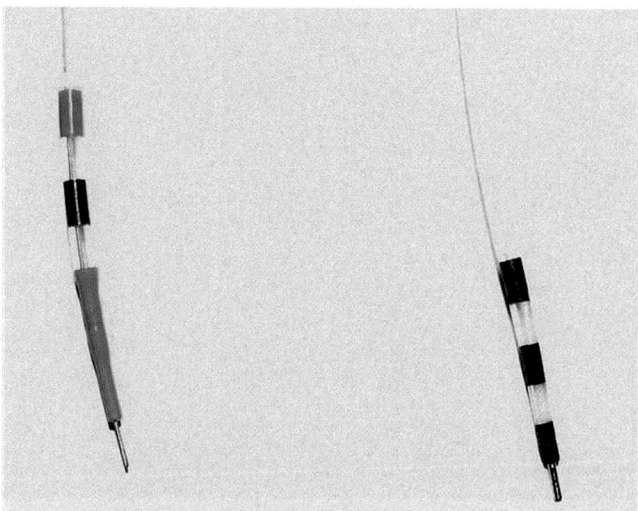

Fig. 48.4 A variety of catheters may be used for cannulation of the minor papilla. Two examples are shown. *On the left,* the contour endoscopic retrograde cholangiopancreatography (ERCP) cannula (Microvasive/Boston Scientific, Watertown, MA) is a catheter tapered to 3-Fr at its distal tip. A 0.018-inch guidewire (Roadrunner; Wilson Cook Medical, Winston-Salem, NC) is passed through the catheter with its tip protruding several millimeters to facilitate cannulation of the minor papilla. An adapter can be fixed to the proximal end of the catheter that allows simultaneous injection of radiopaque contrast material. *On the right,* a metal-tipped catheter (ERCP-LP-23-Lehman; Wilson Cook Medical, Winston-Salem, NC) can be used to facilitate minor papilla cannulation and opacification. A guidewire cannot be passed through this catheter.

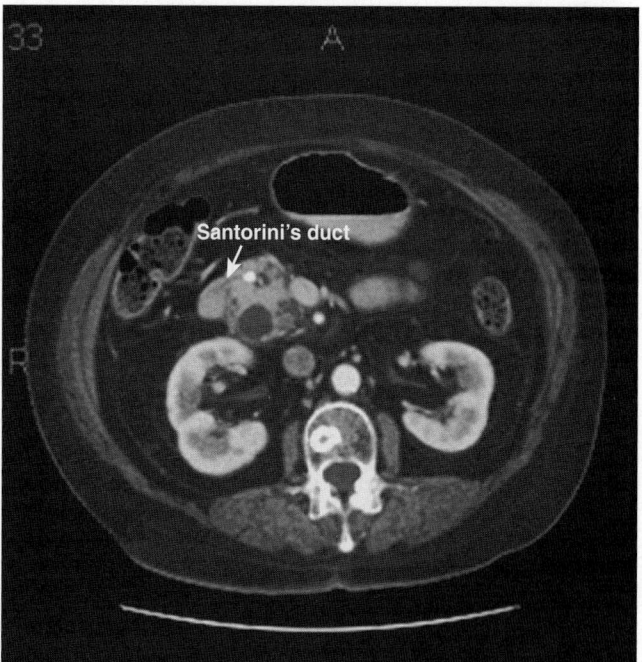

Fig. 48.5 Computed tomography (CT) scan obtained in a patient with acute recurrent pancreatitis disclosed chronic pancreatitis (CP) and pancreas divisum. Santorini's duct is seen *(arrow)* draining into the area of the minor papilla. A large calcified stone is impacted in Santorini's duct, and the dorsal duct proximal to this is dilated. An intraparenchymal pseudocyst is seen below. This patient was treated with minor papilla sphincterotomy, temporary stent placement, hydrostatic balloon dilation, and stone extraction.

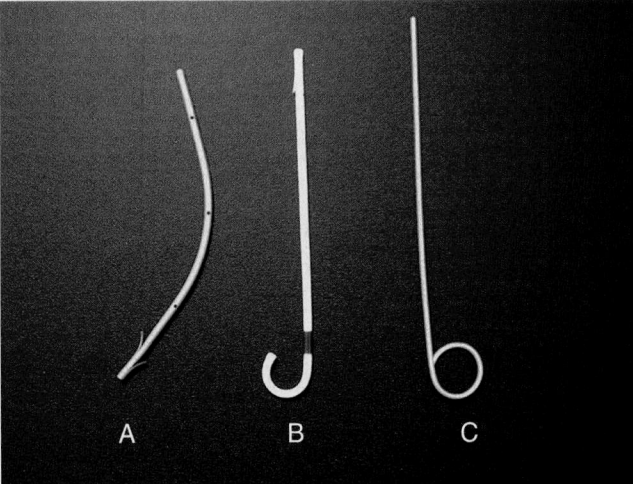

Fig. 48.6 A variety of stents can be placed into the pancreatic duct to treat symptomatic pancreas divisum or as prophylaxis against post–endoscopic retrograde cholangiopancreatography (ERCP) pancreatitis. Stent *A* is the Geenen pancreatic stent (Wilson Cook Medical, Winston-Salem, NC). This example is 5-Fr in diameter and contains a single set of external flaps that allow the stent to migrate out spontaneously over the ensuing days in most patients. A variant of this stent comes with internal flaps, if the stent is intended to stay in the duct for longer periods. Stent *B* is the Freeman Pancreatic Flexi-Stent (Hobbs Medical, Stafford Springs, CT). This is a soft Silastic stent with an internal flange to prevent outward migration and an external pigtail to prevent inward migration. The example shown is 5-Fr in diameter. As with the Geenen stent, multiple side holes are present. Stent *C* is the Zimmon pancreatic stent (Wilson Cook Medical, Winston-Salem, NC). This 3-Fr stent has an external pigtail to prevent inward migration. No side holes are present, and this stent migrates out spontaneously over days in most patients.

intraoperatively or by delayed clearance of dye after dorsal ductography during ERCP, and a positive ultrasound secretin test are the best predictors of outcome after surgical intervention for pancreas divisum.[65]

To avoid laparotomy, numerous endoscopic maneuvers have been applied for the management of symptoms related to pancreas divisum. These have included minor papilla dilation, stent placement, and sphincterotomy. The technique of minor papilla stent placement involves free selective cannulation of the dorsal duct, placement of a guidewire, and advancement of a stent specifically designed for use in the pancreas over the guidewire with a pushing cannula (see Video). These stents are plastic and vary in diameter from 3-Fr to 10-Fr (**Fig. 48.6**). Larger stents (7-Fr and 10-Fr) are reserved for patients with dilated pancreatic ducts or CP. Pancreatic stents 5-Fr and larger have multiple side holes to permit drainage from side branches and have external flanges or pigtails to prevent inward migration. Some stents have internal barbs to prevent outward migration. The number and need for multiple stent exchanges have not been firmly established; the interval necessary for stent exchanges likewise has not been established, although most authors advocate 4 to 8 weeks for stents 5-Fr to 7-Fr in diameter.

Minor papilla dilation may be accomplished with catheter dilators or hydrostatic balloons. Catheter dilators generally vary in diameter from 5-Fr to 10-Fr and are advanced into the dorsal ducts over a preplaced wire. Although balloons vary in diameter, for the sole purpose of dilating the minor papilla,

4-mm over-the-wire hydrostatic balloons are the smallest commercially available devices. Larger balloons should be used with caution, unless concurrent CP exists with need for additional therapy (e.g., stone extraction or stricture dilation; see Chapter 49).

Two techniques have been described for minor papilla sphincterotomy: standard traction papillotomy (see Video) and needle-knife sphincterotomy over a stent. Traction papillotomes with braided or monofilament cutting wires can be used to accomplish traction papillotomy. The papillotome tip in the pancreatic duct usually directs the wire in a 12 o'clock to 2 o'clock direction; the length of the cut depends on the size of the minor papilla mound, usually about 5 mm. Some authors advocate the use of pure cutting current to prevent cautery to the pancreatic parenchyma with resulting stenosis of the outflow tract. It is generally advisable to leave a temporary pancreatic stent, which has been shown to decrease the risk of postprocedure pancreatitis for pancreatic sphincterotomy of the major papilla.[66,67] The needle-knife technique involves placing a pancreatic stent into the dorsal duct and using it as a guide to create an approximately 5-mm cut over the stent. The stent may be left in place temporarily to reduce the risk of post-ERCP pancreatitis. Minor papilla dilation alone has not been studied in a controlled fashion but has been used in combination with stent placement.

Categorizing patients with symptomatic pancreas divisum may help decide management and predict outcome (**Table 48.3**). Two prospective, randomized, controlled trials have evaluated endoscopic therapy for patients with pancreas divisum. One trial looked at the role of stent placement in the minor papilla in patients with pancreas divisum and ARP and reported 90% success over a mean 29-month period.[64] The second trial evaluated the role of minor papillotomy in treating patients with pancreas divisum and chronic abdominal pain and reported symptomatic relief in 44% of patients.[68] Studies looking at dorsal duct stent placement and minor papillotomy summarized in **Table 48.3**[69–72] suggest symptomatic improvement or resolution of ARP in 70% to 80% of patients with pancreas divisum; however, these studies are limited by heterogeneous study populations, varied follow-up, and lack of controls. The response in the setting of CP is less satisfactory and, for chronic abdominal pain, suboptimal and ill-advised in our opinion.

Regarding the choice of therapy, most authorities now favor minor papillotomy over dorsal duct stent placement. The overall success rate of endoscopic therapy (stent placement, dilation, or sphincterotomy) is similar to the results of surgical sphincteroplasty. The restenosis rate in the surgical literature appears to be less than for endoscopic minor papillotomy, although reports suggesting that patients who have restenosis after ES also have restenosis after sphincteroplasty.[73] Endoscopic techniques seem preferable as a first choice because laparotomy can be avoided. The short-term success rates of minor papilla ES and surgical sphincteroplasty may be similar, but long-term follow-up and comparative trials are needed before firmer recommendations regarding procedure choice and cost-effectiveness can be made.

Complications

Complications of stent therapy include acute pancreatitis; the induction of pancreatic ductal changes, many of which may

Table 48.3 Results of Endoscopic Therapy in Patients with Pancreas Divisum

Author (Year)	Study Design	No.	Mean Follow-up (mo)	Intervention	NP	Symptom Relief ARP	CP	CAP	Restenosis	Chronic Duct Changes
Russell et al (1984)[56]	Retro	5	8	MES	1/5	2/2	4/4		NP	
Soehendra et al (1986)[223]	Retro	6	3	MES		5/8			NP	
Liquory et al (1986)[224]	Retro	8	24	MES					3/8	
McCarthy et al (1988)[69]	Retro	19	6–36	Stent	17/19					2/19
Prabhu et al (1989)[70]	Retro	18	12–60	Stent		15/18				NS
Siegel et al (1990)[71]	Retro	31	24	Stent	26/31					NS
Lans et al (1992)[225]	RCT	10 (9 controls)	29	Stent		9/10				0/10
Sherman et al (1994)[68]	RCT	16 (17 controls)	25	MES				7/16	NP	
Lehman et al (1993)[76]	Retro	52	20	MES		13/17	3/11	6/24	10/18	
Coleman et al (1994)[72]	Retro	34	23	Stent		7/9	12/20	2/5	NP	NS
Kozarek et al (1995)[145]	Retro	39	26	MES and/or stent		11/15	6/19	1/5	3/26	10/39
Boerma et al (2000)[226]	Prosp	16	51	Stent			5/16			NS
Ertan (2000)[227]	Prosp	25	24	Stent		19/25				21/25
Heyries et al (2002)[228]	Prosp	24	39	MES or stent		22/24	NS			16/16

ARP, acute recurrent pancreatitis; CAP, chronic abdominal pain; CP, chronic pancreatitis; MES, minor papilla endoscopic sphincterotomy; NP, not provided; NS, not significant; Prosp, prospective uncontrolled trial; RCT, randomized controlled trial; Retro, retrospective review.

be irreversible[74]; stent occlusion or migration; pancreatic duct perforation; and the need for repeated procedures. Complications of minor papilla ES, including bleeding, perforation, and pancreatitis, have been reported and are similar to complications of major papilla ES.[75] Lehman and coworkers[76] reported a 15% procedural complication rate for minor papilla ES, primarily mild pancreatitis. Frequency of restenosis is reported to be 5% to 10%.[77]

Biliary Microlithiasis

Introduction

Many terms have been used interchangeably for biliary microlithiasis including *biliary sludge* and *biliary sand*. The term *biliary microlithiasis* typically refers to finding cholesterol monohydrate crystals and calcium bilirubinate granules on light microscopy of an endoscopically acquired centrifuged sample of bile.[78] The criteria for differentiating between biliary microliths and small stones are unclear, but generally a gallstone is defined as a particle with a diameter greater than 2 to

3 mm that cannot be crushed by digital compression.[78] Biliary sludge is the ultrasound finding of low-level echoes without acoustic shadowing that gravitate toward the dependent portion in the gallbladder[79] and move with positioning. Biliary sludge consists of cholesterol monohydrate crystals and calcium bilirubinate granules suspended in gallbladder mucus. Other calcium salts, proteins, and xenobiotics such as ceftriaxone can also be found.[80]

Epidemiology

Similar to gallstones, the risk of developing biliary microlithiasis is increased in women and in several conditions including pregnancy,[81,82] rapid weight loss,[83] critical illness,[84] prolonged fasting,[85] long-term administration of total parenteral nutrition,[85–88] ceftriaxone[86–91] or octreotide administration,[92–94] and bone marrow or solid organ transplantation.[95–99] The development of ARP in these clinical situations should prompt an aggressive search for microlithiasis (approximately 31%). Approximately 31% of patients with nonalcoholic pancreatitis have biliary microlithiasis, and 74% of patients with "idiopathic" pancreatitis have been shown to have biliary microlithiasis.[11,100] Two prospective studies of consecutive patients with apparently idiopathic pancreatitis found that two-thirds to three-fourths had microlithiasis as the presumed cause, as documented by biliary drainage studies, follow-up ultrasound studies, and ERCP with sphincterotomy or cholecystectomy.[11,100]

Pathogenesis

The clinical significance of biliary microlithiasis is very controversial. Experts remain divided over whether it is a transient phenomenon or a precursor to gallstones. After chemical dissolution of gallstones, gallbladder sludge is usually seen on ultrasound before gallstone recurrence,[101] suggesting that the pathogenesis of sludge is similar to that of gallstones.[102–106] Sludge resolves spontaneously in most cases, and gallstones form in only a few individuals with sludge. There are few studies of the pathogenesis and natural history of biliary sludge, and most are limited by insufficient follow-up.[101,107,108] Three clinical outcomes were noted in one study, including complete resolution, a waxing and waning course, and gallstone formation.[101] Sludge found in patients with abdominal pain seems to disappear spontaneously in about 50% of cases. Asymptomatic persistence is seen in about 20% of cases over 3 years, and symptoms may develop in 10% to 15% of patients. Gallstones develop in 5% to 15%.[109]

Further support for the role of biliary microlithiasis in producing pancreaticobiliary symptoms comes from the observations that symptomatic patients with gallstones receiving ursodeoxycholic acid had resolution of symptoms in 3 months, although the number and size of gallstones remained unchanged.[110] The supposition is that the treatment resolved concurrent biliary microlithiasis, which led to the symptoms. Asymptomatic patients with gallstones who receive shock wave lithotripsy have been reported to develop biliary colic, cholecystitis, or acute pancreatitis.[111–115] In this situation, the therapy may have created sludge, which produced the symptoms.

Hypothetically, microlithiasis can lead to pancreatitis through numerous mechanisms. Small stones may transiently impact at the papilla leading to pancreatic duct obstruction and pancreatitis.[116] Recurrent passage of stones may lead to papillary stenosis or SOD, both of which are associated with pancreatitis.[117]

Diagnosis

The diagnosis of biliary sludge is confirmed by ultrasound. The sensitivity of transabdominal ultrasound for sludge is approximately 55%, whereas the sensitivity of EUS is approximately 96% (see **Fig. 48.2**), compared with duodenal bile collection (67%).[118,119] Although clinically less applicable, microscopic examination of gallbladder contents is considered the diagnostic "gold standard" and allows the chemical composition of sludge to be defined. The sensitivity is 83% when bile is obtained directly from the common bile duct during ERCP.[120] Bile sampling is indicated only if less invasive studies are negative, the clinical suspicion for microlithiasis is high, and the results would guide management. Techniques vary as to the site of bile collection, cholecystokinin use, sample processing, and criteria for a positive test. The

relationship between the quantity of crystals and the clinical outcome remains unproved.

Treatment

Numerous therapeutic options are available to treat symptomatic biliary microlithiasis and include cholecystectomy, ES, and chemical dissolution. The benefit of therapy has been shown by the significant decrease in recurrent episodes of pancreatitis after therapy (<10%) versus a recurrence rate of approximately 66% to 75% in untreated patients.[11,121–126]

Laparoscopic cholecystectomy offers definitive therapy[11,78] and is indicated in good operative candidates of almost any age. Biliary ES is an effective alternative in very elderly patients or patients with significant comorbid illness. The benefits of sphincter ablation[124–130] include enhanced gallbladder motility and reduced stasis, which may persist for years.[131] Biliary ES also reduces bile lithogenicity by modifying the bile composition.

Although there is no demonstrable difference in the clinical benefit of cholecystectomy or biliary ES for microlithiasis-induced pancreatitis, the safety profile of laparoscopic cholecystectomy outweighs the immediate and late complications of biliary ES for an indication of ARP in most clinical situations. Biliary ES may be used as a temporizing measure in patients who have severe acute pancreatitis secondary to microlithiasis in whom cholecystectomy must be deferred for weeks or months. Few studies have examined ursodeoxycholic acid for the treatment of biliary sludge. In patients with rapid weight loss, ursodeoxycholic acid has been shown to decrease the incidence of gallstones by 50% to 100%.[132,133] In patients with idiopathic pancreatitis and sludge,[11] maintenance therapy after initial treatment with ursodeoxycholic acid to dissolve cholesterol crystals successfully prevents the recurrence of sludge and pancreatitis. This form of therapy is a reasonable alternative in poor operative candidates and elderly patients.

Sphincter of Oddi Dysfunction

A detailed description of SOD is provided in Chapter 46. Direct evidence of the involvement of the sphincter of Oddi in the pathogenesis of pancreatitis is lacking. However, experts recognize SOD as a condition that may be associated with ARP. Using probes, surgeons have documented narrowing of the sphincter of Oddi in patients undergoing surgery for ARP. Secretin-stimulated ultrasound studies of the pancreatic duct in patients with SOD have revealed prolonged dilation of the pancreatic duct compared with controls, which is associated with a good outcome after surgical sphincteroplasty.[134] The morphine-Prostigmin test has been used to show an association between SOD and abdominal pain associated with pancreatitis. Likewise, manometric studies have shown an association between SOD and a proportion of patients with ARP, most commonly an abnormally increased sphincter of Oddi basal pressure[135,136]; intuitively, surgeons and endoscopists have devised treatment strategies aimed at relieving obstruction at the sphincter of Oddi.

Earlier surgical literature was characterized by inhomogeneous patient populations and mixed results.[137,138] More recent literature using sphincter of Oddi manometry to guide selection of patients with ARP for open sphincteroplasty and septoplasty reveals cessation of attacks in greater than 90% of patients with manometric stenosis; however, in patients with ARP, manometric evidence of SOD varies widely. SOD can involve either the biliary or the pancreatic segment or both. Pancreatic SOD has been implicated in causing recurrent pancreatitis in patients with prior biliary sphincter ablation.[139,140] More recent literature reveals that pancreatic SOD often coexists with biliary SOD; many centers recommend documentation and ablation of both conditions.[141,142]

Pancreatic sphincterotomy of the major papilla uses the same techniques as described previously for the minor papilla (see Video). Whether concomitant biliary sphincterotomy is required is controversial and currently under investigation. Leaving a temporary pancreatic stent in place after biliary sphincterotomy alone for SOD or after pancreatic sphincterotomy reduces the incidence and severity of postsphincterotomy pancreatitis.[67,143] Most data regarding SOD have evolved from studies of the biliary segment and therapy directed at it. Assumptions regarding manipulation of treatment directed at the pancreatic duct based on such data can be misleading and potentially dangerous. Response of the pancreatic duct to endoscopic stent placement has been used either to treat patients or to select patients for surgery.[144,145] However, long-term outcomes are lacking. In a randomized controlled trial, sphincter of Oddi basal pressure in the biliary tree has been shown to predict who will respond to biliary sphincterotomy among patients with type II biliary SOD.[146] Corresponding studies for pancreatic duct manometry have not been performed in ARP; the ability of pancreatic duct manometry to discriminate between responders and nonresponders to pancreatic duct sphincterotomy among patients with ARP and pancreatic duct SOD has never been shown.

Circumstantial evidence suggests a higher incidence of post-ERCP pancreatitis in patients with ARP undergoing ERCP and sphincter of Oddi manometry.[147] Patients with ARP and a dilated pancreatic duct in the absence of morphologic criteria for CP (type 1 SOD) are considered to have stenosis of the pancreatic sphincter (**Fig. 48.7**),[148] and, analogous to the biliary tract, pancreatic sphincterotomy appears reasonable.

Ampullary and Pancreatic Malignancies

In a small subset of patients, malignant or premalignant obstruction of the pancreatic duct may lead to the development of ARP; this is most commonly due to ductal adenocarcinomas of the pancreas and ampulla but can also be seen with neuroendocrine tumors,[149] metastatic tumors, and ampullary adenomas (**Fig. 48.8**).[150] Intraductal papillary mucinous neoplasms (IPMNs) of the pancreas are a rarer form of premalignant or malignant tumors that typically manifest with ARP. Mucin secretion from hyperplastic ductal cells can obstruct the pancreatic duct and cause ARP. CT scans commonly show a dilated main pancreatic duct (**Fig. 48.9**) or isolated side branch dilation (**Fig. 48.10**). Associated cystic lesions may also be present. At ERCP, a fish-mouth papilla held open with mucus is pathognomonic (**Fig. 48.11**). EUS may show a diffusely enlarged main pancreatic duct with thickened walls and side branch dilation forming small cystic spaces.

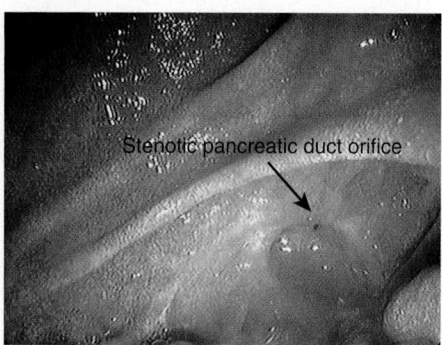

Fig. 48.7 This patient presented with acute recurrent pancreatitis 18 months after a biliary and pancreatic surgical sphincteroplasty for sphincter of Oddi dysfunction. At endoscopic retrograde cholangiopancreatography (ERCP), a grossly stenotic pancreatic duct orifice is seen as a pinpoint opening *(arrow)* within the defect at the site of prior surgery. Treatment with hydrostatic balloon dilation and temporary stent placement was successful.

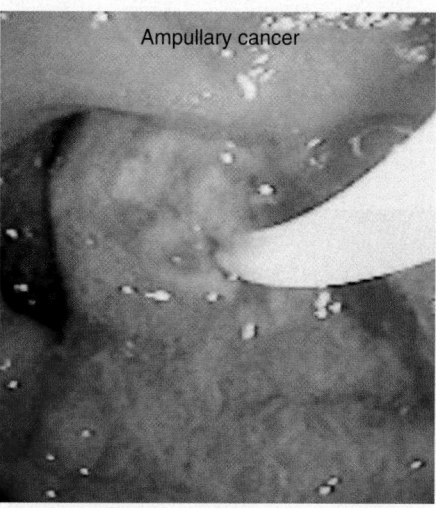

Fig. 48.8 This patient with an ampullary cancer presented with cholestatic liver tests and acute recurrent pancreatitis. The lesion was found to be early stage by endoscopic ultrasound (EUS), and curative Whipple's resection was performed.

IPMNs are categorized into three forms based on areas of involvement: main pancreatic duct (MD), side branch (SB), or combined main duct and side branch.[151] Both ARP and CP have been observed in patients with MD-IPMN; however, the rate of ARP with SB-IPMN is not well established.[152-154] A more recent retrospective study suggested a frequent association (34%) of acute pancreatitis in patients with suspected SB-IPMN.[155] However, additional studies are necessary to determine the natural course of SB-IPMN and frequency of ARP. Pancreatic stents have been used to palliate obstructive pain and to treat ARP in patients with pancreatic malignancies who are not candidates for surgery.[156] Pancreatic duct ES may allow mucus passage and palliate symptoms in patients with IPMNs who are nonoperative candidates. Patients with ARP secondary to ampullary adenomas can be treated with endoscopic or surgical ampullectomy.[157]

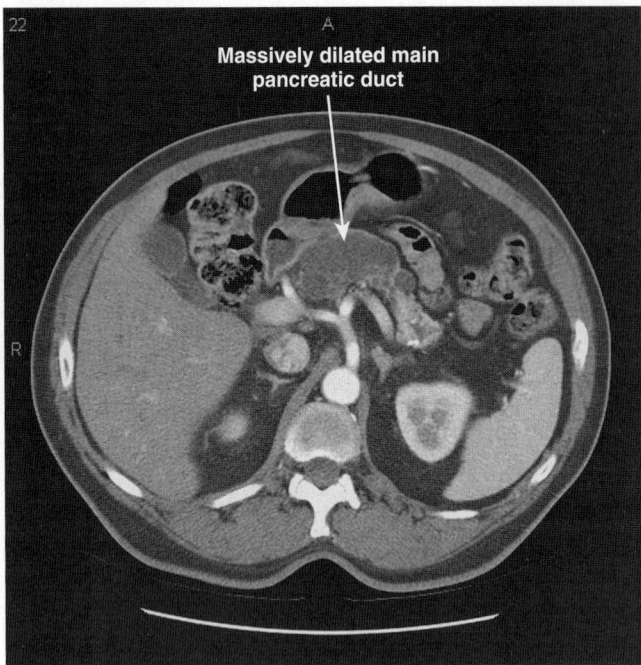

Fig. 48.9 Computed tomography (CT) scan obtained in a patient with intraductal papillary mucin-producing tumor. A massively dilated pancreatic duct filled with low-density material is seen *(arrow)*.

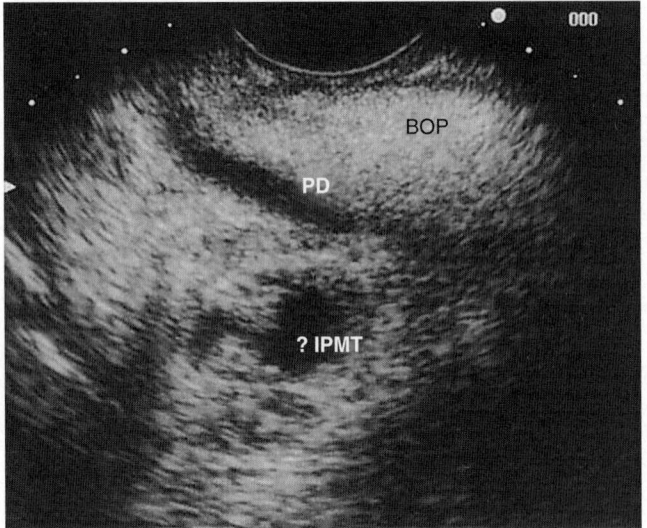

Fig. 48.10 Endoscopic ultrasound (EUS) is performed on a patient with a side branch variant of intraductal papillary mucin-producing tumor (IPMT). A cystic hypoechoic region (IPMT) is seen immediately caudal to the main pancreatic duct (PD). *(Courtesy of Dr. Kevin McGrath, University of Pittsburgh Medical Center.)*

Choledochocysts

Choledochocysts are congenital anomalies of the biliary tract that are most often diagnosed in children and often associated with pancreaticobiliary malunion (**Fig. 48.12**). ARP in children with choledochocysts is usually associated with biliary stones or sludge that forms in the native or retained cyst.[158] Complete surgical excision is the treatment of choice to prevent pancreaticobiliary symptoms and to prevent the development

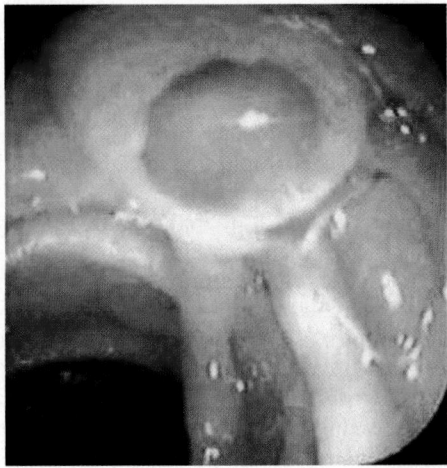

Fig. 48.11 Photograph of the endoscopic appearance of the major papilla of a patient with intraductal papillary mucin-producing tumor shows that the pancreatic orifice is held widely patent with intraductal mucus giving the classic fish-mouth appearance.

of biliary cancer, which is increased in the cysts if left in situ. Type 3 choledochocysts (choledochoceles) have been associated with ARP and can be treated with biliary ES through the cyst or via surgical transduodenal marsupialization.[159] They may be recognized at endoscopy as a suprapapillary submucosal bulge and confirmed fluoroscopically at ERCP.

Periampullary Duodenal Diverticula

Periampullary diverticula have been indicated in the etiology of ARP. These diverticula are more commonly seen in elderly patients and are more often associated with choledocholithiasis and ARP compared with patients without diverticula.[160] Periampullary diverticula are associated with an incompetent sphincter of Oddi with resultant colonization of the bile duct with intestinal bacteria, leading to the generation of mixed pigment bile duct stones.[161] Although direct causative evidence linking periampullary diverticula to ARP are lacking, relative outflow obstruction of bile duct with bacterial colonization and microlith formation or outflow obstruction of exocrine pancreas secretions have been postulated in the pathogenesis of ARP, and a biliary sphincterotomy is generally performed.

Annular Pancreas

Annular pancreas is a rare congenital malformation in which the pancreatic parenchyma encircles the duodenal sweep. It most commonly manifests with obstruction of the duodenum and is best treated with a surgical duodenal bypass. Case reports of ARP associated with annular pancreas exist[4,162]; however, causality has not been confirmed.

Genetic Causes

Introduction

More recent developments in molecular biology have led to the recognition of a strong genetic predisposition for a

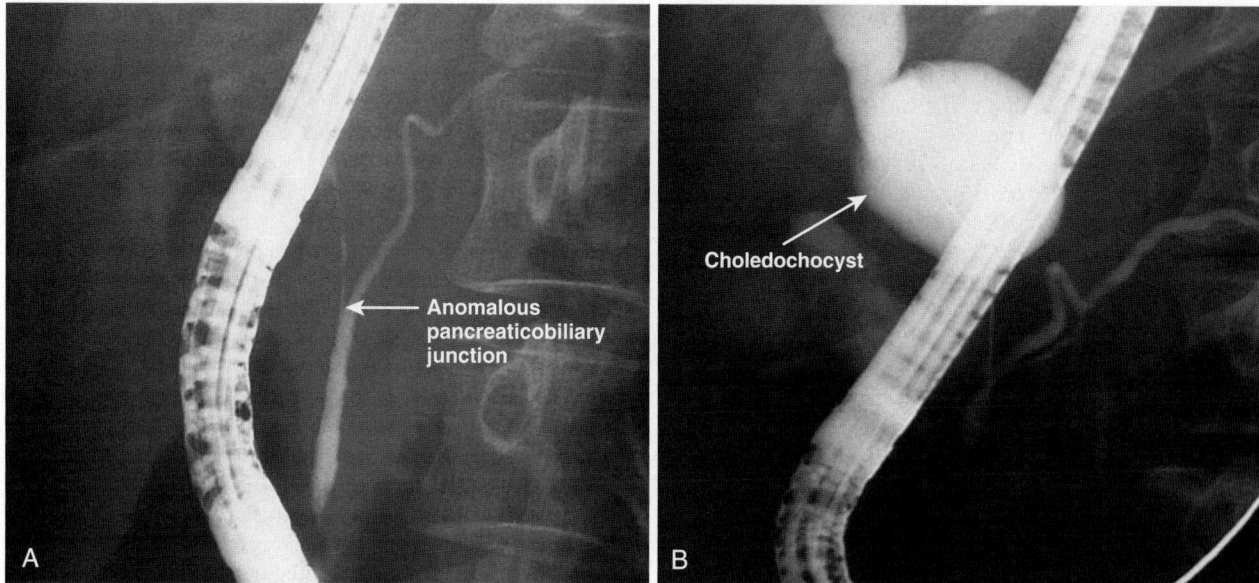

Fig. 48.12 A 22-year-old woman presented with acute recurrent biliary pancreatitis. **A,** At endoscopic retrograde cholangiopancreatography (ERCP), an anomalous pancreaticobiliary junction *(arrow)* is seen. **B,** Filling of the distal bile duct is seen via a strictured segment. Further contrast agent injection into the bile duct fills a classic type I choledochocyst. The patient was taken to surgery and had complete excision of the cyst with a hepaticojejunostomy and has done well without recurrent symptoms.

significant proportion of patients with idiopathic pancreatitis and evidence for gene-environment interactions for other forms of pancreatitis including alcohol-related pancreatitis. The focus of this section is on ARP and associated genetic etiologies.

Hereditary Pancreatitis
Epidemiology

Familial pancreatitis refers to pancreatitis of any etiology occurring in a family with an incidence that is greater than expected by chance. HP specifically refers to unexplained pancreatitis in a member of a family in which a pancreatitis-causing gene mutation is expressed in an autosomal dominant pattern. The phenotypic features of HP encompass the spectrum of pancreatic inflammatory diseases. HP typically manifests as ARP in childhood and progresses to CP by young adulthood in more than half of cases and is associated with an approximately 40% risk of pancreatic cancer by age 71,[163,164] which is exaggerated by smoking.[165]

Pathogenesis

The gene for HP was mapped to chromosome 7q35[166,167] and was identified as the cationic trypsinogen gene (protease, serine, 1; PRSS1; OMIM 276000) by Whitcomb and colleagues in 1996.[168] Two point mutations, R122H and N29I[169] occurring in exon3 and exon2 of cationic trypsinogen, account for most cases. These are the only mutations at the present time for which genetic testing is recommended according to a consensus conference.[170,171] The same consensus also provides guidelines for testing. The R122H mutant cationic trypsin is thought to be resistant to autolysis through elimination of the

arginine or lysine residues recognized by trypsin, which is critical in initiating trypsin autolysis.[172] Trypsin is a proteolytic enzyme that activates most pancreatic digestive enzymes within the intestinal lumen and is maintained in the inactive trypsinogen form within the pancreas. Several mechanisms protect the pancreas from the consequences of prematurely activated trypsinogen. When trypsinogen is activated within the pancreas, the first known protective mechanism is inhibition by pancreatic secretory trypsin inhibitor (PSTI; unigene symbol SPINK1; serine protease inhibitor, Kazal type 1; OMIM 167790), which has the capacity to inhibit approximately 20% of potential trypsin activity.[172]

If trypsin activity overwhelms the SPINK1/PSTI inhibitory capacity, trypsin inactivation occurs via trypsin autolysis. With mutations that eliminate the autolysis site in HP, the second protective mechanism is lost, and pancreatitis occurs. Studies of families with HP reveal mutations in cationic trypsinogen that enhance autoactivation (N29I), mutations in SPINK1/PSTI that likely diminish inhibition of active trypsinogen (e.g., N34S), and mutations in cationic trypsinogen that prevent autolysis (R122H). One-third of families with HP have no mutation in either cationic trypsinogen or SPINK1/PSTI, suggesting that other genes are also important. For reasons that are unclear, HP disease penetrance is incomplete. A review of large kindred groups worldwide revealed a fairly constant rate of penetrance of 80%.[163–176] A study of identical twins with HP[171] suggested that the mechanism of disease penetrance is not one of simple genetics and that the protective element is not a modifier gene or obvious environmental factor. SPINK1/PSTI mutations are common in the general population and are not clearly associated with pancreatitis but may enhance the likelihood of pancreatitis related to other etiologies.[165,176] The most commonly identified mutation in control populations is N34S (1% allele frequency), and the highest frequency is seen in patients with idiopathic CP.

Approximately 10% of familial pancreatitis kindreds have identifiable *SPINK1* mutations. The clinical presentations are varied and include ARP or more commonly CP. The age at first presentation is typically before 20 years. Because less than 1% of patients with a heterozygous *SPINK1* mutation alone ever develop pancreatitis, most experts do not recommend genetic testing or screening.[170]

Tropical Pancreatitis

Tropical pancreatitis is a syndrome of ARP that progresses to CP, which usually develops in children from lower socioeconomic families in tropical regions of Indonesia, Asia, Africa, and South America. There appears to be some variation in presentation; some children have severe calcific CP with late diabetes mellitus, whereas others develop diabetes and pancreatic fibrosis before developing calcification. The etiology of tropical pancreatitis is uncertain, but some clues are beginning to accumulate. First, diet has been eliminated as a cause of this disease. Second, there seems to be genetic susceptibility because a significant minority of patients has mutations in the pancreatic secretory trypsin inhibitor gene *SPINK1*.[177,178] Third, the immune systems and pancreaticobiliary tree of these children are constantly challenged by infectious agents including helminths such as *Ascaris lumbricoides* that are endemic.[179–181] If these infectious agents trigger acute pancreatitis, an altered immune response may drive pancreatic fibrosis in genetically susceptible individuals.[182] Current evidence suggests that tropical pancreatitis is a complex condition with strong environmental trigger factors and genetic susceptibility and modifier factors that eventually result in irreversible pancreatic damage.

Therapy

Endoscopic therapy for ARP secondary to HP is reserved for general complications of CP, including strictures, stones, fistulas, and pseudocysts; this is discussed in detail in Chapter 49.

Cystic Fibrosis
Pathogenesis

CF (OMIM 219700) is the most common lethal autosomal recessive disorder in whites and is caused by a mutation of the *CFTR* gene (OMIM 602421) located on chromosome 7q32.[183] CFTR is a chloride channel located on the luminal surface of the pancreatic duct cell that is tightly linked to bicarbonate secretion.[175–187] Major mutations in both alleles leads to loss of CFTR function and the ability to hydrate mucus resulting in inspissated glands. Based on their functional impact, *CFTR* gene mutations are classified as either severe (class 1 to 3) or mild (class 4 and 5).[187,188] Severe mutations yield little or no functional protein, whereas mild mutations diminish CFTR function.

Pulmonary consequences and abnormal sweat chloride occurs with CFTR function less than 5%; however, pancreatic exocrine function may be maintained down to 1% CFTR function. One or two mild CFTR mutations retaining more than 1% CFTR function may not lead to pancreatic insufficiency despite the overall disease status.[189,190] Such patients are susceptible to ARP, as may be patients with one severe mutation (e.g., delta F508, the most common mutation [approximately 70%]) and a second milder mutation (e.g., CFTR R117H, R334W, R347W) any time the CFTR function becomes less than 10% of normal.[191,192] The pancreas behaves differently from the lung and vas deferens qualitatively depending on the degree of CFTR impairment.

Although the spectrum of pancreatic disease ranges from pancreatic insufficiency to ARP and CP, most of the available data pertain to patients with pancreatic insufficiency and idiopathic CP and are based on a select number of the known mutations; firm recommendations with regard to patients with ARP cannot be made. Patients with ARP resulting from diminished CFTR activity probably reflect an intermediate stage with CP as the result. Studies involving histologic correlation are needed to elucidate this process further. In patients with ARP and suspected *CFTR* gene mutations, diminished CFTR function can be confirmed with nasal bioelectric potential difference measurements because many mild *CFTR* gene mutations are not included in commercial CFTR tests.

Therapy

Endoscopic therapy for ARP in CF is reserved for complications of CP and is discussed in Chapter 49.

Autoimmune Pancreatitis

Pancreatitis associated with hypergammaglobulinemia was first reported in 1965.[193] Since then, evidence for an autoimmune basis for recurrent attacks (but more commonly CP) in a subset of patients has been increasing.[194,195]

Epidemiology and Diagnosis

The clinical findings in autoimmune pancreatitis (AIP) encompass the clinical findings typical of pancreatitis but often with milder symptoms and usually without acute attacks. Obstructive jaundice seems to be a common feature, and a therapeutic response to steroid therapy has been reported.[196] The sex ratio for AIP varies remarkably in the literature, probably because of the small study populations.[197,198] In a more recent major U.S. study, the median age at presentation was 62.5 years (range 23 to 86 years) with 65% male and 88% white.[199] The most common clinical presentations included new-onset mild abdominal pain (65%), jaundice (65%), and weight loss (42%).

Radiologic findings include diffuse or focal pancreatic parenchymal enlargement with a "sausage-shaped" pancreas on abdominal CT (**Fig. 48.13**), diffuse or focal main pancreatic duct narrowing and beading, and a characteristic absence of pancreatic calcifications or cysts.[200,201] EUS typically shows a diffusely hypoechoic, enlarged pancreas or a focal, irregularly shaped mass (**Fig. 48.14**).[202] In the absence of cytologic evaluation, it may be difficult to discern these findings from a malignant pancreatic neoplasm. EUS-guided fine needle aspiration rarely provides an adequate tissue sample for a definitive diagnosis in cases of AIP. More recently, EUS-guided Tru-Cut needle biopsies have enabled core tissue sampling from the pancreas and other organs.[203] Studies have shown

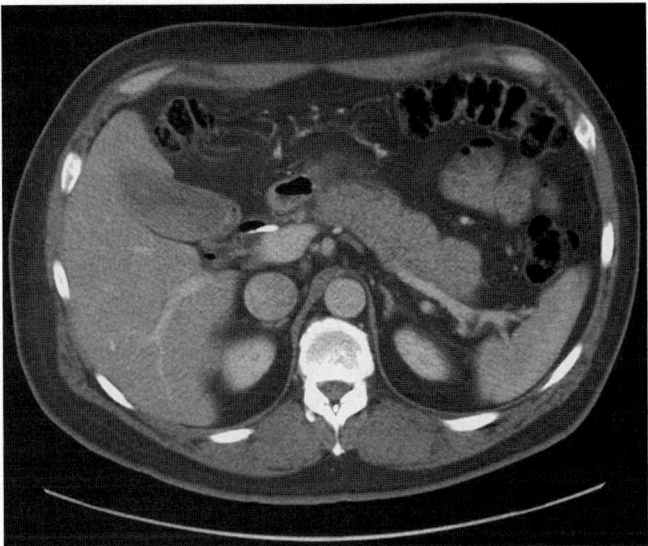

Fig. 48.13 Enlarged, sausage-shaped pancreas observed on abdominal computed tomography (CT) scan in a middle-aged white man with autoimmune pancreatitis (AIP) presenting with mild abdominal pain and new-onset jaundice. The pancreatic body and tail region are enlarged.

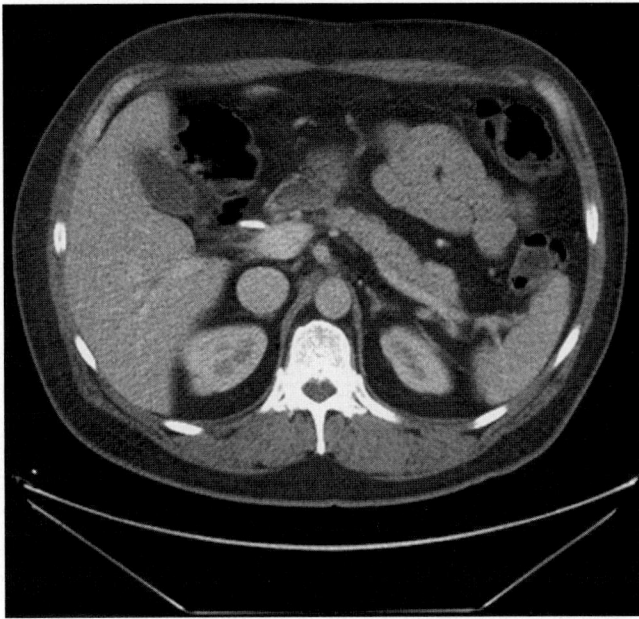

Fig. 48.15 Abdominal computed tomography (CT) image shows response to corticosteroid treatment in a patient with autoimmune pancreatitis (AIP). Compare with Fig. 48.13, which shows an enlarged pancreatic body and tail in the same patient before corticosteroid treatment.

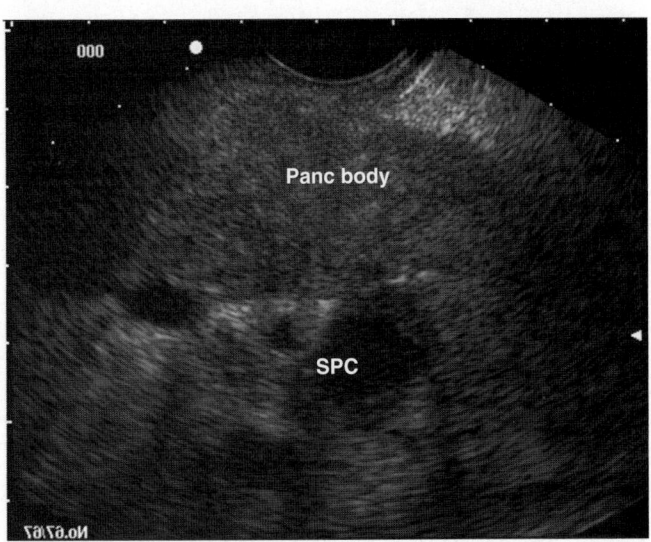

Fig. 48.14 Endoscopic ultrasound (EUS) image of a patient with autoimmune pancreatitis (AIP) shows diffuse hypoechoic changes throughout the pancreas. *SPC,* splenoportal confluence.

Laboratory findings in AIP may differ between isolated AIP and AIP associated with an autoimmune disorder. Both entities are characterized by elevated serum IgG and the presence of autoantibodies including antinuclear, antilactoferrin, and anti–carbonic anhydrase II and less commonly anti–smooth muscle and rheumatoid factor.[201] Elevated IgG4 levels are useful in diagnosing isolated AIP.[200,209] IgG4 is the least common of the IgG subclasses and has been considered a noninflammatory protective antibody,[210] and its secretion along with IgE is regulated by T helper-2 cytokines such as interleukin-4, interleukin-5, and interleukin-13.[1] The antigens driving the elevated IgG4 antibody titers in isolated AIP remain obscure.

Therapy

The finding of elevated IgG4 levels in the appropriate clinical setting may also be useful for deciding on a trial of steroid therapy.[210,211] In addition to the improvement in symptoms and radiographic features, patients with AIP and diabetes mellitus display a trend toward normalizing insulin secretion and glycemic control with steroid therapy.[211] Other regimens have been reported, including the use of additional immunosuppressive therapy such as azathioprine and mycophenolate mofetil. Repeat abdominal CT scan after immunosuppressive therapy may show dramatic improvement in the pancreas (**Fig. 48.15**).

Celiac Disease

A known association between celiac disease and pancreatic insufficiency has been recognized for many years,[212–214] and

that EUS-guided Tru-Cut needle biopsy is a safe and effective technique for obtaining a histologic diagnosis in patients with suspected AIP.[204] Classic histologic findings include a lymphoplasmacytic infiltrate with obliterative venulitis and immunostaining positive for IgG4 plasma cells. Patients with AIP may also have an abundant infiltration of IgG4-positive plasma cells at the major duodenal papilla, and mucosal biopsies may provide an alternative method for helping to establish the diagnosis.[205] Formal diagnostic criteria have been developed for the diagnosis of AIP.[206–208] Strict adherence to these criteria may help to avoid misdiagnosis.

reports exist of improvement in pancreatic function in non-CP cases with gluten-free diet. Postulated mechanisms include malnutrition[215,216] and reduced gallbladder emptying resulting from impaired cholecystokinin release.[217–219] More recently, an association between ARP and celiac disease has been reported, presumably resulting from duodenal inflammation leading to papillary stenosis.[220] In 169 patients referred for suspected SOD, celiac disease was diagnosed in 12 (3 men, 9 women); 10 patients had ARP, and 2 had elevated liver function tests associated with abdominal pain. These patients had manometric evidence of papillary stenosis and histologic evidence of periampullary inflammation and celiac disease. Improvement in duodenal inflammation and symptoms was seen on a gluten-free diet; however, all patients had undergone biliary ES, and the data are difficult to interpret.

Acknowledgments

The authors thank Dr. Asif Khalid for assistance in the preparation of the sections on hereditary and AIP.

References

The complete reference list is available online at www.expertconsult.com.

Chronic Pancreatitis, Stones, and Strictures

Shyam Varadarajulu and Robert H. Hawes

 Video related to this chapter's topics can be found online at expertconsult.com.

Introduction

Chronic pancreatitis is an inflammatory condition that results in permanent structural changes in the pancreas, which can lead to impairment of exocrine and endocrine function.[1] This disorder contrasts with acute pancreatitis in that the latter is nonprogressive, and the gland returns to histologic and functional normalcy once the acute event subsides. Most diagnostic and therapeutic efforts in chronic pancreatitis are directed toward evaluation and management of symptoms, primarily abdominal pain and steatorrhea. Although interpretation of data on the role of endoscopic therapy for management of chronic pancreatitis remains difficult, this area is rapidly expanding and is of great interest and challenge to gastrointestinal endoscopists.

Epidemiology

The incidence of chronic pancreatitis is in the range of 3 to 10 per 100,000 population in many parts of the world.[2] The crude incidence rate for chronic pancreatitis per 100,000 population in Germany is 6.4; in Czech Republic, 7.9; and in Japan, 27.9.[3–5] The peak incidence for chronic pancreatitis in Germany is in the age group 45 to 54 years, which is 10 years older than the peak age group for acute pancreatitis suggesting that chronic pancreatitis develops during this time frame following first attacks of acute pancreatitis. In a prospective study that evaluated patients with alcoholic chronic pancreatitis, an annual incidence of 8.2 cases per year per 100,000 population and an overall prevalence of 27.4 cases per year per 100,000 population were noted.[6] The incidence rates in retrospective European and North American studies range from 2 to 10 per 100,000 cases per year.[7,8] Chronic pancreatitis is more common in male patients[3,5,6]; the male-to-female ratio in Japan is 3.5.[5] Compared with whites, blacks are two to three times more likely to be hospitalized for chronic pancreatitis than for alcoholic cirrhosis.[9] The explanation for this observation is unclear but could be related to racial differences in diet, type or quantity of alcohol consumption, smoking, or ability to detoxify substances harmful to the liver or pancreas. The absence of any screening programs and unresolved debate on the "gold standard" for diagnosis of chronic pancreatitis make epidemiologic studies in this area more difficult and explain the wide range of variations noted among studies.

Pathophysiology

The pathogenesis of chronic pancreatitis seems to be multifactorial and is probably initiated by two distinct events (**Fig. 49.1**). The first event is a decrease in bicarbonate secretion that is due to either a mechanical or a functional ductal obstruction. Mechanical causes include strictures, sphincter of Oddi dysfunction, and tumors. Functional causes include mutations in the cystic fibrosis transmembrane conductance regulator (*CFTR*) gene leading to impaired bicarbonate secretion. This impaired bicarbonate secretion has formed the basis for the secretin pancreatic function test. The second event involves intraparenchymal activation of digestive enzymes within the pancreatic gland. Ischemia, antioxidant stress, and sphincter of Oddi dysfunction are possible later events involved in perpetuating the disease process. This multifactorial model provides an explanation as to why no single therapy works in all patients with chronic pancreatitis.

Pancreatic Duct Obstruction

Proteinaceous plugs are one of the earliest findings noted in patients with chronic pancreatitis.[10] It is theorized that increased glandular secretion of pancreatic proteins causes precipitation of proteinaceous plugs within the pancreatic ductal system. These plugs may act as a nidus for calcification that leads to stone formation. As ductal obstruction progresses, inflammatory changes and cell loss occur. The importance of these proteinaceous plugs in perpetuating changes within the pancreas is emphasized by studies that have shown relief of clinical symptoms after endoscopic removal of these plugs in patients with chronic pancreatitis.[11,12] GP2 is a glycosyl phosphatidylinositol anchored protein that is cleaved

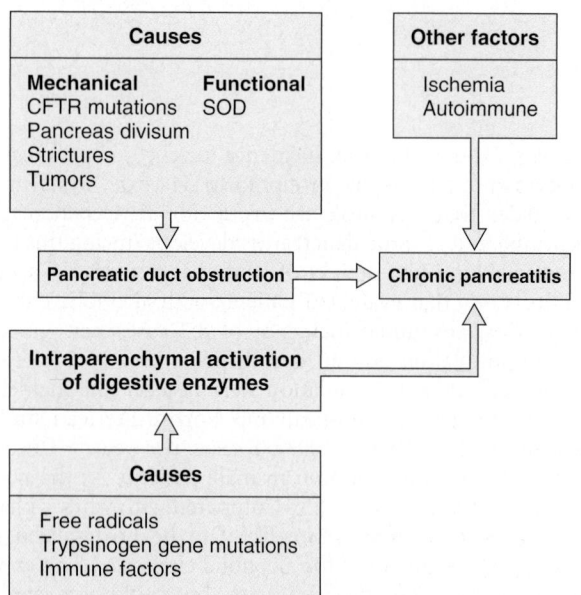

Fig. 49.1 The pathogenesis of chronic pancreatitis is initiated by two distinct events. First, a decrease in bicarbonate secretion is due to either a mechanical or a functional pancreatic duct obstruction. Second, intraparenchymal activation of digestive enzymes occurs within the pancreatic gland. Ischemia and autoimmune factors are postulated to be other important events in this pathway. *CFTR*, cystic fibrosis transmembrane conductance regulator (gene); SOD, sphincter of Oddi dysfunction.

from the zymogen granules and secreted into the pancreatic juice. This protein has been identified as a major component of intraductal plugs.[13] Pancreatic acinar cells release another protein called lithostatine that prevents calcium carbonate precipitation and stone formation in pancreatic juice.[14] Low levels of these proteins in patients with chronic pancreatitis may be another factor involved in stone formation.

Ischemia

Ischemia may be another important event in the pathogenesis of chronic pancreatitis. Animal models have shown that partial pancreatic duct ligation induces ductal hypertension and increased resistance to blood flow within the pancreas.[15,16] Blood flow was found to be 40% of that observed in controls. Secretory stimulus reduced blood flow further as opposed to the normal increase. In patients with chronic pancreatitis, pancreatic interstitial pressure increases to a greater degree than in normal individuals owing to decreased glandular elasticity. The rapid relief of symptoms achieved by ductal decompression procedures suggests that ischemia plays a central role in the complex mechanisms involved in chronic pancreatitis.

Antioxidants

Nutritional depletion is frequently seen in patients with chronic pancreatitis. In particular, antioxidants such as selenium, vitamin C and E, and methionine are depleted.[17,18] An imbalance between a decrease in antioxidants and an increased demand for them in pancreatic cells in chronic pancreatitis may lead to elevation in free radical formation, which is associated with lipid peroxidation and cellular impairment. Increased membrane lipid peroxidation, a marker of oxidative stress and free radical production, can also be seen in alcoholic chronic pancreatitis.[19] It is postulated that alcohol causes a disproportionate increase in the secretion of trypsinogen leading to premature activation of digestive enzymes within the acinar or ductal cell systems.[20]

Autoimmunity

Chronic pancreatitis is also seen in association with autoimmune disorders such as Sjögren's syndrome and primary biliary cirrhosis.[21,22] Autoantibody to pancreatic antigens has been shown in patients with Sjögren's syndrome and idiopathic chronic pancreatitis. Some cases of idiopathic chronic pancreatitis are associated with the expression of novel HLA-DR antigens on duct cells in combination with a localized T-cell inflammatory infiltrate, lending further credibility to an autoimmune pathogenesis.[23]

Interstitial Fibrosis

It is proposed that repeated episodes of acute pancreatitis initiate a sequence of perilobular fibrosis, duct distortion, and altered secretion and flow of pancreatic juice.[24] Studies on the natural history of pancreatitis have shown that more frequent and more repeated attacks of acute pancreatitis lead to chronic changes as seen in the alcoholic type of chronic pancreatitis.[25] The exact mechanisms involved in the pathophysiology of chronic pancreatitis are still elusive and unproven. Multiple exogenous factors may act in a genetically predisposed patient in an appropriate clinical setting, such as alcohol consumption, to trigger a cascade of events culminating in progressive destruction of pancreatic parenchyma and ensuing sequelae. Although the focus of therapies has been the inhibition of acinar cell secretion, further insights into the role of ductal bicarbonate secretion, ductal obstruction, and the relative contribution of ischemia and oxygen-derived free radicals in this process may provide new therapeutic avenues.

Etiology

Alcohol

Alcohol abuse accounts for 70% to 80% of cases of chronic pancreatitis (**Table 49.1**); the mechanism by which this occurs is unclear. The risk seems to be related to the duration and amount of alcohol consumed rather than the type of alcohol or the pattern of consumption.[26] Intake of large amounts of alcohol (>50 g/day) has been shown to be associated with a shortened time to pancreatic calcification and survival.[27] There is considerable variation in individual sensitivity to the toxicity of alcohol making it difficult to define a "safe" level of consumption. Only 5% to 10% of alcoholics develop chronic pancreatitis, suggesting that other unidentified factors may be important in the pathogenesis of the disease.[28] Tobacco, although not important in the pathogenesis of alcoholic pancreatitis,[29,30] has been implicated in the development of calcification in patients who already have chronic pancreatitis.[31] A U.S.-based study showed an association between the presence of calcium-sensing receptor gene polymorphisms and chronic pancreatitis.[32] The risk for developing chronic pancreatitis was significantly higher in patients with these gene polymorphisms who consumed moderate to heavy amounts of alcohol.

Hereditary Pancreatitis

Hereditary pancreatitis is characterized by a young age at onset and prominent pancreatic calcifications. It is transmitted as an autosomal dominant trait, and nearly 80% of patients with the inherited defect develop chronic pancreatitis.[33] Most affected individuals develop symptoms before age 20. In some kindreds, hereditary chronic pancreatitis has been mapped to the long arm of chromosome 7 (7q35), where a cluster of trypsinogen genes is located.[34,35] Several mutations associated with chronic pancreatitis have been identified in this region.

Table 49.1 Etiology of Chronic Pancreatitis

Alcohol	70%
Idiopathic	10%–30%
Other	10%–15%
Pancreatic duct obstruction (trauma, divisum, tumor, fibrosis)	
Hereditary (*CFTR* gene mutation, trypsinogen gene mutation)	
Hyperlipidemia	
Tropical	

CFTR, cystic fibrosis transmembrane conductance regulator.

Although the exact consequences of these mutations on trypsin activity are unclear, they are known to interfere with trypsin inactivation or to enhance its activation, permitting autodigestion of the pancreas.[36,37] Although mutations in the trypsinogen gene are specific for hereditary pancreatitis, not all affected family members develop chronic pancreatitis. The relationship between mutations of other genes associated with chronic pancreatitis, such as the *CFTR* and the trypsinogen genes, needs further elucidation.

Mutations of the Cystic Fibrosis Gene

Cystic fibrosis is due to mutations in the *CFTR* gene. Most patients with cystic fibrosis develop progressive pancreatic damage as a result of defective ductular and acinar pancreatic secretion.[38] In some series, mutations in the *CFTR* gene have been identified in 13% to 37% of patients with idiopathic chronic pancreatitis who have no clinical evidence of cystic fibrosis.[39,40] This percentage range could be an underestimation because currently available genetic screening tests identify only 18 to 23 of the most severe *CFTR* mutations that cause classic, childhood cystic fibrosis.

Tropical Pancreatitis

Tropical pancreatitis is a condition of unknown etiology that is seen commonly in younger individuals in south India and other parts of the tropics, where it is the most common cause of chronic pancreatitis. The pathology is characterized by large intraductal calculi, marked dilation of the pancreatic ducts, atrophy, and fibrosis. Clinically, most patients experience abdominal pain, diabetes mellitus, and fat malabsorption. The etiology of tropical pancreatitis is unknown. The cassava fruit had been implicated as an etiologic factor in this disorder, although it is no longer thought to be related.[41] Mutations in the serine protease inhibitor SPINK1 have been identified in some patients.[42,43]

Ductal Obstruction

Obstruction of the pancreatic duct from any cause can lead to chronic pancreatitis. The histologic abnormalities that are induced may persist after relief of the obstruction. Sphincter of Oddi dysfunction seems to be associated with chronic pancreatitis. In one study of patients with chronic pancreatitis undergoing sphincter of Oddi manometry, more than 60% had sphincter of Oddi dysfunction.[44]

Pancreas divisum may cause chronic pancreatitis by producing a relative obstruction to flow of pancreatic juice at the minor papilla. It is estimated that less than 5% of patients with pancreas divisum develop pancreatic symptoms. The low frequency of symptoms has created controversy as to whether pancreas divisum and its associated small minor papilla orifice are ever a cause of obstructive pancreatitis. The arguments against an association are based on two major observations. First, some studies have found that the incidence of pancreas divisum is the same among patients with and without pancreatitis.[45] Second, symptoms occur infrequently in patients with this anomaly. We believe that there is a group of patients with pancreas divisum who are subject to recurrent bouts of seemingly idiopathic pancreatitis. In these patients, the minor papilla orifice is so small that excessively high intrapancreatic dorsal ductal pressure occurs during active secretion, which may result in inadequate drainage, ductal distention, pain, and, in some cases, pancreatitis. To support this view, greater than 60% of patients with pancreas divisum and otherwise unexplained abdominal pain had relief of pain after surgical sphincteroplasty suggesting that obstruction to flow of secretion was the proximate cause of symptoms in these patients.[46]

Metabolic and Endocrine Causes

Elevation of serum triglycerides greater than 500 mg/dL and hyperparathyroidism are other rare causes of chronic pancreatitis. Recurrent episodes of acute pancreatitis in patients with hypertriglyceridemia lead to chronic glandular damage. The pathophysiology in hyperparathyroidism is thought to be related to increased calcium concentration in pancreatic juice, which leads to precipitation of calcium deposits in the pancreatic ducts.

Idiopathic Chronic Pancreatitis

An etiology for pancreatitis cannot be determined in 10% to 30% of patients with chronic pancreatitis despite extensive investigations. Concealed alcohol ingestion, hypersensitivity to small amounts of alcohol, unreported pancreatic trauma, and mutations in the *CFTR* and the trypsinogen genes may be contributing factors in at least a small proportion of patients with idiopathic chronic pancreatitis.[47,48] Although in the past patients with idiopathic chronic pancreatitis were considered as a single group, data from the Mayo Clinic have defined an early and late onset form of idiopathic chronic pancreatitis.[49] Age distribution at onset of symptoms showed a bimodal distribution of patients with early and late onset idiopathic chronic pancreatitis with a median age of 19.2 years for early onset and 56.2 years for late onset. No gender differences were observed among patients in either group. Pain was the predominant symptom in 96% of patients with early onset idiopathic pancreatitis but was present in only 54% of late onset idiopathic pancreatitis. Regardless of whether patients had early or late onset idiopathic pancreatitis, pain was the presenting symptom, and endocrine and exocrine insufficiency with pancreatic calcification was seen in both forms of the disease.

Clinical Features

Abdominal pain and pancreatic insufficiency are the two cardinal clinical manifestations of chronic pancreatitis.

Abdominal Pain

Abdominal pain in chronic pancreatitis is typically centered in the epigastric area and frequently radiates to the back. The pain is worsened with eating and is sometimes associated with nausea and vomiting. Early in the course of chronic pancreatitis, the pain may occur in discrete attacks; as the condition progresses, pain tends to become more continuous.

The mechanism for abdominal pain is poorly understood. Causes are perhaps multifactorial and include inflammation, duct obstruction, high pancreatic tissue pressure, fibrotic encasement of sensory nerves, and neuropathy characterized

by both increased numbers and sizes of intrapancreatic sensory nerves and by inflammatory injury to the nerve sheaths allowing exposure of the neural elements to toxic substances.[50,51] Pain is not in the spectrum of clinical symptoms in nearly one-fourth of patients with chronic pancreatitis.[52] The view that chronic pain subsides in a substantial number of patients as the disease progresses to the point of organ failure[53] has been widely accepted, but that process may take an unpredictable number of years or may never occur. Some studies suggest that the likelihood of spontaneous pain relief is low.[54] In a study that evaluated the natural history of pain in chronic pancreatitis, pain decreased or disappeared in 67%, 64%, and 77% of early onset idiopathic, late onset idiopathic, and alcoholic pancreatitis over a median time of 25 years, 13 years, and 14 years.[49]

Pancreatic Insufficiency

Patients with severe pancreatic exocrine dysfunction cannot properly digest complex foods or absorb digestive breakdown products. Nevertheless, clinically significant protein and fat deficiencies do not occur until more than 90% of pancreatic function is lost.[55] In a large natural history study, the median time for development of pancreatic insufficiency was 13.1 years in patients with alcoholic chronic pancreatitis, 16.1 years in patients with late onset idiopathic chronic pancreatitis, and 26.3 years in patients with early onset idiopathic chronic pancreatitis.[48] Steatorrhea usually occurs before protein deficiencies because lipolytic activity decreases more quickly than proteolysis.[56,57] Glucose intolerance occurs frequently in chronic pancreatitis, but overt diabetes mellitus usually occurs late in the course of disease. Patients with chronic calcific disease, particularly patients who develop early calcifications, may develop diabetes more frequently than patients with chronic noncalcific disease.[58,59] Nearly 40% to 70% of patients with chronic pancreatitis develop diabetes on prolonged follow-up. In one study, the median time to develop diabetes was 19.8 years, 11.9 years, and 26.3 years in patients with alcoholic, late onset idiopathic, and early onset idiopathic chronic pancreatitis.[49] In chronic pancreatitis, both insulin-producing beta cells and glucagon-producing alpha cells are destroyed. When exogenously administered insulin leads to hypoglycemia, the deficiency in glandular glucagon storage fails to correct the serum glucose levels back to normal leading to prolonged and severe hypoglycemia. The nature of diabetes in this patient population is brittle, and management is more complicated than that of patients with type 1 diabetes.

Pathology

In early stages of chronic pancreatitis, glandular damage is patchy and uneven (**Fig. 49.2**). Areas of irregularly distributed fibrosis, reduced number and size of acini with relative sparing of the islets of Langerhans, and variable degrees of obstruction of pancreatic ducts of all sizes are seen.[60] A chronic inflammatory infiltrate around lobules and ducts is usually present. The interlobular and intralobular ducts are dilated and contain protein plugs in their lumens. The ductal epithelium may be atrophied or hyperplastic or show squamous metaplasia, and ductal concretions may be evident. Remaining islets become embedded in sclerosed tissue or severely damaged lobules

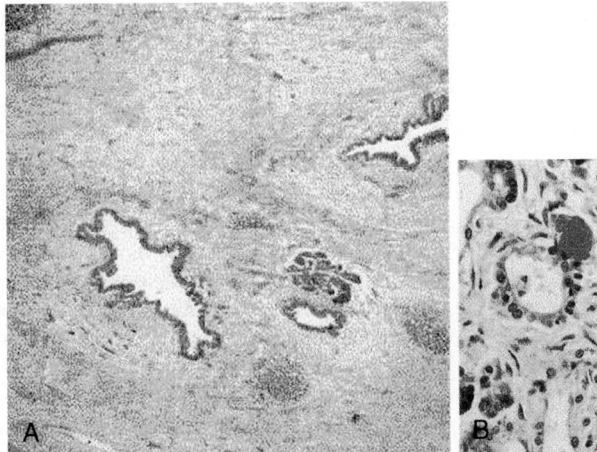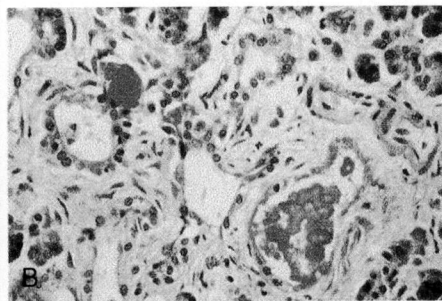

Fig. 49.2 Histopathology of chronic pancreatitis. **A,** Extensive fibrosis and atrophy of the pancreatic parenchyma has left only residual islets and ducts, with occasional chronic inflammatory cells and acinar tissue. **B,** High-power view shows dilated ducts with inspissated eosinophilic ductal concretions.

before they too disappear. Grossly, the gland is hard, sometimes with extremely dilated ducts and grossly visible calcified concretions. Pseudocyst formation is common.

Differential Diagnosis

None of the currently available laboratory and radiologic tests is absolutely diagnostic of chronic pancreatitis. Numerous disorders, such as pancreatic cancer, peptic ulcer disease, irritable bowel syndrome, and symptomatic cholelithiasis, must be considered in the differential diagnosis. A careful history and physical examination coupled with judicious use of tests such as esophagogastroduodenoscopy and transabdominal ultrasound can establish or exclude the diagnosis in most instances. Pancreatic cancer is the principal diagnosis that must be strongly considered in patients suspected to have chronic pancreatitis. Some data suggest that chronic pancreatitis is associated with an increased risk of developing pancreatic carcinoma.

The International Pancreatitis Study Group observed a standardized incidence ratio for pancreatic cancer of 26.3 among patients with chronic pancreatitis compared with an expected ratio of 2.13 that was calculated from country-specific incidence data and adjusted for age and sex.[61] Similar to chronic pancreatitis, patients with pancreatic cancer can present with abdominal pain, weight loss, and jaundice. Findings suggestive of possible pancreatic cancer in a patient thought or known to have chronic pancreatitis include older age, absence of a history of alcohol use, weight loss, a protracted flare of symptoms, and the onset of significant constitutional symptoms. The physician should maintain a high index of suspicion for pancreatic cancer, particularly in any elderly patient presenting with a new-onset pancreatitis when common causes such as alcohol and gallstones have been excluded. Tumor markers such as CA 19.9 (for colorectal and pancreatic carcinomas) and carcinoembryonic antigen (CEA) are helpful if elevated, but normal values do not rule out pancreatic cancer. Computed tomography (CT) or endoscopic ultrasound (EUS)–guided biopsy may be required to establish the diagnosis in some patients.

Table 49.2 Diagnostic Tests for Chronic Pancreatitis

| Structural Tests | Functional Tests | |
	Indirect	*Direct*
X-ray	Serum enzymes (trypsinogen)	Secretin stimulation test
Ultrasound	Fecal tests (fat, elastase, chymoptrysin)	
CT	Urine tests (bentiromide, pancreolauryl)	
MRCP		
ERCP		
EUS		

CT, computed tomography; ERCP, endoscopic retrograde cholangiopancreatography; EUS, endoscopic ultrasound; MRCP, magnetic resonance cholangiopancreatography.

Diagnosis

Tests for chronic pancreatitis can be classified into tests that evaluate the structure of the gland (parenchyma, ductal anatomy, or both) or its exocrine function (**Table 49.2**). The tests most widely used clinically are tests that assess structure. The clinical manifestations of pancreatic insufficiency are usually a late event in the course of chronic pancreatitis when more than 90% of the glandular tissue is not functioning either because of glandular dysfunction or because of fibrotic tissue replacement or proximal pancreatic duct obstruction. The most sensitive and accurate among pancreatic function tests is the secretin stimulation test. However, this test is invasive, its methodology is very time-consuming and demanding, and its diagnostic accuracy is not superior to endoscopic retrograde cholangiopancreatography (ERCP).[62,63] Noninvasive pancreatic function tests yield sufficient diagnostic accuracy only in the advanced stages of the disease, and their sensitivity for detection of early or moderate chronic pancreatitis is low.[64]

Tests that evaluate pancreatic structure, although limited by sensitivity, are advantageous in that they are more widely available and are better standardized for clinical use.

Tests of Pancreatic Function

Invasive or Direct Pancreatic Function Tests (Secretin Stimulation Test)

The "gold standard" for detection of pancreatic functional insufficiency is the secretin stimulation test. The basis for this test is that secretin (with or without cholecystokinin) causes the secretion of bicarbonate-rich fluid from the pancreas. The patient swallows a dual-lumen catheter (Dreiling tube) into the duodenum, allowing sampling of the duodenal contents. Intravenous secretin (1 U/kg) is administered, and duodenal juice is collected. A peak bicarbonate concentration less than 80 mEq/L is consistent with pancreatic exocrine insufficiency.

Some studies have shown the secretin stimulation test to be slightly more sensitive than ERCP for the diagnosis of chronic pancreatitis, but the evaluation of all tests in the diagnosis of chronic pancreatitis is suspect because of the lack of a "gold standard." Sensitivity ranges from 74% to 97%, and specificity ranges from 80% to 90%.[63,65–69] The percentage of patients with an abnormal stimulation test and a normal pancreatogram ranges from 3% to 20%.[66–69] When such patients were followed, two studies found that 90% of patients developed chronic pancreatitis.[69,70] Conversely, these studies also identified a small group of patients (<10% on average) with a normal hormonal stimulation test but an abnormal pancreatogram. On long-term follow-up, chronic pancreatitis developed in 0% to 26% of patients.[69,70] When the results of pancreatic function tests were compared with pancreatic histology, the overall sensitivity, specificity, and accuracy were 67%, 90%, and 81%.[71] Limitations of this test are that it is not well accepted by patients, it is time-consuming and expensive, and it requires specialized equipment and methodology. The test has not been well standardized, and a consensus on the normal ranges for the test results is yet to be reached. The test is available in very few specialized pancreatic centers around the world.

Noninvasive or Indirect Pancreatic Function Tests

There has been great effort and interest to develop noninvasive tests for evaluating pancreatic function. These tests are designed to measure pancreatic enzymes in blood or stool or the effect of pancreatic enzymes on an orally administered substrate by collection of metabolites in blood or urine.

SERUM ENZYMES

Because chronic pancreatitis is a patchy, focal disease with significant parenchymal fibrosis, pancreatic serum enzyme levels (amylase and lipase) are not or only minimally elevated. Very low levels of serum trypsinogen (<20 ng/mL) are reasonably specific for chronic pancreatitis, but levels as low as this are seen only in very advanced stages of the disease where there is accompanying steatorrhea.[55] In clinical practice, serum enzyme levels are helpful to identify an acute attack of chronic

pancreatitis or for monitoring the disease evolution with abnormally low concentration once steatorrhea occurs.

FECAL TESTS

Steatorrhea can be diagnosed qualitatively by Sudan staining of feces or quantitatively by determination of fecal fat excretion over 72 hours while the patient is consuming a 100 g/day fat diet for at least 3 days before the test. Excretion of more than 7 g of fat per day is diagnostic of malabsorption, although patients with steatorrhea often have values greater than 20 g/day. On qualitative analysis, more than six globules per high-power field is considered to be positive, but the patient must be ingesting adequate fat to allow measurable steatorrhea. In a landmark study on exocrine insufficiency, steatorrhea did not occur until more than 90% of the pancreas or more than 85% of pancreatic lipase had been destroyed.[55] Stool fat analysis has limited sensitivity in chronic pancreatitis because patients with mild and moderate and often severe chronic pancreatitis in the absence of steatorrhea would not be detected by this technique. A novel method, near-infrared reflectance analysis (NIRA), may become the procedure of choice for evaluating fat malabsorption.[72–74] NIRA is equally accurate but less time-consuming than a 72-hour fecal fat collection and allows for simultaneous measurement of fecal fat, nitrogen, and carbohydrates in a single sample. NIRA is being increasingly used in Europe and is available in some centers in the United States.

The low diagnostic value of fat malabsorption in chronic pancreatitis led to the discovery of individual pancreatic enzymes in stool specimen that have increased diagnostic sensitivity. Measurement of fecal chymotrypsin is abnormal in most patients with chronic pancreatitis and steatorrhea.[65] Since inception of fecal chymotrypsin measurement into clinical use, its utility has been clearly established only in advanced chronic pancreatitis with exocrine insufficiency. This assay is unavailable in the United States at the present time. More recently, an assay to measure human pancreatic elastase in feces has been developed. The assay detects exclusively human elastase, and so no interference occurs with simultaneous therapeutic pancreatic enzyme supplementation. The diagnostic sensitivity and specificity of the fecal elastase test are superior to the fecal chymotrypsin test, although both tests are most accurate in advanced chronic pancreatitis.[75] The fecal elastase test may be falsely abnormal in other diseases causing steatorrhea, such as short bowel syndrome or small bowel bacterial overgrowth syndrome. This test is available but not widely used in the United States.

URINE TESTS

The principle of urine tests is based on the administration of a complex substrate, which is hydrolyzed by a specific pancreatic enzyme with the release of a pancreatic marker substance. This marker is absorbed from the gut and detected and quantitated either in urine or in serum. The bentiromide (N-benzoyl-L-tyrosyl-p-aminobenzoic acid [NBT-PABA]) test measures the presence of pancreatic chymotrypsin within the gut lumen, and the pancreolauryl test measures the presence of pancreatic arylesterases within the gut lumen. Both tests are accurate in advanced chronic pancreatitis, with sensitivities of 80% to 100%.[65] Limitations of these tests lie in the fact that both tests require anatomic and functional integrity of the digestive systems. Although these tests have reasonable accuracy, they are both unavailable for clinical use in the United States at the present time.

Tests of Pancreatic Structure
Plain Abdominal Radiography

Calcifications within the pancreas are present on plain films in about one-third of patients with chronic pancreatitis (**Fig. 49.3**). Calcifications occur late in the natural history of chronic pancreatitis and may take 5 to 25 years to develop.[49,53] Both anteroposterior and oblique views should be employed because small flecks of calcium can be lost in the spine if oblique views are not obtained. The finding of calcification is pathognomonic of chronic pancreatitis, but the sensitivity of this test is very low.

Abdominal Ultrasound

Ultrasound was the first technique that allowed complete imaging of the pancreas. Several morphologic characteristics of chronic pancreatitis are detectable by ultrasound, including irregular contours in the margin of the gland, dilation and irregularity of the main pancreatic duct, heterogeneity of the gland parenchyma, cysts within or adjacent to the pancreas, and the presence of calcifications.[76] The sensitivity and specificity of ultrasound for the diagnosis of chronic pancreatitis are 60% to 70% and 80% to 90%.[77] However, the detail to which the pancreas can be interrogated depends on the body habitus of the patient, the presence or absence of overlying bowel gas, and the experience and expertise of the sonographer.

Computed Tomography

The sensitivity and specificity of CT for the diagnosis of chronic pancreatitis are 75% to 90% and 85%.[65] The main advantage of CT is that it can be standardized and in virtually all cases can visualize the pancreas in its entirety. CT scan is

the most sensitive test for detecting calcification, is accurate in detecting main pancreatic duct dilation, and can detect an irregular contour of the gland (**Fig. 49.4**).[65,78,79] These features are characteristics of advanced chronic pancreatitis, and CT is quite good at detecting these changes. However, CT is poor at detecting subtle abnormalities in pancreatic parenchyma or changes in side branches of the pancreatic duct, which are commonly seen in milder forms of the disease. CT has good specificity but lacks sensitivity for diagnosis of chronic pancreatitis. The newer spiral CT scanners would be likely to produce better sensitivity.

Magnetic Resonance Cholangiopancreatography

Several small studies have reported on the utility of magnetic resonance cholangiopancreatography (MRCP) in assessing pancreatic duct morphology.[80,81] MRCP agrees with ERCP in 70% to 80% of findings, with higher rates of agreement in studies using the most advanced image analysis techniques (**Fig. 49.5**). In studies that compared MRCP findings with ERCP, MRCP visualized the main pancreatic duct in the head, body, and tail in 79%, 64%, and 53% of cases.[82] Correlation with ERCP with respect to main pancreatic duct dilation, narrowing, and filling defects was 83% to 92%, 70% to 92%, and 92% to 100%. The major disadvantage of MRCP compared with conventional cholangiography is a lower spatial resolution, such that MRCP continues to be partially limited in the assessment of fine detail, such as subtle side branch

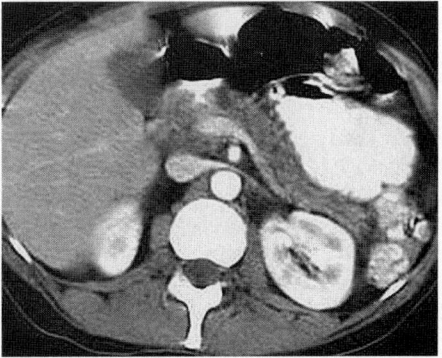

Fig. 49.4 Chronic pancreatitis on computed tomography (CT). CT image shows diffusely decreased enhancement relative to the renal cortices.

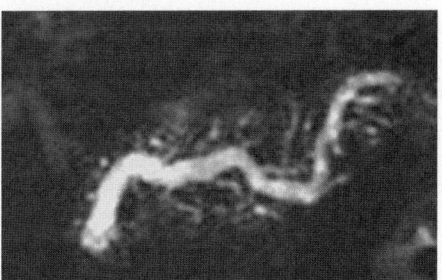

Fig. 49.5 Chronic pancreatitis on magnetic resonance cholangiopancreatography (MRCP). Coronal two-dimensional MRCP shows diffuse, irregular side branch dilation and dilation of the main pancreatic duct.

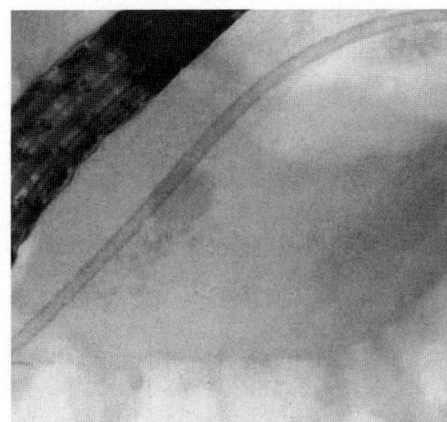

Fig. 49.3 Chronic pancreatitis on digital radiography. Anteroposterior digital radiograph obtained as a scout image during endoscopic retrograde cholangiopancreatography (ERCP) shows multiple calcifications in the expected location of the pancreas.

changes of chronic pancreatitis. Improvements in magnetic resonance (MR) imaging analysis are expected to continue to improve the image quality of MRCP, and image quality could approach ERCP in accuracy in the future.

Endoscopic Retrograde Cholangiopancreatography

ERCP is the most widely used structural test for chronic pancreatitis (**Fig. 49.6**). In 1984, the Pancreatic Society of Great Britain and Ireland reached a consensus on ductographic definitions for chronic pancreatitis, known as "the Cambridge criteria," which have become the most widely accepted criteria for interpreting pancreatography.[83] The criteria are based on abnormalities seen in the main pancreatic duct and side branches (**Table 49.3**). In most studies, the sensitivity of ERCP is 70% to 90%, and specificity is 80% to 100%.[63,65–69] ERCP is highly sensitive and specific in patients with advanced structural disease; less dramatic pancreatographic changes are less definitive.[84,85] The ductographic abnormalities of chronic pancreatitis are not specific; age-related changes, morphologic changes such as in pancreatic cancer or recovery phase of

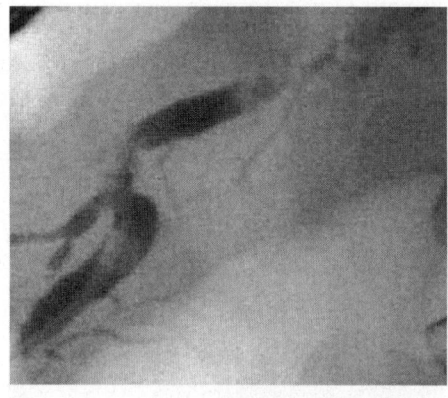

Fig. 49.6 Chronic pancreatitis on endoscopic retrograde cholangiopancreatography (ERCP). ERCP image shows irregular narrowing and dilation of the main pancreatic duct and irregular side branch dilation, most prominent in the body and tail.

acute pancreatitis, and injury induced by stent treatment can mimic chronic pancreatitis.

Chronic pancreatitis can involve the pancreatic parenchyma per se and completely spare the radiographically visible portions of the pancreatic ductal system leading to false-negative studies.[86,87] Also, significant interobserver and intraobserver variability is noted in the interpretation of pancreatography.[88] Much of this variability is related to interpretation of mild pancreatographic changes rather than to severe abnormalities. There are several limitations with ERCP as a diagnostic test for chronic pancreatitis. Reliable interpretation of ERCP depends on adequate filling of the pancreatic duct with dye such that the secondary branches are well visualized. However, inadequate opacification of ducts, especially the secondary ducts, occurs in at least 30% of cases.[84] The procedure is invasive and is associated with a 3% to 7% chance of causing acute pancreatitis.[89] This risk is low in patients with advanced disease and high in patients with mild disease, particularly patients with underlying sphincter of Oddi dysfunction.[90]

Endoscopic Ultrasound

EUS provides a safe, noninvasive method of obtaining detailed structural information on the pancreatic parenchyma and ducts. There are two main advantages for EUS that make it a very sensitive test for chronic pancreatitis. First, the pancreas lies within a few millimeters of the duodenum and stomach obviating the need for deep penetration of the sound waves. Positioning the EUS transducer at this site enables a thorough evaluation of the pancreas in its entirety. Second, positioning of the transducer in the gut lumen eliminates bowel gas being an obstacle for thorough imaging.

Numerous EUS criteria for pancreatic disease have been described (**Fig. 49.7**). Lees and colleagues[91,92] first described EUS findings in patients with clinical and radiologic evidence of chronic pancreatitis and characterized EUS criteria that distinguish normal from abnormal pancreas. Wiersema and associates[93] refined their definitions and found that abnormal EUS changes occurred frequently in patients with abnormal endoscopic pancreatograms and were absent in healthy volunteers. Criteria for chronic pancreatitis that are specific to EUS can be divided into two groups (**Table 49.4**): parenchymal and ductal. Parenchymal criteria include

Table 49.3 Cambridge Grading of Chronic Pancreatitis by Endoscopic Retrograde Pancreatography

Grade	Main Pancreatic Duct	Side Branches
Normal	Normal	Normal
Equivocal	Normal	<3 abnormal
Mild	Normal	>3 abnormal
Moderate	Abnormal	>3 abnormal
Severe	Abnormal, with at least one of the following Large cavity (>10 mm) Duct obstruction Intraductal filling defects Severe dilation or irregularity	>3 abnormal

Adapted from Axon AT, Classen M, Cotton PB, et al: Pancreatography in chronic pancreatitis: International definitions. Gut 25:1107, 1984.

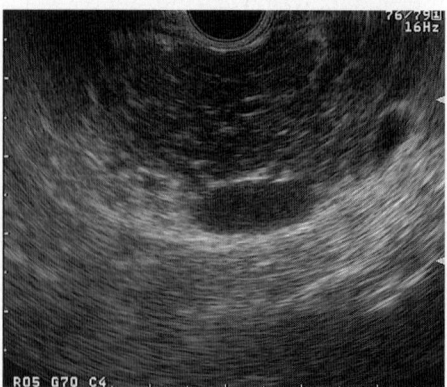

Fig. 49.7 Chronic pancreatitis on endoscopic ultrasound (EUS). EUS shows a pancreatic duct with hyperechoic margins. The pancreatic parenchyma shows stranding, foci, and lobularity.

Table 49.4 **Endoscopic Ultrasound Criteria for Chronic Pancreatitis**	
Parenchymal Changes	**Ductal Changes**
Inhomogeneity	Ductal dilation
Hyperechoic foci	Hyperechoic main duct margins
Hyperechoic strands	Irregular main duct margins
Lobularity	Visible side branches
Pseudocysts	

inhomogeneity, hyperechoic foci, hyperechoic strands, cysts, and lobularity. Ductal criteria specific to EUS include obvious to more subtle ductal dilation (≥3 mm in the head, ≥2 mm in the body, ≥1 mm in the tail), hyperechoic main duct margins, irregular main duct margins, and visible side branches.

Several studies show that the increasing EUS abnormalities correlate with the severity of pancreatographic changes[94–97] and with reductions in secretin-stimulated duodenal bicarbonate.[98] A quantitative analysis[94] with nine possible criteria (hyperechoic foci, hyperechoic strands, lobularity, ductal dilation, ductal irregularity, hyperechoic duct margins, visible side branches, calcifications, and cysts) suggested that in a population at low to moderate risk of chronic pancreatitis EUS is most reliable only when it is either clearly normal (two or fewer criteria) or clearly abnormal (five or more criteria). When the threshold for normal is set at two or fewer criteria and the threshold for abnormal is set at five or more criteria, the predictive values are 85%.[99] Some of the controversy regarding the accuracy of EUS may be due to studies that use three or four criteria (i.e., mild abnormalities) as threshold values to distinguish normal from abnormal EUS. When EUS is only mildly abnormal, endoscopic retrograde pancreatography and functional tests are often normal.

It is unclear whether minimal EUS changes reflect early chronic pancreatic disease. In a prospective study that compared EUS findings of the pancreas with surgical histopathology in 42 patients, there was a significant correlation between the number of EUS criteria and fibrosis score at histology ($r = 0.85$).[100] Because EUS provides higher resolution imaging than previously used imaging methods and provides information on both the ducts and the parenchyma, it is logical to assume that it may detect abnormalities not described previously with tests used traditionally to study pancreatic morphology. Functional testing is said to become abnormal only after greater than 60% to 70% of pancreatic functional reserve is depleted.[101] If this is the case, it may also be reasonable to expect that EUS could detect subtle structural changes that predate functional abnormalities. Finally, even severe chronic pancreatitis can be asymptomatic. EUS may show pancreatic abnormalities in asymptomatic individuals. It has been shown that alcohol consumption is often associated with asymptomatic abnormalities.[102,103]

Treatment

There are three approaches to the treatment of chronic pancreatitis. The first approach strategy endeavors to decrease pancreatic exocrine secretion. The second approach aims to

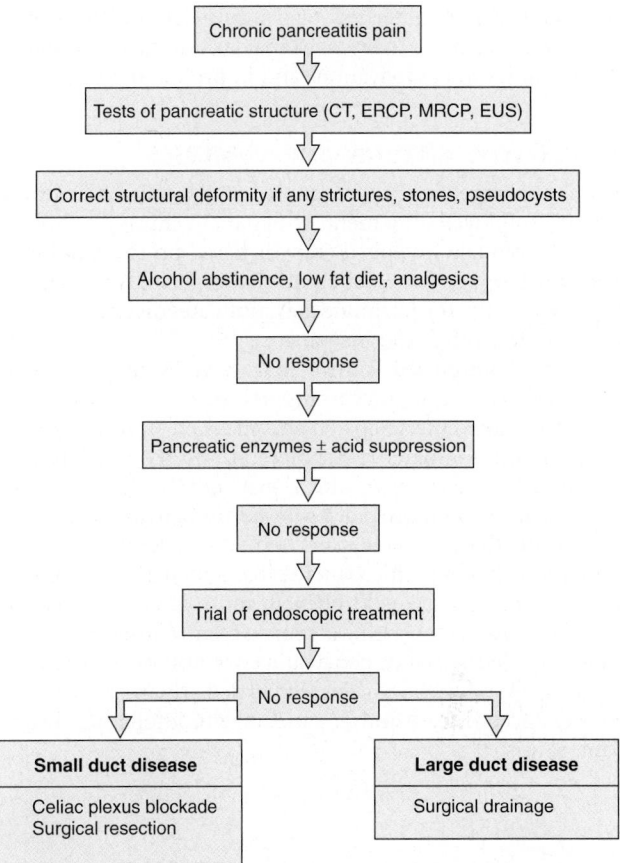

Fig. 49.8 Algorithm for the management of pain in chronic pancreatitis. CT, computed tomography; ERCP, endoscopic retrograde cholangiopancreatography; EUS, endoscopic ultrasound; MRCP, magnetic resonance cholangiopancreatography.

decompress the duct. In the third approach, often employed after the first two fail, partial or complete resection of the gland is performed. The goal of all three strategies is to relieve pain, which is the primary symptom of chronic pancreatitis. Pain management is an integral part of the treatment as well and is usually employed in parallel with the three aforementioned approaches.

Medical Management
Pain Management
ABSTINENCE FROM ALCOHOL

Early in the course of chronic pancreatitis, many patients experience recurrent acute attacks rather than chronic pain (**Fig. 49.8**). In these patients with recurrent attacks, a temporal relationship with alcohol binge can be commonly elucidated. In such patients, abstinence from alcohol may be of substantial benefit, in contrast to patients with end-stage disease and chronic pain. Mortality in chronic pancreatitis has been shown to be related to continued alcohol abuse.[104] In a meta-analysis[105] evaluating the effect of abstinence on pain, a substantial reduction in pain was associated with cessation of alcohol (continued pain in 26% of abstinent patients compared with 53% of patients who continued to consume alcohol). Also, in a large natural history study, continued drinking was associated with a higher risk of painful relapses.[106] Cessation of alcohol seems to have a beneficial effect in preventing alcohol-induced complications and in prolonging life.

PANCREATIC ENZYME SUPPLEMENTS

A trial of pancreatic enzyme supplements should be the initial strategy employed for patients with pain in chronic pancreatitis. The rationale for this therapy is based on suppression of feedback loops in the duodenum that regulate the release of cholecystokinin, the hormone that stimulates digestive enzyme secretion from the exocrine pancreas.[107]

Several randomized control trials have evaluated pancreatic enzymes as a method to provide pain relief. Two of the trials used non–enteric-coated enzymes and showed a reduction in pain compared with placebo.[108,109] Four trials used enteric-coated enzymes (which may not be released until they reach the jejunum) and showed no benefit.[110–113] In the two trials that showed pain reduction, female patients, patients with idiopathic pancreatitis, and patients with less advanced disease seemed to benefit most. Despite the lack of proof of clear-cut benefit, a more recent consensus review recommended a trial of pancreatic enzymes for pain relief.[114] Such a trial should be considered particularly in patients with less advanced disease and in patients with idiopathic chronic pancreatitis.

ANALGESICS

Most patients with painful chronic pancreatitis require analgesics for symptom relief. Although there are no accurate estimates of the risk of narcotic addiction, most experts suggest it occurs in 10% to 20% of patients. This problem is observed to occur more commonly in patients with poor social support and in patients with a history of narcotic addiction. A useful strategy is to begin with nonnarcotic analgesics such as acetaminophen and nonsteroidal antiinflammatory drugs. If these agents fail to provide adequate symptom relief, narcotic agents may be administered. In many patients, coexistent depression lowers the visceral pain threshold, and the addition of an antidepressant is often useful. Also, antidepressants have a direct effect on pain and potentiate the effects of narcotic analgesia.[115,116] Chronic narcotic analgesia may be required in patients with persistent significant pain. Long-acting narcotic agents generally are more effective than short-acting agents, which last only 3 to 4 hours.

ANTIOXIDANTS

In a placebo-controlled double-blind trial of 127 patients randomly assigned to placebo or antioxidants,[117] patients receiving antioxidants had significantly fewer painful days per month compared with the placebo group and required less analgesia for pain control. Also, more patients receiving antioxidants (32%) became pain-free compared with the placebo group (13%). This finding was confirmed by the lower levels of oxidative stress noted in patients receiving antioxidants.

CELIAC PLEXUS NERVE BLOCK

Pancreatic pain is predominantly transmitted through the celiac plexus. Celiac plexus neurolysis, via a surgical or

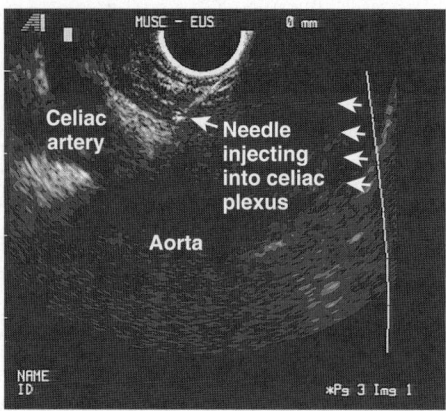

Fig. 49.9 Celiac plexus block is being performed with the curvilinear array echoendoscope. The celiac artery is seen emerging from the aorta, and the needle is shown just above this point.

transcutaneous approach, has been used for many years to manage abdominal pain resulting from advanced malignancy.[118,119] These approaches have had complications such as paralysis that might be overcome by better visualization of the region. The celiac artery is a landmark structure readily visualized on EUS (**Fig. 49.9**). Wiersema and Wiersema[120] performed transgastric EUS-guided celiac plexus neurolysis and found that the success rate was similar to surgical or transcutaneous approaches. An injection of absolute ethanol that permanently destroys the plexus is referred to as a celiac plexus neurolysis, and an injection of corticosteroids that temporarily block the plexus is referred to as a celiac plexus block. EUS-guided celiac plexus block and neurolysis are safe and well-tolerated procedures that can be performed in an outpatient setting with conscious sedation. The procedures can be performed in 10 minutes or less. Mild complications include transient diarrhea (4% to 15%), transient orthostasis (1%), and transient increase in pain (9%). Major complications (2.5%) have included retroperitoneal bleeding and peripancreatic abscess.[121]

In a prospective study, Wiersema and associates[122] evaluated patients with pancreatic malignancy and chronic pancreatitis treated by celiac plexus neurolysis and found that the initial pain scores were similar between the two patient groups. However, after 16 weeks of follow-up, the pain score improvement after celiac plexus neurolysis in patients with chronic pancreatitis was not found to be significant. The malignant disease group had a mean pain score of less than baseline. Celiac plexus neurolysis is not recommended for chronic pancreatitis. Gress and colleagues[123] used injection of triamcinolone in 90 patients with chronic pancreatitis. At 8 weeks after the procedure, 55% of patients had a decreased score; this became 10% of patients by 24 weeks. Based on available data, the technique of performing celiac plexus block does not seem to affect treatment outcomes.[124] In a prospective study of 51 patients with chronic pancreatitis and pain who underwent celiac plexus block at either one side or either side of the celiac trunk, there was no significant difference in short-term pain relief between both cohorts. Of patients, 57% who received a single injection had pain relief compared with 54% who received two injections.

Management of Pancreatic Insufficiency

One approach in patients with steatorrhea is to restrict fat intake to 20 g/day or less. Patients who continue to have steatorrhea after fat restriction require medical therapy.

LIPASE SUPPLEMENTATION

Supplemental oral lipase is effective in preventing steatorrhea. Three tablets of non–enteric-coated pills (total of 30,000 U of lipase) with meals is typically sufficient to improve symptoms. The goal of treatment is control of symptoms rather than restoring fat absorption to normal levels.

Enzyme supplements may be inactivated at an acidic pH. Patients who are not responding to the typical dose of medications may benefit from the addition of a histamine-2 antagonist or a proton pump inhibitor. Alternatively, a micro-encapsulated preparation of pancreatic enzymes with a higher lipase concentration may be effective. There are several explanations for failure of enzyme therapy for steatorrhea. The most common is inadequate dosage, generally owing to patient noncompliance because of the numerous pills that must be taken. Also, patients taking non–enteric-coated preparations must take an acid suppressant to ensure that the enzymes are not denatured by gastric acid or destroyed by proteases. If these measures fail, it is appropriate to search for alternative causes that could cause malabsorption, such as celiac sprue or small intestinal bacterial overgrowth.

MEDIUM-CHAIN TRIGLYCERIDES

Medium-chain triglycerides may provide extra calories in patients with weight loss and a poor response to diet and pancreatic enzyme therapy. In contrast to long-chain triglycerides, which require bile salts and pancreatic lipase, medium-chain triglycerides are readily degraded by gastric and pancreatic lipase and do not require the presence of bile. In addition, medium-chain triglycerides can be directly absorbed by the intestinal mucosa and are less of a stimulant to pancreatic secretion. In a pilot study of eight patients with chronic pancreatitis and postprandial pain, three to four cans of Peptamen (enriched in medium-chain triglycerides and hydrolyzed peptides) per day for 10 weeks resulted in improvement in pain, which in some patients was sustained after stopping this oral supplement.[125] The mechanism of action may relate to the fact that administration of this internal formulation resulted in a minimal increase in plasma cholecystokinin levels or alternatively may be due to its antioxidant effects.

Management of Complications

Chronic pancreatitis may be associated with various complications. Splenic vein thrombosis, pseudoaneurysm formation, and common bile duct or duodenal strictures are occasionally encountered. Other complications such as pseudocyst formation and pancreatic ascites or pleural effusion are discussed in Chapter 47. Pancreatic ductal complications such as pancreatic stones and strictures are discussed subsequently.

SPLENIC VEIN THROMBOSIS

The splenic vein courses along the posterior surface of the pancreas, where it can be affected by inflammation and resultant splenic vein thrombosis. Patients may develop associated gastric varices. Bleeding from gastric varices in this setting is uncommon, and no specific therapy is needed in nonbleeding patients. If bleeding occurs, splenectomy is usually curative.

PSEUDOANEURYSMS

Pseudoaneurysm formation is a rare complication of chronic pancreatitis. The splenic artery is the most commonly involved vessel. Pseudoaneurysms form as a consequence of enzymatic digestion of muscular wall of the artery by a pseudocyst. The presence of unexplained anemia or any degree of gastrointestinal bleeding in a patient with chronic pancreatitis or a known pseudocyst should immediately raise the possibility of a pseudoaneurysm. When bleeding occurs, the mortality is 40% to 60%.[126] Although contrast CT scanning and MR imaging with MR angiography may be diagnostic, mesenteric angiography permits confirmation and provides a means of therapy by embolization. Operative intervention for bleeding pseudoaneurysms is difficult and associated with a high morbidity and mortality.

COMMON BILE DUCT STRICTURES

Intrapancreatic common bile duct strictures have been reported in 2.7% to 45.6% of patients with chronic pancreatitis.[127,128] Common bile duct strictures can have serious sequelae of cholangitis, cholelithiasis, choledocholithiasis, intrahepatic stones, and secondary biliary cirrhosis. Deviere and colleagues[128] evaluated the use of biliary stent placement in patients with biliary strictures secondary to chronic pancreatitis. They reported that endoscopic biliary drainage is an effective therapy for resolving cholangitis or jaundice in this patient subset. However, the long-term efficacy of this therapy was unsatisfactory because stricture resolution rarely occurred. Preliminary results using metal stents for this indication suggest they could be an effective alternative to operative biliary diversion. More than 90% of patients had no recurrence of strictures at 3 years, but longer follow-up and controlled trials are necessary to confirm these findings.[129,130] In a nonrandomized retrospective study that compared surgical drainage procedures with stent insertion, Pitt and coworkers[131] found a significantly higher success rate of 88% in the surgically treated group compared with 55% for patients managed by stent insertion.

DUODENAL OBSTRUCTION

Duodenal stenosis is seen in around 5% of patients with chronic pancreatitis, particularly patients with alcoholic pancreatitis. Coexistent obstruction of the common bile duct may be seen. The diagnosis is made at upper endoscopy or barium swallow. Attempts to dilate the stricture endoscopically are generally futile. The simplest and safest approach is operative drainage via gastrojejunostomy; this may be combined with drainage of the bile duct or pancreatic duct or both.

Surgical Management

Operative therapy for pain relief in chronic pancreatitis should be considered in patients who fail medical therapy. Other indications for operative intervention in chronic pancreatitis include management of pancreatic pseudocyst, abscess, fistula, ascites, fixed common bile duct obstruction, or variceal hemorrhage secondary to splenic vein thrombosis. Because the manifestations of chronic pancreatitis can mimic the manifestations of pancreatic cancer, operative resection is required in some instances to exclude malignancy. The ideal operation for chronic pancreatitis should relieve pain and preserve endocrine and exocrine function. Both pancreatic drainage and resection procedures may relieve pain. Pancreatic duct drainage procedures relieve pancreatic hypertension and pain but without sacrificing functioning glandular tissue. However, long-term success requires that the duct be dilated—greater than 8 mm is desirable. Extensive resections should be avoided to prevent endocrine and exocrine insufficiency. No one particular procedure can be applicable to all patients. The approach is tailored to meet the problems posed in each individual patient.

Pancreatic Duct Decompression

In patients with a dilated pancreatic duct, a Roux-en-Y side-to-side pancreaticojejunostomy is performed to drain the entire pancreatic duct from the tail to the duodenum. When necessary, a partial resection of the head of the gland is performed to ensure complete drainage. Operative mortality for this technique is less than 3%.[132] Substantial improvement in symptoms is seen in 65% to 85% of patients.[133,134] Although some authors reported that improvements in symptoms were durable over a follow-up of 7.9 years,[128] others reported recurrence of symptoms in a substantial number of patients within 1 year.[133–136] The explanation for this decline in effectiveness may be that the secondary ducts, which are not amendable to main duct drainage procedures, may subsequently become obstructed. Although improvement in pancreatic endocrine or exocrine function is not expected after pancreaticojejunostomy, steatorrhea and insulin-dependent diabetes arising as a consequence of surgery are not inevitable.[132] However, some studies have noted progressive loss of endocrine and exocrine pancreatic function despite a lateral pancreaticojejunostomy.[137–139]

Pancreatic Resection

Pancreatic resection involves resection of a portion of the pancreas, usually the tail or head. This procedure is most appropriate when there is focal disease, particularly in the absence of pancreatic ductal dilation. In one series of patients who had no benefit from pancreaticojejunostomy, reoperation to resect the head of the pancreas led to a significant improvement in pain in a select group of patients.[140] The reason for the improvement was unclear because there was no evidence of focal pancreatitis. The choice of distal or proximal pancreatectomy and the magnitude of resection are determined by the location and extent of disease. Distal resection is limited to patients with disease involving the tail, most commonly as a sequela of traumatic pancreatitis. Pancreaticoduodenectomy (Whipple's procedure) has been advocated because the fibrosis

of chronic pancreatitis is often more prominent in the head and uncinate process. This procedure often preserves enough islets in the tail to prevent diabetes. Duodenum-preserving resection of the pancreatic head is another alternative that has alleviated pain with lesser rates of exocrine and endocrine dysfunction.[141]

Steatorrhea can develop in 30% to 40% of patients undergoing simple drainage procedures and in 66% of patients undergoing extensive pancreatic resections.[142–144] Diabetes mellitus can occur after pancreatic resection either as a consequence of surgery or secondarily from ongoing disease process. In a randomized trial that compared extended drainage and resection for pain relief,[144] although there was no difference in pain score between both cohorts (94% vs. 95%), the global quality of life at 2 years was superior for patients who underwent drainage (71%) compared with resection (43%) procedures. However, at a long-term follow-up of 7 years, there was no significant difference in pain relief, quality of life, and pancreatic exocrine or endocrine functions between both cohorts.[145]

Total Pancreatectomy with Islet Cell Autotransplantation

Because chronic pancreatitis is progressive and has an unpredictable clinical course, there is an increasing trend to recommend total pancreatectomy as opposed to partial resection. When partial resections are performed, 30% of patients may require subsequent completion or salvage pancreatectomy. The main goal of total pancreatectomy is to achieve a durable treatment for chronic pain. The main long-term morbidity of total pancreatectomy is related to brittle diabetes. The addition of islet cell autotransplantation has dramatically reduced morbidity related to hypoglycemia and has achieved insulin independence in select patients. In a report of 26 patients who underwent total pancreatectomy and islet cell autotransplantation, 80% of patients reported decreased or eliminated use of narcotics for pain control at 6-month follow-up.[146] However, all patients required a moderate dosage of insulin for management of diabetes. In patients undergoing resection procedures, such as Whipple's procedure, islet cell autotransplantation of the tail can be attempted to decrease the risk of diabetes.[147] Total pancreatectomy with islet cell autotransplantation is currently the only surgical option available for patients with small duct disease variant of chronic pancreatitis who have unremitting pain and without a focal inflammatory mass.

Endoscopic Management

Patients with an established diagnosis of chronic pancreatitis who have failed medical management should undergo ERCP. The goal of ERCP is to evaluate for an obstructive component to the pancreatopathy. Endoscopically treatable causes of obstruction can be at the level of the papilla (papillary stenosis) or along the course of the main pancreatic duct, primarily secondary to stones or strictures or both.

Sphincter of Oddi Dysfunction

The role of sphincter of Oddi dysfunction as a cause of chronic pancreatitis is not completely understood. In a study that evaluated 104 patients with unexplained abdominal pain, 29%

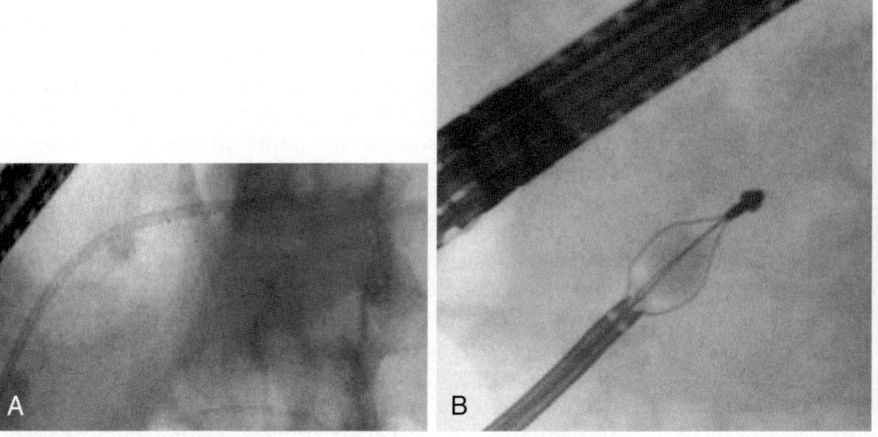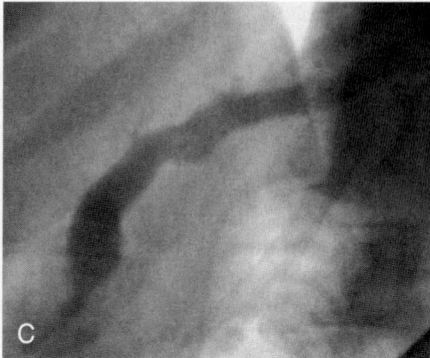

Fig. 49.10 Pancreatic stone removal with endoscopic retrograde cholangiopancreatography (ERCP). ERCP images obtained before (**A**), during (**B**), and after (**C**) stone removal by lithotripsy. **A**, Scout ERCP image reveals a large stone within the main pancreatic duct. **B**, Second image was obtained during basket capture of the stone. **C**, Postprocedural ERCP image reveals absence of the stone within the duct and no evidence of residual obstruction.

of patients diagnosed with sphincter of Oddi dysfunction had structural evidence of chronic pancreatitis.[90] Two other studies made similar observations and found that basal sphincter pressures were elevated particularly in the pancreatic segment of the sphincter of Oddi.[148,149] It is unknown whether the sphincter becomes dysfunctional sometimes as part of the overall general scarring process or has a role in the pathogenesis of chronic pancreatitis. Studies have shown that sphincter ablation therapy benefits 30% to 60% of patients with chronic pancreatitis who have manometrically proven sphincter of Oddi dysfunction.[150,151] Bagley and colleagues[152] reported a series of 67 patients with mild to moderate chronic pancreatitis who underwent empiric sphincterotomy or sphincteroplasty and found that 44% of patients during a 5-year follow-up period had pain relief. The utility of sphincter ablation therapy in patients with chronic pancreatitis awaits further study, probably in randomized controlled trials.

Pancreatic Duct Stones

Approximately one-third of patients with chronic pancreatitis have pancreatic stones. There is no close correlation between the presence of pancreatic duct stones and pain, and many patients with pancreatic duct stones report no pain. It is unclear if pancreatic calculi aggravate the clinical course of chronic pancreatitis or are the consequence of ongoing glandular destruction from persistent disease processes. It is postulated that pain in chronic pancreatitis is related to increased intrapancreatic pressure arising as a consequence of mechanical duct obstruction by pancreatic stones or strictures.[153,154] This notion is supported by studies that show improvement in symptoms after ductal clearance of stones.[155–159] Removal of pancreatic duct stones is recommended in patients with symptomatic chronic pancreatitis.

DIAGNOSIS

Most pancreatic duct stones are readily apparent on plain films of the abdomen because of radiopacity of the calcium component. However, small stones may not be readily seen.

Oblique view on plain films may uncover stones missed because of the overlying spine on anteroposterior films. Many patients have multiple stones of varying diameters in the main and branch pancreatic ducts in association with strictures. High-resolution CT and MRCP provide the best noninvasive mapping of the duct and may help select patients appropriate for therapy. The main benefit of such imaging is the formulation of an efficient treatment algorithm for these patients. In most patients, however, the suitability for endoscopic therapy is best assessed at ERCP.

TREATMENT

The most suitable features for successful endoscopic removal are *small number* of *mobile* stones in the duct *without* significant *strictures*. An impacted stone that impedes injection of contrast material into the pancreatic duct usually requires adjunctive therapy using extracorporeal shock wave lithotripsy (ESWL) or intraductal lithotripsy for clearance. Endoscopic management involves sphincterotomy, stricture dilation, and stone removal by baskets or balloons (**Fig. 49.10**).

Removal of pancreatic stones requires an adequate opening of the pancreatic orifice. There is often thickening and fibrosis or stenosis of the pancreatic orifice in chronic pancreatitis. Cholangiography and pancreatography are performed initially, and the termination of either duct is correctly assessed. Usually a biliary sphincterotomy is performed first to expose the pancreatic septum and to help assess the necessary extent of the pancreatic cut. Pancreatic sphincterotomy can be done using either a standard pull-type sphincterotome or a needle-knife to perform sphincterotomy over a previously placed pancreatic stent. In patients with pancreas divisum, a minor papilla sphincterotomy may be required and is usually performed by using a needle-knife over a previously placed dorsal duct pancreatic stent. The ability to remove a stone by endoscopic methods alone depends on stone size and number, location in the duct, presence of downstream stricture, and degree of impaction.[157] Downstream strictures may require dilation either with catheters or with hydrostatic balloons.

The duct features particular to the pancreas require special consideration. Because of the tortuosity of the main duct and multiple side branches, there is a tendency for the leading tip of a basket to get caught in a side branch. Negotiating around the genu can be particularly difficult because of the sigmoid turn at the junction of the head and body of the pancreas. Soft wire or wire-guided baskets may be necessary to navigate these tortuous areas of the pancreatic duct. Pancreatic stones are very hard because of their crystalline structure. Care must be taken to assess the adequacy of the ductal system downstream from where the stone is entrapped in the basket to avoid getting stuck up the duct with a basket. In a grossly dilated duct, a "through-the-scope" mechanical lithotripsy device can be used, but this is often restricted to stones in the head of the pancreas with a straight line of approach to the stone. Otherwise, the rigidity of this device and its large diameter are restrictive. This device may also be used through a much dilated dorsal duct if it permits a straight approach.

Sherman and coworkers[157] reported that endoscopic therapy was effective in 83% of patients presenting with chronic relapsing pancreatitis compared with 46% of patients presenting with continuous pain alone. Factors favoring successful endoscopic therapy included three or fewer stones, stones confined to head or body of the pancreas, stone size less than 10 mm, absence of impacted stones, and absence of downstream strictures.[151,160] After successful stone removal, 25% of patients had regression of ductographic changes of chronic pancreatitis, and 42% had a decrease in the main pancreatic duct diameter. The only complication was pancreatitis encountered in 8% of patients. Studies have reported success rates with endoscopic therapy of 45% to 79% and improvement in symptoms of 60% to 90%.[157,159,161] One study reported clinical improvement in steatorrhea in 73% of patients after endoscopic management.[159]

Electrohydraulic lithotripsy may be an effective adjunct to endoscopic treatment of pancreatic stones. In this technique, shocks are delivered in a fluid medium under direct visualization because inadvertent firing on tissue can cause perforation or bleeding. This technique requires the use of a baby pancreatoscope that is passed up the pancreatic duct to the stone. Although pancreatoscopy can be used to visualize directly probe contact with the stone and fragmentation, intraductal manipulation remains difficult and very limited.[158,162] These smaller baby scopes have fragile control systems with limited one-way tip deflection, which may hinder accurate placement of the probe. The operating channel diameter in these scopes is 0.75 to 1.0 mm and accepts only specialized ultrathin accessories. The electrohydraulic lithotripsy probe is 1.9-Fr in diameter and can be used, but channels of 1.0 mm or less do not allow for much coaxial perfusion of saline necessary for lithotripsy. The saline is essential for transmission of the shock waves at the stone surface and for irrigation after the shock wave. The debris that is created after the shock waves obscures visibility and must be flushed away. Placement of a nasopancreatic tube (5-Fr) beyond the stone before pancreatoscopy is helpful for irrigation purposes. Advancing the pancreatoscope requires an ample pancreatic sphincterotomy for insertion and may require a guidewire to advance up a tortuous pancreatic duct. A 450-cm wire is placed into the duct beforehand, and the proximal stiffer end is backloaded into the baby scope. The stiff end of the wire should be slightly bent before back-

loading to help negotiate the elbow junction of the accessory port and the scope body.

A new device developed more recently, the frequency-doubled YAG laser (FREDDY), fires with pulses of such short duration that no thermal damage occurs even when the fiber fires directly on the tissue. Clinical experience with this device is limited. More studies are required before the place of FREDDY in the armamentarium against pancreatic stones can be defined.

The main advantage of endoscopic therapy in pancreatic stone management is that recurrence of symptoms secondary to migrated stone can be treated again by endoscopy with or without ESWL. Rate of repeat surgery for recurrent pain is 20% with a striking increase in morbidity and mortality after repeated surgery.[163] Controlled trials comparing surgical and endoscopic therapies are awaited. ESWL has become almost indispensable to specialized centers treating many patients with advanced chronic pancreatitis.

ESWL should be considered when endoscopic procedures fail to remove large or impacted stones and for patients with recurrent attacks of pancreatic pain who have moderate to marked changes in the pancreatic ductal system and obstructive ductal stones. Stones are amendable to ESWL in almost all patients because the biochemical composition of the stones consists of 95% calcium carbonate on a protein matrix. The procedure is contraindicated only in patients who have coagulation disorders or who have bone, calcified aneurysms, or lung tissue in the shock wave path. Lithotripsy works by concentrating focused shock waves on stones, which causes their disruption. Gradual disintegration of the stone is accomplished with application of several hundred to thousand shock waves to the calculi at a focal area. Shock waves can be generated by three methods: spark discharge (Dornier, Germering, Germany), piezoelectric elements (Wolf, Knittlingen, Germany), and electromagnetic deflection of a metal membrane (Siemens, Erlangen, Germany).

Shock wave generation occurs in degassed water. The shock waves are focused by reflection of the primary wave, arraying of the piezoceramic elements on a hemispheric disc, or an acoustic lens. Shock waves are directed to the body via a water cushion or basin. In most patients, a radiologic target system is needed, which can be provided by the placement of a stent. Fluoroscopic focusing of densely calcified stones can be achieved without pancreatography. In other patients, MRCP with secretin or CT can show pancreatic ductal obstruction related to stones. For very small stones or radiolucent stones, visualization can be improved by instillation of contrast material via a nasopancreatic catheter. Patients require sedation, which can range from conscious sedation to general anesthesia. Routine antibiotic prophylaxis is unnecessary. Shock waves are focused first on the distalmost stone and then on other calculi moving from the head to tail, allowing stone fragments to drain downward through the papilla. In one treatment session, 3000 to 5000 shock waves using the highest possible energy levels are delivered. Pancreatic stones are hard and usually require a higher powered shock wave (22 to 24 kV). Each session lasts approximately 45 to 60 minutes.

ESWL is an effective adjunct to the nonsurgical endoscopic approach in chronic calcifying pancreatitis with complete or partial relief of symptoms in 80% of patients, which is comparable to the surgical literature.[164,165] In one study, stones were successfully fragmented in 99% of patients resulting in a

Table 49.5 Technical and Clinical Results of Extracorporeal Shock Wave Lithotripsy for Pancreatic Stones

Reference	No. Patients	Complete or Partial Pain Relief (%)	Fragmentation (%)	Complete Clearance (%)
Dumonceau et al[163]	70	68	58	50
Sherman et al[157]	32	85	99	58
Delhaye et al[164]	123	85	99	59
Sauerbruch et al[165]	24	83	87.5	42
Farnbacher et al[166]	114	93	82	39
Adamek et al[167]	80	76	54	ND
Schneider et al[168]	50	62	86	60
Ohara et al[169]	32	86	100	75
Kozarek et al[172]	40	80	100	ND
Tadenuma et al[160]	117	97	97	56
Inui et al[173]	555	91.1	92.4	73

ND, not determined.

decrease in duct dilation in 90%.[164] The main pancreatic duct was cleared of all stones in 59%. However, one of the challenges in pancreatic duct therapy is evaluating treatment efficacy. Disintegration of a stone can be considered successful when a decrease is seen in the radiographic density of the stone or the stone surface area. Also, the ability to show relief of ductal obstruction at deep cannulation of the pancreatic duct during ERCP is an indicator of treatment efficacy.[164] Using the aforementioned criteria, the success rate of fragmentation has been approximately 76% to 100% in most series regardless of the shock wave system used.[164–167] Most patients require endoscopic extraction of stone fragments after ESWL for complete clearance from the ductal system. Some authorities recommend that pancreatic sphincterotomy should be performed before ESWL to facilitate stone passage.[161,168] With the exception of one report[157] in which successful treatment was more frequent in patients with solitary stones (74% vs. 43% for multiple stones), successful fragmentation and stone clearance was not correlated with the initial size or the number of main pancreatic duct stones by others.[166,169,170]

Repeat ESWL may be required if stones have incompletely disintegrated, which is often the case in patients with large or multiple stones. The reported mean number of treatment sessions required to complete lithotripsy has ranged from 1.3 to 4.1 per patient in most reports.[161,167,168] The radiographic success of ESWL has been associated with clinical improvement (**Table 49.5**). Complete or partial pain relief was observed in 62% to 97% of the patients in the largest series during a mean follow-up ranging from 7 to 44 months.[160,164,168,170–173] However, complete stone clearance was not required for symptom relief. Many patients gained weight because of a reduction in postprandial pain attacks, improvement in pancreatic function, or both. The number and location of stones, the presence of a stricture, or continued alcohol use did not seem to be associated with recurrent pain.[164,168] As a result, ESWL does not have to be restricted to patients without these unfavorable clinical characteristics.

One study[163] identified three independent predictors of pain relapse at long-term follow-up after ESWL therapy: (1) a high frequency of pain attacks before treatment (more than or at least two pain attacks during the 2 months before treatment), (2) a long duration of disease before treatment, and (3) the presence of a nonpapillary stenosis of the main pancreatic duct. This study suggests that ESWL in association with endoscopic therapy should be performed as early as possible in the course of chronic pancreatitis. In another study, pain relapse was noted to occur more frequently in patients who had incomplete removal of stones than in patients in whom ductal clearance was complete.[160] Early ductal decompression of the main pancreatic duct may also help prevent further fibrosis, which can lead to pancreatic insufficiency. In addition, it may improve pancreatic function in patients who have already developed pancreatic insufficiency. Although some studies investigating this issue found that exocrine pancreatic function improved more often after treatment compared with endocrine pancreatic function, others have shown progressive deterioration in both exocrine and endocrine functions at long-term follow-up.[162,164,170–173] In a multicenter study, the rate of recurrence of pancreatic duct stones after ESWL was reported to be 20% to 30%.[173] Factors predictive of stone recurrence included ongoing alcohol use and the presence of pancreatic duct strictures. Complications in series using ESWL were primarily related to the endoscopic procedure.

Pancreatic Strictures

Pancreatic duct strictures (**Fig. 49.11**) may be a complication of previously embedded stone or a consequence of acute inflammatory changes around the pancreatic duct.[174] Pancreatic duct strictures may contribute to pain, recurrent acute pancreatitis, and exocrine insufficiency. Strictures may also be associated with stones, pseudocysts, and pancreatic malignancy.[161,175–177] The mechanism of pain in patients with pancreatic strictures is poorly understood but may be attributable partly to pancreatic duct hypertension from obstruction

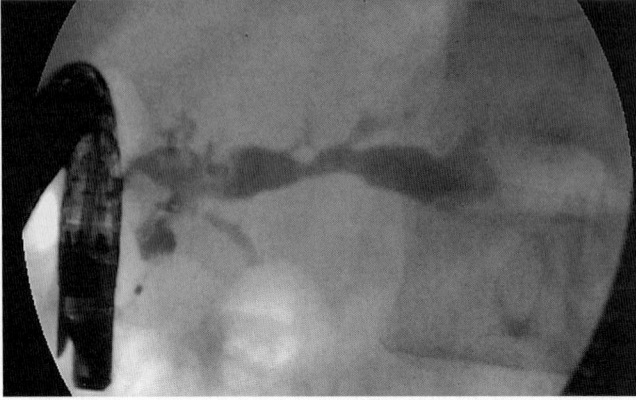

Fig. 49.11 Endoscopic retrograde cholangiopancreatography (ERCP) shows changes of chronic pancreatitis with a stricture in the main pancreatic duct.

caused by the stricture to the flow of pancreatic juice. Pancreatic duct strictures may be present in association with biliary strictures, and liver function test abnormalities, jaundice, and cholangitis may be presenting symptoms.

DIAGNOSIS

The finding of a pancreatic duct stricture often poses a diagnostic dilemma regarding the specific cause of the stricture. The cause of a pancreatic duct stricture may be related to acute or chronic pancreatitis, pancreatic neoplasm, pseudocyst, and traumatic injury. Cancer is the most feared cause and should be considered in all patients with pancreatic duct strictures. When evaluating these patients, background clinical information is paramount. Patients older than 50 years presenting with idiopathic or multiple episodes of acute pancreatitis, with pancreatic duct stricture, must have malignancy included in the differential diagnosis, particularly in the absence of alcohol abuse. Thorough evaluation of pancreatic strictures requires multidisciplinary testing. When evaluating pancreatograms, changes in the ductal anatomy other than strictures should be sought. These changes include irregularity in the contour or dilation of the pancreatic duct or of the secondary radicles. The presence of a single stricture with proximal dilation and normal distal ductal anatomy suggests a neoplastic cause. Changes noted throughout the duct, particularly when they occur downstream to the stricture, in addition to the anticipated upstream changes, suggest chronic pancreatitis. The presence of multiple strictures and dilations in a "chain-of-lakes appearance" is characteristic of chronic pancreatitis. However, the presence of mucous plugs and a patulous papilla should raise the possibility of intraductal papillary mucinous tumor of the pancreas.

No findings on pancreatography are absolutely specific for chronic pancreatitis. At ERCP, complete cutoff of the pancreatic duct implies an abrupt stop in the flow of contrast material at some point along the length of the pancreatic duct. Incomplete filling of the pancreatic duct can also portray a similar picture. Sufficient contrast material must be injected so that the secondary branches of the pancreatic duct can be seen downstream to the blockage; this confirms the presence of a functionally important stricture in the main pancreatic duct because it indicates that the contrast material has taken the path of least resistance into the secondary branches. During ERCP, it is important to attempt to cross the stricture with accessories to allow for complete imaging and tissue sampling by brush cytology, forceps, and needle aspirate. Adjunctive imaging modalities are also important in the differential diagnosis of pancreatic duct strictures. These include conventional studies such as CT and EUS. Both modalities can detect and differentiate chronic pancreatitis and pancreatic neoplasms in advanced stages and may assist in obtaining tissue diagnosis. The role of probe-based optical coherence tomography (OCT) was evaluated in 12 patients with pancreatic duct strictures. All patients underwent ERCP with brush cytology and OCT.[178] Although a three-layer architecture was noted in all patients with nonmalignant strictures, the architecture was totally distorted in patients with malignancy. The accuracy of OCT for diagnosing malignancy was 100% compared with 66.7% for brush cytology. OCT remains an investigational modality at the present time that needs further evaluation.

TREATMENT

Endoscopic therapy for pancreatic duct strictures is primarily indicated for patients presenting with refractory abdominal pain, with or without upstream ductal dilation. The technique for placing a stent in the pancreatic duct is similar to the technique used for inserting a biliary stent. A guidewire is first maneuvered beyond the stricture several centimeters. Hydrophilic, flexible tip wires are generally helpful. Pancreatic stents are similar to biliary stents except for side holes along their length to allow for flow from side branches. Generally, the diameter of the stent should not exceed the size of a normal downstream duct. In small ducts, 3-Fr, 4-Fr, and 5-Fr stents are used commonly, whereas 7-Fr and 10-Fr stents can be used in advanced chronic pancreatitis with dilated pancreatic ducts. Occasionally, in patients with small duct disease who have recurrent strictures, we place multiple 3-Fr stents to dilate the stricture. We believe that stent-induced trauma could be obviated by this method, but data are still forthcoming. Also, the severity of the stricture, location, and duct size influence the choice of stent.

Generally, the best candidates for stent treatment are patients with a distal stricture and upstream dilation. Other therapy, such as pancreatic or biliary sphincterotomy, pancreatic duct stone removal, and dilation of strictures, may be required concomitantly at time of stent placement. Dilation to widen single or multiple strictures of the main pancreatic duct in chronic pancreatitis can be performed successfully. Dilating catheters with graded tips are generally used, although canalization and dilation using the Soehendra stent retriever as an auger can be employed in very tight strictures. After dilation, stents of adequate size are left in place to facilitate drainage and to prevent recurrent stricture formation. If stents larger than 7-Fr are to be used, patients often require biductal sphincterotomy followed by stricture dilation. For optimal results, therapy must address both the pancreatic duct stricture and duct stones if any are present.

The appropriate duration of pancreatic stent placement is currently unknown. Most stents in diagnostic trials or for short-term therapy are left in place for 2 to 4 weeks. In contrast, stents for long-term therapy are left in place for several months. If the patient has improvement in symptoms, the

Table 49.6 Stent Therapy for Chronic Pancreatitis with Dominant Strictures

Reference	No. Patients	Technical Success	No. Patients Improved	Mean Follow-up Duration (mo)
Cremer et al[174]	76	75	41	37
Ponchon et al[181]	28	23	12	26
Smits et al[182]	51	49	40	34
Binmoeller et al[183]	93	84	61	39
Costamagna et al[184]	19	19	16	38
Total	*267*	*231 (94%)*	*154 (64%)*	*35*

stent can be removed and the patient can be followed clinically, stent therapy can be continued for a more prolonged period, or a surgical drainage procedure can be performed. The last option suggests that the results of endoscopic stent treatment would predict the surgical outcome. Two preliminary reports support this concept, but more studies are required.[179,180] Quantitation of the degree of improvement in pancreatic disorders is often poorly defined. Generally, partial or complete symptom improvement indicates that intraductal hypertension was an etiologic factor. Continued improvement in symptoms after stent removal indicates adequate dilation of the narrowing. The results of stent insertion for dominant pancreatic duct strictures (**Table 49.6**) have been favorable, with technical success in 72% to 99%, relief of pain in 75% to 94%, and good long-term outcomes in 52% to 81%.[174,181-183]

Although long-term symptom resolution has been reported in more than 60% of patients, endoscopic resolution of strictures has been documented in only about one-third of patients managed by endoscopic stent placement.[181,182] Although these data suggest that stricture resolution is not a prerequisite for symptom improvement, other concomitant therapies at the time of pancreatic stent placement such as pancreatic sphincterotomy or pancreatic stone removal may account for successful outcomes. It is also likely that pain in chronic pancreatitis tends to decrease over time as glandular destruction of the pancreas progresses in an uninhibited manner.[53]

In a study of 75 patients with pancreatic duct strictures and upstream dilation managed by placement of 10-Fr stents, Cremer and coworkers[174] reported that 71 patients (94%) were improved over a follow-up of 3 years, with 40 patients (53%) symptom-free. Improvement in symptoms was associated with a decrease in the pancreatic duct diameter. Also, in a prospective study of 23 patients, Ponchon and associates[181] reported that disappearance of stenosis at stent removal and a reduction in the pancreatic duct diameter by more than 2 mm were predictive of pain relief after pancreatic duct stent placement. Binmoeller and colleagues[183] made a similar observation in their study of 93 patients with chronic pancreatitis and dominant pancreatic duct strictures managed by pancreatic duct stent placement. Although 74% of the patients experienced complete or partial symptom relief, most patients were found to have a regression of ductal dilation after successful stent treatment.

The placement of multiple stents results in successful obliteration of benign biliary strictures; the role of multiple stent placement in pancreatic duct strictures was evaluated in a more recent study of 19 patients.[184] All patients with a single main pancreatic duct stricture underwent balloon dilation (6 to 10 mm) followed by placement of multiple stents (8.5-Fr to 11.5-Fr) across the stricture site. All stents were retrieved at a mean follow-up of 7 months. The median number of stents placed per patient was three, and the most common stent diameters used were 10-Fr and 11.5-Fr. During a mean follow-up of 38 months, 84% of patients were asymptomatic, and 10.5% developed symptom recurrence. Although all the above-described studies used conventional plastic stents, Cremer and coworkers,[185] in a pilot study, reported their experience with self-expandable metal stents in patients with chronic pancreatitis. Stent placement through the major duodenal papilla was performed in 22 patients with relapsing dominant strictures of the main pancreatic duct. Successful placement, associated with an immediate decrease of pancreatic duct diameter and disappearance of pain, was noted in 100% of cases. Although no immediate complications were encountered, follow-up of these patients showed a high occlusion rate of these metal stents from mucosal hyperplasia.

Another pilot study evaluated the role of covered self-expandable metal stents (8-mm) in patients with refractory main pancreatic duct strictures.[186] The stents were retrieved by endoscopy 3 months after placement. Although the pain scores improved significantly, three of six patients developed recurrent strictures warranting subsequent placement of large-caliber (10-mm) metal stents. Although this concept appears novel, more studies with a larger cohort of patients are needed to evaluate the role of covered metal stents in the management of benign pancreatic duct strictures. Direct comparative studies evaluating the efficacies of surgery and endoscopic therapy are required to identify a subset of patients who would benefit from either treatment modality.

Two prospective, randomized studies comparing surgical and endoscopic therapy in chronic pancreatitis have been reported in the literature.[187,188] In the first study,[187] 140 patients with obstructive chronic pancreatitis were treated either by endoscopic therapy or by surgical resection or drainage procedures. Although immediate relief of symptoms was identical in both groups (51.6% in the endotherapy group vs. 42.1% in the surgical group), at 5 years of follow-up, complete absence of pain was more frequent after surgery (37% vs. 14%), with partial relief of pain being similar (49% vs. 51%). The increase in body weight was also greater by 20% to 25% in the surgical group, whereas new-onset diabetes mellitus developed with similar frequency in both groups (34% in the surgical group vs. 43% in the endotherapy group). In the second randomized trial of 39 patients with chronic pancreatitis and pain, patients managed surgically had lower pain scores and better quality of life at 2-year follow-up.[188] Also,

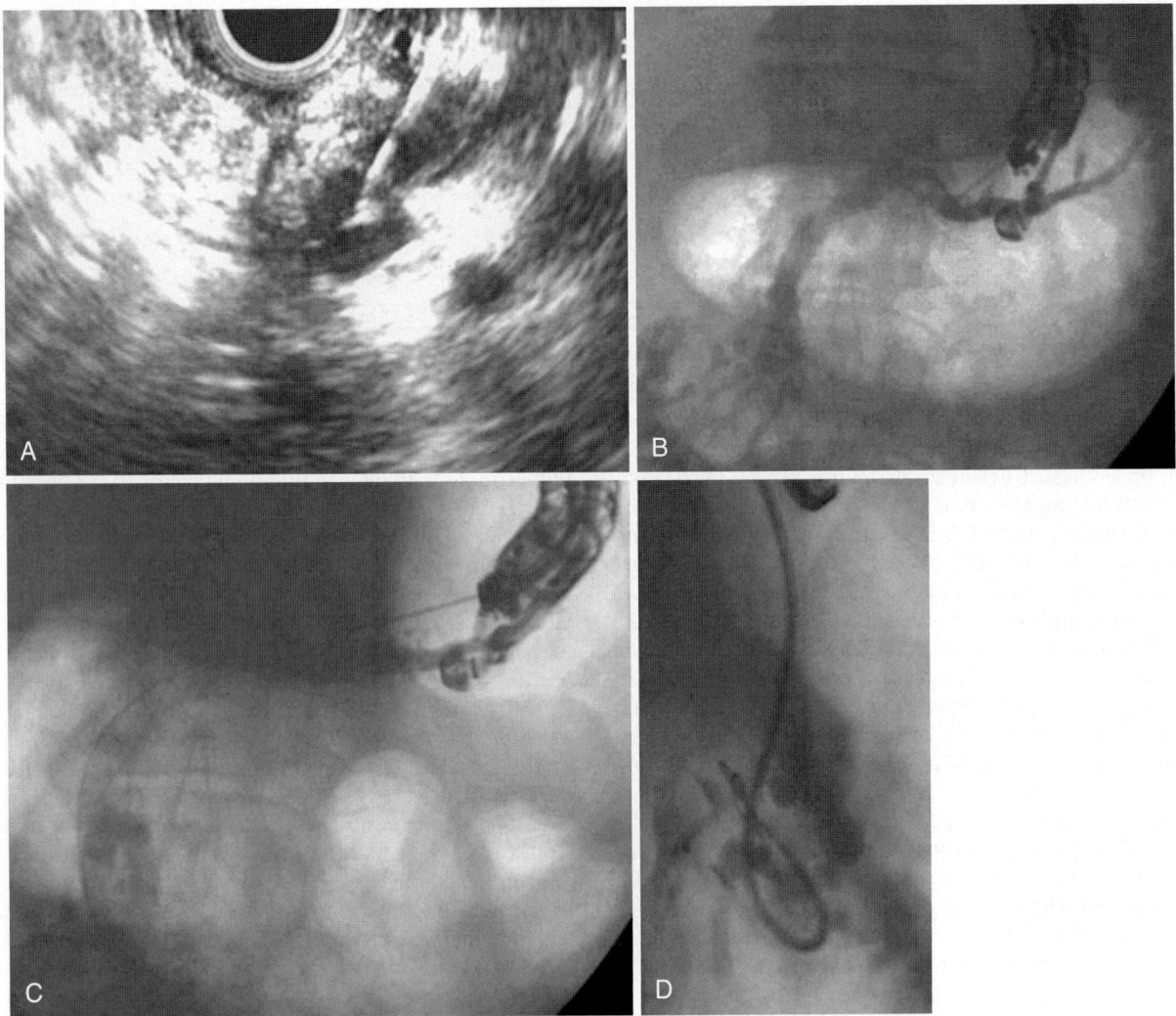

Fig. 49.12 A, Pancreatic duct accessed with a 19-gauge fine needle aspiration under endoscopic ultrasound (EUS) guidance. **B,** EUS-guided pancreatogram. **C,** Passage of a guidewire into the main pancreatic duct. **D,** Placement of a transmural stent into the main pancreatic duct. *(Courtesy of Michel Kahaleh, MD.)*

although only 32% of patients randomly assigned to endoscopy had better or partial pain relief, 75% of patients randomly assigned to surgery had better pain relief. There was no difference in the complications, length of hospital stay, and pancreatic function between both groups; however, patients undergoing endotherapy required more interventions.

Pancreatic stent therapy is not without consequences. Complications related directly to stent therapy include acute pancreatitis, pancreatic infection, pseudocyst formation, duct injury, stone formation, and migration.[154,189] The rate of pancreatic stent occlusion appears similar to that of biliary stents.[180] Most of these occlusions are without adverse clinical events, however, because pancreatic juice may siphon along the sides of the stent. Morphologic changes of the pancreatic duct directly related to stent placement occur in more than 50% of patients.[190–193] It is uncertain what the long-term consequences of these stent-induced ductal changes are in most patients, although permanent new strictures are seen in a few patients. EUS identified parenchymal changes in 68% of patients who underwent short-term pancreatic stent treatment.[85] Although such changes may have significant

long-term consequences in patients with a normal pancreas, the outcomes in patients with advanced chronic pancreatitis seem less certain.

Future Trends

The available diagnostic armamentarium for chronic pancreatitis focuses exclusively on pancreatic structure and function with inability to diagnose the disease in its early stages. The association between *CFTR* mutations and idiopathic chronic pancreatitis raises the possibility of genetic testing to evaluate idiopathic chronic pancreatitis. At the present time, the role of *CFTR* mutation testing is uncertain because no guidelines exist for genetic counseling or altered clinical management of idiopathic chronic pancreatitis based on the results of such testing. As further research clarifies whether patients with idiopathic chronic pancreatitis with *CFTR* mutations differ from other patients with idiopathic chronic pancreatitis, this information may lead to wider use of genetic testing during the evaluation of patients with idiopathic chronic pancreatitis.

Genetic testing may help young patients to seek medical care at an early stage of the disease and may facilitate referral to a specialized center for the management of cystic fibrosis. Although surgery is currently an effective alternative to endoscopic therapy for management of chronic pancreatitis, not all patients are candidates for surgery because of the attendant comorbidity. Often the complex morphologic situation in these patients (inflammatory tumor, ductal obstruction owing to stricture or stones or both) mandates the adoption of alternative techniques for relief of pancreatic duct obstruction.

EUS has been advocated more recently as a means to establish pancreatic ductal drainage in patients after failed ERCP.[194] This treatment can be accomplished either by rendezvous stent placement after passage of a guidewire into the main pancreatic duct and through the ampulla under EUS guidance or by transmural drainage of the main pancreatic duct via the stomach or duodenum (**Fig. 49.12**). However, in addition to technical difficulties, EUS-guided pancreatic duct drainage was associated with a complication rate of nearly 20% that included pancreatitis, perforation, bleeding, and death. Although clinicians have a keen interest in assessing the effects of medical intervention on outcomes related to morbidity and mortality, quality-of-life evaluation remains an area that has long been neglected. Quality of life may be defined as an individual's overall satisfaction with life and one's general sense of well-being.[195] This definition may be focused further by limiting it to just health-related quality of life. Physicians have always attempted to integrate their patients' well-being into therapeutic plans. However, health care providers have repeatedly been shown to be poor proxies for measuring quality of life.[196] By using instruments that measure quality of life, clinicians can learn whether the patient truly benefits from therapeutic interventions, rather than relying solely on clinical indicators. There are currently numerous disease-specific instruments for conditions such as inflammatory bowel disease, arthritis, and cancer, but only one instrument is available for evaluating patients with chronic pancreatitis.[197] Patient-centered outcomes and quality-of-life assessment are important areas in chronic pancreatitis that must be researched further to evaluate the impact of technical and technologic advances in this area.

References

The complete reference list is available online at www.expertconsult.com.

Chapter **50**

Pancreatic Duct Leaks and Pseudocysts

Richard A. Kozarek

Video related to this chapter's topics can be found online at expertconsult.com.

Introduction

The initial manifestations of acute pancreatitis are caused for the most part by local enzyme activation and acute cytokine release. This combination leads to local pain, ileus, peripancreatic burn, systemic inflammatory response syndrome, and early organ failure including acute respiratory distress syndrome. Perpetuation of the disease process may be a consequence of infection of necrotic tissue or ongoing ductal leak.[1-4] Chronic pancreatitis may also result in a pancreatic duct leak or fistula, as may trauma, surgical or otherwise.[1,5] In chronic pancreatitis, the consequence of the leak depends on the etiology, the size of the ductal disruption, the location of the leak relative to anatomic tissue planes, and the body's success in walling off and containing the disruption. In traumatic pancreatitis, there is usually a smoldering acute inflammatory response and an acute leak. This combination can result in a seriously ill patient after penetrating trauma or a patient who remains clinically well after surgical drain placement at the time of splenectomy and inadvertent damage to the pancreatic tail.[6]

Pancreatic duct leaks or fistulas have traditionally been defined as internal or external.[3,7] External leaks (pancreaticocutaneous fistulas) almost always follow percutaneous drainage of internal pancreatic fluid collections or pancreatic surgery. Less commonly, they are the consequence of penetrating abdominal trauma. Internal pancreatic fistulas include pancreaticoenteric fistulas, pseudocysts, pancreatic ascites, and pancreatic pleural effusions.[4,8] Pancreatic necrosis, which is clearly associated with ductal disruption in three-fourths of patients, has not traditionally been defined as the cause or consequence of a pancreatic fistula.[9-11] **Box 50.1** summarizes the current classification of pancreatic fistulas.

Epidemiology

The incidence of pancreatic duct leaks is uncertain and seems to be independent of the cause of the underlying pancreatitis. Whether caused by alcohol, biliary tract disease, metabolic disorders, or medications, an acute leak seems to be related more to disease severity. Multiple reports suggest that 30% to 75% of pancreatic necrosis is associated with ductal disruption, although there is considerable debate whether this disruption is a primary or secondary phenomenon.[7,9,10,12] Also, 40% of patients with acute pancreatitis may develop some peripancreatic fluid collection, although less than 5% of these patients develop a true pseudocyst, and a much smaller percentage have decompression of these fluid collections by formation of a pancreaticoenteric fistula.[13] Chronic pancreatitis predisposes not only to pseudocyst formation but also to pancreatic ascites and high-amylase pleural effusions. High-amylase pleural effusions are chronic and have a distinctly different chemical composition and pathophysiology than the more common acute pleural effusions noted in the setting of severe acute pancreatitis.[3,7]

Box 50.1 Consequences of Pancreatic Duct Leaks

Acute Disruption

Peripancreatic fluid collection
Pseudocyst
Pancreatic necrosis
Smoldering pancreatitis (?)

Chronic Disruption

Internal fistula
Pseudocyst
Pancreatic ascites
High-amylase pleural effusion
Pancreatic-enteric, biliary, or bronchial fistula

External Fistula

Pancreaticocutaneous fistula

Box 50.2 Pathogenesis of Pancreatic Fistulas

Internal Fistula

Pseudocyst
Pancreatic necrosis
Ductal obstruction
    Stone
    Stricture
    Inflammatory
    Malignant

Pancreatic Ascites, High-Amylase, Pleural Effusion
Pancreatic duct stricture, stone, or pseudocyst

Pancreaticoenteric Fistula
Pancreatic necrosis
Percutaneous tube erosion, contiguous bowel loop

External Fistula

Penetrating trauma
Pancreatic resection or trauma
Percutaneous drainage of pseudocyst or pancreatic fluid collection

Pathogenesis

Pancreatic duct leaks are the consequence of enzyme activation with subsequent necrosis of ductal epithelium, the result of increased intraductal pressure often behind a stricture or stone or both.[3,7] Alternatively, leaks may be caused or perpetuated by percutaneous drainage of peripancreatic fluid collections; surgical resection or bypass; tumor disruption of ductal epithelia; or pancreatic trauma, particularly penetrating trauma.[14–25] **Box 50.2** lists some etiologies of pancreatic duct leaks.

Clinical Features

The clinical features of pancreatic duct leaks depend on the cause of the disruption and its size and site. Pancreatic juice follows tissue planes, and the body is variably successful in containing this leak contingent on such factors as rate of leak and presence or absence of superinfection. Superinfection, early cytokine release, bacterial translocation from the gut, endotoxin release, and extraluminal enzyme activation also determine many of the clinical features associated with acute pancreatitis, such as pain, ileus, nausea and vomiting, tachycardia, oliguria, and hypotension.[26,27] From an anatomic standpoint, a leak may be low grade and stay within the confines of the parenchyma leading to smoldering pancreatitis or variable degrees of necrosis, the latter often associated with multisystem organ failure and local and systemic infections.[7,28–32] Necrosis may also lead to internal fistulization into contiguous organs including the C-loop most commonly but also the bile duct, stomach, transverse colon, or jejunum.[3,33–36]

Depending on the degree of leak and its perpetuation by necrosis or downstream ductal obstruction and ongoing oral feeding and pancreatic stimulation, head leaks often are associated with right pararenal fluid collections and can track along the psoas musculature to cause pelvic fluid collections that can track into the scrotum or buttocks.[36] If volumes of juice are sufficient, with resultant pancreatic ascites, I have even seen prolapsed and ulcerated vaginal vaults and uteri because of increased intraabdominal pressure. Pancreatic head leak that is successfully walled off by the body may cause a pseudocyst localized to the right upper quadrant. Although the latter may be asymptomatic, if small, common presentations of larger pseudocysts in this location include postprandial or chronic pain, early satiety or postprandial nausea and vomiting from variable degrees of gastric outlet obstruction, or biliary obstruction. Biliary obstruction may cause jaundice or occasional cholangitis but is more often associated with liver function abnormalities including variable elevations of transaminases and alkaline phosphatase.

Leaks of the pancreatic duct tail have been associated with left upper quadrant or perisplenic pseudocysts,[3,37] if contained and walled off. Alternatively, they may track into the retroperitoneum and cause high-amylase pleural effusions[22,38–40] or acute pararenal or pelvic fluid collections. Fistulization into the ligament of Treitz or the transverse colon or splenic flexure also is occasionally seen but almost exclusively in the setting of active necrosis.[15,34,41] Depending on the rapidity of the leak and the presence or absence of concomitant necrosis, clinical signs and symptoms of a tail leak may include shortness of breath, nausea and postprandial pain, or clinical signs of sepsis because of a pancreaticocolonic fistula.

Leaks that occur from the genu to the distal body or proximal tail area of the pancreas occur most commonly in the setting of necrosis and result in lesser sac fluid collections.[3,14,42–46] Traditionally defined as pseudocysts, these fluid collections are usually more complex, containing considerable saponified fat and tissue debris. The consistency and viscosity of lesser sac fluid collections are routinely misinterpreted by abdominal computed tomography (CT), often leading to therapeutic misadventures with attempts to drain these collections radiographically, endoscopically, or surgically.[4,11,19,47–50] To distinguish these collections from more traditional pseudocysts that can have a similar imaging appearance, Baron and colleagues[50] termed these latter collections *evolving pancreatic necrosis,* a variant of walled-off pancreatic necrosis, and suggested that the patient's clinical course may be more important than traditional abdominal imaging.

The lesser sac is also often a decompressive site for patients with chronic pancreatitis with downstream duct obstruction from a pancreatic stone or stricture. This condition can result in a variably sized pseudocyst or pancreatic pericardial effusion if there is mediastinal involvement. Additional chest manifestations include pancreatic pleural effusion, as noted previously, and pericardial tamponade or pancreaticobronchial fistulas.[3,31] Central pancreatic leaks are usually the cause of pancreatic ascites also.[7,22,39,51] Associated with a concomitant and leaking pseudocyst in 50% of patients, clinical presentation may include increased pain plus abdominal girth, shortness of breath from diaphragmatic compression or concomitant pleural effusions, and occasional spontaneous bacterial peritonitis from bacterial translocation from the gut.

Pathology

Because of the variability of etiology of ductal disruptions, there is no one all-encompassing pathology. Instead, chronic pancreatitis is usually associated with the formation of a leak and its myriad manifestations (pseudocyst, ascites, and pancreatic pleural effusions) by virtue of ductal obstruction by an inflammatory stricture or intraductal calcification.[3,8] In such settings, acute parenchymal inflammation may be negligible. In contrast, the acute inflammatory response seen in acute pancreatitis, particularly pancreatic necrosis, has been claimed by some authors to be the primary event with subsequent lysis of ductal epithelial cells resulting in a leak.[52] There is likely a mixture of scenarios in either setting with the resultant pathology depending on the site and size of the disruption; the presence or absence of activated enzymes; and the body's success at walling off the leak, initially with inflammatory cells but later with formation and organization of collagen. The last-mentioned is perhaps best represented by a pseudocyst that can be broken down further into acute pseudocyst (collection of pancreatic juice enclosed by a wall of nonepithelialized granulation tissue that arises as a consequence of acute pancreatitis, requires at least 4 weeks to form, and is devoid of significant solid debris) and chronic pseudocyst (a collection of pancreatic juice enclosed by a wall of fibrous or granulation tissue that arises as a consequence of chronic pancreatitis).[23,50]

Differential Diagnosis

The etiology and the benign nature of most pancreatic duct leaks are easy to confirm if one considers the diagnosis in the first place because of access to excellent abdominal imaging through ultrasound, CT scanning, magnetic resonance (MR) imaging including secretin-magnetic resonance cholangiopancreatography (S-MRCP), and endoscopic modalities such as endoscopic ultrasound (EUS) and endoscopic retrograde cholangiopancreatography (ERCP).[3,13,23,53–57] Routine aspiration of ascites or pleural effusions for amylase and lipase usually confirms a pancreatic etiology, and a fluid collection in the left upper quadrant after a splenectomy, left nephrectomy, or complicated antireflux procedure can be confirmed as pancreatic in origin if one thinks to check an amylase level

at the time of diagnostic percutaneous aspiration or therapeutic drain placement. In these instances, inadvertent damage to the tail of the pancreas is substantially more common than local perforation of the stomach or splenic flexure of the colon at the time of surgery.

In addition, the diagnosis of a pancreatic duct leak should not be difficult in patients with a persistent fluid output after a pancreatic resection or percutaneous drainage of an acute, amylase-rich fluid collection in the setting of acute or chronic pancreatitis. The major differential diagnostic dilemma occurs in patients without a known history of pancreatitis who present with what appears to be a pseudocyst. There have been multiple approaches to distinguish pseudocysts from cystic neoplasms and benign from potentially malignant cystic tumors. Ultrasound and CT characteristics favoring pseudocyst include parenchymal or ductal calcifications, a uniform appearance to the cyst, and lack of calcifications in the lesion itself. Cysts that show an irregular wall thickness with mass effect, septations, or punctate wall calcification are more likely to be neoplastic. Cyst aspiration for amylase, mucus, carcinoembryonic antigen level, and cytology can be done under CT, ultrasound, or EUS guidance and has been used to distinguish benign and malignant neoplastic cysts from pseudocysts.[58] Pseudocysts are discussed in detail in other chapters.

As noted previously, S-MRCP has occasionally been used to document a pancreatic duct leak, particularly in the setting of pancreatic necrosis.[53] ERCP has been used more commonly not only to diagnose but also to treat pancreatic duct leaks. Leaks may be demonstrable by abnormal flow of contrast material into a pseudocyst, into the peritoneal or thoracic cavity, or into the bile duct or a contiguous loop of bowel in the setting of internal fistulas.[1,3,7] Alternatively, contrast material can often be seen flowing into a surgically or radiologically placed Jackson-Pratt drain in external fistulas.[5,22,36,59] In the setting of central pancreatic necrosis or severe chronic pancreatitis, ERCP may simply document a complete obstruction of the main pancreatic duct. In this setting, the leak occurs upstream from the obstruction or from a disconnected portion of the gland—the disconnected duct syndrome. **Box 50.3**

Box 50.3 Diagnosis of Pancreatic Leaks

External Fistula

Demonstrable pancreatogram through surgically or percutaneously placed Jackson-Pratt drain
Persistent high amylase output through Jackson-Pratt drain

Internal Fistula

Pleural effusion: Chest x-ray, abdominal and thoracic CT
  High amylase with aspiration
Pancreatic ascites: Ground-glass appearance, loss of psoas shadow on flat film; confirmation via ultrasound, abdominal CT, or MR imaging
  High amylase with aspiration
Pseudocyst ± ductal stone and dilated duct: CT, MR imaging, EUS, ERCP
Duct disruption ± obstruction: ERCP, S-MRCP

CT, computed tomography; ERCP, endoscopic retrograde cholangiopancreatography; EUS, endoscopic ultrasound; MR, magnetic resonance; S-MRCP, secretin-magnetic resonance cholangiopancreatography.

Box 50.4 **Therapy of Pancreatic Duct Leaks**

Minimize Pancreatic Secretion

Clear liquids vs. NPO and hyperalimentation
Somatostatin or its analogues

Treat Ductal Disruption

Transpapillary stent
Downsize and reposition external catheter
Surgery (disconnected gland syndrome)

Treat Consequences of Ductal Disruption

Ascites and pleural effusion: Paracentesis or thoracentesis
Pseudocyst: Endoscopic, radiographic, or surgical drainage

NPO, nil per os (nothing by mouth).

summarizes some diagnostic tests available for pancreatic duct leaks.

Treatment

Therapy for pancreatic duct leaks does not occur in an endoscopic vacuum. Strategies include preventing a leak in the first place, using good surgical technique, and possibly using intraoperative fibrin glue or stent placement or postoperative octreotide after partial pancreatectomy or decompressive pancreatic surgery.[5,60-64] The ability to place a transpapillary stent does not mean that this modality is suitable for all patients. Individuals with leaks are best approached by a team consisting of an interventional radiologist, a pancreaticobiliary surgeon, and an endoscopist capable of performing both diagnosis and therapy (**Box 50.4**).[1,3,65]

Pseudocysts

Pseudocysts were historically treated surgically, usually by cyst-enteric or cyst-gastric anastomoses, although pancreatic resection has occasionally been used for pseudocysts in the pancreatic tail.[25,66-69] Likewise, complex cysts with significant internal septations or debris have been treated with external drainage. Morbidity and 30-day mortality rates for open surgery have approximated 25% to 30% and 2% to 5% with recurrence rates of 10% to 20%.[25,57,69,70] These statistics have led some centers to approach surgical decompression laparoscopically and to insist on preoperative MRCP or ERCP to delineate better the ductal anatomy as a guide to type of surgery (decompression vs. resection).[25,56,71,72] No randomized trials have compared surgical with nonsurgical management of pseudocysts; instead, retrospective reviews are available in which 30 patients with pseudocysts were treated with surgery (49%), endoscopy (39%), or percutaneously (11%). There were no differences in pseudocyst resolution or complications in patients treated surgically or endoscopically.[73]

A series by Melman and colleagues[66] defined higher initial success rates for laparoscopic versus open pseudocyst drainage, although comparable success rates were noted with endoscopic, radiologic, or salvage surgical drainage. In many centers, percutaneous drainage of pseudocysts with long-term

catheter placement has become the standard of care by which other treatment modalities have been judged. Individual series and meta-analyses of the literature suggest 85% successful resolution rates, although catheter occlusions with subsequent bacterial seeding and iatrogenic infection with need for urgent catheter exchange remain problematic particularly if the cyst is filled with debris.[7,36,74] In addition, in individuals who develop a disconnected gland syndrome from trauma or necrosis, placement of a percutaneous drain may result in a chronic pancreatic external fistula that may necessitate Jackson-Pratt drainage for months or years. Alternatively, percutaneous injection of glue or fibrin has been used in an attempt to close the fistulous tract, and surgery may be required to resect the distal (tail), disconnected portion of the gland.[75]

Endoscopic pseudocyst drainage was first described by Rogers and coworkers[76] in 1978 using a needle placement through the gut wall to drain a pseudocyst that rapidly recurred. The first successful electrocautery fistulization into a pseudocyst was done more than 2 decades ago and resulted in permanent cure in three of the first four patients in whom it was undertaken.[77] Although the procedure has been refined to take advantage of abdominal CT, EUS, and MR imaging and MRCP, large pseudocysts still require some form of access, either by needle-knife sphincterotome or transgastric or transenteric injection with a Seldinger needle followed by placement of one or more guidewires into the cavity proper (**Fig. 50.1**).[78-97] Historically, the incisions were enlarged using some form of electrocautery (conventional or needle-knife sphincterotomy or an overtube that conducted cautery), but 6- to 10-mm hydrostatic balloons are used in most cases at the present time to enlarge the communication to the stomach or duodenum. A variation of this procedure is use of a transluminal balloon accessotome.[98] Although various stents have been used to maintain the fistulous communication between the gut and pseudocyst, most endoscopists currently use 7-Fr to 10-Fr double-pigtail stents to minimize migration, leaving them in place for 6 to 8 weeks or until abdominal imaging has confirmed pseudocyst resolution.

Although the need for preprocedure antibiotics has not changed, other things have. With the advent of therapeutic EUS scopes, it is no longer necessary to see a "bulge" on the stomach or duodenal wall to ensure that one is entering the fluid collection.[83,89-91,94,95,99-102] Therapeutic duodenoscopes are not required; concomitant ERCP is usually employed to define ductal anatomy including the presence of an ongoing leak or disconnected duct and gland syndrome.[1,7] A leak can be treated with transpapillary stents (**Fig. 50.2**) allowing resolution of small pseudocysts without need for concomitant drainage[102]; disconnected duct and gland syndrome can signal the need for ultimate surgery or long-term indwelling pseudocyst stents in patients who are a very poor surgical risk.[103]

Many case reports or series have described transpapillary stents or transenteric or transgastric fistulization into pseudocysts with their attendant resolution; however, one of the better ones has been by Baron and colleagues.[50] These authors looked at endoscopic drainage techniques and outcomes in acute versus chronic pseudocysts and in pancreatic necrosis. Historically, endoscopic attempts at drainage of necrosis were fraught with bleeding and infectious complications because of increased vascularity at the necrosis–viable tissue interface and because it has proven difficult to drain extremely thick

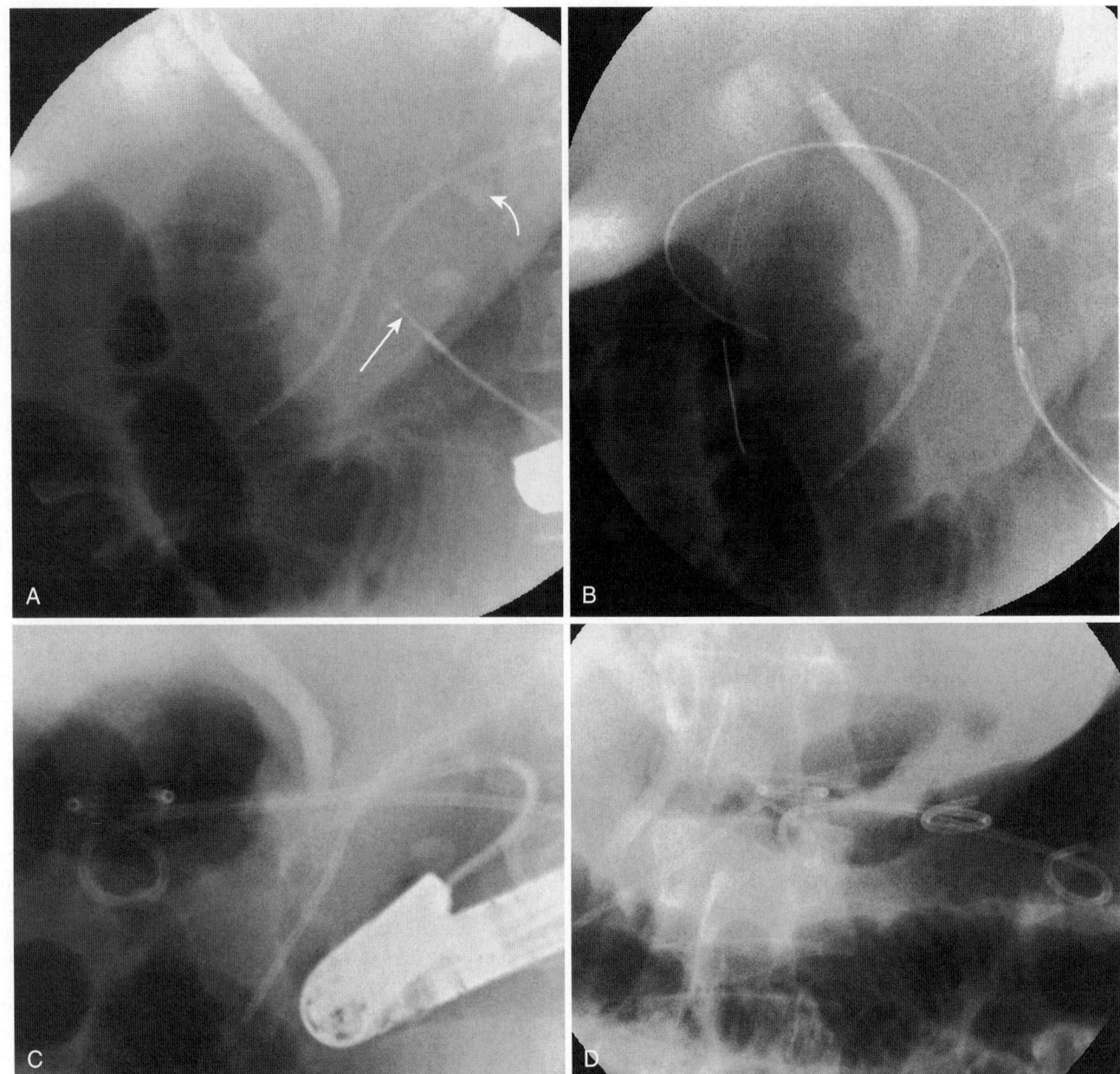

Fig. 50.1 A, Transgastric puncture *(small arrow)* in a patient with ductal leak and pseudocyst because of an obstructing ductal stone *(curved arrow).* Note the transpapillary stent. **B–D,** Guidewire placement within the pseudocyst (**B**) is followed by placement of two double-pigtail stents (**C** and **D**).

and viscous debris through small-diameter, endoscopically placed stents. Baron and colleagues[50] instead placed nasocystic tubes and performed irrigation with large-volume saline for prolonged periods (3 to 6 weeks) of irrigation in an attempt to break up the necrotic debris and flush it into the lumen of the gut. Ultimately, they achieved complete resolution of the various pancreatic fluid collections in 113 of 138 (82%) patients, although resolution was more frequent in patients with chronic pseudocyst (59 of 64 [92%]) than in patients with acute pseudocyst (23 of 31 [74%]; $P = .02$) or pancreatic necrosis (31 of 43 [72%]; $P = .006$). In addition, complications were more common in patients with necrosis who had endoscopic drainage (16 of 43 [37%]) than patients with acute pseudocysts (6 of 31 [19%]; P = not significant) or chronic pseudocysts (11 of 64 [17%]; $P = .02$). At a median follow-up

of 2.1 years, recurrent fluid collections were more common in patients with necrosis (9 of 31 [29%]) than patients with acute pseudocysts (2 of 23 [9%]; $P = .07$) or chronic pseudocysts (7 of 59 [12%]; $P = .047$) (**Table 50.1**).

In more recent reports, necrosis is treated more aggressively by means of retroperitoneal endoscopic débridement after initial fistulization through, and balloon dilation of, the stomach wall[104–108]; whether this becomes the standard of care remains to be seen and is discussed in detail in another chapter. What is certain, however, is that pseudocyst and necrosis drainage are not risk-free, and these therapies must be used alongside other treatment modalities including open and laparoscopic surgery and percutaneous drainage. Because it is unlikely that a randomized prospective trial would be done comparing these individual modalities or that the results

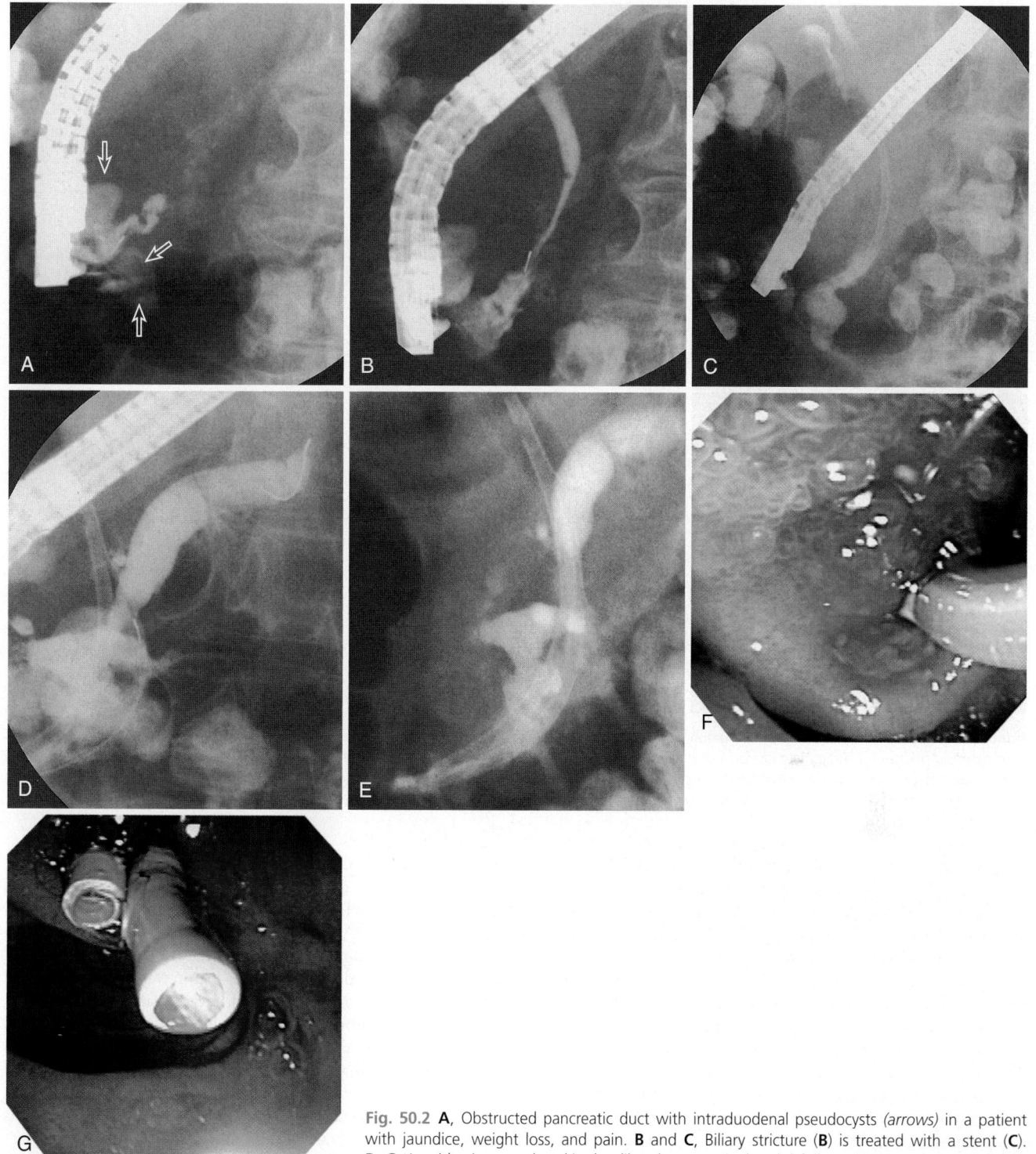

Fig. 50.2 A, Obstructed pancreatic duct with intraduodenal pseudocysts *(arrows)* in a patient with jaundice, weight loss, and pain. **B** and **C**, Biliary stricture (**B**) is treated with a stent (**C**). **D–G**, A guidewire was placed in the dilated pancreatic duct (**D**) followed by stent insertion (**E–G**).

could be generalized to institutions with different levels of subspecialty strengths and skills, it is imperative for physicians who care for such patients to work with a team that includes endoscopists, surgeons, and interventional radiologists.

Numerous series have looked at either EUS or standard luminal endoscopy or surgery for pseudocyst drainage.[66,73,93,109] Varadarajulu and associates[110] randomly assigned patients to various endoscopic techniques of pseudocyst drainage and

concluded that EUS procedures were more successful. The same group showed that EUS-facilitated procedures had efficacy and complications comparable to surgery, although patients with endoscopic treatment had statistically significant decreased costs and resource use compared with patients treated surgically.[84] Our group previously reported 133 patients with severe necrosis (Balthazar score ≥ 6) treated with multimodality therapy (**Fig. 50.3**).[9] We showed that 76% of

Table 50.1 Outcomes after Attempted Endoscopic Drainage of Pancreatic Fluid Collections

	Acute Pancreatitis	Chronic Pancreatitis	Pancreatic Necrosis	Necrotic Pancreatitis vs. Acute Pancreatitis	Acute Pancreatitis vs. Pancreatic Necrosis	Chronic Pancreatitis vs. Pancreatic Necrosis
Successful resolution	24/31 (74%)	59/64 (92%)	31/43 (72%)	P = .02	NS	P = .006
Complications	6/31 (19%)	11/64 (17%)	16/43 (37%)	NS	NS	P = .02
Hospital days	9	3	20	P = .0003	NS	P = .0001
Recurrence	2/23 (9%)	7/59 (12%)	9/31 (29%)	NS	NS	P = .047

NS, not significant.

Modified from Baron TH, Harewood GC, Morgan DE, et al: Outcome differences after endoscopic drainage of pancreatic necrosis, acute pancreatic pseudocysts, and chronic pancreatic pseudocysts. Gastrointest Endosc 56:7–17, 2002.

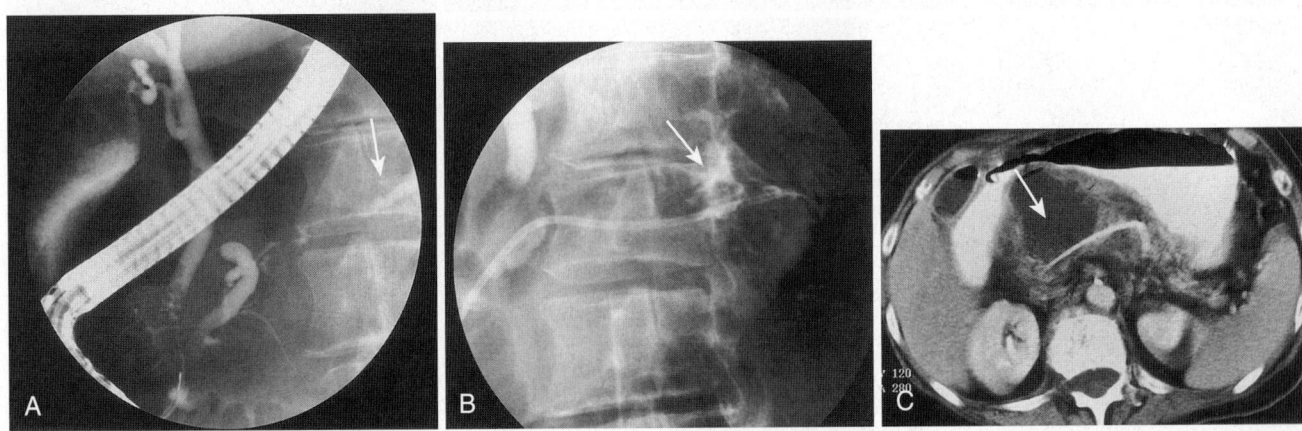

Fig. 50.3 A, Endoscopic retrograde cholangiopancreatography (ERCP) in a patient with multisystem failure from pancreatic necrosis. Arrow shows tight extrinsic stricture of the pancreatic duct. Note distal common bile duct stones. **B,** A leak at the junction of the body and tail *(arrow)* was treated with biliary sphincterotomy and transpapillary stent placement. **C,** Massive necrosis *(arrow)* (treated percutaneously) and a stent are visible in the residual pancreatic duct. The patient responded to conservative management and required only elective cholecystectomy.

these patients had ductal disruption including side branch or major ductal leak and disconnected gland syndrome. Of the 115 patients to undergo ERCP, 70 (61%) had stent placement, 15 (13%) had cyst-gastrostomy or cyst-duodenotomy, 11 (9.6%) had a nasopancreatic drain, and 11 (9.6%) had a nasobiliary drain. In addition, 98 of 133 (74%) had placement of one or more large Jackson-Pratt drains, and 75 patients ultimately required elective surgery including pancreatic resection in 47 (33%) for glandular disconnection. Mean hospital days approximated 1 month, and there was a 9% mortality rate in this exceptionally sick group of patients, many with multisystem organ failure. These results equal or exceed previously reported outcomes in surgical series using routine or selective débridement.[4,111–115]

Pancreatic Ascites and Pleural Effusions

Historically, pancreatic ascites was treated by resting the pancreas to minimize flow and leak. Patients were given nothing by mouth, were given parenteral nutrition, and were started on somatostatin analogues.[65,116–120] Diuretics and large-volume thoracentesis and paracentesis were commonly used before "salvage" operations—usually pancreatic resection or Roux-en-Y cyst-jejunostomy if a concomitant pseudocyst was present. Medical therapy was effective at best in half of the

patients, and the subsequent surgical approach, usually predicated on anatomy as defined by preoperative ERCP, was associated with an 8% to 15% periprocedural mortality and a 15% recurrence rate.[116–121] More than a decade ago, we showed that stent placement beyond a ductal disruption, with or without concomitant pseudocyst decompression, was effective therapy in a small group of patients with pancreatic ascites, particularly when combined with large-volume paracentesis (**Figs. 50.4, 50.5,** and **50.6**).[51,121] Bracher and coworkers[122] confirmed our original findings, and 91% of patients had resolution of ascites without major complications. There were no recurrences in the two series at 60 months and 14 months. This approach apparently works by relieving upstream duct hypertension by bypassing the sphincter or an obstructing stone or inflammatory stenosis. It does not work with a disconnected gland syndrome in which most of the pancreatic juice enters the peritoneal or thoracic cavity from a disconnected tail; this condition is ultimately treated better with surgery.

Pancreaticoenteric Fistula and Acute Pancreatic Trauma

Our group previously reported successful healing of eight patients with pancreaticoduodenal (five patients) or pancreaticocutaneous (three patients) fistulas.[59] Three patients

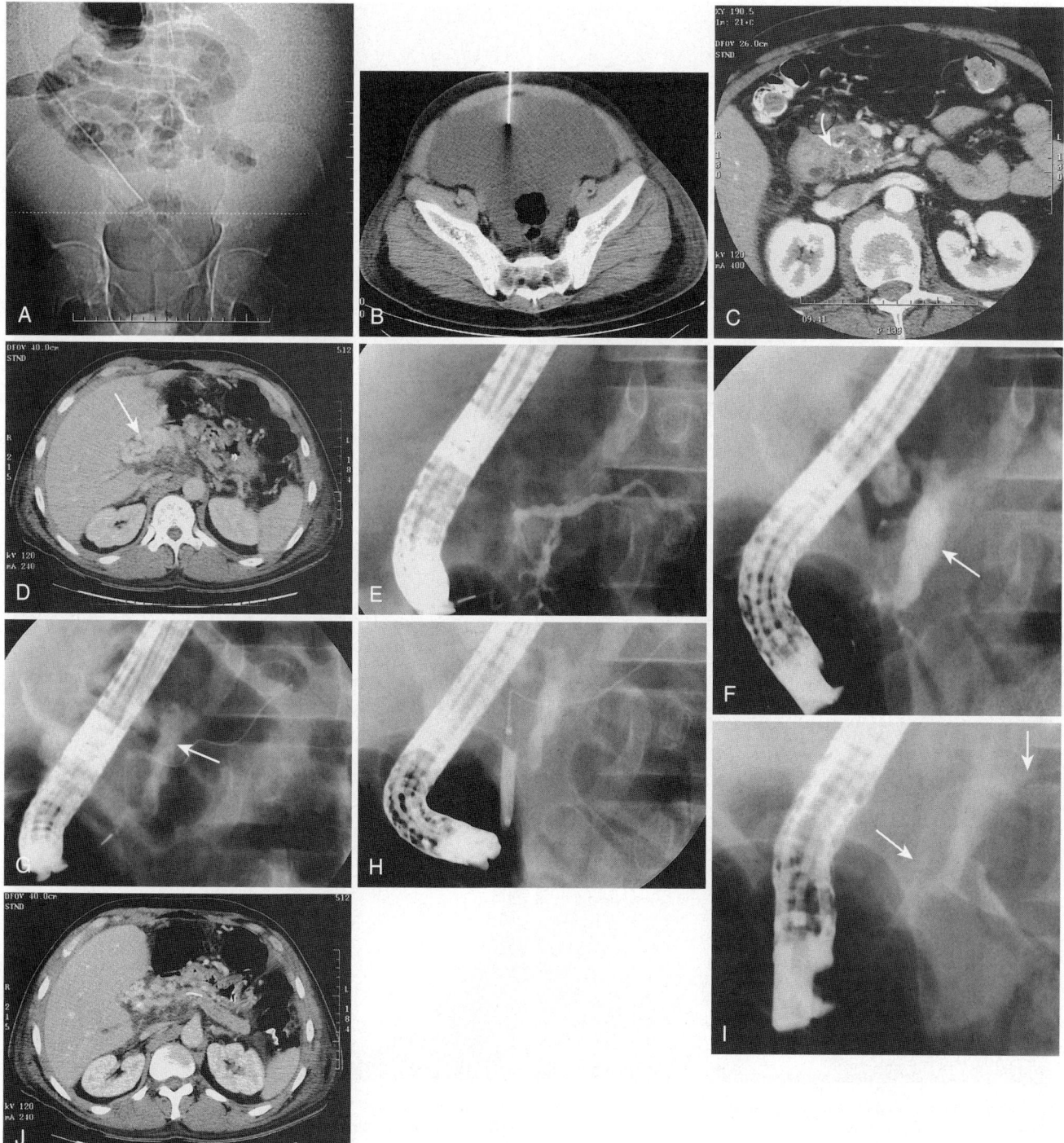

Fig. 50.4 Ground-glass appearance in a patient with pancreatic ascites (**A**) initially treated with repeated paracentesis (**B**). Abdominal computed tomography (CT) scan shows a complex cystic inflammatory mass in the head of the pancreas (**C**) with portal vein thrombosis (**D**). Porta hepatis varices are present. Endoscopic retrograde cholangiopancreatography (ERCP) shows stricture and ductal leak *(arrows)* (**E–G**) initially treated with balloon dilation (**H**) and placement of an 8-cm, 3-Fr stent (**I**). **J**, Resolution of small pseudocyst on subsequent CT scan.

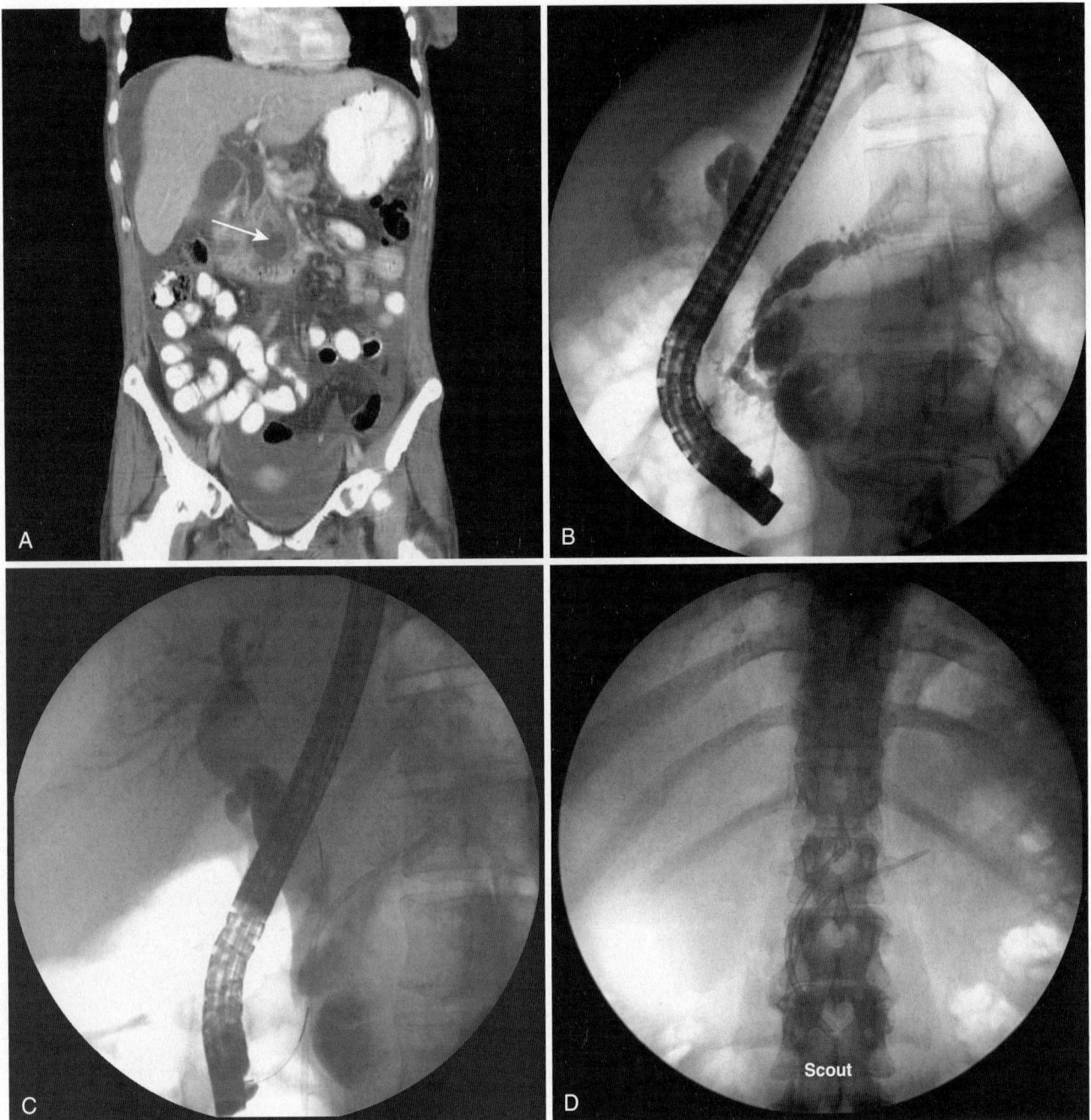

Fig. 50.5 A patient with pancreatic ascites (*arrow* denotes pseudocyst) (**A**). Endoscopic retrograde cholangiopancreatography (ERCP) shows pancreatic duct stricture and two pseudocysts (**B**) treated with pancreatic (**C**) and biliary (**D**) stents for concomitant biliary obstruction.

healed after downsizing or removal of an external drain, three patients had healing of their fistulas with transpapillary stent placement, and two patients ultimately required pancreatic resection. An additional six patients with pancreaticobiliary fistulas all were successfully treated using a combination of biliary sphincterotomy and pancreaticobiliary stent placement.[9] ERCP has also been used to treat internal fistulas associated with acute pancreatic trauma.[6] Kim and colleagues[21] noted injury to the pancreatic duct in 14 of 23 patients, including 8 patients who had leakage into the pancreatic parenchyma that resolved spontaneously. An additional three patients had a leak from the main pancreatic duct and

responded to transpapillary stent placement. These authors believed that early ERCP with directed therapy (i.e., medical, endoscopic, surgical) was advantageous in the setting of acute pancreatic trauma and potential ductal leak.

External Fistulas

As previously noted, external pancreatic fistulas are usually iatrogenic. Etiologies include surgical or percutaneous drainage of a pancreatic fluid collection with an ongoing ductal disruption as a consequence of a disconnected gland or downstream obstruction from a stone or stricture. Fistulas

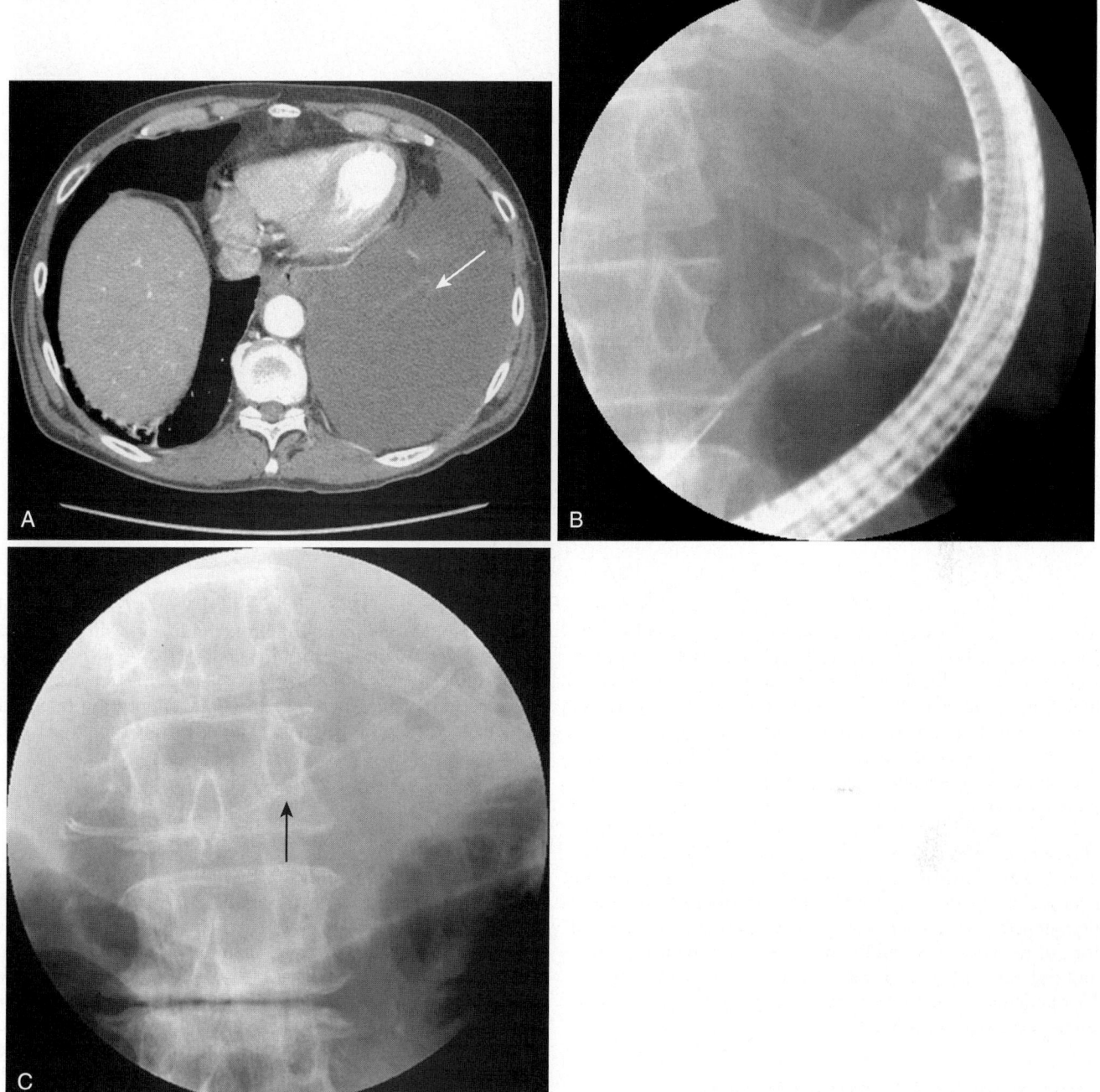

Fig. 50.6 A, Large right pleural effusion *(arrow)*. **B**, Endoscopic retrograde cholangiopancreatography (ERCP) shows a leak in the pancreatic duct tail in this patient with high-amylase pancreatic pleural effusion. **C**, The leak responded to placement of two pancreatic duct stents and thoracentesis without reaccumulation of effusion.

may also follow partial pancreatic resection or bypass or result from penetrating abdominal trauma.[1,3,7,65,123] Since our initial report using variable length prostheses bridging ductal disruptions for head or body leaks and placing short transpapillary stents alone in postoperative tail disruptions without downstream obstruction,[124] multiple additional series have been published.[125–127] Of 58 patients with an average fistulous output of 200 mL/day, 50 (86%) had successful stent placement, 46 of whom (92%) had resolution of the fistula within 5 weeks. Several patients experienced minor flares of pancreatitis, and two deaths occurred in one of the series, unrelated

to the fistula or endotherapy. Contingent on the series, there were no recurrences in follow-up ranging from 12 to 36 months. More recently, Pelaez-Luna and colleagues[2] at the Mayo Clinic looked at their experience with the disconnected pancreatic duct syndrome in several subsets of patients with acute pancreatitis, including patients with external fistulas. Endoscopy improved manifestations of leakage in 19 of 26 patients in whom it was attempted. For patients who successfully avoided surgery, pancreatic atrophy of the disconnected portion was common and associated with development of diabetes in 10%.

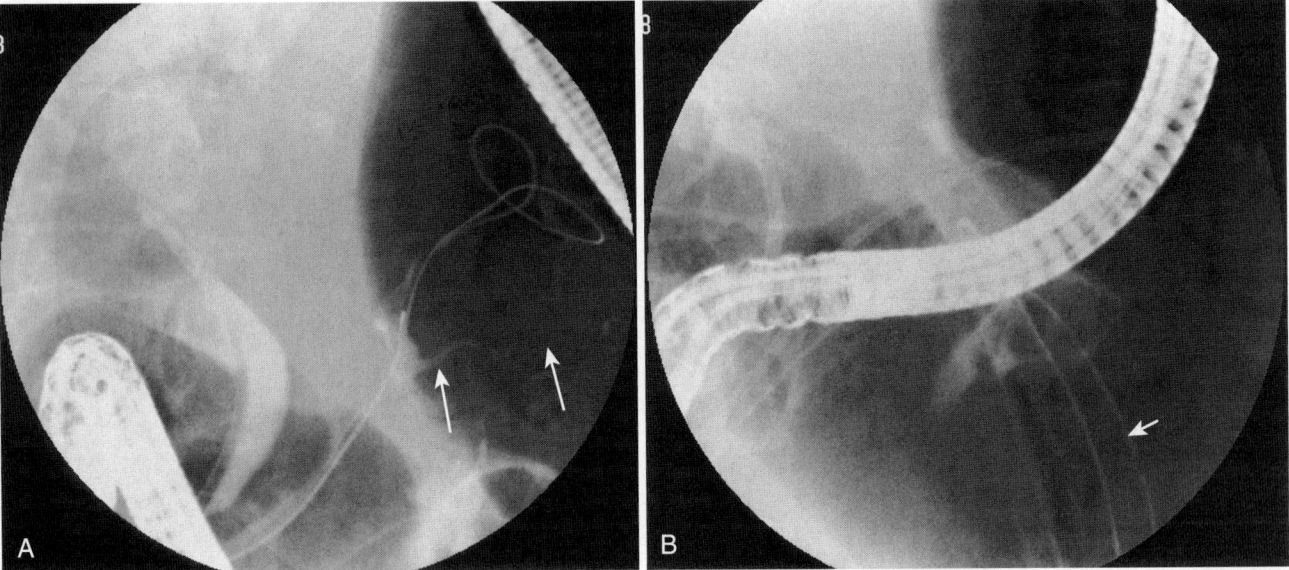

Fig. 50.7 **A,** Course of the pancreatic duct in a patient with acute blowout, pancreaticocutaneous fistula *(arrows)*. A guidewire is curled in the cavity. **B,** The leak was treated with a transpapillary stent and percutaneous drain *(arrow)*.

It is our practice to treat patients with enteral nutrition using formula diets or total parenteral nutrition when the patient is acutely ill with pancreatic necrosis, usually adding a somatostatin analogue if there is persistent high-amylase, high-volume Jackson-Pratt drain output.[128–132] We may also treat postoperative patients with a persistent external fistula this way. However, if there is not dramatic and immediate decrease in fistulous output, our group is now studying these patients earlier in the course (<1 week) and attempting to place a transpapillary prosthesis if the anatomy is amendable (**Fig. 50.7**). Alternatively, in patients who remain unwell after 2 to 3 weeks, our group places transgastric stents into the necrotic cavity in conjunction with concomitant large-bore percutaneous drain placement in an attempt to preclude need for tail resection.[132] In addition, there are individual reports and case series approaching a subset of such patients, particularly patients with disconnected glands, with various interventional radiologic techniques.[123,132–134]

Indications and Contraindications

The indications for treating a pancreatic duct leak are (1) persistence of an external fistula, (2) inability to refeed a patient without developing recurrent pain or pancreatitis, (3) enlarging pancreatic fluid collection (pseudocyst, pancreatic ascites, high-amylase, pleural effusion), or (4) symptomatic fluid collection. A fifth indication may be uncertainty about diagnosis, which is usually an issue only when attempting to differentiate pseudocysts from cystic neoplasms of the pancreas.[1] Many more recent publications tend to lump the many manifestations of pancreatic duct leak together recognizing that evolving fluid collections in acute pancreatitis may have considerable necrotic debris and be better defined as walled-off pancreatic necrosis.[5,135,136] Pseudocysts can leak, obstruct, or erode, causing manifestations such as concomitant pancreatic ascites, gastric outlet obstruction, or pseudoaneurysm or pancreaticoenteric fistula. Hookey and colleagues[135] from

Brussels lumped 116 patients, reporting an 87.9% successful treatment rate endoscopically and finding no difference in patients with acute or chronic pancreatitis. There was a significantly higher failure rate in patients with pancreatic necrosis. For all patients, there was an 11% complication rate, and 6 patients died within 30 days, with one death directly related to the drainage.

A comprehensive look at EUS-directed drainage of various pancreatic fluid collections was published in a 2008 EUS Working Group document (**Table 50.2**).[48] From my perspective, the major contraindication to studying a patient is inability to apply therapy. It is potentially dangerous to perform ERCP in the setting of pancreatic necrosis or pseudocyst because of the potential of iatrogenic infection unless one is prepared to treat this leak. As noted previously, treatment can be directed at either the leak (transpapillary stent) or the consequences of the leak (see **Box 50.4**). Other contraindications are relative and include inability to give informed consent, anaphylaxis with iodinated contrast agents, and a patient so unstable that endoscopic diagnosis or therapy entails prohibitive procedural risk. In this setting, S-MRCP may define anatomy and leak site so that percutaneous drainage may initially be preferable to stabilize the patient.

Preoperative History and Consideration

The presence of a pancreatic fluid collection or internal or external fistula does not by itself demand therapy. Important considerations include whether duct disruption occurs in the setting of acute or chronic pancreatitis, whether necrosis is present or absent, or whether the patient has a controlled or uncontrolled leak. An example of the latter is a low-volume fistula through a surgically placed Jackson-Pratt drain after distal pancreatectomy. Most of these fistulas resolve within days or weeks. An example of the last-mentioned consideration would occur in a patient with rapidly accruing pancreatic ascites or an enlarging pancreatic pseudocyst. What is the

Table 50.2 Results of Endoscopic Ultrasound–Guided Drainage from Large Series

Study	No. Patients	Type of Fluid Collection (No. Cases)	Technical Success (%)	Treatment Success (%)	Complication Rates
Pfaffenbach et al, 1998[96]	11	Pseudocyst	91	82	0
Giovannini et al, 2001[97]	35	Pseudocyst (15)	100	100	3% (1 pneumoperitoneum)
		Abscess (20)	90	80	
Seewald et al, 2005[105]	13	Abscess (80), necrosis (5)	100	85	31% (4 minor bleeding)
Kahaleh et al, 2006[93]	46	Pseudocyst	100	93, short-term; 84, long-term	20% (2 bleeding, 1 stent migration, 4 infection, 2 pneumoperitoneum)
Hookey et al, 2006[135]	51/116	Pseudocyst (94), abscess (9), necrosis (8), acute fluid collection (5)	96	93	Without EUS, 11.7%; with EUS, 10.8%; total 11.2% (6 bleeding, 4 pneumoperitoneum, 1 systemic infection, 1 post-ERCP pancreatitis, 1 duodenal or surgical drain communication)
Antillon et al, 2006[138]	33	Pseudocyst	94	82, complete resolution; 12, partial resolution	Major 6% (1 perforation, 1 major bleeding), minor 9% (2 minor bleeding, 1 asymptomatic pneumoperitoneum)
Azar et al, 2006[141]	23	Pseudocyst	91	82	4% (1 pneumoperitoneum)
Kruger et al, 2006[94]	35	Pseudocyst 30, abscess 5	94	88	Immediate complications 9%, delayed infection 31% (4 stent occlusion, 3 ineffective drainage, 4 secondary infection)
Ahlawagt et al, 2006[95]	11	Pseudocyst	100	82	18% (2 stent migration)
Charnley et al, 2006[106]	13	Necrosis	100	92	0 (note: 2 unrelated mortalities after successful treatment and resolution)
Lopes et al, 2007[91]	51	Pseudocyst (36), abscess (26) (51 patients with 62 collections)	100	94	Immediate 3% (1 pneumoperitoneum, 1 stent migration), delayed 18% (3 stent occlusion, 8 stent migration)
Voermans et al, 2007[107]	25	Necrosis	100	93	Severe 7% (1 perforation, 1 major bleeding), minor 30% (8 minor bleeding)
Seifert et al, 2007[108]	60	Necrosis	100	73	13% (2 perforation, 5 bleeding, 1 pneumoperitoneum, with 1 mortality)
Varadarajulu et al, 2008[110]	60	Pseudocyst (36), abscess (15)	95	93	0%

ERCP, endoscopic retrograde cholangiopancreatography.

From Seewald S, Ang TL, Kida M, et al: EUS 2008 Working Group document: Evaluation of EUS-guided drainage of pancreatic-fluid collections (with video). Gastrointest Endosc 69(2 Suppl):S13–21, 2009.

etiology of the pancreatic fistula? Is the patient symptomatic? Is there a possibility of infection? Is it certain that the fluid collection in question is not neoplastic? What are the alternatives to diagnosis? Can EUS be performed? Can MR imaging–MRCP be performed? What are the alternatives to treatment, and have these been thoroughly discussed with the patient and family? Does the patient and endoscopist have immediate access to a team that includes a pancreaticobiliary surgeon and an interventional radiologist? If not, perhaps the patient would be better served in a setting with these capabilities.

Description of Technique

Placement of a pancreatic duct stent to bridge a ductal disruption is comparable to biliary stent placement for a cystic duct leak but with subtle differences. It should be undertaken only over a hydrophilic wire passed beyond the leak proper.[3,7,136] Broad-spectrum antibiotic coverage should be routine. Biliary sphincterotomy would help access by exposing the pancreaticobiliary septum and the pancreatic orifice at the 5 o'clock position at the lower edge of the incision.[8,137] I use pure cutting current if a pancreatic duct sphincterotomy is needed to improve access to the duct. Stent size is important, and one usually chooses 3-Fr, 5-Fr, 6-Fr, or 7-Fr pancreatic duct stents depending on the diameter of the duct and lengths that are 2 to 3 cm longer than the leak to be bridged (see Video). Depending on the situation, balloon or catheter dilation of concomitant strictures or stone removal may be necessary. Alternatively, in patients with ductal leaks in the tail, a short transpapillary stent usually is effective. Stents usually play no or a limited role in patients with central pancreatic necrosis and a disconnected gland syndrome. In the latter situation, most of the ongoing leak is from the tail, and small-caliber drains or stents are ineffective in removing the large chunks of necrotic debris often present.

Transgastric stents can be used as a placeholder to preclude formation of a chronic external fistula in patients who have undergone percutaneous catheter drainage in the setting of a disconnected duct syndrome.[65,138] When stent placement is done for pancreatic ascites or pleural effusions, a large-volume paracentesis or thoracentesis under ultrasound guidance speeds the healing process considerably. As previously noted, endoscopic drainage of pseudocysts can be done in a transpapillary fashion, as described previously.[7,8] Very large or complex pseudocysts are best drained by fistulizing into the collection using a duodenoscope with therapeutic capabilities.[4,66,73,80,90] Pseudocysts can be localized by defining an extrinsic bulge on the stomach or duodenum or by more precise localization with EUS.[2,48,83,91,92,94,95,99–101,109,138–141] EUS also has the advantage of Doppler capabilities to define vasculature, particularly in the setting of splenic vein thrombosis and gastric varices. I use a needle-knife sphincterotome with a 0.035-inch wire after initial localization by transgut injection of contrast material using a long sclerotherapy needle. Alternatively, localization and access can be accomplished using the Seldinger technique with a needle alone.[50] When access has been gained into the cavity, I add a second guidewire, curling both deep within the pseudocyst proper (see Video). A 6- to 10-mm biliary dilating balloon is used to enlarge the tract followed by placement of at least two 7-Fr to 10-Fr double-pigtail stents of variable length. The latter not only prevent migration into or out of the pseudocyst but also allow drainage between the stents if stent occlusion should occur. I routinely aspirate fluid from the cyst for Gram stain, culture and sensitivity, amylase level, and cytology at the time of drainage, and I routinely perform ERCP and place an additional transpapillary stent if an amendable ongoing ductal leak is shown.

Variations and Unusual Situations

The most common scenario that one encounters when draining pseudocysts is considerable necrotic debris interspersed with a liquid interface (walled-off pancreatic necrosis or abscess); this occurs because abdominal CT scan routinely underestimates debris in pancreatic fluid collections.[15] When this scenario occurs, options are to use even larger balloons and perform a retroperitoneal necrosectomy with a therapeutic endoscope,[97,100,106–108] add multiple large-diameter percutaneous catheters,[36] or leave one or more nasocystic drains in place and perform large-volume and repeated irrigations (see Video).[10] Surgery (débridement) may also be necessary, particularly if one inadvertently infects a necrotic cavity and the cavity is inaccessible for percutaneous drainage.[9]

Other variations may occur depending on the location and the consequences of the leak. Ductal disruptions tend to follow anatomic tissue planes; our institution has had to place concomitant drains in scrotal sacs, buttocks, and inverted vaginal vaults and to perform pericardial windows for pericardial tamponade as a result of an ongoing leak. Variations also occur with anatomy, and often one finds that the easiest or only access into the pancreas is the accessory papilla in patients with incomplete or complete pancreas divisum.

Postoperative Care and Complications

The most common acute complications when using endoscopy to treat pancreatic fistulas are exacerbation of pancreatitis and iatrogenic infection,[7,8,50,135,141] although the full range of potential procedural problems (e.g., aspiration, drug reaction, bleeding, perforation) must be discussed with the patient and family. Postoperative care must be anticipatory with routine measurement of pulse, temperature, and constitutional complaints and blood studies including a complete blood count, amylase, lipase, and a liver profile. Pancreatitis flare is more common with otherwise normal pancreatic ducts and is contingent on the amount of manipulation and the success of the procedure. It approximates 10% in my practice, is close to 0 in patients with extensive chronic pancreatitis, and is usually of the mild variety. Iatrogenic infection often follows placement of small catheters or stents in large, debris-filled cavities, and proactive treatment with larger percutaneous Jackson-Pratt drains and a 7- to 10-day course of oral antibiotics is usually indicated. I have also learned to minimize use of antisecretory drugs (i.e., proton pump inhibitors, histamine-2 blockers) because these are associated with significantly higher intraluminal gastric bacteria counts and seem to increase the risk of bacterial translocation and cavity infection. Finally, pancreatic duct stent placement by itself is associated with the colonization of bacteria within the duct proper. We have noted that pancreatic sepsis, previously thought to be uncommon because of the inhibitory effect of pancreatic enzymes, is noted in a small subset of patients even without a ductal disruption and seems to be more common in patients who have occlusion of prostheses.[142]

Longer term complications of transpapillary stent placement include iatrogenic ductitis, such as focal strictures and side branch ectasis.[143] It is prudent to remove prostheses as soon as feasible after placement; this is easy to define in patients with an external fistula. In this setting, stents can be removed 5 to 7 days after fistula closure, removal of the external Jackson-Pratt drain, and abdominal CT scan to ensure that there has been no recurrence of an undrained fluid collection. I usually leave stents in place for internal fistulas for 4 to 6 weeks, but 8.5-Fr to 10-Fr stents can be left in place for 3 to 4 months in patients with chronic pancreatic leaks and downstream stones or strictures. Transgastric or transenteric stents are usually left in place for 4 to 6 weeks after ensuring resolution of the pseudocyst at follow-up CT examination. An exception may be a high-risk surgical patient with a disconnected pancreas in whom stent retrieval is usually associated with recurrent pseudocyst.[103] In this setting, and only this setting, a long-term indwelling pancreatic stent is occasionally justified.

Future Trends

Although one can speculate that prostheses will be developed that have prolonged patency and cause minimal ductitis obviating the urgency of removal, there are numerous trends in diagnosis and treatment that are likely to continue in the future. One trend is the use of S-MRCP to define the presence or absence of a pancreatic fistula and its location. Another trend is likely earlier use of ERCP in patients with pancreatic necrosis with placement of transpapillary prostheses to limit further necrosis and to prevent additional local complications and the use of concomitant pancreatic stents in necrotic cavities being treated percutaneously to prevent external fistulas in patients with the disconnected duct syndrome. Although our group has currently adopted this practice model, prospective multicenter trials are needed before I would recommend widespread acceptance of this approach. Superglue (cyanoacrylate) or fibrin injection to occlude a disconnected duct either percutaneously or by EUS may also gain more acceptance in the treatment of disconnected pancreatic duct tail as a means to avoid distal pancreatectomy. In addition, the endo-

scopic approach to the débridement of pancreatic necrosis may be standardized. This standardization would require new endoscopic accessories, a change in mindset such that multiple endoscopic procedures are the expectation as opposed to the exception, and an even closer working relationship with surgical colleagues. There have been case reports more recently using a per os stapler to effect a pseudocyst gastrostomy,[107] a device classically limited to open or laparoscopic surgery.

Finally, one hopes that many patients with ductal disruption will be sent to centers with expertise in their treatment. Similar to all techniques and procedures, data clearly show that endoscopists who have drained more than 20 pseudocysts have significantly better results draining pancreatic fluid collections than endoscopists who have drained fewer than 20.[30,144] In other words, endoscopists who dabble in drainage probably should not.

References

The complete reference list is available online at www.expertconsult.com.

Chapter 51

Palliation of Malignant Pancreaticobiliary Obstruction

Marco J. Bruno

Video related to this chapter's topics can be found online at expertconsult.com.

Introduction

Pancreaticobiliary malignancies include pancreatic head cancer; gallbladder carcinoma; and proximal cholangiocarcinomas, also referred to as Klatskin's tumors. Pancreatic head carcinoma comprises tumors that may originate from various tissues and include pancreatic adenocarcinoma, distal cholangiocarcinoma, carcinoma of the ampulla of Vater, and duodenal carcinoma. Although there are marked differences in biologic behavior and clinical outcome among these tumors, the overall prognosis is dismal. At the time of presentation, more than 90% of patients have local unresectable disease or distant metastases, leaving only a few patients as suitable candidates for curative resection. Other treatment modalities such as chemotherapy and radiotherapy have little to no effect on survival. Most of these patients can be offered only palliative treatment. More than 85% of patients with pancreaticobiliary malignancies develop obstructive jaundice in the course of their disease, and it is often a presenting symptom. The main indications for palliative therapy are relief of jaundice and pain management. In the past, the "gold standard" treatment was surgical biliary diversion, which was associated with morbidity and mortality. Since the introduction of endoscopic retrograde cholangiopancreatography (ERCP) in 1980, endoscopic stent placement has challenged surgical treatment. Endoscopic biliary drainage has become the palliative treatment of choice to relieve biliary obstruction in pancreaticobiliary malignancies.

Epidemiology

Of all pancreaticobiliary malignancies, pancreatic adenocarcinoma has the highest incidence, with around 30,000 new cases annually in the United States. It ranks fifth among the leading causes of cancer-related deaths.[1,2] Only 10% of patients are suitable candidates for resection, and the overall 5-year survival rate is less than 4%.[3,4] The incidence of gallbladder carcinomas is 1 per 100,000 person-years. The survival rate is only slightly higher than that of pancreatic carcinoma.[2] Patients most likely to survive are patients in whom early cancer was detected in a postcholecystectomy specimen. Klatskin's tumors also have a poor prognosis, with less than 10% of patients surviving 5 years after being diagnosed and most patients dying in the first year.[5] The number of potentially resectable tumors is low, ranging from 10% to 20%. In ampullary carcinoma, biliary obstruction usually develops early in the course of the disease. Tumors are usually small, and radical resection is possible in most cases, with an overall 5-year survival rate of 50%.[6]

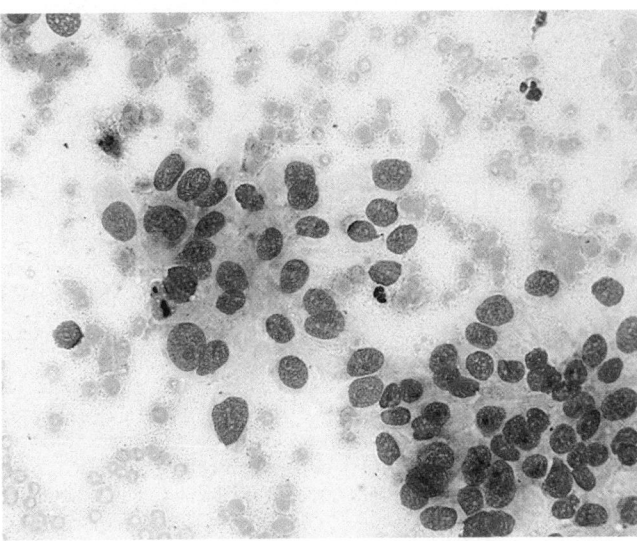

Fig. 51.1 Brush cytology of ductal adenocarcinoma of the pancreatic head (Giemsa staining).

Pathogenesis

A detailed discussion of the pathogenesis of pancreaticobiliary malignancies is beyond the scope of this chapter; however, several epidemiologic studies have identified risk factors for the development of pancreaticobiliary malignancies. Tobacco smoking doubles the risk of pancreatic cancer.[7,8] Patients with chronic pancreatitis have an increased risk for developing pancreatic cancer that is estimated at 4% per 20 years.[9] The risk of developing pancreatic cancer in patients with hereditary pancreatitis is 50%, with smoking as an important risk modifier.[10,11] Etiologic factors for cholangiocarcinoma include primary sclerosing cholangitis and hepatolithiasis.[12,13] Gallstone disease is the most important risk factor for gallbladder cancer.[14]

Clinical Features

The most common presenting symptoms of pancreaticobiliary malignancies are painless jaundice with anorexia and weight loss, which are seen in most patients. If pain occurs, it is most often located in the epigastric region or right upper quadrant and may radiate to the back. Back pain usually indicates retroperitoneal infiltration with tumor and unresectability. Other symptoms may include dark urine, pale stools, and pruritus. At the time of presentation, 80% of patients with pancreatic cancer have impaired glucose tolerance or frank diabetes mellitus. Carcinoma of the body and tail of the pancreas manifests with similar features, although jaundice is usually absent or develops very late in the course of the disease.

Pathology

About 90% of pancreaticobiliary malignancies are ductal adenocarcinomas (**Fig. 51.1**). Most of these tumors arise from the pancreatic head. Other exocrine malignancies are mucinous cyst adenocarcinoma and acinar cell carcinomas. Endocrine tumors include gastrinoma and insulinoma. Metastases of a primary tumor (mammary, lung, and melanoma) and lymphoma should be considered because of important treatment implications (e.g., chemotherapy). Mesenchymal tumors are extremely rare.

The definitive diagnosis of malignancy depends on obtaining a tissue diagnosis. Although many patients receive palliation without definite confirmation of the tumor, a cytologic or histologic biopsy-proven malignancy is a prerequisite in cases of adjuvant therapies such as radiotherapy or chemotherapy. To reduce the number of costly and cumbersome ultrasound-guided or computed tomography (CT)–guided punctures, it is advisable to attempt to obtain a tissue diagnosis during the same ERCP procedure in which a biliary endoprosthesis is inserted for palliation of jaundice. Various techniques can be used to obtain tissue specimens during ERCP, including cytologic brushings, forceps biopsy, needle aspiration cytology, and fluid collection from the bile or pancreas or both.

Cytologic brushings are easy to obtain and widely used. Specificity approaches 100%, but sensitivity is 30% to 60%.[15,16] The sensitivity in cholangiocarcinoma is greater than in pancreatic carcinoma. Forceps biopsy requires endoscopic sphincterotomy and is associated with a slightly increased risk of complications.[17] Biopsy specimens of ampullary tumors can be obtained directly. Sampling of ductal fluid is a simple method, but the sensitivity is very low, and it is not used very often. Several studies have shown that sensitivity can be increased by combining different techniques of tissue sampling.[16,18] Endoscopic ultrasound (EUS)–guided fine needle aspiration biopsy has an excellent sensitivity of 85% to 90% and specificity of virtually 100%.[19] Although these tests may be useful in making the diagnosis of carcinoma, a negative test cannot rule out malignant disease. Percutaneous fine needle aspiration biopsy is another accurate method for confirmation of malignancy, with a sensitivity of 60% to 90%.[20] However, needle tract seeding has been described, and this technique should be used only for tissue confirmation in the case of unresectable disease.

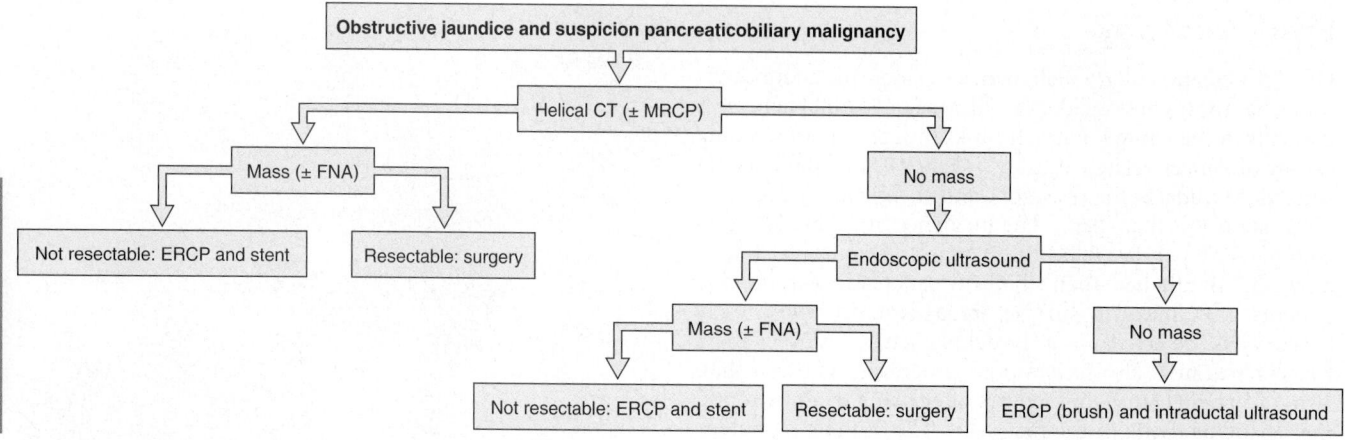

Fig. 51.2 Algorithm for diagnosis of pancreaticobiliary cancer. CT, computed tomography; ERCP, endoscopic retrograde cholangiopancreatography; FNA, fine needle aspiration; MRCP, magnetic resonance cholangiopancreatography.

Differential Diagnosis

The most important discrimination is the differential diagnosis between benign and malignant lesions. In the case of the former, surgery may not be indicated and may cause harm to the patient. In the latter case, surgery is the treatment of choice if a lesion is resectable.

An enlarged pancreatic head may be caused either by pancreatitis or by carcinoma. The patient's history and clinical presentation contribute to making a diagnosis. Autoimmune pancreatitis is an increasingly recognized condition and may mimic a malignant tumor. Differential diagnosis is based on a distinct clinical picture with a diffusely enlarged pancreas with a nondilated pancreatic duct, elevated IgG4 levels, and a prompt response to corticosteroid therapy with improvement of clinical symptoms including jaundice and resolution of morphologic abnormalities on cross-sectional imaging.[21] Cystic lesions of the pancreas may be benign (pancreatic pseudocyst or serous cystadenoma), premalignant (mucinous cystadenoma), or malignant (cystadenocarcinoma). Radiologic imaging is used to characterize these lesions. EUS in combination with fine needle aspiration and fluid analysis may increase accuracy of the diagnosis further. In the case of a suspicious stricture in the mid–bile duct or proximal bile duct, a gallbladder carcinoma should be included in the differential diagnosis. It is important to exclude benign causes of strictures, such as Mirizzi's syndrome, primary and secondary sclerosing cholangitis, and postoperative conditions. An algorithm for the diagnosis of pancreaticobiliary cancer is presented in **Fig. 51.2**.

Treatment

Since the introduction of endoscopic biliary stent therapy in 1980, the palliative treatment of pancreaticobiliary malignancies has changed considerably. At the present time, endoscopic stent placement to relieve jaundice is well established and is considered the preferred treatment (**Fig. 51.3**). Compared with percutaneous and surgical drainage, endoscopic biliary stent therapy is associated with lower morbidity and mortality rates.[22–24] The main problem of endoscopic biliary drainage is late stent occlusion, which necessitates stent exchange. The technical success rate of endoscopic biliary drainage is 70% to

90% and is higher for distal tumors compared with more proximal malignancies involving the bifurcation. The complication rate of therapeutic ERCP is 5% to 10%.[25,26]

Indications and Contraindications

The indications for ERCP with a drainage procedure by stent placement include jaundice, fever, and pruritus. Biliary stent placement has also been shown to improve symptoms of anorexia and quality of life.[27,28] It has been suggested that preoperative biliary drainage may improve surgical outcome after pancreaticoduodenectomy, but this has not been substantiated in clinical trials.[29,31] In a randomized study comprising 202 patients with pancreatic head carcinoma comparing direct surgery with delayed surgery after biliary drainage, surgical outcome and complication rates were not affected by preoperative stent placement. The overall complication rate in the delayed surgery group with preoperative stent placement was significantly increased, mainly owing to stent-related complications. The outcome of this study strongly argues against standard preoperative drainage in patients with pancreatic head cancer in whom immediate surgery is planned. Preoperative drainage is indicated, however, when operative resection is not imminent. One common example is preoperative drainage performed with neoadjuvant chemotherapy. Some authors argue for preferential insertion of an expandable metal stent owing to their comparable durable patency.[32,33] There are no absolute contraindications. Coagulation disorders are a relative contraindication and should be corrected before ERCP.

Overview of Stents for Biliary Drainage

Plastic Stents

The median patency of a conventional 10-Fr plastic stent is 3 to 6 months. The incidence of stent occlusion is 20% to 50%.[34–36] The initial event in stent blockage is adherence of proteins and bacteria to the inner wall of the stent and subsequent formation of a biofilm. Bacteria are introduced into the

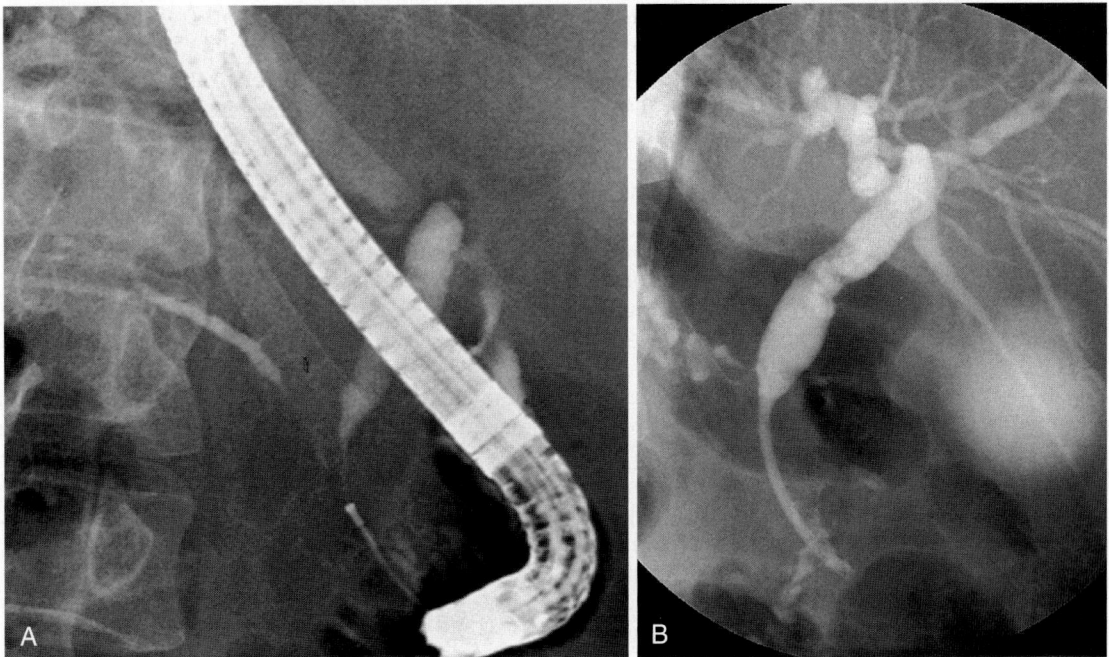

Fig. 51.3 A, Stenosis of both the common bile duct and the pancreatic duct, also called a *double-duct sign,* caused by pancreatic adenocarcinoma. **B,** A 10-Fr, 9-cm plastic endoprosthesis inserted through a distal bile duct stricture.

biliary system during transpapillary placement of the stent. Sludge forms from the accumulation of bacteria, which produce β-glucuronidase and form calcium bilirubinate and calcium palmitate.[37–39] Many efforts have been made to prolong stent patency, some of which are discussed in the following paragraphs.

Stent Diameter

The first biliary stents that were placed were only 7-Fr or 8-Fr in diameter because of limitations of the diameter of the working channel of the endoscope (2.8 mm). When side-viewing endoscopes with large-diameter working channels (4.2 mm) were introduced in 1980, it became possible to insert large-bore plastic stents.[40] Larger stents (10-Fr) perform better than smaller stents (7-Fr)[41] apparently because of the higher flow rate, as predicted by Poiseuille's law, and less stasis with larger diameter stents. Theoretically, bile flow rate is proportional to the internal diameter raised to the fourth power; even a small increase in diameter results in a substantial increase in flow capacity.[42] In contrast to this hypothesis, the use of larger diameter plastic stents of 11.5 Fr or 12 Fr did not result in further improvements in stent patency.[43–45]

Stent Design

The first biliary stents had a pigtail configuration at the proximal end to provide better anchorage. Straight stents were developed because of their improved bile flow characteristics compared with pigtail stents (**Fig. 51.4**).[42,46,47] Huibregtse and Tytgat[48] developed the Amsterdam-type stent—a straight design with two side holes to facilitate biliary drainage and two side flaps to prevent dislocation—which has been the standard type of stent since 1980.

Sludge in plastic stents mainly accumulates around side holes.[37,49] This accumulation seems to be the result of higher

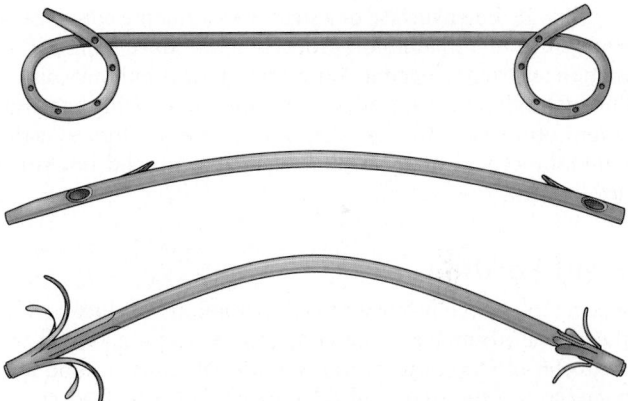

Fig. 51.4 Different types of plastic endoprosthesis *(from top downward):* double-pigtail stent, Amsterdam-type stent (one side hole and one side flap at each end), and Tannenbaum-type stent (without side holes and multiple side flaps at each end).

intraluminal flow turbulence and decreased flow rates.[42] Soehendra and others[50,51] postulated that elimination of side holes might improve patency rates and designed the so-called Teflon Tannenbaum stent (a straight stent without side holes and with multiple proximal and distal side flaps to prevent dislocation). At first, uncontrolled results were encouraging, with patency rates comparable to metal stents, but randomized trials could not confirm these initial results.[52–54] Omitting side holes in a standard-design polyethylene stent also did not improve stent patency.[55]

Stent Material

Different materials have been used for stent construction, including polyethylene, polyurethane, and polytef (Teflon). In vitro studies have shown a direct relationship between the coefficient of friction and the amount of encrusted material. Teflon has the lowest friction coefficient and the best potential for preventing stent clogging.[37] Initially, Teflon Tannenbaum stents showed a favorable patency rate.[50,51] A randomized study comparing Amsterdam-type stents made from polyethylene and Teflon did not show a difference in stent patency.[56] Other controlled clinical trials also could not confirm the superiority of Teflon material in a Tannenbaum-design stent.[52–54]

Scanning electron microscopy of out-of-package biliary stents has shown that the inner surface smoothness of plastic stents is highly variable. This variability is possibly a result of the manufacturing process of plastic stents by extrusion. Only the polyurethane stent was found to have an extremely smooth surface.[57] Two new polymers were introduced with an ultrasmooth surface, Vivathane and Hydromer. Both materials have been shown to reduce bacterial adherence in vitro.[58,59] In addition, the Hydromer stent has not only a smooth texture but also a coating that absorbs water and provides a hydrophilic sheath. Because bacteria initially attach by hydrophobic interactions, this coating could potentially lower bacterial adhesion and increase stent patency. However, the encouraging results of in vitro studies could not be confirmed in prospective clinical trials.[60,61]

Stent Coating

Priming the inner surface of a stent with a coating comprising some form of antiadhesion property may reduce biofilm formation and stent clogging. Antibiotics, antithrombotics, silver, and hydrophilic coating all were effective in reducing bacterial colonization in vitro.[59,62,63] However, clinical studies using antibiotic-coated or hydrophilic-coated stents did not show any benefit.[61]

Stent Position

Placing the stent entirely within the common bile duct has the theoretical advantage of preserving the barrier function of the sphincter of Oddi; this prevents duodenal reflux of food and bacteria into the stent and biliary tree. This so-called inside stent approach can be performed only when a free margin of 1 to 2 cm is maintained between the distal end of the stricture and the papilla. With this parameter in mind, about one-third of patients with malignant obstructive jaundice are potential candidates for such treatment.[64] However, no difference was found in stent performance in a randomized trial. In the inside stent group, stent migration occurred significantly more often.[65]

Antibiotics

Bacteria can enter the bile duct through the portal circulation but more easily directly from the duodenum. When an endoprosthesis is placed, the barrier function of the sphincter of Oddi is lost, and bacteria enter the biliary tract freely. Sludge may form because these bacteria produce β-glucuronidase and form calcium bilirubinate and calcium palmitate. To prolong stent patency, prophylactic treatment with antibiotics seemed a logical step.

In vitro studies showed that antibiotic treatment reduced bacterial adherence to plastic stents.[66] In a prospective randomized study with ciprofloxacin, no difference in stent patency was found.[67] In another study, rotating antibiotics (cycles of 2 weeks of ampicillin, metronidazole, and ciprofloxacin) were combined with ursodeoxycholic acid, and no difference in stent patency was shown.[68] Only one small pilot study showed a reduced rate of stent blockage with norfloxacin plus ursodeoxycholic acid.[69] Other studies combining antibiotics and bile salts (ofloxacin and ursodeoxycholic acid, ciprofloxacin, and Rowachol) did not show a longer duration of stent patency.[70,71] There is no compelling evidence that stent patency benefits from antibiotic prophylaxis.

Aspirin

Animal studies in prairie dogs showed that aspirin inhibits mucous glycoprotein secretion by blocking prostaglandin synthesis.[72] In a clinical study, the use of aspirin reduced the content of all sludge components, although no effect was shown on stent patency.[73] No further studies using aspirin have been performed.

Bile Salts

Bile salts have a potent antibacterial effect and may stimulate bile flow. Because bacteria attach by hydrophobic interactions, hydrophobic bile salts (deoxycholate, taurodeoxycholate) inhibit initial bacterial attachment, as was shown in experimental studies.[74] However, hydrophobic bile salts are not well tolerated. Hydrophilic bile salts such as ursodeoxycholate, which are better tolerated, have a minimal effect on bacterial adhesion. Except for one small pilot study, different prospective clinical studies using ursodeoxycholic acid alone or combining ursodeoxycholic acid with antibiotics could not show a difference in stent patency.[68–71]

Stent Exchange

Some endoscopists prefer to schedule patients for elective stent exchange every 3 to 4 months. The optimal time interval is unknown.[75,76] Prophylactic stent exchange requires a repeat (clinically not indicated) endoscopy and has to be compared with the risks of watchful waiting and the risk of (severe) cholangitis. Because most patients do not develop stent occlusion before dying of the underlying disease, most endoscopists favor an expectant management strategy.

Stent Cleaning

Some endoscopists have proposed leaving an occluded stent in situ and cleaning the obstructed lumen with a cytology brush or flushing with saline instead of performing stent replacement.[77] However, stent cleaning carries the risk of inducing biliary sepsis by actively introducing the biofilm of the stent and bacteria from the duodenum into the biliary tract. Stent cleaning is not recommended.

Self-Expanding Metal Stent

The diameter of biliary stents was restricted by the size of the instrumentation channel of the endoscope until the development of self-expanding metal stents. All currently available expandable stents are made of metal. They differ in the way they are braided, the size of the mesh, the metal used, and their rigidity. At the present time, different types of self-expanding metal stents are available from various manufacturers (**Fig. 51.5**). To date, the most experience has been gained with the self-expanding Wallstent (Boston Scientific, Natick, MA). This stent is delivered in a collapsed configuration on an 8-Fr delivery system. When deployed, it expands to a final diameter of 30 Fr (approximately 10 mm) and shortens about 30% in length. The final diameter is achieved after 1 week, when equilibrium is achieved between the dilating force of the stent and the resistance of the bile duct wall and tumor. These large-caliber self-expanding metal stents of 30 Fr remain patent for longer than plastic stents but do not prevent blockage indefinitely. Metal stents with a 6-mm diameter occlude significantly more frequently than 10-mm (30-Fr) metal stents, showing that size is the most important determining factor for stent patency.[78]

Because of their design, self-expanding metal stents have much less surface to which bacteria can adhere. The mechanism of stent blockage differs from that seen in plastic stents and includes tumor ingrowth through the interstices of the stent or overgrowth of the end of the stent and intima hyperplasia. Several studies have shown a median stent patency of about 6 to 9 months (**Table 51.1**).[35,36,76,79,80] Self-expanding metal stents are more difficult to insert, uncovered metal stents cannot be removed after deployment, and initial costs are high (about $1000). Various types of self-expanding metal stents are available to date.

Wallstent

The initial endoscopic placement experience was reported in 1989.[81] The Wallstent is made from stainless steel alloy filaments braided in a tubular mesh configuration. In the early phase of development, technical problems mainly involved the restraining membrane failing to retract completely, but this is now rarely seen.[82] The first randomized trial comparing plastic stents and the Wallstent was performed by Davids and coworkers.[35] Wallstent patency was superior to patency of plastic stents, with a median duration of 9 months. These results were confirmed in several other studies.[36,76,83] The Wallstent is offered in two diameters (8 mm and 10 mm) and various lengths (40 mm, 60 mm, 80 mm, and 100 mm). The Wallstent is also available with a covering designed to resist tumor ingrowth.

WallFlex Biliary Stent

The WallFlex biliary stent (Boston Scientific) has a Platinol wire construction for enhanced full-length radiopacity designed to facilitate stent placement. Its radial force is similar to the Wallstent. Enhanced flexibility should make the stent better suited for placement across strictures in tortuous and kinked bile ducts (e.g., in Klatskin's strictures). It is also available with a covering to resist tissue ingrowth. The WallFlex stent is available in an uncovered, a partially covered, and a fully covered version. The stent is available in two diameters (8 mm and 10 mm) and four different lengths (40 mm, 60 mm, 80 mm, and 100 mm).

Zilver Biliary Self-Expanding Stent

The Zilver biliary self-expandable stent (Wilson-Cook Medical, Winston-Salem, NC) has a slotted tube design and is made from nitinol. It has gold markers for enhanced visibility under fluoroscopy while deploying the stent. A particular advantage of this stent is that it does not foreshorten on expansion. It is available in lengths of 4 cm, 6 cm, and 8 cm and diameters of 6 mm, 8 mm, and 10 mm.

Hanaro Biliary Stent

The Hanaro biliary stent (MI Tech Corporation, Seoul, South Korea) is a metal stent with both ends flare-shaped to prevent migration. It has radiopaque gold markers on both ends and the center of the stent for enhanced visibility under fluoroscopy. It is available in a diameter of 10 mm and lengths of 60 mm, 80 mm, and 100 mm. The covered version is marketed as the Shin-Hanaro stent.

Niti-S Biliary Stent

The Niti-S biliary stent (Taewoong Medical Co. Ltd., Kyonggi-Do, South Korea) is a flexible, fine mesh tubular prosthesis made of Nitinol wire. It is available in various design shapes and coverings (e.g., Teflon, silicone). The silicone-covered version features a retrieval suture for ease of removal. Available sizes are 8 mm and 10 mm diameter and lengths range from 40 to 120 mm. A specialty type Niti-S stent is the Y-type and T-type uncovered stent used for hilar obstruction (see also the section on intrahepatic biliary obstruction).

Covered Self-Expanding Metal Stent

Tissue ingrowth through the meshes of the stent is responsible for stent occlusion in about 22% to 33% of patients.[35,36] To overcome this problem, self-expanding metal stents have been covered with a polyurethane or silicone membrane. Results of various stents in studies are contradictory.[84–86] At first, many prospective cohort studies could not confirm a lower rate of tumor ingrowth while using covered metal stents.[87,88] However, in a prospective comparative study, stent obstruction owing to tumor ingrowth occurred significantly less frequently with covered stents compared with uncovered stents.[89] Data with regard to the risk of complications are scarce, but stent migration, cholecystitis, and pancreatitis seem to occur at a slightly higher rate.[88–90] There seems to be no benefit from endoscopic papillotomy before deployment of covered metal stents with regard to the prevention of pancreatitis, whereas migration rates may increase.[91] Covered stents should not be used intrahepatically because of occlusion of hepatic side branches by the covering membrane.

Plastic versus Metal Stent

Self-expanding metal stents have a longer duration of patency than plastic stents and ideally should be placed in all patients. The high initial costs have limited their use in different health care settings worldwide. In a cost-effective approach, the choice between a plastic and metal stent depends mainly on an estimate of patient survival. Tumor size seems to be a reliable predictor of survival. Prat and coworkers[92] claimed that in the case of a tumor greater than 30 mm, a polyethylene stent should be placed because of shorter expected survival. The presence and number of liver metastases have also been

Fig. 51.5 Different types of self-expanding metal stents. **A**, Wallstent (Boston Scientific, Natick, MA). **B**, Uncovered Hanaro stent (MI Tech Corporation, Seoul, South Korea). **C**, Fully covered WallFlex biliary stent (Boston Scientific). **D**, Zilver stent (Wilson-Cook Medical, Winston-Salem, NC). **E**, Covered Niti-S biliary stent (Taewoong Medical Co. Ltd., Kyonggi-Do, South Korea). **F**, Uncovered Niti-S biliary Y-type stent (Taewoong Medical Co. Ltd.).

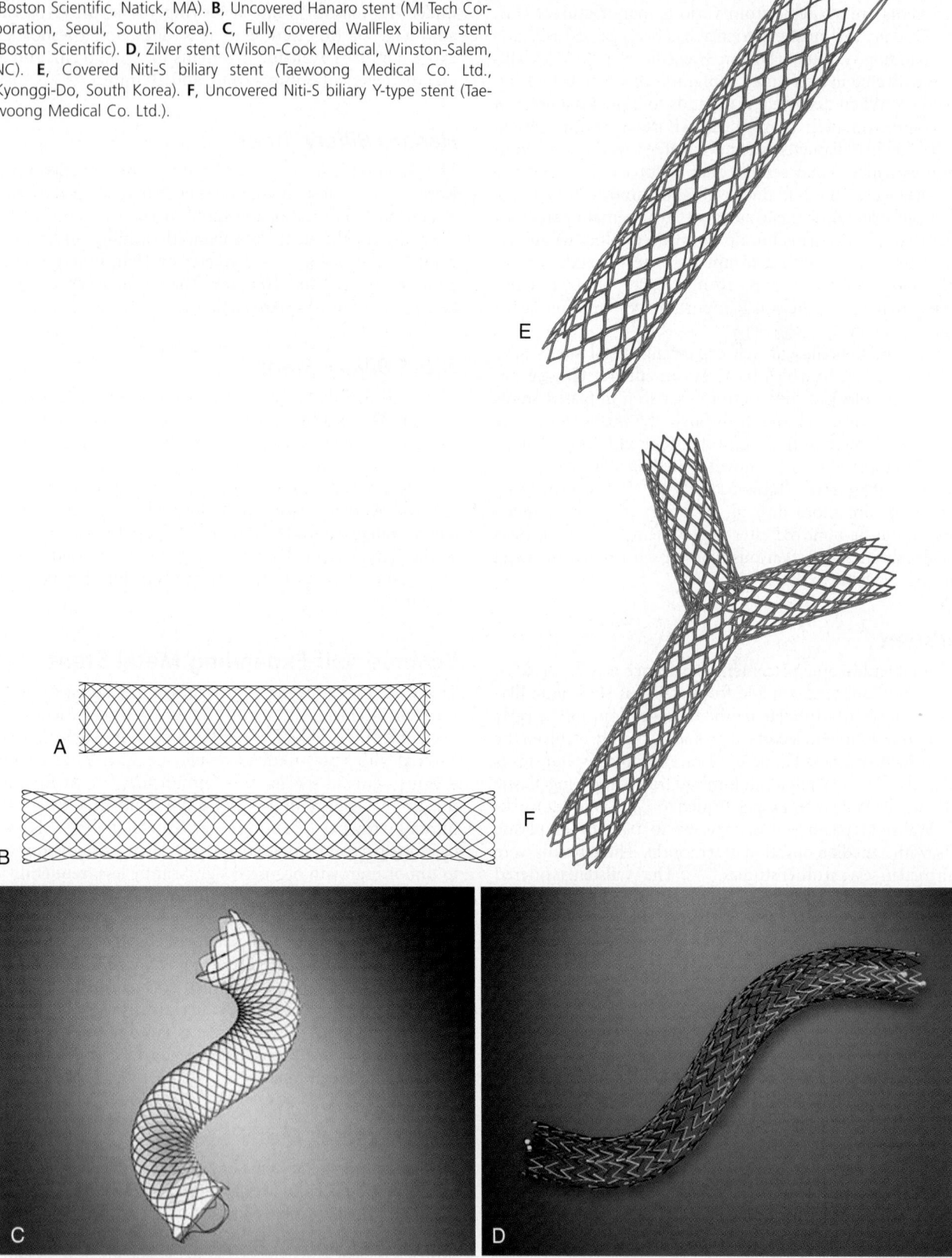

Table 51.1 Results of Trials Comparing Self-Expandable Stents with Plastic Stents

Reference	No. Patients		Drainage (%)		Occlusion Rate (%)		Median Stent Patency (days)	
	PE	SEMS	PE	SEMS	PE	SEMS	PE	SEMS
Davids et al[35]	49	56	95	96	54	33	126	273
Carr-Locke et al[80]	78	86	95	98	13	13	62	111
Knyrim et al[36]	31	31	100	100	43	22	140*	189*

*Mean.
PE, polyethylene stent; SEMS, self-expanding metal stent.

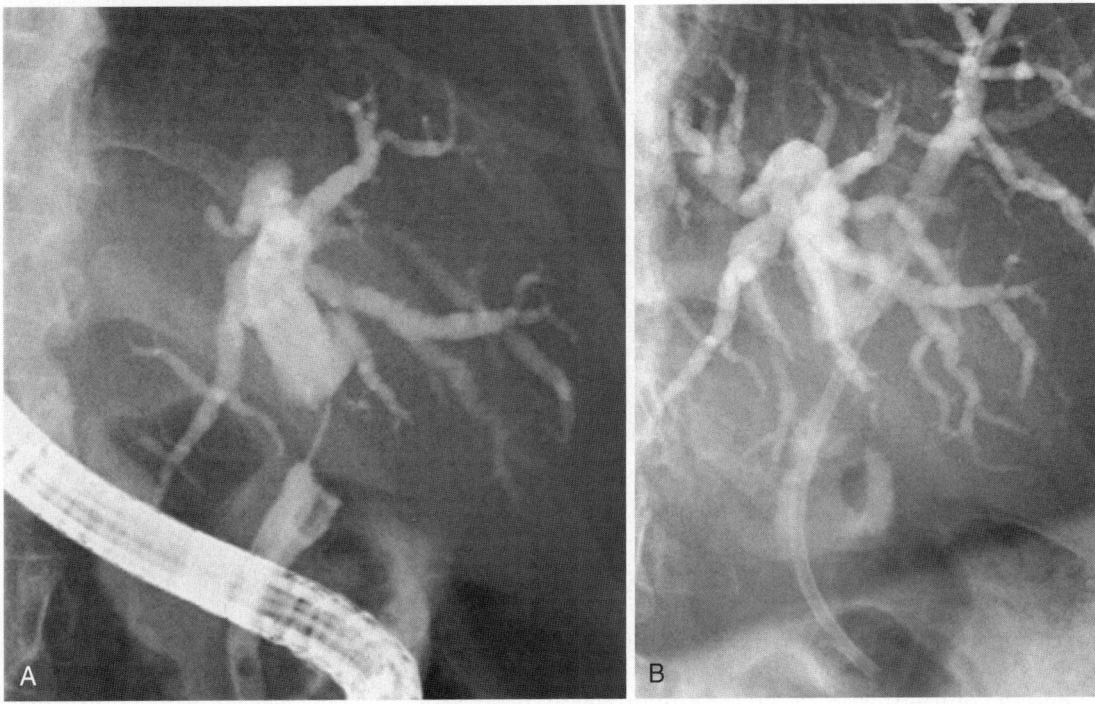

Fig. 51.6 **A**, Mid–common bile duct stricture caused by gallbladder carcinoma. **B**, An 11-cm, 10-Fr plastic endoprosthesis has been inserted.

shown to be independently related to prognosis.[93,94] Comparative studies did not show any benefit of self-expanding metal stents compared with polyethylene stents in the first 3 months after insertion.[35,76] It seems reasonable to insert a polyethylene stent in patients with a life expectancy of less than 3 months (**Fig. 51.6**). If expected survival is 3 to 6 months, a self-expanding metal stent should be considered (**Fig. 51.7**). Different authors have shown this strategy to be cost-effective.[35,95–98] Patients who present with early clogging of a polyethylene stent (within 1 month) should also receive a self-expanding stent, regardless of their life expectancy, although this has not been proved in prospective studies.[99]

Antibiotics before Stent Placement Procedure

Drainage of the biliary tree is the mainstay of therapy for patients with cholangitis. There is controversy about the routine use of preprocedure antibiotic prophylaxis.[100–102] Preoperative administration of antibiotics should definitely be started in a patient with fever. Because failure to drain the entire biliary tree is the most important risk factor associated with cholangitis after ERCP, antibiotic prophylaxis should also be administered in a highly selective group of patients in whom incomplete drainage is anticipated, such as patients with a hilar malignancy or primary sclerosing cholangitis.[103,104] Prophylaxis can be given as a single, adequate dose shortly before the procedure. If contrast agent is injected in the biliary tract but obstruction cannot be relieved, antibiotic therapy should be continued (or started) until drainage is established.

Gram-negative bacteria are consistently the most common organisms in bile (*Escherichia coli* and to a lesser extent *Klebsiella* species and gram-positive *Enterococcus* species). Antibiotics in these cases should be bactericidal and aimed at gram-negative bacteria with good penetration in liver tissue and bile. Ciprofloxacin is currently the first choice of antibiotic in our unit with the caveat that it does not cover enterococci. In cases of fever despite ciprofloxacin, the addition of amoxicillin or a switch to piperacillin/tazobactam is advisable.

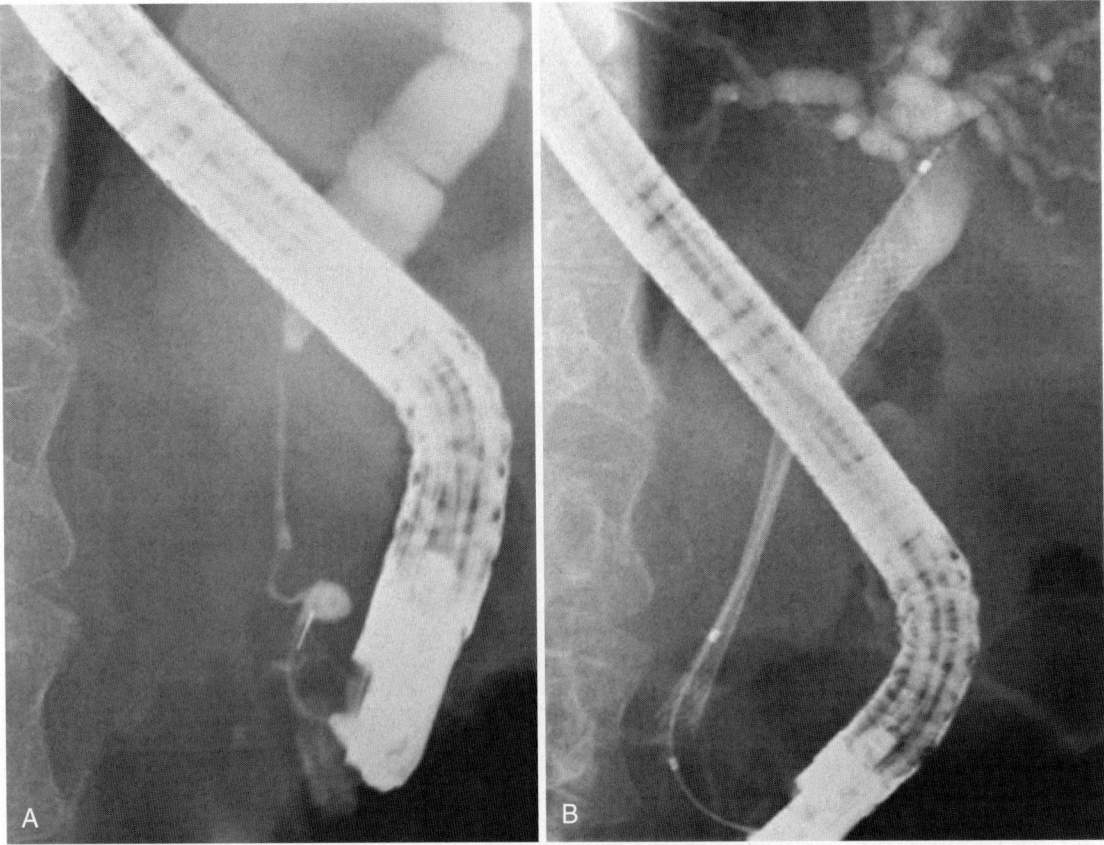

Fig. 51.7 A, Distal common bile duct stricture caused by pancreatic adenocarcinoma. **B,** Self-expanding metal stent has been inserted.

Technique of Stent Placement

A large-channel (4.2-mm) side-viewing therapeutic endo-scope is introduced into the second portion of the duodenum. Standard cannulation of the papilla of Vater is performed by a ball-tip or cone-tip catheter; eventually cannulation can be attempted with a guidewire inserted in the ball-tip catheter. If this approach fails, a double-lumen sphincterotome with a guidewire (cannulatome) should be used. Use of this device may aid in achieving an optimal angle for bile duct cannula-tion. If a sphincterotome is unsuccessful, a precut sphincter-otomy is performed to obtain biliary access.[105] With the use of all these different techniques, deep cannulation is achieved in up to 95% of patients.

After a diagnostic catheter is inserted into the bile duct, contrast agent is injected. It is essential to define the exact anatomy, location, and nature of the stenosis. To avoid post-procedural cholangitis in patients with complex hilar stric-tures, contrast filling of segments that would not be drained should be avoided. The next step is to pass a guidewire through the stricture to facilitate introduction of the catheter and enable exchange for other instruments. When passage of a guidewire through the stricture cannot be accomplished, the direction of the guidewire can be changed by manipulating its position with movements of the endoscope similar to move-ments made for standard cannulation. The assistant can help to cross the stricture by moving the guidewire in and out of the catheter. The endoscopist can manipulate the guidewire by moving the guiding catheter.

Various guidewires are available with different flexibility, diameter, and tip shape. On the one hand, rigid guidewires facilitate introduction of instruments (e.g., an intraductal ultrasound probe) and small-diameter stents. On the other hand, very slippery guidewires with a hydropolymer coating follow bends easily and are used to pass asymmetric stric-tures. After the guidewire is passed through the stricture, a catheter can be advanced, and more complete filling can be achieved. A sphincterotomy is not routinely necessary for introduction of one biliary stent. Previously, it was believed that a sphincterotomy was necessary to facilitate introduction of different devices and to avoid occlusion of the pancreatic duct by the endoprosthesis; however, this did not prove to be a problem in clinical practice. A sphincterotomy is indicated only in cases in which more than one prosthesis is placed.

Plastic Stents

After the stricture is passed with a guidewire, a stent can usually be inserted. First, a catheter is introduced over the guidewire through the stricture to ensure a more rigid intro-ductory system to facilitate stent placement. If appropriate, the guidewire can be exchanged for a cytology brush to obtain tissue samples. The endoprosthesis is positioned over the guiding catheter and inserted into the instrumentation channel. With a pusher tube, the stent is advanced further toward the tip of the endoscope with the elevator bridge closed. When the prosthesis reaches the tip of the instrumentation channel, the elevator bridge is opened, and the stent is pushed out of the endoscope by the pusher tube under endoscopic and fluoroscopic control.

During further advancement of the stent, it is important to keep the endoscope tip close to the papilla. The stent should be advanced one step at a time by pushing it a little bit further each time into the duodenum. The stent is raised by closing the elevator bridge, and the tip of the endoscope is moved closer to the papilla with the up and down knob, introducing the stent. These steps are repeated until the distal side flap has reached the papilla. Finally, the assistant pulls out the catheter and guidewire while the endoscopist keeps the prosthesis in position with the pusher tube. In most distal common bile duct and mid–common bile duct strictures, it is usually possible to insert a 10-Fr endoprosthesis without prior dilation. However, in proximal strictures, the stricture may have to be dilated to allow stent placement; this can be achieved with the use of progressively dilating catheters, which are introduced over a rigid guidewire. Balloon catheters can be used as well to accomplish this goal. If it is still impossible to insert a 10-Fr stent, a smaller caliber prosthesis (7-Fr) should be inserted; this can be exchanged for a 10-Fr prosthesis at a later stage. When both right and left liver lobes have to be drained, it is usually more convenient to place the endoprosthesis draining the left side first, followed by the right side.

The required length of the endoprosthesis can be determined by using the guidewire as a measuring device. First, under fluoroscopic control, the proximal tip of the guidewire is positioned at the level at which the proximal tip of the endoprosthesis is projected. The endoscopy nurse fixes the guidewire between finger and thumb where it exits the catheter. Subsequently, under fluoroscopic control, the guidewire is withdrawn from the catheter until the proximal tip reaches the duodenum. The distance between finger and thumb and the distal margin of the catheter is the required length of the endoprosthesis. Plastic stents are available in various widths (range 5-Fr to 12-Fr) and lengths (range 5 to 20 cm).

Management of Plastic Stent Occlusion

A clogged plastic stent can be removed with the use of a snare or dormia basket. It is important to keep the position of the endoscope in line with the common bile duct. When a snare is used, the stent is caught in the snare and removed through the instrumentation channel of the endoscope. When a dormia basket is used, the stent is pulled close to the endoscope, and both the endoscope and the stent are withdrawn. When massive tumor invasion is present in the duodenum, and difficult stent exchange is anticipated because of a nonoptimal scope position, it can be helpful to leave the occluded stent in place and use it as a guide for common bile duct cannulation and introduction of a second stent. Soehendra and coworkers[106] described a technique that enables the removal of a clogged stent while maintaining the original pathway to the bile duct. A ball-tip catheter is positioned at the distal end of the stent, and the stent is cannulated with the guidewire. A Soehendra retriever is introduced over the guidewire, and the tip is screwed into the distal end of the stent. The retriever is pulled out along with the stent, leaving the guidewire in place.

Self-Expanding Metal Stents

For introduction of a self-expanding metal stent, a stiff guidewire is positioned through the stricture by standard techniques. The insertion device with the constrained stent is inserted through the instrumentation channel over the guidewire. When the insertion device is in position, with the help of radiopaque markers, the prosthesis can be released by removing the outer catheter while keeping the inner catheter in place. Deployment follows gradually as the outer catheter is withdrawn and can be followed fluoroscopically. If deployment is not proceeding according to plan and repositioning is required, the expanding stent may be constrained again by pushing the outer catheter inward, provided that the point of no return has not yet been passed. This point may vary with stent type but may extend to 83% of total stent deployment and is indicated by a marker.

Deployment reduces the length of certain self-expanding metal stents up to about 30%. It is important to correct the position of the expanding stent constantly under fluoroscopic control, which usually means that one has to pull the insertion device outward while deploying the stent. When the expanding metal stent bridges the papilla, in the case of a distal stenosis, the endoscopic image is used to keep a fixed distance of about 1 cm between the papillary orifice and the distal margin of the stent. Stent diameter expands to 8 to 10 mm, and the available deployed lengths are 40 mm, 60 mm, 80 mm, and 100 mm. In case of a complex hilar stricture in which both liver lobes are drained by two or more self-expanding endoprostheses, the procedure is as follows.[107] First, two stiff guidewires are introduced, one in each liver lobe. If appropriate, dilation of a stricture is performed over one of the guidewires. An expanding metal stent is inserted over the guidewire into the left system and deployed. Finally, an expanding metal stent is inserted into the right system alongside the first stent and deployed under fluoroscopic control (**Fig. 51.8**). Although technically difficult, it is also possible to insert a second self-expanding metal stent through the meshes of a formerly placed self-expanding stent.[108] In such a case, a guidewire is introduced, and the mesh is dilated using a balloon catheter before passing the second constrained stent and deploying it.

Management of Occlusion of a Self-Expanding Metal Stent

A noncovered self-expanding metal stent can be removed without problems within the first days after deployment by grasping it with a forceps or a snare. After this time, the stent becomes embedded in the tumor tissue, and extraction can become extremely difficult, although successful removal has been reported after months.[109] Stent obstruction is mainly due to tumor ingrowth through the interstices of the stent or overgrowth of the ends of the stent. Management of stent occlusion consists of placement of a polyethylene stent or a second self-expanding metal stent through the occluded self-expanding metal stent. Another strategy is mechanical cleaning by using a balloon and flushing, but this is effective only in cases of sludge formation. Covered stents can be removed more easily for a much longer period compared with uncovered stents.[109,110] Covered stents can be grasped at their distal end with a snare or with a forceps in case a retrieval loop is present.

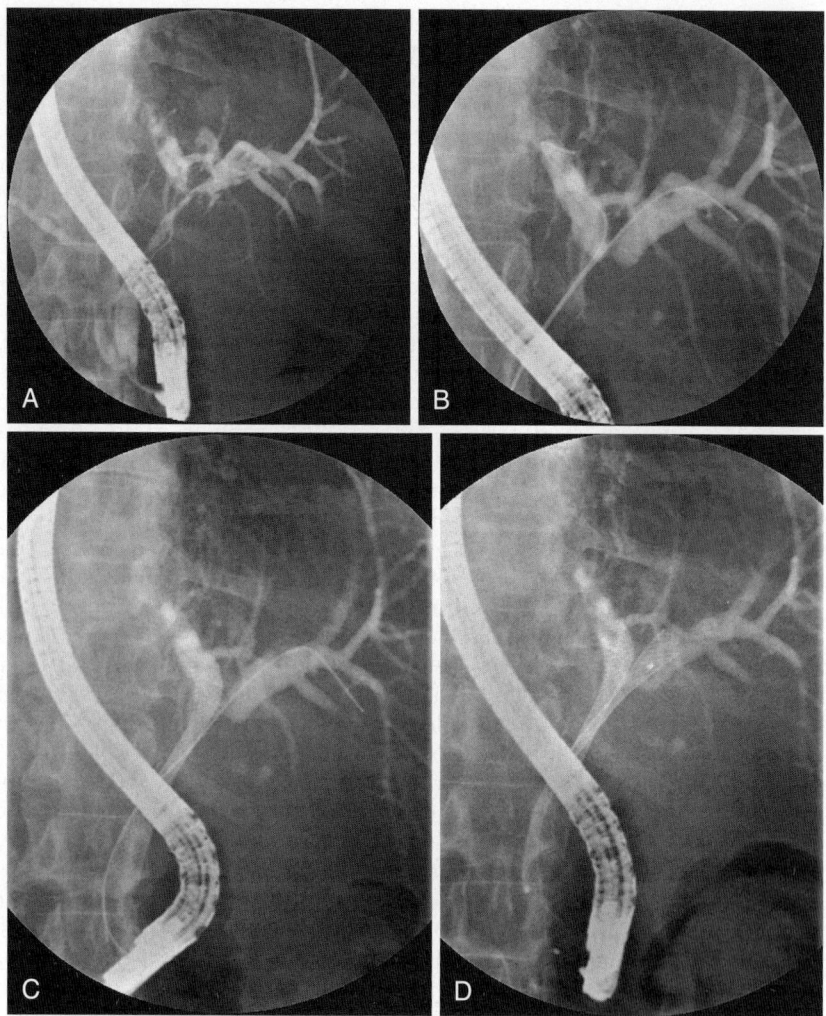

Fig. 51.8 **A**, Klatskin type II tumor (unresectable because of vascular involvement). **B**, Guidewires inserted to both the left and the right biliary system. **C**, Self-expanding metal stent has been inserted into the left system and deployed. **D**, Bilateral self-expanding metal stent drainage.

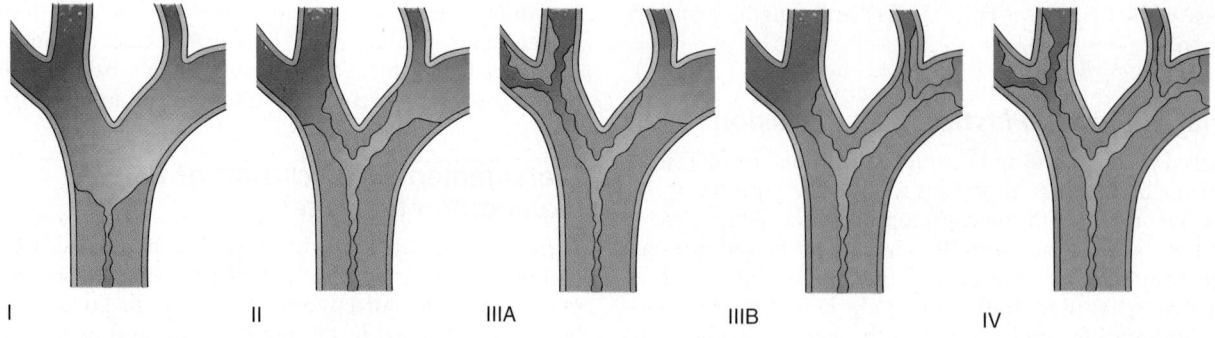

Fig. 51.9 Bismuth classification. *I:* Stricture involving the common hepatic duct. *II:* Stricture involving both the right and the left hepatic duct. *IIIA:* Stricture extending proximally to the right secondary intrahepatic ducts. *IIIB:* Stricture extending proximally to the left secondary intrahepatic ducts. *IV:* Stricture involving secondary intrahepatic ducts bilaterally.

Intrahepatic Biliary Obstruction

Strictures at the level of the hepatic confluence account for about 20% of malignant bile duct obstruction and mainly consist of primary cholangiocarcinoma, gallbladder neoplasms, and metastatic spread to hilar nodes. Cholangiocarcinoma arising at the hilar level is also referred to as Klatskin's tumor and is classified according to the degree of involvement of the intrahepatic bile ducts (**Fig. 51.9**).[111] Stent placement in the proximal biliary tree is more challenging and is associated with lower success rates than stent placement for distal common bile duct stenosis. Drainage can be achieved either endoscopically (retrograde) or percutaneously (antegrade). Procedure-induced cholangitis caused by contrast agent injection in undrained biliary branches is the main complication and occurs in 30% of cases.[112–114] The current management strategy (depending on local services available) is first to attempt endoscopic drainage; when this strategy is unsuccessful, percutaneous drainage offers additional opportunities.[115–117] When internal drainage fails, an external drain can be left in situ, minimizing the risk of cholangitis.

Unilateral versus Bilateral Drainage

There is controversy whether to drain one or both liver lobes in Bismuth type II, III, and IV strictures. In Bismuth type I, one stent always suffices because the left and right ducts communicate, and drainage is complete. Theoretically, at least 25% of the liver volume must be drained to achieve biochemical improvement and relief of symptoms.[118] Concerns about unilateral drainage include the inability to relieve jaundice and the potential for bacterial contamination in the undrained lobe. The worst treatment results seem to be obtained in patients with cholangiographic opacification of both lobes but drainage of only one.[119]

In a prospective randomized trial comparing unilateral with bilateral hepatic duct drainage, the latter procedure was associated with a significantly higher rate of complications because of the higher rate of early cholangitis.[120] In per-protocol analysis, the rates of successful drainage, complications, and mortality did not differ between the two groups. Magnetic resonance cholangiopancreatography (MRCP)–guided endoscopic stent placement in Bismuth III and IV malignancies was associated with a low morbidity and mortality in an uncontrolled study.[121] The intention was to place a unilateral stent in one of both lobes, guided by the MRCP picture, and to avoid entry and contrast agent injection in the contralateral lobe. In patients in whom, by accident, guidewire entry (50%) or contrast agent injection (20%) occurred in the contralateral liver lobe, stents were placed bilaterally. This treatment strategy resulted in a very low cholangitis rate of only 6%. A more recent study evaluated selective unilateral MRCP-targeted or CT-targeted drainage, and no episodes of cholangitis were observed.[122] The message seems to emerge that unilateral drainage is appropriate when unilateral cannulation and opacification has been achieved. If the contralateral lobe is (unintentionally) opacified or probed, it should also be drained to avoid cholangitis.

Plastic versus Self-Expanding Metal Stent

By design, expandable stents may be more suitable than plastic stents for draining hilar tumors. The stent lumen is much wider, and, more importantly, intrahepatic side branches can drain through the metal meshes. Self-expanding metal stents that were inserted via the percutaneous route showed a higher rate of treatment efficacy than plastic stents.[115,123] No randomized studies comparing endoscopic and percutaneous insertion of self-expanding metal stents in hilar strictures are available. Additional proof of the superiority of self-expanding metal stents over plastic stents is suggested by a retrospective series of patients with nonresectable hilar cholangiocarcinoma in whom plastic stents were replaced by metal expandable stents during stent treatment.[124] Successful palliation without the need for further biliary reintervention was achieved in most patients (69%). In a prospective multicenter observational cohort study in patients with a malignant hilar biliary obstruction, it was observed that metallic stent performance was superior to plastic stent performance for hilar tumor palliation with respect to short-term outcomes (30 days), independent of disease severity, Bismuth class, or drainage quality.[125]

For primary bilobar drainage, a specialty "Y" stent has been introduced consisting of two uncovered Niti-S Y-type biliary stents (TaeWoong Medical Co. Ltd.). The first self-expanding metal stent has a radiologically marked segment with wider mesh holes in its middle part, through which the second stent is advanced into the contralateral liver lobe.[126] A potential drawback of the placement of a metal stent is that introduction of additional stents in the case of treatment failure may become difficult. However, a technique for introducing a second stent through the wire mesh of the first stent has been described.[108]

Duodenal Stenosis

Duodenal stenosis resulting from pancreaticobiliary malignancies occurs in 10% to 20% of patients.[127] Presenting symptoms include nausea and vomiting resulting from gastric outlet obstruction. Duodenal stenosis is usually a late event and occurs in patients in poor general condition who have already received a biliary endoprosthesis.[128] Surgical bypass has a significant procedure-related mortality of 10% and related morbidity and prolonged hospital stay.[24,129,130] Endoscopic stent treatment for duodenal obstruction with bile duct stent placement may be an effective alternative. Placement of duodenal stents has a high technical success rate without major procedure-related complications.[131–134] Stent placement is performed under simultaneous endoscopic and fluoroscopic control. Patients are usually able to tolerate a liquid diet immediately after stent placement. Full stent deployment may take a few days, during which time soft foods are allowed.

The results of a retrospective study in 95 patients suggest that duodenal stent placement is associated with better short-term outcomes, and gastrojejunostomy is associated with better long-term outcomes.[135] The choice of treatment modality may depend on the life expectancy of the patient. One study reported simultaneous endoscopic decompression of biliary and duodenal obstruction with similar success rates compared with duodenal stent placement alone.[136] Because of the difficulty of accessing the biliary tree endoscopically through the mesh wall of a duodenal stent, an expanding metal biliary stent should preferably be placed before the duodenal stent is introduced (**Fig. 51.10**). In expert hands, however, it seems also feasible to drain the biliary tree endoscopically through the meshes of a metal duodenal stent.[137] If endoscopic biliary stent treatment fails, the remaining treatment options are percutaneous stent placement, combined percutaneous and endoscopic management, and surgical bypass.

Postprocedural Care

General measures after conscious sedation include observation in a day care unit for several hours with monitoring of blood pressure and oxygen saturation. When a patient develops fever after ERCP, specimens should be obtained for

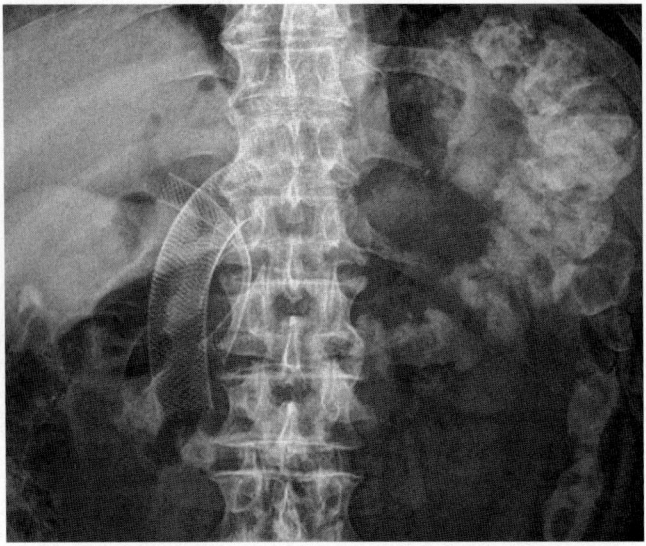

Fig. 51.10 Pancreatic adenocarcinoma growing into the duodenum with a self-expanding metal stent (not yet fully deployed) in the biliary tract and a self-expanding metal stent in the duodenum.

culture, and antibiotics should be administered. If fever does not subside, the accuracy of biliary drainage should be reassessed, and migration and early stent occlusion should be excluded. In the case of a complex malignant hilar stricture, it is important to check for undrained dilated intrahepatic segments and to rule out abscesses by transabdominal ultrasound or CT. Depending on the findings, ERCP should be reattempted or percutaneous drainage should be achieved.

Complications

Early Complications

Early complications are defined as complications that occur less than 1 week after the conclusion of the procedure. The rate of complications is 5% to 10% for therapeutic ERCP with a mortality rate of up to 1%.[25,26,138] Cotton and coworkers[25] introduced a grading system in which complications are graded as mild, moderate, and severe, and these guidelines are still widely used. The most frequent early complication is cholangitis, probably resulting from introduction of bacteria into the biliary tract during the procedure. Cholangitis is reported in approximately 10% to 15% of patients in most series. It occurs more often after endoscopic procedures for complex hilar strictures when incomplete drainage is achieved. The same holds true for patients with primary sclerosing cholangitis. In these high-risk procedures, antibiotics should be administered prophylactically and continued for a few days after the procedure.

Pancreatitis develops after ERCP in about 5% to 7% of patients. It is defined as new-onset or increased abdominal pain lasting at least 24 hours after ERCP, with associated elevation in serum amylase or lipase to at least three to five times normal.[25,26,139] Most cases are mild, are self-limiting, and require only intravenous fluids and gut rest. Serious cases may evolve into (infected) necrotizing pancreatitis with multiorgan failure.

The rate of postsphincterotomy bleeding is about 0.2% to 5% with an associated mortality rate less than 1%.[140] Bleeding is usually obvious immediately after sphincterotomy but can be delayed for hours or several days. Most episodes of delayed bleeding are managed successfully by conservative measures and blood transfusions if the hemoglobin level decreases significantly. Postsphincterotomy bleeding usually occurs at the apex of the sphincterotomy site and can be managed endoscopically with injection of epinephrine.

Retroperitoneal perforation occurs in less than 1% of cases in most series. It may be caused by standard sphincterotomy, precut sphincterotomy, or guidewire manipulation. Most cases are diagnosed or suspected during ERCP. These perforations mostly heal with conservative measures and do not usually result in clinical symptoms.[141] Conservative treatment measures consist of giving nothing by mouth, antibiotic treatment, and nasogastric suction. About 20% to 30% of patients require surgery. In cases of peritoneal perforation caused by the duodenoscope, prompt exploratory laparotomy, with repair or oversewing of the defect in the duodenal wall, is mandatory.[142]

Late Complications

The primary late complication of stent placement is occlusion of the endoprosthesis, which can occur in 50% of cases.[35,36] These patients present clinically with a flulike syndrome with cholestasis, frank cholangitis, or jaundice. Treatment consists of exchange of the occluded stent or, in the case of an occluded self-expanding metal stent, insertion of a polyethylene stent or second self-expanding metal stent (see sections on management of plastic stent occlusion and management of self-expanding metal stent occlusion) through the obstructed expanding stent. Plastic stent migration, either proximally or distally, may occur in 10% of cases.[143]

Future Trends

Photodynamic Therapy

Photodynamic therapy (PDT) involves the administration of a photosensitizer, which is activated with a laser light and causes necrosis of the exposed tissue. Preliminary results suggest prolonged survival and stent patency for PDT in cholangiocarcinoma at the hilum.[144–146] Controlled trials are under way. Previously, it was thought that PDT was incompatible with uncovered expanding stents because stents may occlude by necrotic tumor tissue.[147] However, this does not seem to be a major issue, although the light dose should be adjusted to counteract the reduction of light transmittance caused by the metal.[148] PDT has also been used successfully to recanalize metal stents that were blocked by tumor ingrowth.[149]

Drug-Coated Biliary Stents

Covering biliary stents with chemotherapeutic agents, delivering chemotherapy directly to the tumor tissue, at least in theory should give protection against tumor ingrowth, overgrowth, or both. For optimal therapeutic effects, these drugs should be released over a longer time with good penetration in tissue and without systemic toxicity. Carboplatin and paclitaxel have been shown to inhibit cell proliferation in vitro.[150,151] Carboplatin-coated plastic stents have been used with promising preliminary results in a few patients.[151] Placement of a metallic stent covered with a paclitaxel-incorporated membrane in patients with malignant biliary obstruction proved to be feasible, safe, and effective.[152] Median patency was 270 days (range 68 to 810 days), and cumulative patency rates at 3 months, 6 months, and 12 months were 100%, 71%, and 36%. Whether drug-eluting stents represent an advancement in the treatment of patients with malignant biliary strictures remains to be proven in prospective comparative trials.

Transgastric Endoscopic Ultrasound–Guided Biliary Drainage

EUS-guided hepaticogastrostomy has been reported by several groups as an alternative treatment to percutaneous biliary drainage or surgical bypass in the case of failed ERCP.[153,154] A dilated biliary duct in the left lobe is punctured by a 19-gauge needle under EUS guidance. Next, a guidewire is advanced, and the needle is removed. A cytotome is introduced over the wire to create a fistulous tract by the use of electrocautery. Successful long-term drainage has been reported with plastic stents and covered metal stents.

Endoscopic Ultrasound–Guided Plexus Neurolysis

Celiac plexus neurolysis is used to control pain in patients with pancreatic cancer. The injected agent usually includes a local anesthetic (bupivacaine or lidocaine) and a neurolytic (phenol or alcohol). Comparative studies with conventional pain management (uptitration of opioids) or percutaneous celiac plexus neurolysis are lacking. Side effects occur in about 3% of cases and are usually mild, the most frequent being asymptomatic hypotension.[155] Bilateral injection of the neurolytic agent (i.e., right and left sides of the celiac trunk) has shown to be more effective than central injection (i.e., in the midline and anterior to the celiac artery).[156] Reliable data with regard to the efficacy of EUS-guided celiac plexus neurolysis in cancer are unavailable, but a meta-analysis of percutaneous celiac plexus neurolysis showed long-lasting benefit for 70% to 90% of patients.[157] For the best results, it is recommended to perform celiac plexus neurolysis not too late in the course of the disease when pain has become unbearable. The central effects of chronic pain lead to hypersensitization and unresponsiveness to pain treatments. EUS may reduce neurologic complications (because of the anterior approach) compared with the percutaneous technique, although no comparative studies have been performed.[158]

References

The complete reference list is available online at www.expertconsult.com.

Section IV

Emerging Endoscopy

Gregory G. Ginsberg

Chapter **52**

Endoscopic Management of Post–Bariatric Surgery Complications

Elizabeth Rajan

Video related to this chapter's topics can be found online at expertconsult.com.

Introduction

As the field of bariatric surgery continues to grow in pace with the increasing prevalence of obesity, an increasing number of patients are referred for endoscopic evaluation after bariatric surgery. Endoscopic findings may represent the normal post-surgical appearance or a complication. A basic understanding of the anatomic changes and potential complications associated with bariatric procedures is essential for optimal endoscopic assessment and appropriate management. A thorough review of the surgical report and any relevant imaging studies are key elements for a successful endoscopic procedure.[1] Recognizing that certain complications are unique to specific types of bariatric surgery allows for accurate diagnosis and therapy. Close communication and collaboration with the bariatric surgeon is strongly recommended before endoscopy, particularly when therapy is contemplated.

Roux-en-Y Gastric Bypass

Marginal or Stomal Ulcers

Marginal or stomal ulcers are ulcerations at the gastrojejunostomy that frequently occur on the jejunal side of the anastomosis (**Fig. 52.1**). Marginal ulcers may be seen in 16% of patients after Roux-en-Y gastric bypass (RYGB).[2] Many ulcers remain subclinical, and the true incidence is likely higher. Ulceration can occur at any time but patients usually present within 3 months of surgery with pain, nausea, bleeding, or perforation.[3,4] Several potential and controversial inciting factors are implicated, including gastrogastric fistula, large gastric pouch with inclusion of parietal cells and resultant acid exposure, ischemia, foreign body reaction to staples or non-absorbable sutures at the anastomosis, *Helicobacter pylori*, nonsteroidal anti-inflammatory drugs (NSAIDs), and gastric pouch orientation.[5–7] The etiology is probably multifactorial with ischemia the likely culprit. Preoperative *H. pylori* testing and eradication is not routinely recommended because of conflicting data that this practice reduces the incidence of marginal ulceration.[8,9] During upper endoscopy, the gastric pouch should be closely inspected for a gastrogastric fistula, and biopsy specimens should be obtained for *H. pylori*. Patients usually respond to treatment with proton pump inhibitors, liquid sucralfate, and *H. pylori* eradication therapy when appropriate.[10,11] NSAIDs should be avoided, and smoking should be discontinued. Endoscopic removal of foreign material, such as nonabsorbable suture or staples, may help ulcer resolution. In cases of symptomatic refractory ulceration, surgical revision may be required.

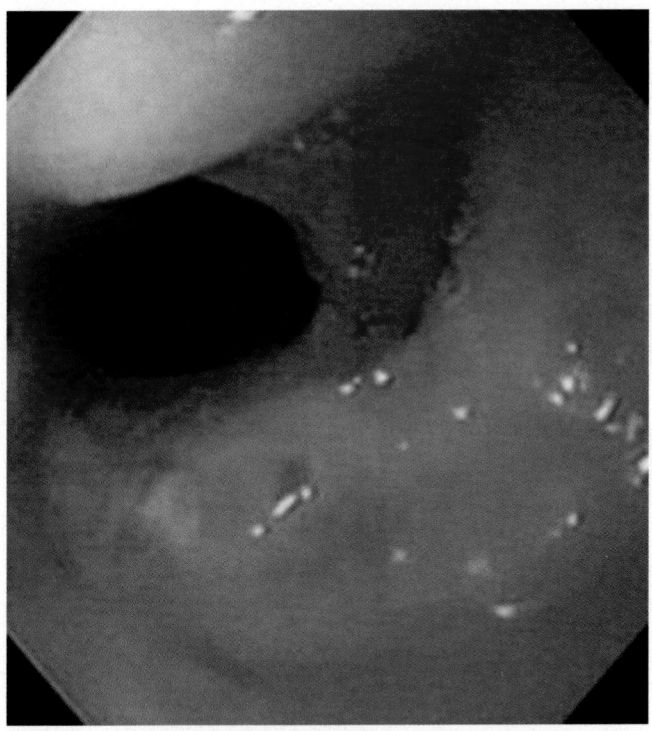

Fig. 52.1 Marginal ulceration on the gastric side of the gastrojejunostomy.

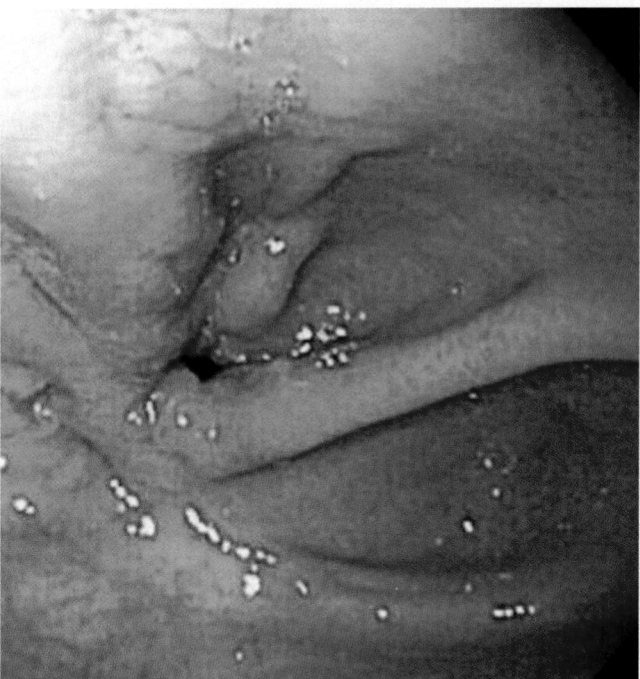

Fig. 52.2 Stomal stenosis.

Stomal Stenosis

Stomal stenosis is an important complication that occurs in approximately 3% to 12% of patients after open RYGB and in 11% to 27% of patients after laparoscopic RYGB.[2,4] Most strictures occur within the first year after surgery, with a mean time interval of 2 to 3 months to diagnosis.[12,13] Patients present with nausea, vomiting, pain, or dysphagia. The exact mechanism for stricture formation is unknown, but ischemia, ulceration, subclinical anastomotic leak, circular stapler size, and surgical expertise are potential contributing factors.[13,14] The gastrojejunostomy is intentionally created to be 11 to 15 mm in diameter. Although there is no clear definition for stomal stenosis, the latter is diagnosed when the luminal diameter is less than 10 mm or when passage of a standard upper endoscope through the anastomosis is met with resistance (**Fig. 52.2**).

In cases of symptomatic strictures, serial dilation using a through the scope balloon dilation catheter is preferred with the goal of achieving a stomal diameter of 10 to 12 mm. Dilation should not exceed 15 mm. The initial balloon size is based on the estimated diameter of the anastomotic stricture. Three sequential sizes may be inflated during one session, in keeping with the recommended "rule of 3's" for stricture dilation. An effective dilation results in partial disruption of the anastomotic wall. Caution is warranted in the setting of coexistent marginal ulceration because of increased risk of perforation. Overzealous dilation, which can result in perforation or an overstretched anastomosis with resultant dumping syndrome and regain of weight, should be avoided. When a tight stricture precludes traversal with the endoscope and impairs visualization of the postanastomotic jejunal limbs, wire-guided through the scope balloon dilation under fluoroscopy is recommended. The reported perforation rate after balloon

dilation approximates 2% to 3%.[13,15] Small perforations can be managed conservatively.

Most (>90%) strictures are responsive to endoscopic balloon therapy.[12,16] Most strictures can be effectively dilated in one or two sessions, but tight strictures may require several sessions. The time interval between sessions ranges from 1 to 3 weeks.[15,16] The successful use of bougie dilators has been reported, but this technique requires guidewire placement within the jejunal Roux limb before dilation.[17] Although temporary placement of a fully covered stent in selected patients with refractory strictures may be successful at achieving long-term stoma patency, a high rate of stent migration (>50%) has been observed in some studies (**Fig. 52.3**).[18] If stent placement is contemplated, it is best to avoid dilating the stricture before stent placement to minimize the risk of migration. The duration of stent placement is typically 3 months. Other therapeutic techniques, including needle-knife electroincision of the anastomosis (which carries an increased risk of perforation) and intralesional steroid injection after balloon dilation, have been reported with some success.[19,20] In the rare case in which endoscopic therapy is ineffective, surgical revision may be necessary. Patients with a modified RYGB with a Silastic ring around the proximal pouch to prevent dilation of the gastrojejunostomy may require surgical removal or replacement of the band.

Gastrogastric Fistula

The reported incidence of staple line dehiscence with resultant gastrogastric fistula varies with the extent of division of the excluded stomach and is greater than 20% when the gastric pouch and bypassed stomach are undivided or partially divided to less than 5% when the segments are completely transected.[21,22] Gastrogastric fistula denotes an abnormal communication between the neogastric pouch and the bypassed

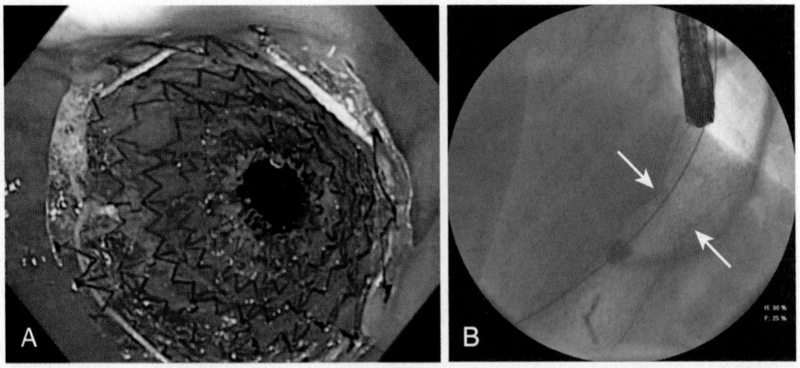

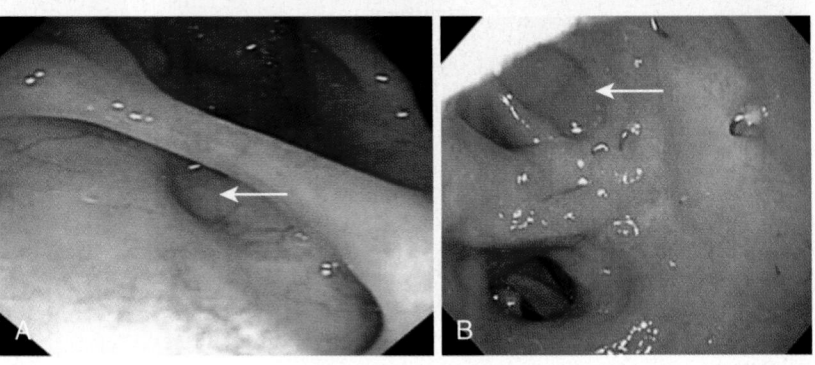

Fig. 52.3 **A,** Enteral stent across gastrojejunostomy stricture. **B,** Fluoroscopic image shows fully covered stent traversing the gastrojejunostomy stricture immediately after deployment; *arrows* indicate the waist of the stricture.

Fig. 52.4 **A,** Small diverticulumlike gastrogastric fistula *(arrow).* **B,** Large gastrogastric fistula *(arrow).*

stomach. There are several postulated reasons for the development of fistulas, including surgical technique without complete division of the gastric pouch, marginal ulceration, anastomotic leak, and foreign body erosion.[21,23] Even when the pouch is completely transected, a gastrogastric fistula can occur if the pouch is situated in close proximity to the bypassed stomach. Surgical interposition of omentum or a loop of jejunum between the segments may reduce this complication.[24] Patients usually present with regain of weight, abdominal pain, or reflux symptoms. When a gastrogastric fistula is suspected, diagnosis is confirmed by upper endoscopy, upper gastrointestinal (GI) series, or in some instances abdominal computed tomography scan with oral contrast agent.

Gastrogastric fistulas are frequently small and easily overlooked. Endoscopically, a small gastrogastric fistula can appear as a diverticulum in the gastric pouch; larger fistulas allow endoscope passage into the excluded stomach (**Fig. 52.4**). When gastrogastric fistulas are associated with marginal ulceration, gastric biopsy specimens for *H. pylori* should be obtained. Barium studies are helpful in diagnosing small dehiscences. Most symptomatic patients require surgical intervention. However, in patients with small gastrogastric fistulas and associated marginal ulcers, an initial conservative approach consisting of proton pump inhibitor therapy, liquid sucralfate, or *H. pylori* eradication, as appropriate, may be effective.[21,23] NSAID use and smoking should be strictly avoided. Patients are reevaluated after 4 to 8 weeks; if the fistula is healed, long-term use of a proton pump inhibitor is advised.[21,23] In patients with small gastrogastric fistulas (<5 mm) who are unresponsive to medical therapy, endoscopic therapy, in the form of endoscopic suturing, argon plasma coagulation, fibrin glue injection, hemoclip application, or a combination thereof, may be considered given the reported successful outcome in small case series.[23,25,26]

Long-term follow-up data are awaited before any particular endoscopic therapy can be formally recommended for this select group of patients.

Gastrointestinal Bleeding

Early bleeding is uncommon after open bariatric surgery (<1%) compared with laparoscopic RYGB (1% to 4%).[27–30] Bleeding is generally from the gastrojejunostomy. Endoscopic management of an early postoperative bleed is challenging because of the risk of perforation at the surgical anastomosis. In this setting, air insufflation should be minimized, and the use of nonthermal hemostatic devices, such as endoscopic clips, is preferred. Close collaboration with the surgeon is key for a successful outcome. Hematemesis is the most common clinical presentation in early bleeds.[31] GI bleeding that occurs beyond the early postoperative period tends to occur from staple lines at the gastrojejunostomy (e.g., marginal ulcers), jejunojejunostomy, or bypassed stomach. Most patients are managed successfully with appropriate endoscopic therapy. Endoscopic therapy is achieved by standard hemostatic interventions such as injection, thermal, or mechanical modalities. Discontinuation of NSAIDs and testing for *H. pylori* serology are advised. Deep enteroscopy (e.g., balloon-assisted enteroscopy) is generally required to access the jejunojejunal anastomosis and enable retrograde examination of the bypassed stomach and duodenum. Patients presenting with obscure GI bleeding should be investigated for causes not related to the surgery, such as colonic pathology.

Food Impaction

Inadequate chewing and rapid ingestion of large food boluses, stomal stenosis, and motility disturbances result in food impaction.[32,33] Retrosternal or abdominal pain and dysphagia are presenting symptoms. Food disimpaction is usually achieved by cautious push of the impacted food with the tip of the scope into the jejunal limb. Otherwise, piecemeal extraction through an overtube becomes necessary using accessories such as snares, nets, and grasping forceps. Care must be exercised not to traumatize the gastric pouch, anastomosis, or jejunal limbs. Gastric bezoars are a rare complication.[34]

Choledocholithiasis

Rapid weight loss predisposes bariatric patients to cholesterol gallstones. Within 6 months of surgery, 36% of patients develop new gallstones, and an additional 10% develop biliary sludge.[5,35–37] Several causative factors have been suggested, including altered bile composition, cholesterol supersaturation of bile, gallbladder dysmotility, and loss of duodenal induced stimulation of gallbladder emptying.[35–39] Although gallstones are prevalent in morbidly obese individuals, there is no consensus on the need for prophylactic cholecystectomy. Cholecystectomy is generally performed in open RYGB but is not standard practice in laparoscopic RYGB, unless gallstones are diagnosed preoperatively. Elective cholecystectomy during bariatric surgery may contribute further to the symptoms of diarrhea and intolerance to fatty foods, and the occurrence of postoperative bile leaks poses a considerable challenge in these patients, in whom endoscopic retrograde cholangiopancreatography (ERCP) is unsafe in the immediate postoperative period and a transhepatic approach is difficult in the absence of biliary dilation.[19,40]

Although new gallstones may be common, symptomatic gallstones occur infrequently (7%), and subsequent cholecystectomy is usually well tolerated in these patients.[41,42] Choledocholithiasis after gastric bypass is uncommon. Diagnosis is usually based on abnormal liver tests, transabdominal ultrasound, or magnetic resonance cholangiopancreatography. Performing ERCP in these patients is a challenging and arduous task. The procedure may be attempted by using a pediatric colonoscope, a balloon-assisted enteroscope, or a duodenoscope back-loaded onto a guidewire. Alternatively, a duodenoscope may be passed through a surgical, radiologic, or endoscopically guided gastrostomy or through a gastrogastric fistula.[43,44] Laparoscopy-assisted transgastric ERCP allows quick access to the common bile duct with visualization of the papilla in the usual anatomic orientation.[45]

Anastomotic Leaks

Reported rates of anastomotic leaks are 0 to 5.6%.[46,47] Endoscopy should be avoided in early anastomotic leaks, which can be life-threatening and may be associated with signs of toxicity such as tachycardia, fever, and leukocytosis. There is an increased risk of leak exacerbation or wound dehiscence with endoscopy. The mainstay of treatment is sepsis control and supportive care or surgical exploration in patients who are unstable.[19,48] If the leak develops late with no signs of toxicity, endoscopic approaches may be considered. Enteral stents are an alternative therapeutic option with reported success.[49] Data on the use of temporary enteral stent placement, fibrin glue, and hemoclips to seal leaks are limited.[50,51] Additional long-term outcomes data are required before firm

recommendations can be made on the efficacy and safety of these procedures in this setting.

Laparoscopic Adjustable Gastric Banding

Band Erosion

Band erosion occurs in 1% to 11% of patients.[2,52] Patients can present with infection at the access port site, pain, vomiting, bleeding, abdominal abscess, fistula, or sudden weight gain. Endoscopic removal of a near-complete penetration of a gastric band has been described, but surgical removal is strongly recommended.[53] Caution must be exercised if endoscopic removal of a gastric band is considered, especially when the penetration through the gastric wall is incomplete because this carries a high risk of gastric perforation and peritonitis.

Pouch Dilation

The gastric pouch may dilate in approximately 12% of patients after laparoscopic adjustable gastric banding owing to proximal herniation of the stomach.[5,54] Deflation of the band resolves this problem in most cases. Endoscopy is of no therapeutic value in this setting.

Gastroesophageal Reflux Disease

Acid reflux is common with a reported increase in acid regurgitation from 13% to 69% after band placement.[55] The prevalence of postoperative esophagitis was 75% in one study.[55] Initial management consists of acid suppression therapy combined with sucralfate; surgical revision is considered in unresponsive patients.

Vertical Banded Gastroplasty

Band Erosion

Approximately 1% to 2% of patients with vertical banded gastroplasty develop band erosion.[2,56] Patients tend to present with weight gain and to a lesser extent abdominal pain. Surgical consultation should be sought in these patients, who generally require reoperation or conversion to RYGB.

Staple Line Dehiscence

Staple line disruption in vertical banded gastroplasty results in failure to lose weight rather than ulceration. Staple line dehiscence has been described after blunt abdominal trauma.[57] Endoscopy is helpful in diagnosing and evaluating the disruption. Patients should be referred for surgical revision to RYGB.

Pouch Dilation

Pouch dilation can occur as a consequence of band erosion, stomal obstruction, or staple line dehiscence. Endoscopy is the modality of choice for diagnosis before surgical intervention.

Table 52.1 Indications for Endoscopy after Roux-en-Y Gastric Bypass (RYGB) and Laparoscopic Vertical Banded Gastroplasty (LVBG)

	RYGB	LVBG
Abdominal pain	30%–53%	42%
Nausea and vomiting	35%–62%	50%
Dysphagia	4%–16%	13.2%
GI bleed	12%	9.2%
Weight regain	6%	—
Heartburn	2%	29%

GI, gastrointestinal.

Table 52.2 Endoscopic Findings after Roux-en-Y Gastric Bypass (RYGB) and Laparoscopic Vertical Banded Gastroplasty (LVBG)

	RYGB	LVBG
Normal	43%–44%	41.4%
Marginal ulcer	27%–36%	7.2%
Stomal stenosis	13%–19%	9.9%
Staple line dehiscence	4%–16%	—
Esophagitis	3%	18%

Sleeve Gastrectomy and Duodenal Switch

Anastomotic Leaks

Data are limited on the endoscopic management of anastomotic leaks after sleeve gastrectomy alone or in combination with duodenal switch. Similar to leaks seen with other bariatric procedures, operative treatment is the mainstay for patients with signs of sepsis and hemodynamic instability unresponsive to conservative management. Successful treatment of gastric leaks at the gastroesophageal junction using temporary coated self-expanding stents in stable patients was reported in a small study.[58]

Fistulas

A study using partially covered self-expanding metal stents to treat gastrocutaneous and duodenocutaneous fistulas reported a success rate in 66% of patients.[59] More than one stent was required in some cases to achieve fistula closure.

Gastric Sleeve Stricture

Endoscopic balloon dilation and temporary placement of covered self-expanding stents are options for therapy. However, experience is limited, and there is a paucity of data regarding the long-term success of these approaches.[58]

Indications for Endoscopy

Tables 52.1 and 52.2 summarize findings from studies that have evaluated indications for endoscopy and endoscopic findings after RYGB and laparoscopic vertical banded gastroplasty.[24,32,60] After RYGB, 20% to 30% of patients developed upper GI symptoms that prompted endoscopy; 15% of endoscopic procedures performed within the first 6 months were normal compared with 53% of procedures performed beyond 6 months. Upper GI bleeding and dysphagia were more likely to be associated with endoscopic abnormalities, whereas normal endoscopic findings were more commonly reported with epigastric pain.

Experimental Therapies

Gastric pouch or gastrojejunostomy dilation after RYGB can result in weight regain. There is a 5% to 13% rate of major complications after reoperation for weight regain.[61] Early promising data on the use of StomaphyX (EndoGastric Solutions, Redmond, WA) showed reduction in gastric pouch size with resultant weight loss.[62] Minor self-limiting complications of sore throat and epigastric pain were noted. The device uses polypropylene H-fasteners to create full-thickness, serosa-to-serosa tissue apposition. Successful use of the StomaphyX device to repair gastric pouch leaks was reported in a small case series.[63] Data from a small pilot study suggest that endoscopic suturing using the EndoCinch device (C.R. Bard, Murray Hill, NJ) to tighten dilated gastrojejunal anastomoses is technically feasible and safe and may lead to weight loss in some patients.[64] Prospective controlled trials are essential to validate efficacy, safety, and durability of emerging endoscopic therapies before use in clinical practice.

References

The complete reference list is available online at www.expertconsult.com.

Emerging Endoluminal Bariatric Techniques

Jacques Devière

Introduction

Obesity is the pandemic of the 21st century and is associated with considerable morbidity and mortality.[1] Management of obesity depends on body mass index (BMI) and the presence of comorbidities, including heart disease, diabetes, hypertension, dyslipidemia, osteoarthritis, and sleep apnea.[2] Approximately 1.6 billion adults are overweight; at least 400 million adults are obese. The World Health Organization further projects that by 2015, approximately 2.3 billion adults will be overweight, and more than 700 million will be obese. Previously considered a problem only in high-income countries, overweight and obesity are now dramatically increasing in low-income and middle-income countries, particularly in urban settings.[3]

The only effective therapy at the present time for morbid obesity, as defined by BMI of 40 kg/m^2 or more or by BMI of 35 kg/m^2 or more in the presence of comorbidities, is surgery.[4] Bariatric surgery has been shown to be effective in the long-term and significantly reduces the risk of mortality associated with morbid obesity. In the United States, the indications for bariatric surgery increased by 80% during the period 1998–2004,[5] and in terms of health care demand, morbid obesity clearly represents the pandemic of the 21st century.

Bariatric surgery for morbidly obese patients has shown significant clinical benefits. It induces and maintains satisfactory weight loss while decreasing comorbidities in the patient associated with overweight.[6] Efficacy varies with the type of procedure, which can be divided into restrictive (lap band, vertical gastroplasty, sleeve gastrectomy), malabsorptive (biliopancreatic diversion), or a combination of both (gastric bypass). The first and second types of operations are the most frequently performed sometimes as an optional two-step procedure starting with gastric restriction. Although very effective, laparoscopic and surgical bariatric procedures have complication rates of 3% to 20% and mortality rates of 1%.[7] Cardiopulmonary events and anastomotic leaks are the major sources of severe morbidities.

The demand in recent years for less invasive therapy for obesity led to the emergence of endoscopic technology potentially characterized by less invasiveness and fewer postprocedure complications. Endoluminal surgery, performed entirely through a natural orifice, offers the potential for a less invasive weight loss procedure, possibly performed on an ambulatory basis, and might find its place in the current armamentarium for morbid obesity treatment, extending indications for treatment to patients with severe comorbidities and older age and even to non–morbidly obese patients. We review the various endoluminal techniques that are either in routine use or in clinical evaluation at the present time and address the role of endoscopy in management of complications occurring after bariatric surgery.

Endoscopic Options for Endoluminal Primary Treatment of Obesity

Intragastric Balloon

The use of an intragastric device to induce weight loss in obese patients was first described in 1982.[8] Since then, numerous intragastric balloons have been in use worldwide, and several have been withdrawn from the market. The BioEnterics Intragastric Balloon (BIB; Allergan, Irvine, CA) has a spherical shape and larger capacity than earlier models and has been the most extensively studied device. Among the more recently improved minimally invasive procedures, the intragastric balloon has been one temporary nonsurgical option that can promote weight loss in obese patients by partially filling their stomach and inducing a sense of early satiety.[9,10] One of the major drawbacks of balloon implantation is weight regain after balloon removal. Two more recent studies help clinicians to understand better what can be expected from balloon implantation.

In the first study, Mathus-Vliegen and Tytgat[11] included patients who had participated in a randomized controlled trial comparing a balloon with a sham for a 3-month period in an additional trial including 9 months of balloon treatment and follow-up for 1 year after removal. The authors excluded eight patients who had not met the weight loss goal during the first 3 months (five patients) or who did not tolerate the balloon (three patients). Although there was no difference between the sham and balloon during the first 3 months, after 1 year of balloon treatment, a mean weight loss of 21.3 kg (17.1%) was achieved in all patients; 12.6 kg (9.9%) was maintained at the end of the second balloon-free year. Overall, 47% of patients sustained a 10% weight loss at the end of 2 years of follow-up. Although this study could not show an independent benefit of balloon treatment beyond diet, exercise, and behavioral therapy in the first treatment, balloon treatment for 1 year, in the patients who tolerated the treatment, resulted in substantial weight loss, a significant part of which was maintained during the first year after removal of the balloon.

The second study looked at the long-term outcome after treatment with an intragastric balloon for 6 months, with no structured weight maintenance program after balloon removal. After BIB placement, 100 consecutive morbidly obese individuals were prospectively followed; 97 patients completed the final follow-up at a mean of 4.8 years. After 6 months, 63% of patients had more than 10% baseline weight loss, whereas there were only 28% at final follow-up. At that time, 35 patients had undergone bariatric surgery, and 34 patients had no significant weight change from baseline.[12]

These studies confirm further that balloon implantation may be helpful for long-term weight loss in a few patients. It is a potential option for patients who are unwilling to undergo bariatric surgery or are not candidates for bariatric surgery. Balloon implantation could also be used as a temporary measure in superobese patients to induce weight loss and decrease the risk of complications associated with further bariatric surgery.[13]

Gastric Restriction
Endoluminal Vertical Gastroplasty Using EndoCinch

The EndoCinch suturing system (C.R. Bard, Murray Hill, NJ) was initially designed for endoscopic treatment of gastroesophageal reflux disease. This system allows the placement of a series of stitches in the lower esophagus to create a pleat in the sphincter. This pleat alters the gateway between the stomach and the esophagus and potentially prevents acid from flowing out of the stomach. Although associated with encouraging early results, use of the EndoCinch for the treatment of gastroesophageal reflux disease has been called into question because of the lack of retention of plications in the long-term.[14]

Fogel and colleagues[15] first described the use of this technology for the treatment of obesity in 64 patients. Their technique comprised the deployment of seven sutures in a continuous and cross-linked design from the proximal fundus to the distal body. The result of the treatment is suggested to be a significant decrease in distensibility of the stomach. The procedure was performed as an ambulatory procedure, and of the 59 patients followed for 12 months, the percentage excess weight loss reported was 21% at 1 month and 58% at 12 months. Only a few patients ($n = 14$) underwent repeated endoscopy in the follow-up period. In 11 patients, the suture line was reported as completely or partially intact. A randomized controlled trial is ongoing in the United States to investigate this technique further. It is hoped that this trial will also provide long-term data that are relevant both clinically and anatomically.

Transoral Gastroplasty

Transoral gastroplasty (TOGa System; Satiety, Inc., Palo Alto, CA) has emerged as a new and apparently safe technique for endoluminal surgical treatment of obesity. It uses the first endoscopic stapling device to create a full-thickness plication in the proximal stomach with a strictly endoluminal approach. Similar to other restrictive procedures, the purpose is to induce an early satiety owing to the reduction of the stomach capacity.

The system consists of the TOGa Sleeve Stapler, a flexible 18-mm diameter shaft device, which rides over a guidewire for introduction. It is specifically designed for the procedure and accommodates a standard endoscope up to 8.6 mm in diameter and creates full-thickness plications of the anterior and posterior walls of the stomach, which are acquired using vacuum pots located parallel to the staple line (**Fig. 53.1**). The stapling allows a serosa-to-serosa apposition and is performed via two successive applications of staple lines of 5 cm each.

In the first evaluation, this procedure was completed by the placement of restriction in the distal part of the pouch, using a dedicated stapling device also based on vacuum acquisition of the tissues. Only two series in humans have been published so far as full articles. The first series[16] comprised 21 patients with a mean BMI of 43.3 kg/m^2. The mean excess weight loss was 16%, 23%, and 25% at 1 month, 3 months, and 6 months after treatment. No severe adverse events were reported; endoscopy at 6 months showed gaps between the two staple lines in 13 of 21 patients. After this first evaluation, the technique was improved, especially concerning the successive application of the two staple lines, and the device was modified. A second human pilot series[17] was subsequently reported in 11 patients, showing better results with mean excess weight loss of 19%, 34%, and 46% at 1 month, 3 months, and 6 months. A 1-year follow-up on a larger multicenter European study has confirmed these data.[17a] Although the TOGa technique is performed under general anesthesia, recovery is very fast, and the procedure could be performed within 30 to 45 minutes on an outpatient basis, suggesting that this technique might have become a high ideal first step for bariatric treatment strategy. A multicentric randomized sham-controlled study was performed in 11 centers comparing the active and sham procedure (2:1 ratio) in a series of more than 200

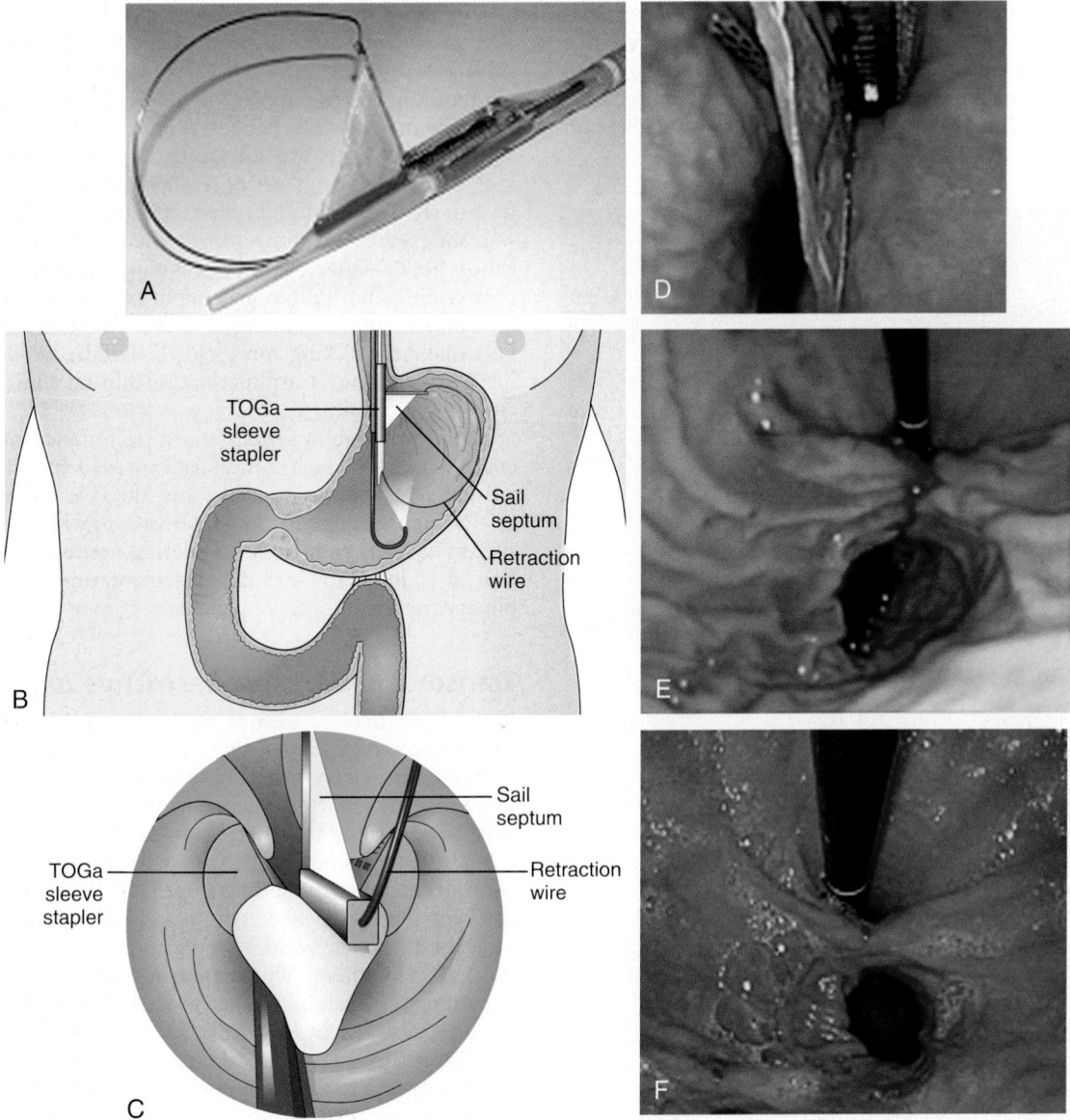

Fig. 53.1 Transoral gastroplasty procedure.

patients. This randomized controlled trial showed significant but modest differences between the two groups and therefore the FDA required additional data. In shortage of financing, the company (Satiety Inc., Palo Alto) closed and sold its assets.

Duodenojejunal Bypass Sleeve

The bypass technique has to be put in line with the development of metabolic surgery and particularly with the clinical observation that bypassing the proximal bowel improves type 2 diabetes and induces weight loss, a feature that partly explains the greater improvement of diabetes observed in patients undergoing a laparoscopic RYGB for the same weight loss compared with a pure restrictive procedure.[19] The first strictly endoluminal device used to bypass the proximal small intestine is the duodenojejunal bypass sleeve (DJBS), also

called the EndoBarrier (GI Dynamics Inc., Watertown, MA). It is composed of a self-expanding implant that is placed in the duodenum and has antimigration features. It is attached to a 60-cm plastic sleeve that extends into the proximal jejunum and works by creating a physical barrier between food that has been ingested and the intestinal wall and biliopancreatic secretions (**Fig. 53.2**). The device is left in place for a maximum of 3 to 6 months and is removed with a dedicated and relatively easy system.

Three trials showed the potential benefit of the DJBS. In the first trial,[20] the DJBS was successfully deployed in 12 patients in less than 30 minutes (and required approximately 40 minutes to be removed). With the exception of pain prompting early removal, it was associated with a significant decrease in hemoglobin A_{1c} compared with a control group. A second multicenter trial from Chile showed a weight loss significantly greater in 24 patients treated with the

EndoBarrier system at 12 weeks compared with the diet control group in a preoperative setting.[21] The last available study is a sham-controlled trial with a 12-week study design comprising 24 patients treated and 13 patients undergoing the sham procedure. Excess weight loss (11.9% vs. 2.7%) and

loss of more than 10% excess weight (62% of patients vs. 17% of patients) were in favor of the DJBS. However, seven subjects terminated the study earlier because of gastrointestinal bleeding (three patients) or device intolerance (pain or vomiting or both, four patients), showing that some technologic developments are still needed.[22] Although these techniques have disadvantages of requiring the implantation of a foreign body and the limited duration of indwell, they warrant further technical improvement and clinical investigation because they could be techniques that have the most impact on comorbidities and might be of particular interest in diabetic obese patients.[19] Other implantable devices, potentially mimicking more closely RYGB, are in development (Valentx Inc., Carpinteria, CA), but no clinical data are currently available.

Table 53.1 summarizes current techniques of bariatric endotherapy for which clinical data are available. Further data are likely to become available, and the role of endotherapy in the management of obese patients undergoing bariatric surgery is likely to increase, rendering necessary the integration of endotherapy into the armamentarium of multidisciplinary treatment of these patients.

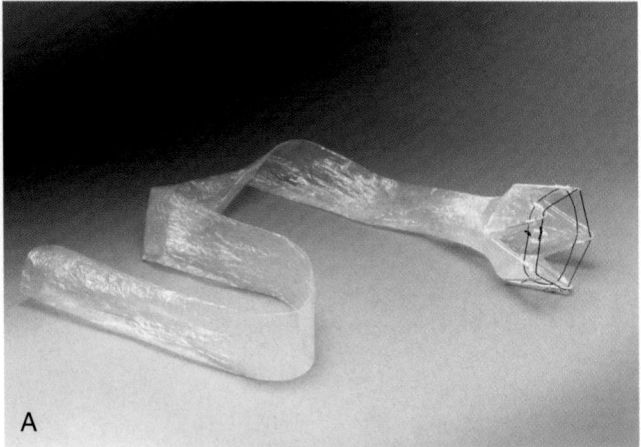

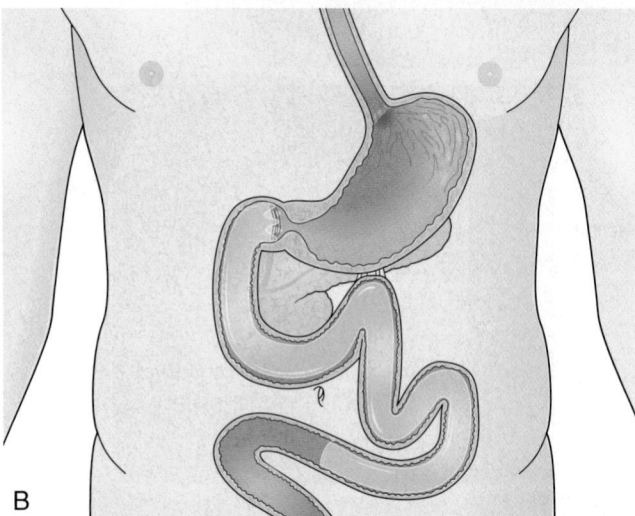

Fig. 53.2 A, Duodenojejunal sleeve. **B,** Schematic representation of the sleeve in place in the proximal jejunum. (**A,** *Photo used with permission of GI Dynamics, Inc., Lexington, MA.*)

Transoral Endoscopic Restrictive Implant

If the DJBS may be seen as the endoscopic counterpart of RYGB, and the TOGa may be seen as the endoscopic counterpart of sleeve gastrectomy or vertical banded gastroplasty, a more recently reported endoscopic implantable device (Transoral Endoscopic Restrictive Implants System [TERIS]; Barosense, Redwood City, CA) may be seen as an endoscopic equivalent to gastric banding (**Fig. 53.3**). A phase I pilot trial has been reported.[23] Successful placement has been achieved in 12 of 13 patients with complications (including perforation) in 3 of them. This system is technically demanding (22-mm insertion tube, median procedural time 142 minutes), but an excess weight loss of 28% was observed at 3 months, suggesting that with technical improvements, it could become another option in the endoscopic armamentarium. This procedure is associated with the placement of an implant, which means that it offers the potential advantage of being removable (the drawback being, similar to other implants, the long-term durability of the procedure, which can be shown only by long-term follow-up).

Table 53.1 Available Bariatric Endotherapy Technology

Endoscopic Procedures	Mechanism	Human Applications	Limitations
Intragastric balloon	Restrictive	Prospective crossover study; >2000 cases reported	Patient tolerance Limited effect (6 mo)
EndoCinch vertical gastroplasty	Restrictive	One prospective study (64 patients)	Long-term efficacy Depth of suture
TOGa	Restrictive	Limited human studies (33 patients); multicentric sham-pivotal trial completed	Long-term efficacy Restrictive procedure Gap consequences
DJBS	Malabsorptive	12 patients investigated	Patient tolerance Long-term safety and efficacy Reversibility

DJBS, duodenojejunal bypass sleeve.

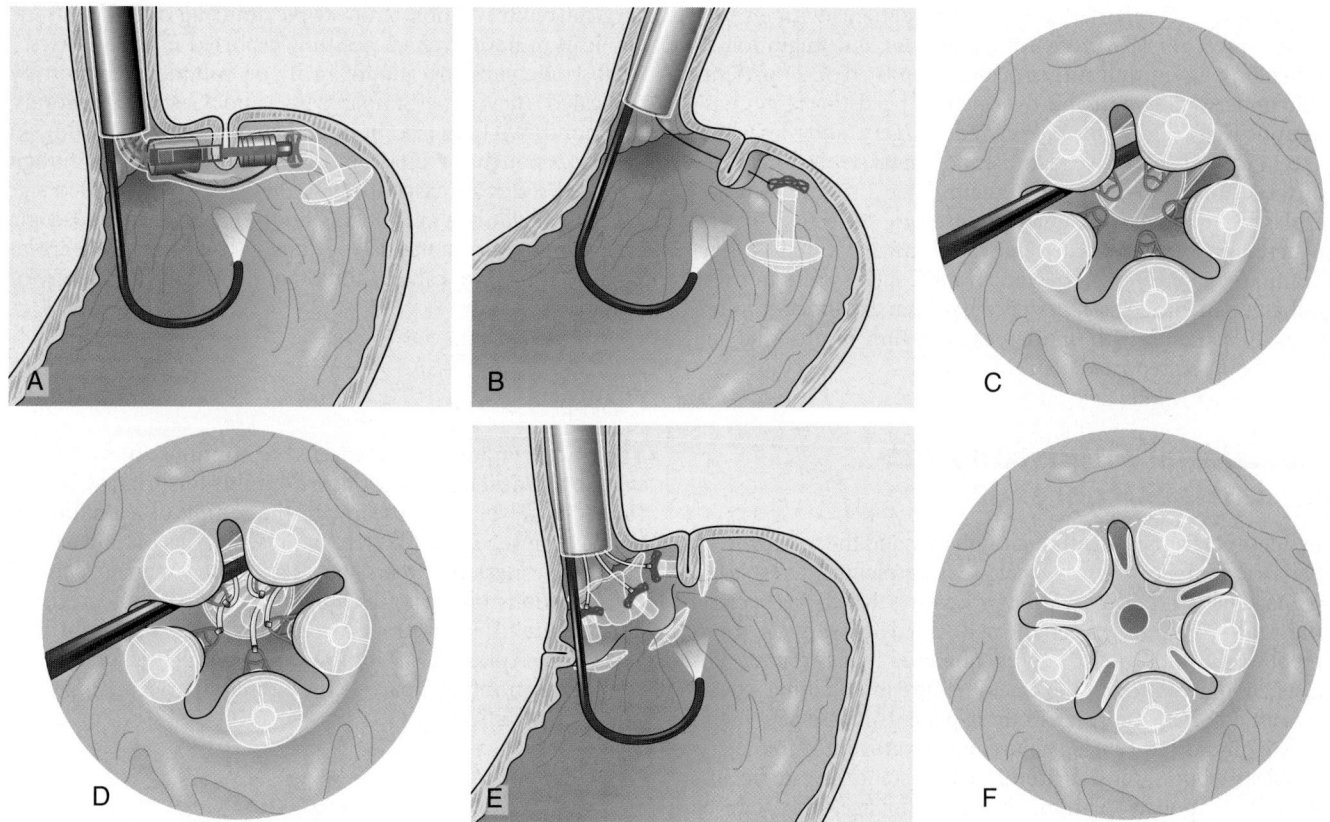

Fig. 53.3 Schematic representation of the various steps of Transoral Endoscopic Restrictive Implants System (TERIS) placement. *(Redrawn from original courtesy of P. Fockens.)*

Endoscopy for Managing Complications after Bariatric Surgery

The dramatic increase in indications for bariatric surgery is associated with a similar increase in complications. Endoscopy is also playing a major emerging role in the management of these complications. It is crucial to identify complications early and to propose adequate treatment, potentially choosing a less invasive option. Major complications occurring after RYGB or a restrictive procedure and amendable to endotherapy include stomal ulceration, stomal stenosis, band erosion, and postoperative fistula.

Stomal ulceration usually occurs within the first 3 months after the procedure with a decreased incidence thereafter. Although the exact cause is unclear, management consists of proton pump inhibitor therapy, liquid sucralfate, eradication of *Helicobacter pylori* if present, and elimination of ulcerogenic medications.[24] Ulcers may also occur as a result of foreign body reaction to nonabsorbable suture. In this case, endoscopic removal of this foreign material may induce the resolution of the ulcer and symptoms.[25]

Stomal stenosis represents a different problem and may occur at the gastrojejunal anastomosis of RYGB or at the level of the gastric band in restrictive procedure. The treatment consists of dilation, which must be performed cautiously, usually at a diameter of 15 mm, which represents a good balance between efficacy and risk of complication.[26]

Gastric band erosion represents a more difficult problem that is traditionally approached by surgical revision. This latter can be difficult, however, and may compromise further bariatric surgery if needed. The need to avoid potential gastrostomies and disruption of blood supply is an argument for endoscopic management of these complications. Blero and coworkers[27] reported their experience in removing partially migrated lap bands or vertical banded gastroplasty rings by using a technique combining the placement of self-expandable plastic stents for a limited duration to induce the more complete migration of the band and a technique of section of the foreign bodies to allow their endoscopic removal. Using this original technique, these authors were able to remove all but one partially migrated band in their first series. With the past proliferation of vertical banded gastroplasty and the associated complication of decompensated proximal pouch owing to stenosis at the level of the band and the current increase of the use of adjustable gastric banding, this less invasive approach could provide an elegant way of managing this complication in the setting of a multidisciplinary team.

Anastomotic leaks are probably the most severe complications occurring after RYGB and sleeve gastrectomies. The use of sealants and sclerosing agents has been described in small series and in attempts to close staple line dehiscence. Use of endoclips has also been reported in a small group of patients with unequal results. The largest experience has been reported in treating post–bariatric surgery gastrocutaneous leaks in two more recent series using self-expandable metal stents. Salinas and colleagues[28] reported a series of 17 patients with 16 successes and 3 complications (mucosal tears and migration to the colon). Eisendrath and associates[29] reported on 21 patients who underwent endoscopic treatment of persisting large anastomotic leaks before considering redo surgery. They described a technique of successive placement of metal stents for closure of the fistula followed by placement, after 2 to 4 months, of a plastic stent, which induces by pressure a necrosis of the hyperplasia and allows the removal of the metal stent. Eisendrath and associates[29] reported an 80% success rate in these difficult patients. This experience has been expanded to more than 70 patients with similar encouraging results that are expected to be reported soon.

Revisional Endoscopy after Bariatric Surgery

Besides the primary treatment of obesity and the treatment of bariatric complications, another area of growing interest is the management of failed bariatric procedures. RYGB has become the most common procedure performed for surgical treatment of morbid obesity and encountered by gastroenterologists. Reintervention in the case of failure in obtaining weight loss after bariatric surgery in these patients is associated with very high morbidity. This failure may be attributed to dietetic problems, but several anatomic factors, such as staple line disruption, pouch dilation, or band slippage, also may be partially responsible.

Staple line disruption resulting in gastrogastric fistula is a classic cause of weight regain in patients. Besides the classic surgical reintervention, endoscopic suturing and fibrin glue application have been successfully reported in small series.[30] Endoscopic suturing (EndoCinch) or volume reduction by dedicated devices (StomaphyX; EndoGastric Solutions, Redmond, WA) has also been reported in patients having an enlarged pouch or anastomosis after RYGB.[31,32] Although reported series are uncontrolled, they have documented significant weight loss at 6- to 12-month follow-up. Endoscopic interventions are potential options for patients who are at high risk of complications and often desperate after failure of bariatric surgery.

Conclusion

The role of endoscopy is expected to continue to evolve, not only in the development of novel options for primary bariatric therapy, where endoscopy, in the setting of a multidisciplinary approach, is likely to represent a classic alternative within the next few years, but also in the management of complications occurring after bariatric surgery and revision after failure of a bariatric procedure in terms of weight loss. With the explosion of indications, therapeutic endoscopy should be an integral part of multidisciplinary care for morbidly obese patients.

References

The complete reference list is available online at www.expertconsult.com.

Gastroenterologic Perspectives on Natural Orifice Transluminal Endoscopic Surgery (NOTES)

Marvin Ryou and Christopher C. Thompson

Introduction

Through opposite trends of invasiveness, gastrointestinal (GI) endoscopy and laparoscopic surgery have converged to produce an intriguing but still largely experimental field termed *natural orifice transluminal endoscopic surgery (NOTES)*. Since the publication in 2004 by Kalloo and colleagues[1] on transgastric peritoneoscopy in the porcine model, NOTES continues to develop as a minimally invasive, "scarless" technique for intraperitoneal and more recently intrathoracic surgeries. The theoretical advantages of NOTES include cosmesis; decreased anesthesia time; shortened postoperative recovery; and elimination of postsurgical complications associated with transabdominal and transthoracic incisions, such as skin infections, wound dehiscence, and hernias. Early questionnaire studies indicated that patients would prefer a NOTES approach over a traditional laparoscopic approach primarily because of issues surrounding pain and visible scars.[2]

The definition of the NOTES concept is in flux and currently spans a continuum. Initially, the concept referred to surgeries performed purely via a natural orifice; and these procedures are referred to in this chapter as *pure NOTES*. More recently, the concept of *hybrid NOTES* has evolved to allow for concomitant assistance provided by laparoscopy as a bridge to pure NOTES. In addition, the concept of NOTES now also encompasses single-incision laparoscopic surgery (SILS) (i.e., single-port laparoscopy or transumbilical laparoscopy), which technically is not surgery via an orifice but rather the coalescing of several laparoscopic ports into a single multilumen transabdominal trocar accommodating rigid laparoscopic instruments.

Moving forward, how might gastroenterologists fit within the broad and shifting NOTES landscape? Which NOTES procedures might become realistic procedures for GI endoscopists? An analysis of the published literature provides clues to factors that may influence the answer.

Current State of Natural Orifice Transluminal Endoscopic Surgery (NOTES) Research

Since the first NOTES publication by Kalloo and colleagues in 2004,[1] there has been progress toward human NOTES in numerous international centers but only a handful of U.S. centers. As of July 2009, the Natural Orifice Surgery Consortium for Assessment and Research NOTES registry had 166 human cases from eight U.S. sites and two international sites, 162 of which were approved by an institutional review board.[3] SILS cases were not included in this registry. Most of these natural orifice cases were performed via the transvaginal route because of the historical precedent of culdoscopy performed by gynecologists, a reduced concern regarding sterility, and a decreased need for "secure" closure of the posterior fornix access point compared with enteral closure. Most of these cases also required laparoscopic assistance and would be more accurately categorized as hybrid NOTES procedures. Of the few pure NOTES procedures, Swanstrom and coworkers[4] succeeded in performing transgastric cholecystectomy. Other pure NOTES procedures on closer examination have been hybrid transgastric procedures. There have been two small published case series of transgastric cholecystectomies assisted by the use of one to three transabdominal trocars.[5,6] There has also been a series of 10 diagnostic transgastric peritoneoscopies performed after laparoscopic exploration before Whipple's surgery,[7] but the challenge of access closure was not directly addressed. Generally, most pure NOTES publications to date have been animal and human cadaveric studies.

Of the eight fundamental obstacles to NOTES identified in the original 2005 White Paper (**Box 54.1**),[8] the most challenging obstacles to pure NOTES human studies have been the ones heavily dependent on device development.[9] Two specific areas of technical need are highlighted here. First, current closure devices remain in various stages of development with none emerging as the clear favorite. Viscerotomy closure must be 100% secure and ideally be easy to perform and reproducible for any chance of clinical adoption of NOTES. No device has yet fulfilled all of these requirements. The second and probably the most rate-limiting step in the clinical adoption of NOTES is the commercial development of a robust, flexible, versatile multitasking platform. Complex surgical maneuvers, even in surgeries as commonplace as cholecystectomies, have

technical requirements that cannot be met by a double-channel endoscope, such as triangulation of instruments, aggressive traction and countertraction of tissue, position fixation, and reliable force transmission over instruments. The NOTES platform should be versatile enough to manage iatrogenic intraperitoneal complications, such as hemorrhage, perforation, or organ injury. It is not surprising that there has been such a preponderance of hybrid NOTES studies and a general tendency to retain the laparoscopic paradigm insofar as SILS is concerned.

Future Indications for the Gastroenterologist

Despite the many limitations on the translation of NOTES from animal and cadaveric studies to actual human trials, endoluminal GI endoscopy has steadily grown bolder in procedures involving and sometimes traversing the gut wall in ways not heretofore considered as NOTES per se. Endoscopic mucosal resection (EMR) and endoscopic submucosal dissection (ESD) have naturally evolved to attempts at endoscopic full-thickness resection (EFTR) for early GI cancers. Endoscopic treatment of pancreatic disease has expanded from endoluminal treatment of the pancreatic duct (endoscopic retrograde pancreaticocholangiography [ERPC]) to transgastric or transduodenal needle puncture for sampling of pancreatic lesions (endoscopic ultrasound [EUS]–guided fine-needle aspiration) and for endoscopic pseudocyst drainage. Transgastric retroperitoneal necrosectomies have also been increasingly performed.

This chapter elaborates on five areas we believe are potential NOTES procedures that will be performed by gastroenterologists in the future (**Box 54.2**). These procedures share one or more of the following characteristics: (1) surgical sites more easily reached using a flexible endoscope or flexible NOTES platform compared with a laparoscope or via open access, (2) surgical procedures of low to medium complexity, and (3) probable improved outcomes from adjunct use of EUS for access or directed biopsies or resections.

Endoscopic Full-Thickness Resection

EFTR represents the next step in the natural evolution of endoscopic procedures aimed at removing GI cancers and cancerous precursor lesions. EFTR follows in the line of

---

Box 54.1 Fundamental Problems for Natural Orifice Transluminal Endoscopic Surgery (NOTES) Identified in Original 2005 White Paper

Access to peritoneal cavity
Gastric (intestinal) closure
Prevention of infection
Development of suturing or anastomotic device
Maintenance of spatial orientation
Development of a multitasking platform
Management of iatrogenic intraperitoneal complications
Identifying physiologic untoward events

Box 54.2 Potential Natural Orifice Transluminal Endoscopic Surgery (NOTES) Procedures for Gastroenterologists

Endoscopic full-thickness resection
Diagnostic peritoneoscopy with or without lymph node resection (sentinel node sampling)
Liver biopsies
Bariatric surgery
Anastomosis

polypectomy, EMR, and ESD. For early stage gastric cancers, ESD cures certain T1, N0 adenocarcinomas. EFTR may find a role in the treatment of T2, N0 adenocarcinoma and small GI stromal tumors.[10] In 2006, Kaehler and associates[11] reported EFTR in two patients (one with early gastric cancer and the other with carcinoid tumor) using a flexible stapler. There have been other case reports of gastric and duodenal EFTR but with laparoscopic assistance.[12,13] In these cases, resection was performed endoscopically, but closure was performed laparoscopically. A full-thickness suturing device has been used to close comparably smaller gastric defects during or after EMR of gastric tumors[14] and a perforation resulting from GI stromal tumor resection using ESD.[15]

Although experience of EFTR in other organs has been reported mostly in animal studies, human studies are likely to be performed in the near future. Successful EFTR has been reported in an animal survival study.[16] Colonic full-thickness resection has also been successfully shown in the animal model using various closure strategies, including but not limited to T-tags,[17] clips,[18] nitinol compression clamps,[19] and staplers.[20]

Diagnostic Peritoneoscopy and Lymph Node Harvesting

NOTES peritoneoscopy with lymph node harvesting has potential as a minimally invasive and accurate means of intraabdominal cancer staging. In patients in whom operability is uncertain, NOTES peritoneoscopy and lymph node mapping may be preferable to staging laparoscopy. In pancreatic, biliary, or gynecologic cancers, transgastric peritoneoscopy could be used to assess quickly for peritoneal and liver implants.[21] Diagnostic transgastric endoscopic peritoneoscopy has already been performed in humans for staging of pancreatic head masses. In this particular study, transgastric peritoneoscopy corroborated laparoscopic findings for surgical decision making in 19 of 20 patients.[22]

NOTES locoregional sentinel node sampling could potentially be combined with EFTR in the same procedure.[9] In early stage gastric cancer, gastric EFTR could be performed with perigastric lymph node harvesting. In early stage colon cancer, direct NOTES sentinel node sampling could potentially save a patient from radical mesenteric lymphadenectomy.[23] Cahill and colleagues[24,25] reported the technical feasibility of lymphatic mapping and node biopsy by NOTES in a porcine model. They performed transvaginal endoscopic peritoneoscopy for gastric lymphatic mapping[24] and transgastric endoscopic peritoneoscopy for lymphatic mapping in the sigmoid colonic mesentery.[25] Methylene blue was injected into the submucosal layer for identification of lymphatic channels and lymph nodes. Excisional biopsy was performed using a coagulating electrode and an endoscopic grasper.

Finally, lymph node harvesting is of particular interest for staging of neoplasias of the chest and mediastinum as an alternative to thoracoscopy and mediastinoscopy, which can be quite painful.[26] The adjunctive use of EUS is likely to be important for safe mediastinal entry. In addition to lymph node harvesting, more recent human cadaveric studies have shown that other procedures may be possible, such as pleural biopsy, vagotomy, thymectomy, thoracic duct ligation, thymectomy, and pericardial window formation.[27]

Liver Biopsies

When directed core liver biopsies are required, the transgastric approach may play a role. Steele and coworkers[28] showed transgastric liver biopsy in three patients undergoing laparoscopic gastric bypass surgery, adding only 4 to 6 minutes to the primary procedure. Segments II, III, IVb, V, and VI (partial) were able to be visualized. Self-limited minor bleeding was encountered after obtaining liver biopsy specimens using standard endoscopic biopsy forceps. Because this study protocol was added to gastric bypass surgeries, gastrostomy closure was not specifically addressed. In another study evaluating liver biopsies in a porcine model, animals were randomly assigned to liver biopsy by laparotomy, laparoscopy, and transgastric NOTES. Both the incidence and the severity of adhesions were lowest with transgastric NOTES.[29]

Bariatric Surgery

Natural orifice bariatric procedures may not be transluminal per se but are likely to represent a significant opportunity for therapeutic gastroenterologists in the future given both the obesity pandemic and the need for a safe and durable alternative to bariatric surgery. Ultimately, avoidance of the transabdominal route makes intuitive sense in morbidly obese patients. Numerous strategies are available for endoluminal treatment of obesity, including suturing, stapling, implantable polymers and prostheses (e.g., sleeves), electrical stimulation, and mucosal ablation.[30] These strategies have been developed to replicate the understood mechanisms of bariatric surgery, classically described as restrictive, malabsorptive, or both.[31] Preclinical studies have shown promising early data regarding safety and efficacy (percent excess weight loss 24% to 58% depending on the device).[32,33] Understanding of the pathophysiology of obesity and the mechanisms of bariatric surgery is in its infancy. The complex interplay between anatomic alterations and neurohormonal modulation remains to be worked out, but the elucidation of critical mechanisms promises to yield bariatric devices and procedures for the gastroenterologist's armamentarium.[32]

Anastomosis

Creation of an endoscopic anastomosis has been a goal of NOTES since its inception. Endoscopic gastrojejunostomy for palliation of malignant gastric outlet obstruction would theoretically be a superior alternative to surgical gastrojejunostomy at the end of life. Similarly, endoscopic creation of a cholecystogastrostomy could enable direct endoscopic treatment of gallbladder disease or allow for prophylactic gallstone removal and mucosal ablation. Early feasibility work in endoscopic anastomosis creation has featured the use of T-tags or endoscopic suturing devices.[34,35] Additional work is under way in our laboratory featuring injectable, self-assembling magnets, which could significantly simplify endoscopic anastomotic creation (unpublished data).

Table 54.1 Natural Orifice Transluminal Endoscopic Surgery (NOTES) Access Points: Relative Advantages and Disadvantages

	Transgastric	Transcolonic	Transvaginal	Transesophageal
Upper abdominal organs well accessed	No	Yes	Yes	NA
Lower abdominal organs well accessed	Yes	No	No	NA
Larger caliber lumen for instrument insertion and specimen extraction	No	Yes	Yes	No
Easily reachable for repair by rigid instrument or by hand	No	Yes	Yes	No
Concerns over sterility	No	Yes (peritonitis)	No	Yes (mediastinitis)

NA, not applicable.

Equipment

The evolution of NOTES depends on technical development. The most pressing need is a safe and reproducible means of closing perforations. Several strategies are available for perforation closure—suturing, tissue anchors, staples, clips, occluding devices.[36] Requirements would differ depending on the tissue involved (e.g., gastric vs. colonic vs. esophageal). Similarly, there is still a need for robust, flexible, multitasking platforms. Promising prototypes of direct drive systems and multitasking flexible endoscopes are now being tested, and it is hoped that these new tools would enable more complex surgical maneuvers.[37]

Anatomic Considerations

The transgastric approach provides excellent access to the lower abdomen and pelvis (**Table 54.1**). To view the upper abdomen from a transgastric access point, the endoscope must be retroflexed, which can limit maneuverability and reach. Peritoneal access is targeted along the anterior gastric body guided by transabdominal palpation. When creating the gastrostomy, the endoscopist should be mindful of the gastroepiploic arteries running along the greater curvature, the left lobe of the liver, and the anterior abdominal wall. The most frequently used technique for access involves using a needle-knife attached to cautery. A wire is passed through the needle-knife into the peritoneal cavity. An endoscopic dilating balloon is advanced over the wire to dilate the gastrostomy tract. The endoscope is advanced into the peritoneal cavity. Alternatively, the gastrostomy can be created using the percutaneous endoscopic gastrostomy tube technique whereby a transabdominal needle delivers the wire over which a balloon is advanced to dilate the gastrostomy. Another option is to use the tunneling method whereby a 5- to 15-cm submucosal tunnel is created before serosal exit to create a gastric flap that self-approximates and seals more easily (**Figs. 54.1, 54.2, and 54.3**).

In contrast to the transgastric approach, the transcolonic approach provides excellent access to the upper abdominal organs, but it requires retroflexion to visualize and engage the lower abdominal organs (see **Table 54.1**). Usually an entry point is chosen in the proximal anterior rectum, just proximal to the superior valve of Houston, because the proximal third

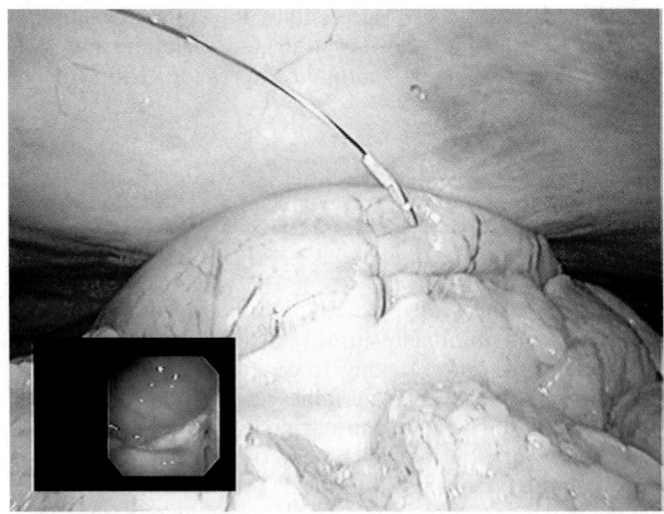

Fig. 54.1 Natural orifice transluminal endoscopic surgery (NOTES) gastrostomy creation. Laparoscopic view with endoscopic view *(inset)* in human cadaver.

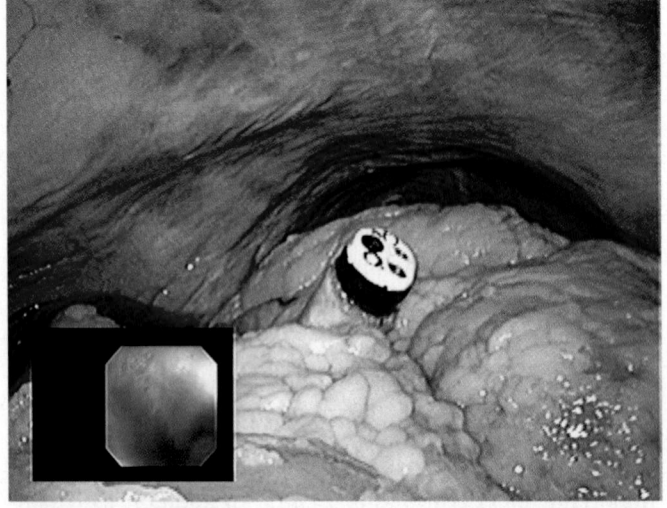

Fig. 54.2 Natural orifice transluminal endoscopic surgery (NOTES) gastrostomy access. Laparoscopic view in human cadaver.

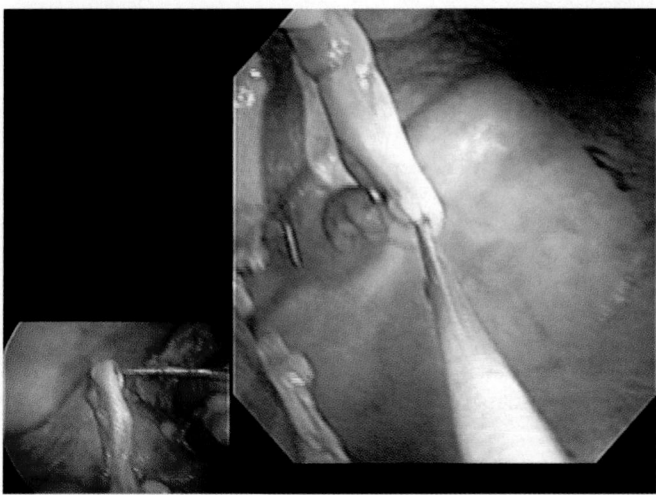

Fig. 54.3 Transgastric appendectomy. Endoscopic view with laparoscopic view *(inset)* in human cadaver.

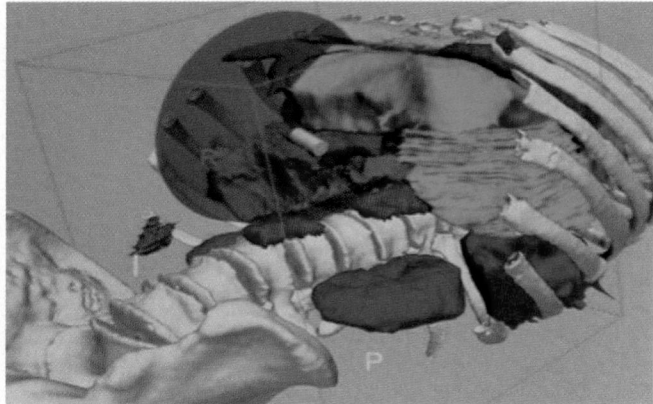

Fig. 54.4 Image registered gastroscopic ultrasound (IRGUS) system.

of the rectum is covered by visceral peritoneum.[38] The peritoneal reflection is generally 7 to 9 cm from the anal verge in men and 5 to 7.5 cm from the anal verge in women. This anterior peritonealized space is the rectovesicle pouch in men and the rectouterine pouch in women. As with transgastric access, the needle-knife is used to create the initial transmural cut. However, there is usually no need to balloon dilate as in transgastric access because of the comparatively thinner colonic wall. Other sites of inferior access include transvaginal and transvesicular, which are briefly mentioned here. As described previously, most recent NOTES literature has used the transvaginal route given a historical precedent in the form of culdoscopy, decreased concerns of sterility, and the adequacy of hand-sewn sutures for closure of the posterior fornix. However, this technique is available only to female patients, and gastroenterologists would likely not be involved in this approach. The transvesicular approach has not seen much clinical use.

The transesophageal approach (see **Table 54.1**) is usually guided by the use of EUS to identify an area of the mediastinum beyond the esophageal wall that appears suitable for entry, with no vessels. For viscerotomy creation, most published studies (all in animals or cadavers) use either the direct needle-knife technique or a modified tunneling method for "flap" access. As with the transcolonic approach, the transesophageal approach is associated with concerns of infection (i.e., mediastinitis). Closure methods for transesophageal access in animal studies have included clips and a T-tag suturing system, but a more fail-safe closure method is likely required before embarking on human trials.

Peritoneal and mediastinal anatomy would initially be foreign to the endoscopist accustomed to endoluminal navigation. To "recalibrate" the endoscopist to new anatomic perspectives, part of the answer may lie in a formal NOTES training fellowship.[39] Although such a fellowship would incorporate fundamentals of surgical training (e.g., surgical exposure, understanding tissue planes during dissection), NOTES would cover new ground even for the surgeon. NOTES allows for full prone positioning of the patient, which in the porcine model has shown full exposure of the retroperitoneum, a view not seen even by laparoscopic surgeons.

Additionally, part of the answer may lie with complementary, real-time image-guided navigational systems to compensate for difficulties with spatial positioning and orientation, identification of anatomy, and localization of pathology.[40] A real-time three-dimensional CT guidance system has been employed for navigational assistance during colonoscopy, ERCP and EUS, and NOTES procedures in human cadaveric studies.[41] This system can track endoscope position with a three-dimensional volumetric reconstruction of a preoperative computed tomography scan (**Fig. 54.4**).

Case Preparation

It is unlikely that patient preparation for NOTES procedures would be greatly different from preparation protocols for current endoscopic procedures. For upper GI procedures, patients would likely be placed on nothing by mouth (NPO) status for 6 to 12 hours and may be required to undergo an additional purge preparation depending on the intended procedure (e.g., NOTES bypass). Intravenous antibiotics would likely be administered. Early NOTES procedures would also probably require patients to undergo general anesthesia to satisfy institutional review board requirements. Sedation protocols may transition to intravenous conscious sedation as the body of safety data accumulates.

During the procedure, carbon dioxide insufflation would likely be required to replicate laparoscopic insufflation conditions. Intraperitoneal pressures would require monitoring, either through an endoscope-based system or via a transabdominal Veress needle connected to a laparoscopic insufflator.

Precautions

The concern regarding infection is paramount in NOTES. More recent studies in patients have shown that intravenous antibiotics are sufficient in preventing peritonitis after transgastric peritoneoscopy.[42,43] However, the mean intraperitoneal time in these studies was less than 21 minutes. Transmural breach involving longer durations, organs with greater microbial load (e.g., transcolonic or even transesophageal), and prosthetic implantation may require additional mucosal antiseptics, such as chlorhexidine or povidone-iodine, which have been shown to reduce mucosal microbial burden to near zero when used in conjunction with intravenous antibiotics.[44]

Conclusion

The arrival of NOTES allowed therapeutic endoscopy to move beyond the GI lumen. Breaching the gut wall—previously a forbidden act to the endoscopist and a reflexive, urgent call to the surgeon—now opens doors to intraperitoneal endoscopic procedures. It became conceivable and reasonable that gastroenterologists could be outside the GI tract. Looking ahead, the following NOTES surgeries have potential as procedures performed by interventional gastroenterologists: (1) EFTR, (2) diagnostic peritoneoscopy with or without lymph node resection, (3) directed liver biopsies, (4) bariatric procedures, and (5) anastomosis creation. These procedures share the following characteristics: (1) surgical sites more easily reached using a flexible endoscope or flexible NOTES platform compared with a laparoscope or via open access, (2) surgical procedures of low to medium complexity, and (3) probable improved outcomes from adjunct use of EUS for access or directed biopsies.

From a technical perspective, the advancement of NOTES depends on technical developments in the areas of viscerotomy closure and multitasking flexible platforms. From a training perspective, gastroenterologists are likely to need to undergo formalized training incorporating the fundamentals of extraluminal anatomy, dissection techniques, and management of complications. Infection control is of paramount importance. Still in its infancy, human NOTES research needs to be performed under oversight of institutional review boards to allow for data collection and safety evaluation in a rigorous manner.

References

The complete reference list is available online at www.expertconsult.com.

Surgical Perspectives on Natural Orifice Transluminal Endoscopic Surgery (NOTES)

Juliane Bingener and Erica A. Moran

Introduction

Surgical procedures have been performed since Neolithic times with advances in the field marked by key events.[1] In 1809, McDowell completed the first successful abdominal operation without the use of general anesthetic.[2] The invention and use of inhaled ether as a form of general anesthetic marks the first great advance in surgical therapy (**Fig. 55.1**), followed by the introduction of antisepsis by Lister.[3] In the centuries that followed, large abdominal incisions were required to permit the surgeon's hands and instruments access to the disease process. More recently, disease processes have been accessed with smaller incisions (as in laparoscopy) or by a different route entirely (endoscopy or endovascular), decreasing the pain and infection risk of the abdominal incision and improving patient outcomes.

Natural orifice transluminal endoscopic surgery (NOTES) is an experimental surgical technique whereby scarless abdominal operations can be performed with an endoscope passed through a natural orifice (mouth, anus, vagina, or urethra) and then through an internal incision in the stomach, colon, posterior vaginal fornix, or bladder, avoiding any external incisions or scars (**Fig. 55.2**). Similar to the introduction of laparoscopy, surgical opinions of this new approach vary widely. This chapter briefly reviews NOTES and examines current surgical opinions.

History of Minimally Invasive Surgery

The advent of minimally invasive surgery brought with it an opportunity to decrease postoperative pain with resultant shorter hospital stays and quicker returns to normal activity and to shrink surgical scars, providing a more pleasing cosmetic outcome.[4] The minimally invasive surgery concept influenced the next paradigm shift in intervention, NOTES, which may eliminate the anterior abdominal wall approach altogether (**Fig. 55.3**).

History of Natural Orifice Transluminal Endoscopic Surgery

The history of NOTES begins in 1901, when Ott performed the first endoscopic examination of the peritoneal cavity through the vagina.[5] He termed the procedure *ventroscopy* and became the pioneer of natural orifice access. The feasibility of a peroral transgastric flexible endoscopic approach to the peritoneal cavity with long-term survival in a porcine model was reported by the Apollo Group in 2004 (**Fig. 55.4**).[4] Since this publication, NOTES has continued to evolve. Success in early animal studies led to the initiation of human trials.[6–11] Rao and Reddy performed the first flexible endoscopic transgastric appendectomy in humans in Hyderabad, India; although this report remains unpublished, a description of their technique and videos have become widely dispersed throughout the research community.[12,13] Since that time, this group has successfully attempted the transluminal approach for 17 cases, including appendectomy, liver biopsy, and tubal ligation.[14] Multiple transvaginal and transgastric NOTES procedures have been published by other NOTES teams, including transgastric appendectomy, cholecystectomy, fallopian tube ligation, and transvaginal cholecystectomy with active clinical trials ongoing.[15–20] Currently, the number of successful NOTES procedures (with or without laparoscopic assistance) around the world is greater than 3000 cases.

Advantages of Natural Orifice Transluminal Endoscopic Surgery

Abdominal incisions elicit a pain reaction that results in a stress response from the body, initiated through the inflammatory cytokine cascade. Theoretical advantages of NOTES include the avoidance of this pain reaction and stress response. A possible development can be imagined with procedures under conscious sedation rather than general anesthesia. This development has already occurred for several procedures that used to be the domain of open surgery, such as endoscopic retrograde cholangiopancreatography for choledocholithiasis or pancreatic pseudocyst drainage. As is shown with the percutaneous endoscopic gastrostomy rescue report by Marks and colleagues,[21] transluminal procedures may avoid additional insults to ill patients. In addition to the esthetic improvements offered by incisionless surgery, NOTES would also decrease the risk of wound infection and postoperative incisional hernias. NOTES may be ideally suited for patients who have conditions that preclude an open or laparoscopic procedure, such as patients with large areas of burn, scar, or infection of the anterior abdominal wall. Additionally, the NOTES team and equipment are portable allowing procedures to be done in an intensive care unit, multipurpose procedure room, outpatient setting, and battlefield.

These potential advantages, if realized, would have a significant economic impact in health care. These advantages are also appealing to developing countries where complex laparoscopic equipment and sterile operating environments may not be consistently available. There is also the potential for decreased length of hospital stay, faster return of bowel function, and increase in overall patient satisfaction. Perhaps the biggest advantage of NOTES would be the improvements in laparoscopic and endoscopic surgery,

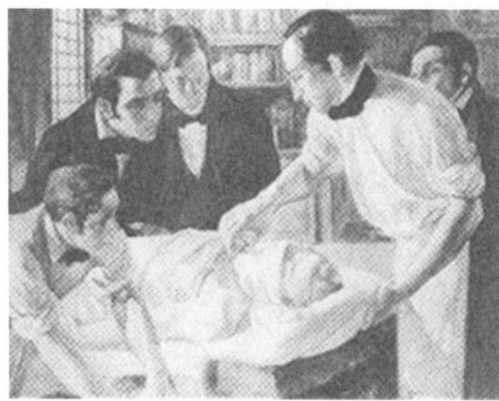

Fig. 55.1 Artist's conception of Dr. Crawford Long demonstrating for the first time the use of ether as an inhaled anesthetic on March 30, 1842. *(From Boland F: The first anesthetic: The story of Crawford Long, Athens, 1950, University of Georgia Press.)*

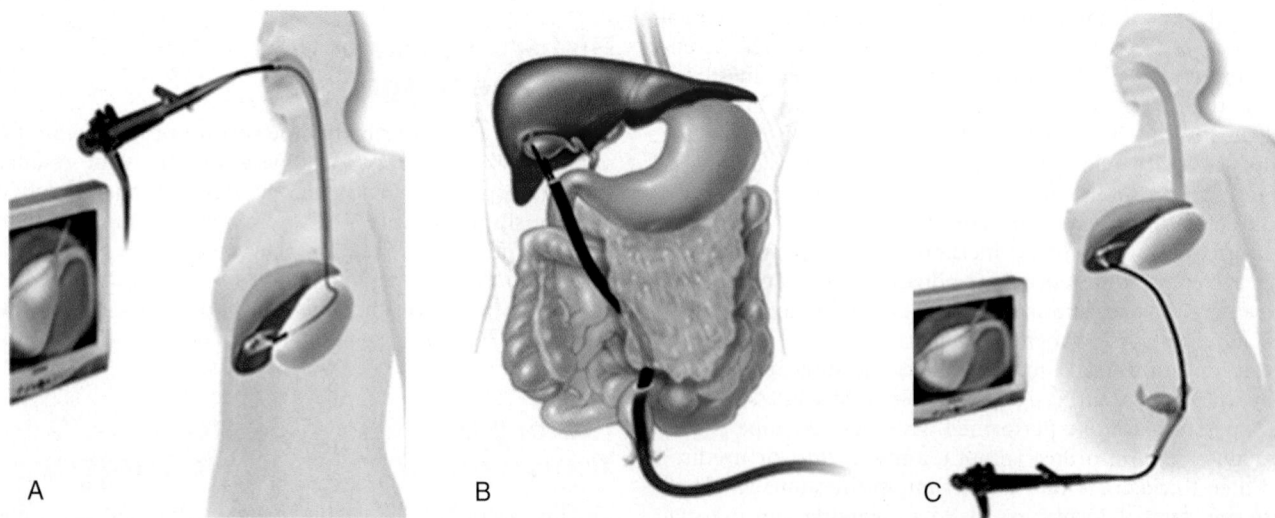

A B C

Fig. 55.2 **A–C,** Renderings of natural orifice access through transgastric (**A**), transcolonic (**B**), and transvaginal (**C**) routes. *(From Bessler M, Stevens P, Milone L, et al: Transvaginal laparoscopically assisted endoscopic cholecystectomy: A hybrid approach to natural orifice surgery. Gastrointest Endosc 66:1243–1245, 2007.)*

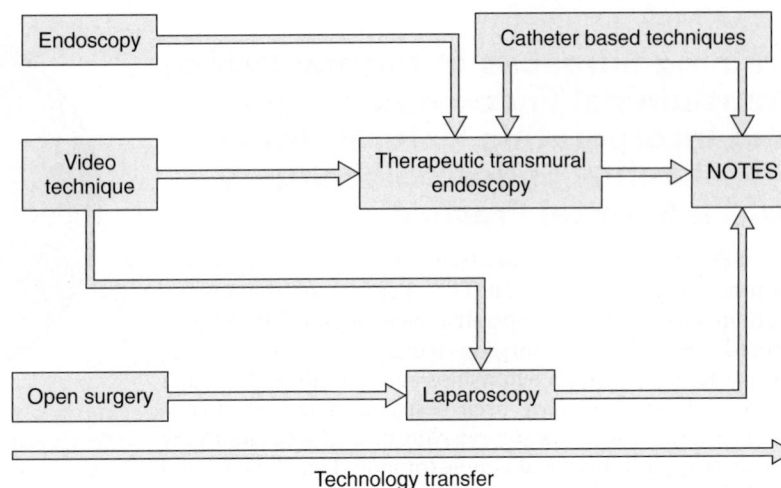

Fig. 55.3 Depiction of the transfer of advances in technology between specialties leading to decreased invasiveness.

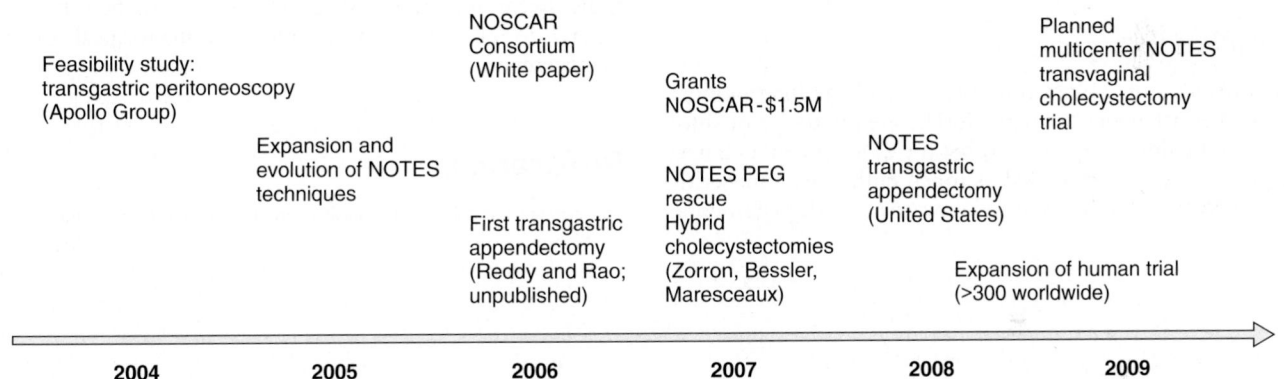

Fig. 55.4 Timeline for the development of natural orifice transluminal endoscopic surgery (NOTES) from the first feasibility studies to more advanced animal studies.

including the tool sets used in each and the skills of the surgeons involved.

Disadvantages of Natural Orifice Transluminal Endoscopic Surgery

Not all surgeons support the concept of NOTES. Although studies have shown the feasibility of a NOTES approach, significant constraints also have been identified with the use of a flexible endoscopy platform, including a relative inability to apply off-axis forces, mechanical stability, inadequate triangulation, and limits in passing multiple instruments simultaneously into the peritoneal cavity. Surgeons have also expressed concerns for the risk of postoperative leak and infection. Data from pilot clinical trials have not supported these concerns. Surgeons have also stated that although there is significant research work focused on intestinal closure systems for NOTES access sites, it is doubtful that 100%

safety can be achieved. Many current procedures involve the vagina, which avoids the need for intestinal or bladder closure. There is concern that current instrumentation for grasping, dissection, and suction are substandard compared with laparoscopy. Additionally, concerns have surfaced that the operative near-field view using an endoscope is more limited than with a laparoscope, and steering of the endoscopic instrumentation by endoscopic movement leads to poor visualization of the instrument tip.

Industry developments have answered many of these concerns with the design of new operative endoscopes that permit independent instrument and optical movement and development of grasping, dissecting, and closure tools. Many of these tools are expected to evolve over time much as open and laparoscopic instrumentation has evolved from first introduction. One of the greatest challenges faced by NOTES is changing the view of currently practicing surgeons whose training and practice decreed not to perforate otherwise healthy hollow viscus organs. Changes in surgery and health care require surgeons to look at patient care in a new way.

Training Surgeons in Natural Orifice Transluminal Endoscopic Surgery and Incorporating Natural Orifice Transluminal Endoscopic Surgery into a Surgical Practice

As with any new technique, training is important for the clinical incorporation of NOTES. Because of the unique equipment used and the operative view obtained in NOTES procedures, a NOTES surgeon requires specialty training similar to other surgical fellowships and specialties. Although no formal programs have been designed, it is likely that a NOTES surgeon would require an education in general surgery concepts and advanced endoscopic training (**Fig. 55.5**). Several procedures in the vascular environment are now performed by either vascular surgeons or radiologists and training for both types of specialists has evolved to combine more of both specialties. A similar training model could be applied for training of NOTES surgeons.

Conclusion

The prospects of evolution of NOTES and the international research effort associated with NOTES are exciting. Not since the introduction of laparoscopy has the development of a new surgical technique generated as much enthusiasm and criticism as NOTES. Surgeons must be aware of the developmental

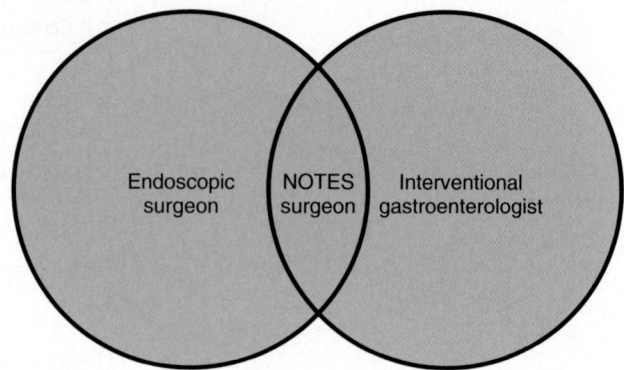

Fig. 55.5 Depiction of the training for a surgeon in natural orifice transluminal endoscopic surgery (NOTES), which requires both general surgery and interventional endoscopic training.

nature of these techniques and proceed with appropriate caution in the setting of institutional review board–approved studies. NOTES also needs to be assessed in larger multicenter trials. Regardless of the surgeon's opinion of NOTES, it is crucial to be informed of advances in surgical disease management.

References

The complete reference list is available online at www.expertconsult.com.

Emerging Intramural and Transmural Endoscopy

Kazuki Sumiyama, Christopher J. Gostout,* and Hisao Tajiri

Video related to this chapter's topics can be found online at expertconsult.com.

Introduction

Limitless possibilities exist for the endoscope to serve as a sophisticated diagnostic probe and a platform for endoluminal therapeutic interventions. Flexible gastrointestinal (GI) endoscopy has achieved major accomplishments so far, which include inspection of the total digestive canal, detection of grossly invisible minute mucosal abnormalities, reliable hemostasis for GI bleeding, pancreaticobiliary intervention, ultrasound staging of neoplasms, and radical excision of mucosal malignancies. Despite these practical technologic accomplishments, the working space for flexible endoscopy has been confined to the gut lumen. The gut wall has always been the great barrier for flexible endoscopy, instilling a tradition of respect to maintain its integrity and limiting intervention. Both gastroenterologists and surgeons are now exploring the new frontier through the gut wall to achieve incisionless surgery.[1] More recent research has approached the gut wall as an opportunity and showed that an artificially created intramural space could become a working space for novel endoscopic interventions.[2,3]

Techniques for Creation of a Submucosal Working Space: Submucosal Endoscopy with Mucosal Safety Valve Technique

The submucosal endoscopy with mucosal flap (SEMF) "safety valve" technique represents a global concept of using a submucosal space as a practical working space for endoscopic intervention.[4] Using the SEMF technique, major technical challenges to standard endoscopic intervention may be overcome by using the endoscope and surgical devices inserted into the intramural space—formally the submucosa. It was hypothesized that the technique may offer safe (offset) access into the peritoneal cavity for natural orifice transluminal endoscopic surgery (NOTES) by using the submucosal space as a tunneled portal and the isolated free overlying mucosa as a protective sealant flap to minimize the potential for contamination of the extraluminal anatomic cavity (**Fig. 56.1**).[3] Also, mucosal resection could be safely performed in an "inside-out" manner, directing intervention toward the lumen with a greatly reduced risk of perforation, regardless of the size for a mucosal based lesion.[5]

In the original SEMF technique,[6] the submucosal layer was mechanically dissected by a combination of high-pressure

*Christopher J. Gostout is a member of the Apollo Group, which owns and operates Apollo Endoscopy, Austin, Texas.

743

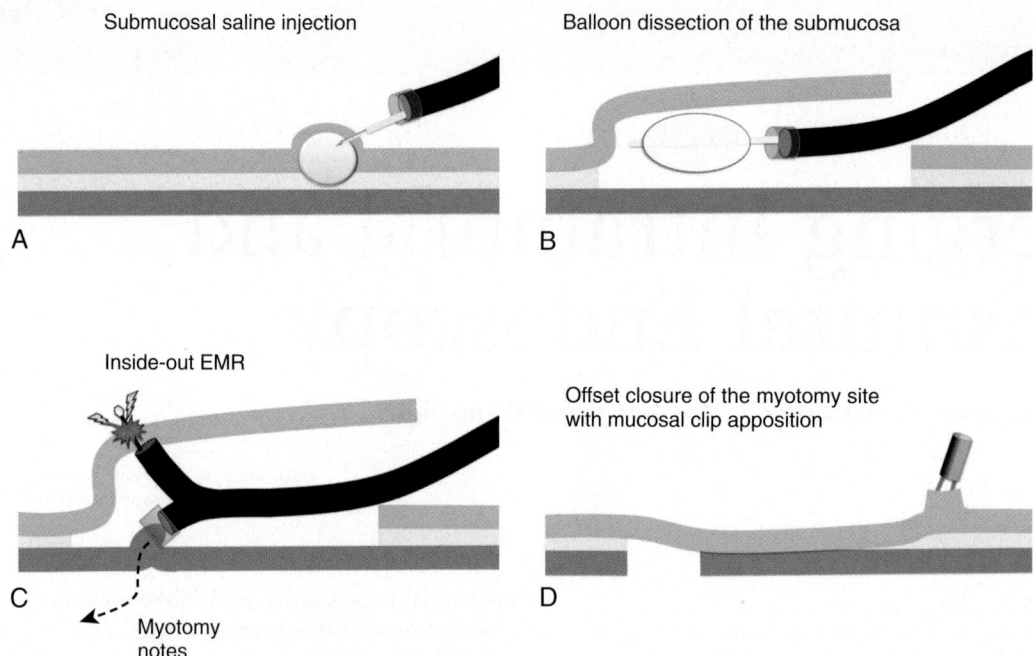

Submucosal saline injection

Balloon dissection of the submucosa

Inside-out EMR

A

B

Offset closure of the myotomy site
with mucosal clip apposition

C

Myotomy
notes

D

Fig. 56.1 Schematic presentation of submucosal endoscopy with mucosal flap (SEMF) technique. **A,** A small submucosal saline bleb is made to identify the submucosal tissue plane. **B,** After pretreatment of the submucosa with high-pressure carbon dioxide (CO_2) or mesna, balloon dissection is performed to create an open space within the submucosal tissue plane. **C,** The submucosal space is used as a working space for interventions such as inside-out submucosal endoscopy with mucosal resection (SEMR), intramural myotomy, and offset access for natural orifice transluminal endoscopic surgery (NOTES) procedures. **D,** The muscular defect after myotomy is sealed with an overlying mucosal flap, and the submucosal tunnel is closed with mucosal clip apposition.

carbon dioxide (CO_2) and balloon dissection. The procedure was initiated by a submucosal injection of a small amount of saline to identify the submucosal tissue plane (see **Fig. 56.1A**). Millisecond bursts of high-pressure CO_2 (100 psi on average) were injected into the bleb to create a gas-filled giant submucosal bleb and gas-dissected submucosa. This gas dissection technique allows instant isolation of a large area of the mucosa as desired, greater than 10 cm in diameter. An injection of 1.5% hydroxypropyl methylcellulose into this dissected plane prevents gas escape and maintains the large bleb. A mucosal incision (10 mm) made with a needle-knife at one margin of the combination bleb and fluid cushion allows entry below the mucosa. With persistent submucosal tissue stranding present, balloon dissection using a 15-mm biliary retrieval balloon can be performed to disrupt the tissue strands to transform the submucosa into an intramural free space (see **Fig. 56.1B**). Instead of the combination of gas and balloon dissections, blunt dissection with a grasping forceps also could be used for the mechanical disruption of the submucosal layer. In contrast to the SEMF technique and long preceding it, Japanese endoscopists have used repetitive time-consuming needle-knife dissection directed into the submucosal plane using one of a series of needle-knives specially designed for endoscopic submucosal dissection (ESD) technique.

Chemically Assisted Submucosal Dissection Technique

The original gas dissection SEMF technique was developed with the intent of rapidly creating an open submucosal space. This technique can be slow because of tedious balloon

dissection in the setting of a resilient submucosa. The large mucosal flap can be susceptible to necrosis because of inadvertent mechanical trauma and, perhaps, microvascular ischemia. To preserve blood supply of the free mucosal flap, it is necessary to identify an optimal width and length of the submucosal tunnel or space matched to the specific intervention. In an effort to minimize mechanical trauma to the mucosal flap, we have discovered mesna ($C_2H_5NaO_3S_2$) as a practical pretreatment of the submucosa before the blunt dissection. Mesna can chemically soften the submucosa by dissolving disulfide bonds in connective tissues that play an important role in the folding and stability of proteins.[7] Mesna is clinically used as a mucolytic agent for patients with respiratory disorders and is better known in oncology as a uroprotective drug to prevent ifosfamide-induced and cyclophosphamide-induced hemorrhagic cystitis. Drug safety has been shown from these clinical experiences.

The concept of chemically assisted surgical dissection with mesna was initially introduced to assist blunt dissection of the facial planes in the field of otorhinolaryngology. The benefits of mesna have been confirmed in other surgical interventions. In the chemically assisted SEMF technique, 4 to 8 mL of 10% mesna solution is injected into the saline submucosal bleb before initiating balloon dissection. A randomized porcine study using this method showed that a longitudinal submucosal tunnel greater than 5 cm could be created within 10 minutes in porcine stomachs with significantly less tissue resistance to insertion of a balloon catheter and subsequent mechanical balloon dissection. Clinical experience has subsequently been obtained using mesna to facilitate excision of colon polyps and gastric neoplasms.[8] The preliminary clinical experiences in the stomach and colon support the benefits of mesna in "softening" the submucosa.

Intramural Endoscopy (Submucosal Endoscopic Procedures)

In Vivo Histologic Imaging of the Muscularis Propria

Abnormalities of the muscularis propria occur in diseases such as GI stromal tumors, achalasia, and GI motility disorders. Although ex vivo conventional histologic evaluation of sampled tissues has been the reference standard for the diagnosis of GI disease, muscle layer sampling and subsequent histologic analysis are used primarily for diagnosis of suspected neoplastic disease. Muscle layer tissue acquisition for motility-related and functional clinical disorders is especially challenging for both diagnosis and etiologic analysis but nevertheless very appealing. We are trying to establish a minimally invasive advanced endoscopic imaging method for in vivo histologic imaging of the muscularis propria.

We have so far applied two imaging technologies for muscle layer imaging in an animal study using porcine models,[9] both of which have been newly introduced into flexible endoscopy in a clinical setting. These imaging technologies are endocytoscopy (EndoCytoscope, Olympus, Tokyo, Japan), which is a catheter-style ultrahigh-magnifying endoscopy with optical magnification greater than 1000× and confocal microscopy (**Fig. 56.2**). The chemically assisted SEMF technique was used to access the muscularis propria in esophageal and gastric locations. Nissl stains and two types of neuronal molecular stains were topically applied onto the exposed muscularis propria within the SEMF submucosal space. The muscular layer was imaged in vivo 2 minutes after the muscular staining with the endocytoscope inserted into the SEMF submucosal space. A sample of the muscularis propria was stained with

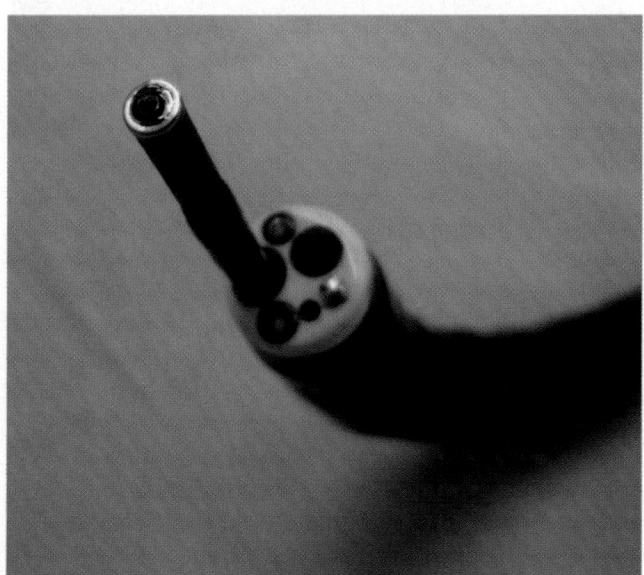

Fig. 56.2 The endocytoscope (Olympus, Tokyo, Japan), a flexible catheter-type contact magnifying videoendoscope, provides optical magnification more than 1000×.

molecular-based stains and evaluated, ex vivo after necropsy by confocal microscopy. Endocytoscopy revealed cellular microstructures resembling spindle-shaped smooth muscle cells comparable to bench microscopy (**Fig. 56.3A**). Confocal microscopy performed after necropsy showed that the in vivo topical application of neuronal molecular stains successfully stained the muscularis and highlighted neuronlike cells (**Fig. 56.3B**).

These results showed that in vivo endoscopic histologic evaluation of the muscularis propria is technically feasible and easy. Minimally invasive advanced endoscopic imaging may be useful for the diagnosis and study of neuroenteric disorders at the level of the muscularis propria, avoiding surgical full-thickness tissue sampling. The introduction of confocal endoscopic imaging technology with biologic markers might allow anatomic and functional analysis of the muscularis propria and its neural elements, providing an opportunity for optical assessment of GI motility disorders.

Submucosal Endoscopic Myotomy

In addition to muscularis propria imaging, full-thickness sampling of the muscularis propria has been achieved with the SEMF technique combined with the cap endoscopic mucosal resection (EMR) technique to obtain the muscle sample from within the SEMF submucosal space. The suction and snare myotomy with the cap EMR technique provides a myotomy specimen greater than 2 cm in size. This technique is theoretically safer than direct electrosurgical resection of a muscle sample because it minimizes the risk of collateral coagulation injury to surrounding organs by blind insertion of a cutting tool. The technical feasibility of this technique has been confirmed in the stomach and esophagus by a series of porcine animal studies (**Fig. 56.4**).[10,11] The free overlying mucosa over the myotomy has been sufficiently durable to maintain the integrity of the gut wall. We anticipated that this method for a full-thickness myotomy would be desirable for histologic and etiologic analysis of GI motility disorders, for safe access for NOTES procedures, and as an alternative to the Heller myotomy in the treatment of achalasia.

Pasricha and the Apollo group[12] showed that selective subtotal needle-knife incision of only the circular layer of the muscularis propria from within the submucosal working space reduced lower esophageal sphincter pressure in a porcine model. The efficacy and safety of the SEMF-based myotomy technique was subsequently confirmed by a Japanese group in patients with achalasia.[13] In this experience, repetitive electrosurgical dissection with a needle-knife was used to create a working space for the myotomy in the lower esophagus. Although successful, this dissection method would be intuitively less appealing from a safety perspective compared with blunt dissection.

Submucosal Endoscopy with Mucosal Resection

In Japan and other Asian countries with a high incidence of gastric cancer, a widespread EMR technique, ESD, has become front-line treatment for mucosal cancers associated with a negligible risk of lymph node metastasis. In ESD, tedious repetitive needle-knife dissection is used to isolate the mucosal lesion from the deeper gastric wall layers. Although the concept

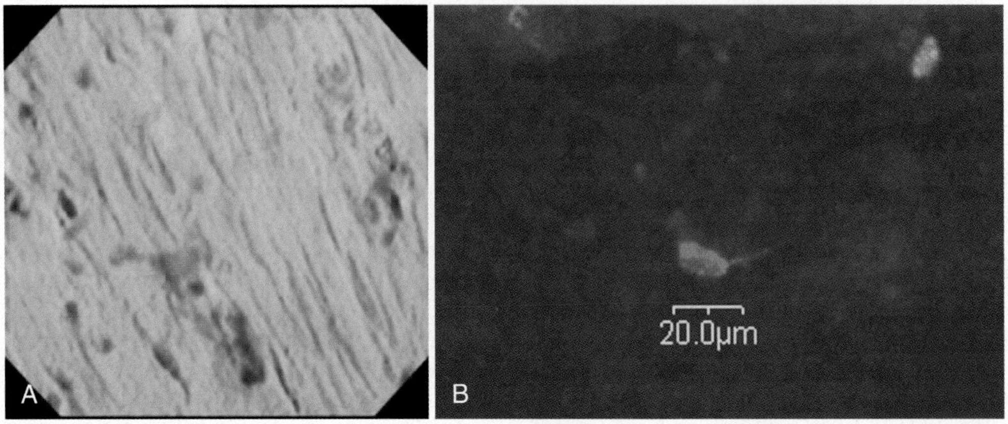

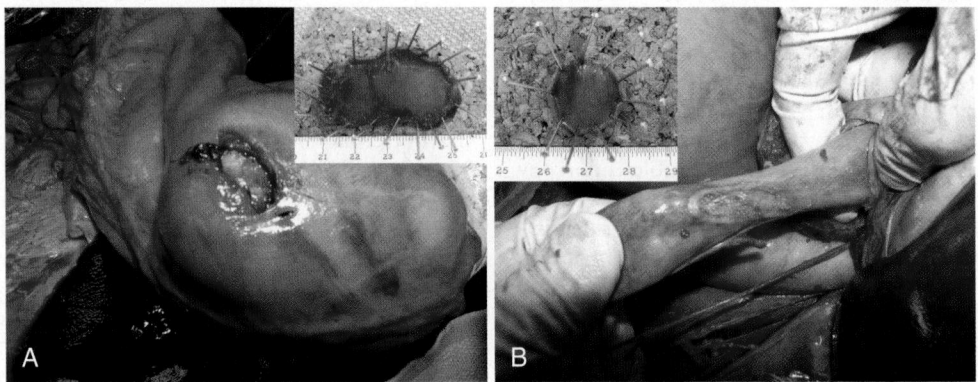

Fig. 56.3 A, In vivo muscularis propria imaged with endocytoscopy in the submucosal endoscopy with mucosal flap (SEMF) submucosal space. **B,** A myenteric neuron–like cell stained in vivo in the SEMF submucosal space with topically applied neuronal molecular probes.

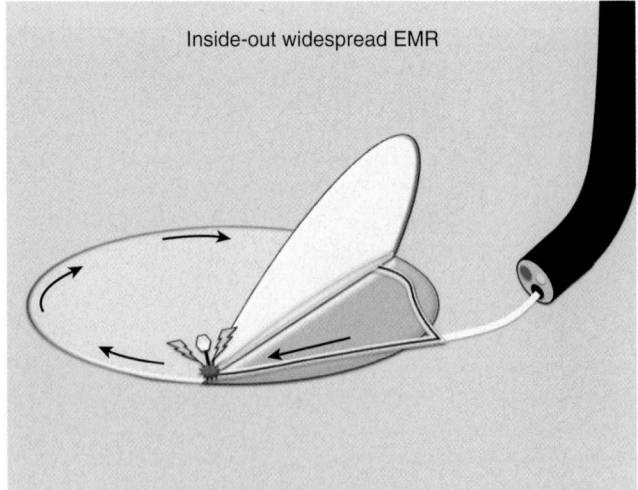

Fig. 56.4 A muscular defect 1 week after myotomy with an aspiration cap endoscopic mucosal resection (EMR) technique in the submucosal endoscopy with mucosal flap (SEMF) submucosal space and a sampled muscular layer. The defect was sealed with an overlying mucosa in the stomach (**A**) and in the esophagus (**B**).

of ESD providing en bloc excision of malignancy is appealing, the electrosurgical dissection is overwhelmingly labor-intensive and time-consuming and is associated with significant risk for perforation and bleeding. It is anticipated that transformation of the submucosa into a working space by SEMF could be applied to the undermining of mucosally based disease offering a safer and more expedient alternative for the isolation and resection of diseased mucosa, redirecting the most hazardous aspect of tissue resection, electrosurgical cutting, toward the lumen.[14] The Apollo Group has developed a unique tool set designed to perform submucosal endoscopy with mucosal resection (SEMR), an inside-out widespread EMR, using uniquely designed, highly compliant balloons to undermine targeted diseased mucosa safely and accommodate a simple en bloc excision of the freed-up area of diseased mucosa (**Fig. 56.5**).

Transmural Procedures with Submucosal Endoscopy with Mucosal Flap Approach

As described previously, one of the main aims of SEMF was to offer a protective tunneled space for offset entry into extraluminal anatomic cavities from the lumen to prevent

Inside-out widespread EMR

Fig. 56.5 A schema of inside-out widespread submucosal endoscopy with mucosal resection (SEMR). The isolated free mucosa after the submucosal balloon dissection is unroofed with a specially designed loop cutter placed along the contour of the submucosal space. An insulated-tip electrosurgical needle-knife is stowed within the looped cartridge of the device. The overlying mucosa is circumferentially excised with the deployed knife running on the loop (Apollo Endosurgery, Austin, TX).

contamination by luminal contents. This method has been adopted as a safe access technique for NOTES with various NOTES procedures having been performed using this offset transmural approach.

Transgastric Cholecystectomy via a Cephalad Submucosal Tunnel

The organs in the lower half of the peritoneal cavity and pelvis are easily accessible regardless of any anterior gastrostomy technique. Conversely, there are technical challenges to performing surgical procedures in the upper abdominal cavity (e.g., cholecystectomy) using the currently designed flexible endoscope from a standard anterior gastrostomy. To access the organs located higher than the level of the stomach, retroflexion of the endoscope is mandatory. This access is restrictive because of the potential target organ distance and the angle of approach after exiting from a typical anterior gastrostomy. The gallbladder may not be consistently identified. Pai and colleagues[15] reported that the gallbladder was visualized in only 55.6% of cases in their porcine model study. Using the SEMF technique from a retroflexed position, the submucosal tunnel can be directed cephalad and can effectively create a biologic endoscope and instrument guide into the upper abdominal cavity.[16] This cephalad access using the SEMF technique allowed visualization of the gallbladder in all eight attempts in our experiments with NOTES unassisted transgastric cholecystectomy using the porcine model (**Fig. 56.6**).

Transesophageal Thoracic Natural Orifice Transluminal Endoscopic Surgery

The transesophageal SEMF technique may provide the most appealing platform to allow safe access to important thoracic organs including the cardiovascular system.[11,17] For transesophageal SEMF, a long submucosal tunnel (8 to 10 cm) is longitudinally created with a 15-mm biliary occlusion balloon after preliminary CO_2 gas dissection, water dissection, or a "softening" mesna submucosal cushion over this length. Because the esophageal mucosa is thin, the mucosal entry site can be securely and simply closed by clip application. To access the thoracic cavity safely via the esophagus, a myotomy must be located in the distal esophagus because of the position of critical organs within the thoracic cavity. The muscularis propria is snare resected by cap EMR providing access to the posterior mediastinum (**Fig. 56.7** and see **Fig. 56.4**), which contains the descending thoracic aorta, the esophagus, the azygos vein, and the autonomic ganglia and nerves. These structures can be easily visualized with a SEMF transesophageal approach. The pleural cavity can be accessed through a pleural incision using a hook knife (Hook knife; Olympus, Tokyo, Japan) inserted through the endoscope retroflexed at the level of transesophageal entry.

We have accessed the epicardium using the transesophageal SEMF technique and successfully created a pericardial window. This approach has allowed endoscopic contact and coagulation of the epicardial surface testing the technical feasibility of cardiac interventions. After visual identification of the heart within the pleural cavity, our method included a pericardial puncture (2 to 3 mm) created with the hook knife followed by creation of a pericardial window (approximately 3 cm in length) with an insulated-tip needle-knife (IT knife; Olympus) (see **Fig. 56.5**). A point coagulation was performed on the exposed epicardium through the pericardial window with a heat probe (Olympus), with two to four pulses of 30 J, and a hook knife, with a monopolar coagulation current (30 W) while monitoring the cardiac rhythm. There were no rhythm disturbances. After a period of survival, no gross contamination or signs of contamination in the thoracic cavity were identified on necropsy. The pericardial space was normal in

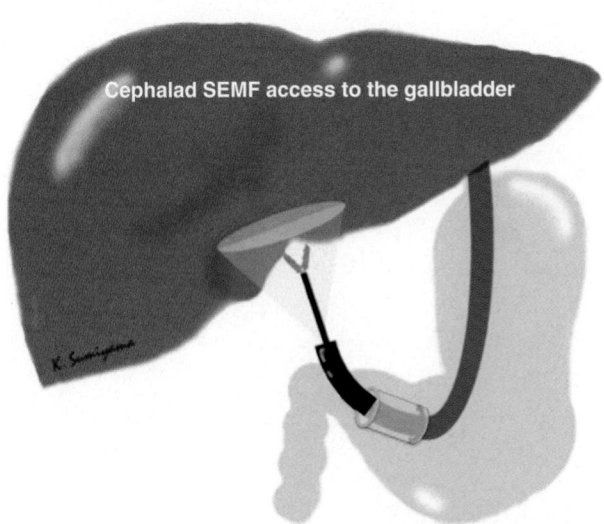

Fig. 56.6 Access to the gallbladder from the stomach with a cephalad submucosal endoscopy with mucosal flap (SEMF) technique. The submucosal tunnel can be directed cephalad, effectively creating a biologic endoscope and instrument guide into the upper abdominal cavity.

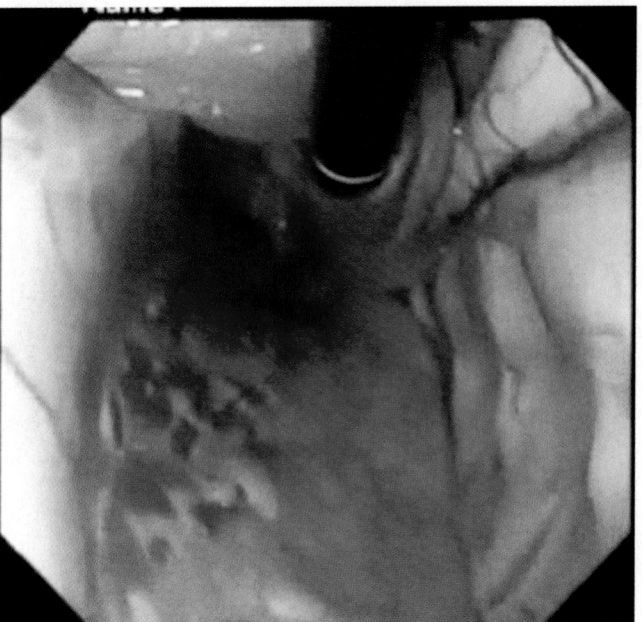

Fig. 56.7 Posterior mediastinum endoscopically accessed from the esophagus with the submucosal endoscopy with mucosal flap (SEMF) technique.

appearance. The epicardial coagulation sites were healing, without exudative ulceration.

Transgastric Peritoneoscopy for Preoperative Staging of Pancreatic Cancer

SEMF transgastric access to the peritoneal cavity has been clinically evaluated as a less invasive alternative to diagnostic peritoneoscopy for preoperative staging of pancreatic cancer.[18] The clinical procedure used a cephalad submucosal tunnel within the anterior gastric wall. The gastric access site was identified by transillumination and finger palpation over the anterior abdominal wall. A 3-cm long submucosal tunnel was created using an ESD technique. A small needle-knife incision of the seromuscular layer was made at the distal end of the tunnel and enlarged with a 15-mm dilation balloon for endoscopic access to the peritoneal cavity. Peritoneal exploration and biopsy were performed. The gastrostomy was closed with mucosal clip apposition of the tunnel entry site. This experience with five transgastric peritoneoscopies has been published.[19] The SEMF-based transgastric peritoneoscopy was negative in all cases, followed by radical surgical excision of the primary tumor. There were no procedure-related complications. Secure closure of the gastrostomy without leakage and the absence of peritoneal contamination were confirmed during the open portion of the operation.

Conclusion

The novel techniques described in this chapter have advanced flexible endoscopy into and beyond the gut wall. GI diseases involving the deeper wall layers hidden by an overlying normal mucosa and diseases in the extraluminal anatomic cavities can be potentially managed via a natural orifice SEMF approach exclusively using a flexible endoscope. Although further innovations are needed to establish these revolutionary methods firmly within standard medical practice, a door has been opened allowing a potentially exciting journey for flexible endoscopy as a result of these promising early efforts and experiences.

References

The complete reference list is available online at www.expertconsult.com.

Gastroduodenal and Colonic Endoprostheses

Gregory A. Coté and Steven A. Edmundowicz

Introduction

Since the 1990s, the development of self-expanding metal stents (SEMS) has increased the role of palliative and therapeutic endoscopy. Initially designed to address biliary and esophageal obstruction, enteral stents are now increasingly used to manage malignant upper intestinal and colonic obstruction. Before the advent of stent technology, nonsurgical options for patients with malignant bowel obstruction were limited to balloon dilation and intraluminal tumor debulking with thermal techniques such as neodymium:yttrium-aluminum-garnet (Nd:YAG) laser photoablation, bipolar ablation, and argon plasma coagulation. In the best circumstances, these interventions provided transient palliation of symptoms, but repeat procedures were required to maintain luminal patency. Surgical options such as resection and bypass are inherently more invasive and often limited by malnutrition in the patient and other comorbidities that limit the ability of the patient to recover successfully from the intervention.

With evolving stent technology, the potential indications for SEMS placement are steadily increasing. To avoid surgical intervention, endoscopists have extended the use of SEMS for many other indications with variable success. There are reports using SEMS for bowel obstruction from extraluminal malignancies, anastomotic leaks, benign colonic strictures, perforations, and fistulas. Although SEMS offer a potentially simpler alternative to surgery, there are important risks associated with the deployment and durability of these devices. Despite extensive experience using enteral stents for upper intestinal and colonic obstruction, prospective data comparing stents with surgical options are limited. This chapter reviews the technical characteristics of SEMS available for gastroduodenal and colonic obstruction. Available data for enteral stents in the management of upper intestinal and colonic obstruction are also reviewed. In reviewing the evidence, we focus on three fundamental outcomes associated with SEMS placement: rates

of technical success, clinical success, and complications. Technical success is defined as successful deployment of a stent across an obstructing stricture. Clinical success is defined as significant improvement or resolution of obstructive symptoms after stent placement.

Technical Review

Stent designs and deployment systems are evolving rapidly worldwide, with new devices arriving frequently on the market. Three SEMS for gastroduodenal use and two for colonic obstruction have been approved by the U.S. Food and Drug Administration (FDA) and are available in the United States (**Table 57.1**). These are all uncovered to reduce the risk of migration. Over time, uncovered SEMS are expected to be incorporated into the surrounding tissues.[1] These devices become permanent shortly after placement and require surgical resection for removal once there is significant tissue ingrowth through the mesh. No uncovered SEMS are approved by the FDA for benign disease at this time. Endoscopists should become familiar with several important characteristics of enteral stents, including their composition, lattice pattern and width, flexibility, expandability, deployment mechanism, and degree of foreshortening after placement in the bowel.[2]

The flexibility and expandability of a stent are directly related to its primary composition.[3] Most SEMS are made from shape-memory alloys such as nitinol (nickel-titanium) and Elgiloy (cobalt-chromium-nickel), which balance the need for strong radial forces to expand a malignant stricture while maintaining enough flexibility to minimize the risk of bowel perforation and allow for deployment in tortuous segments of the bowel. SEMS are made in one of two general designs. Stents with large delivery systems that cannot be passed through a therapeutic endoscope are often referred to

Table 57.1 Colonic and Enteral Stents Available in the United States in 2010

Name	Composition	Deployment Mechanism	Unconstrained Outer Diameter Body/Flare (mm)	Unconstrained Lengths (cm)	Foreshortening (%)
GASTRODUODENAL					
WallFlex Duodenal (Boston Scientific, Natick, MA)	Nitinol	TTS	22/27 proximal 25/30 proximal	6, 9, 12	30–38
Wallstent Duodenal (Boston Scientific)	Elgiloy	TTS	20/no flare 22/no flare	6, 9	39–49
COLONIC					
Colonic Z stent (Cook Medical, Bloomington, IN)	Stainless steel	Fluoroscopic	25/35 proximal and distal	4, 6, 8, 10, 12	None
Ultraflex Precision Colonic (Boston Scientific)	Nitinol	Fluoroscopic	25/30	6, 9, 12	23
WallFlex Colonic (Boston Scientific)	Nitinol	TTS	22/27 proximal 25/30 proximal	6, 9, 12	30–38

TTS, through the scope.

as over the wire enteral SEMS. These are typically designed for obstructions in the rectum and sigmoid colon and have a larger internal diameter when fully deployed. Most newer models are designed for through the scope (TTS) deployment, in which the stent is contained within a sheath that can be fitted into the working channel of a therapeutic endoscope (3.7-mm).

As additional stent designs from various manufacturers become commercially available, it is convenient to describe all stents by their characteristics: stent type (TTS or over the wire), design (woven or laser cut), covering, deployed length and diameter, shortening percentage at deployment, potential for reconstrainability during deployment, and size of the endoscope channel required to accommodate the deployment system. SEMS design allows stent placement under endoscopic and fluoroscopic visualization even in cases where the endoscope cannot traverse the stricture, provided that a guidewire and stent deployment system can be advanced into the correct position (**Fig. 57.1**). In this setting, a guidewire is advanced across the stricture, which may be facilitated by using a standard endoscopic retrograde cholangiopancreatography (ERCP) catheter or a multilumen biliary extraction balloon catheter. Contrast agent injection and fluoroscopy can be helpful in delineating the anatomy. Once the stenosis is engaged and passed with the guidewire, the balloon catheter can be advanced beyond the stenosis, and the length of the stricture can be measured using the inflated balloon and fluoroscopic image. The guidewire is left in place, and the initial catheter is exchanged for an appropriately sized SEMS system. The stent and sheath mechanism can be advanced over the guidewire without having to remove the endoscope. Once correctly positioned across the stricture, the stent can be released by an assistant as the stent position is carefully maintained by the endoscopist. Several stent deployment systems allow recapturing of the partially deployed stent if the position is suboptimal. Currently available TTS enteral stents continue to expand and foreshorten over several days after being released until the full external diameter is achieved. The

endoscopist should account for this in choosing the length and position of the stent before its deployment.

Exceptions to the TTS design are the Colonic Z stent (Cook Medical, Bloomington, IN) and the Ultraflex Precision Colonic stent (Boston Scientific, Natick, MA), which are released over a guidewire under fluoroscopic guidance. The endoscopist may choose to advance the endoscope alongside the stent mechanism, although this is more cumbersome, to visualize deployment endoscopically.

Malignant Gastroduodenal Obstruction

Tumors of the periampullary region, distal stomach, and proximal duodenum often manifest with symptoms of nausea and vomiting secondary to gastric outlet obstruction (GOO). Because most of these patients have unresectable disease, symptom palliation is typically the primary goal. Before the advent of SEMS, surgical gastrojejunostomy had been used to bypass the obstruction. Despite limiting surgical decompression to good surgical candidates, this option would still be associated with significant morbidity and mortality.[4]

Among patients with GOO, clinical success is typically defined as resolution of symptoms (nausea, vomiting) and tolerance of a soft diet. Comparative trials have shown the superiority of SEMS compared with surgical bypass in palliation of symptoms, length of hospitalization, and cost-effectiveness.[5–9] A systematic review of 606 cases of GOO reported technical success and clinical response rates to enteral stent placement of 97% and 87%.[10] Newer stent designs such as the WallFlex Enteral stent (Boston Scientific) and the Niti-S Enteral Colonic stent (Taewoong Medical Co., Ltd., Kyonggi-Do, South Korea) are promoted for their greater flexibility while maintaining sufficient radial forces to open strictures.[11–13] These stents have blunt woven ends theoretically to reduce the risk of wire penetration and subsequent

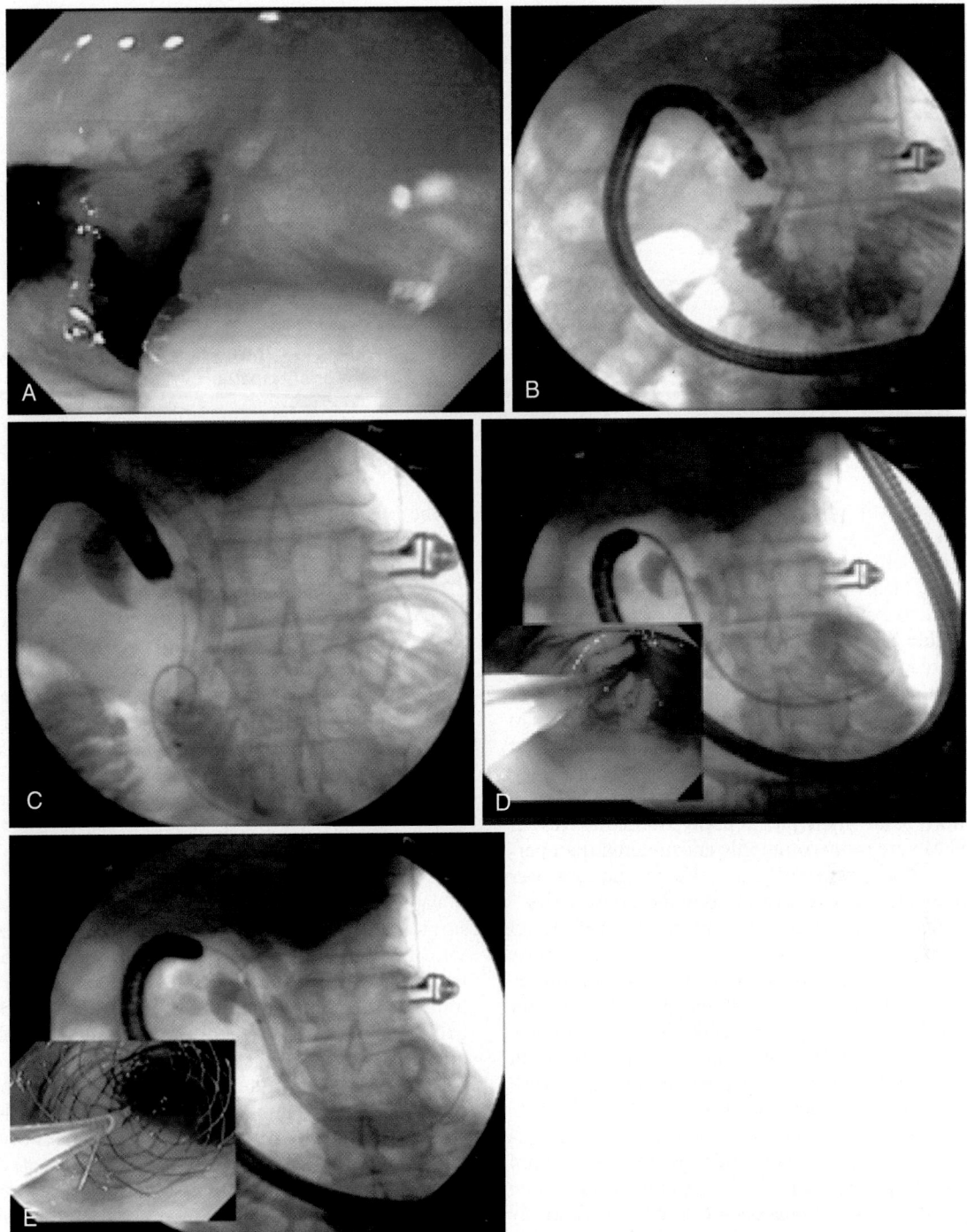

Fig. 57.1 Through the scope placement of an enteral stent across a duodenal stricture. **A** and **B,** Obstructing malignant stricture is visualized in the duodenal sweep (**A**) and demarcated using fluoroscopy (**B**). A previous biliary metallic stent is seen only on fluoroscopy. **C,** A balloon catheter is used to advance a 0.035-inch stiff guidewire across the stricture, aided by a combination of endoscopy and fluoroscopy. **D,** The endoscope is withdrawn to the antrum, where the stent catheter is advanced over the guidewire and centered across the stricture. **E,** The stent is deployed by slowly withdrawing its sheath, allowing its proximal margin to flare in the antrum.

perforation. As a result of its woven design, the Niti-S stent has less foreshortening (23%) compared with other TTS enteral stents, but the clinical significance of this characteristic is unclear.[12] Although there are no comparative trials available, case series using these stents suggest their equivalence to older devices. A multicenter, randomized study comparing the Enteral WallFlex stent with surgical gastrojejunostomy suggested better short-term (<2 months) clinical improvement after stent placement but more favorable long-term results with surgical bypass.[14] Although stent placement was associated with lower initial inpatient costs, the differences in long-term costs and incremental cost-effectiveness of either approach are minimal.[15] When deciding between endoprosthetic placement and surgery, the patient's comorbidities and

Table 57.2 Potential Complications of Enteral Stenting

Complication	Frequency by Location		Notes
	Gastroduodenal	*Colonic*	
Perforation	+	++	Perforation may occur early (<7 days) or late (>7 days)
			Sites are usually within malignant stricture or at stent margin
Migration	++	++	Migration rates highest among patients undergoing chemotherapy
Bleeding	+	+	
Recurrent obstruction	+++	++	Recurrent obstruction may develop as a result of restenosis secondary to tumor or hyperplastic tissue ingrowth and food or fecal impaction
			Rates expected to increase over time
Biliary obstruction	+	NA	Placement of a biliary metallic stent before a duodenal stent is recommended if biliary obstruction is present or anticipated

NA, not applicable.

anticipated long-term prognosis are the most important considerations.

Complications of stent placement for GOO include perforation, bleeding, stent migration, restenosis, biliary obstruction, and failure to expand fully, despite technically successful placement (**Table 57.2**).[10,16] Perforation (0.7%) and bleeding (0.5%) rates are low, but these are potentially life-threatening complications that warrant discussion with the patient. Newer stent designs advertise greater flexibility and blunt ends to reduce the rate of perforation, but there are no data to support these claims.[11,12]

Stent migration and restenosis secondary to tumor ingrowth or granulation tissue hyperplasia between the lattices of uncovered SEMS are more commonly encountered than perforation. As expected, restenosis rates steadily increase over time, with an incidence of 18% reported in the largest series.[10] Given the limited life expectancy of many patients with GOO secondary to malignant obstruction, stent restenosis is more likely to occur in patients who are likely to survive beyond the limited life expectancy of patients with malignant GOO. Stent migration may be more likely in patients who are treatment-naïve and expected to undergo systemic chemotherapy. Both stent migration and restenosis can often be managed with placement of additional endoprostheses.

There are limited cases where an enteral stent is appropriately deployed but fails to expand fully across the stricture because of inadequate radial forces pushing against the obstructing tumor. If symptoms persist despite a technically successful procedure, an upper gastrointestinal series using Gastrografin solution (if a perforation is also suspected) or barium may clarify the luminal diameter and expansion of the stent.

Covered SEMS have been considered to address the issue of tumor ingrowth. However, migration rates of 10% to 20% have limited their use.[17,18] Kim and associates[19] published their series of 213 patients with GOO who underwent placement of a layered dual nitinol endoprosthesis composed of a partially covered outer stent overlying an inner, uncovered stent. The reported migration rate of 4% was markedly lower than rates reported in other series of covered SEMS, and the mean patency period was 324 days. Although the rate of biliary obstruction in this series was low (2%), biliary obstruction may occur more frequently with covered SEMS, and access

to the biliary tree is significantly limited after deployment. Generally, because access to the papilla is limited by duodenal stents, placement of a biliary SEMS before a duodenal SEMS is recommended for patients with impending or concurrent biliary obstruction.[3] In a series of 176 patients who underwent enteral stent placement, the rate of cholangitis after stent placement was 6% (9 patients); all patients with cholangitis had received an enteral stent that traversed the major papilla.[20] Endoscopic drainage of the bile duct was technically successful in only two of six patients who underwent attempted ERCP.

Colonic Obstruction

Malignant obstruction of the large bowel was traditionally a surgical emergency that required urgent decompression. Historically, surgeons performed a Hartmann's procedure, in which the primary tumor was resected and a diverting colostomy was created to decompress the proximal colon.[21] Patients had to wait at least 8 weeks for colostomy reversal, although many had to wait longer or never underwent the procedure because of age and underlying comorbidities.[22] The presence of a colostomy is unquestionably associated with a significantly lower quality of life.[23] The management of these cases has significantly changed with the advent of endoscopic devices for colonic decompression. Stents placed for malignant colonic obstruction can serve as a bridge to a single-stage surgical resection or as a palliative measure in patients with advanced disease.

With successful placement of a stent, patients can receive a full bowel preparation before undergoing a single-stage resection with reanastomosis. In addition to avoiding a colostomy, a prepared colon may be inspected to rule out a synchronous tumor at the time of surgery. No randomized, controlled trials have compared emergency surgery with endoscopic placement of a stent as a bridge to surgery in acute malignant colonic obstruction. However, in a meta-analysis of the published literature comparing stent placement with open surgery, stent placement was associated with a shorter hospital stay, lower mortality, fewer medical complications, and reduced rate of stoma formation.[24] In a pooled analysis of 1198 patients who underwent placement of a colonic stent for acute malignant obstruction, the technical and clinical success rates were 94% and 91%.[25] Comparable success rates were reported in multiple case series using newer stent designs.[26–31] In a multicenter series of 36 patients, 94% were successfully bridged to a single-stage resection within 2 weeks of stent placement.[27]

In the largest published series of colonic stents, technical and clinical failure rates were highest in patients with right-sided colonic lesions and patients with large bowel obstruction secondary to extrinsic compression.[25] Subsequent publications reporting on the use of colonic stents for obstruction secondary to extrinsic lesions confirmed a significantly lower success rate.[32,33] Stent placement in the proximal colon has become more feasible with the TTS design, provided that the endoscope can be straightened before advancing the stent sheath through the working channel.[29] Distal rectal strictures within several centimeters of the anal verge are also problematic because the stent is more likely to cause significant perianal discomfort.[34] Decision models based on available data suggest colonic stent placement is a dominant strategy compared with emergency surgery because it reduces the number of operations, the need for a stoma, and costs.[35,36] An ongoing clinical trial is comparing a surgery-first with stent-first approach to acute, left-sided malignant colonic obstruction.[37]

Although the feasibility of colonic stents as a bridge to surgery is well established, data are conflicting on the use of stents for long-term palliation. A randomized trial comparing surgical palliation with endoscopic stent placement (WallFlex Colonic) was closed after only 21 patients were enrolled because of a high rate of perforation in the stent group.[38] Although no perforations occurred during stent placement, six of nine patients returned with perforations during the follow-up period. The authors speculated the perforations might be related to the particular stent used in this trial because three of six patients developed perforations related to erosions through normal colonic wall. However, other open-label and registry studies have not shown such a dramatic perforation rate.[39–42] A case series of 50 patients who underwent placement of a different colonic stent (Ultraflex Precision Colonic) for palliation led to durable relief in symptoms in 81% after 6 months of follow-up.[28] No perforations were reported in this series.

Perforation is observed more frequently with colonic compared with gastroduodenal stents, with a reported rate of 3.8% in the largest compilation.[25] The risk seems to be highest in patients who undergo balloon dilation of the malignant stricture before stent deployment.[25,26] Delayed perforations have been reported several months after deployment.[38] Stent migration most commonly occurs within the first week after placement and is observed more frequently with right-sided lesions. In addition, recurrent obstruction may occur 1 year after decompression, often related to tumor ingrowth or fecal impaction. Newer designs have incorporated a wider proximal flare to facilitate passage of stool, although data supporting this theory are lacking.[26] Tumor ingrowth does not seem to occur more frequently with stents that have a wider mesh.[26]

Covered stents have a lower rate of recurrent obstruction (4.7% vs. 7.8%), but migration rates of 30% compared with approximately 11% with uncoated stents have precluded their widespread adoption.[25] A dual nitinol stent was designed to address the issue of migration associated with covered devices.

This stent combines an inner, bare nitinol stent with an outer device that is bare nitinol at its margins but nylon in the middle (S&G Biotech, Seongnam, Korea). Song and colleagues[43] published their experience with this device in 147 patients with malignant colon obstruction. Overall, technical and clinical success rates were greater than 90%, comparable with other series. Although the rates of tumor ingrowth and stent migration were favorable, the perforation rate was 22% in the bridge to surgery group and 5% in the palliative group. Further developments in covered stent technology are necessary before their widespread use for long-term palliation of colonic obstruction becomes standard practice.

Alternative Indications

As SEMS have become widely available, physicians have investigated their role in the management of benign diseases. The absence of a durable, safe, and removable enteral stent precludes the use of stents in benign disease at the present time. Potential applications for SEMS in the colon may include strictures related to radiation, inflammatory bowel disease, or previous diverticulitis and ischemic colitis.[44–46] In the largest series of 23 patients, delayed (defined as >7 days after deployment) complications occurred more frequently.[44] Five patients in this series had colonic fistulas complicating their benign strictures, all of which responded to stent therapy.

Covered stent technology also offers the potential for treating anastomotic leaks. Initial experience was limited to esophageal pathology such as fistulas, anastomotic leaks, and perforations.[47–51] Most reports described off-label use of self-expanding plastic stents designed and approved by the FDA for subsequent removal from the esophagus. As expected, these stents have a significantly higher risk of migration.[47] Nevertheless, gastroenterologists have emerged in an area that was previously dominated by interventional radiologists and thoracic surgeons.[52] More recently, coated stents have also been applied successfully in the management of anastomotic leaks after Roux-en-Y gastric bypass surgery, with success rates approaching 80%.[50,53–55] To facilitate removal of a partially covered metallic stent, Eisendrath and coworkers[54] inserted a self-expanding plastic stent through the SEMS to induce necrosis of the granulation tissue that had developed along the margins of the SEMS. Eleven patients returned several weeks later for removal of both devices. No rigorous clinical trials comparing SEMS with surgical alternatives for the management of benign diseases have been reported to date. The widespread application of SEMS for benign indications depends on the development of a stent that is effective (having adequate flexibility and expandability), durable (low migration rate with prolonged follow-up), and removable (associated with minimal tumor and granulation tissue ingrowth).

Conclusion

Endoscopic placement of enteral stents is an established alternative to surgical decompression. For many patients with malignant gastrointestinal obstruction, SEMS may be their only prospect for symptom palliation and resumption of oral intake. The benefit of colonic stents as a bridge to a single-stage resection for obstructing left-sided colon cancers is unquestionable. The durability and efficacy of SEMS for long-term palliation of upper intestinal and colonic obstruction should improve as enteral stent technology evolves. For patients with benign disease, removable devices may reduce the need for surgical or percutaneous interventions. Although endoscopic stent placement is safe, patients and physicians should be well informed of the potential complications associated with their deployment.

References

The complete reference list is available online at www.expertconsult.com.

Electronically Enhanced Endoscopic Imaging

Anna M. Buchner

Introduction

Detection and prevention of gastrointestinal (GI) malignancies is a primary goal of endoscopy that is achieved through identification and eradication of preneoplastic lesions. Emerging electronically enhanced endoscopic imaging technologies aim not only at the detection of early and precursor preneoplastic lesions but also their accurate characterization and confirmation during endoscopy.

Although *ex vivo histology* remains the current standard of confirming all lesions, the concept of real-time *in vivo histology* of lesions or *optical biopsies* during ongoing endoscopy has been introduced.[1] In vivo histology could play an important role in a busy GI endoscopy practice not only in diagnosing small lesions of otherwise unknown significance before making a decision regarding their necessary resection but also in targeting biopsies and directing treatment decisions during surveillance endoscopic evaluation, such as in inflammatory bowel disease or Barrett's esophagus.

Electronically enhanced endoscopy is also expected to improve lesion detection rates. Conventional white light videoendoscopy was found to be associated with alarming miss rates for subtle lesions (e.g., flat and depressed adenomas).[2] Even experienced gastroenterologists can miss 6% of advanced adenomas and 30% of all adenomas.[3,4] Some studies confirmed the development of colorectal cancer, especially in the right site of the colon, despite a surveillance colonoscopy program.[5,6] Because subtle dysplastic and early neoplastic lesions are often not easily recognized during regular standard white light endoscopy, electronically enhanced endoscopic technologies are intended to improve their detection. These electronically enhanced imaging technologies including broad field and point fields (**Table 58.1**) combined together are expected to improve diagnostic yield and to allow in vivo

histology diagnosis, minimize the burden of unnecessary biopsies, and lead to immediate decisions for definitive management.

Broad Field Image Enhancement Techniques: High-Resolution Endoscopy, Virtual Chromoendoscopy, and Other Optical Techniques

Broad image enhanced endoscopy (IEE) technologies include traditional dye-based IEE with chromoendoscopy and optical methods including equipment-based IEE with narrow band imaging (NBI), electronically based IEE with spectral estimation technologies such as Fuji Intelligent Chromo Endoscopy (FICE) and i-Scan, and autofluorescence imaging (AFI).[7] These technologies are used with more recently developed high-resolution endoscopes.

High-Resolution and High-Definition Endoscopy

The key element of all videoendoscopes is a charge-coupled device (CCD)—an integrated electrical circuit that is composed of photosensitive silicone semiconductors. The CCD surface consists of photosensitive elements (pixels) that generate an electrical charge in proportion to light exposure and then generate an analog signal that is digitalized by the computer videoprocessor. CCDs in standard videoendoscopes have 100,000 to 300,000 pixels. These standard endoscopes have a focal distance of 1 to 9 cm, and images appear out of

Table 58.1 Methods of Enhanced Endoscopic Imaging

Methods	Technology	Aims
Broad field electronic enhancement technologies	Virtual chromoendoscopy: NBI, i-Scan, AFI	Increased mucosal contrast and detection of flat and depressed lesions
Point field electronic enhancement technologies	Endoscope-based CLE, probe-based CLE	In vivo histology

AFI, autofluorescence imaging; CLE, confocal laser endomicroscopy; NBI, narrow band imaging.

focus if they are beyond this range. Over the last decade, endoscopes with high-density CCDs (600,000 to 1 million pixels per CCD) have been developed, and they are referred to as high-resolution endoscopes. High-resolution endoscopes are capable of producing high-magnification images with increased spatial resolution for the detection of minute abnormalities in mucosal glandular and vascular structures. In conjunction with a movable lens for magnification endoscopy, the focal distance may be controlled to allow detailed examination of the mucosal surface at close range (<3 mm). In addition, high-resolution endoscopes can provide enlargement of the image up to 150× compared with 30× with standard endoscopes.

High-definition (HD) systems can display 1080 scanning lines on a screen compared with standard definition analog systems, which can generate 576 scanning lines. These HD endoscopes with high-density couple charge devices, combined with HD 1080-line television monitors, produce images with increased spatial resolution. A high-definition imaging system was used in more recent trials and showed very high adenoma detection rates greater than 50% in screening patients with average colorectal cancer risk.[8–11]

The use of HD colonoscopy was associated with a higher adenoma detection rate compared with SD colonoscopy in a large cohort study of 2430 patients.[12] This higher rate was most apparent for smaller adenomas (<10 mm) and adenomas in the left colon. Other colonoscopic studies comparing standard definition white light endoscopy with HD white light endoscopy have revealed mixed results.[11,13–15] In a study by East and colleagues[11] of 132 patients undergoing routine screening colonoscopies by one dedicated and highly experienced endoscopist, adenoma detection rate was higher with HD colonoscopy (71% vs. 60%), but this trend did not reach statistical significance in the group of 58 HD patients and 72 standard definition patients. Pellise and coworkers[13] showed no statistically significant advantage in detection of adenomas (HD, 26%; standard definition, 25%) and all polyps (HD, 43%; standard definition, 38%) using a HD colonoscope versus a standard definition colonoscope in 639 patients undergoing routine screening colonoscopy. However, this study was underpowered to detect small differences between groups in a population with a prevalence of adenomas of less than 30%, which is typical of average-risk individuals.

Further studies are needed to determine whether the use of a HD system independently increases neoplasia detection in a general endoscopy practice. The additional advantage of a HD system is that it can be used with any wide field image enhancement technologies such as virtual chromoendoscopy NBI, FICE, i-Scan, and AFI or point field image enhancement techniques such as confocal laser endomicroscopy (CLE), and all techniques combined may lead to better detection of subtle lesions and differentiation between neoplastic and nonneoplastic lesions.

Narrow Band Imaging

NBI (Olympus Corp, Tokyo, Japan) is a method of virtual chromoendoscopy that has a potential to improve detection of mucosal abnormalities without time-consuming and impractical application of chromic agents. NBI is currently the most investigated advanced endoscopic imaging technique for the detection of Barrett's dysplasia and colorectal polyps (**Fig. 58.1**). Conventional white light endoscopy uses the full visible wavelength range (400 to 700 nm) to produce a red/green/blue image, whereas NBI combined with magnification endoscopy illuminates the tissue surface using special filters that narrow the red/green/blue bands and simultaneously increases the relative intensity of the blue band.

The technology was developed by Gono and associates[16] in 1999 as a joint project of the Japanese National Cancer Center Hospital East and Olympus Corporation. The investigators studied variations of conventional endoscopy that potentially could visualize early changes of angiogenesis associated with the development of dysplasia and superficial neoplasia. Using light filters, the contribution of blue light is increased by narrowing the band widths of the red, green, and blue components of the excitation light and reducing the amount of green light and eliminating the red light. The resulting "narrow band" blue/green light improves imaging of mucosal patterns because of the limited optical scattering and shallow penetration depth. This blue light is also absorbed by hemoglobin (because the hemoglobin absorption band [Soret band] lies at 415 nm) for optimal detection of mucosal glandular and vascular patterns and the presence of abnormal blood vessels that are associated with the development of dysplasia.

Numerous studies have shown the value of this technology in the evaluation of patients with upper GI lesions including Barrett's esophagus dysplasia and gastric lesions.[17,18] The systematic review by Curvers and associates[18] summarized performance and clinical utility of NBI in upper GI endoscopy with a focus on the primary detection of premalignant lesions and the differentiation between neoplastic and nonneoplastic lesions.

A prospective, blinded, tandem study in 65 patients referred for evaluation of Barrett's dysplasia by Wolfsen and colleagues[17] showed that in patients evaluated for Barrett's esophagus with dysplasia, NBI detected significantly more patients with dysplasia and higher grades of dysplasia with fewer biopsy samples compared with standard resolution endoscopy. Specifically, NBI-targeted biopsies found dysplasia in more patients (37 patients [57%]) compared with standard resolution endoscopy with targeted plus random biopsies (28 patients [43%]; $P < .001$). NBI also found higher grades of dysplasia in 12 patients (18%) compared with no cases in which standard resolution endoscopy with targeted and random biopsies detected a high grade of histology (0%; $P < .001$). In addition, more biopsy samples were taken using

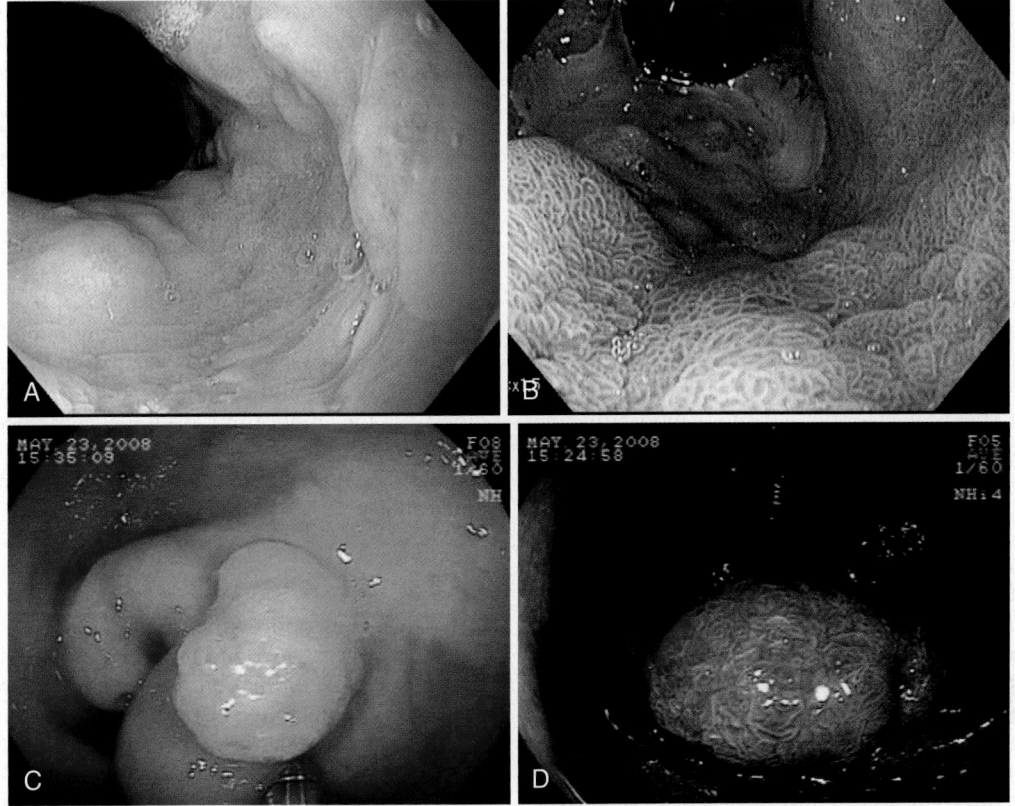

Fig. 58.1 A–D, High-definition (HD) white light image and HD narrow band imaging (NBI) of Barrett's esophagus with focal high-grade dysplasia and intramucosal adenocarcinoma (**A** and **B**) and large tubulovillous adenoma of the colon (**C** and **D**).

standard resolution endoscopy with targeted plus random biopsies (mean 8.5 biopsy samples per case) compared with NBI-directed biopsies (mean 4.7 biopsy samples per case; $P <$ .001). This ability of high-resolution endoscopy combined with NBI to detect dysplasia in significantly more patients with Barrett's esophagus using fewer biopsy specimens supports the role of this technology in surveillance evaluation.

NBI technology was also evaluated for the detection of colorectal lesions.[19,20] More recent studies revealed conflicting results with overall no improvement of adenoma detection rates.[9,21,22] In a study by Adler and coworkers[23] of 401 patients randomly assigned to undergo either standard definition colonoscopy or NBI colonoscopy, a higher adenoma detection rate in the NBI group compared with the standard group (23% vs. 17%) was shown in the initial phase of the study, suggesting a learning effect with the introduction of a new method influencing the conventional technology as well.

The use of NBI for the detection of dysplasia in long-standing ulcerative colitis has not led to improvement of neoplasia detection.[24] East and colleagues[25] showed that NBI improved adenoma detection in high-risk patients with hereditary nonpolyposis colorectal cancer syndrome, in whom a second additional colonoscopic examination with NBI doubled the total number of adenomas detected. A systematic review by van den Broek and coworkers[22] summarized data on the performance and clinical utility of NBI during colonoscopy. Their review did not show a significant improvement in adenoma detection using NBI, but it confirmed the value of NBI for differentiation of neoplastic from nonneoplastic colonic polyps when used by experts.

The main advantage of NBI seems to be not detection but rather characterization because NBI has a high sensitivity of 90% to 95% and a specificity of 80% to 85% for differentiation of neoplastic from nonneoplastic lesions.[26] Based on available studies, this level of accuracy is comparable to that of expert chromoendoscopists.[27,28] It is anticipated that with appropriate training, NBI will be used routinely for lesion discrimination and management.

More recent trials confirmed very high accuracy of NBI for the diagnosis of small colorectal lesions (<10 mm) in selected cases of high-quality and high-confidence stored images interpreted offline.[29,30] Rex[29] introduced the concept of confidence levels to the endoscopic interpretation of colorectal polyp histology. This concept allowed sufficient accuracy (>91%) for the use of NBI to identify distal hyperplastic polyps that do not need resection and to plan postpolypectomy surveillance without pathologic evaluation of polyps 5 mm or smaller.[29]

Ignjatovic and colleagues[30] showed that for polyps less than 10 mm, in vivo optical diagnosis using NBI as virtual chromoendoscopy or in a few cases dye-based chromoendoscopy can be an acceptable approach for polyp characterization. Wada and associates[31] showed that both NBI and chromoendoscopy can be useful in distinguishing between neoplastic and nonneoplastic colorectal lesions based on analysis of pit pattern and vascular patterns.

Rastogi and coworkers[32] also showed that using a simple surface mucosal and vascular pattern classification, NBI without magnification was highly accurate and significantly superior to high-definition white light imaging for prediction of adenomas. It is anticipated that with appropriate training,

NBI will be used routinely for better lesion discrimination and characterization.

Fluorescence and Trimodal Imaging

Fluorescence imaging endoscopy uses techniques that distinguish tissue types based on their differences in fluorescence emission. When the tissue is exposed to short-wavelength light, endogenous fluorophores are excited leading to emission of fluorescent light of a longer wavelength (AFI). Because of changes of endogenous fluorophores in normal, dysplastic, and neoplastic mucosa, the altered autofluorescence is reflected by a pseudocolored image of normal mucosa (green color) and images of dysplasia or neoplasia of varying tones of red/purple color. AFI has been incorporated into trimodal imaging endoscopes that combine high-resolution white light endoscopy and virtual chromoendoscopy with NBI.

In a prospective randomized study, AFI endoscopy significantly increased the diagnostic yield of surveillance endoscopy to detect intraepithelial neoplasia in high-risk patients with ulcerative colitis.[33] However, AFI has not been shown to enhance the diagnostic yield of screening colonoscopy in a tandem colonoscopy trial by the same group.[34]

Curvers and colleagues[35] published the initial results of four expert endoscopy centers using trimodal imaging for the evaluation of 84 patients with Barrett's dysplasia in their uncontrolled trial. The use of AFI increased the number of patients found to have high-grade dysplasia from 53% to 90%. The use of NBI reduced the false-positive rate of AFI from 81% to 26%. The same group more recently published their subsequent randomized crossover trial evaluating endoscopic trimodal imaging (ETMI), which combines high-resolution endoscopy, NBI, and AFI for the detection of high-grade dysplasia and early cancer of Barrett's esophagus.[36] The ETMI system improved the targeted detection of high-grade dysplasia and early cancer compared with standard white light endoscopy, although NBI was found to have a limited value in characterizing the mucosal changes. Based on these results, ETMI cannot replace random biopsies for the detection of lesions and targeted biopsies for characterization of the lesions.

A subsequent study by the same group[37] compared the role of ETMI with standard definition endoscopy for the detection of neoplasia in 99 patients with Barrett's esophagus in their community practice. ETMI had a significantly higher targeted histologic yield because of additional detection of 22 lesions with low-grade intraepithelial neoplasia, high-grade intraepithelial neoplasia (HGIN), or carcinoma by AFI. There was no significant difference in the overall histologic yield (targeted plus random) between ETMI and standard definition endoscopy. HGIN or carcinoma was diagnosed only by random biopsies in 6 of 24 patients and 7 of 24 patients with ETMI and standard definition endoscopy. ETMI performed in a community-based setting did not improve the overall detection of dysplasia compared with standard definition endoscopy. The diagnosis of dysplasia still required identification of a significant number of patients with dysplasia by random biopsies.

Overall studies on AFI for colorectal adenoma have shown very mixed results. Matsuda and colleagues[38] showed that AFI detected more polyps in the right-sided colon compared with white light colonoscopy. van den Broek and coworkers[39] evaluated interobserver agreement and accuracy for differentiation of polyps among experienced and nonexperienced gastroenterologists and confirmed that AFI had higher interobserver agreement and accuracy for diagnosing polyps than NBI. In a randomized prospective study, Takeuchi[40] showed that AFI colonoscopy with a transparent hood detected significantly more colorectal neoplasms than conventional colonoscopy without a hood. Overall, studies on AFI have shown very mixed results, and the future application of AFI is still to be determined.

The experience with trimodal endoscopy systems combining AFI, high-resolution endoscopy, and NBI is based so far on expert endoscopists evaluating their use for detection of dysplasia and carcinoma and seems very promising. However, the application of these combined technologies has not been yet studied in routine endoscopy practice settings. Further studies are needed to determine clinical applicability.

FICE and i-Scan

NBI depends on optical filters within the light source, whereas the FICE system, introduced by Fujinon, is based on a computed spectral estimation technology processing of the reflected photons to reconstruct virtual images with a choice of different wavelengths. A similar system, i-Scan, has been developed by Pentax. Both of these systems are based on physical principles similar to NBI, but they are not dependent on optical filters. These systems lead to enhancement of the tissue microvasculature as a result of the differential optical absorption of light by hemoglobin in the mucosa.

The FICE system was used to evaluate esophageal neoplasia and showed improvement in detection of early neoplasia.[41] In this prospective crossover randomized pilot study, the detection of HGIN or early cancer in 57 patients with Barrett's esophagus was compared using conventional chromoendoscopy with acetic acid with the FICE system. The sensitivity of targeted biopsies for HGIN or early cancer on a "per lesion" basis was 87% (26 of 30) for chromoendoscopy and FICE. Computed virtual chromoendoscopy is a helpful adjunct for surveillance of Barrett's esophagus and seems to be as accurate as conventional chromoendoscopy in the detection of HGIN or early cancer.

The FICE system can be useful in evaluation of colorectal neoplasia. However, in the prospective randomized trial of tandem colonoscopy by Chung and associates,[42] there was also no objective advantage of the FICE technique over conventional high-resolution endoscopy in terms of improved adenoma detection rate. The adenoma miss rate with FICE showed no significant difference compared with white light colonoscopy (6.6% vs. 8.3%; $P = .59$).

In a prospective randomized trial, Pohl and associates[43] compared a computed virtual chromoendoscopy system (FICE) with other modalities such as standard colonoscopy and conventional chromoendoscopy with indigo carmine in low-magnification and high-magnification modes for determination of colonic lesion histology. Based on this study, the FICE system was able to identify morphologic details that efficiently predict adenomatous histology and was superior to standard colonoscopy and equivalent to conventional chromoendoscopy. The same investigators were also able to show that computed virtual chromoendoscopy is a helpful adjunct

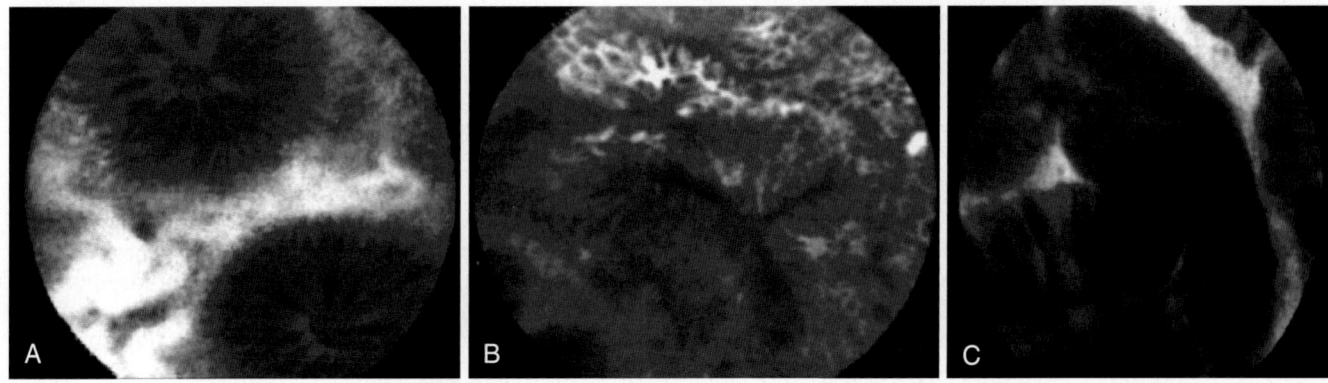

Fig. 58.2 **A–C,** Confocal endomicroscopy image (probe-based confocal laser endomicroscopy) of normal colonic mucosa, hyperplastic polyp, and tubular adenoma.

for surveillance of Barrett's esophagus, and it seems to be as accurate as traditional chromoendoscopy in the detection of HGIN or early cancer.[41]

Hoffman and coworkers[44] showed that high-definition endoscopy combined with i-Scan is significantly superior in detecting colorectal neoplasia compared with standard videocolonoscopy, and it allows prediction of histology of the identified lesions and surface enhancement. In their study, high-definition endoscopy plus colonoscopy with i-Scan identified significantly more patients with at least one neoplasm compared with standard resolution endoscopy (38% vs. 13%; $P < .001$). The histology of polyps was predicted accurately with i-Scan with a sensitivity of 98% and a specificity of 100% (95% confidence interval sensitivity 90.6 to 99.6, specificity 92.8 to 100.) Although the techniques of NBI, FICE, and i-Scan are very promising, further studies are needed to evaluate their final application not only in tertiary referral centers but also in routine endoscopy practices in terms of efficiency and cost-effectiveness in both detection and characterization of malignant GI lesions.

Confocal Laser Endomicroscopy

CLE is a novel tool that allows real-time imaging of GI mucosa at cellular and subcellular levels during endoscopy and yields in vivo histopathology. It can replace conventional biopsies with in vivo optical biopsies. CLE can be performed using one of two devices approved by the U.S. Food and Drug Administration (FDA): endoscope-based CLE endomicroscopy (Pentax, Fort Wayne, NJ) and a probe-based CLE system (Cellvizio; Mauna Kea Technologies, Paris, France). Confocal systems have been used in combination with virtual chromoendoscopy (NBI, i-Scan, FICE) for detection and characterization of subtle mucosal abnormalities and circumscribed lesions. When the targeted lesion or mucosal abnormality is detected, it can be interrogated by the confocal system for in vivo histology.

The principle of CLE is based on tissue illumination with a low-power laser allowing a better spatial resolution with 1000× magnification. Because both illumination and detection systems are on the same plane, images are not contaminated by light scattering from other planes. To obtain images, exogenous fluorescence contrast is required with agents such as fluorescein (10% solution, intravenous application),

acriflavine hydrochloride (topical application), or cresyl violet (topical application).

Intravenous fluorescein (1.0 to 5.0 mL of 10% solution) distributes throughout the capillary network and connective matrix, whereas acriflavine accumulates in superficial epithelial cells and nuclei, which raised a concern for a potential mutagenic risk and limited its broader use. In a cross-sectional survey of 16 international medical centers with active research protocols involving 2272 patients, no serious adverse events were reported with the use of intravenous fluorescein.[45]

Numerous studies have supported the application of both CLE systems, endoscope-based and probe-based, as novel tools for in vivo histopathology in various clinical settings, including colorectal neoplasia (**Fig. 58.2**), Barrett's esophagus, and ulcerative colitis.[46–49] The CLE systems have been shown to distinguish accurately dysplastic Barrett's esophagus from nondysplastic Barrett's esophagus.[46,50] In the initial pilot study, Kiesslich and colleagues[46] developed criteria for gastric mucosa, intestinal metaplasia, and neoplastic epithelium based on the confocal vascular and cellular features. It enabled prediction of Barrett's esophagus dysplasia versus nondysplasia with a sensitivity of 93% and specificity of 98%.

These initial results have been validated further in a prospective randomized crossover study comparing standard endoscopy with random biopsy and endomicroscopy (endoscope-based CLE) with targeted biopsies.[51] CLE with targeted biopsy almost doubled the diagnostic yield for endoscopically inapparent Barrett's esophagus neoplasia (from 17% to 33%) in 16 patients. Two-thirds of 23 patients in the surveillance group did not need any mucosal biopsies at all because no neoplasia was present during endomicroscopic imaging. CLE with targeted biopsy also greatly reduces the number of biopsies needed per patient and allows some patients without neoplasia to forgo mucosal biopsy.[15]

The other confocal system—probe-based CLE—has been also tested in Barrett's esophagus. Pohl and colleagues[43] developed probe-based CLE criteria for neoplastic Barrett's esophagus that included irregular epithelial lining, variable width of epithelial lining, fusion of glands, presence of dark areas, and an irregular vascular pattern. These criteria were established based on 95 biopsy specimens from 15 patients and were validated prospectively in 23 patients with assessment of not only accuracy of probe-based CLE but also interobserver agreement. The overall sensitivity, specificity, positive predictive value, and negative predictive value were 80%, 94%, 44%, and

99%, with good interobserver agreement ($\kappa = 0.6$). Subsequently, Wallace and colleagues[50] evaluated the accuracy of probe-based CLE for prediction of dysplasia and dysplastic Barrett's esophagus among endoscopists and estimated overall sensitivity of 88% and specificity of 96% with good interobserver agreement ($\kappa = 0.72$).

The probe-based CLE criteria also have been validated more recently in a large multicenter randomized controlled trial (DON'T BIOPCE trial) that used blinded endoscopists to perform tandem endoscopic procedures to evaluate the sensitivity and specificity of probe-based CLE, in addition to white light endoscopy, for the detection of high-grade dysplasia and early adenocarcinoma in Barrett's esophagus.[52] Preliminary data on 39 patients with Barrett's esophagus and 51 suspicious lesions and 245 random locations showed sensitivity of white light endoscopy, white light endoscopy plus NBI, and probe-based CLE to be 0.32, 0.46, and 0.59 and specificity to be 0.92, 0.91, and 0.89.

Both systems have been shown to improve accuracy in diagnosing colorectal neoplasia.[47,49] Kiesslich and colleagues[47] published the first report of the use of endoscope-based CLE in 42 patients during ongoing colonoscopy in diagnosing intraepithelial neoplasia and colorectal cancer. After staining with methylene blue, 134 small lesions (mean size 4 mm) were identified during colonoscopy. With the help of the confocal endoscope, intraepithelial neoplasia could be predicted with a sensitivity of 97% and a specificity of 99% (accuracy 99%). Buchner and associates[49] compared virtual chromoendoscopy systems (NBI, FICE) with probe-based CLE for classification of colorectal polyps and confirmed higher sensitivity of probe-based CLE with similar specificity in accurate differentiation between neoplastic and nonneoplastic lesions. Sanduleanu and colleagues[53] showed that endoscope-based CLE can reliably distinguish low-grade dysplasia from high-grade dysplasia in colorectal lesions with very good interobserver and intraobserver agreement.

The chromoendoscopy-guided endomicroscopy technique also has been evaluated in patients with long-term ulcerative colitis.[48] The results confirmed that the presence of dysplastic changes could be predicted by endomicroscopy with high accuracy (sensitivity 94.7%, specificity 98.3%, accuracy 97.8%). Endomicroscopy has the potential to determine if ulcerative colitis lesions identified by chromoscopy should undergo biopsy examination and increase the diagnostic yield and reduce the need for biopsy examinations. Chromoscopy-guided endomicroscopy may lead to significant improvement in the long-term with clinical management of ulcerative colitis. Despite these promising results, CLE is used mainly as a research tool in academic centers.

Summary

The electronically enhanced endoscopic imaging modalities discussed in this chapter represent novel technologies that may assist in the detection, characterization, and in vivo diagnosis of precursor and malignant lesions during endoscopy. However, they still have only limited use in general GI practice, with use limited to large academic centers that can offer training. Virtual chromoendoscopy techniques can be easily used in surveillance of high-risk patients based on ease of use. CLE combined with broad field technologies such as NBI, FICE, and i-Scan further can provide histopathology in vivo (diagnosis confirmation) and direct immediate therapeutic decisions. CLE could also lead to replacement of random, untargeted biopsies required in surveillance evaluation with targeted, "smart" biopsies. This approach could revolutionize enhanced image–based GI endoscopy.

References

The complete reference list is available online at www.expertconsult.com.

Index

Page numbers followed by "f" indicate figures, "t" indicate tables, and "b" indicate boxes.